PRENTICE HALL

Pediatric
Drug Guide

Ruth McGillis Bindler, RNC, PhD
Associate Professor, Washington State University,
Intercollegiate College of Nursing, Spokane, Washington

Linda Berner Howry, RN, MS
Associate Professor,
College of the Canyons, Santa Clarita, California

Billie Ann Wilson, RN, PhD
Professor and Director, Department of Nursing,
Loyola University New Orleans, New Orleans, Louisiana

Margaret T. Shannon, RN, PhD
Professor Emeritus of Nursing, Our Lady of
Holy Cross College, New Orleans, Louisiana

Carolyn L. Stang, PharmD
Vice President, Clinical Program Development,
Caremark Inc., Northbrook, Illinois

PEARSON
Prentice Hall

Upper Saddle River, New Jersey 07458

Library of Congress Cataloging-in-Publication Data

Pediatric drug guide / Ruth McGillis Bindler . . . [et al.].
   p. ; cm.
   Includes index.
   ISBN 0-13-119615-4
   1. Pediatric pharmacology—Handbooks, manuals, etc. 2. Pediatric
nursing—Handbooks, manuals, etc.
   [DNLM: 1. Drug Therapy—Child. 2. Drug Therapy—Infant.
3. Pediatric Nursing—methods. WS 366 P3686 2005] I. Title: Also
known as: Prentice Hall's pediatric drug guide. II. Bindler, Ruth
McGillis.

  RJ560.P388 2005
  615.5′8′083—dc22

                       2004024418

Notice: The authors and the publisher of this volume have taken care to make certain that the doses of drugs and schedules of treatment are correct and compatible with the standards generally accepted at the time of publication. Nevertheless, as new information becomes available, changes in treatment and in the use of drugs become necessary. The reader is advised to carefully consult the instruction and information material included in the package insert of each drug or therapeutic agent before administration. This advice is especially important when using, administering, or recommending new and infrequently used drugs. The authors and publisher disclaim all responsibility for any liability, loss, injury, or damage incurred as a consequence, directly or indirectly, of the use and application of any of the contents of this volume.

07 08 09 / 10 9 8 7 6 5

Pearson Education Ltd.
Pearson Education Australia Pty, Limited
Pearson Education Singapore, Pte. Ltd.
Pearson Education North Asia Ltd.
Pearson Education Canada, Ltd.
Pearson Educación de Mexico, S.A. de C.V.
Pearson Education—Japan
Pearson Education Malaysia, Pte. Ltd.

ISBN: 0-13-119615-4

PRINTED IN THE UNITED STATES OF AMERICA

CONTENTS

CONTENTS

ABOUT THE AUTHORS

Dr. Ruth Bindler received her Bachelor of Science in Nursing degree from Cornell University—New York Hospital School of Nursing in New York. She worked in oncology nursing at Sloan Kettering Cancer Center in New York, and then moved to Wisconsin and became a public health nurse there in Dane County. Thus began her commitment to work in pediatrics as she visited children and their families at home, and served as a school nurse for several elementary, middle, and high schools. Due to this interest in child health care needs, she earned a Master of Science degree in Child Development from the University of Wisconsin.

A move to Washington State was accompanied by a new job as a faculty member at the Intercollegiate Center for Nursing Education in Spokane. Ruth has been fortunate to be involved for 30 years in the growth of this nursing education consortium, which is a combination of public and private universities and colleges and is now the Washington State University Intercollegiate College of Nursing. She teaches theory and clinical courses in child health and a graduate research course, and serves as lead faculty for the maternal and child health courses. Her first professional book, *Pediatric Medications,* was published with co-author Linda Howry in 1981, and she has continued to publish articles and books in the areas of pediatric medications and pediatric health. Her research interests focus on cardiovascular risk factors and type 2 diabetes in children, topics that were the focus of her Doctor of Philosophy work in Human Nutrition at Washington State University. Ethnic diversity has been another theme in Ruth's work. She facilitates international and other diversity experiences for students, performs research with culturally diverse children, and works with underserved populations.

Ruth believes that her role as a faculty member has enabled her to learn continually, to foster the development of students in nursing, and to participate fully in the profession of nursing. In addition to teaching, research, publication, and leadership, she enhances her life by activities with her family, and by service in professional and community organizations.

Linda Howry received a diploma in nursing from Lincoln General Hospital School of Nursing in Lincoln, Nebraska. She worked in medical surgical nursing at Lincoln General and at a 30-bed community hospital in Nebraska. Linda received her Bachelor of Nursing from Northern Illinois University in DeKalb, Illinois. Her interest in pediatrics began when she worked at Children's Hospital in St. Louis, Missouri. She taught pediatrics to diploma nursing students rotating to Children's Hospital. Because of her work with children and family health, she was motivated to earn a Master of Science degree in Maternal and Child Health from the University of Colorado.

Linda taught at the University of Virginia where she was actively involved in teaching. She helped establish a multidiscipline child abuse team. Linda was commissioned as a captain in the army reserve and served two years at Tripler Army Hospital in Hawaii. Because of family moves Linda's teaching and work experience has been diverse including teaching nursing at the Intercollegiate College of Nursing, Spokane, and Messiah College, Grantham, Pennsylvania, and pediatric staff nursing and teaching community courses in childbirth preparation.

Currently Linda teaches at College of the Canyons in Santa Clarita, California. Her teaching responsibilities include teaching fundamentals theory, pharmacology, and a theory and clinical course in maternal, newborn, and child health. *Pediatric Medications* was published with co-author Ruth Bindler in 1981. Her interests focus on child abuse, diabetes, pharmacology, and obesity in children. Linda is committed to teaching and stimulating the intellectual and professional growth of her students. She is grounded in life by her husband and sons.

Billie Ann Wilson is currently professor and director of the Department of Nursing at Loyola University in New Orleans, Louisiana. Prior to entering nursing, she taught natural and physical sciences at the secondary and collegiate levels. She holds a B.S. in biology from Boston College, an M.S. in biology from Purdue University, a B.S. in nursing from Northwestern State University of Louisiana, a master of nursing from Louisiana State University Health Sciences Center, and a Ph.D. in curriculum and instruction from the University of New Orleans.

Margaret T. Shannon is Professor Emeritus of Nursing at Our Lady of Holy Cross College, New Orleans, Louisiana, Her educational preparation includes a B.S. in chemistry and an M.S. in chemistry, both from Saint Louis University; an M.A. in teaching biology from Saint Mary's College, a B.S. in nursing from Northwestern State University of Louisiana, a master of nursing from

Louisiana State University Health Sciences Center, and a Ph.D. in curriculum and instruction from the University of New Orleans. Prior to entering nursing, she taught physical science, natural science, and mathematics at the secondary and collegiate levels.

Carolyn L. Stang is currently vice president for clinical program development at Caremark Inc. She has worked in hospital and community pharmacies, home health care, and the pharmaceutical industry. Dr. Stang has been a freelance medical writer and an assistant professor at Rutgers University College of Pharmacy. She holds a B.S. in pharmacy from The Ohio State University and a doctor of pharmacy from the University of Tennessee, Memphis, completed a fellowship in family medicine at the Medical University of South Carolina, Charleston.

PREFACE

The important field of pediatric pharmacology continues to grow, and nurses need resources in order to apply this body of knowledge to the administration of medications to children. *Prentice Hall's Pediatric Drug Guide* is based on the book previously titled *Pediatric Drugs & Nursing Implications* and is the only resource currently in print that addresses the specialty of pediatric pharmacology in the context of nursing care. While our primary users are expected to be practicing pediatric nurses and student nurses, we are confident it will be an asset to nurse practitioners, pharmacists, and other health professionals as well. We are all partners together in providing safe and effective medications for children.

Organization

Part One focuses on the knowledge needed to administer drugs to children. The *Physiological Considerations* section describes physiological characteristics of children that influence pharmacokinetics. The *Developmental Considerations* section includes approaches that nurses can apply to explain and administer drugs to children at various ages. Major developmental theories are included with examples to assist the nurse in applying these theories to medication administration. Throughout the book, the child is viewed in the context of the family and community. These concepts of development and family teaching needs are also integrated in nursing implication sections throughout the drug monographs. In the *Techniques of Administration* section, concepts needed to successfully perform the skills of administration are described and illustrated. Contemporary techniques that have grown in use during the last few years are included, such as patient-controlled analgesia, regional pain blocks, and parenteral nutrition. The book also presents and explains sample drug calculation problems.

Part Two contains drug monographs for most medications that are administered to children. Traditional information is included with an emphasis on nursing implications and teaching for children and families. Pediatrics encompasses age ranges from the newborn to the adolescent. Dosing and other implications for these wide age ranges are described, including newborn, infant, child, and adult. In most cases children metabolize drugs similarly to adults from approximately 12 years of age. Thus, infant, child, and adult doses (or 12 years and over) are all included when pertinent. Pregnancy categories in the monographs can be consulted when working with teens who are pregnant. For further information about the drug monographs, read the section titled How to Use *Prentice Hall's Pediatric Drug Guide.*

The appendixes contain much useful information. They include information about the drug classifications, controlled substances, antineoplastics, resuscitation medications, immunizations, ocular medications, inhaled corticosteroids, intravenous drug compatibility, corticosteroids, pregnancy categories, key terms, and abbreviations. The reader is encouraged to review them in order to be aware of their content and therefore able to refer to them regularly.

How to Use *Prentice Hall's Pediatric Drug Guide*

Each drug monograph in Part Two of this handbook follows the same consistent format, making the drug information easy to access and use. For every drug presented, you will find the following sections in the monograph:

Drug Name

Drugs are listed alphabetically by generic name throughout the book. The generic name is in capital, **bold** letters, followed by pronunciation, then current trade names. Trade names for drugs only marketed in Canada are noted by a maple leaf, and combination products are indicated if they are applicable. Drug classification follows by pharmacologic and therapeutic categories, as described by the American Hospital Formulary System (see Appendix C). Drugs are listed in the index by generic and trade names and under their drug classifications. Prototype drugs are indicated by the icon when pertinent, and are identified in the index in **bold.** These are characteristic and early drugs developed in a class. Later drugs exhibit many of the same characteristics so prototype drug monographs can be consulted for additional detail.

Pregnancy Category

Pregnancy categories of A, B, C, D, or X are indicated when available. These data should be combined with developmental variations when caring for pregnant adolescents. See Appendix A–2 for further information.

Controlled Substance

Controlled substances, as regulated by the U.S. Food and Drug Administration, are indicated by Schedules I through V. See Appendix A–1 for a full description of these schedules.

Availability

The available dosage forms and amounts are listed. These include oral forms such as tablets, capsules, suspensions, and elixirs; rectal suppositories; inhaled forms; otic, ophthalmic, and topical forms; and parenteral forms for subcutaneous (SC), intramuscular (IM), intravenous (IV), and intrathecal routes.

Actions and Therapeutic Effects

The drug's action in the body is described. This includes available information at the cellular to organ levels. The nurse can also read about the actions of prototype drugs for additional detail. The specific therapeutic effects of the drug are described.

Uses and Unlabeled Uses

The uses of the drug are described. These include both those uses for which the drug is approved and, when common, unlabeled or additional uses described in medical literature.

Contraindications and Cautious Use

Absolute contraindications such as pregnancy or certain disease states or reactions exist for specific drugs. In addition, caution is needed at times. For example, a drug may not have been adequately tested yet in children so caution is urged. Disease states such as renal disease or cardiovascular problems may necessitate lower doses or additional assessments. Developmental variations may dictate cautious use at young ages.

Route and Dosages

The recommended dosages for each drug are listed in this section along with corresponding routes of administration. When different doses are recommended for different ages, they begin with newborn doses (birth to 1 month), infant (generally >1 month to 1 year), child (generally >1 to 12 years), and adult, which are those generally recommended for children 12 years of age and older. If the age range recommendations differ from these guidelines, the specific ages are listed. Dosages for new-borns and premature infants are not established for many drugs so when working with these groups, nurses are urged to consult specialized references and resources. Dosage routes are indicated using the abbreviations PO, SC, IM, IV, and PR and the terms intrathecal, inhalation, otic, ophthalmic, and topical. Other abbreviations used in the route and dosage section include accepted forms such as b.i.d., t.i.d., q.i.d., mg/kg/day, and mg/m^2/day. See Appendix E–1 for a complete list of abbreviations. Always have other nurses, pharmacists, or physicians check doses whenever orders are not clear or seem unusual.

Storage

The temperature and other storage requirements are stated as appropriate. The amount of time that oral or IV medications can be used after mixing is included. Consult package inserts and pharmacists for additional information.

Administration

Administration instructions for oral, parenteral, and other drug forms are noted in each monograph. Preparation for oral suspensions and IV medications is followed by administration recommendations. For IV drugs that can be administered both by direct and intermittent or continuous infusion, administration rates for each are noted. Incompatibilities with IV fluids and other drugs are listed.

Adverse Effects

Adverse or side effects are undesirable effects that can occur in response to drugs. Some may create only minor discomfort, whereas others can be life threatening. The most common adverse effects are *italicized* and the life-threatening ones are underlined. Idiosyncratic effects can occur with any drug so report assessment data, even if it is not listed here.

Diagnostic Test Interference

Sometimes, drugs will interfere with the results of laboratory and diagnostic tests. Misinterpretation of test results can interfere with proper treatment of the child. Thus, each monograph identifies the possible effects of the drug on diagnostic tests and alerts the nurse of any interference. The specific altered element is highlighted in the ***bold italic*** type.

Interactions

In each monograph, the drug's interactions with other medications, with herbal products, and/or food are noted in this section. Such information will help you monitor for interference with or enhancement of drug actions, and will suggest questions that the nurse can ask the child and family about the use of complementary therapies during the health history. Generic drugs are given in **bold** type and drug classes are in SMALL CAPITAL LETTERS.

Pharmacokinetics

The body's handling of drugs is complex. This section describes the absorption, time to onset of action, peak level, duration of action, distribution in the body, metabolic pathway, elimination process, and half-life. Total pharmacokinetics are not known for every drug and may vary in young children, pregnant females, and those with certain disease states, especially those affecting the liver or kidneys. See Part One of this book for an overview of pharmacokinetic variations in children.

Nursing Implications

This important section translates drug information to nursing interactions with infants, children, adolescents, and their families. The section under *Assessment & Drug Effects* describes nursing assessments to note regarding desired actions and adverse effects of the medication. Gather baseline assessment data before administration and as indicated throughout treatment. Ensure that necessary laboratory studies are completed. Therapeutic and toxic levels are indicated in boldface italics. The *Patient & Family Education* section lists information that should be provided to the child or adolescent when able to understand and/or to the family members. Nurses and families are partners in the health care of the child, so encourage family members to share honestly and openly all concerns, questions about administration, and the use of complementary therapies such as over-the-counter medications and herbal or supplemental products. Work together to solve problems in medication administration and to ensure safety for children. Include children and adolescents to the level of their ability, gradually increasing their responsibility for own self-medication. See Part One of this book for further detail on developmental and teaching approaches.

ACKNOWLEDGMENTS

This book has been written with support and assistance from many people. The authors of the *Prentice Hall Nurse's Drug Guide 2005,* Billie Ann Wilson, RN, PhD, Margaret T. Shannon, RN, PhD, and Carolyn L. Stang, PharmD, graciously allowed us to access their drug monographs from the *Prentice Hall Nurse's Drug Guide 2005* for detailed information. Jason Blauwet, PharmD, reviewed monographs for pediatric data and served as consultant throughout the project. Beth Richardson, DNS, RN, CPNP, revised, updated, and added new information to Part One and the appendixes. Sladjana Repic, assistant editor at Prentice Hall Health, tirelessly provided information needed, served as liaison between all contributors, and ably assisted with every request. Maura Connor, editor-in-chief, displayed her visionary leadership in proposing novel ways to complete this drug book. Lorretta Palagi and Karen Ettinger provided meticulous attention in the editing process. Our students and colleagues and the children and families with whom we work are truly the sparks that inspired the writing of this drug book. We value their questions, knowledge, and the partnerships we all form to integrate wise use of medications within health care. Our families provide support and love in our personal and professional lives. We thank them for supporting and sustaining us.

Ruth McGillis Bindler
Linda Berner Howry

PART ONE

ADMINISTRATION OF PEDIATRIC MEDICATIONS

▶ **Physiological Considerations**

I. Pharmacokinetic Principles

A. Pharmacokinetics
1. Pharmacokinetics is the study of the processes of absorption, distribution, and excretion of drugs. These processes involve a constantly dynamic interaction between the drugs and the human body.
2. Because of the unique characteristics of a child, pediatric pharmacokinetics is a distinct field. The child may tolerate drugs differently than would an adult depending on age and developmental characteristics.

B. Pharmacodynamic/Pharmacokinetic Concepts
1. The *therapeutic level* or *index* is the concentration of a drug that is needed to elicit the desired clinical response without causing toxic effects.
2. *Serum concentration* is the level of drug present in the serum, as measured on a blood sample in the laboratory. Knowing the serum concentration can be helpful in establishing the dosage needed to reach the therapeutic level, thus avoiding toxic effects. Serum concentration levels are not available for all drugs due to limitations in assay techniques and the inability to predict pharmacologic response from the levels of some drugs. In the latter case, clinical response rather than serum levels is used to establish therapeutic dosages.
3. *Trough level* is the lowest concentration of the drug reached between dosages (Figure I–1).
4. *Peak serum level* is the highest concentration of the drug reached after administration of dosages (Figure I–2).
5. The *steady-state concentration* is reached when the drug's distribution is in equilibrium in the body, that is, when the amount of drug taken into the body equals the amount excreted. This is attained after repetitive dosing and is dependent on the half-life of the drug. A longer half-life requires a longer time to reach the steady state (Figure I–3).

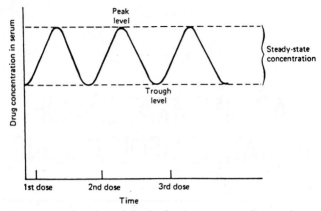

Figure I-1. Peak and trough levels of a drug in serum when steady-state concentration is achieved.

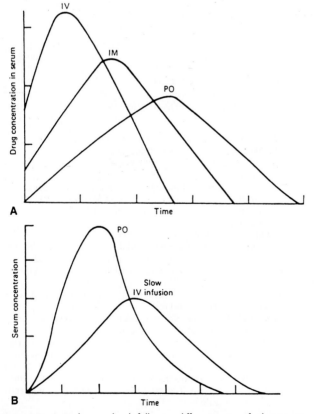

Figure I-2. A. Peak serum levels following different routes of administration. **B.** Differences in peak serum concentrations after oral administration and during slow IV infusion.

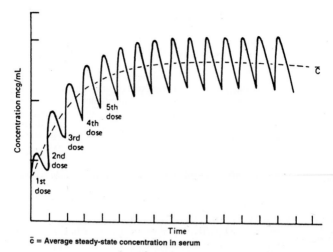

Figure I–3. Achievement of steady-state concentration after repetitive dosing. When the fixed dose of a drug is given repeatedly at intervals approximating the half-life of the drug, a steady-state concentration results after about five half-lives of the drug; hence, the longer the half-life of a drug, the longer the time required for steady-state concentration to occur (*dotted line*). If a loading dose is used, the process is shortened considerably.

6. The *half-life* of a drug is the time required for 50% of a dose to be excreted. It is used to determine frequency of drug dosages. To avoid accumulation and toxic effects, drugs are given at intervals close to their half-lives.

7. The *loading dose* is a large dose used with some drugs to begin therapy and shorten the time it takes for the body to reach the steady-state concentration. The loading dose is sometimes referred to as a *bolus,* or in the case of digitalis, a *digitalizing dose.* Once the loading dose is given, the patient is given a smaller *maintenance dose* on a scheduled basis.

8. *Minimum inhibitory concentration (MIC)* is the sensitivity of a particular organism to various antimicrobial agents. This is the minimum amount of drug needed to inhibit the organism's growth in the laboratory. Antibiotics that kill the organism with a concentration that is not toxic are considered for treatment. A serum level greater than the MIC at the site of the infection is the goal.

II. Pediatric Variations

A. Height, Weight, and Body Surface Area
   1. The proportions between height and weight in children are different from those in adults. These differences are most marked in newborns, infants, and young children.

2. The differences in proportions can cause inaccurate dosages to be administered if a pediatric dose is calculated by adapting an adult dose and altering it based on a child's weight.
3. Body surface area, measured by the relationship between height and weight, increases about 7 times between birth and adulthood.
4. Body surface area, measured in square meters, is a good reflection of many physiological processes significant in metabolizing, transporting, and eliminating drugs, such as metabolic rate, extracellular fluid and total fluid volumes, cardiac output, and glomerular filtration rate. See the nomogram of Figure I–4 for an example of a computation of body surface area in square meters.
5. Body surface area and weight are generally used to calculate pediatric dosages of medications. Pediatric dosages are usually stated in terms of milligrams per kilogram (mg/kg) or milligrams per square meter (mg/m^2). These methods are more accurate than calculating a drug dose based on age or by using another method.

B. Muscle Mass
1. Muscle makes up 25% of body weight in infancy and 50% in adulthood (Table I–1).
2. Infants and young children have little muscle tissue available for injection and may have erratic blood flow to muscle tissue, thus decreasing medication absorption.

C. Fat
1. Fat makes up 16% of an infant's body weight, 22 to 24% of a 1-year-old's, 12% of a preschooler's, and 15% of an adult's (Table I–1).
2. Blood levels of lipid-soluble drugs are dependent on the amount of fat tissue in the body, because the fat must get saturated with these drugs before blood levels begin to increase (e.g., diazepam, barbiturates).
3. The variable fat percentages observed throughout childhood as well as among individual children may lead to a need for different milligram per kilogram dosages to achieve therapeutic blood levels.
4. Increased adipose tissue of adolescence, particularly in females, increases storage of and decreases availability of lipid-soluble drugs. Consider this potential effect in children who are obese.

D. Body Fluid
1. Eighty-five percent of body weight in premature infants is fluid, 70–80% in term infants, and 60% in 4-year-olds and throughout childhood (Figure I–5 and Table I–1).
2. Forty-five percent of body weight in infancy is extracellular fluid; about 35% is intracellular. Fifteen to twenty percent of body weight in the adult is extracellular; 40 percent is intracellular.
3. Greater milligram per kilogram dosages of aqueous- (water)-soluble drugs (e.g., sulfisoxazole) are needed in young children, because their total body fluid levels, especially extracellular (circulating) volumes, are greater.
4. The greater proportion of extracellular fluid in young children makes them more prone to dehydration. Dehydration states can alter needed dosages and response to medications.

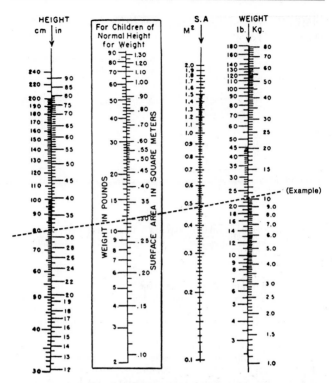

Alternative calculation: Mosteller's formula

$$\text{Surface area (m}^2) = \sqrt{\frac{\text{Height (cm)} \times \text{Weight (kg)}}{3600}}$$

Figure I–4. The body surface area is indicated at the intersection of a straight line connecting the height and weight column with the surface area column; if the patient is of roughly average size, it is determined by the weight alone (*enclosed area*). *Adapted from Behrman, R. E., Kliegman, R. M., Jenson, T. B. (Eds.):* Nelson textbook of pediatrics. *17th ed. Philadelphia, W. B. Saunders, copyright 2004 and Briars, G., and Bailey, B.: "Surface area estimation: Pocket calculator v nomogram."* Archives of Disease in Children, *1994, 70, 246 with permission from Elsevier.*

E. Skin
    1. *Variations in children:*
        a. Large body surface area and, therefore, more skin surface;
        b. Thin dermis and epidermis (especially the stratum corneum, or outer layer of epidermis);
        c. Relatively inactive sebaceous glands before puberty.
    2. Variations result in a tendency to absorb topical medications (e.g., hexachlorophene, boric acids, steroids) through the skin, creating systemic effects.

TABLE I-1 Percentage of Body Weight Made Up of Water, Muscle, and Fat

	Muscle	Fat	Total Body Water	Extracellular Water	Intracellular Water
Premature	*	1	85	*	*
Birth	25	16	70–80	45–47	32–35
12 months	*	22–24	58–60	25–27	41
4 years	*	12	60	24	41
10–11 years	40	18–20	60	17	41
Adult	50	15	50–60	15	40

*Not determined.

3. Skin of young children, especially infants, is prone to irritation and allergy. Diaper rash, hives, eczema, and contact dermatitis are not uncommon.

F. Eye
   1. Eye medications, especially those in solution form, create systemic effects when they pass through the nasolacrimal duct, become absorbed through the nasal mucous membranes, or get swallowed and absorbed from the gastrointestinal tract. Ointments are often used in children rather than solutions to minimize this effect (e.g., atropine).
   2. It may be difficult to administer eye medications to young children. Caution and correct techniques are advised.
   3. Oxygen used therapeutically in newborns may lead to retinopathy of prematurity, which causes blindness. Premature infants administered high levels of oxygen over prolonged periods are most at risk of this complication.

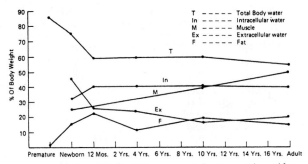

Figure I-5. Percentage of body weight composed of water, muscle, and fat.

G. Gastrointestinal System
1. *Variations in children:*
   a. Gastric emptying time is prolonged (6 to 8 hours) in newborns as compared with children in the second year (2 hours).
   b. Peristalsis is irregular in infants.
   c. The gastrointestinal tract is long in proportion to the body size.
   d. Some substances needed for active transport of certain drugs are not yet produced in infants.
   e. The gastric pH of newborns is neutral, falls to 1 to 3 a few hours after birth, varies a good deal in the first month of life, and gradually nears the more adult pH of 0.9 to 1.5 by 3 to 4 months of age. Gastric pH is elevated in premature infants, leading to higher serum levels of acid-labile drugs such as ampicillin and nafcillin and lower concentrations of weakly acidic drugs such as phenobarbital.
   f. Pepsin and other factors influencing drug absorption vary in relation to gastric acid levels.
   g. Infants eat every 2 to 4 hours, therefore, food is in their stomachs much of the time; food and digestive enzymes may interfere with drug absorption.
2. Variations result in slower, more erratic absorption of oral medications, especially in newborns and infants in the first half year of life. Acidic drugs, such as the penicillins, may be more readily absorbed in newborns and very young infants because of their lower gastric pH. In contrast, basic drugs, such as diazepam and theophylline, may have delayed absorption.
3. Sublingual administration to children younger than adolescence is generally avoided because of their inability to carry out this route of administration correctly.

H. Liver
1. Enzyme systems are less well developed in infants and young children. Enzymes used for drug binding are, therefore, at lower levels (Table I–2).
2. The neonate has some substances that compete with medications for plasma protein binding sites, such as maternal hormones and free and fatty acids. Therefore, proportionately smaller doses of some drugs that bind to plasma proteins, such as phenytoin and salicylate, are needed.
3. The lower levels of many liver enzymes also decrease biotransformation rates of many drugs. Toxic effects of such drugs may be reached more readily; for example, chloramphenicol leads to the "gray baby" syndrome.
4. Monitoring for side and toxic effects and sometimes blood levels is particularly important in infants and young children.

I. Respiratory System
1. *Variations in children:*
   a. Children have a proportionately small lung size and high metabolic rate.
   b. The alveoli of newborn are immature and not fully functional.

TABLE I–2   Serum Protein Values*

Group	Total Protein	Albumin	α_1-Globulin
At birth	4.6–7.0	2.6–3.6	0.1–0.3
3 months	4.5–6.5	2.6–3.6	0.1–0.3
1 year	5.4–7.5	3.4–4.2	0.1–0.3
>4 years	5.9–8.0	3.7–5.6	0.1–0.3

Group	α_2-Globulin	β-Globulin	λ-Globulin
At birth	0.2–0.3	0.3–0.6	0.6–1.2
3 months	0.3–0.7	0.3–0.7	0.2–0.7
1 year	0.5–1.1	0.4–1.0	0.2–0.9
>4 years	0.4–0.8	0.5–1.0	0.4–1.3

*Values are for cellulose acetate electrophoresis and are in grams per deciliter. SI conversion factor: g/L × 10 = g/dL.

From Ball, J., Bindler, R.: Pediatric nursing: Caring for children. *4th ed.* Upper Saddle River, NJ: Prentice Hall, 2005.

    c. The upper respiratory passages (e.g., nose, trachea, bronchi, eustachian tube) are shorter and narrower in infants and young children.

    d. Infants breathe almost totally through the nose to facilitate breathing while nursing.

    e. The lower respiratory passages (bronchioles, alveoli) are shorter and narrower in infants and young children.

    f. The immune system is immature in young children.

2. Variations result in:

    a. More rapid respiratory rates in young children (Table I–3),

    b. More frequent respiratory infections,

TABLE I–3   Respiratory Rates

Age	Range (breaths/min)
Newborn	30–80
6 months	24–36
1 year	20–40
3 years	20–30
6 years	16–22
10 years	16–20
17 years	12–20

From Ball, J., Bindler, R.: Pediatric nursing: Caring for children. *4th ed.* Upper Saddle River, NJ: Prentice Hall, 2005.

TABLE I-4   Average Pulse Rates

Age	Pulse Rate (beats/min)
Newborn	100–170
6 months–1 year	90–130
3 years	65–110
5 years	70–110
10–14 years	60–95

Adapted from Behrman, R. E., Kliegman, R. M., Jenson, T. B. (Eds.): Nelson textbook of pediatrics. *17th ed. Philadelphia: W. B. Saunders, copyright 2004 with permission from Elsevier.*

    c. The inability of the infant to breathe and nurse simultaneously when nasal passages are compromised from a respiratory infection,

    d. Upper respiratory infections frequently followed by middle ear infections (otitis media).

J. Cardiovascular System

    1. Poorly developed peripheral circulation in the infant may cause intramuscular and subcutaneous injections to be absorbed slowly or erratically. Vasoconstriction due to a cold environment can further decrease or slow the absorption (Tables I–4 and I–5).

    2. Intravenous and oral routes are more often used in young children because of a greater predictability of drug action by these routes.

TABLE I-5   Median Blood Pressure Values*

Age	Systolic (mm Hg)	Diastolic (mm Hg)
Newborn	73	55
1 month	86	52
6 months	90	53
1 year	90	56
3 years	92	55
6 years	96	57
9 years	100	61
12 years	107	64
15 years	114	65
18 years	121	70

*Readings show 50th percentile. Normal blood pressure readings for girls are very similar to those for boys at all age groups.

Adapted from the Normal Blood Pressure Readings for Boys from the Second Task Force on Blood Pressure Control in Children, National Heart, Lung, and Blood Institute (1987), Bethesda, MD.

3. A proportionately large amount of circulating extracellular fluid creates the need for relatively high doses of water-soluble drugs.

K. Neurological System
1. The blood–brain barrier is not mature in the first 2 years of life; therefore, encephalopathy is more commonly seen as a toxic drug effect.
2. Central nervous system stimulants and depressants more often cause unpredictable results in children (e.g., phenobarbital leads to excitement; amphetamines cause decreased hyperactivity).

L. Endocrine System
1. Increased level of sex steroids in adolescence can compete for enzymes that may be necessary for drug metabolism.
2. Androgens in adolescent males may increase binding of some drugs.
3. Rate of elimination of some drugs (e.g., aminophylline) is related to sexual maturity.
4. Genetic makeup can influence enzyme systems and the ability to metabolize and excrete some drugs.

M. Renal System (Tables I–6 and I–7)
1. *Variations in children:*
   a. Glomerular filtration rates in the young infant are 30 to 50% that of adults; mature rates are reached in the first half year of life.
   b. Tubular secretion is less in the infant because of a smaller number of tubular cells, shorter tubules, reduced blood flow, and less active transport systems; mature rates are reached by 7 months of age.

TABLE I–6   Daily Water Requirements at Various Ages

Age	Average Body Weight (kg)	Total Water Requirements per 24 h (mL)	Water Requirements per kg per 24 h (mL)
3 days	3.0	250–300	80–100
10 days	3.2	400–500	125–150
3 months	5.4	750–850	140–160
6 months	7.3	950–1100	130–155
9 months	8.6	1100–1250	125–145
1 year	9.5	1150–1300	120–135
2 years	11.8	1350–1500	115–125
4 years	16.2	1600–1800	100–110
6 years	20.0	1800–2000	90–100
10 years	28.7	2000–2500	70–85
14 years	45.0	2200–2700	50–60
18 years	54.0	2200–2700	40–50

TABLE I–7   Daily Urine Output

Age	Output (mL/24 hours)
Newborn	50–300
Infant	350–550
Child	500–1000
Adolescent	700–1400

Note: These are average expected output amounts. Fluid intake totals, medications, diseases and infections can alter levels for particular children.

Data from Behrman, R.E., Kliegman, R.M. & Jenson, H.B. (2004). Nelson textbook of pediatrics, 17th ed. Philadelphia: Saunders, p 2415.

   c. Urinary pH of the newborn is more acidic and remains the same over 24 hours of the day. (Older children and adults have a more basic urine during the daytime and a more acidic urine at night.)

   d. Children have little ability to concentrate or dilute urine.

  2. Variations result in:

    a. Longer half-life in infants for drugs excreted by glomerular filtration (e.g., kanamycin, streptomycin, gentamicin, digoxin),

    b. Longer half-life in infants for drugs excreted by tubular secretion (e.g., penicillins),

    c. Increased reabsorption of acidic drugs in the infant (e.g., sulfisoxazole),

    d. Increased incidence of dehydration and overhydration.

    e. Oliguria or anuria, which necessitates close observation for drug toxic effects as well as decreased dosages of drugs excreted by the kidneys.

N. Immune System

  1. The immune system is immature because of a low exposure to and slow response to infections. A greater number of infections (particularly respiratory and gastrointestinal) are seen.

  2. Allergies, for example, of the skin and respiratory system, are common.

  3. Allergy to medication should be carefully described and recorded.

  4. Medication allergy is caused by a Type I IgE-mediated hypersensitivity when an antigen (in this case a medication) interacts with IgE antibodies bound to cells and creates an antigen–antibody reaction with release of histamine and several other chemical mediators. Anaphylaxis is an acute and life-threatening reaction to an antigen and usually begins in seconds or minutes after exposure to a causative medication. Symptoms include vasovagal collapse, laryngeal edema and bronchospasm, urticaria, angioedema, gastrointestinal reactions, and shock. Children with a previous

allergic response to medication must not be given the medication again. Allergies are documented on medical records, hospital wristbands, and other important places. Parents and children must inform all health care providers of the known allergies to medications. Health care providers must be able to give basic life support in case of allergic or anaphylactic reactions. Epinephrine 1:1000 and other drugs and equipment should be readily available when medications are administered. Some common medication allergies involve:

- Amphotericin B
- Aspirin
- Cephalosporins
- Codeine
- Dextran
- Ibuprofen
- Indomethacin
- Local anesthetics
- Meperidine
- Morphine
- Naproxen
- Nitrofurantoin
- Radiographic iodine contrast media
- Penicillins

Note: Parents and care providers sometimes confuse a side effect of a medication with true allergy. For example, a rash or gastrointestinal effects may occur as side effect of some medications and do not indicate allergy to the medication. The prescriber or an allergy specialist can clarify if a reaction is a true allergy. Teach families the difference between allergy and side effect.

III. Principles of Pediatric Dosages

A. Solutions
1. Intravenous (IV) flow rates are most frequently calculated in microdrops in pediatrics. For all companies, 60 microdrops equals 1 mL of solution. Note the number of drops (gtt) required to administer 1 mL of IV fluid using tubing manufactured by different companies.

Company	Number of Drops (gtt/1 mL)
Baxter	10 drops (gtt)
Lifeline	10 drops (gtt)
Travenol	10 drops (gtt)
Abbot	15 drops (gtt)
Braun/McGaw	15 drops (gtt)
All companies	60 microgtt (mcgtt) = 1 milliliter (mL)

Flow rate is calculated using the following formula:

$$\text{Drops/min} = \frac{\text{Total volume ordered} \times \text{gtt/mL}}{\text{Total infusion time (min)}}$$

For example, if 250 mL of fluid were to be administered by microdrop over 3 hours, the drops per minute would be calculated as follows:

$$\text{Drops/min} = \frac{250 \times 60}{180}$$
$$= \frac{15,000}{180}$$
$$= 83.3$$

The IV flow rate in this example would be adjusted to administer 83 drops/min.

2. When microdrip tubing is used, because 60 drops = 1 mL and there are 60 minutes in an hour, the formula to use is drops/min = mL/h. For example, if a child needed 250 mL to be delivered in 6 hours, the problem would be calculated as follows:

$$\frac{250\,\text{mL}}{6\,\text{h}} = 41.67\,\text{mL/h}$$

Therefore, the rate is set at 42 drops/min.

3. Intravenous pumps are generally used in pediatrics. Regulation of dosage is easier and safer with use of these pumps. Pumps usually calculate the required flow rate in milliliters per hour. So if 500 mL of IV fluid needed to be delivered in 8 hours:

$$\frac{500\,\text{mL}}{8\,\text{h}} = 62.5\,\text{mL/h}$$

Therefore, the pump would be set at 62 or 63.

B. Methods of Measurement
   1. *Metric system.* The basic units are a *gram* for measuring the weight of solids, a *liter* for measuring the volume of liquids, and a *meter* for measuring length. Prefixes indicate the division or multiplication by 10 of the basic unit as follows:
   deci- = 0.1 of the basic unit
   centi- = 0.01 of the basic unit
   milli- = 0.001 of the basic unit
   micro- = 0.00001 of the basic unit = 0.001 of milli-
   nano- = 0.000000001 of the basic unit
   deka- = 10 of or times the basic unit
   hecto- = 100 of or times the basic unit
   kilo- = 1000 of or times the basic unit

Metric System

Weight
   mcg = microgram
   mg = milligram
   g or gm = gram
   kg = kilogram

Volume
   mL = milliliter
   L = liter
   cc = cubic centimeter

Length
    m = meter

Commonly Used Metric Equivalents

Weight
    1 milligram (mg) = 1000 micrograms (mcg)
    1 milligram (mg) = 0.001 gram (g or gm)
    1 gram = 1000 milligrams (mg)
    1 kilogram (kg) = 1000 grams (g or gm)

Volume
    1 milliliter (mL) = 1 cubic centimeter (cc)
    1 liter (L) = 1000 milliliters (mL)
              = 1000 cubic centimeters (cc)

2. *Apothecaries' system.* Measures of weight in this system are the *grain, dram, ounce,* and *pound.* Volume is measured by the *minim, fluid ram, fluid ounce, pint,* and *quart.* Formerly symbols were frequently used but are avoided now to minimize chance of error in interpretation of dosages. The quantity or weight or volume follows the symbol and is indicated by Roman numbers. Thus:

$$15\,\text{grains} = \text{gr xv or gr}\,\overline{\text{xv}}$$
$$2\,\text{drams} = \text{ʒII or ʒII}$$

Apothecaries' System

Note: Symbols are often misinterpreted so words should be written out. Clarify whenever necessary. The metric system is preferred for all medication orders.

Weight
    gr = grain
    dr or ʒ = dram
    oz or ʒ = ounce
    lb = pound

Volume
    m or *m* = minim
    fl dr or *f*ʒ = fluid dram
    fl oz or *f*ʒ = fluid ounce
    O or pt = pint
    qt = quart

Commonly Used Apothecary Equivalents

Weight
    1 dram (dr or ʒ) = 60 grains (gr)
    1 ounce (oz or ʒ) = 8 drams (dr or ʒ) = 480 grains (gr)
    1 pound (lb) = 12 ounces (oz or ʒ) = 5760 grains (gr)

Volume
    1 fluid dram (fl dr or *f*ʒ) = 60 minims (m or *m*)
    1 fluid ounce (fl oz or ʒ) = 8 fluid drams (fl dr or *f*ʒ)
        = 480 minims (m or *m*)
    1 pint (O or pt) = 16 fluid ounces (fl oz or ʒ)
    1 quart (qt) = 2 pints (O or pt) = 32 fluid ounces (fl oz or ʒ)

3. *Household system.* Volume measurements used include the *teaspoon, tablespoon, cup,* and *glass.* Volume measured by household

implements varies greatly; therefore, their use to administer medications should be discouraged.

Household System
gtt = drop
t or tsp = teaspoon
T or tbsp = tablespoon
c = cup

Commonly Used Household Equivalents

Volume
1 teaspoon (t or tsp) = 5 cubic centimeters (cc)
1 tablespoon (T or tbsp) = 3 teaspoons (t or tsp) (or 15 cc)
1 cup (c) = 6 fluid ounces (fl oz or ℥) = 180 cubic centimeters (cc)
1 glass = 8 fluid ounces (fl oz or ℥) = 240 cubic centimeters (cc)

4. Conversion between systems is also a nursing responsibility. Equivalents for transfer among metric, apothecaries', and household systems are as follows:

	Metric	Apothecaries'	Household
Weight	1 milligram (mg)	1/60–1/65 grain (gr)	
	60–65 milligrams (mg)	1 grain (gr)	
	1 gram (g)	15/16 grains (gr)	
	30 grams (g)	1 ounce (oz)	
	1 kilogram (kg)	2.2 pounds (lb)	

	Metric	Apothecaries'	Household
Volume	0.06 milliliter (mL)	1 minim (*m*)	
	1 milliliter (mL) or 1 cubic centimeter (cc)	15–16 minims (*m*)	
	4–5 milliliters (mL)	1 fluid dram (fl dr)	1 teaspoon (tsp)
	15 milliliters (mL)	4 fluid drams (fl dr)	1 tablespoon (tbsp)
	30 milliliters (mL)	1 fluid ounce (fl oz)	
	180 milliliters (mL)	6 fluid ounces (fl oz)	1 cup (c)
	240 milliliters (mL)	8 fluid ounces (fl oz)	1 glass
	473.2 or 500 milliliters (mL)	1 pint (pt)	
	1000 milliliters (mL) or 1 liter or 1000 cubic centimeters (cc)	1 quart (qt)	

These approximate equivalents of weights and volumes among metric, apothecaries', and household systems are useful in giving medications. It is important to remember that these are approximate and not exact equivalents. Some loss of accuracy occurs whenever one system of measure is converted to another. The metric system should be used whenever possible.

C. Dosage Calculation
1. A certain number of milligrams of a drug is specified for each kilogram of body weight. This is commonly written as *mg/kg*.
2. A certain number of milligrams of a drug is specified for each square meter of body surface area. This is commonly written as *mg/m²*.
3. Rules for calculation of pediatric dosages by using adult doses and considering the age or weight of the child have sometimes been used in the past. These are not considered safe or accurate and should not be used.
4. Some common types of dosage calculation problems follow.

Example 1
The prescriber has ordered 20 mg of a liquid oral medication for a child. The medication is available in an elixir with 5 mg/mL. What amount should be administered?

Answer

$$\frac{\text{Dose desired}}{\text{Dose on hand}} \times \text{Quantity (mL)} = \text{Volume to be administered}$$

$$\frac{20 \text{ mg}}{5 \text{ mg}} \times 1 \text{ mL} = 4 \text{ mL to be administered}$$

Note: This is a very small volume and will need to be measured in a syringe for accuracy and then administered via oral syringe or other desired device.

Example 2
A physician has ordered morphine 2 mg IV q4h PRN for a child with a weight of 25 kg. Morphine is available as 10 mg/mL and the recommended dose for children is 0.05–0.1 mg/kg q4h PRN. What amount of medication is to be administered? Is this a safe dose?

Answer

$$\frac{\text{Dose desired}}{\text{Dose on hand}} \times \text{Quantity (mL)} = \text{Volume to be administered}$$

$$\frac{2 \text{ mg}}{10 \text{ mg}} \times 1 \text{ mL} = 0.2 \text{ mL to be administered}$$

$$\text{Recommended dose} \times \text{Weight} = \text{Dose for patient}$$

$$\frac{0.05 \text{ mg}}{\text{kg}} \times 20 \text{ kg} = 1 \text{ mg}$$

$$\frac{0.1 \text{ mg}}{\text{kg}} \times 20 \text{ kg} = 2 \text{ mg}$$

The child can receive 1–2 mg so the dose ordered is within recommended levels.

D. Guidelines for Medication Administration
1. Before giving any medication to a child, ask yourself these questions:
a. How will the drug be absorbed, metabolized, and excreted?

    b. How will the child's illness and developmental physiology influence the absorption, metabolism, and excretion of the drug?

    c. Is the child taking other drugs that will interact or compete with this drug for utilization and excretion?

    d. What dose should be given?

    e. What are the child's pulse, temperature, respiratory rate, blood pressure, skin color and condition, fluid status, and behavior? (Document in the medical record.)

2. After giving any medication to a child, ask these questions:

    a. What time, route, amount, and site (for injections) were used for medication administration? (Document in the medical record.)

    b. What pertinent physical findings, such as changes in condition, lack of expected results, side effects, or unusual effects of the drug are observed? (Document in the medical record.)

    c. Would it be useful to obtain blood levels of the drug for establishing the therapeutic dose?

    d. How can results of this therapy be shared with other health professionals?

IV. Problems in Pediatric Dosing

A. Lack of approved drugs for use in children results from:

1. Difficulty in controlling experimental conditions to test drugs adequately with children;

2. Risk of potential unique side effects and long-term developmental effects, leading to ethical considerations;

3. Difficulty in obtaining informed parent and child consent and assent;

4. High experimental costs (e.g., small samples of blood often require special equipment and assay techniques);

5. Unusual, unique response to some drugs that is sometimes observed in children (e.g., chloramphenicol causes toxic effects in newborns);

6. Lack of incentives for drug companies to test drugs on children.

B. This lack of approved drugs for use in children results in:

1. Depriving children of some drugs that may be useful for them,

2. Off-label use of drugs in children when there are no clearly established dosages for various age groups. (In this book, in the dosage section, a dosage established by clinicians is sometimes given rather than one recommended by drug companies. This indicates that the drug is used in pediatrics even though the manufacturer has not been licensed to label the drug as safe and effective in children and to provide pediatric dosages.)

C. The child has been referred to as a "therapeutic orphan" due to the lack of information about pharmacokinetics of many drugs in pediatric bodies.

D. The United States government has taken steps to encourage drug testing on children. Examples include the following:

1. The Pediatric Rule of 1994 allows labeling of some drugs for pediatric use based on efficacy in adults and some study of pharmacokinetics and safety in children. The course of disease for these treatments is similar in adults and children.

2. The Food and Drug Administration Modernization Act (FDAMA) of 1997 provides 6 months of exclusive drug marketing for specific drugs if the manufacturers conduct pediatric clinical trials.
3. In the Best Pharmaceutical for Children Act (BPCA) of 2002, the secretary of the Department of Health and Human Services and director of the National Institutes of Health were mandated to establish a program for drug development that identifies drugs needing study in children and conducting the needed clinical studies. They first identified a list of high-priority drugs for pediatric study in 2003 and plan annual updates. Clinical trials are being designed and requests for proposals for testing are being released.

▶ Developmental Considerations

I. Child Development

A. Areas of Development
1. Psychosocial development influences the child's interaction with the person giving a medication.
2. Cognitive development determines the child's understanding of the need for a medication. It is important to assess the child's intellectual understanding of medications to plan effective interactions and teaching.
3. Physical growth characteristics may influence the child's medication experience.

II. Methods of Communicating with Children

A. Communications Strategies
It is important to consider children's development when speaking with them about medications and general health care. Table I–8 provides strategies about how best to communicate with children/adolescents using developmental considerations.

B. Drawings
1. Body line drawings (Figure I–6) can be used as assessment tools to determine the child's understanding of anatomy or medication effects. The health care provider gives the child an appropriate picture and asks the child questions such as "What is in the chest? Draw it on the picture" or "Where does this medicine go when you swallow it?"
2. Children often display feelings about medication administration in drawings. The child may draw spontaneously or can be encouraged to do so by asking "Will you draw a picture of a little girl in the hospital like you?" Open-ended statements are used to encourage children to explain their drawings.
3. The nurse can use body line drawings to teach the child about the body and the effects of medicines.

C. Stories
1. Pictures of children in health care settings or receiving medicine can be shown and the child asked to make up a story about what is happening in a particular picture. Anxiety may be displayed in this fantasy experience that is not evident in direct conversation.

TABLE I–8   Methods of Communicating with Children

Age Group	Developmental Stages	Nursing Applications
Infant (birth to 1 year)	Oral stage (Freud): The baby obtains pleasure and comfort through the mouth.	When a baby is NPO, offer a pacifier if not contraindicated. After painful procedures, offer a baby a bottle or pacifier or have the mother breast-feed.
	Trust versus mistrust stage (Erikson): The baby establishes a sense of trust when basic needs are met.	Hold the hospitalized baby often. Offer comfort after painful procedures. Meet the baby's needs for food and hygiene. Encourage parents to room in. Manage pain effectively with use of pain medications and other measures.
	Sensorimotor stage (Piaget): The baby learns from movement and sensory input.	Use crib mobiles, manipulative toys, wall murals, and bright colors to provide interesting stimuli and comfort. Use toys to distract the baby during procedures and assessments.
Toddler (1–3 years)	Anal stage (Freud): The child derives gratification from control over bodily excretions.	Ask about toilet training and the child's rituals and words for elimination during admission history. Continue child's normal patterns of elimination in the hospital. Have potty chairs available in hospital and child care centers.
	Autonomy versus shame and doubt stage (Erikson): The child is increasingly independent in many spheres of life.	Allow self-feeding opportunities. Encourage child to remove and put on own clothes, brush teeth, or assist with hygiene. If restraint for a procedure is necessary, proceed quickly, providing explanations and then comfort.

continued

TABLE I–8 (continued)

Age Group	Developmental Stages	Nursing Applications
	Sensorimotor stage (end); preoperational stage (beginning) (Piaget): The child shows increasing curiosity and explorative behavior. Language skills improve.	Ensure safe surroundings to allow opportunities to manipulate objects. Name objects and give simple explanations.
Preschooler (3–6 years)	Phallic stage (Freud): The child initially identifies with the parent of the opposite sex but by the end of this stage has identified with the same-sex parent.	Be alert for children who appear more comfortable with male or female nurses, and attempt to accommodate them. Encourage parental involvement in care. Plan for playtime and offer a variety of materials from which to choose.
	Initiative versus guilt stage (Erikson): The child likes to initiate play activities.	Offer medical equipment for play to reduce anxiety about strange objects. Assess children's concerns as expressed through their drawings. Accept children's choices and expressions of feelings.
	Preoperational stage (Piaget): The child is increasingly verbal but has some limitations in thought processes. Causality is often confused, so the child may feel responsible for causing an illness.	Offer explanations about all procedures and treatments. Prepare the child right before the procedure/ treatment. Clearly explain that the child is not responsible for causing the illness.
School age (6–12 years)	Latency stage (Freud): The child places importance on privacy and understanding the body.	Provide gowns, covers, and underwear. Knock on door before entering. Explain treatments and procedures to the child before they occur.
	Industry versus inferiority stage (Erikson): The child gains a sense of self-worth from involvement in activities.	Encourage the child to continue school work while hospitalized. Encourage child to bring favorite pastimes to the hospital.

TABLE I-8 *(continued)*

Age Group	Developmental Stages	Nursing Applications
		Help child adjust to limitations on favorite activities.
	Concrete operational stage (Piaget): The child is capable of mature thought when allowed to manipulate and see objects.	Give clear instructions about details of treatment. Show the child equipment that will be used in treatment.
Adolescent (12–18 years)	Genital stage (Freud): The adolescent's focus is on genital function and relationships.	Ensure access to gynecologic care for adolescent girls. Provide information on sexuality. Ensure privacy during health care. Have brochures and videos available for teaching about sexuality.
	Identity versus role confusion stage (Erikson): The adolescent's search for self-identity leads to independence from parents and reliance on peers.	Provide a separate recreation room for teens who are hospitalized. Take health history, perform examinations, and give medications without parents present unless the teen requests their presence. Introduce adolescent to other teens with same health problem who have received similar treatments.
	Formal operational stage (Piaget): The adolescent is capable of mature, abstract thought.	Give clear and complete information about health care and treatments. Offer both written and verbal instructions. Continue to provide education about the disease to the adolescent with a chronic illness, because mature thought now leads to greater understanding.

Adapted from Ball, J., Bindler, R., DeWitt, J.: Pediatric nursing: Partnering with children and their families. Upper Saddle River, Pearson, 2005.

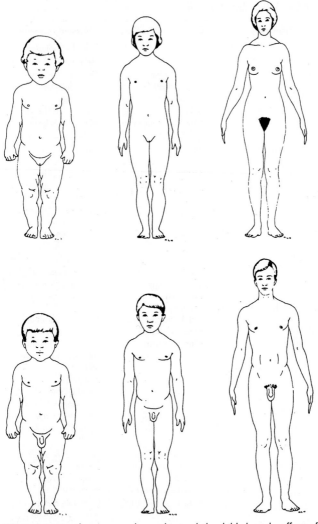

Figure 1–6. Line drawings can be used to teach the child about the effects of medication on the body.

2. The nurse can tell stories to convey necessary information, a technique that works particularly well with preschoolers. For example, "Susie was a four-year-old girl who had to get a shot every week for an allergy. She was very afraid of the shots and wondered why she had to get them. Then the nurse told Susie all about what the shots would do. Do you know what she told Susie? She told her that. . . ."

3. Books written for various age groups are available to explain health conditions or procedures as well as the medications required for treatment. The nurse can read these stories to the child to enhance understanding.

D. Toy Boxes
   1. The health care provider who wishes to discover which events about the medication experience are important to the child can put together a toy box with items such as medication cups, syringes without needles, various sizes and sexes of dolls, bandages, medicine bottles, gauze squares, and alcohol preps. The care provider brings the toy box to the child and allows supervised play for a period of time such as 20 minutes. Much information can be elicited regarding the feelings of the child by observing the items chosen for play, the content of the dramatic play in which the child engages, and the behavior manifested by the child during the play session. Remember to remain with the child during play and to take the items as you leave in order to ensure the safety of the child.
   2. Playing with items used to administer medications can help the child feel more in control and less fearful of such equipment. The nurse can demonstrate intravenous equipment, for example, and allow the child time to handle tubing and bags. Medication administration techniques can be demonstrated by use of a doll. By attaching intravenous tubing and a bag to a doll and performing a medication lock insertion or an intravenous discontinuation procedure, the child will learn what to expect. The child must be closely and individually supervised when using any potentially dangerous equipment in play with dolls.

E. Puppets
   Puppets are another effective tool used to impart information. The child believes in the identity of the puppet, forgets that the adult is actually playing the part of the character portrayed, and listens attentively to what is being discussed.

F. Music/Videos/CDs
   Music or favorite videos/CDs can be used to soothe and calm children after medication administration. This may be particularly effective with infants after uncomfortable procedures or with toddlers and preschoolers at sleep time. If children listen to tapes or watch videos/CDs at home, they can be brought to the hospital as an important link to provide security.

G. Discussion
   1. The older school-age child and the adolescent often respond best to clear explanations regarding their medications. They may also like to meet other children with the same condition. An adolescent coping with the disfiguring effects of antineoplastic drugs may gain much from a relationship with a similar adolescent who adjusted successfully to the same situation. The nurse should introduce such children to each other to encourage helpful relationships.
   2. Feedback is needed to determine if explanations are understood.

H. Learning Resources
   1. Audiovisual aids, such as pictures and key words, assist in capturing attention and increasing clarity during teaching sessions.

2. A number of videotapes/CDs are available for children of various ages to provide information on certain health conditions.
3. Health information can be provided by computer programs in the form of games or fun activities to assist children/adolescents to learn about their medical condition. Websites with accurate information are useful and can be provided to the patient and family.

▶ Techniques of Administration

I. General Principles

A. Information on administering medications to children is built on general knowledge and methods of giving medication to adults. Therefore, if administrative techniques are similar to those for adults they will not be discussed here.

B. Use of the nursing process when administering medications:
1. Assessment
   a. Conduct a thorough patient assessment including baseline data such as height and weight.
   b. Take a medication history including prescription, over-the-counter, and herbal medications.
   c. Ask about medication allergies.
   d. Assess for readiness to learn about medications.
   e. Assess need for medication (e.g., checking the pulse before giving a medication to slow the heart).
   f. Assess need for medication ordered as needed (PRN)

2. Diagnosis
   Some examples of nursing diagnoses related to medications include these:
   a. Risk for infection related to inadequate primary defenses (e.g., broken skin, traumatized tissue).
   b. Deficient knowledge of medications related to lack of prior experience.
   c. Acute pain related to surgery.
   d. Risk for injury related to effects of pharmaceutical agents.

3. Planning
   a. Set schedule for administration that is convenient for the client.
   b. Plan time for medication education.

4. Implementation
   a. Administer medications according to the Five Patient Rights of Medication Administration (see page 26).
   b. Deliver medication education.
   c. Begin medication schedule.

5. Evaluation
   a. Is the medication effective in relieving signs and symptoms?
   b. Does the schedule work well for the client and family?
   c. What side effects are observed?

C. The child needs well-planned, careful administration of medication to prevent physical and psychosocial trauma.
1. Consideration of the child's physiological variations, growth and development, and disease condition is important for understanding

of and accuracy in pediatric drug administration. Medication dosages for some drugs are based on Tanner stages of pubertal sexual maturation (Table I–9).

2. The care provider must possess knowledge of each drug's therapeutic effect on the child's body. Know the specific reason why the drug is prescribed for the specific child.

3. After accurate calculation of drug dose and individual assessment of the child, and discussion with the parent about how the child

TABLE I–9 Tanner Stages of Pubertal Sexual Maturation

Female Breast Development

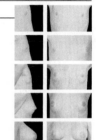

Stage 1 Prepubertal, no change in the size of the breast

Stage 2 Breast bud stage with areolar enlargement

Stage 3 Further enlargement of the areola and breast with no separation of their contours

Stage 4 Projection of areola with papilla forming a secondary mound above the level of the breast

Stage 5 Adult-like areola is recessed to the contour of the breast with the overall size of the breast increasing

Pubic Hair

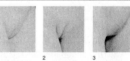
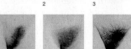

Stage 1 No pubic hair present

Stage 2 Sparse pubic hair primarily along the labia

Stage 3 Coarser, darker and more curly, spreading to the middle of the pubic bone

Stage 4 Appears adult-like but has not spread to the thighs

Stage 5 Adult-like and extends onto the thighs

Male Sexual Maturation

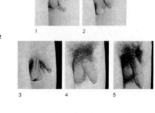

Stage 1 Prepubertal with no pubic hair; penis, scrotum, and testes are child-like in size

Stage 2 Enlargement of the scrotum and testes; scrotal area reddens; sparse hair appears along the base of the penis

Stage 3 Enlargement of penis mostly in length; pubic hair is coarser, darker, and curlier and extends over the middle of the pubic bone

Stage 4 Penis, scrotum, and testes are adult-like in size and appearance; pubic hair is adult-like in appearance

Stage 5 Continued growth of the testes and scrotum; penis grows in width; pubic hair extends to thighs and up to umbilicus

takes medication, the care provider is ready to begin drug administration.

D. Good hand washing technique should always be used before preparing and giving medications to the child. Use Standard Precautions whenever contact with the child's bodily secretions is possible.

E. Confirm correct drug and dose with every medication given and properly document procedure.
  1. Always check dosage prescribed against safe dosage ranges. Nurses are liable legally for any drug they administer. Use the Five Patient Rights of Medication Administration (see below).
  2. Identify each child carefully to avoid giving a medication to the wrong child. In the hospital, check identification bands, and in the office or outpatient setting, have the parent or child provide verbal identification. Verify allergy history.
  3. Use the Five Patient Rights of Medication Administration. Nurses should follow these five rights when administering medications to help prevent errors:
    a. The Right Drug
    b. In the Right Dose
    c. To the Right Patient
    d. At the Right Time
    e. By the Right Route
  4. After administration, use a sixth right which is correct documentation. Document the drug, dose, time, route and site, as well as the name and title of the person who administered the medication. Check the child's response to the medication and document the response as needed.
  5. In patient-specific documentation, including clinical documentation, order forms, progress notes, and consultation and operative reports, certain abbreviations should not be used because of the potential problem of misinterpretation. Additional recommendations about abbreviations to avoid can be found on the Joint Commission on Accreditation of Healthcare Organizations (JCAHO) website referenced following the table and on the ISMP Medication Safety Alert website.

Abbreviation to Avoid	Preferred Term
U (unit)	Unit
IU (international unit)	International unit
QD (daily)	Daily
QOD (every other day)	Every other day
Trailing zero (X.0 mg)	Omit a zero by itself after a decimal point (X mg)
Lack of leading zero (.X mg)	Always use a zero before a decimal point (0.X mg)
MS, MSO$_4$, MgSO$_4$	Morphine sulfate or magnesium sulfate in words.

From JCAHO, retrieved May 11, 2004, from http://www.jcaho.org/ accredited+organizations/patient+safety/04+npsg/04_faqs.htm.

6. The American Academy of Pediatrics has adopted a policy statement titled "Prevention of Medication Errors in the Pediatric Inpatient Setting." The statement lists recommendations regarding hospital-wide system actions and guidelines, prescriber actions and guidelines, prescriber education and communication, pharmacy action and guidelines, nursing actions and guidelines, nursing education and communication, and patients and families. The nursing actions and guidelines follow:

- Check medication calculations with another professional member of the health care team.
- Confirm patient identity before administration of each dose.
- Be familiar with medication ordering and dispensing systems.
- Verify drug orders before medication administration.
- Unusually large or small volumes or dosage units for a single patient dose should be verified.
- When a patient or parent or caregiver questions whether a drug should be administered, listen attentively, answer questions, and double-check the medication order.
- Remain familiar with the operation of medication administration devices and the potential for error with such devices, particularly patient-controlled analgesia or infusion pumps.

Data from Committee on Drugs and Committee on Hospital Care. (2003). Prevention of medication errors in the pediatric inpatient setting. *Pediatrics, 112,* 431–436.

II. Oral Administration

A. Liquid Preparations
   1. The child under 5 years of age usually experiences difficulty in swallowing tablets and capsules; thus, most medications for pediatric use are also available in the form of elixirs, syrups, or suspensions. Your pharmacy may be able to compound products into liquid preparations if the products are unavailable commercially.
   2. Liquid preparations contain the active drug (dissolved or suspended in a liquid base) and a flavoring agent to disguise the drug's taste. Syrups and elixirs contain drugs in a homogeneous solution and are clear in appearance. Syrups are sugar based (some contain aspartame®) and elixirs contain differing percentages of alcohol. Suspensions are not homogeneous solutions; the active drug is suspended in a liquid base, giving the solution a cloudy appearance.
   3. Liquid medications are supplied in a unit dose of drug; for example, milligram or microgram per cubic centimeter or milliliter of fluid (e.g., 5 mg/0.5 mL). Medication is usually prescribed in the metric system for administration in the medical setting (e.g., 125 mg every 6 hours) and in household measurements for administration by parents (e.g., 1 tsp every 6 hours).
   4. In 1903, the American Medical Association defined the standard teaspoon as containing 5 cc or mL. Research has demonstrated that the average household teaspoon may hold between 2.5 mL and 7.8 mL, thus only calibrated devices (e.g., plastic medicine cups, spoon-like devices, droppers, or syringes) should be used.

A medication dose that computes to less than 5 mL or to an uneven number, such as 7 mL, needs to be measured with a calibrated dropper or syringe to ensure accuracy of the dose. Some medications come with scored droppers and these should only be used to measure and give that particular medication.

5. Some medications that smell good may taste quite unpleasant; odor is not a reliable index of the taste.
6. Check expiration date of liquid medications before each dosage.
7. Many liquid medications must be refrigerated and some must be kept out of light. Read labels and follow instructions carefully for correct storage. Instruct parents about proper storage of medications at home.

B. Tablets and Capsules
1. Tablets and capsules are often available in doses appropriate for children. Before deciding on this route of administration, carefully assess the individual child's ability to swallow this form of medication.
2. If medication is only available in a tablet or capsule form and the child is unable to swallow it, the tablet may have to be crushed or the powder, "spansules," or liquid removed from the capsule for administration.
   a. Factors to consider when crushing a tablet:
      1. Is the dose required accurately measurable from the form of drug available? If not, can a particular tablet or capsule be accurately divided in half? Tablets are extremely difficult to divide into thirds or fourths and, therefore, this practice should be avoided. If a very small dose is required, the pharmacy may be able to put the drug into solution so that the correct dose can be administered. This is especially important when the drug has a narrow therapeutic index.
      2. Enteric-coated tablets (e.g., bisacodyl [Dulcolax]) have a special coating so that the tablet will dissolve in the duodenum and not be destroyed by stomach acidity. Such tablets should not be crushed because the drug would then be dissolved in the stomach, resulting in undesirable effects. Certain liquids, such as milk, may also destroy the enteric coating of a tablet.
      3. Sustained-release tablets are formulated with the drug embedded inside the tablet in such a manner that gradual release of the drug in the gastrointestinal tract is achieved. Crushing these tablets causes improper release of the drug.
      4. If the child cannot swallow the desired medication and it cannot be crushed, notify the prescriber so that a decision to change the medication's route or form can be made.
   b. Crushed tablets and contents taken from capsules usually have a bitter or unpleasant taste, therefore, they need to be mixed with something to disguise their flavor. When choosing a vehicle, consider if the drug will alter the food's taste; essential foods or fluids (e.g., orange juice) should be avoided, in case the child does not like the taste and refuses to accept the food or fluid again (aversion). Some commonly used vehicles are

jelly, honey, chocolate syrup, apple sauce, and fruit-flavored drinks. Pharmacies can provide syrups.

1. Applesauce is primarily used in young infants because it is a nonessential food; it is one of the first foods given to infants, and allergic reaction to it is rare. Honey is not recommended in the child under 12 months of age, because there is evidence that some honey contains *Clostridium botulinum* spores and can cause infants to develop botulism. Data demonstrate that the use of honey is not unsafe for the older child with normal intestinal microflora and immunities. Always check for drug–food interactions between the medication and chosen vehicle for administration.

2. Jelly and honey have a very high sugar content and should be avoided in a child whose sugar intake is restricted. Good oral care after intake of medication in these sweet foods helps prevent dental caries. Some medications are sweetened with aspartame®. Avoid use of these preparations in children with phenylketonuria (PKU).

3. Elixirs have alcohol content and may cause choking. Administer them slowly, aiming toward the inside of the cheek to minimize this effect. For infants, a nipple can be placed in the mouth and the medication placed in that so the baby can suck it out. The medication may be diluted in a small amount of another fluid. However, a very small amount, such as 5 to 10 mL, is used because the child will have to drink it all. Avoid use of essential foods such as milk because the medication may alter the taste and cause the child to develop an aversion to the food. Another fluid may be given after medication administration to wash the flavoring from the mouth.

4. Medication should be placed in the smallest amount of liquid or food possible to ensure that the child will take the entire amount.

c. With chewable tablets, chewing affects the disintegration of these tablets and is important in ensuring proper absorption of the drug from the gastrointestinal tract. The child losing deciduous teeth needs to take care not to inadvertently dislodge and swallow a loose tooth while chewing the tablet.

d. Most capsules can be safely separated, although the powder or liquid contents may be unpalatable and may need to be placed in a disguising vehicle. Capsules that contain sustained-release particles can be safely opened for administration because the coating on each particle will control its release in the gastrointestinal tract. The child, however, should be instructed not to chew the particles, which would destroy the protective coating.

e. Gelatin capsule containers can be used to disguise the taste of bitter tablets for the child who can safely swallow a capsule. The crushed or safely divided tablet can be placed in the empty capsule.

C. Positioning the Child and Administering Medication

The most important point in positioning the child for oral medication administration is to prevent aspiration of the drug. The child must be placed in an upright position and should never lie flat. The medication should be given in small amounts (0.2 to 0.5 mL) to prevent choking.

1. *Premature infant:* Assess for sucking reflex; if weak, the infant may need to receive oral medications by nasogastric or gastrostomy tube. Assess for tube placement and patency before instillation. Follow agency procedure. Be sure to flush the tube of medication after instillation to ensure that the dosage is delivered into the infant's stomach. If giving orally, take great care to prevent aspiration.

2. *Infant*
   a. The infant should be positioned or held comfortably with the head elevated to 45 degrees and the extremities restrained as necessary.
   b. An infant less than 3 to 4 months of age with a normal sucking and rooting reflex will usually suck medication from a nipple, dropper, or syringe. The baby will take the medication more readily if hungry. If a nipple is placed in the mouth, the medication can be poured in small amounts directly into the nipple. The infant of this age does not have a good sense of taste and, therefore, will usually take the medication without difficulty. Support the child's head and back.
   c. An infant less than 5 or 6 months of age will push anything solid out of the mouth and off the tongue because of the normal tongue movements used in sucking. This may interfere with giving crushed tablets disguised in solid food. The medication may need to be mixed in a liquid rather than a solid and administered by syringe instead of by a teaspoon. A child this age has good grasping abilities and, therefore, hands may need to be restrained while giving medication.
   d. An infant of 6 to 12 months can spit things out of the mouth. An oral syringe or medicine cup may work more effectively than a nipple. The plastic medicine cup can be bent slightly so that it fits into the infant's mouth and can deliver the medication in small amounts. A dropper, syringe, or medication spoon can also be used. The oral syringe or injectable syringe without a needle works effectively when it is placed across the tongue and directed toward the side of the mouth rather than the throat. This prevents aspiration or eliciting of the cough reflex. The child cannot spit out the medication because the syringe is across the tongue. This method works best with a child who will not take the medication from a cup. If the infant will not swallow the medication, the throat may be lightly stroked in a downward motion. This technique may be used effectively with infants or older children who have difficulty swallowing.

3. *Toddler:* The approach to use with the toddler directly affects the medication experience in a positive or a negative manner. Be positive and approach the child appropriately for developmental level. If the child will drink the medication from a cup or hollow-handled medication spoon, use this method. Either have the child hold the cup and drink from it or have the care provider give the medication in small amounts. If the child refuses to take the medication in this manner, it can be given in a syringe. Seat the child

across your lap facing the hand that will be used to give the medication. Put the child's arm that is nearer to your body along your side and under your arm. Grasp the child's free arm in the hand not giving the medication. To control the child's head place it against your shoulder. Use your free hand to give the medication. The medication can be given by the syringe method as described for the infant. Prevent aspiration.

4. *Preschooler:* Most preschoolers will take oral medications without much difficulty. This child can reason and with the use of appropriate developmental approaches, medication administration is usually successful. If not, the technique described for the toddler may be used. The use of play enables the preschooler to vent fears and frustrations.

5. *School-age child:* This child takes medication well. The child sometimes procrastinates in taking medication. This can be effectively dealt with by imposing time limits.

6. *Child who refuses medication:*
   a. A child from any age group may refuse to take oral medications because of a negative experience with medications or a desire to be independent. Work with this child to alleviate this negative experience first and then to gain cooperation. Try to involve the parents or significant others to see if they can get the child to take the medication.
   b. Sometimes a child will spit out medication. The best way to prevent this is to place the syringe across the tongue. If the child refuses to swallow, stroke the throat as described in the infant section. If the child spits out all the medication, readminister it immediately. If more than half but not all of the dose is spit out, repeat half of the dose. If the child spits out less than half the dose, if it is difficult to estimate how much has been spit, or if the care provider has any questions about repeating the medication, the prescriber should be consulted.

D. Special Considerations
   1. The child who is unable to retain oral medication because of vomiting needs careful evaluation by the prescriber. The medication treatment may need to be reassessed and another route of administration selected (rectal, intramuscular [IM] or intravenous [IV]). It is important to note that drug dose may vary among these different routes. For example, the oral dose may need to be higher to achieve the same therapeutic blood level maintained by IV administration. Consult drug dosage references when routes of administration are changed.
   2. The child who is taking daily medication for chronic illness requires careful evaluation of medication needs if receiving nothing by mouth (NPO) or vomiting. If the child is taking vitamins or laxatives daily, these can usually be omitted for 24 to 48 hours without negative effects. Cardiac medications and anticonvulsants are examples of drugs that usually need to be administered by another route if the child is NPO more than 12 hours.

E. Gastrostomy Tubes
   1. The child who has a gastrostomy tube in place for nutritional intake generally is given medications by this route. It is best to

administer the medications separately rather than adding them to the enteral formula in the feeding bag. If the child is on continuous feedings, they may need to be stopped for a period of time before medications to allow for adequate absorption. Verify that the medication is recommended to be given on an empty stomach.

2. Verify proper location of the tube in the stomach. Flush the tube with water to remove any residual feeding and flush it again after the medication to ensure that none is left in the tubing. These fluids must be added to the child's intake totals.

3. Liquid medications are easiest to give. If a pill or capsule is used, it must be crushed or opened and the contents added to a small amount of water (5 to 10 mL) for administration. The same principles that pertain to oral medications must be followed when using crushed medications. For example, sustained-release or enteric-coated tablets should not be crushed. Gastric irritants such as aspirin should not be given through the tube. Medications with the potential to irritate the stomach are sometimes diluted with water or enteral feeding for administration. Bulk-forming medications such as some laxatives should not be given through the tube because they may harden and clog it.

III. Rectal Administration

Rectal medications are not usually the most desirable type of drug to use with children because of erratic and unpredictable absorption from the colon. Fecal matter present in the rectum may cause part or all of the drug not to be absorbed. The rectal route occasionally becomes the method of choice if a child is vomiting or is NPO. This route, however, may be contraindicated in the child prone to rectal abscesses (e.g., a child being treated with certain antineoplastic agents).

A. Suppositories
1. Suppositories are the most frequent form of drug used rectally in the child. The drug is usually combined in a base of glycerin or lanolin that melts at body temperature.
2. Splitting or quartering of a suppository is difficult and does not guarantee that the child will receive the proper dose; therefore, it is best to give suppositories only as manufactured, especially when using drugs with a narrow therapeutic index.
3. In an infant or toddler, the suppository is inserted with an adult's fifth digit. For children older than 3 years, the rectum can usually accommodate an adult's index finger.
4. Because a child dislikes having a suppository inserted, proper restraint is necessary. The preschool child can become extremely upset by this procedure because of age-related fear of body entry. For these reasons, pay particular attention to giving adequate explanations to the child older than 2 years of age and use developmental approaches to decrease the child's fears.

B. Positioning the Child and Administering Suppositories
1. Follow manufacturer's recommendations regarding the need to lubricate the suppository before inserting it. When indicated, a water-soluble lubricating jelly can be used.

2. The child is usually placed in Sims' position or a knee–chest position for rectal administration.

3. The suppository is inserted gently into the rectum and is pushed past the internal sphincter toward the child's umbilicus. The child may be instructed to breath deeply or to pant like a puppy to provide distraction from the procedure. This also helps to discourage defecation. The buttocks should be held together firmly for 5 to 10 minutes after drug administration or until the child loses the urge to defecate.

4. If the child has a stool within 10 to 30 minutes after the insertion of the suppository, it should be examined for the presence of the suppository. If the suppository was not given for its laxative action and all of it is expelled with the stool, the prescriber should be contacted.

5. Chart the expulsion of the suppository and the subsequent course of action in the child's record.

C. Drug Administration by Enema
   1. Occasionally drugs are administered in an enema. Follow agency procedure for the administration of an enema to a child.
   2. The child, especially during infancy, is very susceptible to fluid overload and electrolyte imbalances; thus, the vehicle and the amount of solution for the enema should be carefully evaluated.

IV. Ophthalmic Administration

A. *Special considerations.* Sterile technique is essential when instilling medication into a child's eyes to prevent the introduction of pathogens into this delicate organ. The child should have an individually dispensed container of ophthalmic medication, and care must be taken even with individual medications to prevent contamination. If contaminated, the solution or ointment should be discarded.

B. Some factors that affect the absorption of a medication from the eye are child cooperation, gravity, blinking, and lid closure.
   1. The young child greatly fears having anything placed in the eyes, and even in infancy the child is able to close the eyelids so tightly that the care provider has difficulty opening them. When the child is old enough to comprehend the procedure, an explanation of ophthalmic instillation may help gain cooperation. Play also assists in dissipating fear and anxiety caused by eye instillations.
   2. Most ophthalmic preparations come in liquid or ointment form. Solutions at room temperature cause less discomfort and decrease blinking.
   3. Crying during the instillation of eye drops causes the solution to have little or no contact with the eye and the drug's therapeutic value may be lost. Thus, the child's cooperation greatly affects the therapy.
   4. Positioning of the child for administration of either liquid or ointment ophthalmic medication is the same. Hyperextend the child's neck over an adult's lap or put pillows under the shoulders. The child's head will then be lower than the body and gravity will help to disperse the medication over the cornea.

5. Proper restraint of the child is necessary to prevent injury to the eye. More than one individual may be required to accomplish this task, especially when dealing with an infant or a toddler. A mummy restraint can be used so that the child's extremities will not impede the instillation. Some individuals prefer to place the child's arms alongside the head to stabilize the drug during instillation. Either of these methods is effective as long as head control is achieved.

6. Because fear appears to be increased when the child actually sees the dropper coming toward the eye, the care provider can suggest that the child close the eyes while the lower lid is retracted for instillation. A demonstration of how the eyelid will be retracted can further understanding and reduce fear. When eyes are closed the cornea naturally deviates upward, preventing discomfort that could result in blinking or head movement. When the child blinks, the outflow of the medication from the eye increases, thereby decreasing the therapeutic value of the medication.

7. Stabilize the hand used for instilling medication by resting it on the child's forehead. Retract the lower lid to form a sac; apply medicine without touching the conjunctiva. To ensure sterility and to prevent blinking or ocular injury, do not allow the dropper to touch the child's eyelashes or the eye itself.

8. After instillation, keep the child in position for 1 to 3 minutes so that the medicine will have maximal contact with the eye. The child should close the eyes gently and keep them closed for several minutes to allow the medication greater contact time with the ocular area.

9. To minimize systemic absorption of eye drops immediately after instillation, apply a finger to the periphery of the nasolicrimal sac using light pressure for 1 to 2 minutes. Blot any excess medication with clean tissue.

10. If the ointment has been used previously, the care provider can prepare the ointment for instillation by squeezing a small amount of medication onto a sterile gauze pad and discarding it before instillation. This clears the end of the tube that may have been inadvertently contaminated during previous instillation or storage.

11. Technique for administration of an ophthalmic ointment is similar to that of placement of ophthalmic drugs. Squeeze a small line of ointment into the sac-like areas along conjunctiva. To stop ointment flow, rotate the tube with a twisting motion. Close the lid margin and have the child remain for several minutes in a hyperextended position with the eyes closed. Ointments usually blur vision for several minutes after instillation.

V. Otic Administration

A. Some medications are available in a liquid form to be placed in the external ear canal by dropper. Because the external auditory canal is not sterile, the ear is not treated in a sterile manner. If, however, the eardrum is ruptured and draining, the ear canal should be treated with sterile technique. Separately dispensed ear medication should be used for each individual child. Sometimes physicians prescribe eye drops to be placed in the ears because eye drops may be more comfortable.

B. The child should be placed in a side-lying position with the affected ear exposed. Two people may be needed to restrain a young child to prevent turning of the head during instillation. An older child needs an explanation to gain cooperation.

C. Sometimes a child's ears may need to be cleaned if a large amount of cerumen is present in the outer ear canal. The prescriber may use otic drops designed for this purpose or may order gentle water irrigation of the ear. If the ear is draining, only the outer aspect of the ear should be cleansed, with care taken to prevent fluid from entering the canal. Drainage from the ear is usually quite irritating to the skin. It should be cleansed frequently and the outer ear should be closely observed for skin breakdown.

D. In a child younger than 3 years, structures surrounding the ear canal area are cartilaginous and straight. To separate the walls of the canal effectively for drop instillation in such a child, the pinna is gently pulled down and back.

E. In a child older than 3 years, the ear canal has more ossification and the canal angles slightly. To instill drops in this child, pull the pinna up and back. Direct drops toward the ear canal rather than toward the eardrum. Drops directly hitting the eardrum may produce pain; if they are cold, they may induce nausea or vertigo. Drops should be at room temperature or body temperature when administered.

F. Immediately after instillation of the eardrops, massage the anterior ear gently to ease entry of the drops into the ear. The child should remain in a side-lying position for a few minutes so the drops can permeate to the tympanic membrane.

G. Cotton pledgets are occasionally used to prevent medication from escaping from the ear canal. They are also used if the ear canal is draining. A child should be instructed not to play with the ears or with the pledgets.

VI. Nasal Administration

A. Instillation of medication into the nares is a clean but not sterile procedure. The nares drain into the back of the mouth and throat, and instillation of medication may produce sensations of difficulty in breathing, tickling, or bad taste. Oil-based drops should be avoided because this solution may be aspirated into the lungs and produce aspiration pneumonia.

B. A child often reacts negatively to the experience of having drops placed in the nares. The infant, who breathes primarily through the nose, will squirm and attempt to get away, whereas the older child may violently protest. Proper restraint of the child is important to accomplish nasal instillation and to prevent injury.

C. A small infant may be placed in the care provider's lap with the head hyperextended over the care provider's knees. If the child's extremities are bound, the head can be controlled effectively.

D. An older child's head can be hyperextended by placing pillows under the shoulders. It may be necessary for two individuals to restrain a child.

E. After instillation of drops, the child should remain in the instillation position for several minutes to facilitate the action of the drops. The child should be closely observed for choking or vomiting during or after nasal drop instillation.

F. The young infant who has a respiratory ailment may receive saline nose drops before feedings to clear the nasal passages and aid in breathing during feeding. Outer nares may need to be cleansed first if mucus has crusted over the nares.

VII. Aerosol Therapy

A. An aerosol is a suspension of solid particles or liquid droplets in air. This method of drug administration may be desired because of its direct effect on lung passages. While systemic absorption is not generally as marked as with drugs taken by oral or parenteral routes, it is good to remember that medications can be absorbed systemically from the lungs and that both local and systemic side effects may occur.

B. Intermittent positive-pressure breathing (IPPB) treatments with a machine are usually given by a respiratory therapist or by specially trained nurses. The care provider delivering treatment must be knowledgeable about the machine's operation. The prescriber will order the medication dose, amount of pressure to be exerted during therapy, duration of the treatment, and number of treatments in a 24-hour period.

   1. The infant and the young child are usually frightened by the IPPB machine itself, whereas an older child may fear being unable to breathe during the treatment. Many of the aerosol medications have an unpleasant smell and the child may be overwhelmed by the combination of machines and medication. The child who can comprehend directions needs careful instructions to increase understanding of the treatment.

   2. With an infant and a young child, a facial mask is used to deliver the IPPB treatment, so both the nose and the mouth are covered.

      a. If a mouthpiece is used and the child is having difficulty triggering the machine, nose plugs may aid in complete breathing into the machine and thus make the treatment effective.

      b. The young child will usually respond more positively if held during IPPB treatment.

   3. To prevent contamination, each child should have an individual mask or mouthpiece and tubing for the machine. These pieces of equipment should be cleansed according to agency policy after each treatment.

C. Small-volume nebulizers are sometimes used to administer respiratory medications to children. Nebulizers may be hooked to an air and oxygen supply in the hospital or may be part of a small machine that uses room air for administration at home. The medication is placed in a reservoir, turns to mist as the air passes through it, and is breathed in by the child. The medicated mist can be delivered by a mask placed near the nose and mouth of a young child or can be breathed in through a mouthpiece when the child is old enough to cooperate. The equipment used should be cleaned as agency policy dictates or as the manufacturer suggests because the moisture in the tubing and reservoir can become a medium for growth of microbials.

D. Metered-dose inhalers are small handheld devices consisting of a canister containing a drug and a device for inhalation. The canister is inserted into the mouthpiece and the child is instructed to inhale and exhale fully. Then the mouthpiece is inserted into the mouth and the lips are closed tightly around it. The head is tilted back slightly and the child is told to inhale slowly and deeply through the mouth. By depressing the canister one time, one dose of medication is delivered and immediately inhaled. The child holds the breath for about 10 seconds. The small particles dispersed by the metered-dose inhaler reach deep into the lungs when directions are followed correctly. Children can easily carry the inhaler in a fanny pack when they need to take the medication on a regular basis or during emergencies. Teaching and demonstration are required to ensure that the child can use the inhaler correctly. When children are not old enough or have difficulty using a metered-dose inhaler correctly, a holding chamber may be used to capture the mist until the child breathes it in. These may include a reservoir, spacer, or extender. Another option for the child having difficulty with this type of administration is to use a breath-activated metered-dose inhaler, which releases the medication once the child begins to inhale.

VIII. Topical Agent Administration

A. Careful assessment of the area of skin to be treated and charting of observations is necessary before application of the topical agent. This provides a point of reference for determining the progress of healing or development of undesirable effects.

B. The care provider must be aware of the ingredients present in the topical drug being applied. If undesirable reactions to compounds occur, a careful assessment must be made to identify which ingredient is causing the reaction.

C. Topical agents are applied to a clean skin surface. Cleansing of the involved skin is accomplished from inner to outer aspects using a clean technique.
   1. If the skin is broken, sterile technique should be used. The exception to this may be the diaper area, where clean rather than sterile technique is usually employed.
   2. Lotions are usually applied to the skin with sterile applicators; they need frequent reapplication because of drying and flaking of residues.
   3. Ointments are usually rubbed on with gloved hands or are applied with sterile applicators. Thin-coat applications are preferred unless otherwise directed.
   4. After the medication is applied to the skin, careful assessment of the area is once again necessary. Any new skin irritation,

breakdown, or rashes should be noted, reported to the prescriber immediately, and use stopped until further direction is received.

D. The child usually does not understand the necessity to refrain from scratching an infected area even with repeated reminders and explanations.
1. The child's hands may need to be restrained or wrapped with clean cotton mittens, especially when the child is sleeping.
2. All nails, including toenails, should be kept short and clean to prevent introduction of bacteria to the affected site.
3. Drugs to relieve itching may be necessary.
4. The child's toys must be carefully selected to prevent trauma or infection. Fuzzy stuffed toys are usually not recommended, especially if the child's skin is broken or draining. Washable cotton or plastic toys are a better choice.

IX. Vaginal Administration

Vaginal medication is rarely used in the young female child or infant; adolescent girls more commonly receive this form of medication.

A. When a toddler or a preschool child receives vaginal medication, great care must be taken to reduce psychological trauma. Because these age groups have great fear of body entry, it is necessary to assess their developmental level carefully.

B. The school-age child and adolescent usually understands explanations of the vaginal administration process. A child this age, however, needs sensitive assessment of the understanding of the vaginal area and its functions. Because the vagina is a sexual organ, it is important to ascertain the beliefs with respect to sexuality and family values and what cultural influences affect the beliefs. It is also important to assess parental views.

C. Vaginal medications commonly come in suppository, cream, or irrigation form. These medications are instilled in the same manner as for the adult woman. Because the vaginal opening is small, good visualization of the area is necessary to prevent trauma. The medication should be inserted gently to reduce fear and possible discomfort. Adolescents usually can be instructed to administer their own vaginal medication.

D. Applicators should be cleansed after each administration, and separate applicators should be used with each child receiving vaginal drugs.

X. Parenteral Medication Administration

A. Care providers must be sensitive to the needs of the child and should administer injections in a manner that will decrease the physical as well as the psychosocial trauma.
1. Syringes should be prepared out of visual range of the child, to prevent anxiety created by viewing a needle. Needles may seem to get larger and more frightening if the child has to look directly at them for an extended time. Occasionally, an older child may wish to look at the needle just before the injection.

2. Structured play with needles and syringes has been found to reduce anxiety associated with injections.
3. Best results occur if play is performed several hours in advance of the injection or after an injection, rather than at the time of injection.
4. It is important to assist every child receiving an injection in relieving feelings through appropriate developmental approaches.

B. Reconstitution of Injectable Medications
1. Follow drug manufacturer's recommendations for the amount and types of solutions to reconstitute. When a newborn or premature infant requires extremely small doses of medication, further dilution of the drug may be needed. The pharmacist can provide the necessary dilution information. Do not reconstitute medications for this age group using solutions containing benzyl alcohol because of its potential to cause fatal toxicity (gasping syndrome).
2. Store injectable medications according to manufacturers' recommendations to ensure stability of the drug.
3. Refrigerated injectables should be stored in a refrigerator that is used only for medications. The vials should not be stored in the refrigerator door because frequent opening of the door may cause significant temperature variations. The measles vaccine is one medication affected by temperature changes that can result in loss of its therapeutic value.
4. Injectable drugs must be properly labeled as to when they were opened or reconstituted and the total amount of solution in which the drug is dissolved, the solution strength, date and time it was prepared, and initials or name of the individual who prepared the solution. The labels of reconstituting solutions, such as sterile water or normal saline, indicate whether preservatives are present in solution. Solutions that do not have preservatives should be used immediately. Solutions with preservatives (e.g., bacteriostatic water) should be discarded after 7 days, or immediately if contaminated. Expiration dates of all injectables should be checked before each injection preparation.
5. Mathematical calculations of drug dose should be checked by each person giving an injectable medication, even if the pharmacist has made the calculation. This ensures accuracy and prevents errors.
6. After injections are given, it is important to chart medication correctly and according to agency policy, always including the site in which the injection was administered. This not only is a legal requirement but also assists the care provider who gives the next injection in rotating injection sites, thereby reducing tissue irritation.

C. Subcutaneous Injections
Subcutaneous injections are placed in subcutaneous fat layers of a child's body. A child's fat deposits differ from those of an adult. Preferred sites are the anterior thighs, buttocks, upper arms, and abdomen.
1. The subcutaneous layer can be lifted to isolate the site and avoid injecting a muscle; this is especially helpful if the child is thin and has very little subcutaneous tissue. The injection is given as for an adult.
2. Restrain the child as necessary.

TABLE I–10   Guidelines for Maximal Amounts of Solutions to Be Injected into Muscle Tissues

Muscle Group	Birth to 1.5 Years (mL)	1.5 to 3 Years (mL)	3 to 6 Years (mL)	6 to 15 Years (mL)	15 Years to Adulthood (mL)
Deltoid	Not recommended	Not recommended unless other sites are not available 0.5	0.5	0.5	1
Gluteus maximus	Not recommended	Not recommended unless other sites are not available 1	1.5	1.5–2	2–2.5
Ventrogluteal	Not recommended	Not recommended unless other sites are not available	1.5	1.5–2	2–2.5
Vastus lateralis	0.5–1	1	1.5	1.5–2	2–2.5

D. Intramuscular Injections
  1. Giving IM injections to a child requires understanding of anatomy and physiology, careful site selection, and adequate restraint of the child.
  2. The total volume of solution that can be injected into an injection site for each dose must be carefully assessed. Factors to be considered are size of the muscle, tissue integrity, and the child's age and development. Table I–10 shows maximal amounts of solutions to be injected into muscle tissues.
  3. Assess the amount of subcutaneous fat over the injection site. This determines the appropriate needle length for delivery of medication into a muscle mass. Most 1- to 1½-inch needles, gauge 20, 21, or 22, are appropriate for the child. Use the smallest gauge needle available to deliver a drug into the muscle mass.
  4. Physiologically, the gluteus maximus muscle mass is not well developed until the child has walked for at least 1 full year. The authors recommend that the gluteus maximus never be used for an injection site in a child who has not walked for at least 1 year and that in the child younger than 4 to 6 years this site be used only if other sites are contraindicated (Figure I–7). Always approach this site with great care because the sciatic nerve is large and runs through the medial portion of the muscle mass. Identify the greater trochanter and posterior iliac spine and inject superior and lateral to the imaginary line connecting these landmarks.

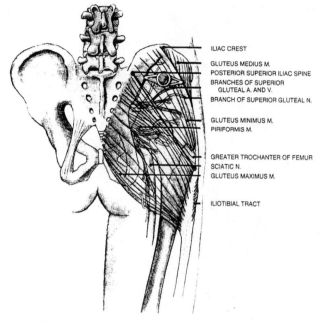

ILIAC CREST

GLUTEUS MEDIUS M.
POSTERIOR SUPERIOR ILIAC SPINE
BRANCHES OF SUPERIOR
GLUTEAL A. AND V.
BRANCH OF SUPERIOR GLUTEAL N.

GLUTEUS MINIMUS M.
PIRIFORMIS M.

GREATER TROCHANTER OF FEMUR
SCIATIC N.
GLUTEUS MAXIMUS M.

ILIOTIBIAL TRACT

Figure I–7. Dorsogluteal injection site.

5. The vastus lateralis muscle is the preferred site for injection because it is the largest muscle mass in a child younger than 3 years and is free of major nerves and vessels. The injection site is the medial outer aspect in the center one-third portion of the thigh. This muscle can be isolated for injections by pinching up the muscle mass. Insert the needle at a right angle, directing it toward the knee (Figure I–8).

6. The ventrogluteal site is also relatively free of major nerves and vessels. This makes it an ideal site in a child older than 3 who has been walking for some years. Place the child on one side and flex the top leg at the knee to relax the muscle site. Locate the greater trochanter and place the heal of the hand on this landmark while pointing fingers toward the child's head. Place the index finger over the anterior superior iliac tubercle and with the middle finger spread to the iliac crest, forming a "V" with the fingers. Make the injection into the center of the triangle formed with the fingers, placing the needle at a right angle but slightly canted toward the iliac crest. This site must be correctly identified to prevent injection into the bone or hip joint (Figure I–9).

7. The deltoid muscle is rarely used in children younger than 4 or 5 years because of its small muscle mass. It is used for immunizations in the child older than 1.5 years, because of the small amount of solution to be injected. This site also requires careful

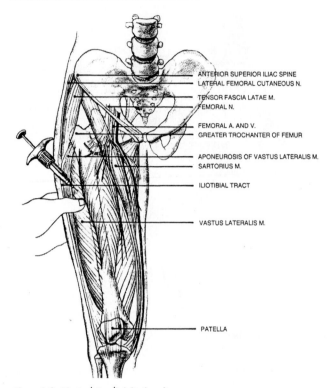

Figure I–8. Vastus lateralis injection site.

identification because of the position of the nerves. Find the acromion process and give the injection into the upper one third of the muscle located about two fingers' length below the acromion. Insert the needle at a right angle slightly canted toward the shoulder (Figure I–10).

8. Topical anesthetics such as EMLA and Numbys can be applied prior to injection at an IM site to decrease injection pain. Giving infants oral sucrose solutions during injections also decreases pain.

9. Because the child may move during an injection, be sure to have a firm grip on the lower portion of the syringe (to ensure that the drug is injected at the site of aspiration) and have a second needle available in case the first one becomes contaminated.

10. The child may need to be distracted during injection to facilitate relaxation of the muscle and thus permit ready needle entry. This can be accomplished by having the child pant, count, or wiggle or point toes during the injection. Use developmental approaches to assist in gaining the child's cooperation and in allaying fears.

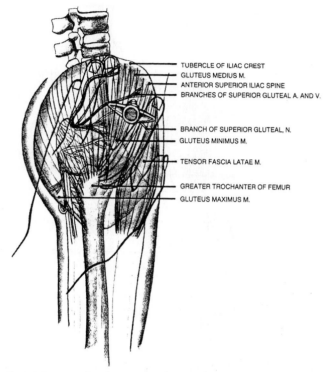

TUBERCLE OF ILIAC CREST
GLUTEUS MEDIUS M.
ANTERIOR SUPERIOR ILIAC SPINE
BRANCHES OF SUPERIOR GLUTEAL A. AND V.

BRANCH OF SUPERIOR GLUTEAL, N.
GLUTEUS MINIMUS M.

TENSOR FASCIA LATAE M.

GREATER TROCHANTER OF FEMUR
GLUTEUS MAXIMUS M.

Figure I–9. Ventrogluteal injection site.

11. Remember that overuse, frequent injections, or large volumes of drugs injected into IM sites can cause muscle wasting and atrophy.

12. Dispose of used injection materials safely, following agency policy. Do not recap needles before discarding because that increases the likelihood of a needle-stick injury for the health care provider. Gloves may be used if the provider has open lesions or may come in contact with body fluids from the child.

E. The child must be securely restrained to avoid giving the injection in the wrong site or having the needle become dislodged or broken.

1. The child younger than 6 months can easily be restrained by one person. A care provider can be positioned horizontally above the infant, facing the legs, using body or arms as a gentle but effective restraint. Then the exact site can be selected, the muscle lifted with one hand, and the injection given with the other.

2. When an infant can turn over or is particularly strong, a second person may be needed during an injection. The second person should restrain the infant's arms and the leg not being injected.

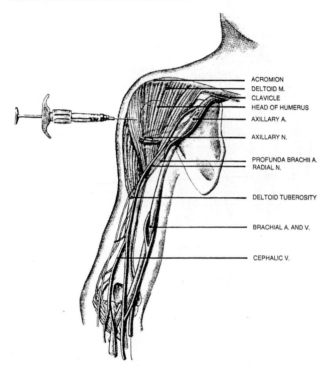

ACROMION
DELTOID M.
CLAVICLE
HEAD OF HUMERUS
AXILLARY A.

AXILLARY N.

PROFUNDA BRACHII A.
RADIAL N.

DELTOID TUBEROSITY

BRACHIAL A. AND V.

CEPHALIC V.

Figure I-10. Deltoid injection site.

The professional giving the injection then has more control over the needle and syringe and over the site being injected.

3. It is always best to have two adults present for injection administration to toddlers and preschoolers.

4. The care provider may need someone to help hold a school-age child still during the injection. This is best accomplished by a parent or by another health care worker. On the other hand, a school-age child may prefer having only the professional who is giving the injection present.

5. The child who is combative may need more than two adults for restraint. If the child wants parents to help restrain, they must be carefully assessed for their ability to support and restrain their child during an injection. Some parents are invaluable and can assist not only by restraining but also by comforting the child. Other parents become upset by the thought of an injection and their anxiety only increases the child's anxiety. These parents need the care provider's understanding and assistance to learn how to support the child during future injections.

F. Intravenous Medication

The IV route is often preferred over the IM route for administration of certain drugs, such as antibiotics, especially with premature babies, infants, and toddlers. With the IV route, therapeutic blood levels of the drug are achieved quickly because of direct access into the systemic circulation.

G. Insertion and Regulation of Intravenous Line

1. Maintenance of pediatric IV drug therapy poses many problems owing to the child's psychological makeup and cognitive level. Recognition of the child's level of development and individual needs can assist the care provider in reducing the fear and trauma of IV therapy.

2. Adverse reactions can be seen in a matter of seconds to minutes. Knowledge of each drug's therapeutic actions, calculation of dosage, and close monitoring of the child are imperative.

3. The veins of a child are small and fragile, requiring skilled insertions. Also, most individuals who start IV infusions in pediatric clients prefer to insert them in a treatment room rather than at the child's bedside so that the child does not view the bed as a place of punishment. Gloves must be worn and used equipment discarded according to agency policy.

4. Methods for starting IV infusions are not discussed in this book because the technique is similar to the technique used for adults. The child's veins are smaller and need small-gauge needles, and in the infant, scalp veins are also used as infusion sites. Anesthetic creams such as EMLA and Numbys can be used to reduce pain when IVs are started.

5. A young child requires restraint by one or more adults while an IV infusion is started.

6. Intravenous lines must be securely anchored. Assess the child for tape allergies and use hypoallergenic tape when necessary. Stabilize the IV site so that the child can move freely and infiltration is avoided.

   a. Opsite dressings or other IV protective devices are used to stabilize and protect the site.

   b. Parents need explanations about their child's limitations with IV therapy to prevent them from inadvertently dislodging the IV line or stopping the flow.

   c. Explaining the reason for the IV treatment promotes cooperation.

7. The IV fluid and medication need close monitoring in the child because fluid overload can occur easily (Table I–11).

   a. A younger child is most susceptible to fluid overloads. Most institutions regulate the maximal volumes that can be used with various age groups (see Table I–6 for average fluid needs).

   b. Careful regulation of the rate of fluid infusion also prevents fluid overload. The IV drip rate should be monitored every 15 to 30 minutes. Hourly IV infusion rates and amounts should be recorded on an IV flowchart.

   c. A safeguard for pediatric clients is a measured volume chamber. Most of these measured chambers also have microdrip drop mechanisms. When using these chamber devices, no more than twice the amount of solution a child is to receive in an hour should be placed into the chamber at any one time. This prevents fluid overload.

TABLE I-11   Fluid Requirements as Determined by Weight

Weight (kg)	Fluid Requirements
0–10	100 mL/kg/24 h
10–20	1000 mL + 50 mL/kg/24 h for each kilogram between 11 and 20
20–70	1500 mL + 20 mL/kg/24 h for each kilogram between 21 and 70
Over 70	2500 mL/24 h (adult requirement)

    d. Frequent checking of the IV line and site helps detect flow stoppage due to a change in the child's position, kinks in tubing, or other causes.

    e. Medication infused by constant drip also requires close monitoring of the IV site for potential infiltration, skin breakdown, or phlebitis. Infiltrations can occur suddenly and are usually noted by symptoms of edema at the needle site, changes in skin color or temperature, or complaints of pain at the needle site.

    f. Most institutions recommend that IV tubing be changed every 24 to 48 hours.

8. The IV medications can be placed in the entire bottle of solution for infusion over an extended time, in a special holding device attached to the intravenous tubing, in a second bag attached by piggyback to the main IV line, administered by IV push directly into the line, or by syringe pump. With every drug given, the care provider must know the drug's dose range, side effects, interaction, compatibility with the IV solution, and safe infusion rate.

    a. If the drug is placed in a measured chamber, the chamber should be flagged in some manner to inform other care providers that no more fluid should be placed in the chamber until the drug has been completely infused.

    b. Parents and the child need to be instructed not to tamper with either the fluid levels in the measured chamber or the IV infusion rate.

    c. Drugs given by the IV push method should not be injected quickly but should be administered according to the manufacturer's maximal rate of drug infusion.

9. Immediately before injecting the drug, the site should be inspected to ensure the integrity of the infusion.

10. When drugs are given by constant infusion, it is important to keep the flow rate on schedule. Constant-infusion pumps deliver the solution into the vein at a constant and controlled rate and are usually used with pediatric patients. Syringe pumps can be used for very small infusions or when several drugs are being given. Small volumes of solution (2 to 3 mL/h) can be infused while keeping the infusion patent.

    a. Infusion pumps are not infallible and need to be observed for dry chambers, air in the tubing, and improper pump rates.

    b. Battery-powered infusion pumps and syringe pumps allow the child greater freedom of movement.

    c. Patient-controlled analgesia (PCA) is delivered by programmable pumps that are set to administer a continuous infusion as well as a bolus dose at determined times and amounts. The bolus dose is delivered when the child or parent pushes a button. This route enables steady blood concentrations of analgesia and facilitates pain relief.

11. The medication lock is a needle or catheter with a specially designed cap through which a heparin or saline solution is injected to maintain needle patency.

    a. Medication locks are maintained as they are for adults. The heparinized solution most hospitals use for pediatric flush is 50 to 100 U/mL. Many agencies use normal saline to maintain line patency because research has shown this technique to be effective in most cases.

    b. The child and family must be cautioned not to tamper with the medication lock.

H. Central Venous Catheters

1. Central venous catheters are long catheters placed through a vein (such as the subclavian vein) and threaded into the right atrium. Catheters may also be inserted through a peripheral intravenous site and threaded centrally into the superior vena cava; these are called PICC lines. Catheters may have one, two, or three lumens. These lines are inserted when a child needs long-term intravenous therapy such as antibiotic therapy or chemotherapy. Some children are discharged with these lines, and parents learn to clean and maintain them at home.

2. The catheter site is covered with a clear occlusive dressing and is usually cleaned and redressed two to three times weekly. Sterile technique with gloves and mask is used. The site is cleaned with half-strength hydrogen peroxide and then povidone-iodine swabs. Assessment of the site and the marking on the catheter at the insertion site are performed before reapplying the dressing. Problems with a central line can be similar to those for other intravenous sites: clot or thrombus formation, phlebitis, leakage, malposition, and sepsis. Assess the site according to agency policy and the patient's condition.

3. If the catheter is not used for continuous intravenous therapy, it is maintained by periodic flushes with normal saline or heparin solution. Follow agency policy for maintaining patency of the line.

I. Implanted Ports

Some children who will need intravenous therapy over time will have a port implanted under the skin of the chest wall or arm. The disk-shaped port has a catheter that is inserted into a vein leading to the right atrium. The skin and self-healing rubber surface of the disk are punctured when an infusion is needed, and when finished the needle is removed and the port reseals. Sterile technique with gown, mask, and gloves is used to access the port.

J. Intraosseous Administration

In critical situations when access to circulation is not possible, intraosseous administration of fluids and medication has been used. A needle (such as a bone marrow needle) is inserted into the medullary cavity of the femur or tibia and fluids and medication given, similar to intravenous administration. Specialized protocols should be developed for agencies utilizing this route of administration.

K. Intrathecal Administration
A catheter is placed in the cerebrospinal canal, fluid is removed so that medication can be accommodated, and medications (such as chemotherapeutic agents or opioids with or without anesthetics) are administered. Specialized protocols should be developed for agencies utilizing this route of administration.

L. Epidural Administration
A catheter is placed in the epidural space of the spinal canal and used for continuous or intermittent analgesic administration. This method is used postoperatively or for pain control. It provides steady drug levels, long-lasting analgesia, and less risk of respiratory depression and other side effects than systemic administration. Specialized protocols should be developed for agencies utilizing this route of administration.

M. Regional Blocks
Regional blocks may be used during surgery with a catheter left in place so that pain medication can be administered via pump after surgery. Some common locations for regional blocks are popliteal or axillary regions. Nurses generally monitor regional block infusion after surgery. Specialized protocols should be developed for agencies utilizing this route of administration.

N. Sedation for Diagnostic and Therapeutic Procedures
Moderate sedation is a medically controlled state of minimally depressed consciousness that allows protective reflexes to be maintained, retains the patient's ability to maintain a patent airway independently and continuously, and permits appropriate response by the patient to physical stimulation and/or verbal command. This level of sedation was formerly called *conscious sedation* and is commonly used for diagnostic and therapeutic procedures that are more easily and painlessly carried out when the child is sedated. In contrast with moderate sedation, *mild sedation* is equivalent to anxiolysis, and *deep sedation* is characterized by reflex activity but inability to respond to pain or verbal command.
The following guidelines for sedation should be followed:
1. *Before procedure:*
   a. Obtain informed consent. This includes written and/or verbal instructions to the responsible person.
   b. Obtain age; weight; health history, including allergies, drugs, diseases, hospitalizations, prior complications with sedation, family history; family physician; review of systems; vital signs; physical examination; physical status evaluation by trained anesthetist or anesthesiologist. A focused airway examination must be included.
   c. Evaluate food and fluid intake. Desired time to be NPO for foods is 8 hours; for fluids, 4 to 6 hours.

    d. Prepare emergency drugs, equipment, and personnel and have them ready. Equipment and drugs must be appropriate for age and size of the child. At least one person must be trained in pediatric life support, preferably in pediatric advanced life support.

    e. Sedative or anxiolytic drugs should not be given at home prior to travel to a facility for a procedure.

2. *During procedure:*

    a. The practitioner using sedation must be trained in use of the medications and in airway management. An additional support person must be present to monitor the child. Personnel should be trained in advanced life support in emergency situations.

    b. Record all drugs, routes, doses, and times.

    c. Monitor oxygen saturation and heart rate continuously, and record them as well as level of sedation, respiration and blood pressure, regularly and frequently. A specific person must be assigned solely to monitoring for deep sedation, and vital signs must be recorded at least every 5 minutes.

    d. Check restraints and head position frequently.

    e. Have suction present and functional.

3. *After procedure:*

    a. Maintain monitoring in presence of suction and emergency services such as ventilatory support and drugs.

    b. Monitor oxygen saturation and heart rate continuously until recovered.

    c. Take vital signs frequently, usually every 5 minutes until awake and then every 15 minutes until discharge. Record according to agency protocol.

    d. Discharge criteria must be followed and include:

        1. Satisfactory and stable cardiovascular function and airway patency.

        2. Easily arousable, protective reflexes intact.

        3. Can sit up unassisted if old enough to do so.

        4. If child is very young or handicapped, discharge state is the same as admission state.

        5. Hydration is adequate.

Data from: Committee on Drugs (1992). Guidelines for monitoring and management of pediatric patients during and after sedation for diagnostic and therapeutic procedures. *Pediatrics 89,* 1110–1115 and Committee on Drugs (2002). Guidelines for monitoring and management of pediatric patients during and after sedation for diagnostic and therapeutic procedures: addendum. *Pediatrics 110,* 836–838.

4. Common Medications for Sedation

    a. Chloral hydrate: 25 to 100 mg/kg PO or PR (maximum 2 g)

    b. Demerol-Phenergan-Thorazine: 2–1–1 mg/kg IM

    c. Pentobarbital: 2 to 6 mg/kg PO, PR, IM; 0.5 to 1.0 mg/kg IV

    d. Diazepam: 0.15 to 0.3 mg/kg PO or 0.05 to 0.1 mg/kg IV

    e. Midazolam: 0.035 to 0.4 mg/kg PO, PR, nasal, IV intermittent infusion with 0.4 mcg/kg/min usually effective or 0.035 to 0.1 mg/kg (maximum total of 2.5 mg)

      f. Morphine: 0.05 to 0.1 mg/kg IV

      g. Fentanyl: 0.5 to 1 mcg/kg IV to begin, titrate upward as needed for desired response

5. Suggested Emergency Drugs

- Oxygen
- 50% glucose
- Atropine
- Epinephrine
- Phenylephrine
- Dopamine
- Diazepam
- Isoproterenol
- Calcium chloride or gluconate
- Sodium bicarbonate
- Lidocaine
- Naloxone
- Diphenhydramine
- Hydrocortisone
- Succinylcholine
- Aminophylline
- Racemic epinephrine
- Inhalation albuterol
- Insulin
- Maricon.

6. See also the following references:

    1. American Academy of Pediatric Dentistry. Policy statement on the use of deep sedation and general anesthesia in the pediatric dental office. http://www.aapd.org.

    2. American Society of Anesthesiologists. Continuum and depth of sedation: Definition of general anesthesia and levels of sedation/analgesia. http://www.asahq.org/standards/20.htm.

    3. Joint Commission on Accreditation of Healthcare Organizations. Standards and intents for sedation and anesthesia care. http://www.jcaho.org/standard/aneshap.html.

O. Total Parenteral Nutrition

Total parenteral nutrition (TPN) infusions require skillful monitoring and maintenance. The physician inserts the catheter surgically, under sterile conditions, into the subclavian vein, the jugular vein, or the umbilical vein of the newborn or premature infant. The site is then covered with a sterile dressing that is changed every 24 to 48 hours under sterile conditions according to agency policy.

1. The child must be instructed not to touch or play with the catheter dressing; the young child may need to be restrained to prevent contamination of the site.

2. The infusion rate is maintained with an infusion pump. Extreme care in recording the infusion rate and volume of fluid infused is imperative, as are strict input and output measurements and daily weighings to detect fluid imbalances.

3. Special tubing and filters designed for TPN administration are used; tubing and filters are changed down to the catheter site every 24 to 48 hours, depending on agency policy.

4. Medication should not be administered through the hyperalimentation fluid, nor blood be drawn through this central line. The pharmacist must be consulted before any drugs are added to this fluid. If drugs are given intravenously, they are usually administered through another IV infusion site and using a different infusion pump.

5. TPN fluid is prepared in the pharmacy under sterile conditions to prevent contamination. It is ideally made no more than 8 hours in advance of the infusion time; a bottle should be considered safe for infusion for only 24 hours after preparation. Most TPN fluids should be refrigerated in the medication refrigerator until needed, but should be allowed to come to room temperature before infusion.

6. Before each new bottle of fluid is hung, carefully check the contents of the solution against the prescriber's orders.

7. If fluid begins to leak from the tubing, the tubing should be changed immediately; tape should not be placed over the tubing.

8. The catheter site and the patient should be carefully observed for any signs of infection and reaction during therapy.

P. Lipid Emulsions

Lipid emulsions are infused through a central venous line. These emulsions have a milky appearance because of the suspended fat globules in the solution.

1. The appearance of this solution may frighten a child and the parents; therefore, explanations are necessary.

2. Lipid emulsions are refrigerated and then brought to room temperature by standing for 30 minutes before infusion.

3. Nothing should ever be added to the emulsion mixture, and it should be checked for consistency, texture, and color.

4. Rates of infusion need to be confirmed by the physician and pharmacist before infusion.

5. Observe for signs of adverse reaction, especially in the first 30 minutes. The infusion rate should not exceed 1 mL/min.

6. The child receiving this infusion should be monitored constantly during the infusion and should be observed for delayed symptoms after the infusion.

Q. Recommendations for Controlling Occupational Exposure to Hazardous Drugs

Adapted from Section VI, Chapter 2, "Controlling Occupational Exposure to Hazardous Drugs" OSHA Technical Manual (2003), http://www.osha.org.gov/dts/osta/otm/otm_VI/otm_VI_Z.html.

Hazardous drugs are those that can cause genotoxicity, carcinogenicity, teratogenicity or fertility impairment, serious organ or other toxic manifestation at low doses in experimental animals or treated patients. While most antineoplastic or cytotoxic agents are considered hazardous drugs, other drugs are also included in this classification. Investigational products should be considered hazardous until information on their safety is demonstrated. Each agency should develop a list of potentially hazardous drugs used in its facility and which require hazardous drug handling protocols. Lists should be reviewed and updated regularly. Examples of noninvestigational hazardous drugs included in this book are listed next. This is not intended to be a complete list of hazardous drugs nor to indicate that all other drugs are safe to handle. Wise handling and minimized exposure are recommended for all drug products.

- Asparaginase
- Bleomycin
- Busulfan
- Carboplatin
- Carmustine
- Chlorambucil
- Chloramphenicol
- Cisplatin
- Cyclophosphamide
- Cyclosporin
- Cytarabine
- Dacarbazine
- Dactinomycin
- Daunorubicin
- Doxorubicin
- Etoposide
- Fluorouracil
- Gancyclovir
- Hydroxyurea
- Idarubicin
- Ifosfamide
- Interferon A
- Isotretinoin
- Leuprolide
- Lomustine
- Mechlorethamine
- Medroxyprogesterone
- Mercaptopurine
- Methotrexate
- Pentamidine
- Procarbazine
- Ribavirin
- Tamoxifen
- Teniposide
- Thioguanine
- Thiotepa
- Uracil mustard
- Vidarabine
- Vinblastine
- Vincristine
- Zidovudine

Health personnel can be exposed to hazardous drugs during preparation, administration, and disposal of these drugs. The aim is to minimize exposure and consequent risks from these drugs. Direct cutaneous contact as well as airborne absorption from all products (not only aerosolized) can occur. Home health care personnel are using these drugs with increasing frequency. All precautions must still be taken when giving these drugs in patient homes, and spill kits, emergency procedures, and phone numbers must be available. Develop procedures for transport based on OSHA guidelines.

Although recommended precautions are listed next, each agency should develop its own policy for specific hazardous drug handling. Potentially exposed personnel are monitored regularly for adverse health effects via agency policy. Spontaneous abortion and congenital malformation have been documented in health care workers exposed to hazardous drugs, whether male or female. Agencies need policies about reproductive toxicity of its hazardous drugs. Exposure during pregnancy, especially early months, and during breast feeding are generally prohibited. Employee information and training are important parts of agency policy. All training must be identified and recorded in employee records.

1. Preparation of Hazardous Drugs
   a. General Guidelines
      Although pharmacists generally prepare hazardous drugs, in some small hospitals and in office practice, trained nurses may be engaged in drug preparation. Therefore, general guidelines for preparation are included here.
      - Perform in a restricted, central area in a Class II or III biological safety cabinet.
      - The cabinet should have downward airflow and high-efficiency particulate air filters.
      - The exhaust fan should be on at all times.
      - Cabinets without air recirculation are most protective.
      - If vented outside, keep away from air intake units.
      - Use continuous monitoring devices to confirm air flow and cabinet performance.
      - Place cabinet in area with minimal air turbulence and limited traffic; post signs restricting access by nonauthorized personnel.
      - Follow manufacturers' recommendations for cleaning, decontamination, and service.
      - Eating, drinking, smoking, chewing gum, applying cosmetics, and storing food in the area are prohibited.
      - Personnel wear protective garments and respirators for cleaning the cabinet as well as when preparing drugs.
      - Post signs for spill and emergency procedures.
   b. Protective Equipment
      - *Gloves.* Latex gloves that are thick (0.007 to 0.009 inch thick) and long enough to cover gown cuff and have no powder are used. Double gloving is recommended. Change hourly or immediately if torn or contaminated, and when beginning any new batch of medicine. Wash hands before and after glove application. Remove using proper technique before leaving area and dispose of properly.
      - *Gowns.* Disposable, lint-free with low permeability and closed front, long sleeves, elastic or knit cuffs. Place inner glove under cuff and outer glove over cuff. Remove before leaving area and dispose of properly.

- *Eye and face protection.* Recommended if splashes, spray, or aerosol exposure could occur. Chemical-barrier protection devices are needed. Eye wash facility should be immediately available.
- *Respiratory protection.* If an approved biological safety cabinet is not available for drug preparative, an approved respirator should be used.

c. Equipment and Procedures
- Place liner with plastic back on all work surfaces.
- Use syringes and intravenous sets with Luer-locks.
- Do not fill syringes full.
- Cover excess solution during work.
- Use covered sharps container; do not clip or cap needles.
- Prime intravenous tubing in the cabinet prior to adding drug.
- Use venting devices or other procedures to minimize negative pressure and resultant drips from vials.
- Tap medication out of neck of ampules before opening and use gauze around neck when opening.
- Wipe outside of containers and entry ports after preparation.
- Transport in sealed plastic bags.
- Label all containers of hazardous drugs.
- Dispose of used syringes and needles in hazardous chemical master disposal containers.
- Above procedures apply to counting of tablets or capsules as well as preparation of injectable medications.

2. Administration of Hazardous Drugs
   a. General Guidelines
   Keep hazardous drugs in an area with entry restricted to authorized personnel. Label the area and all hazardous drugs. Post the agency hazardous drug list and protocols. No other drugs should be kept in this area.
   b. Protective Equipment
   - Gowns
   - Latex gloves
   - Chemical splash goggles
   - Respirator for aerosolized products (type approved by the National Institute for Occupational Safety and Health).

   c. Equipment and Procedures
   See recommendations in preparation section for washing hands, use of gown and gloves, and infusion devices used. In addition:
   - Place plastic backed absorbent pad under tubing during administration.
   - Use sterile gauze around intravenous push sites.
   - Tape intravenous tubing connections.
   - Prime tubing with plain solution before adding tubing primed with drug.
   - Clean any drug or container with sterile gauze and dispose of properly.
   - Return unused drug to pharmacy.
   - Use only in defined patient care area.

- Material Safety Data Sheets must be immediately available for personnel.
- Administration and spill kits must be available (see listing of contents later in this section).
- See specialized drug administration recommendations for aerosolized drugs such as pentamidine and ribavirin.
- Recognize manipulations that can lead to splatters or sprays of medication, including withdrawal of needle from vial, drug transfer with needles and syringes, opening ampules, and expelling air from syringe with drug.

d. Patient Care
- Use universal precautions in caring for all patients receiving hazardous drugs.
- Handle urine and other excretion within 48 hours of drug administration with hand washing, latex gloves, and disposable gowns.
- Eye protection should be used if splashes are possible.
- Handle contaminated linen and eating utensils with blood-borne pathogen guidelines.

3. Waste Disposal
a. General Guidelines
- Thick, colored bags are used to collect disposable materials in a hazardous-waste-only container. These are segregated from other wastes. Place needles, syringes, breakables in sharps container first, then in bag. Do not clip or break needles; discard intact. Seal bags before completely full and tape. Policies for handling and disposal of hazardous material are followed.

b. Spills
- Clean immediately.
- Post warning signs to limit access.
- Complete incident report of spill and those exposed.
- Remove gloves and gown during the spill and cleanse skin with soap and water.
- Flood eye with water or eyewash for 15 minutes.
- Obtain medical evaluation.
- Document in medical record. Maintain record for the period of employment plus 30 years.

   1. *Small spills (under 5 mL):*
   - Clean up immediately by personnel with gown, double latex gloves, splash goggles, respirator if aerosol exposure is possible.
   - Use absorbent gauze pad or a wet pad if the spill is a solid.
   - Clean the surface three times with detergent solution and water.
   - Clean up glass fragments with a scoop rather than gloved hand.

   2. *Large spills (over 5 mL):*
   - Isolate the location.
   - Avoid aerosol production of the spill by covering gently with absorbent sheets for liquids or damp cloths for powder; cloths used should be incinerable.

- Only trained individuals should conduct the cleanup.
- Use all equipment listed for small spills; respirators must also be used.

Administration Kit Contents
- Protective equipment
- Sterile gauze for cleanup
- Alcohol wipes
- Disposable plastic-back absorbent liner
- Sharps container
- Hazardous waste plastic bags
- Warning labels.

Spill Kit Contents
All items listed for administration plus:
- Splash goggles
- Respirator
- Two absorbent plastic-back sheets (12 × 12 inches)
- Scoop for glass fragments
- Spill control pillows (250 mL and 1 L)
- Two pairs of disposable gloves
- Disposable protective garments
- Two thick plastic hazardous waste disposable bags.

PART TWO

PEDIATRIC MEDICATIONS

ABACAVIR SULFATE
(a-ba′ca-vir)
Ziagen
Classifications: ANTI-INFECTIVE; ANTIVIRAL; ANTIRETROVIRAL AGENT; NUCLEOSIDE REVERSE TRANSCRIPTASE INHIBITOR (NRTI)
Prototype: Zidovudine
Pregnancy Category: C

AVAILABILITY 300 mg tablets; 20 mg/mL strawberry-banana flavored oral solution
Combination Products: Trizivir (in combination with lamivudine/zidovudine)

ACTIONS Abacavir is a synthetic nucleoside analog with inhibitory activity against HIV. It inhibits the activity of HIV-1 reverse transcriptase (RT) both by competing with the natural DNA nucleoside and by incorporation into viral DNA.

THERAPEUTIC EFFECTS Abacavir prevents the formation of viral DNA replication. Therefore, the viral load decreases as measured by an increased CD_4 lymphocyte cell count and suppression of HIV RNA, indicated by decreased HIV RNA copies, in HIV-positive individuals with little or no exposure to zidovudine (AZT).

USES Treatment of HIV infection in combination with other antiretroviral agents.

CONTRAINDICATIONS Hypersensitivity to abacavir; pregnancy (category C); HIV-positive mothers should be counseled not to breast feed.
CAUTIOUS USE Prior resistance to another nucleoside reverse transcriptase inhibitor; hepatic dysfunction; infants.

ROUTE & DOSAGE

HIV Infection
Child: **PO** 3 mo–16 y, 8 mg/kg b.i.d. (max 300 mg b.i.d.); although safety is not yet established, infants from 1–3 mo are now being treated with 8 mg/kg b.i.d.
Adult: **PO** 300 mg b.i.d.

STORAGE

Store tablets and oral solution at room temperature (20°–25° C or 68°–77° F); oral solution may be refrigerated. Expiration date for tablets and solution is 18 mo after manufacture.

ADMINISTRATION

Oral

- Tablets and oral solution are interchangeable on a milligram-for-milligram basis. Always given in combination with other medications to treat HIV.

ADVERSE EFFECTS Body as a Whole: Hypersensitivity reactions (including fever, skin rash, fatigue, nausea, vomiting, diarrhea, abdominal pain); malaise; lethargy; myalgia; arthralgia; paresthesia; edema; shortness of breath. **CNS:** Insomnia, *headache, fever.* **CV:** Hypotension (associated with hypersensitivity reaction). **GI:** Hepatomegaly with steatosis, *nausea, vomiting, diarrhea, anorexia,* pancreatitis, increased GGT, increased liver function tests. **Skin:** *Rash.* **Other:** Lactic acidosis, renal insufficiency.

INTERACTIONS Drug: Alcohol may increase abacavir blood levels. Abacavir increases amprenavir levels. Zidovudine resistance does not confer abacavir resistance.

PHARMACOKINETICS Absorption: Rapidly absorbed, 83% bioavailable. **Distribution:** Distributes into extravascular space and erythrocytes; 50% protein bound. **Metabolism:** Metabolized by alcohol dehydrogenase and glucuronyl transferase to inactive metabolites. **Elimination:** 84% excreted in urine, primarily as inactive metabolites; 16% excreted in feces. **Half-Life:** 1.5 h.

NURSING IMPLICATIONS

Assessment & Drug Effects

- Monitor for S&S of hypersensitivity: fever, skin rash, fatigue, GI distress (nausea, vomiting, diarrhea, abdominal pain). Withhold drug immediately and notify physician if hypersensitivity develops.
- Lab tests: Periodically monitor liver function, BUN and creatinine, CBC with differential, triglyceride levels, and blood glucose, especially in diabetics.
- Withhold drug and notify physician for S&S of acidosis, hepatotoxicity, or renal insufficiency.

Patient & Family Education

- Take drug exactly as prescribed at indicated times. Missed dose: Take immediately, then resume dosing schedule. Do not double a dose.
- Withhold drug immediately and notify physician at first sign of hypersensitivity reaction (see Assessment & Drug Effects).
- Carry warning card provided with drug at all times.
- Do not breast feed while taking this drug.
- Store this medication out of reach of children.

ACETAMINOPHEN, PARACETAMOL ⊕
(a-seat-a-mee'noe-fen)

Abenal ♣, **A'Cenol, Acephen, Anacin-3, Anuphen, APAP, Atasol** ♣, **Campain** ♣, **Datril Extra Strength, Dolanex, Exdol** ♣, **Halenol, Liquiprim, Panadol, Pedric, Robigesic** ♣, **Rounox** ♣, **Tapar, Tempra, Tylenol, Valadol**

Classifications: CENTRAL NERVOUS SYSTEM AGENT; NONNARCOTIC ANALGESIC; ANTIPYRETIC
Pregnancy Category: B

AVAILABILITY 80 mg, 120 mg, 125 mg, 300 mg, 325 mg, 650 mg suppositories; 80 mg, 160 mg, 325 mg, 500 mg tablets; 80 mg/0.8 mL, 80 mg/2.5 mL, 80 mg/5 mL, 120 mg/5 mL, 160 mg/5 mL, 500 mg/5 mL liquid
Combination Products: Available in combination with numerous products, such as acetaminophen with codeine, with aspirin and codeine, with diphenhydramine, with oxycodone, with propoxyphene, and others.

ACTIONS Produces analgesia by unknown mechanism, perhaps by action on peripheral nervous system. Reduces fever by direct action on hypothalamus heat-regulating center with consequent peripheral vasodilation, sweating, and dissipation of heat. Unlike aspirin, acetaminophen has little effect on platelet aggregation, does not affect bleeding time, and generally produces no gastric bleeding.
THERAPEUTIC EFFECTS Provides temporary analgesia for mild to moderate pain. In addition, acetaminophen lowers body temperature in individuals with a fever.

USES Fever reduction. Temporary relief of mild to moderate pain. Because aspirin is generally not recommended for children, acetaminophen (or ibuprofen) is the drug of choice for fever or mild to moderate pain.

CONTRAINDICATIONS Hypersensitivity to acetaminophen or phenacetin; G6PD deficiency.
CAUTIOUS USE Children <3 y unless directed by a physician; repeated administration to patients with anemia or hepatic disease; arthritic or rheumatoid conditions affecting children <12 y; alcoholism; malnutrition; thrombocytopenia. Safety during pregnancy (category B) or lactation is not established.

ROUTE & DOSAGE

Mild to Moderate Pain, Fever
Neonate: **PO** 10–15 mg/kg q6–8h
Child: **PO** 0–3 mo, 40 mg q4–6h; 4–11 mo, 80 mg q4–6h; 1–2 y, 120 mg q4–6h; 2–3 y, 160 mg q4–6h; 4–5 y, 240 mg q4–6h; 6–8 y, 320 mg q4–6h; 9–10 y, 400 mg q4–6h; 11–12 y, 480 mg q4–6h (max 5 doses/day).

Common adverse effects in *italic;* life-threatening effects <u>underlined</u>; generic names in **bold;** drug classifications in SMALL CAPS; ♣ Canadian drug name; ⊕ Prototype drug.

Alternatively, 10–15 mg/kg q4h can be used. This weight-based dosage is preferred for children who are in upper or lower percentiles for age becuase dosing based on weight is more accurate than dosing based on age.

PR Equivalent to PO dosing.

Adult: **PO** 325–650 mg q4–6h (max 4 g/day) **PR** 650 mg q4–6h (max 4 g/day)

STORAGE
Store in light-resistant containers at room temperature, preferably between 15°–30° C (59°–86° F).

ADMINISTRATION

Oral
- Administer tablets or caplets whole or crushed and give with fluid of patient's choice.
- Chewable tablets should be thoroughly chewed and wetted before they are swallowed.
- Do not coadminister with a high carbohydrate meal; absorption rate may be retarded.

Rectal
- Insert suppositories beyond the rectal sphincter.

ADVERSE EFFECTS Body as a Whole: Negligible with recommended dosage; rash. **Acute poisoning:** Anorexia, nausea, vomiting, dizziness, lethargy, diaphoresis, chills, epigastric or abdominal pain, diarrhea; onset of <u>hepatotoxicity</u>—elevation of serum transaminases (ALT, AST) and bilirubin; hypoglycemia, <u>hepatic coma, acute renal failure</u> (rare). **Chronic ingestion:** neutropenia, pancytopenia, leukopenia, thrombocytopenic purpura, *hepatotoxicity in alcoholics,* renal damage.

DIAGNOSTIC TEST INTERFERENCE False increases in ***urinary 5-HIAA*** (5-hydroxyindoleacetic acid) by-product of serotonin; false decreases in ***blood glucose*** (by ***glucose oxidase–peroxidase procedure***); false increases in ***urinary glucose*** (with certain instruments in glucose analyses); and false increases in ***serum uric acid*** (with ***phosphotungstate method***). High doses or long-term therapy: hepatic, renal, and hematopoietic function (periodically).

INTERACTIONS Drug: Cholestyramine may decrease acetaminophen absorption. With chronic coadministration, BARBITURATES, **carbamazepine, phenytoin,** and **rifampin** may increase potential for chronic hepatotoxicity. Chronic, excessive ingestion of **alcohol** will increase risk of hepatotoxicity.

PHARMACOKINETICS Absorption: Rapid and almost complete absorption from GI tract; less complete absorption from rectal suppository. **Peak:** 0.5–2 h. **Duration:** 3–4 h. **Distribution:** Well distributed in all body fluids; crosses placenta. **Metabolism:** Extensively metabolized in liver. **Elimination:** 90–100% of drug excreted as metabolites in urine; excreted in breast milk. **Half-Life:** 1–3 h.

NURSING IMPLICATIONS

Assessment & Drug Effects

- Monitor for S&S of hepatotoxicity, even with moderate acetaminophen doses, especially in individuals with poor nutrition or who have ingested alcohol over prolonged periods; poisoning, usually from accidental ingestion or suicide attempts; potential abuse from psychological dependence (withdrawal has been associated with restless and excited responses). Do not divide suppositories.

Patient & Family Education

- Do not take other medications (e.g., cold preparations) containing acetaminophen without medical advice; overdosing and chronic use can cause liver damage and other toxic effects.
- Do not self-medicate adults for pain more than 10 days (5 days in children) without consulting a physician.
- Do not use this medication without medical direction for fever persisting longer than 3 days, fever over 39.5° C (103° F), or recurrent fever.
- Keep the drug safely locked away because it is a common source of poisoning in children.
- Do not give children more than 5 doses in 24 h unless prescribed by physician.
- Do not breast feed while taking this drug without consulting prescriber.

ACETAZOLAMIDE ⊘

(a-set-a-zole′a-mide)

Acetazolam ♦, AkZol, Apo-Acetazolamide ♦, Dazamide, Diamox, Diamox Sequels

ACETAZOLAMIDE SODIUM

(a-set-a-zole_a-mide)

Diamox Parenteral

Classifications: EYE PREPARATION: CARBONIC ANHYDRASE INHIBITOR; DIURETIC; CENTRAL NERVOUS SYSTEM AGENT; ANTICONVULSANT

Pregnancy Category: C

AVAILABILITY 125 mg, 250 mg tablets; 500 mg sustained-release capsules; 500 mg powder for injection

ACTIONS The mechanism of anticonvulsant action with acetazolamide is unknown but thought to involve inhibition of CNS carbonic anhydrase, which retards abnormal paroxysmal discharge from CNS neurons. Diuretic effect is due to inhibition of carbonic anhydrase activity in proximal renal tubule, preventing formation of carbonic acid. Inhibition of carbonic anhydrase in eye reduces rate of aqueous humor formation with consequent lowering of intraocular pressure.

THERAPEUTIC EFFECTS Reduces seizure activity and intraocular pressure. Additionally, Diamox has a diuretic effect.

USES Treatment of seizures: absence or petit mal, generalized tonic-clonic (grand mal), and focal; hydrocephalus; reduction of intraocular

Common adverse effects in *italic;* life-threatening effects <u>underlined</u>; generic names in **bold;** drug classifications in SMALL CAPS; ♦ Canadian drug name; ⊘ Prototype drug.

61

pressure in open-angle glaucoma and secondary glaucoma; preoperative treatment of acute closed-angle glaucoma; drug-induced edema and as adjunct in treatment of edema due to congestive heart failure; acute high-altitude sickness.

UNLABELED USES Prevent uric acid or cystine renal calculi; to treat acute pancreatitis, premenstrual syndrome (PMS), metabolic alkalosis, and hypokalemic and hyperkalemic forms of familial periodic paralysis; to increase secretion of phenobarbital or lithium; hydrocephalus.

CONTRAINDICATIONS Hypersensitivity to sulfonamides and derivatives (e.g., thiazides); marked renal and hepatic dysfunction; Addison's disease or other types of adrenocortical insufficiency; hyponatremia, hypokalemia, hyperchloremic acidosis; prolonged administration to patients with hyphema or chronic noncongestive angle-closure glaucoma. Safety during pregnancy (category C) or lactation is not established.

CAUTIOUS USE History of hypercalciuria; diabetes mellitus, gout, patients receiving digitalis, obstructive pulmonary disease, respiratory acidosis.

ROUTE & DOSAGE

Glaucoma

Child: **PO** 8–30 mg/kg/day divided into 3 doses or 300–900 mg/m^2/day divided into 3 doses **IV** 5–10 mg/kg q6h
Adult: **PO** 250 mg 1–4 times/day, 500 mg sustained release b.i.d. **IM/IV** 500 mg, may repeat in 2–4 h

Epilepsy

Child/Adult: **PO** 8–30 mg/kg/day in 1–4 doses Max.: 1 g/24 h.

Edema

Child: **PO/IM/IV** 5 mg/kg or 150 mg/m^2 every a.m.
Adult: **PO** 250–375 mg every a.m. (5 mg/kg)

High-Altitude Sickness

Adult: **PO** 250 mg q8–12h or 500 mg sustained release q12–24h, starting 24–48 h before climb and continuing for 48 h at high altitude

Hydrocephalus

Neonate/Infant: **PO/IV** 5 mg/kg q6h, may increase by 25 mg/kg/day (max 100 mg/kg/day); used in combination with furosemide

Renal Impairment

Cl$_{cr}$:
Adult: 10–50 mL/min: dose q 12h; <10 mL/min: use not recommended

STORAGE

Store oral preparations at 15°–30° C (59°–86° F) unless otherwise directed.

ADMINISTRATION

Oral

- Administer diuretic dose in morning to avoid interrupted sleep.
- Give with food or meals to minimize GI upset.

- Note: If tablet(s) cannot be swallowed, soften tablet(s) (not sustained-release form) in 2 tsp of hot water and add to 2 tsp of syrup or fruit jelly to disguise bitter taste; avoid syrups containing alcohol or glycerin that will not disguise taste. Alternately crush tablet(s) and suspend in syrup (250–500 mg/5 mL syrup). Prepare just before administration. Drug does not dissolve in fruit juices.

Intramuscular

- Reconstitute as for IV administration. See PREPARE Direct.
- Give IM for rapid lowering of intraocular pressure or in patients unable to take oral dosage.
- Note: The intramuscular dosage is not the route of choice because the alkalinity of the solution makes the injection painful.

Intravenous

- IV administration to neonates, infants, and children: Verify correct IV concentration and rate of infusion/injection with physician.
PREPARE Direct: Reconstitute each 500-mg vial with at least 5 mL of sterile water for injection. **IV Infusion:** Reconstituted solution may be further diluted with D5W or NS. Use within 24 h of reconstitution.
ADMINISTER Direct: Give at a rate of 500 mg or fraction thereof over 1 min. **IV Infusion:** Give as a continuous infusion over 4–8 h.

ADVERSE EFFECTS CNS: Paresthesias, sedation, malaise, disorientation, depression, fatigue, muscle weakness, <u>flaccid paralysis</u>. **GI:** Anorexia, nausea, vomiting, weight loss, dry mouth, thirst, diarrhea. **Hematologic:** Bone marrow depression with <u>agranulocytosis, hemolytic anemia, aplastic anemia</u>, leukopenia, <u>pancytopenia</u>. **Metabolic:** Increased excretion of calcium, potassium, magnesium, and sodium; metabolic acidosis; hyperglycemia; hyperuricemia. **Urogenital:** Glycosuria, urinary frequency, polyuria, dysuria, hematuria, crystalluria that can lead to kidney stones. **Other:** Exacerbation of gout, hepatic dysfunction.

DIAGNOSTIC TEST INTERFERENCE Monitor for false-positive *urinary protein* determinations; falsely high values for *urine urobilinogen;* depressed *iodine uptake* values (exception: hypothyroidism)

INTERACTIONS Drug: Renal excretion of AMPHETAMINES, **ephedrine, flecainide, quinidine, procainamide,** TRICYCLIC ANTIDEPRESSANTS may be decreased, thereby enhancing or prolonging their effects. Renal excretion of **lithium** is increased. Excretion of **phenobarbital** may be increased. **Amphotericin B** and CORTICOSTEROIDS may accelerate **potassium** loss. DIGITALIS GLYCOSIDES may predispose persons with hypokalemia to **digitalis** toxicity; puts patients on high doses of SALICYLATES at high risk for SALICYLATE toxicity.

PHARMACOKINETICS Absorption: Well absorbed from GI tract. **Onset:** 1 h regular release; 2 h sustained release; 2 min IV. **Peak:** 2–4 h reg; 8–18 h sustained; 15 min IV. **Duration:** 8–12 h reg; 18–24 h sustained; 4–5 h IV. **Distribution:** Distributed throughout body, concentrating in RBCs, plasma, and kidneys; crosses placenta. **Elimination:** Excreted primarily in urine. **Half-Life:** 2.4–5.8 h.

Common adverse effects in *italic;* life-threatening effects <u>underlined</u>; generic names in **bold;** drug classifications in SMALL CAPS; ♣ Canadian drug name; ⊘ Prototype drug.

63

NURSING IMPLICATIONS

Assessment & Drug Effects

- Establish baseline weight before initial therapy and weigh daily thereafter when used to treat edema.
- Monitor for S&S of mild to severe metabolic acidosis; potassium loss, which is greatest early in therapy.
- Monitor I&O especially when used with other diuretics.
- Lab tests: Blood pH, blood gases, urinalysis, CBC, and serum electrolytes (initially and periodically during prolonged therapy or concomitant therapy with other diuretics or digitalis).

Patient & Family Education

- Maintain adequate fluid intake for age and weight to reduce risk of kidney stones.
- Report any of the following: numbness, tingling, burning, drowsiness, and visual problems, sore throat or mouth, unusual bleeding, fever, skin or renal problems.
- Eat potassium-rich diet and take potassium supplement when taking this drug in high doses or for prolonged periods.
- Do not breast feed while taking this drug without consulting prescriber.
- Store this medication out of reach of children.

ACETYLCYSTEINE ℗ℱ
(a-se-til-sis′tay-een)
Airbron ♦, Mucomyst, Mucosol, *N*-Acetylcysteine
Classifications: SKIN AND MUCOUS MEMBRANE AGENT; MUCOLYTIC; ANTIDOTE
Pregnancy Category: B

AVAILABILITY 10%, 20% solution

ACTIONS Acetylcysteine probably acts by disrupting disulfide linkages of mucoproteins in purulent and nonpurulent secretions.
THERAPEUTIC EFFECTS Acetylcysteine lowers viscosity and facilitates the removal of secretions.

USES Adjuvant therapy in patients with abnormal, viscid, or inspissated mucous secretions in acute and chronic bronchopulmonary diseases, and in pulmonary complications of cystic fibrosis and surgery, tracheostomy, and atelectasis. Also used in diagnostic bronchial studies and as an antidote for acute acetaminophen poisoning.
UNLABELED USES As an ophthalmic solution for treatment of dry eye (keratoconjunctivitis sicca); as an enema to treat bowel obstruction due to meconium ileus.

CONTRAINDICATIONS Hypersensitivity to acetylcysteine; patients at risk of gastric hemorrhage. Safety during pregnancy (category B) or lactation is not established.
CAUTIOUS USE Patients with asthma, older adults, debilitated patients with severe respiratory insufficiency.

Common adverse effects in *italic;* life-threatening effects <u>underlined;</u> generic names in **bold;** drug classifications in SMALL CAPS; ♦ Canadian drug name; ℗ Prototype drug.

ROUTE & DOSAGE

Mucolytic

Infant: **Inhalation** 1–2 mL 20% solution or 2–4 mL of 10% solution 3–4 times/day
Child: **Inhalation** 3–5 mL of 20% solution or 6–10 mL of 10% solution 3–4 times/day
Adult: **Inhalation** 1–10 mL of 20% solution 3–4 times/day or 2–20 mL of 10% solution 3–4 times/day **Direct instillation** 1–2 mL of 10–20% solution q1–4h

Acetaminophen Toxicity

Child/Adult: **PO or NG** 140 mg/kg of 20% solution diluted 1:4 in carbonated beverage (cola) or orange juice as loading dose, followed by 70 mg/kg q4h for 17 doses. Use a 5% solution, or if using 10%, dilute 1:1 with cola or orange juice.)

STORAGE

- Store opened vial in refrigerator to retard oxidation; use within 96 h.
- Store unopened vial at 15°–30° C (59°–86° F), unless otherwise directed.

ADMINISTRATION

Inhalation and Instillation

- Prepare dilution within 1 h of use; drug does not contain an antimicrobial agent to deter growth of microorganisms. A light purple discoloration does not significantly impair drug's effectiveness.
- Dilute the 20% solution with NS or water for injection. The 10% solution may be used undiluted.
- Give by direct instillation into tracheostomy (1–2 mL of 10–20% solution).
- Instruct patient to clear airway, if possible, coughing productively prior to aerosol administration to ensure maximum effect.

ADVERSE EFFECTS CNS: Dizziness, drowsiness. **GI:** Nausea, *vomiting,* stomatitis, hepatotoxicity (urticaria). **Respiratory:** <u>Bronchospasm</u>, rhinorrhea, burning sensation in upper respiratory passages, epistaxis.

PHARMACOKINETICS Onset: 1 min after inhalation or instillation. **Peak:** 5–10 min. **Metabolism:** Deacetylated in liver to cysteine and subsequently metabolized.

NURSING IMPLICATIONS

Assessment & Drug Effects

- Nausea and vomiting may occur, particularly when face mask is used, due to unpleasant odor and taste of drug; premedicate with metoclopramide to prevent this effect. Monitor for S&S of aspiration of excess secretions, and for bronchospasm (unpredictable); withhold drug and notify physician immediately if either occurs.
- Lab tests: Monitor ABGs, pulmonary functions and pulse oximetry as indicated. Monitor plasma or serum acetaminophen when being used to treat overdose.

- Have suction apparatus immediately available. Increased volume of respiratory tract fluid may be liberated; suction or endotracheal aspiration may be necessary to establish and maintain an open airway.
- Nausea and vomiting may occur, particularly when face mask is used, due to unpleasant odor and taste of drug and excess volume of liquefied bronchial secretions; premedicate with metoclopramide to prevent this effect.

Patient & Family Education

- Report difficulty with clearing the airway or any other respiratory distress.
- Report nausea, because an antiemetic may be indicated (see nursing administration section).
- Note: Unpleasant odor of inhaled drug becomes less noticeable with continued use.
- Do not breast feed while taking this drug without consulting prescriber.

ACYCLOVIR, ACYCLOVIR SODIUM ◐

(ay-sye′kloe-ver)
Acycloguanosine, Zovirax
Classifications: ANTI-INFECTIVE; ANTIVIRAL
Pregnancy Category: C

AVAILABILITY 200 mg capsules; 400 mg, 800 mg tablets; 200 mg/5 mL suspension; 50 mg/mL injection; 5% ointment

ACTIONS Acyclovir is a synthetic acyclic purine nucleoside analog, derived from guanine. It reduces viral shedding and formation of new lesions and speeds healing time. Acyclovir triphosphate preferentially interferes with DNA synthesis of herpes simplex virus types 1 and 2 (HSV-1 and HSV-2) and varicella-zoster virus, thereby inhibiting viral replication.

THERAPEUTIC EFFECTS Acyclovir demonstrates antiviral activity against herpes virus simiae (B virus), Epstein–Barr (infectious mononucleosis), varicella-zoster and cytomegalovirus, but does not eradicate the latent herpes virus.

USES Parenterally for treatment of initial and recurrent mucosal and cutaneous herpes simplex virus (HSV-1 and HSV-2) infections in immunocompromised adults and children and for severe initial episodes of herpes genitalis in immunocompetent (normal immune system) patients. Used orally for treatment of initial episodes of genital herpes, for management of selected patients with severe recurrent episodes, and for prophylaxis to reduce frequency and severity of recurrent infections. Also used orally in varicella-zoster (chickenpox) in immunocompetent children and adolescents. Used topically for initial episodes of herpes genitalis and in non-life-threatening mucocutaneous herpes simplex virus infections in immunocompromised patients.

UNLABELED USES Treatment of eczema herpeticum caused by HSV; localized and disseminated herpes zoster.

Common adverse effects in *italic;* life-threatening effects <u>underlined</u>; generic names in **bold**; drug classifications in SMALL CAPS; ◆ Canadian drug name; ◐ Prototype drug.

CONTRAINDICATIONS Safety during pregnancy (category C) or in children is not established.
CAUTIOUS USE Lactation, renal insufficiency, dehydration.

ROUTE & DOSAGE

Genital Herpes Simplex

Child: **IV** <12 y, 250 mg/m^2 q8h, 80 mg/kg/day in 2–5 doses
Adult: **PO** 200 mg q4h 5 times/day, 400 mg t.i.d. for
7–10 day cycle **IV** 5 mg/kg q8h **Topical** Apply q3h 6 times/day
for 7 days

Herpes Simplex Immunocompromised Patient

Child: **IV** <1 y, 15–30 mg/kg/day divided into doses given q8h for
7–14 day cycle; ≥1y, 750–1500 mg/m^2/day, *or* 15–30 mg/kg/day
divided into doses given q8h for 7–14 day cycle
Adult: **IV** 15 mg/kg/day divided into doses given q8h for 5–7 day
cycle

Prophylaxis for Genital Herpes Simplex

Child: **PO** 80 mg/kg/day given in 2–5 divided doses
Adult: **PO** 200 mg divided into doses given 2–5 times/day, *or* 400 mg
t.i.d., *or* 800 mg b.i.d.

Herpes Zoster

Child: **PO** 80 mg/kg/day divided into 5 doses
Adult: **PO** 800 mg/day divided into 5 doses

Herpes Simplex Encephalitis

Premature Neonate: **IV** 20 mg/kg/day divided into doses given q12h
for 14–21 day cycle
Neonate: **IV** 30 mg/kg/day divided into doses given q8h for 14–21
day cycle
Child/Adult: **IV** 15 mg/kg q8h for 14–21 day cycle

Varicella Zoster

Child/Adolescent: **PO** 20 mg/kg (max 800 mg) q.i.d. for 5 day cycle
initiated within 24 h of onset of rash

Renal Impairment

Cl$_{cr}$: 25–50 mL/min: same dose q12h; 10–25 mL/min: same
dose q24h

STORAGE

Store capsules, topical preparations, injectable powder, and concentrate
in tight, light-resistant containers at 15°–25° C (59°–78° F) unless otherwise directed.

ADMINISTRATION

Oral

- Shake suspension well prior to use.

Topical

- Wash hands thoroughly before and after treatment of lesions and after
  handling and disposition of secretions.

Common adverse effects in *italic;* life-threatening effects underlined; generic names
in **bold;** drug classifications in SMALL CAPS; ♣ Canadian drug name; ❻ Prototype drug.

67

- Apply approximately ½ inch of ointment ribbon for each 4 square inches of surface area. Use sufficient ointment to completely cover lesions.
- Apply topical preparation with finger cot or surgical glove.

Intravenous

- Verify correct IV concentration and rate of infusion with physician for neonates, infants, children. ▪ Note: Solutions containing benzyl alcohol are toxic to neonates. ▪ Directions for administration to adults follow.

PREPARE **Intermittent:** Reconstitute by adding 10 mL sterile water for injection to 500-mg vial to yield 50 mg/mL. Shake well. Use reconstituted solution within 12 h. Dilute to ≤7 mg/mL to reduce risk of renal injury and phlebitis. Example: Add 1 mL of reconstituted solution to 9 mL of diluent to yield 5 mg/mL. Use standard electrolyte and glucose solutions (e.g., NS, RL, D5W) for dilution. Diluted solution should be used within 24 h.

ADMINISTER **Intermittent:** Administer over at least 1 h to prevent renal tubular damage. Rapid or bolus IV administration must be avoided. Monitor IV flow rate carefully; infusion pump or microdrip infusion set preferred.

INCOMPATIBILITIES **Solution/Additive: Bacteriostatic water for injection, albumin, hetastarch, dopamine, dobutamine. Y-Site: Foscarnet, TPN.**

- Refrigerate reconstituted solution; although it may precipitate, crystals will redissolve at room temperature.

ADVERSE EFFECTS Body as a Whole: Generally minimal and infrequent. **CNS:** *Headache,* light-headedness, lethargy, fatigue, tremors, confusion, seizures, dizziness. **GI:** *Nausea, vomiting, diarrhea.* **Urogenital:** Glomerulonephritis, renal tubular damage, <u>acute renal failure</u>. **Skin:** Stevens-Johnson syndrome, rash, urticaria, pruritus, burning, stinging sensation, irritation, sensitization. **Other:** Inflammation or phlebitis at IV injection site, sloughing (with extravasation), <u>thrombocytopenic purpura/hemolytic uremic syndrome</u>.

INTERACTIONS Drug: Probenecid decreases acyclovir elimination; **zidovudine** may cause increased drowsiness and lethargy.

PHARMACOKINETICS Absorption: Oral dose is 15–30% absorbed. **Peak:** 1.5–2 h after oral dose. **Distribution:** Distributes into most tissues with lower levels in the CNS; crosses placenta. **Metabolism:** Drug is primarily excreted unchanged. **Elimination:** Renally eliminated; also excreted in breast milk. **Half-Life:** 2.5–5 h.

NURSING IMPLICATIONS

Assessment & Drug Effects

- Observe infusion site during infusion and for a few days following infusion for signs of tissue damage.
- Monitor I&O and hydration status.
- Keep patient adequately hydrated during first 2 h after infusion to maintain sufficient urinary flow and thus prevent precipitation of drug

Common adverse effects in *italic;* life-threatening effects <u>underlined</u>; generic names in **bold**; drug classifications in SMALL CAPS; ✦ Canadian drug name; ✪ Prototype drug.

in renal tubules. Consult physician about amount and length of time oral fluids need to be pushed after IV drug treatment.

- Monitor for S&S of reinfection in pregnant patients; acyclovir-induced neurologic symptoms in patients with history of neurologic problems; drug resistance in immunocompromised patients receiving prolonged or repeated therapy; acute renal failure with concomitant use with other nephrotoxic drugs or preexisting renal disease.
- Lab tests: Monitor baseline and periodic renal function studies, particularly with IV administration. Elevations of BUN and serum creatinine and decreases in creatinine clearance indicate need for dosage adjustment, discontinuation of drug, or correction of fluid and electrolyte balance.
- Monitor for adverse effects and viral resistance with long-term prophylactic use of the oral drug.

Patient & Family Education
- Start therapy as soon as possible after onset of S&S for best results.
- Affected pregnant women can infect their babies; herpes status of pregnant women must be carefully monitored by physician.
- Do not exceed recommended dosage, frequency of drug administration, or specified duration of therapy. Contact physician if relief is not obtained or adverse effects appear.
- Store this medication out of reach of children.
- Cleanse affected areas with soap and water 3–4 times daily prior to topical application; dry well before application. With application to genitals, wear loose fitting clothes over affected areas.
- Report immediately worsening of lesions or additional symptoms such as lethargy in babies. Teach parents to recognize lesions in their children and report them immediately so treatment can begin. Infection of the CNS with the virus is a major, serious, and life-threatening possibility in newborns, infants, and young children.
- Note: Even after HSV infection is controlled, latent virus can be activated by stress, trauma, fever, exposure to sunlight, sexual intercourse, menstruation, treatment with immunosuppressive drugs.
- Refrain from sexual intercourse if either partner has S&S of herpes infection; neither topical nor systemic drug prevents transmission to other individuals.
- Avoid topical drug contact in or around eyes. Report unexplained eye symptoms to physician immediately (e.g., redness, pain); untreated infection can lead to corneal keratitis and blindness.
- Do not breast feed while taking this drug without consulting physician.

ADENOSINE

(a-den′o-sin)
Adenocard, Adenoscan
Classifications: CARDIOVASCULAR AGENT; ANTIARRHYTHMIC, CLASS IA
Prototype: Procainamide
Pregnancy Category: C

Common adverse effects in *italic;* life-threatening effects <u>underlined</u>; generic names in **bold**; drug classifications in SMALL CAPS; ◆ Canadian drug name; ◍ Prototype drug.

69

AVAILABILITY 3 mg/mL in 2, 5, and 30 mL vials

ACTIONS Slows conduction through the atrioventricular (AV) and sinoatrial (SA) nodes. Can interrupt the reentry pathways through the AV node. Depresses left ventricular function, but effect is transient due to short half-life.
THERAPEUTIC EFFECTS Restores normal sinus rhythm in patients with paroxysmal supraventricular tachycardia.

USES Conversion to sinus rhythm of paroxysmal supraventricular tachycardia (PSVT) including PSVT associated with accessory bypass tracts (Wolff-Parkinson-White syndrome). "Chemical" thallium stress test.
UNLABELED USES Afterload-reducing agent in low-output states; to prevent graft occlusion following aortocoronary bypass surgery; to produce controlled hypotension during cerebral aneurysm surgery.

CONTRAINDICATIONS AV block, preexisting second- and third-degree heart block or sick sinus rhythm without pacemaker, because a heart block may result. Also contraindicated in atrial flutter, atrial fibrillation, and ventricular tachycardia because the drug is ineffective.
CAUTIOUS USE Asthmatics, pregnancy (category C), hepatic and renal failure.

ROUTE & DOSAGE

Supraventricular Tachycardia

Neonate/Infant/Child: **IV** 0.05 mg/kg; may increase dose by 0.05 mg/kg in q2 min increments (max 0.25 mg/kg/dose or 12 mg/dose)
Adult: **IV** 6 mg rapid IV bolus (over 1–2 sec); may repeat in 1–2 min with 12 mg IV push, 2 times (total of 3 doses with max 12 mg/dose)

Stress Thallium Test

Adult: **IV** 140 mcg/kg/min × 6 min (max 0.84 mg/kg total dose)

STORAGE

Store at room temperature 15°–30° C (59°–86° F). Do not refrigerate, because crystallization may occur. If crystals do form, dissolve by warming to room temperature.

ADMINISTRATION

Intravenous

- Make sure solution is clear at time of use. ▪ Discard unused portion (contains no preservatives).
PREPARE **Direct:** No dilution is required.
ADMINISTER **Direct:** Administer directly into vein as a rapid bolus over 1–2 sec. If given by IV line, administer as proximally as possible, and follow with a rapid saline flush.
- Note: If high-level block develops after one dose, do not repeat dose.

ADVERSE EFFECTS CNS: Headache, light-headedness, dizziness, tingling in arms (from IV infusion), apprehension, blurred vision, burning sensation (from IV infusion). **CV:** *Transient facial flushing,* sweating, palpitations, chest pain, atrial fibrillation or flutter. **Respiratory:** Shortness of breath, bronchoconstriction, transient *dyspnea,* chest pressure. **GI:** Nausea, metallic taste, tightness in throat. **Other:** Irritability in children.

INTERACTIONS Drug: Dipyridamole can potentiate the effects of adenosine; **theophylline and caffeine** block the electrophysiologic effects of adenosine, thus antagonizing its effect; **carbamazepine** may increase risk of heart block.

PHARMACOKINETICS Absorption: Rapid uptake by erythrocytes and vascular endothelial cells after IV administration. **Onset:** 20–30 sec. **Metabolism:** Rapid uptake into cells; degraded by deamination to inosine, hypoxanthine, and adenosine monophosphate. **Elimination:** Route of elimination unknown. **Half-Life:** 10 sec.

NURSING IMPLICATIONS

Assessment & Drug Effects

- Monitor for S&S of bronchospasm in asthma patients. Notify physician immediately.
- Use a hemodynamic monitoring system during administration; monitor BP and heart rate and rhythm continuously for several minutes after administration.
- Note: Adverse effects are generally self-limiting due to short half life (10 sec).
- Note: At the time of conversion to normal sinus rhythm, PVCs, PACs, sinus bradycardia, and sinus tachycardia, as well as various degrees of AV block, are seen on the ECG. These usually last only a few seconds and resolve without intervention.

Patient & Family Education

- Note: Flushing may occur along with a feeling of warmth as drug is injected.
- Report shortness of breath, dyspnea, or light-headedness because they may signal bronchospasm.

ALBENDAZOLE

(al-ben′da-zole)
Albenza
Classifications: ANTI-INFECTIVE; ANTHELMINTIC AGENT
Prototype: Mebendazole
Pregnancy Category: C

AVAILABILITY 200 mg tablets

ACTIONS Albendazole is a broad spectrum oral anthelmintic agent. It is the only anthelmintic drug active against all stages of the helminth life cycle (ova, larvae, and adult worms). Its mechanism of action is unclear, but it appears to cause selective degeneration of cytoplasmic microtubules in the intestinal cells of the helminths and larvae.

THERAPEUTIC EFFECTIVENESS Albendazole ultimately causes decreased ATP production in the helminths, resulting in energy depletion, which kills the worms.

USES Treatment of neurocysticercosis caused by the larval form of pork tapeworm (*Taenia solium*), hydatid disease caused by the larval form of dog tapeworm (*Echinococcus granulosus*).

CONTRAINDICATIONS Hypersensitivity to the benzimidazole class of compounds or any components of albendazole; pregnancy (category C). **CAUTIOUS USE** Retinal lesions, lactation.

ROUTE & DOSAGE

Neurocysticercosis

Child/Adult: **PO** >6 y, weight <60 kg, 15 mg/kg/day divided into doses given b.i.d. for 8–30 day cycle (max 800 mg/day); weight ≥60 kg, 400 mg b.i.d. for 8–30 day cycle

Hydatid Disease

Child/Adult: **PO** >6 y, weight <60 kg, 15 mg/kg/day divided into doses given b.i.d. (max 800 mg/day); weight ≥60 kg, 400 mg b.i.d. for 28 day cycle (then 14 day without drug and repeat regimen for 3 cycles)

STORAGE
Store at 20°–25° C (68°–77° F).

ADMINISTRATION

Oral

- Give with meals. Absorption is significantly increased with a fatty meal.
- Do not exceed maximum total daily dose of 800 mg.

ADVERSE EFFECTS Body as a Whole: Hypersensitivity reactions. **CNS:** *Headache,* dizziness, vertigo, increased intracranial pressure, meningeal signs, alopecia (reversible), fever. **GI:** *Abnormal liver function tests,* abdominal pain, nausea, vomiting. **Hematologic:** (Rare) Leukopenia, granulocytopenia, pancytopenia, <u>agranulocytosis</u>. **Skin:** Rash, urticaria.

INTERACTIONS Drug: Cimetidine, dexamethasone, praziquantel increase albendazole levels.

PHARMACOKINETICS Absorption: Poorly absorbed from GI tract, absorption enhanced with a fatty meal. **Peak:** 2–5 h. **Distribution:** 70% bound to plasma proteins; widely distributed throughout body including CSF; secreted into breast milk. **Metabolism:** Metabolized in liver to active metabolite, albendazole sulfoxide. **Elimination:** Excreted in bile. **Half-Life:** 8–12 h.

NURSING IMPLICATIONS

Assessment & Drug Effects

- Lab tests: Monitor WBC count, absolute neutrophil count, and liver function tests at start of each 28 day cycle and q2 wk during cycle.

- Withhold drug and notify prescriber if WBC count falls below normal or liver enzymes are elevated.
- Note: Patients should be concurrently treated with appropriate steroid and anticonvulsant therapy.

Patient & Family Education
- Take with meals (see ADMINISTRATION).
- Do not become pregnant during or for at least 1 mo after therapy.
- Do not breast feed while taking this drug without consulting prescriber.
- Store this medication out of reach of children.

ALBUMIN (NORMAL SERUM), HUMAN ⓟ

(al-byoo'min)

Albuminar, Albutein, Buminate, Plasbumin

Classifications: BLOOD FORMERS, COAGULATORS, AND ANTICOAGULANTS; BLOOD DERIVATIVE; PLASMA VOLUME EXPANDER

Pregnancy Category: C

AVAILABILITY 5%, 25% injection

ACTIONS Obtained by fractionating pooled venous and placental human plasma, which is then sterilized by filtration and heat to minimize possibility of transmitting hepatitis B virus or HIV. Risk of sensitization is reduced because it lacks cellular elements and contains no coagulation factors, Rh factor, or blood group antibodies.

THERAPEUTIC EFFECTS Expands volume of circulating blood by osmotically shifting tissue fluid into general circulation.

USES To restore plasma volume and maintain cardiac output in hypovolemic shock; for prevention and treatment of cerebral edema; as adjunct in exchange transfusion for hyperbilirubinemia and erythroblastosis fetalis; to increase plasma protein level in treatment of hypoproteinemia; and to promote diuresis in refractory edema. Also used for blood dilution prior to or during cardiopulmonary bypass procedures. Has been used as adjunct in treatment of adult respiratory distress syndrome (ARDS).

CONTRAINDICATIONS Severe anemia; cardiac failure, patients with normal or increased intravascular volume, burn patients first 24 h postburn, latex allergies. Safety during pregnancy (category C) or lactation is not established. 25% solutions contraindicated in preterms.

CAUTIOUS USE Low cardiac reserve, pulmonary disease, absence of albumin deficiency; liver or kidney failure, dehydration, hypertension, restricted sodium intake.

ROUTE & DOSAGE

Volume Replacement

Neonates: **IV** 0.5 g/kg/dose of 5% solution
Infant, Child: **IV** 0.5–1 g/kg/dose of 5% solution, may repeat as necessary
Adult: **IV** 25 g, may repeat in 15–30 min if necessary (max 250 g/48 h or 6 g/kg/24 h)

Common adverse effects in *italic;* life-threatening effects <u>underlined;</u> generic names in **bold;** drug classifications in SMALL CAPS; ♣ Canadian drug name; ⓟ Prototype drug.

73

Hyperbilirubinemia, Erythroblastosis Fetalis
Child: **IV** 1 g/kg of 25% solution 1–2 h before transfusion
Hypoproteinemia
Neonates/Infant/Child: **IV** 0.5–1 g/kg/dose given over 30–120 min depending on patient's condition, may repeat every 1–2 day (25% solution used)

STORAGE
Store not to exceed 37° C (98.6° F).

ADMINISTRATION
Intravenous

Note: 5% solution = 5 g/100 mL; 25% solution = 25 g/100 mL.
***PREPARE* IV Infusion:** Normal serum albumin, 5%, is infused without further dilution. Normal serum albumin, 25%, may be infused undiluted or diluted in NS or D5W (with sodium restriction). Use filter size according to institutional policy. Use solution within 4 h, once container is opened, because it contains no preservatives or antimicrobials. Discard unused portion.
***ADMINISTER* IV Infusion: Hypovolemic Shock:** Give initially as rapidly as necessary to restore blood volume. As blood volume approaches normal, rate should be reduced to avoid circulatory overload and pulmonary edema. Give 5% albumin at rate not exceeding 2–4 mL/min. Give 25% albumin at rate not to exceed 1 mL/min. **With Normal Blood Volume:** Give 5% albumin at rate not to exceed 5–10 mL/min; give 25% albumin at rate not to exceed 2 or 3 mL/min. **Children:** Usual rate is ¼–½ the adult rate. 25% solutions contraindicated in preterms because of risk of intraventricular hemorrhage.
***INCOMPATIBILITIES* Solution/Additive:** Verapamil. **Y-Site:** Midazolam, vancomycin, verapamil.

ADVERSE EFFECTS Body as a Whole: Fever, chills, flushing, increased salivation, headache, back pain. **Skin:** Urticaria, rash. **CV:** Hypernatremia, circulatory overload, pulmonary edema (with rapid infusion); hypotension, hypertension, dyspnea, tachycardia. **GI:** Nausea, vomiting.

DIAGNOSTIC TEST INTERFERENCE False rise in *alkaline phosphatase* when albumin is obtained partially from pooled placental plasma (levels reportedly decline over period of weeks).

INTERACTIONS No clinically significant interactions established.

NURSING IMPLICATIONS
Assessment & Drug Effects
- Monitor BP, pulse and respiration, and IV albumin flow rate. Adjust flow rate as needed to avoid too rapid a rise in BP.
- Lab tests: Monitor dosage of albumin using plasma albumin (normal): 3.5–5 g/dL; total serum protein (normal): 6–8.4 g/dL; Hgb; Hct; and serum electrolytes.

- Observe closely for signs and symptoms of circulatory overload and pulmonary edema (see Appendix D-1). If signs and symptoms appear, slow infusion rate just sufficiently to keep vein open, and report immediately to physician.
- Observe for bleeding points that did not bleed at lower BP with injuries or surgery and as BP rises.
- Monitor I&O ratio and pattern. Report changes in urinary output. Increase in colloidal osmotic pressure usually causes diuresis, which may persist 3–20 h.
- Withhold fluids completely during succeeding 8 h, when albumin is given to patients with cerebral edema.

Patient & Family Education
- Report chills, nausea, headache, or back pain to physician immediately.
- Do not breast feed while taking this drug without consulting physician.

ALBUTEROL ⊕
(al-byoo′ter-ole)
Accuneb, Novosalmol ♣, Proventil, Proventil HFA, Proventil Repetabs, Salbutamol, Ventolin, Ventolin Rotocaps, Volmax
Classifications: AUTONOMIC NERVOUS SYSTEM AGENT; BETA-ADRENERGIC AGONIST (SYMPATHOMIMETIC); BRONCHODILATOR (RESPIRATORY SMOOTH MUSCLE RELAXANT)
Pregnancy Category: C

AVAILABILITY 2 mg, 4 mg tablets; 4 mg, 8 mg extended-release tablets; 2 mg/5 mL syrup; 200 mcg capsules for inhalation; 0.083%, 0.5% solution for inhalation

ACTIONS Synthetic sympathomimetic amine and moderately selective beta$_2$-adrenergic agonist with comparatively long action. Acts more prominently on beta$_2$ receptors (particularly smooth muscles of bronchi, uterus, and vascular supply to skeletal muscles) than on beta$_1$ (heart) receptors. Minimal or no effect on alpha-adrenergic receptors. Inhibits histamine release by mast cells.
THERAPEUTIC EFFECTS Produces bronchodilation, regardless of administration route, by relaxing smooth muscles of bronchial tree. This decreases airway resistance, facilitates mucous drainage, and increases vital capacity.

USES To relieve bronchospasm associated with acute or chronic asthma, bronchitis, or other reversible obstructive airway diseases. Also used to prevent exercise-induced bronchospasm.
UNLABELED USES Adjunct in treatment of refractory heart failure and to stimulate intracellular transport of potassium in hyperkalemic familial periodic paralysis.

CONTRAINDICATIONS Pregnancy (category C), lactation. Use of oral syrup in children <2 y.
CAUTIOUS USE Cardiovascular disease, hypertension, hyperthyroidism, diabetes mellitus, hypersensitivity to sympathomimetic amines or to fluorocarbon propellant used in inhalation aerosols.

ROUTE & DOSAGE

Bronchospasm

Child: **PO** 2–6 y, 0.1–0.2 mg/kg t.i.d. (max 4 mg/dose); 6–12 y, 2 mg 3–4 times/day; **Inhaled** 6–12 y, 1–2 inhalations q4–6h
Adult: **PO** 2–4 mg 3–4 times/day, 4–8 mg sustained release 2 times/day **Inhaled** 1–2 inhalations q4–6h

STORAGE

- Store tablets and syrup between 2°–25° C (36°–77° F) in tight, light-resistant container.
- Store inhalation canisters between 15°–30° C (59°–86° F) away from heat and direct sunlight.

ADMINISTRATION

Oral

- Do not crush extended-release tablets. Scored tablets may be broken in half.

Inhalation

- Administer albuterol 20–30 min before concomitant beclomethasone (Vanceril) or other corticosteroid or long-acting beta-2 agonist treatments to allow deeper penetration of beclomethasone into lungs, unless otherwise directed by physician.

ADVERSE EFFECTS Body as a Whole: Hypersensitivity reaction. **CNS:** *Tremor*, anxiety, nervousness, restlessness, convulsions, weakness, headache, hallucinations. **CV:** Palpitation, tachycardia, hypertension, hypotension, bradycardia, reflex tachycardia. **Special Senses:** Blurred vision, dilated pupils. **GI:** Nausea, vomiting. **Other:** Muscle cramps, hoarseness.

DIAGNOSTIC TEST INTERFERENCE: Transient small increases in *plasma glucose* may occur.

INTERACTIONS Drug: With **epinephrine,** other SYMPATHOMIMETIC BRONCHODILATORS, possible additive effects; MAO INHIBITORS, TRICYCLIC ANTIDEPRESSANTS potentiate action on vascular system; BETA-ADRENERGIC BLOCKERS antagonize the effects of both drugs.

PHARMACOKINETICS Onset: Inhaled: 5–15 min; PO 30 min. **Peak:** Inhaled: 0.5–2 h; PO 2.5 h. **Duration:** Inhaled: 3–6 h; PO 4–6 h (8–12 h with sustained release). **Metabolism:** Metabolized in liver; may cross the placenta. **Elimination:** 76% of dose eliminated in urine in 3 days. **Half-Life:** 2.75 h.

NURSING IMPLICATIONS

Assessment & Drug Effects

- Monitor therapeutic effectiveness, which is indicated by significant subjective improvement in pulmonary function within 60–90 min after drug administration.

- Monitor peak expiratory flow rate and teach families to measure and record at home.
- Monitor for S&S of fine tremor in fingers, which may interfere with precision handwork; CNS stimulation, particularly in children 2–6 y, (hyperactivity, excitement, nervousness, insomnia), tachycardia, GI symptoms. Report promptly to physician.
- Lab tests: Periodic ABGs, pulmonary functions, and pulse oximetry.
- Consult physician about giving last albuterol dose several hours before bedtime if drug-induced insomnia is a problem.

Patient & Family Education
- Review directions for correct use of medication and inhaler (see ADMINISTRATION). Have child demonstrate correct use of inhaler.
- Avoid contact of inhalation drug with eyes.
- Do not increase number or frequency of inhalations without advice of physician.
- Notify physician if albuterol fails to provide relief, because this can signify worsening of pulmonary function, and an evaluation of condition/therapy may be indicated.
- Note: Albuterol can cause dizziness or vertigo. Take necessary precautions.
- Do not use OTC drugs without prescriber approval. Many medications (e.g., cold remedies) contain drugs that may intensify albuterol action.
- Do not breast feed while taking this drug without consulting prescriber.
- Store this medication out of reach of children.

ALLOPURINOL
(al-oh-pure′i-nole)
Alloprin A ✦, Alloprim, Apoallopurinol-A ✦, Lopurin, Novopurinol A, Purinol ✦, Zyloprim
Classifications: ANTIGOUT AGENT; ANTILITHIC
Prototype: Colchicine
Pregnancy Category: C

AVAILABILITY 100 mg, 300 mg tablets; 500 mg vial

ACTIONS Allopurinol reduces endogenous uric acid by selectively inhibiting action of xanthine oxidase, the enzyme responsible for converting hypo-xanthine to xanthine and xanthine to uric acid (end product of purine catabolism). Has no analgesic, anti-inflammatory, or uricosuric actions.
THERAPEUTIC EFFECTS Urate pool is decreased by the lowering of both serum and urinary uric acid levels, and hyperuricemia is prevented.

USES To control primary hyperuricemia that accompanies severe gout and to prevent possibility of flare-up of acute gout attack; to prevent recurrent calcium oxalate stones; prophylactically to reduce severity of hyperuricemia associated with antineoplastic and radiation therapies, both of which greatly increase plasma uric acid levels by promoting nucleic acid degradation.
UNLABELED USES To reduce hyperuricemia secondary to Lesch–Nyhan syndrome, polycythemia vera, G6PD deficiency, sarcoidosis, and therapy with thiazides or ethambutol.

CONTRAINDICATIONS Hypersensitivity to allopurinol; as initial treatment for acute gout attacks; idiopathic hemochromatosis (or those with family history); children (except those with hyperuricemia secondary to neoplastic disease and chemotherapy or those with genetic purine metabolic disease). Safety during pregnancy (category C) or lactation is not established. **CAUTIOUS USE** Impaired hepatic or renal function, history of peptic ulcer, lower GI tract disease, bone marrow depression.

ROUTE & DOSAGE

Treatment Hyperuricemia

Child: **PO** ≤*10 y,* 10 mg/kg/day given in 2–3 divided doses (max 800 mg/day) **IV** 200 mg/m^2/day divided into 2–4 doses
Adult: **PO** 100 mg/day, may increase by 100 mg/wk (max 800 mg/day), divide doses >300 mg/day **IV** 200–400 mg/m^2/day (max 600 mg/day) in 1–4 divided doses

Treatment Secondary Hyperuricemia

Child: **PO** *6–10 y,* 100 mg t.i.d., *<6 y,* 50 mg t.i.d.
Adult: **PO** 200–800 mg/day for 2–3 day or longer, divide doses >300 mg/day

Renal Impairment

Cl$_{cr}$: 80 mL/min: 250 mg/day; 60 mL/min: 200 mg/day; 40 mL/min: 150 mg/day; 20 mL/min: 100 mg/day; 10 mL/min: 100 mg q2d; 0 mL/min: 100 mg q3d; OR Cl$_{cr}$ 10–50 mL/min: reduce dose by 50%; Cl$_{cr}$ <10 mL/min: reduce dose by 70%

STORAGE

Store at 15°–30° C (59°–86° F) in a tightly closed container.

ADMINISTRATION

Oral

- Give after meals for best toleration; tablet may be crushed and taken with fluid or mixed with food.

Intravenous

PREPARE **Intermittent:** Reconstitute a single-dose vial (500 mg) with 25 mL of sterile water for injection to yield 20 mg/mL. Further dilute with NS or D5W to a concentration of ≤6 mg/mL.
- Note: Adding 2.3 mL of diluent yields 6 mg/mL.
ADMINISTER **Intermittent:** Usually administered over 30–60 min.

INCOMPATIBILITIES **Solution/Additive: Amikacin, amphotericin B, carmustine, cefotaxime, chlorpromazine, cimetidine, clindamycin, cytarabine, dacarbazine, daunorubicin, doxycycline, droperidol, floxuridine, gentamicin, haloperidol, hydroxyzine, idarubicin, imipenem-cilastatin, mechlorethamine, meperidine, metoclopramide, methylprednisolone, minocycline, nalbuphine, netilmicin, ondansetron, prochlorperazine, promethazine, sodium bicarbonate, streptozocin, tobramycin, vinorelbine.**

ADVERSE EFFECTS CNS: Drowsiness, headache, vertigo. **GI:** Nausea, vomiting, diarrhea, abdominal discomfort, indigestion, malaise. **Hematologic:** (Rare) <u>Agranulocytosis, aplastic anemia, bone marrow depression</u>, thrombocytopenia. **Skin:** Urticaria or pruritus, pruritic maculopapular rash, toxic epidermal necrolysis. **Other:** <u>Hepatotoxicity</u>, renal insufficiency.

DIAGNOSTIC TEST INTERFERENCE Possibility of elevated blood levels of *alkaline phosphatase* and *serum transaminases (AST, ALT),* and decreased blood *Hct, Hgb, leukocytes.*

INTERACTIONS Drug: Alcohol may inhibit renal excretion of uric acid; **ampicillin, amoxicillin** increase risk of skin rash; enhances anticoagulant effect of **warfarin;** toxicity from **azathioprine, mercaptopurine, cyclophosphamide, cyclosporin** increased; increases hypoglycemic effects of **chlorpropamide;** THIAZIDES increase risk of allopurinol toxicity and hypersensitivity (especially with impaired renal function).

PHARMACOKINETICS Absorption: 80–90% absorbed from GI tract. **Onset:** 24–48 h. **Peak:** 2–6 h. **Metabolism:** 75–80% metabolizes to the active metabolite oxypurinol. **Elimination:** Slowly excreted in urine; excreted in breast milk. **Half-Life:** 1–3 h; oxypurinol, 18–30 h.

NURSING IMPLICATIONS

Assessment & Drug Effects
- Monitor for therapeutic effectiveness, which is indicated by normal serum and urinary uric acid levels usually by 1–3 wk (aim of therapy is to lower serum uric acid level gradually to about 6 mg/dL), gradual decrease in size of tophi, absence of new tophaceous deposits (after approximately 6 mo), with consequent relief of joint pain and increased joint mobility.
- Monitor for S&S of an acute gout attack, which is most likely to occur during first 6 wk of therapy.
- Lab tests: Monitor serum uric acid levels q1–2 wk to check adequacy of dosage. Perform baseline CBC, liver, and kidney function tests before therapy is initiated and then monthly, particularly during first few months. Check urinary pH at regular intervals.
- Monitor patients with renal disorders more often; they tend to have a higher incidence of renal stones and drug toxicity problems.
- Report onset of rash or fever immediately to physician; withdraw drug. Life-threatening toxicity syndrome can occur 2–4 wk after initiation of therapy (more common with impaired renal function) and is generally accompanied by malaise, fever, and aching, a diffuse erythematous, desquamating rash, hepatic dysfunction, eosinophilia, and worsening of renal function.

Patient & Family Education
- Drink enough fluid to produce generous urinary output for age and weight. Report diminishing urinary output, cloudy urine, unusual color or odor to urine, pain or discomfort on urination.
- Report promptly the onset of itching or rash. Stop drug if a skin rash appears, even after 5 or more wk (and reportedly as long as 2 y) of therapy.

- Minimize exposure of eyes to ultraviolet or sunlight, which may stimulate the development of cataracts.
- Do not drive or engage in potentially hazardous activities until response to drug is known.
- Remain under medical supervision while taking allopurinol (generally continued indefinitely); drug can cause severe adverse reactions.
- Do not breast feed while taking this drug without consulting physician.
- Store this medication out of reach of children.

ALPROSTADIL (PGE₁)

(al-pross'ta-dil)
Prostin VR Pediatric, Caverject
Classification: PROSTAGLANDIN
Prototype: Dinoprostone
Pregnancy Category: C

AVAILABILITY 500 mcg/mL injection; 5 mcg/mL, 10 mcg/mL, 20 mcg/mL, 40 mcg/mL powder for injection; 125 mcg, 250 mcg, 500 mcg, 1000 mcg pellets

ACTIONS Actions include vasodilation, inhibition of platelet aggregation, and stimulation of intestinal and uterine smooth muscles.
THERAPEUTIC EFFECTS Preserves ductal patency by relaxing smooth muscle of ductus arteriosus. Used to treat penile erection dysfunction in adults.

USES Temporary measure to maintain patency of ductus arteriosus in infants with ductal-dependent congenital heart defects until corrective surgery can be performed.

CONTRAINDICATIONS Ductus arteriosus respiratory distress syndrome (hyaline membrane disease); hypersensitivity to alprostadil.
CAUTIOUS USE Ductus arteriosus; bleeding tendencies; hypersensitivity to alprostadil; sickle cell anemia or trait; patients on anticoagulants, vasoactive or antihypertensive drugs.

ROUTE & DOSAGE

To Maintain Patency of Ductus Arteriosus
Neonate: **IV/Intra-Arterial/Intra-Aortic** 0.05–0.1 mcg/kg/min, may increase gradually (max 0.4 mcg/kg/min if necessary)

STORAGE
Store at 2°–8° C (36°–46° F) unless otherwise directed by manufacturer. Protect from freezing.

ADMINISTRATION

Intravenous

PREPARE **Continuous:** Dilute 500 mg alprostadil with NS or D5W to volume appropriate for pump delivery system. Prepare fresh solution q24h. Discard unused portions. A 500 mg ampule diluted in 250 mL yields a concentration of 2 mg/mL.

Common adverse effects in *italic;* life-threatening effects <u>underlined</u>; generic names in **bold;** drug classifications in SMALL CAPS; ◆ Canadian drug name; ● Prototype drug.

***ADMINISTER* Continuous:** Infuse at rate of 0.05–0.1 mg/kg/min up to a maximum of 0.4 mg/kg/min.
- Reduce infusion rate immediately if arterial pressure drops significantly or if fever occurs.
- Discontinue promptly, if apnea or bradycardia occurs.

ADVERSE EFFECTS CNS: *Fever,* seizures, lethargy. **CV:** *Flushing,* bradycardia, hypotension, syncope, tachycardia; CHF, <u>ventricular fibrillation, shock</u>. **GI:** Diarrhea, gastric regurgitation. **Hematologic:** <u>Disseminated intravascular coagulation (DIC)</u>, thrombocytopenia. **Respiratory:** Apnea. **Skin:** Rash on face and arms, alopecia. **Other:** Leg pain.

INTERACTIONS Drug: May increase anticoagulant properties of **warfarin;** ANTIHYPERTENSIVE AGENTS increase risk of hypotension.

PHARMACOKINETICS Onset: 15 min to 3 h. **Metabolism:** Rapidly metabolized in lungs. **Elimination:** Metabolites excreted through kidneys. **Half-Life:** 5–10 min.

NURSING IMPLICATIONS

Assessment & Drug Effects Ductus Arteriosus
- Monitor therapeutic effectiveness, which is indicated by increase in blood oxygenation (PO_2), usually evident within 30 min, in infants with cyanotic heart disease (restricted pulmonary blood flow). Normal PO_2 for neonates is 60–70 mm Hg. Indicated by increased pH in those with acidosis, increased systemic BP and urinary output, return of palpable pulses, and decreased ratio of pulmonary artery to aortic pressure in infants with restricted systemic blood flow. Redue to lowest effective dosage to reduce incidence of side effects.
- Monitor for arterial pressure, ECG, heart rate, BP, respiratory rate, and rectal temperature, intermittently throughout the infusion.
- Lab tests: Monitor arterial blood gases and arterial blood pH intermittently throughout the infusion.
- Monitor systemic BP, pulmonary artery and descending aorta pressures, femoral pulse, and urinary output.

Patient & Family Education
- Explain purpose of therapy and child's condition and expected treatment.

ALTEPLASE RECOMBINANT ☻
(al'te-plase)
Actilyse, Activase, Cathflo Activase
Classifications: BLOOD FORMERS, COAGULATORS, AND ANTICOAGULANTS; THROMBOLYTIC ENZYME
Pregnancy Category: C

AVAILABILITY 50 mg, 100 mg vials

ACTIONS This recombinant DNA-derived form of human tissue-type plasminogen activator (t-PA) is a thrombolytic agent.

Common adverse effects in *italic*; life-threatening effects <u>underlined</u>; generic names in **bold**; drug classifications in SMALL CAPS; ◆ Canadian drug name; ☻ Prototype drug.

81

THERAPEUTIC EFFECTS The agent t-PA promotes thrombolysis by forming the active proteolytic enzyme plasmin. Plasmin is capable of degrading fibrin, fibrinogen, and factors V, VIII, and XII.

USES Indicated in selective cases of acute MI, preferably within 6 h of attack for recanalization of the coronary artery; lysis of acute pulmonary emboli; acute ischemic stroke or thrombotic stroke (within 3 h of onset); treatment of acute coronary artery thrombosis in the setting of percutaneous coronary intervention (PCI); reestablishing patency of occluded IV catheter.

UNLABELED USES Lysis of arterial occlusions in peripheral and bypass vessels; DVT; restoration of patency in central venous catheters occluded by blood clot.

CONTRAINDICATIONS Active internal bleeding, history of cerebrovascular accident, recent (within 2 mo) intracranial or interspinal surgery or trauma, intracranial neoplasm, arteriovenous malformation, bleeding disorders, severe uncontrolled hypertension, likelihood of left heart thrombus, acute pericarditis, bacterial endocarditis, severe liver dysfunction, pregnancy (category C), septic thrombophlebitis, current use of oral anticoagulants.

CAUTIOUS USE Recent major surgery (within 10 day), cerebral vascular disease, recent GI or GU bleeding, recent trauma, hypertension, lactation, hemorrhagic ophthalmic conditions. Safety and effectiveness in children are not established.

ROUTE & DOSAGE

Acute MI

Adult: **IV** ≥65 kg: 60 mg over first hour, with 6–10 mg infused over first 1–2 min; then 20 mg over the second hour and 20 mg over the third hour (100 mg over 3 h); <65 kg: Infuse 1.25 mg/kg over 3 h (60% h 1; 20% h 2, 20% h 3); *accelerated schedule:* 15-mg bolus, then 0.75 mg/kg (up to 50 mg) over 30 min, then 0.5 mg/kg (up to 35 mg) over 60 min

Acute Ischemic Stroke/Thrombotic Stroke

Adult: **IV** 0.9 mg/kg over 60 min with 10% of dose as an initial bolus over 1 min (max 90 mg)

Pulmonary Embolism

Child: 0.1–0.6 mg/kg/h × 6 h
Adult: **IV** 100 mg infused over 2 h

Reopen Occluded IV Catheter

Child: >2 y, 10–29 kg **IV** Instill 110% of internal lumen volume with 1 mg/mL concentration (max 2 mg). May repeat if function not restored within 2 h. *<2 y, <10 kg:* **IV** 0.5 mg diluted in a volume to fill the lumen of the catheter
Child/Adult (>30 kg): **IV** Instill 2 mg/2 mL into dysfunctional catheter for 2 h. May repeat once if needed

STORAGE

- Store powder for injection or intracatheter instillation at room temperature of 15°–30° C (59°–86° F) or refrigerated at 2°–8° C (36°–46° F); lyophilized powder for intracatheter instillation is refrigerated at 2°–8° C (36°–46° F). Protect all preparations from light.
- Store reconstituted solutions at room temperature 2°–30° C (36°–86° F) for no longer than 8 h. Discard any unused solution after that time.

ADMINISTRATION

Intravenous

***PREPARE* IV Infusion:** Reconstitute the 50-mg vial as follows: Do not use if vacuum in vial has been broken. Use a large-bore needle (e.g., 18 gauge) and do not prime needle with air. ■ Dilute contents of vial with sterile water for injection supplied by manufacturer. ■ Direct stream of sterile water into the lyophilized cake. Slight foaming is usual. Allow to stand until bubbles dissipate. Resulting concentration is 1 mg/mL. ■ Reconstitute the 100-mg vial as follows: The 100-mg vial does not contain a vacuum. Use supplied transfer device for reconstitution and follow manufacturer's directions.

***ADMINISTER* IV Infusion:** Start IV infusion as soon as possible after the thrombolytic event, preferably within 6 h. ■ Administer drug as reconstituted (1 mg/mL) or further diluted with an equal volume of NS or D5W to yield 0.5 mg/mL. ■ **Pulmonary embolism:** Administer entire dose over a 2 h period. ■ **Acute ischemic stroke:** Give 5 mg as an initial bolus over 1 min, then give the remainder of the 0.75 mg/kg dose over 60 min. ■ Do not exceed a total dose of 100 mg. Higher doses have been associated with intracranial bleeding. ■ Follow infusion of drug by flushing IV tubing with 30–50 mL of NS or D5W. ■ Reconstituted drug is stable for 8 h in above solutions at room temperature (2°–30° C; 36°–86° F). Because there are no preservatives, discard any unused solution after that time.

ADVERSE EFFECTS Hematologic: Internal and superficial bleeding (cerebral, retroperitoneal, GU, GI).

PHARMACOKINETICS Peak: 5–10 min after infusion completed. **Duration:** Baseline values restored in 3 h. **Metabolism:** Metabolized in liver. **Elimination:** Excreted in urine. **Half-Life:** 26.5 min.

NURSING IMPLICATIONS

Assessment & Drug Effects

- Monitor for S&S of excess bleeding q15 min for the first hour of therapy, q30 min for second to eighth hour, then q8h. Monitor neurologic checks throughout drug infusion q30 min for the first 8 h after infusion.
- Protect patient from invasive procedures because spontaneous bleeding occurs twice as often with alteplase as with heparin. IM injections are contraindicated. Also prevent physical manipulation of patient during thrombolytic therapy to prevent bruising.

- Lab tests: Coagulation tests including APTT, bleeding time, PT, TT, INR, must be done before administration of drug. Also check *baseline* Hct, Hgb, and platelet counts, in case of bleeding. Draw Hct following drug administration to detect possible blood loss.
- Keep patient in bed while receiving this medication.
- Check vital signs frequently. Be alert to changes in cardiac rhythm.
- Stop therapy immediately if dysrhythmias occur.
- Report signs of bleeding: gum bleeding, epistaxis, hematoma, spontaneous ecchymoses, oozing at catheter site, increased pain from internal bleeding. Stop the infusion, then resume when bleeding stops.
- Use the radial artery to draw ABGs. Pressure to puncture sites, if necessary, should be maintained for up to 30 min.
- Continue monitoring vital signs until laboratory reports confirm anticoagulant control; patient is at risk for post-thrombolytic bleeding for 2–4 days after intracoronary alteplase treatment.

Patient & Family Education
- Report immediately a sudden severe headache.
- Report blood in urine and bloody or tarry stools.
- Report any signs of bleeding or oozing from cuts or places of injection.
- Remain quiet and on bedrest while receiving this medicine.

AMANTADINE HYDROCHLORIDE

(a-man'ta-deen)
Symmetrel
Classifications: ANTI-INFECTIVE; ANTIVIRAL; AUTONOMIC NERVOUS SYSTEM AGENT; ANTICHOLINERGIC (PARASYMPATHOLYTIC); ANTIPARKINSONIAN AGENT
Prototype: Acyclovir
Pregnancy Category: C

AVAILABILITY 100 mg capsules; 50 mg/5 mL syrup

ACTIONS Because it does not suppress antibody formation, it can be administered for interim protection in combination with influenza A virus vaccine until antibody titer is adequate or to augment prophylaxis in a previously vaccinated individual.
THERAPEUTIC EFFECTS Active against several strains of influenza A virus; not effective against influenza B infections. Also provides anticholinergic effects.

USES In therapy for all forms of parkinsonism. Used for prophylaxis and symptomatic treatment of influenza A infections.
UNLABELED USES Primary enuresis, pseudosclerosis, neuroleptic malignant syndrome (NMS), management of cocaine dependency and withdrawal.

CONTRAINDICATIONS Safety during pregnancy (category C), lactation, and in children <1 y is not established.
CAUTIOUS USE History of epilepsy or other types of seizures; CHF, peripheral edema, orthostatic hypotension; recurrent eczematoid dermatitis;

psychoses, severe psychoneuroses; hepatic disease; renal impairment; older adults with cerebral arteriosclerosis.

ROUTE & DOSAGE

Influenza A Treatment and Prophylaxis

Child: **PO** *1–9 y,* 4.4–8.8 mg/kg divided into 2–3 equal doses (preferable dose is 5 mg/kg with max 150 mg/day) *9–12 y,* 100 mg b.i.d.
Adult: **PO** 200 mg daily or 100 mg q12h

STORAGE

Store in tightly closed container preferably at 15°–30° C (59°–86° F) unless otherwise directed by manufacturer. Avoid freezing.

ADMINISTRATION

Oral

- Give with water, milk, or food.
- Use supplied calibrated device for measuring syrup formulation.
- Influenza prophylaxis: Drug should be initiated when exposure is anticipated and continued for at least 10 days.
- Note: Used in conjunction with influenza A vaccine (generally in high-risk patients who have not been vaccinated previously) until protective antibodies develop (10–21 day) after vaccine administration.
- Schedule medication in the morning or, with q12h dosing, schedule second dose several hours before bedtime. If insomnia is a problem, suggest patient limit number of daytime naps.

ADVERSE EFFECTS CNS: *Dizziness, light-headedness,* headache, ataxia, irritability, anxiety, *nervousness, difficulty in concentrating,* mood or other mental changes, confusion, visual and auditory hallucinations, *insomnia,* nightmares, convulsions. **CV:** Orthostatic hypotension, peripheral edema, dyspnea. **Special Senses:** Blurring or loss of vision. **GI:** Anorexia, *nausea,* vomiting, dry mouth. **Hematologic:** Leukopenia.

INTERACTIONS Drug: Alcohol enhances CNS effects; may potentiate effects of ANTICHOLINERGICS. Cotrimoxazole may reduce renal clearance of amantadine.

PHARMACOKINETICS Absorption: Readily and almost completely absorbed from GI tract. **Onset:** Within 48 h. **Peak:** 1–4 h. **Distribution:** Distributed to saliva, nasal secretions, breast milk, placenta, CSF. **Metabolism:** Not metabolized. **Elimination:** 90% excreted unchanged in urine. **Half-Life:** 9–37 h (prolonged in renal insufficiency).

NURSING IMPLICATIONS

Assessment & Drug Effects

- Treatment may be preceded with diagnostic tests for influenza and RSV.
- Monitor vital signs for at least 3 or 4 day after increases in dosage; also monitor urinary output.
- Monitor for signs of influenza.
- Lab tests: pH and serum electrolytes.

Patient & Family Education

- Note: For influenza take within 24 h but no later than 48 h after onset of symptoms for effective response; continue for 24–48 h after symptoms disappear; contact prescriber if no improvement within this time.
- Make all position changes slowly, particularly from recumbent to upright position, in order to minimize dizziness.
- Report any of the following: shortness of breath, peripheral edema, significant weight gain, dizziness or light-headedness, inability to concentrate, and other changes in mental status, difficulty urinating, and visual impairment to prescriber.
- Do not drive and exercise caution with potentially hazardous activities until response to the drug is known.
- Do not breast feed while taking this drug without consulting prescriber.
- Store this medication out of reach of children.

AMIKACIN SULFATE

(am-i-kay'sin)
Amikin
Classifications: ANTI-INFECTIVE; AMINOGLYCOSIDE ANTIBIOTIC
Prototype: Gentamicin
Pregnancy Category: C

AVAILABILITY 250 mg/mL, 50 mg/mL injection

ACTIONS Semisynthetic derivative of kanamycin with broad range of antimicrobial activity that includes many strains resistant to other aminoglycosides. Pharmacologic properties are essentially the same as those of gentamicin. Appears to inhibit protein synthesis in bacterial cell and is usually bactericidal.

THERAPEUTIC EFFECTS Effective against a wide variety of gram-negative bacteria including *Escherichia coli, Enterobacter, Klebsiella pneumoniae,* most strains of *Pseudomonas aeruginosa,* and many strains of *Proteus species, Serratia, Providencia stuartii, Citrobacter freundii, Acinetobacter.* Also effective against penicillinase- and non-penicillinase-producing *Staphylococcus* species, and against *Mycobacterium tuberculosis* and atypical mycobacteria.

USES Primarily for short-term treatment of serious infections of respiratory tract, bones, joints, skin, and soft tissue, CNS (including meningitis), peritonitis burns, recurrent urinary tract infections (UTIs).

UNLABELED USES Intrathecal or intraventricular administration, in conjunction with IM or IV dosage.

CONTRAINDICATIONS History of hypersensitivity or toxic reaction with an aminoglycoside antibiotic. Safety during pregnancy (category C), lactation, neonates and infants, or use for period exceeding 14 days is not established.

CAUTIOUS USE Impaired renal function; eighth cranial (auditory) nerve impairment; preexisting vertigo or dizziness, tinnitus, or dehydration, fever; older adults, premature infants, neonates and infants; myasthenia gravis; parkinsonism; hypocalcemia.

ROUTE & DOSAGE

Note: All doses based on ideal body weight.

Moderate to Severe Infections

Neonate: **IV/IM** 10 mg/kg loading dose, then 7.5 mg/kg q12–24h; neonates of <37 wk gestational age: 7.5 mg/kg q24h
Child: **IV/IM** 5–7.5 mg/kg loading dose, then 5 mg/kg q8h or 7.5 mg/kg q12h
Adult: **IV/IM** 5–7.5 mg/kg loading dose, then 7.5 mg/kg q12h

Uncomplicated UTI

Adult: **IV/IM** 250 mg q12h

STORAGE

Store injection solution between 15°–30° C (59°–86° F) and protect from freezing. Once the amikacin and ADD-Vantage vial has been entered, it must be discarded in 4 h. Once these vials have been activated for dilution, use within 24 h.

ADMINISTRATION

Intramuscular

Use the 250 mg/mL vials for IM injection. Calculate the required dose and withdraw the equivalent number of milliliters from the vial.

- Give deep IM into a large muscle according to child's age and developmental level; rotate and record sites (see Part I).

Intravenous

Verify correct IV concentration and rate of infusion with physician for neonates, infants, and children.
PREPARE **Intermittent:** Add contents of 500-g vial to 100 or 200 mL D5W, NS injection, or other diluent recommended by manufacturer.
- For pediatric patients, volume of diluent depends on patient's fluid tolerance. ▪ Note: Color of solution may vary from colorless to light straw color or very pale yellow. Discard solutions that appear discolored or that contain particulate matter.
ADMINISTER **Intermittent:** Give over 60 min by IV infusion; must not be given IV push because ototoxicity risk is high. ▪ Increase infusion time to 1–2 h for infants. ▪ Monitor drip rate carefully; maximum concentration 5 mg/mL. A rapid rise in serum amikacin level can cause respiratory depression (neuromuscular blockade) and other signs of toxicity.
INCOMPATIBILITIES **Solution/Additive: Aminophylline, amphotericin B,** CEPHALOSPORINS, **chlorothiazide, erythromycin, heparin, oxytetracycline,** PENICILLINS, **phenytoin, thiopental, vitamin B complex with C, warfarin. Y-Site: Amphotericin B, heparin, phenytoin, thiopental.** Manufacturer recommends that amikacin sulfate injection not be mixed with other drugs.

ADVERSE EFFECTS CNS: Neurotoxicity: drowsiness, unsteady gait, weakness, clumsiness, paresthesias, tremors, convulsions, peripheral neuritis. **Special Senses:** *Auditory–ototoxicity,* high-frequency hearing loss, complete hearing loss (occasionally permanent); tinnitus; ringing or buzzing in ears. *Vestibular:* dizziness, ataxia. **GI:** Nausea, vomiting, hepatotoxicity. **Metabolic:** Hypokalemia, hypomagnesemia. **Skin:** Skin rash, urticaria, pruritus, redness. **Urogenital:** Oliguria, urinary frequency, hematuria, tubular necrosis, azotemia. **Other:** Superinfections.

INTERACTIONS Drug: ANESTHETICS, SKELETAL MUSCLE RELAXANTS have additive neuromuscular blocking effects; **acyclovir, amphotericin B, bacitracin, capreomycin, cephalosporins, colistin, cisplatin, carboplatin, methoxyflurane, polymyxin B, vancomycin, furosemide, ethacrynic acid** increase risk of ototoxicity and nephrotoxicity.

PHARMACOKINETICS Peak: 30 min IV; 45 min to 2 h IM. **Distribution:** Does not cross blood–brain barrier; crosses placenta; accumulates in renal cortex. **Elimination:** 94–98% excreted renally in 24 h, remainder in 10–30 days. **Half-Life:** 2–3 h in adults, 4–8 h in neonates.

NURSING IMPLICATIONS

Assessment & Drug Effects

- Baseline tests: Before initial dose, C&S; renal function and vestibulo-cochlear nerve function (and at regular intervals during therapy; closely monitor in those with documented ear problems, renal impairment, or during high-dose or prolonged therapy).
- Monitor peak and trough amikacin blood levels: Draw blood 1 h after IM or immediately after completion of IV infusion; draw trough levels immediately before the next IM or IV dose.
- Lab tests: Periodic serum creatinine and BUN, complete urinalysis. With treatment over 10 days, daily tests of renal function, weekly audiograms, and vestibular tests are strongly advised.
- Monitor serum creatinine or creatinine clearance (generally preferred) more often, in the presence of impaired renal function and in neonates; note that prolonged high **trough** (>8 mg/mL) or **peak** (>30–35 mg/mL) **levels** are associated with toxicity.
- Monitor for S&S of ototoxicity (primarily involves the cochlear [auditory] branch; high-frequency deafness usually appears first and can be detected only by audiometer); indicators of declining renal function; respiratory tract infections and other symptoms indicative of superinfections and septicemia and notify physician immediately should they occur.
- Monitor for and report auditory symptoms (tinnitus, roaring noises, sensation of fullness in ears, hearing loss) and vestibular disturbances (dizziness or vertigo, nystagmus, ataxia).
- Monitor and report any changes in I&O, oliguria, hematuria, or cloudy urine. Keeping patient well hydrated reduces risk of nephrotoxicity; consult physician regarding optimum fluid intake.

Patient & Family Education

- Report immediately any changes in hearing or unexplained ringing/roaring noises or dizziness, and problems with balance or

Common adverse effects in *italic;* life-threatening effects underlined; generic names in **bold;** drug classifications in SMALL CAPS; ✚ Canadian drug name; ❷ Prototype drug.

coordination. Encourage parents to be aware of the infant's or young child's hearing.

■ Do not breast feed while taking this drug without consulting physician.

AMILORIDE HYDROCHLORIDE

(a-mill'oh-ride)
Midamor
Classifications: ELECTROLYTE AND WATER BALANCE AGENTS; DIURETICS, POTASSIUM SPARING
Prototype: Spironolactone
Pregnancy Category: B

AVAILABILITY 5 mg tablets

ACTIONS Potassium-sparing diuretic with mild diuretic and antihypertensive action. Diuretic action is independent of aldosterone and carbonic anhydrase.
THERAPEUTIC EFFECTS Induces urinary excretion of sodium and reduces excretion of potassium and hydrogen ions by direct action on distal renal tubules.

USES Potassium sparing effect in prevention or treatment of diuretic-induced hypokalemia in patients with CHF, hepatic cirrhosis, or hypertension. Also used in management of primary hyperaldosteronism. Usually combined with a potassium-wasting (kaliuretic) diuretic such as a thiazide or loop diuretic.
UNLABELED USES With hydrochlorothiazide for recurrent calcium nephrolithiasis, lithium-induced polyuria.

CONTRAINDICATIONS Elevated serum potassium (>5.5 mEq/L), concomitant use of other potassium-sparing diuretics; anuria, acute or chronic renal insufficiency; evidence of diabetic nephropathy; type 1 diabetes mellitus; metabolic or respiratory acidosis; hepatic function impairment. Safety during pregnancy (category B), lactation, or in children is not established.
CAUTIOUS USE Debilitated patients; diet-controlled or uncontrolled diabetes mellitus; cardiopulmonary disease; the older adult. Some clinicians have used amiloride in children between 6–20 kg; caution should be used in these cases.

ROUTE & DOSAGE

Diuretic
Child: Weight between 6–20 kg: 0.625 mg/kg/day
Adult: **PO** 5 mg/day, may increase up to 20 mg/day in 1–2 divided doses

STORAGE
Store at 15°–30° C (59°–86° F) in a tightly closed container unless otherwise directed.

Common adverse effects in *italic;* life-threatening effects <u>underlined</u>; generic names in **bold;** drug classifications in SMALL CAPS; ♣ Canadian drug name; ✪ Prototype drug.

89

ADMINISTRATION

Oral

- Give once-a-day dose in the morning and schedule the second b.i.d. dose early to avoid interrupting sleep.
- Give with food to reduce possibility of gastric distress.

ADVERSE EFFECTS Body as a Whole: Generally well tolerated. **CNS:** *Headache,* dizziness, nervousness, confusion, paresthesias, drowsiness. **CV:** Cardiac arrhythmias. **Metabolic:** Hyperkalemia, hyponatremia, positive Coombs' test. **Hematologic:** Aplastic anemia. **Special Senses:** Tinnitus; nasal congestion. Visual disturbances, increased intraocular pressure. **GI:** *Diarrhea* or constipation, anorexia, *nausea,* vomiting, abdominal cramps, dry mouth, thirst. **Urogenital:** Polyuria, dysuria, bladder spasms, urinary frequency. Impotence, decreased libido. **Respiratory:** Dyspnea, shortness of breath. **Skin:** Rash, pruritus, photosensitivity reactions. **Other:** Weakness, fatigue, muscle cramps.

DIAGNOSTIC TEST INTERFERENCE Manufacturer advises discontinuing amiloride in patients with diabetes mellitus at least 3 days before *glucose tolerance* test.

INTERACTIONS Drug: Blood from blood banks, ACE INHIBITORS (e.g., **captopril**), **spironolactone, triamterene,** POTASSIUM SUPPLEMENTS may cause hyperkalemia with cardiac arrhythmias; possibility of increased **lithium** toxicity (decreased renal elimination); possibility of altered **digoxin** response; NSAIDS may attenuate antihypertensive effects. **Food:** POTASSIUM-CONTAINING SALT SUBSTITUTES increase risk of hyperkalemia.

PHARMACOKINETICS Absorption: 50% absorbed from GI tract. **Onset:** 2 h. **Peak:** 6–10 h. **Duration:** 24 h. **Elimination:** 20–50% excreted unchanged in urine, 40% in feces. **Half-Life:** 6–9 h.

NURSING IMPLICATIONS

Assessment & Drug Effects

- Monitor for signs and symptoms of hyperkalemia and hyponatremia (see Appendix D-1). Hyperkalemia occurs in about 10% of patients receiving amiloride and serum potassium can rise suddenly and without warning. It is more common in patients with diabetes or renal disease.
- Lab tests: Serum potassium levels, particularly when therapy is initiated, whenever dosage adjustments are made, and during any illness that may affect kidney function. Intermittent evaluations of BUN, creatinine, and ECG for patients with renal or hepatic dysfunction, diabetes mellitus or the debilitated.

Patient & Family Education

- Learn signs and symptoms of hyperkalemia and hyponatremia (see Appendix D-1) and report to physician immediately.
- Do not take potassium supplements, salt substitutes, high intake of dietary potassium unless prescribed by physician.
- Do not drive or engage in potentially hazardous activities until response to drug is known.

Common adverse effects in *italic;* life-threatening effects underlined; generic names in **bold;** drug classifications in SMALL CAPS; ♣ Canadian drug name; ● Prototype drug.

- Do not breast feed while taking this drug without consulting physician.
- Store this medication out of reach of children.

AMINOCAPROIC ACID ℗

(a-mee-noe-ka-proe'ik)
Amicar, EACA (epsilon-aminocaproic acid)
Classifications: BLOOD FORMERS, COAGULATORS, AND ANTICOAGULANTS; HEMOSTATIC
Pregnancy Category: C

AVAILABILITY 250 mg/mL injection; 500 mg tablets; 250 mg/mL syrup

ACTIONS Synthetic hemostatic with specific antifibrinolysis action. Acts principally by inhibiting plasminogen activator substance; to a lesser degree slightly inhibits activity of plasmin (fibrinolysin), which is concerned with destruction of clots. Does not control bleeding caused by loss of vascular integrity.
THERAPEUTIC EFFECTS Acts as an inhibitor of fibrinolytic bleeding.

USES To control excessive bleeding resulting from systemic hyperfibrinolysis, a pathologic condition that may accompany heart surgery, portocaval shunt, abruptio placentae, aplastic anemia, and carcinoma of lung, prostate, cervix, and stomach. Also used in urinary fibrinolysis associated with severe trauma, anoxia, shock, urologic surgery, and neoplastic diseases of GU tract.
UNLABELED USES To prevent hemorrhage in hemophiliacs undergoing dental extraction; as a specific antidote for streptokinase or urokinase toxicity; to prevent recurrence of subarachnoid hemorrhage, especially when surgery is delayed; for management of amegakaryocytic thrombocytopenia; and to prevent or abort hereditary angioedema episodes.

CONTRAINDICATIONS Severe renal impairment; active disseminated intravascular clotting (DIC); upper urinary tract bleeding. Avoid use in neonates. Safety during pregnancy (category C) is not established.
CAUTIOUS USE Cardiac, renal, or hepatic disease; history of pulmonary embolus, or other thrombotic diseases.

ROUTE & DOSAGE

Hemostatic
Child: **PO/IV** 100–200 mg/kg during first hour, then 33.3 mg/kg q.h. or 100 mg/kg/dose q4–6h (max 30 g/24 h)
Adult: **PO/IV** 4–5 g during first hour, then 1–1.25 g q.h. for 8 h or until bleeding is controlled (max 30 g/24 h)
Dosage reduced in oliguria or end stage renal disease.

STORAGE
Store in tightly closed containers at 15°–30° C (59°–86° F) unless otherwise directed. Avoid freezing.

Common adverse effects in *italic;* life-threatening effects <u>underlined;</u> generic names in **bold;** drug classifications in SMALL CAPS; ♣ Canadian drug name; ℗ Prototype drug.

ADMINISTRATION

Oral

- Note: May need to give adult-sized patient as many as 10 tablets or 4 tsp for a 5-g dose during the first hour of treatment (each tablet contains 500 mg, syrup contains 250 mg/mL)

Intravenous

PREPARE IV Infusion: Dilute parenteral aminocaproic acid before use. Each 4 mL (1 g) is diluted with 50 mL of NS, D5W, or RL.

ADMINISTER IV Infusion: Physician orders specific IV flow rate. Usual rate is 5 g or a fraction thereof over first hour (5 g/250 mL). Give each additional gram over 1 h. Avoid rapid infusion to prevent hypotension, faintness, and bradycardia or other arrhythmias.

ADVERSE EFFECTS CNS: Dizziness, malaise, headache, seizures hypercoagulation when given to someone taking oral contraceptives. **CV:** Faintness, orthostatic hypotension; <u>dysrhythmias</u>; thrombophlebitis, thromboses, hyperkalemia. **Special Senses:** Tinnitus, nasal congestion, conjunctival erythema. **GI:** Nausea, vomiting, cramps, diarrhea, anorexia. **Urogenital:** Diuresis, dysuria, anuria urinary frequency, oliguria, reddish-brown urine (myoglobinuria), <u>acute renal failure</u>, prolonged menstruation with cramping. **Skin:** Rash.

DIAGNOSTIC TEST INTERFERENCE *Serum potassium* may be elevated (especially in patients with impaired renal function).

INTERACTIONS Drug: ESTROGENS, ORAL CONTRACEPTIVES may cause hypercoagulation.

PHARMACOKINETICS Absorption: Rapidly absorbed from GI tract. **Peak:** 2 h. **Distribution:** Readily penetrates RBCs and other body cells. **Elimination:** 80% excreted as unmetabolized drug in 12 h.

NURSING IMPLICATIONS

Assessment & Drug Effects

- Check IV site at frequent intervals for extravasation.
- Observe for signs of thrombophlebitis. Change site immediately if extravasation or thrombophlebitis occurs (see Appendix D-1).
- Monitor and report S&S of myopathy: muscle weakness, myalgia, diaphoresis, fever, reddish-brown urine (myoglobinuria), oliguria, as well as thrombotic complications: arm or leg pain, tenderness or swelling, Homan's sign, prominence of superficial veins, chest pain, breathlessness, dyspnea. Drug should be discontinued promptly.
- Monitor vital signs and urine output.
- Lab tests: With prolonged therapy, monitor creatine phosphokinase activity and urinalyses for early detection of myopathy.

Patient & Family Education

- Report difficulty urinating or reddish-brown urine.
- Report arm or leg pain, chest pain, or difficulty breathing.

Common adverse effects in *italic;* life-threatening effects <u>underlined</u>; generic names in **bold**; drug classifications in SMALL CAPS; ✦ Canadian drug name; ❂ Prototype drug.

AMINOPHYLLINE (Theophylline Ethylenediamide)
(am-in-off'i-lin)
Corophyllin ♣, Paladron ♣, Phyllocontin, Somophyllin, Somophyllin-DF, Truphylline
Classifications: BRONCHODILATOR (RESPIRATORY SMOOTH MUSCLE RELAXANT); XANTHINE
Prototype: Theophylline
Pregnancy Category: C

AVAILABILITY 100 mg, 200 mg tablets; 225 mg sustained-release tablets; 105 mg/5 mL oral liquid; 250 mg/10 mL injection; 250 mg, 500 mg suppositories

ACTIONS Aminophylline is a salt of theophylline with effects similar to those of other xanthines (e.g., caffeine and theobromine). Action is dependent on theophylline content (approximately 80%) and is measured as theophylline in the serum.
THERAPEUTIC EFFECTS It is a respiratory smooth muscle relaxant that results in bronchodilation.

USES To prevent and relieve symptoms of acute bronchial asthma and treatment of bronchospasm associated with chronic bronchitis and emphysema.
UNLABELED USES As a respiratory stimulant in Cheyne-Stokes respiration; for treatment of apnea and bradycardia in premature infants; as cardiac stimulant and diuretic in treatment of CHF.

CONTRAINDICATIONS Hypersensitivity to xanthine derivatives or to ethylenediamine component; cardiac arrhythmias. Safety during pregnancy (category C) or lactation is not established.
CAUTIOUS USE Severe hypertension, cardiac disease, arrhythmias; impaired hepatic function; diabetes mellitus; hyperthyroidism; glaucoma; prostatic hypertrophy; fibrocystic breast disease; history of peptic ulcer; neonates and young children, COPD, acute influenza or patients receiving influenza immunization.

ROUTE & DOSAGE

Bronchospasm
Neonate: **PO/IV** 0.16-0.2 mg/kg/h
Infant: **PO/IV** *6–11 mo,* 0.87 mg/kg/h; *2–6 mo,* 0.5 mg/kg/h
Child: **IV Loading Dose** 6 mg/kg IV over 30 min **IV Maintenance Dose** *1–9 y,* 1–1.2 mg/kg/h; *>9–12 y and young adult smokers:,* 0.9 mg/kg/h; *>12 y and nonsmokers,* 0.7 mg/kg/h **PO** *1–9 y,* 27 mg/kg/24 h divided into 4–6 doses; *9–12 y,* 20 mg/kg/24 h divided into 4–6 doses; *12–16 y,* 16 mg/kg/24 h divided into 4–6 doses
Adult: **IV Loading Dose** 6 mg/kg over 30 min **IV Maintenance Dose** *nonsmoker,* 0.5 mg/kg/h; *smoker,* 0.75 mg/kg/h; *CHF or cirrhosis,* 0.25 mg/kg/h **PO** *nonsmoker,* 0.5 mg/kg/h times 24 h in 4 divided doses; *smoker,* 0.75 mg/kg/h times 24 h divided into 4 doses; *CHF or cirrhosis,* 0.25 mg/kg/hr times 24 h divided into 4 doses

Neonatal Apnea
Neonate: **PO/IV Loading Dose** 5–6 mg/kg **PO/IV Maintenance Dose** 1–2 mg/kg/dose given q6–8h

STORAGE
- Store at 15°–30° C (59°–86° F) in tightly closed containers unless otherwise directed.
- Follow manufacturer's directions regarding storage of suppositories; some can be stored at room temperature; others must be refrigerated.

ADMINISTRATION
Note: All doses based on ideal body weight.

Oral
- Give with a generous amount of water 1/2–1 h before or 2 h after meals for faster absorption; can be given with food if GI irritation occurs because absorption is delayed but not reduced with food.
- Do not chew or crush extended-release preparations before swallowing; however, if tablet is scored, it can be broken in half, then swallowed.
- Do mix contents of extended-release capsules with soft, moist food to promote swallowing.

Suppository
- Note: Rectal preparations may be ordered when patient must fast or cannot tolerate the drug orally; absorption is enhanced if rectum is empty.

Intravenous

Verify correct IV concentration and rate of infusion with physician for neonates, infants, and children.
PREPARE IV **Infusion:** Dilute loading dose in 100–200 mL NS to a concentration of 1 mg/mL (for fluid restricted patients, up to 25 mg/mL may be used), D5W, D5/NS, or RL. For continuous or intermittent infusion, dilute in 500–1000 mL. Do not use aminophylline solutions if discolored or if crystals are present.
ADMINISTER **IV Infusion:** Infuse at a rate not to exceed 25 mg/min.
INCOMPATIBILITIES **Solution/Additive: Amikacin, bleomycin,** CEPHALOSPORINS, **chlorpromazine, ciprofloxacin, clindamycin, codeinephosphate, dimenhydrate, dobutamine, dopamine, doxapram, doxorubicin epinephrine, hydralazine, hydroxyzine, insulin, isoproterenol, levor phanol, meperidine, methadone, methylprednisolone, morphine, nafcillin, norepinephrine, oxytetracycline, papaverine, penicillin G, pentazocine, procaine, prochlorperazine, promazine, promethazine, tetracycline, verapamil, vitamin B complex with C. Y-Site: Amiodarone, codeine phosphate, ciprofloxacin, clindamycin,** PHENOTHIAZINES **(chlorpromazine, prochlorperazine, etc.), epinephrine, dobutamine, dopamine, levorphanol, morphine, meperidine, methadone, norepinephrine, verapamil.**

ADVERSE EFFECTS CNS: *Nervousness,* restlessness, depression, insomnia, irritability, headache, dizziness, muscle hyperactivity, convulsions. **CV:** Cardiac arrhythmias, tachycardia (with rapid IV), hyperventilation, chest pain, <u>severe hypotension, cardiac arrest</u>. **GI:** *Nausea, vomiting, anorexia,* hematemesis, diarrhea, epigastric pain.

INTERACTIONS Drug: Increases **lithium** excretion, lowering **lithium** levels; **cimetidine,** high-dose **allopurinol** (600 mg/day), **alcohol, beta blockers, calcium channel blockers, disulfiram, ephedrine, esmolol, influenza virus vaccine, interferon, isoniazid, methotrexate, mexiletine, oral contraceptives, propafenone, propranolol, tacrine, thiabendazole, thyroid homones, verapamil, zileuton, ciprofloxacin, erythromycin, troleandomycin** can significantly increase **aminophylline** levels. **Carbamazepine, isoproterenol, nevirapine, phenobarbital, phenytoin, rifampin, ritonavir,** and **sypathomimetics** decrease **aminophylline** levels.

PHARMACOKINETICS Absorption: Most products are 100% absorbed from GI tract. **Peak:** IV 30 min; uncoated tablet 1 h; sustained release 4–6 h. **Duration:** 4–8 h; varies with age, smoking, and liver function. **Distribution:** Crosses placenta. **Metabolism:** Extensively metabolized in liver. **Elimination:** Parent drug and metabolites excreted by kidneys; excreted in breast milk.

NURSING IMPLICATIONS

Assessment & Drug Effects

- Monitor for S&S of toxicity (generally related to theophylline serum levels over 20 mg/L). ***Therapeutic level for asthma:*** 10–20 mg/L; ***neonatal apnea:*** 6–13 mg/L. When drawing blood for therapeutic level, use the following schedule: 30 min after IV bolus, 12–24 h after initation of continuous IV, 1 h after liquid of immediate-release tablet, 4 h after sustained-release tablet. Trough levels are drawn just before a scheduled dose.
- Observe patients receiving parenteral drug closely for signs of hypotension, arrhythmias, and convulsions until serum theophylline stabilizes within the therapeutic range.
- Note: High incidence of toxicity is associated with rectal suppository use due to erratic rate of absorption.
- Monitor and record vital signs and I&O. A sudden, sharp, unexplained rise in heart rate may indicate toxicity.
- Lab tests: Monitor serum theophylline levels.
- Note: Acutely ill children and those with severe respiratory problems, liver dysfunction, or pulmonary edema are at greater risk of toxicity due to reduced drug clearance.
- Note: Children appear more susceptible to CNS stimulating effects of xanthines (nervousness, restlessness, insomnia, hyperactive reflexes, twitching, convulsions). Dosage reduction may be indicated.

Patient & Family Education

- Note: Use of tobacco tends to increase elimination of this drug (shortens half-life), necessitating higher dosage or shorter intervals than in nonsmokers.
- Report excessive nervousness or insomnia. Dosage reduction may be indicated.
- Note: Dizziness is a relatively common side effect; take necessary safety precautions.

Common adverse effects in *italic;* life-threatening effects <u>underlined;</u> generic names in **bold;** drug classifications in SMALL CAPS; ♣ Canadian drug name; ❶ Prototype drug.

95

- Do not take OTC remedies for treatment of asthma or cough unless approved by prescriber.
- Do not breast feed while taking this drug without consulting physician.
- Store this medication out of reach of children.

AMINOSALICYLIC ACID (*PARA*-Aminosalicylic Acid)

(a-mee-noe-sal-i-sil′ik)
Paser
Classifications: ANTI-INFECTIVE; ANTITUBERCULOSIS AGENT
Prototype: Isoniazid
Pregnancy Category: C

AVAILABILITY 4 g packets

ACTIONS Aminosalicylic acid and salts are highly specific bacteriostatic agents that suppress growth and multiplication of *Mycobacterium tuberculosis* by preventing folic acid synthesis. Their mechanism of action resembles that of sulfonamides. Aminosalicylates also reportedly have potent hypolipemic action.

THERAPEUTIC EFFECTS Aminosalicylates are an effective anti-infective alone or in combined therapy and reduce serum cholesterol and triglycerides by lowering LDL and VLDL.

USES In combination with streptomycin or isoniazid or both in treatment of pulmonary and extrapulmonary tuberculosis to delay emergence of strains resistant to these drugs.
UNLABELED USES Documented for lipid-lowering effect.

CONTRAINDICATIONS Hypersensitivity to aminosalicylates, salicylates, or to compounds containing *para*-aminophenyl groups (e.g., sulfonamides, certain hair dyes), G6PD deficiency, use of the sodium salt in patients on sodium restriction or CHF. Safety during pregnancy (category C) or lactation is not established.
CAUTIOUS USE Impaired renal and hepatic function; blood dyscrasias; goiter; gastric ulcer.

ROUTE & DOSAGE

Tuberculosis
Child: **PO** 150 mg/kg/day divided into 3–4 doses
Adult: **PO** 10–12 g/day divided into 2–3 doses (max 12 g/day)

STORAGE
Store in tight, light-resistant containers in a cool, dry place, preferably at 15°–30° C (59°–86° F), unless otherwise directed.

ADMINISTRATION

Oral
- Give with or immediately following meals to reduce irritative gastric effects. Prescriber may order an antacid to be given concomitantly. Generally, GI adverse effects disappear after a few days of therapy.

Common adverse effects in *italic;* life-threatening effects <u>underlined</u>; generic names in **bold**; drug classifications in SMALL CAPS; ◆ Canadian drug name; ◐ Prototype drug.

ADVERSE EFFECTS Body as a Whole: Fever, chills, generalized malaise, joint pain, rash, fixed-drug eruptions, pruritus; vasculitis; Loeffler's syndrome. **CNS:** Psychotic reactions. **GI:** *Anorexia, nausea, vomiting, abdominal distress, diarrhea,* peptic ulceration, acute hepatitis, malabsorption. **Hematologic:** Leukopenia, <u>agranulocytosis</u>, eosinophilia, lymphocytosis, thrombocytopenia, <u>hemolytic anemia</u>; G6PD deficiency, prothrombinemia. **Urogenital:** Renal (irritation), crystalluria. **Other:** With long-term administration, goiter.

DIAGNOSTIC TEST INTERFERENCE Aminosalicylates may interfere with urine ***urobilinogen*** determinations (using ***Ehrlich's reagent***), and may cause false-positive ***urinary protein*** and ***VMA*** determinations (with ***diazoreagent***); false-positive ***urine glucose*** may result with ***cupric sulfate tests***, e.g., ***Benedict's solution***, but reportedly not with ***glucose oxidase reagents***, e.g., ***TesTape, Clinistix.*** Reduces ***serum cholesterol***, and possibly ***serum potassium, serum PBI***, and 24-h ***I-131 thyroidal uptake*** (effect may last almost 14 days).

INTERACTIONS Drug: Increases hypoprothrombinemic effects of ORAL ANTIACOAGULANTS; increased risk of crystalluria with **ammonium chloride, ascorbic acid;** decreased intestinal absorption of **cyanocobalamin, folic acid, rifampin;** may decrease absorption of **digoxin;** ANTIHISTAMINES such as **diphenhydramine** may inhibit PAS absorption; may increase or decrease **phenytoin** levels; **probenecid, sulfinpyrazone** decrease PAS elimination.

PHARMACOKINETICS Absorption: Readily and almost completely absorbed from GI tract; aminosalicylate sodium is more rapidly and completely absorbed than the acid. **Peak:** 1.5–2 h. **Duration:** 4 h. **Distribution:** Well distributed to most tissue and body fluids except CSF unless meninges are inflamed. **Metabolism:** Metabolized in liver. **Elimination:** >80% excreted in urine in 7–10 h. **Half-Life:** 1 h.

NURSING IMPLICATIONS

Assessment & Drug Effects

- Monitor for abrupt onset of fever, particularly during the early weeks of therapy, and clinical picture resembling that of infectious mononucleosis (malaise, fatigue, generalized lymphadenopathy, splenomegaly, sore throat), as well as minor complaints of pruritus, joint pains, and headache, which strongly suggest hypersensitivity; report these symptoms promptly.
- Monitor I&O and encourage fluids. High concentrations of drug are excreted in urine, and this can cause crystalluria and hematuria.
- Note: To minimize crystalluria, keep urine neutral or alkaline with adjunctive drugs, such as antacids or with diet.

Patient & Family Education

- Rinse mouth with clear water or chew sugar-free gum or candy to relieve the mildly sour or bitter aftertaste of aminosalicylic acid.
- Note: Hypersensitivity reactions may occur after a few days, but most commonly in the fourth or fifth week; report promptly.
- Notify prescriber if sore throat or mouth, malaise, unusual fatigue, bleeding or bruising occurs (symptoms of blood dyscrasia).

- Note: Therapy generally lasts about 2 y. Doses may need adjustment as child grows older and gains weight. Long-term therapy may be difficult so arrange periodic health care visits for monitoring of adherence and understanding. Adhere to the established drug regimen, and remain under close medical supervision to detect possible adverse drug effects during the treatment period. Resistant TB strains develop more rapidly when drug regimen is interrupted or is sporadic.
- Note: Urine may turn red on contact with bleach used in commercial toilet bowl cleaners.
- Do not take aspirin or other OTC drugs without prescriber's approval.
- Discard drug if it discolors (brownish or purplish); this signifies decomposition.
- Do not breast feed while taking this drug without consulting physician.
- Store this medication out of reach of children.

AMIODARONE HYDROCHLORIDE ◉

(a-mee'oh-da-rone)
Cordarone, Amio-Aqueous, Pacerone
Classifications: CARDIOVASCULAR AGENT; ANTIARRHYTHMIC, CLASS III
Pregnancy Category: D

AVAILABILITY 200 mg tablets; 50 mg/mL injection

ACTIONS Structurally related to thyroxine. Class III antiarrhythmic; also has antianginal and antiadrenergic properties. Totally unrelated to other antiarrhythmics. Acts directly on all cardiac tissues. Prolongs duration of action potential and refractory period without significantly affecting resting membrane potential.
THERAPEUTIC EFFECTS By direct action on smooth muscle, decreases peripheral resistance and increases coronary blood flow. Blocks effects of sympathetic stimulation.

USES Prophylaxis and treatment of life-threatening ventricular arrhythmias and supraventricular arrhythmias, particularly with atrial fibrillation.

CONTRAINDICATIONS Hypersensitivity to amiodarone, cardiogenic shock, severe sinus bradycardia, advanced AV block unless a pacemaker is available; severe liver disease, children. Safety during pregnancy (category D) or lactation is not established.
CAUTIOUS USE Hashimoto's thyroiditis, goiter, or history of other thyroid dysfunction; CHF; electrolyte imbalance; preexisting lung disease; open heart surgery; history of hypersensitivity to iodine. Safety in children is not established. Used mainly in children for ectopic atrial tachycardia and junctional ectopic tachycardia. Solutions contain benzyl alcohol and should be avoided in neonates whenever possible. (A preservative-free IV solution is available.)

Common adverse effects in *italic*; life-threatening effects underlined; generic names in **bold**; drug classifications in SMALL CAPS; ✦ Canadian drug name; ◉ Prototype drug.

ROUTE & DOSAGE

Arrhythmias

Child: **PO Loading Dose** 10–15 mg/kg/day or 600–800 mg/1.73 m^2/day divided into 2 doses for 4–14 day or until adequate control of arrhythmia. **PO Maintenance Dose** 5 mg/kg/day or 200–400 mg/1.73 m^2/day. May be able to reduce to 2–5 mg/kg/day given 5 days per week. Dosage has not been clearly established and may vary considerably. **IV:** IV dose is not established for children. Some clinicians have used 5 mg/kg IV over several minutes to 2 h.

Adult: **PO Loading Dose** 800–1600 mg/day in 1–2 doses for 1–3 wk **PO Maintenance Dose** 400–600 mg/day in 1–2 doses **IV Loading Dose** 150 mg over 10 min followed by 360 mg over next 6 h **IV Maintenance Dose** 540 mg over 18 h (0.5 mg/min), may continue at 0.5 mg/min **Convert IV to PO** duration of infusion <1 wk use 800–1600 mg PO, 1–3 wk use 600–800 mg PO, >3 wk use 400 mg PO

STORAGE

Store at 15°–30° C (59°– 86° F) protected from light, unless otherwise directed.

ADMINISTRATION

Note: Correct hypokalemia and hypomagnesemia prior to initiation of therapy.

Oral

- Give consistently with respect to meals.
- Note: Only a physician experienced with the drug and treatment of life-threatening arrhythmias should give loading doses.
- A pediatric cardiologist should be consulted before this drug is administered to children.
- Note: GI symptoms commonly occur during high-dose therapy, especially with loading doses. Symptoms usually respond to dose reduction or divided dose given with food, including milk.

Intravenous

PREPARE **IV Infusion:** *Adult:* **First rapid loading dose infusion:** Add 150 mg (3 mL) amiodarone to 100 mL D5W to yield 1.5 mg/mL. **Second infusion during first 24 h (slow loading dose and maintenance infusion):** Add 900 mg (18 mL) amiodarone to 500 mL D5W to yield 1.8 mg/mL. **Maintenance infusions after the first 24 h:** Prepare concentrations of 1–6 mg/mL amiodarone. Note: Dilute with D5W; use central line to give concentrations >2 mg/mL).

ADMINISTER **IV Infusion:** *Adult:* Rapidly infuse initial 150 mg dose over the first 10 min at a rate of 15 mg/min. Over next 6 h, infuse 360 mg at a rate of 1 mg/min. Over the remaining 18 h, infuse 540 mg at a rate of 0.5 mg/min. After the first 24 h, infuse maintenance doses of 720 mg/24 h at a rate of 0.5 mg/min. Do not exceed peripheral infusion rate of 2 mg/mL. Use glass or polyolefin bottles for infusion that lasts >2 h.

INCOMPATIBILITIES **Solution/Additive: Sodium bicarbonate. Y-site: Aminophylline, cefamandole, cefazolin, heparin; mezlocillin, sodium bicarbonate.**

ADVERSE EFFECTS CNS: Peripheral neuropathy (*muscle weakness,* wasting numbness, tingling), *fatigue,* abnormal gait, dyskinesias, *dizziness,* paresthesia, headache. **CV:** Bradycardia, *hypotension* (IV), sinus arrest, cardiogenic shock, CHF, arrhythmias; AV block. **Special Senses:** *Corneal microdeposits,* blurred vision, optic neuritis, optic neuropathy, permanent blindness, corneal degeneration, macular degeneration, photosensitivity. **GI:** *Anorexia, nausea, vomiting, constipation,* hepatotoxicity. **Metabolic:** Hyperthyroidism or hypothyroidism; may cause neonatal hypo- or hyperthyroidism if taken during pregnancy. **Respiratory:** (Pulmonary toxicity) Alveolitis, pneumonitis (fever, dry cough, dyspnea), interstitial pulmonary fibrosis, fatal gasping syndrome with IV in children. **Skin:** Slate-blue pigmentation, *photosensitivity,* rash. **Other:** With chronic use, angioedema.

INTERACTIONS Drug: Significantly increases **digoxin** levels; enhances pharmacologic effects and toxicities of **disopyramide, procainamide, quinidine, flecainide, lidocaine;** anticoagulant effects of ORAL ANTICOAGULANTS enhanced; **verapamil, diltiazem,** BETA-ADRENERGIC BLOCKING AGENTS may potentiate sinus bradycardia, sinus arrest, or AV block; may increase **phenytoin** levels 2- to 3-fold; **cholestyramine** may decrease amiodarone levels; **fentanyl** may cause bradycardia, hypotension, or decreased output; may increase **cyclosporine** levels and toxicity; **cimetidine** may increase amiodarone levels; **ritonavir** may increase risk of amiodarone toxicity, including cardiotoxicity. **Herbal: Echinacea** possible increase in hepatotoxicity.

PHARMACOKINETICS Absorption: Approximately 50% absorbed (22–86%); food increases absorption. **Onset:** 2–3 day to 1–3 wk. **Peak:** 3–7 h. **Distribution:** Concentrates in adipose tissue, lungs, kidneys, spleen; crosses placenta. **Metabolism:** Extensively hepatically metabolized; undergoes some enterohepatic cycling. **Elimination:** Excreted chiefly in bile and feces; also excreted in breast milk. **Half-Life:** Biphasic, initial 2.5–10 days, terminal 40–55 days.

NURSING IMPLICATIONS

Assessment & Drug Effects

- Monitor BP carefully during infusion and slow the infusion if significant hypotension occurs; bradycardia should be treated by slowing the infusion or discontinuing if necessary. Monitor heart rate and rhythm and BP until drug response has stabilized; report promptly symptomatic bradycardia. Sustained monitoring is essential because drug has an unusually long half-life.

- Monitor for S&S of adverse effects, particularly conduction disturbances and exacerbation of arrhythmias, in patients receiving concomitant antiarrhythmic therapy (reduce dosage of previous agent by 30–50% several days after amiodarone therapy is started); drug-induced hypothyroidism or hyperthyroidism, especially during early treatment period; pulmonary toxicity (progressive dyspnea, fatigue, cough, pleuritic pain, fever) throughout therapy.

- Lab tests: Baseline and periodic assessments should be made of liver, lung, thyroid, neurologic, and GI function. Drug may cause thyroid function test abnormalities in the absence of thyroid function impairment.
- Monitor for elevations of AST and ALT. If elevations persist or if they are 2–3 times above normal baseline readings, reduce dosage or withdraw drug promptly to prevent hepatotoxicity and liver damage.
- Auscultate chest periodically or when patient complains of respiratory symptoms. Check for diminished breath sounds, rales, pleuritic friction rub; observe breathing pattern. Drug-induced pulmonary function problems must be distinguished from CHF or pneumonia. Keep physician informed.
- Anticipate possible CNS symptoms within a week after amiodarone therapy begins. Proximal muscle weakness, a common side effect, intensified by tremors presents a great hazard to the ambulating patient. Assess severity of symptoms. Supervision of ambulation may be indicated.

Patient & Family Education
- Check pulse daily once stabilized, or as prescribed. Report a pulse <60 and report falling pulse rate.
- Take oral drug consistently with respect to meals.
- Become familiar with potential adverse reactions and report those that are bothersome to the physician.
- Use dark glasses to ease photophobia; some patients may not be able to go outdoors in the daytime even with such protection.
- Follow recommendation for regular ophthalmic exams, including funduscopy and slit-lamp exam.
- Wear protective clothing and a barrier-type sunscreen that physically blocks penetration of skin by ultraviolet light (e.g., titanium oxide or zinc formulations) to prevent a photosensitivity reaction (erythema, pruritus); avoid exposure to sun and sunlamps.
- Do not breast feed while taking this drug without consulting physician.
- Store this medication out of reach of children.

AMITRIPTYLINE HYDROCHLORIDE
(a-mee-trip′ti-leen)
Amitril, Apo-Amitriptyline ◆, Elavil, Emitrip, Endep, Enovil, Levate ◆, Meravil, Novotriptyn ◆, SK-Amitriptyline
Classifications: CENTRAL NERVOUS SYSTEM AGENT; PSYCHOTHERAPEUTIC; TRICYCLIC ANTIDEPRESSANT
Prototype: Imipramine
Pregnancy Category: C

AVAILABILITY 10 mg, 25 mg, 50 mg, 75 mg, 100 mg, 150 mg tablets; 10 mg/mL injection

ACTIONS Among the most active of the tricyclic antidepressants (TCAs) in inhibition of serotonin uptake from synaptic gap; also inhibits norepinephrine reuptake to a moderate degree. Restoration of the levels of these neurotransmitters is a proposed mechanism of antidepressant action.

Common adverse effects in *italic;* life-threatening effects <u>underlined;</u> generic names in **bold;** drug classifications in SMALL CAPS; ◆ Canadian drug name; ⊙ Prototype drug.

101

THERAPEUTIC EFFECTS Interference with the reuptake of serotonin and norepinephrine results in the antidepressant activity of amitriptyline.

USES Endogenous depression.

UNLABELED USES Prophylaxis for cluster, migraine, and chronic tension headaches; intractable pain, peptic ulcer disease, to increase muscle strength in myotonic dystrophy, to treat pathologic weeping and laughing secondary to forebrain disease, for eating disorders associated with depression (anorexia or bulimia), and as sedative for nondepressed patients.

CONTRAINDICATIONS Acute recovery period after MI, history of seizure disorders, narrow-angle glaucoma, MAO inhibitor within last 14 days, pregnancy (category C), lactation, children <12 y.

CAUTIOUS USE History of urinary retention or obstruction; diabetes mellitus; hyperthyroidism; patient with cardiovascular, hepatic, or renal dysfunction; patient with suicidal tendency, electroshock therapy; elective surgery; schizophrenia; respiratory disorders; adolescents.

ROUTE & DOSAGE

Antidepressant

Adolescent: **PO** 25–50 mg/day in divided doses, may gradually increase to 100 mg/day (max 200 mg/day)
Adult: **PO** 40–100 mg/24 h, may gradually increase to 150–300 mg/24 h (use lower doses in outpatients) **IM** 20–30 mg q.i.d. until patient can take PO

STORAGE

Store drug at 15°–30° C (59°–86° F) and protect from light unless otherwise directed by manufacturer.

ADMINISTRATION

Oral

- Give with or immediately after food to reduce possibility of GI irritation. Tablet may be crushed if patient is unable to take it whole; administer with food or fluid.
- Give increased doses preferably in late afternoon or at bedtime due to sedative action that precedes antidepressant effect.
- Give as single dose at bedtime to promote sleep or for patients with dizziness or when daytime sedation interferes with work productivity.
- Note that dose is usually tapered over 2 wk at discontinuation to prevent withdrawal symptoms (headache, nausea, malaise, musculoskeletal pain, panic attack, weakness).

Intramuscular

- Reserve IM injections for patients unable or unwilling to take oral drug.
- Inject deep IM into a large muscle.

ADVERSE EFFECTS CNS: *Drowsiness, sedation, dizziness,* nervousness, restlessness, fatigue, headache, insomnia, abnormal movements (extrapyramidal symptoms), seizures. **CV:** *Orthostatic hypotension,* tachycardia, palpitation, ECG changes. **Special Senses:** Blurred vision, mydriasis. **GI:** *Dry mouth,* increased appetite especially for sweets, *constipation,* weight gain, sour or metallic taste, nausea, vomiting. **Urogenital:** *Urinary retention.* **Other:** (Rare) <u>Bone marrow depression</u>.

Common adverse effects in *italic;* life-threatening effects <u>underlined</u>; generic names in **bold;** drug classifications in SMALL CAPS; ♣ Canadian drug name; ♥ Prototype drug.

INTERACTIONS Drug: ANTIHYPERTENSIVES may decrease some antihypertensive response; CNS DEPRESSANTS, **alcohol,** HYPNOTICS, BARBITURATES, SEDATIVES potentiate CNS depression; ANTICOAGULANTS, ORAL, may increase hypoprothombinemic effect; **ethchlorvynol,** transient delirium; **levodopa,** SYMPATHOMIMETICS (e.g., **epinephrine, norepinephrine**), possibility of sympathetic hyperactivity with hypertension and hyperpyrexia; MAO INHIBITORS, possibility of severe reactions, toxic psychosis, cardiovascular instability; **methylphenidate** increases TCA levels; THYROID DRUGS may increase possibility of arrhythmias; **cimetidine** may increase plasma TCA levels. **Herbal: Ginkgo** may decrease seizure threshold, **St. John's wort** may cause serotonin syndrome.

PHARMACOKINETICS Absorption: Rapidly absorbed from GI and injection sites. **Peak:** 2–12 h. **Distribution:** Crosses placenta. **Metabolism:** Metabolized in liver to active metabolite. **Elimination:** Primarily excreted in urine; enters breast milk. **Half-Life:** 10–50 h.

NURSING IMPLICATIONS

Assessment & Drug Effects

- ***Therapeutic level*** is 100–250 ng/mL; obtain serum for sample after 4–5 days of treatment and 8 h after PO dose.
- Monitor therapeutic effectiveness. It may take 1–6 wk to reduce attacks when used for migraine prophylaxis, or at least 2 wk for antidepressant effect.
- Monitor for S&S of drowsiness and dizziness (initial stages of therapy); institute measures to prevent falling. Also monitor for overdose or suicide ideation in patients who use excessive amounts of alcohol.
- Antidepressants increase risk of suicidal thinking and behavior in children and adolescents with major depressive disorder, obsessive compulsive disorder, and other psychiatric disorders. Observe closely for worsening of condition, suicidality, and behavior changes. Instruct family and caregivers to monitor for these symptoms and discuss with prescriber. A MedGuide describing risks and stating whether the drug is approved for the child's/adolescent's condition should be provided for all families when antidepressants are prescribed.
- Lab tests: Baseline and periodic leukocyte and differential counts; renal and hepatic function tests; eye examinations (including glaucoma testing); recommended particularly for older adults, adolescents, and patients receiving high-doses/prolonged therapy. Monitor ECG, BP, and CBC at start of therapy and when changing doses. Have ECG changes monitored by cardiologist. Monitor BP and pulse rate more frequently in patients with preexisting cardiovascular disease. Assess for orthostatic hypotension. Withhold drug if there is a rise or fall in systolic BP (by 10–20 mm Hg), or a sudden increase or a significant change in pulse rate or rhythm. Notify physician.
- Monitor I&O, including bowel elimination pattern.

Patient & Family Education

- Monitor weight; drug may increase appetite or a craving for sweets.
- Understand that tolerance/adaptation to anticholinergic actions usually develops with maintenance regimen. Keep prescriber informed.
- Relieve dry mouth by taking frequent sips of water and increasing total fluid intake.

- Make position change slowly and in stages to prevent dizziness.
- Do not drive or engage in potentially hazardous activities until response to drug is known.
- Do not use OTC drugs without consulting prescriber while on TCA therapy; many preparations contain sympathomimetic amines.
- Note: Amitriptyline may turn urine blue-green.
- Do not breast feed while taking this drug.
- Store this medication out of reach of children because tablets are small and brightly colored and resemble candy.

AMMONIUM CHLORIDE
(ah-mo'ni-um)
Classifications: ELECTROLYTIC BALANCE AND WATER BALANCE AGENTS
Pregnancy Category: B

AVAILABILITY 26.75% or 5 mEq/mL solution; 500 mg tablets; 486 mg enteric-coated tablets

ACTIONS Acidifying property is due to conversion of ammonium ion (NH^{4+}) to urea in liver with liberation of H^+ and Cl^-. Potassium excretion also increases acid, but to a lesser extent. Tolerance to diuretic effect occurs within 2–3 days.
THERAPEUTIC EFFECTS Systemic acidifier in metabolic alkalosis by releasing H^+ ions which lower pH.

USES Treatment of hypochloremic states and metabolic alkalosis. Diuretic or urinary acidifying agent.

CONTRAINDICATIONS Severe renal or hepatic insufficiency; primary respiratory acidosis. Safety during pregnancy (category B) or lactation is not established.
CAUTIOUS USE Cardiac edema, pulmonary insufficiency, infancy.

ROUTE & DOSAGE

Urine Acidifier, Diuretic
Child: **PO** 75 mg/kg/day divided into 4 doses
(max 6 g/24 h)
Adult: **PO** 4–12 g/day divided into doses given q4–6h

Metabolic Alkalosis and Hypochloremic States
Child/Adult: **IV** Dose calculated on basis of CO_2 combining power or serum Cl deficit, 50% of calculated deficit is administered slowly (not to exceed 50 mg/kg/h or 1 mEq/kg/h)

STORAGE
Store in airtight container.

ADMINISTRATION

Oral
- Give after meals for best tolerance or use enteric-coated tablets. Tablets should be swallowed whole.

Intravenous

Check with physician for slower rate for infants.

***PREPARE* Intermittent:** Dilute each 20-mL vial in 500 mL NS. Do not exceed a concentration of 1–2%.

***ADMINISTER* Intermittent:** Give slowly to avoid serious adverse effects (ammonia toxicity) and local irritation and pain. Give at a rate not to exceed 5 mL/min or 50 mg/kg/h.

***INCOMPATIBILITIES* Solution/Additive: Codeine phosphate, levorphanol, methadone, nitrofurantoin, warfarin.**

- Avoid freezing. ▪ Concentrated solutions crystallize at low temperatures. ▪ Crystals can be dissolved by placing intact container in a warm water bath and warming to room temperature.

ADVERSE EFFECTS Body as a Whole: Most secondary to ammonia toxicity. **CNS:** Headache, depression, drowsiness, twitching, excitability; EEG abnormalities. **CV:** Bradycardia and other arrhythmias. **GI:** Gastric irritation, nausea, vomiting, anorexia. **Metabolic:** Metabolic acidosis, hyperammonia. **Respiratory:** Hyperventilation. **Skin:** Rash. **Urogenital:** Glycosuria **Other:** Pain and irritation at IV site.

DIAGNOSTIC TEST INTERFERENCE Ammonia chloride may increase ***blood ammonia*** and ***AST,*** decrease ***serum magnesium*** (by increasing urinary magnesium excretion), and decrease urine ***urobilinogen.***

INTERACTIONS Drug: Aminosalicylic acid may cause crystalluria; increases urinary excretion of AMPHETAMINES, **flecainide, mexiletine, methadone, ephedrine, pseudoephedrine;** decreased urinary excretion of SULFONYLUREAS, SALICYLATES.

PHARMACOKINETICS Absorption: Completely absorbed in 3–6 h. **Metabolism:** Metabolized in liver to HCl and urea. **Elimination:** Primarily excreted in urine.

NURSING IMPLICATIONS

Assessment & Drug Effects

- Assess IV infusion site frequently for signs of irritation. Change site as needed.
- Monitor for S&S of metabolic acidosis (mental status changes including confusion, disorientation, coma, respiratory changes including increased respiratory rate and depth, exertional dyspnea); ammonium toxicity (cardiac arrhythmias including bradycardia, irregular respirations, twitching, seizures).
- Monitor I&O ratio and pattern. The diuretic effect of ammonium chloride is compensatory and lasts only 1–2 days.
- Lab tests: Baseline and periodic determinations of CO_2 combining power, serum electrolytes, and urinary and arterial pH during therapy to avoid serious acidosis.

Patient & Family Education

- Report pain at IV injection site.
- Do not breast feed while taking this drug without consulting physician.
- Store this medication out of reach of children.

AMOXICILLIN

(a-mox-i-sill'in)

Amoxil, Apo-Amoxi ♣, Larotid, Novamoxin, Polymox, Sumox, Trimox, Utimox, Wymox

Classifications: ANTI-INFECTIVE; ANTIBIOTIC; AMINOPENICILLIN
Prototype: Ampicillin
Pregnancy Category: B

AVAILABILITY 125 mg, 250 mg, 500 mg, 875 mg tablets; 250 mg, 500 mg capsules; 50 mg/mL, 125 mg/5 mL, 250 mg/5 mL powder for suspension

ACTIONS Broad-spectrum, acid stable, semisynthetic aminopenicillin and analog of ampicillin. Acts by inhibiting mucoprotein synthesis in cell wall of rapidly multiplying bacteria. It is bactericidal and is inactivated by penicillinase.
THERAPEUTIC EFFECTS Active against both aerobic gram-positive and aerobic gram-negative bacteria including *Enterococcus faecalis, Streptococcus pneumoniae, Escherichia coli, Haemophilus influenzae, Helicobacter pylori.*

USES Infections of ear, nose, throat, GU tract, skin, and soft tissue caused by susceptible bacteria. Also used in uncomplicated gonorrhea. Available in combination with potassium clavulanate, which extends antibacterial spectrum of amoxicillin to include beta-lactamase-producing strains.

CONTRAINDICATIONS Hypersensitivity to penicillins; infectious mononucleosis.
CAUTIOUS USE History of or suspected atopy or allergy (hives, eczema, hay fever, asthma); severely impaired renal function; history of cephalosporin allergy; pregnancy (category B) or lactation.

ROUTE & DOSAGE

Mild to Moderate Infections

Child: **PO** 25–50 mg/kg/day (max 60–80 mg/kg/day) divided into doses given q8h *or* 200–400 mg q12h
Adult: **PO** 250–500 mg q8h

Otitis Media

(Due to resistant strains of *S. pneumoniae*) 80–90 mg/kg/day divided into doses b.i.d. (max 875 mg b.i.d.)

Endocarditis Prophylaxis

50 mg/kg × 1 dose 1 h prior to procedure (max 2 g)

Gonorrhea

Child: **PO** ≥2 y, 50 mg/kg as single dose with probenecid 25 mg/kg
Adult: **PO** 3 g as single dose with 1 g probenecid

Postexposure Inhalational Anthrax

45 mg/kg/day divided into doses given t.i.d. (max 1500 mg/day)

Common adverse effects in *italic;* life-threatening effects underlined; generic names in **bold;** drug classifications in SMALL CAPS; ♣ Canadian drug name; ❷ Prototype drug.

STORAGE

Store in tightly covered containers at 15°–30° C (59°–86° F) unless otherwise directed. Reconstituted oral suspensions are stable for 7 day at room temperature.

ADMINISTRATION

Oral

- Ensure that chewable tablets are chewed or crushed before being swallowed with a liquid.
- Place reconstituted pediatric solution directly into child's mouth or add to a small amount of food or fluid (see Part I). Have child take all of the dose promptly.

ADVERSE EFFECTS Body as a Whole: As with other penicillins. Hypersensitivity (rash, <u>anaphylaxis</u>), superinfections. **GI:** Diarrhea, nausea, vomiting, <u>pseudomembranous colitis</u> (rare). **Hematologic:** Hemolytic anemia, eosinophilia, <u>agranulocytosis</u> (rare). **Skin:** Pruritus, urticaria, or other skin eruptions. **Special Senses:** Conjunctival ecchymosis.

INTERACTIONS TETRACYCLINES may inhibit activity of amoxicillin; **probenecid** prolongs the activity of amoxicillin.

PHARMACOKINETICS Absorption: Rapid and nearly complete absorption. **Peak:** 1–2 h. **Distribution:** Diffuses into most tissues and body fluids, except synovial fluid and CSF (unless meninges are inflamed); crosses placenta; distributed into breast milk in small amounts. **Metabolism:** Metabolized in liver. **Elimination:** 60% of dose excreted in urine in 6–8 h. **Half-Life:** 1–1.3 h.

NURSING IMPLICATIONS

Assessment & Drug Effects

- Determine previous hypersensitivity reactions to penicillins, cephalosporins, and other allergens prior to therapy.
- Lab tests: Baseline C&S tests prior to initiation of therapy, start drug pending results; periodic assessments of renal, hepatic, and hematologic functions should be made during prolonged therapy.
- Monitor for S&S of an urticarial rash (usually occurring within a few days after start of drug) suggestive of a hypersensitivity reaction. If it occurs, look for other signs of hypersensitivity (fever, wheezing, generalized itching, dyspnea), and report to physician immediately.
- Report onset of generalized, erythematous, maculopapular rash (ampicillin rash) to physician. Ampicillin rash is not due to hypersensitivity; however, hypersensitivity should be ruled out.
- Closely monitor diarrhea to rule out pseudomembranous colitis.

Patient & Family Education

- Take drug around the clock, do not miss a dose, and continue therapy until all medication is taken, unless otherwise directed by prescriber.
- Encourage generous amount of fluid intake for age.
- Report onset of diarrhea and other possible symptoms of superinfection to physician (see Appendix D-1).
- Do not breast feed while taking this drug without consulting prescriber.
- Store this medication out of reach of children.

AMOXICILLIN AND CLAVULANATE POTASSIUM
(a-mox-i-sill'in)
Augmentin, Augmentin-ES600 Clavulin ✚
Classifications: ANTI-INFECTIVE; BETA-LACTAM ANTIBIOTIC; AMINOPENICILLIN
Prototype: Ampicillin
Pregnancy Category: B

AVAILABILITY 250 mg, 500 mg, 875 mg tablets; 125 mg, 200 mg, 400 mg chewable tablets; 125 mg/5 mL, 200 mg/5 mL, 250 mg/5 mL, 400 mg/5 mL, 600 mg/5 mL oral suspension

ACTIONS Used alone, clavulanic acid antibacterial activity is weak. In combination, it inhibits enzyme (beta-lactamase) degradation of amoxicillin and by synergism extends both spectrum of activity and bactericidal effect of amoxicillin against many strains of beta-lactamase-producing bacteria resistant to amoxicillin alone.
THERAPEUTIC EFFECTS Semisynthetic broad-spectrum antibiotic with fixed combination of amoxicillin, an aminopenicillin, and the potassium salt to clavulanic acid, a competitive beta-lactamase inhibitor. Active against gram-positive bacteria including *Staphylococcus aureus, Streptococcus pneumoniae, Clostridium, Peptococcus, Bacteroides fragilis* group, and many gram-negative organisms including *Branhamella catarrhalis* (formerly *Neisseria catarrhalis*), *Haemophilus influenzae, Proteus mirabilis; Salmonella, Shigella,* and *Klebsiella sp.* Generally inactive against *Pseudomonas.*

USES Infections caused by susceptible beta-lactamase-producing organisms: lower respiratory tract infections, otitis media, sinusitis, skin and skin structure infections, and UTI.

CONTRAINDICATIONS Combination shares toxic potential of ampicillin. Hypersensitivity to penicillins; infectious mononucleosis.
CAUTIOUS USE Pregnancy (category B), lactation.

ROUTE & DOSAGE

Mild to Moderate Infections
Neonate/Infant: **PO** *<3 mo*, 30 mg/kg/day (amoxicillin) divided into doses given q12h
Child: **PO** *<40 kg*, 20–40 mg/kg/day (based on amoxicillin component) divided into doses q8–12h; *>3 mo*, 90 mg/kg of 600 mg/5 mL ES divided into doses given q12h × 10 day (max 2 g/24 h)
Adult: **PO** 250 or 500 mg tablet (each with 125 mg clavulanic acid) q8–12h or 875 mg tablet b.i.d.

STORAGE
Store tablets in tight containers at <24° C (71° F). Reconstituted oral suspension should be refrigerated at 2°–8° C (36°–46° F), then discarded after 10 days

Common adverse effects in *italic;* life-threatening effects <u>underlined;</u> generic names in **bold;** drug classifications in SMALL CAPS; ✚ Canadian drug name; ◑ Prototype drug.

108

ADMINISTRATION

Oral

- Give at start of a meal to minimize GI upset and enhance absorption.
- Note that both 250- and 500-mg tablets contain the exact amount of clavulanic acid (125 mg and potassium salt); therefore, two 250-mg tablets are not equivalent to one 500-mg tablet.
- Reconstitute oral suspension by adding amount of water specified on container to provide a 5-mL suspension. Tap bottle before adding water to loosen powder, then add water in 2 portions, agitating suspension well before each addition.
- Agitate suspension well just before administration of each dose.
- Give dialysis patient an additional 2 doses on the day of dialysis; one dose before and another dose after dialysis.

ADVERSE EFFECTS GI: *Diarrhea,* nausea, vomiting. **Skin:** Rash, urticaria. **Other:** Candidal vaginitis; moderate increases in serum ALT, AST; glomerulonephritis; <u>agranulocytosis</u> (rare).

DIAGNOSTIC TEST INTERFERENCE May interfere with **urinary glucose** determinations using **cupric sulfate, Benedict's solution, Clinitest;** does not affect glucose oxidase methods (e.g., **Clinistix, TesTape**). Positive direct **antiglobulin (Coombs')** test results may be reported, a reaction that could interfere with **hematologic studies** or with **transfusion cross-matching** procedures.

INTERACTIONS Drug: Tetracyclines may inhibit activity of amoxicillin; **probenecid** prolongs the activity of amoxicillin.

PHARMACOKINETICS Absorption: Rapid and nearly complete absorption. **Peak:** 1–2 h. **Distribution:** Diffuses into most tissues and body fluids, except synovial fluid and CSF (unless meninges are inflamed); crosses placenta; distributed into breast milk in very small amounts. **Metabolism:** Metabolized in liver. **Elimination:** 50–73% of the amoxicillin and 25–45% of the clavulanate dose excreted in urine in 2 h. **Half-Life:** Amoxicillin 1–1.3 h, clavulanate 0.78–1.2 h.

NURSING IMPLICATIONS

Assessment & Drug Effects

- Determine previous hypersensitivity reactions to penicillins, cephalosporins, and other allergens prior to therapy.
- Lab tests: Baseline C&S tests prior to initiation of therapy; start drug pending results.
- Monitor for S&S of an urticarial rash (usually occurring within a few days after start of drug) suggestive of a hypersensitivity reaction. If it occurs, look for other signs of hypersensitivity (fever, wheezing, generalized itching, dyspnea), and report to prescriber immediately.
- Note: Generalized, erythematous, maculopapular rash (ampicillin rash) is not due to hypersensitivity. It is usually mild, but can be severe. Report onset of rash to prescriber, since hypersensitivity should be ruled out.

Patient & Family Education

- Female patients should report onset of symptoms of *Candida vaginitis* (e.g., moderate amount of white, cheesy, nonodorous vaginal

discharge; vaginal inflammation and itching; vulvar excoriation, inflammation, burning, itching). Therapy may have to be discontinued.
- Encourage generous amount of fluid intake for age.
- Note: Use Clinistix or TesTape when monitoring urinary glucose to avoid false readings with diabetes mellitus.
- Do not breast feed while taking this drug without consulting prescriber.
- Store this medication out of reach of children.

AMPHETAMINE SULFATE ⊕
(am-fet′a-meen)
Racemic Amphetamine Sulfate, Adderall, Adderall XR
Classifications: CENTRAL NERVOUS SYSTEM AGENT; CEREBRAL STIMULANT; ANOREXIANT
Pregnancy Category: C
Controlled Substance: Schedule II

AVAILABILITY 5 mg, 10 mg tablets; **Adderall** 5 mg, 10 mg, 20 mg, 30 mg tablets; 5 mg, 15 mg, 20 mg, 25 mg, 30 mg sustained-release capsules

ACTIONS Indirect-acting synthetic sympathomimetic amine with peripheral alpha- and beta-adrenergic activity. Marked stimulant effect on CNS thought to be due to action on cerebral cortex and possibly the reticular activating system. Acts indirectly on adrenergic receptors by increasing synaptic release of norepinephrine and dopamine in brain and by blocking reuptake at presynaptic membranes.

THERAPEUTIC EFFECTS CNS stimulation results in increased motor activity, diminished sense of fatigue, alertness, wakefulness, and mood elevation. In hyperkinetic children, it exerts a paradoxic sedative effect by unclear mechanism. Anorexigenic effect thought to result from direct inhibition of hypothalamic appetite center, as well as mood elevation.

USES Narcolepsy, attention deficit disorder in children (hyperkinetic behavioral syndrome, minimal brain dysfunction). Use as short-term adjunct to control exogenous obesity not generally recommended because of its potential for abuse.

UNLABELED USES In combination with other drugs for treatment-resistant depression.

CONTRAINDICATIONS Hypersensitivity to sympathomimetic amines; history of drug abuse; severe agitation; hyperthyroidism; diabetes mellitus; moderate to severe hypertension, advanced arteriosclerosis, angina pectoris or other cardiovascular disorders; Gilles de la Tourette disorder; glaucoma; during or within 14 days after treatment with MAOIs. Safety during pregnancy (category C) or lactation is not established.

CAUTIOUS USE Mild hypertension.

ROUTE & DOSAGE

Narcolepsy
Child: **PO** >12y, 10 mg/day, may increase by 10 mg at weekly intervals; 6–12 y, 5 mg/day, may increase by 5 mg at weekly intervals

Common adverse effects in *italic;* life-threatening effects <u>underlined;</u> generic names in **bold;** drug classifications in SMALL CAPS; ◆ Canadian drug name; ⊕ Prototype drug.

Adult: **PO** 5–60 mg/day divided q4–6h into 2–3 doses

Attention Deficit Disorder

Child: **PO** 6 y, 5 mg 1–2 times/day, may increase by 5 mg at weekly intervals (max 40 mg/day); *3–5 y,* 2.5 mg 1–2 times/day, may increase by 2.5 mg at weekly intervals; 10 mg extended release once daily in a.m.; may increase by 5–10 mg at weekly intervals if needed to max 30 mg/day

Adolescent/Adult: **PO** 10 mg extended release once daily in a.m.; may increase by 5–10 mg at weekly intervals if needed to max 30 mg/day

Obesity

Adult: **PO** 5–10 mg 1 h before meals

STORAGE

Store at 15°–30° C (59°–86° F) unless otherwise directed.

ADMINISTRATION

Oral

- Give first dose on awakening or early in a.m. when prescribed for narcolepsy.
- Give last dose no later than 6 h before patient retires to avoid insomnia.
- Ensure that sustained-release capsules are not crushed or chewed.
- Give drug on an empty stomach 30–60 min before meal to suppress appetite when prescribed for obesity.

ADVERSE EFFECTS Body as a Whole: Allergy, urticaria. **CNS:** *Irritability,* psychosis, *restlessness,* nervousness, headache, *insomnia* weakness, *euphoria,* dysphoria, drowsiness, trembling hyperactive reflexes. **CV:** *Palpitation,* elevated BP; tachycardia, vasculitis. **Urogenital:** Impotence and change in libido with high doses. **GI:** Dry mouth, anorexia, weight loss, nausea, vomiting, diarrhea, or constipation.

DIAGNOSTIC TEST INTERFERENCE Elevations in *serum thyroxine (T_4)* levels with high amphetamine doses.

INTERACTIONS Drug: Acetazolamide, sodium bicarbonate decrease amphetamine elimination; **ammonium chloride, ascorbic acid** increase amphetamine elimination; effects of both amphetamine and BARBITURATE may be antagonized if given together; **furazolidone** may increase BP effects of amphetamines, and interaction may persist for several weeks after furazolidone is discontinued; **guanethidine, guanadryl** antagonize antihypertensive effects; because MAO INHIBITORS, **selegiline** can precipitate hypertensive crisis (fatalities reported), do not administer amphetamines during or within 14 days of these drugs; PHENOTHIAZINES may inhibit mood elevating effects of amphetamines; TRICYCLIC ANTIDEPRESSANTS enhance amphetamine effects through increased **norepinephrine** release; BETA AGONISTS increase cardiovascular adverse effects.

PHARMACOKINETICS Absorption: Rapid. Peak effect: 1–5 h. **Duration:** Up to 10 h. **Distribution:** All tissues, especially CNS. **Metabolism:** Metabolized in liver. **Elimination:** Renal elimination; excreted into breast milk. **Half-Life:** 10–30 h.

NURSING IMPLICATIONS

Assessment & Drug Effects

- Monitor for therapeutic effectiveness. Tolerance to the mood elevating effects commonly occurs within a few weeks. Drug is usually discontinued when tolerance develops. Generally, tolerance does not occur when used for attention deficit disorder or narcolepsy.
- Monitor for S&S of toxicity in children. Response to this drug is more variable in children than adults; acute toxicity has occurred over a wide range of dosage.
- Monitor for S&S of insomnia or anorexia. Report complaints to prescriber. Dosage reduction may be required.
- Monitor diabetics closely for loss of glycemic control.
- Monitor growth in children; drug may be discontinued periodically to allow for catch up to normal growth.
- Note: Drug's excitatory and euphoric effects are associated with a high abuse potential.

Patient & Family Education

- Keep prescriber informed of clinical response and persistent or bothersome adverse effects. This drug exerts a stimulating effect that masks fatigue; after exhilaration disappears, fatigue and depression are usually greater than before, and a longer period of rest is needed.
- Report insomnia or undesired weight loss.
- Take dose early in day and do not take after noon.
- Do not drive or engage in potentially hazardous tasks until response to drug is known.
- Rinse mouth frequently with clear water, especially after eating, to relieve mouth dryness; increase fluid intake, if allowed; chew sugarless gum or sourballs.
- Note: Meticulous oral hygiene is required because decreased saliva encourages demineralization of tooth surfaces and mucosal erosion. Use of a commercially available oral lubricant, such as Moi-Stir or Xero-Lube, can relieve soft tissue problems and reduce the potential of tooth decay.
- Note: Appetite suppression usually lessens within a few weeks and appetite increases; dose increase is not indicated.
- Avoid caffeine-containing beverages because caffeine increases amphetamine effects.
- Note that drug is usually tapered gradually following prolonged administration of high doses. Abrupt withdrawal may result in lethargy, profound depression, or other psychotic manifestations that may persist for several weeks.
- Drug has high abuse potential so keep locked and be sure it is taken only by intended patient.
- Do not breast feed while taking this drug without consulting prescriber.
- Store this medication in locked area out of reach of children; this is a Scheduled II drug.

Common adverse effects in *italic*; life-threatening effects <u>underlined</u>; generic names in **bold**; drug classifications in SMALL CAPS; ✦ Canadian drug name; ☻ Prototype drug.

AMPHOTERICIN B ⊖Ⓟ

(am-foe-ter'i-sin)
Amphocin, Fungizone

AMPHOTERICIN B LIPID-BASED

Abelcet, Amphotec, AmBisome
Classifications: ANTI-INFECTIVE; ANTIFUNGAL ANTIBIOTIC
Pregnancy Category: B

AVAILABILITY Abelcet 100 mg/20 mL suspension for injection **Amphotec** 50 mg, 100 mg powder for injection **AmBisome** 50 mg powder for injection **Fungizone** 50 mg powder for injection; 100 mg/mL suspension; 3% cream, lotion, ointment

ACTIONS Fungistatic antibiotic produced by *Streptomyces nodosus*. Fungicidal at higher concentrations, depending on sensitivity of fungus. **THERAPEUTIC EFFECTS** Exerts antifungal action on both resting and growing cells at least in part by selectively binding to sterols in fungus cell membrane.

USES Used intravenously for a wide spectrum of potentially fatal systemic fungal (mycotic) infections including *aspergillosis, blastomycosis, coccidioidomycosis, cryptococcosis, disseminated candidiasis, histoplasmosis, paracoccidioidomycosis, sporotrichosis,* and others. Has been used to potentiate antifungal effects of flucytosine (*Ancobon*) and to provide anticandidal prophylaxis in certain susceptible patients receiving immunosuppressive therapy. Used topically for cutaneous and mucocutaneous infections caused by *Candida* (monilia). *Abelcet:* aspergillosis.
UNLABELED USES Treatment of candiduria, fungal endocarditis, meningitis, septicemia; fungal infections of urinary bladder and urinary tract; amebic meningoencephalitis, and paracoccidioidomycosis.

CONTRAINDICATIONS Hypersensitivity to amphotericin.
CAUTIOUS USE Severe bone marrow depression or renal function impairment. Safety during pregnancy (category B) or lactation is not established.

ROUTE & DOSAGE

Systemic Infections [Amphocin, Fungizone]

Child: **IV Test Dose** 0.1 mg/kg up to 1 mg dissolved in 20 mL of D5W by slow infusion (over 10–30 min) **IV Maintenance Dose** 0.4 mg/kg/day infused over 4–6 h, may increase by 0.25 mg/kg/day to target dose of 0.25–1 mg/kg/day infused over 2–6 h
Adult: **IV Test Dose** 0.1 mg/kg up to max of 1 mg dissolved in 20 mL of D5W by slow infusion (over 10–30 min) **IV Maintenance Dose** 0.25–0.5 mg/kg/day infused over 4–6 h, may gradually increase by 0.5–0.75 mg/kg/day up to 1–1.5 mg/kg/day

[Abelcet]

Child/Adult: **IV** 3–5 mg/kg/day infused at 2.5 mg/kg/h

[Amphotec]

Child/Adult: **IV Test Dose** 10 mL (1.6–8.3 mg) of initial dose infused over 10–30 min **IV Maintenance Dose** 3–4 mg/kg/day (max 7.5 mg/kg/day) infused at 1 mg/kg/h

[AmBisome]

Child/Adult: **IV** 3–5 mg/kg/day infused over 1–2 h

Cryptococcal Meningitis in HIV [AmBisome]

Adult: **IV** 6 mg/kg/day infused over 2 h

Candiduria [Amphocin, Fungizone]

Adult: **Irrigation** 5–50 mg/1000 mL sterile water instilled continuously into the bladder via a 3-way closed drainage catheter system at a rate of 1000 mL/24 h

Oral Candidiasis [Fungizone]

Child/Adult: **PO** 100 mg swish & swallow q.i.d.

Cutaneous Candidiasis [Fungizone]

Infant/Child/Adult: **Topical** Apply to lesions 2–4 times/day for 1–4 wk

---

STORAGE
- Store topical forms in well-closed containers at room temperature, 15°–30° C (59°–86° F), unless otherwise directed.
- Store powder for injection at 2°–8° C (35°–46° F). Protect from light.
- Many preparations are available, so check manufacturer's directions carefully for specific product storage.

ADMINISTRATION

Oral
- Instruct patient not to swallow drug immediately, but swish carefully to coat lesions.

Topical Application
- Do not cover with plastic wrap, plastic cloth, rubber, or other occlusive dressings. Ask prescriber to specify when and how lesions are to be washed.
- Discontinue topical treatment promptly if signs of hypersensitivity, irritation, or worsening of lesions occurs.

Intravenous

PREPARE: Each brand of amphotericin is prepared differently according to manufacturer's directions. Refer to specific manufacturer's guidelines for preparation of IV solutions. Read medicine labels and package inserts carefully to identify particular product used and recommendations for dosing and preparation.
***ADMINISTER* Abelcet Intermittent:** Flush existing IV line with D5W before infusion. ▪ Use 5-micron in-line filter. Infuse total daily dose at

2.5 mg/kg/h. ▪ Shake IV bag at least q2h to evenly mix solution.
Amphotec Intermittent: Do not use an in-line filter. ▪ Infuse total daily dose at 1 mg/kg/h. Infusion time may be shortened but should never be <2 h. Infusion time may also be extended for better tolerance.
AmBisome Intermittent: Do not use an in-line filter. ▪ Infuse total daily dose over 2 h. Infusion time may be shortened but should never be <1 h.
Fungizone Intermittent: Use a 1-micron filter. Infuse total daily dose over 2–6 h. Use longer infusion time for better tolerance. ▪ Alert: Rapid infusion of any amphotericin can cause cardiovascular collapse. If hypotension or arrhythmias develop, interrupt infusion and notify physician. ▪ Protect IV solution from light during administration. ▪ Note incompatibilities. ▪ When given through an existing IV line, flush before and after with D5W. ▪ Initiate therapy using the most distal vein possible and alternate sites with each dose if possible to reduce the risk of thrombophlebitis. ▪ Check IV site frequently for patency.

INCOMPATIBILITIES **Solution/Additive:** Any **saline**-containing solution (precipitate will form), PARENTERAL NUTRITION SOLUTIONS, **calcium chloride, calcium gluconate, cimetidine, edetate calcium disodium, metaraminol, methyldopa, polymyxin, potassium chloride, ranitidine, verapamil. Y-Site:** AMINOGLYCOSIDES, PENICILLINS, PHENOTHIAZINES, **clindamycin, cotrimoxazole, diphenhydramine, dobutamine, dopamine, heparin** (flush lines with D5W, not NS), **lidocaine, procaine, tetracycline, fluconazole, vitamins, TPN.**
▪ Do not mix Abelcet or Amphotec with any other drugs.

ADVERSE EFFECTS Body as a Whole: *Hypersensitivity* (pruritus, urticaria, skin rashes, fever, dyspnea, <u>anaphylaxis</u>); *fever, chills.* **CNS:** Headache, sedation, muscle pain, arthralgia, weakness. **CV:** Hypotension, <u>cardiac arrest</u>. **Special Senses:** Ototoxicity with tinnitus, vertigo, loss of hearing. **GI:** Nausea, vomiting, diarrhea, epigastric cramps, anorexia, weight loss. **Hematologic:** Anemia, thrombocytopenia. **Metabolic:** *Hypokalemia, hypomagnesemia.* **Urogenital:** <u>Nephrotoxicity</u>, urine with low specific gravity. **Skin:** Dry, erythema, pruritus, burning sensation; allergic contact dermatitis, exacerbation of lesions. **Other:** Pain; arthralgias, thrombophlebitis (IV site), superinfections.

INTERACTIONS Drug: AMINOGLYCOSIDES, **capreomycin, cisplatin, carboplatin, colistin, cyclosporine, furosemide, mechlorethamine, vancomycin** increase the possibility of nephrotoxicity; CORTICOSTEROIDS potentiate hypokalemia; with DIGITALIS GLYCOSIDES, hypokalemia increases the risk of **digitalis** toxicity.

PHARMACOKINETICS Peak effect: 1–2 h after IV infusion. **Duration:** 20 h. **Distribution:** Minimal amounts enter CNS, eye, bile, pleural, pericardial, synovial, or amniotic fluids; similar plasma and urine concentrations. **Elimination:** Excreted renally; can be detected in blood up to 4 wk and in urine for 4–8 wk after discontinuing therapy. **Half-Life:** 24–48 h.

NURSING IMPLICATIONS

Assessment & Drug Effects

- Lab tests: Baseline C&S tests prior to initiation of therapy; start drug pending results. Baseline and periodic BUN, serum creatinine, creatinine clearance; during therapy periodic CBC, serum electrolytes (especially K^+, Mg^{2+}, Na^+, Ca^{2+}), and liver function tests.
- Monitor for S&S of local inflammatory reaction or thrombosis at injection site, particularly if extravasation occurs.
- May premedicate with acetaminophen and diphenhydramine 30 min prior to the start of infusion to minimize chance of infusion reaction.
- Monitor cardiovascular and respiratory status and observe patient closely for adverse effects during initial IV therapy. If a test dose (1 mg over 20–30 min) is given, monitor vital signs every 30 min for at least 4 h. Febrile reactions (fever, chills, headache, nausea) occur in 20–90% of patients, usually 1–2 h after beginning infusion, and subside within 4 h after drug is discontinued. The severity of this reaction usually decreases with continued therapy. Keep physician informed.
- Monitor I&O and weight. Report immediately oliguria, any change in I&O ratio and pattern, or appearance of urine (e.g., sediment, pink or cloudy urine [hematuria]), abnormal renal function tests, unusual weight gain or loss. Generally, renal damage is reversible if drug is discontinued when first signs of renal dysfunction appear.
- Report to prescriber and withhold drug, if BUN exceeds 40 mg/dL or serum creatinine rises above 3 mg/dL. Dosage should be reduced or drug discontinued until renal function improves.
- Consult prescriber about the appearance of mild erythema surrounding topical application to skin lesions. This may be an indication to reduce frequency of topical application.
- Consult prescriber for guidelines on adequate hydration and adjustment of daily dose as a possible means of avoiding or minimizing nephrotoxicity.
- Report promptly any evidence of hearing loss or complaints of tinnitus, vertigo, or unsteady gait. Tinnitus may not be a complaint in the very young. Other signs of ototoxicity (i.e., vertigo or hearing loss) are more reliable indicators of ototoxicity in this age group. Also ask parents if they notice symptoms of hearing loss.

Patient & Family Education

- Notify physician if improvement does not occur within 1–2 wk or if lesions appear to worsen. Nail infections usually require several months or longer to improve.
- Wash towels and clothing that were in contact with affected areas after each treatment.
- Note: Topical cream slightly discolors the skin. Generally, lotion and ointment do not stain skin when rubbed in, but nail lesions may be stained.
- Do not breast feed while taking this drug without consulting physician.
- Store this medication out of reach of children.

Common adverse effects in *italic;* life-threatening effects <u>underlined</u>; generic names in **bold**; drug classifications in SMALL CAPS; ♣ Canadian drug name; ❂ Prototype drug.

AMPICILLIN ⊕

(am-pi-sill'in)

Amcill, Ampicin, Novo-Ampicillin ♣, Omnipen, Penbritin ♣, Pfizerpen-A, Polycillin, Principen, SK-Ampicillin, Totacillin

AMPICILLIN SODIUM

Ampicin ♣, Omnipen-N, Penbritin ♣, Polycillin-N, SK-Ampicillin-N, Totacillin-N

Classifications: ANTI-INFECTIVE; ANTIBIOTIC; AMINOPENICILLIN
Pregnancy Category: B

AVAILABILITY 250 mg, 500 mg capsules; 125 mg/5 mL, 250 mg/5 mL oral suspension; 125 mg, 250 mg, 500 mg, 1 g, 2 g vials

ACTIONS A broad-spectrum semisynthetic aminopenicillin; is highly bactericidal even at low concentrations, but is inactivated by penicillinase (beta-lactamase).

THERAPEUTIC EFFECTS Active against gram-positive microorganisms such as *alpha-* and *beta-Hemolytic streptococci, Diplococcus pneumoniae,* non-penicillinase-producing *Staphylococci,* and *Listeria.* Major advantage over penicillin G is enhanced action against most strains of *Enterococci* and several gram-negative strains including *Escherichia coli, Neisseria gonorrhoeae, N. meningitidis, Haemophilus influenzae, Proteus mirabilis, Salmonella* (including typhosa), and *Shigella.* Inactive against *Mycoplasma,* rickettsiae, fungi, and viruses.

USES Infections of GU, respiratory, and GI tracts and skin and soft tissues; also gonococcal infections, bacterial meningitis, otitis media, sinusitis, and septicemia and for prophylaxis of bacterial endocarditis. Used parenterally only for moderately severe to severe infections.

CONTRAINDICATIONS Hypersensitivity to penicillin derivatives; infectious mononucleosis.

CAUTIOUS USE History of severe reactions to cephalosporins; pregnancy (category B) or lactation.

ROUTE & DOSAGE

Systemic Infections

Neonate: **IV/IM** ≤7 *day & ≤2000 g,* 50–100 mg/kg/day divided into doses q12h; ≤7 *day & >2000 g,* 75 mg/kg/day divided into doses q8h; >7 *days,* 50–200 mg/kg/day divided into doses q6–12h
Child: **PO** 25–50 mg/kg/day divided into doses q6h **IV/IM** 25–100 mg/kg/day divided into doses q6h
Adult: **PO** 250–500 mg q6h **IV/IM** 250 mg–2 g q6h

Meningitis

Neonate: **IV/IM** ≤7 *days & <2000 g,* 100 mg/kg/day divided into doses q12h; ≤7 *days & >2000 g,* 150 mg/kg/day divided into doses q8h; >7 *days,* 100–200 mg/kg/day divided into doses q6–12h

---

Child/Adult: **IV** 150–200 mg/kg/day divided into doses q4–6h

Gonorrhea

Adult: **PO** 3.5 g with 1 g probenecid times 1 **IV/IM** 500 mg q8–12h

STORAGE

Store capsules and unopened vials at 15°–30° C (59°–86° F) unless otherwise directed. Keep oral preparations tightly covered.

ADMINISTRATION

Oral

- Give with a full glass of water or generous amount of water for age on an empty stomach (at least 1 h before or 2 h after meals) for maximum absorption. Food hampers rate and extent of oral absorption.

Intramuscular

- Reconstitute each vial by adding the indicated amount of sterile water for injection or bacteriostatic water for injection (1.2 mL to 125 mg; 1 mL to 250 mg; 1.8 mL to 500 mg; 3.5 mL to 1 g; 6.8 mL to 2 g). All reconstituted vials yield 250 mg/mL except the 125-mg vial, which yields 125 mg/mL. Administer within 1 h of preparation.
- Withdraw the ordered dose and inject deep IM into a large muscle appropriate for age (see Part I).

Intravenous

Verify correct IV concentration and rate of infusion with physician for administration to neonates, infants, and children.

PREPARE **Direct/Intermittent:** Reconstitute each 500 mg or less with at least 5 mL of sterile water for injection. ■ Final concentration must be ≤30 mg/mL; thus may be further diluted in 50 mL or more of NS, D5W, D5/NS, D5W/0.45NS, or RL. ■ Stability of solution varies with diluent and concentration of solution. ■ Solutions in NS are stable for up to 8 h at room temperature; other solutions should be infused within 2–4 h of preparation. ■ Give direct IV within 1 h of preparation. ■ Wear disposable gloves when handling drug repeatedly; contact dermatitis occurs frequently in sensitized individuals.

ADMINISTER **Direct/Intermittent:** Slowly over at least 15 min. ■ With solutions of 100 mL or more, set rate according to amount of solution, but no faster than direct IV rate. ■ Convulsions may be induced by too rapid administration.

INCOMPATIBILITIES **Solution/Additive:** Do not add to a dextrose-containing solution unless entire dose is given within 1 h of preparation. **Y-Site: Clindamycin, erythromycin,** AMINOGLYCOSIDES, **lidocaine, verapamil.** Incompatible with **TNA/TPN;** alkalinity of the ampicillin causes calcium/phosphate precipitation from the solution even at the Y-site.

ADVERSE EFFECTS Body as a Whole: Similar to those for penicillin G. Hypersensitivity (pruritus, urticaria, eosinophilia, hemolytic anemia, interstitial nephritis, <u>anaphylactoid reaction</u>); superinfections. **CNS:** Convulsive seizures with high doses. **GI:** *Diarrhea,* nausea, vomiting, <u>pseudomembranous colitis</u>. **Other:** Severe pain (following IM); phlebitis (following IV); **Skin:** *Rash.*

DIAGNOSTIC TEST INTERFERENCE Elevated *CPK* levels may result from local skeletal muscle injury following IM injection. **Urine glucose:** High urine drug concentrations can result in false-positive test results with Clinitest or Benedict's (enzymatic glucose oxidase methods, e.g., Clinistix, Diastix, TesTape are not affected). *AST* may be elevated (significance not known).

INTERACTIONS Drug: Allopurinol increases incidence of rash. Effectiveness of the AMINOGLYCOSIDES may be impaired in patients with severe end-stage renal disease. **Chloramphenicol, erythromycin,** and **tetracycline** may reduce bactericidal effects of ampicillin; this interaction is primarily significant when low doses of ampicillin are used. Ampicillin may interfere with the contraceptive action of ORAL CONTRACEPTIVES. Female patients should be advised to consider nonhormonal contraception while on antibiotics. **Food:** Food may decrease absorption of ampicillin, so it should be taken 1 h before or 2 h after meals.

PHARMACOKINETICS Absorption: Oral dose is 50% absorbed. Peak effect: 5 min IV, 1 h IM, 2 h PO. **Duration:** 6–8 h. **Distribution:** Most body tissues; high CNS concentrations only with inflamed meninges; crosses the placenta. **Metabolism:** Minimal hepatic metabolism. **Elimination:** 90% excreted in urine; excreted into breast milk. **Half-Life:** 1–1.8 h.

NURSING IMPLICATIONS

Assessment & Drug Effects

- Determine previous hypersensitivity reactions to penicillins, cephalosporins, and other allergens prior to therapy.
- Lab tests: Baseline C&S tests prior to initiation of therapy; start drug pending results. Baseline and periodic assessments of renal, hepatic, and hematologic functions, particularly during prolonged or high-dose therapy.
- Note: Sodium content of drug must be considered in patients on sodium restriction.
- Inspect skin daily and instruct patient to do the same. The appearance of a rash should be carefully evaluated to differentiate a nonallergenic ampicillin rash from a hypersensitivity reaction. Report rash promptly to physician.
- Note: Incidence of ampicillin rash is higher in patients with infectious mononucleosis or other viral infections, *Salmonella* infections, lymphocytic leukemia, or hyperuricemia or in patients taking allopurinol.

Patient & Family Education

- Note: Ampicillin rash is believed to be nonallergenic and therefore its appearance is not an absolute contraindication to future therapy. Rash usually disappears in 6–14 days but if severe, drug may need to be discontinued. Take drug for entire prescribed course.
- Take medication around the clock; do not miss a dose; continue taking medication until it is all gone (usually 10 days) unless otherwise directed by prescriber or pharmacist.
- Report diarrhea to prescriber; do not self-medicate. Give a detailed report to the prescriber regarding onset, duration, character of stools, associated symptoms, temperature and weight loss (if any) to help rule

out the possibility of drug-induced, potentially fatal pseudomembranous colitis (see Appendix D-1).

- Report S&S of superinfection (onset of black, hairy tongue; oral lesions or soreness; rectal or vaginal itching; vaginal discharge; loose, foul-smelling stools; or unusual odor to urine).
- Notify prescriber if no improvement is noted within a few days after therapy is started.
- Do not breast feed while taking this drug without consulting physician.
- Store this medication out of reach of children.

AMPICILLIN SODIUM AND SULBACTAM SODIUM

(am-pi-sill'in/sul-bak'tam)
Unasyn
Classifications: ANTI-INFECTIVE; ANTIBIOTIC; AMINOPENICILLIN
Prototype: Ampicillin
Pregnancy Category: B

AVAILABILITY 1.5 g, 3 g vials

ACTIONS Antibiotic agent with broad spectrum of activity resulting from beta-lactamase inhibition. Sulbactam inhibits beta-lactamases most frequently responsible for transferred drug resistance. Because of this action, a wide range of beta-lactamases found in organisms resistant to penicillins and cephalosporins are inhibited.
THERAPEUTIC EFFECTS Effective against both gram-positive and gram-negative bacteria including those that produce beta-lactamase and non-beta-lactamase producers. Ampicillin without sulbactam is not effective against beta-lactamase-producing strains.

USES Treatment of infections due to susceptible organisms in skin and skin structures (e.g., *Klebsiella pneumoniae, Staphylococcus aureus*) and intra-abdominal infections (e.g., *Escherichia coli*) and for gynecologic infections (e.g., *Bacteroides* sp. including *B. fragilis*). Also used for infections caused by ampicillin-susceptible organisms.

CONTRAINDICATIONS Hypersensitivity to penicillins; mononucleosis.
CAUTIOUS USE Hypersensitivity to cephalosporins; pregnancy (category B) or lactation.

ROUTE & DOSAGE

Child: 100–200 mg/kg/h in divided doses q6h
Adult: 1–2 g (ampicillin) q6–8h (max 8 g ampicillin/day)
Systemic Infections
Child: **IV** ≥1 y, 300 mg/kg/day (200 mg/kg ampicillin and 100 mg/kg sulbactam) divided into doses given q6h
Adult: **IV/IM** ≥40 kg, 1.5 g (1 g ampicillin, 0.5 g sulbactam) to 3 g (2 g ampicillin, 1 g sulbactam) q4–6h (max 4 g sulbactam/day)

STORAGE
Store powder for injection at 15°–30° C (59°–86° F) before reconstitution. Storage times and temperatures vary for different concentrations of reconstituted solutions; consult manufacturer's directions.

ADMINISTRATION

Intramuscular

- Reconstitute solution with sterile water for injection by adding 6.4 mL diluent to a 3-g vial. Each mL contains 250 mg ampicillin and 125 mg sulbactam.
- Give deep IM into a large muscle appropriate for age (see Part I). Rotate injection sites.

Intravenous

PREPARE **Direct/Intermittent:** Reconstitute each 1.5 g with 3.2 mL of sterile water for injection to yield 375 mg/mL (250 mg ampicillin/125 mg sulbactam); further dilute with NS, D5W, D5/NS, D5W/0.45NS, or RL to a final concentration within the range of 3–45 mg/mL.

ADMINISTER **Direct/Intermittent:** Give slowly over at least 15 min. ■ With solutions of 100 mL or more, set rate according to amount of solution but no faster than direct IV rate. ■ Convulsions may be induced by too rapid administration. ■ Use only freshly prepared solution; administer within 1 h after preparation.

INCOMPATIBILITIES **Solution/Additive:** Do not add to a dextrose-containing solution unless entire dose is given within 1 h of preparation. **Y-Site: Clindamycin, erythromycin,** AMINOGLYCOSIDES, **lidocaine, verapamil.** Incompatible with **TNA/TPN;** alkalinity of the ampicillin causes calcium/phosphate precipitation from the solution, even at the Y-site.

ADVERSE EFFECTS Body as a Whole: Hypersensitivity (rash, itching, <u>anaphylactoid reaction</u>), fatigue, malaise, headache, chills, edema. **GI:** *Diarrhea, nausea,* vomiting, abdominal distention, candidiasis. **Hematologic:** Neutropenia, thrombocytopenia. **Urogenital:** Dysuria. **CNS:** Seizures. **Other:** Local pain at injection site; thrombophlebitis.

INTERACTIONS Drug: Allopurinol increases incidence of rash; effectiveness of the AMINOGLYCOSIDES may be impaired in patients with severe end-stage renal disease; **chloramphenicol, erythromycin, tetracycline** may reduce bactericidal effects of ampicillin—this interaction is primarily significant when low doses are used; ampicillin may interfere with the contraceptive action of ORAL CONTRACEPTIVES —female patients should be advised to consider nonhormonal contraception while on antibiotics.

PHARMACOKINETICS Peak: Immediate after IV. **Duration:** 6–8 h. **Distribution:** Most body tissues; high CNS concentrations only with inflamed meninges; crosses placenta; appears in breast milk. **Metabolism:** Minimal hepatic metabolism. **Elimination:** Excreted in urine. **Half-Life:** 1 h.

NURSING IMPLICATIONS

Assessment & Drug Effects

- Determine previous hypersensitivity reactions to penicillins, cephalosporins, and other allergens prior to therapy.
- Lab tests: Baseline C&S tests prior to initiation of therapy; start drug pending results.
- Report promptly unexplained bleeding (e.g., epistaxis, purpura, ecchymoses).
- Monitor patient carefully during the first 30 min after initiation of IV therapy for signs of hypersensitivity and anaphylactoid reaction (see Appendix D-1). Serious anaphylactoid reactions require immediate use of emergency drugs and airway management.
- Observe for and report symptoms of superinfections (see Appendix D-1). Withhold drug and notify prescriber.
- Monitor I&O ratio and pattern. Report dysuria, urine retention, and hematuria.

Patient & Family Education

- Report chills, wheezing, pruritus (itching), respiratory distress, or palpitations to physician immediately.
- Do not breast feed while taking this drug without consulting prescriber.

AMPRENAVIR

(am-pre'na-vir)
Agenerase
Classifications: ANTI-INFECTIVE; ANTIRETROVIRAL AGENT; PROTEASE INHIBITOR
Prototype: Saquinavir
Pregnancy Category: C

AVAILABILITY 50 mg, 150 mg capsules; 15 mg/mL oral solution

ACTIONS Amprenavir inhibits the activity of HIV-1 protease enzyme and thus prevents the cleavage of viral polyproteins essential for the maturation and proliferation of the HIV-1 virus.
THERAPEUTIC EFFECTS The protease inhibitor activity results in the formation of immature, noninfectious viral particles. Amprenavir results in reduction of the viral load (HIV-RNA) in the plasma and an increase in the CD$_4$ lymphocyte cell count.

USES Treatment of HIV infection in combination with other antiretroviral agents.

CONTRAINDICATIONS Prior sensitivity to amprenavir; pregnancy (category C); lactation.

CAUTIOUS USE History of hypersensitivity to other protease inhibitors (e.g., indinavir, ritonavir, saquinavir); hypersensitivity to sulfonamides; hepatic dysfunction; diabetes mellitus; hemophilia A and B; vitamin K deficiencies; oral contraceptives; coadmistration with rifampin or sildenafil.

ROUTE & DOSAGE

HIV Infection
Child: **PO** *4–12 y or <50 kg,* 20 mg/kg b.i.d. capsules or 15 mg/kg t.i.d. capsules (max 2400 mg/day); 22.5 mg/kg b.i.d. oral solution or 17 mg/kg t.i.d. oral solution
Adolescent/Adult: **PO** 1200 mg capsules b.i.d.

Hepatic Impairment
Child-Pugh Score of 5–8: Give 450 mg b.i.d.;
Child-Pugh Score of 9–12: Give 300 mg b.i.d.

STORAGE
Store tablets at 20°–25° C (68°–77° F). Do not refrigerate.

ADMINISTRATION

Oral
- Give without regard to food, but not with high-fat meal.
- Capsules & oral solution are not interchangeable on mg-for-mg basis.

ADVERSE EFFECTS CNS: *Oral/perioral paresthesia,* peripheral paresthesia, depression, mood disorders. **GI:** *Nausea, vomiting, diarrhea,* taste disorders, increased triglycerides, hyperglycemia. **Skin:** *Rash,* <u>Stevens-Johnson syndrome</u>.

INTERACTIONS Drug: Administration with **amiodarone, astemizole, bepridil, cisapride, dihydroergotamine, ergotamine, lidocaine, midazolam, quinidine, triazolam,** and TRICYCLIC ANTIDEPRESSANTS may cause life-threatening reactions; **rifampin, rifabutin** decrease **amprenavir** concentrations; **amprenavir** may increase **sildenafil** concentrations; **phenobarbital, phenytoin, carbamazepine** may decrease **amprenavir** levels; monitor INR with **warfarin. Food:** Decreased absorption with high-fat meal. **Herbal: St. John's wort** may decrease antiretroviral activity.

PHARMACOKINETICS Absorption: Oral solution is less absorbed than capsules. **Peak:** 1–2 h. **Distribution:** 90% bound to plasma proteins. **Metabolism:** Metabolized in liver by CYP3A4. **Elimination:** 14% excreted in urine, 75% excreted in feces as metabolites. **Half-Life:** 7.1–10.6 h.

NURSING IMPLICATIONS

Assessment & Drug Effects
- Monitor for therapeutic effectiveness which is indicated by elevated CD$_4$ count & decreased HIV RNA copies.
- Monitor for & promptly notify prescriber of severe skin rash.

- Lab tests: Monitor blood glucose & HbA$_{1c}$, Hgb & Hct, and lipid profile at periodic intervals.
- Note: Monitor blood levels for coadministered drugs including amiodarone, lidocaine, phenobarbital, phenytoin, quinidine, tricyclic antidepressants; monitor PT and INR with warfarin.

Patient & Family Education
- Follow directions for taking this drug (see ADMINISTRATION).
- Take drug exactly as prescribed at the indicated times. Missed dose: If less than 4 h, wait until the next scheduled dose; otherwise, take immediately.
- Do not take supplemental vitamin E with this drug unless approved by physician, because the drug contains large amounts of vitamin E.
- Notify physician promptly about skin rash, nausea, vomiting, diarrhea, numbness or tingling around mouth or hands & feet.
- Inform physician of all other prescription/nonprescription drugs being taken. Serious interactions can occur.
- Use alternative barrier contraceptives rather than hormonal contraceptives while taking this drug.
- Note: Redistribution/accumulation of body fat may occur.
- Note: Diabetics may experience loss of glycemic control.
- Do not breast feed while taking this drug.
- Store this medication out of reach of children.

AMYL NITRITE
(am'il)
Amyl Nitrite
Classifications: CARDIOVASCULAR AGENT; NITRATE VASODILATOR; ANTIDOTE
Prototype: Nitroglycerin
Pregnancy Category: C

AVAILABILITY 0.3 mL ampules

ACTIONS Short-acting vasodilator and smooth muscle relaxant with actions similar to those of nitroglycerin. Action in treatment of cyanide poisoning based on ability of amyl nitrite to convert hemoglobin to methemoglobin, which forms a nontoxic complex with cyanide ion.
THERAPEUTIC EFFECTS Used for vasodilation of the cardiac vessels and immediate treatment of cyanide poisoning.

USES To relieve pain of renal and gallbladder colic. Also used as an adjunct antidote in the immediate treatment of cyanide poisoning. (Because of adverse effects, unpleasant odor, and expense, infrequently used to treat angina pectoris.)
UNLABELED USES Change intensity of heart murmurs.

CONTRAINDICATIONS Hypersensitivity to nitrites or nitrates; cerebral hemorrhage, head trauma; hypotension; glaucoma; severe anemia; hyperthyroidism; recent MI; acute alcoholism. Safety during pregnancy (category C) and lactation is not established.

Common adverse effects in *italic;* life-threatening effects <u>underlined</u>; generic names in **bold;** drug classifications in SMALL CAPS; ♦ Canadian drug name; ☉ Prototype drug.

ROUTE & DOSAGE

Cyanide Poisoning

Child/Adult: **Inhalation** 0.3 mL perle crushed every minute and inhaled for 15–30 sec until sodium nitrite infusion is ready

STORAGE

Store at 8°–15° C (46°–59° F), unless otherwise directed. Protect from light.

ADMINISTRATION

Inhalation

- Crush ampule between fingers to prepare (amyl nitrite is available in 0.18-mL and 0.3-mL perles, which are thin, friable glass ampules enveloped in a woven fabric cover).
- Instruct patient to sit a while immediately after drug is administered.
- Note: Amyl nitrite is volatile and highly flammable; when mixed with air or oxygen, it forms a mixture that can explode if ignited.

ADVERSE EFFECTS Body as a Whole: Transient flushing, weakness. **CV:** Orthostatic hypotension, palpitation, <u>cardiovascular collapse</u>, tachycardia. **GI:** Nausea, vomiting. **Hematologic:** <u>Methemoglobinemia</u> (<u>large doses</u>). **CNS:** *Headache,* dizziness, syncope. **Respiratory:** <u>Respiratory depression</u>.

PHARMACOKINETICS Absorption: Rapidly absorbed from mucous membranes. **Onset:** 10–30 sec. **Duration:** 3–5 min.

NURSING IMPLICATIONS

Assessment & Drug Effects

- Monitor for S&S of syncope, due to a sudden drop in systolic BP, which sometimes follows drug inhalation, particularly in older adults.
- Monitor vital signs until stable. Rapid pulse, which usually lasts for a brief period, is an expected response to the fall in BP produced by the drug.

Patient & Family Education

- Note: Drug has a strongly fruity odor.
- Do not breast feed while taking this drug without consulting physician.
- Store this medication out of reach of children.

ASCORBIC ACID (VITAMIN C)

Apo-C ♣, Ascorbicap, Cebid, Cecon, Cenolate, Cemill, C-Span, Cetane, Cevalin, Cevi-Bid, Ce-Vi-Sol ♣, Cevita, Flavorcee, Redoxon ♣, Schiff Effervescent Vitamin C, Vita-C.

ASCORBATE, SODIUM

(a-skor′bate)
Cenolate, Cevita
Classification: VITAMIN
Pregnancy Category: C

Common adverse effects in *italic;* life-threatening effects <u>underlined</u>; generic names in **bold;** drug classifications in SMALL CAPS; ♣ Canadian drug name; ❷ Prototype drug.

125

AVAILABILITY 25 mg, 50 mg, 100 mg, 250 mg, 500 mg, 1000 mg tablets; 250 mg/mL, 500 mg/mL injection

ACTIONS Water-soluble vitamin essential for synthesis and maintenance of collagen and intercellular ground substance of body tissue cells, blood vessels, cartilage, bones, teeth, skin, and tendons. Unlike most mammals, humans are unable to synthesize ascorbic acid in the body; therefore, it must be consumed daily.

THERAPEUTIC EFFECTS Increases protection mechanism of the immune system, thus supporting wound healing. Necessary for wound healing and resistance to infection.

USES Prophylaxis and treatment of scurvy and as a dietary supplement.

UNLABELED USES To acidify urine; to prevent and treat cancer; to treat idiopathic methemoglobinemia; as adjuvant during deferoxamine therapy for iron toxicity; in megadoses unproven to reduce severity and duration of common cold. Widely used as an antioxidant in formulations of parenteral tetracycline and other drugs.

CONTRAINDICATIONS Use of sodium ascorbate in patients on sodium restriction; use of calcium ascorbate in patients receiving digitalis. Safety during pregnancy (category C) or lactation is not established.

CAUTIOUS USE Excessive doses in patients with G6PD deficiency; hemochromatosis, thalassemia, sideroblastic anemia, sickle cell anemia; patients prone to gout or renal calculi.

ROUTE & DOSAGE

Therapeutic
Child: **PO/IV/IM/SC** 100–300 mg/day given in 1–2 doses
Adult: **PO/IV/IM/SC** 150–500 mg/day divided into 1–2 doses

Prophylactic
Child: **PO/IV/IM/SC** 30–60 mg/day
Adult: **PO/IV/IM/SC** 45–60 mg/day

Urinary Acidifier
Child: **PO/IV/IM/SC** 500 mg q6–8h
Adult: **PO/IV/IM/SC** 4–12 g/day given in 1–2 doses

STORAGE

- Store in airtight, light-resistant, nonmetallic containers, away from heat and sunlight, preferably at 15°–30° C (59°–86° F), unless otherwise specified by manufacturer. Contact with air will result in oxidation.
- Open ampules with caution. After prolonged storage, decomposition may occur with release of carbon dioxide and resulting increase in pressure within ampule.

ADMINISTRATION

Oral

- Give oral solutions mixed with food.
- Dissolve effervescent tablet in a glass of water immediately before ingestion.

Common adverse effects in *italic*; life-threatening effects <u>underlined</u>; generic names in **bold**; drug classifications in SMALL CAPS; ♣ Canadian drug name; ❷ Prototype drug.

Intramuscular, Subcutaneous

- Be aware that ascorbic acid injection may gradually darken on exposure to light; slight coloration reportedly does not affect its therapeutic action.

Intravenous

Intramuscular route is preferred over intravenous. Verify correct IV concentration and rate of infusion for children with prescriber.

PREPARE **Direct/Continuous/Intermittent:** Give undiluted or diluted in solutions such as NS, D5W, D5/NS, RL. Be aware that parenteral vitamin C is incompatible with many drugs. ▪ Consult pharmacist for compatibility information.

ADMINISTER **Direct:** Give undiluted at a rate of 100 mg or a fraction thereof over 1 min. **Continuous/Intermittent:** Give at ordered rate determined by volume of solution to be infused.

INCOMPATIBILITIES **Solution/Additive: Aminophylline, bleomycin, cephapirin, erythromycin, nafcillin, sodium bicarbonate, warfarin. Y-Site: Cefazolin, doxapram, sodium bicarbonate.**

ADVERSE EFFECTS GI: Nausea, vomiting, heartburn, diarrhea, or abdominal cramps (high doses). **Hematologic:** Acute hemolytic anemia (patients with deficiency of G6PD); sickle cell crisis. **CNS:** Headache or insomnia (high doses). **Urogenital:** Urethritis, dysuria, crystalluria, hyperoxaluria, or hyperuricemia (high doses). **Other:** Mild soreness at injection site; dizziness and temporary faintness with rapid IV administration.

DIAGNOSTIC TEST INTERFERENCE High doses of ascorbic acid can produce false-negative results for *urine glucose* with *glucose oxidase* methods (e.g., **Clinitest, TesTape, Diastix**); false-positive results with *copper reduction methods* (e.g., Benedict's solution, Clinitest); and false increases in *serum uric acid* determinations (by *enzymatic methods*). Interferes with *urinary steroid* (17-OHCS) determinations (by modified *Reddy, Jenkins, Thorn procedure*), decreases in *serum bilirubin,* and may cause increases in *serum cholesterol, creatinine,* and *uric acid* (methodologic inferences). May produce false-negative tests for *occult blood* in stools if taken within 48–72 h of test.

INTERACTIONS Drug: Large doses may attenuate hypoprothombinemic effects of ORAL ANTICOAGULANTS; SALICYLATES may inhibit ascorbic acid uptake by leukocytes and tissues, and ascorbic acid may decrease elimination of SALICYLATES; chronic high doses of ascorbic acid may diminish the effects of **disulfiram.**

PHARMACOKINETICS Absorption: Readily absorbed PO; however, absorption may be limited with large doses. **Distribution:** Widely distributed to body tissues; crosses placenta; distributed into breast milk. **Metabolism:** Metabolized in liver. **Elimination:** Rapidly excreted from body in urine when plasma level exceeds renal threshold of 1.4 mg/dL.

NURSING IMPLICATIONS

Assessment & Drug Effects

- Lab tests: Periodic Hct & Hgb, serum electrolytes.
- Monitor for S&S of acute hemolytic anemia, sickle cell crisis.

Patient & Family Education

- High doses of vitamin C are not recommended during pregnancy or in chidhood.
- Teach RDAs for particular age of child, as well as food sources.
- Take large doses of vitamin C in divided amounts because the body uses only what is needed at a particular time and excretes the rest in urine.
- Megadoses can interfere with absorption of vitamin B_{12}.
- Note: Vitamin C increases the absorption of iron when taken at the same time as iron-rich foods.
- Do not breast feed while taking this drug without consulting prescriber.
- Store this medication, as well as all vitamin preparations, out of reach of children.

ASPARAGINASE

(a-spar′a-gi-nase)
Colaspase, Elspar, Kidrolase A, L-asparaginase
Classification: ANTINEOPLASTIC ENZYME
Pregnancy Category: C

AVAILABILITY 10,000 international units vial

ACTIONS A highly toxic drug with a low therapeutic index. Catalyzes hydrolysis of asparagine to aspartic acid and ammonia, thus depleting extracellular supply of an amino acid essential to synthesis of DNA and other nucleoproteins.
THERAPEUTIC EFFECTS Reduced availability of asparagine causes death of tumor cells, because, unlike normal cells, tumor cells are unable to synthesize their own supply. Resistance to cytotoxic action develops rapidly; therefore, this is not an effective treatment for solid tumors and not recommended for maintenance therapy.

USES Primarily in combination regimens with other antineoplastic agents to treat acute lymphocytic leukemia (ALL).
UNLABELED USES Other leukemias, lymphosarcoma, and (intra-arterially) treatment of hypoglycemia due to pancreatic islet cell tumor.

CONTRAINDICATIONS History of/or existing pancreatitis; chickenpox (existing or recent illness or exposure), herpetic infection. Safety during pregnancy (category C) or lactation is not established.
CAUTIOUS USE Liver impairment; diabetes mellitus; infections; history of urate calculi or gout; antineoplastic or radiation therapy.

ROUTE & DOSAGE

Induction Agent

Child/Adult: **IM:** 6000–10,000 international units/mL in 1 dose 3 times/wk **IV** 200 international units/kg/day for 28 days, inject over at least 30 min into running IV

STORAGE

- Store sealed vial of lyophilized powder below 8° C (46° F) unless otherwise directed by manufacturer.

Common adverse effects in *italic;* life-threatening effects <u>underlined</u>; generic names in **bold**; drug classifications in SMALL CAPS; ♦ Canadian drug name; ❷ Prototype drug.

- Store reconstituted solutions and solutions diluted for IV infusion at 2°–8° C (36°–46° F) for up to 8 h; then discard.

ADMINISTRATION

Child: Must be given under the care and direction of a pediatric oncology specialist. Use recommended handling techniques for hazardous medications (see Part I).

Intravenous

An intradermal skin test is usually performed prior to initial dose and when drug is readministered after an interval of a week or more; allergic reactions are unpredictable. ▪ Observe test site for at least 1 h for evidence of positive reaction (wheal, erythema). A negative skin test, however, does not preclude possibility of an allergic reaction. ▪ Administer test dose and IV infusion under constant supervision by clinician experienced in cancer chemotherapy. ▪ Use only clear solutions.

PREPARE **Intermittent:** Reconstitute with sterile water or with 0.9% NaCl. ▪ Each 10,000-international units vial is diluted with 5 mL of diluent to yield 2000 IU/mL. ▪ Shake vial well to promote dissolution of powder. Avoid vigorous shaking. Ordinary shaking does not inactivate the enzyme or cause foaming of content.

ADMINISTER **Intermittent:** Further dilute reconstituted solution with NS or D5W by administration into tubing of an already free-flowing infusion of one of these solutions. ▪ Give over a period of not less than 30 min. ▪ Use a 5-mm filter to remove gelatinous fiber-like particles that can develop in solutions on standing.

ADVERSE EFFECTS Body as a Whole: Hypersensitivity (*skin rashes, urticaria,* respiratory distress, <u>anaphylaxis</u>), chills, fever, <u>fatal hyperthermia</u>, perspiration, weight loss. **CNS:** Depression, fatigue, lethargy, drowsiness, confusion, agitation, hallucinations, dizziness, Parkinson-like syndrome with tremor and progressive increase in muscle tone. **GI:** *Severe vomiting, nausea,* anorexia, abdominal cramps, diarrhea, acute pancreatitis, liver function abnormalities. **Urogenital:** Uric acid nephropathy, azotemia, proteinuria, <u>renal failure</u>. **Hematologic:** *Reduced clotting factors* (especially V, VII, VIII, IX), *decreased circulating platelets and fibrinogen,* leukopenia. **Metabolic:** Hyperglycemia, glycosuria, polyuria, hypoalbuminemia, hypocalcemia, hyperuricemia. **Other:** Flank pain, infections.

DIAGNOSTIC TEST INTERFERENCE Asparaginase may interfere with *thyroid function* tests: decreased total *serum thyroxine* and increased *thyroxine-binding globulin index;* pretreatment values return within 4 wk after drug is discontinued.

INTERACTIONS Drug: Decreased hypoglycemic effects of SULFONYL-UREAS, **insulin;** increased potential for toxicity if asparaginase is given concurrently or immediately before CORTICOSTEROIDS, **vincristine;**

methotrexate's antitumor effect is blocked if asparaginase is given concurrently or immediately before it.

PHARMACOKINETICS Distribution: Distributed primarily into intravascular space (80%) and lymph; low levels in CSF and pleural and peritoneal fluids. **Metabolism:** Unknown. **Elimination:** Small amounts found in urine. **Half-Life:** 8–30 h.

NURSING IMPLICATIONS

Assessment & Drug Effects

- Assess immunization status prior to beginning therapy in order to be alert for diseases that pose risk.
- Have immediately available: Personnel, drugs, and equipment for treating allergic reaction (which may range from urticaria to anaphylactic shock) whenever drug is administered, including skin testing.
- Monitor for S&S and be alert to evidence of hypersensitivity or anaphylactoid reaction during drug administration. Anaphylaxis usually occurs within 30–60 min after dose has been given and is more likely with intermittent administrations, particularly at intervals of ≥7 days.
- Monitor I&O and maintain adequate fluid intake.
- Evaluate CNS function (general behavior, emotional status, level of consciousness, thought content, motor function) before and during therapy.
- Note: Toxicity potential is increased when giving drug immediately before a course of prednisone and vincristine; toxicity appears less when given after these drugs.
- Lab tests: Periodic serum amylase, serum calcium blood glucose, coagulation factors, ammonia and uric acid levels, hepatic and renal function tests, peripheral blood counts, and bone marrow function; liver function tests at least twice weekly during therapy.
- Monitor diabetics for loss of glycemic control.
- Monitor for and report S&S of hyperammonemia: Anorexia, vomiting, lethargy, weak pulse, depressed temperature, irritability, asterixis, seizures, coma.
- Anticipate possible prolonged or exaggerated effects of concurrently given drugs or their toxicity because of potential serious hepatic dysfunction that reduces enzymatic detoxification of other drugs. Report incidence promptly.
- Watch for neurotoxic reaction (25% of patients), which usually appears within the first few days of therapy. It is manifested by tiredness and changing levels of consciousness (ranging from confusion to coma).
- Note: Protect from infection during first several days of treatment when circulating lymphoblasts decrease markedly and leukocyte counts may fall below normal. Report promptly S&S of infection: Chill, fever, aches, sore throat.
- Report sudden severe abdominal pain with nausea and vomiting, particularly if these symptoms occur after medication is discontinued (may indicate pancreatitis).

Patient & Family Education

- Note: Therapeutic response will most likely be accompanied by some toxicity in all patients; toxicity is reportedly greater in adults than in children.

- Notify physician of continued loss of weight or onset of foot and ankle swelling.
- Notify physician without delay if nausea or vomiting make it difficult to take all prescribed medication.
- Report onset of unusual bleeding, bruising, petechiae, melena, skin rash or itching, yellowed skin and sclera, joint pain, puffy face, or dyspnea. Avoid contact with persons with infections such as colds, influenza, and chickenpox.
- Do not drive or operate equipment that requires alertness and skill. Exercise caution with potentially hazardous activities. These effects can continue several weeks after last dose of the drug.
- Do not breast feed while taking this drug without consulting physician.

ASPIRIN (ACETYLSALICYLIC ACID) 🅿

(as′pe-ren)
Alka-Seltzer, A.S.A., Aspergum, Astrin ♣, Bayer, Bayer Children's, Cosprin, Easprin, Ecotrin, Empirin, Entrophen ♣, Halfprin, Measurin, Novasen ♣, St Joseph Children's, Supasa, Triaphen-10 ♣, ZORprin

Classifications: CENTRAL NERVOUS SYSTEM AGENT; ANALGESIC, SALICYLATE; ANTIPYRETIC
Pregnancy Category: D

AVAILABILITY 81 mg chewable tablets; 325 mg, 500 mg tablets; 81 mg, 165 mg, 325 mg, 500 mg, 650 mg, 975 mg enteric-coated tablets; 650 mg, 800 mg sustained-release tablets; 120 mg, 200 mg, 300 mg, 600 mg suppositories

ACTIONS Major actions appear to be associated primarily with inhibiting the formation of prostaglandins involved in the production of inflammation, pain, and fever. **Anti-inflammatory action:** Inhibits prostaglandin synthesis. As an anti-inflammatory agent, aspirin appears to be involved in enhancing antigen removal and in reducing the spread of inflammation in ground substances. These anti-inflammatory actions also contribute to analgesic effects. **Analgesic action:** Principally peripheral with limited action in the CNS, possibly on the hypothalamus; results in relief of mild to moderate pain. **Antipyretic action:** In addition to inhibiting prostaglandin synthesis, aspirin lowers body temperature in fever by indirectly causing centrally mediated peripheral vasodilation and sweating. **Antiplatelet action:** Aspirin (but not other salicylates) powerfully inhibits platelet aggregation. High serum salicylate concentrations can impair hepatic synthesis of blood coagulation factors VII, IX, and X, possibly by inhibiting action of vitamin K.

THERAPEUTIC EFFECTS Reduces inflammation, pain, and fever. Also inhibits platelet aggregation, reducing ability of blood to clot.

USES To relieve pain of low to moderate intensity. Also for various inflammatory conditions, such as acute rheumatic fever, Kawasaki disease, systemic lupus erythematosis, juvenile rheumatoid arthritis, osteoarthritis, bursitis, and calcific tendonitis, and to reduce fever in selected febrile conditions. Used to reduce risk and recurrence of TIA and stroke due to

---

fibrin platelet emboli; to prevent recurrence of MI; for anticoagulation in heart disease.

UNLABELED USES As prophylactic against thromboembolism; to prevent cataract and progression of diabetic retinopathy; and to control symptoms related to gluten sensitivity.

CONTRAINDICATIONS History of hypersensitivity to salicylates including methyl salicylate (oil of wintergreen); sensitivity to other NSAIDS; patients with "aspirin triad" (aspirin sensitivity, nasal polyps, asthma); chronic rhinitis; chronic urticaria; history of GI ulceration, bleeding, or other problems; hypoprothrombinemia, vitamin K deficiency, hemophilia, or other bleeding disorders; CHF. Do not use aspirin during pregnancy (category D), especially in third trimester; lactation; or in prematures, neonates, or children under 2 y, except under advice and supervision of physician. Do not use in children or teenagers with chickenpox or influenza-like illnesses because of possible association with Reye's syndrome. Because cause of illness in children is often not known, aspirin is not recommended for treatment of mild illness in case it is influenza or chickenpox; acetaminophen or ibuprofen preferred.

CAUTIOUS USE Otic diseases; gout; children with fever accompanied by dehydration; hyperthyroidism; cardiac disease; renal or hepatic impairment; G6PD deficiency; anemia; preoperatively; Hodgkin's disease.

ROUTE & DOSAGE

Mild to Moderate Pain, Fever
Child: **PO/PR** 10–15 mg/kg in 4–6 h (max 3.6 g/day)
Adult: **PO/PR** 350–650 mg q4h (max 4 g/day)

Arthritic Conditions
Child: **PO** 80–100 mg/kg/day divided into 4–6 doses (max 130 mg/kg/day)
Adult: **PO** 3.6–5.4 g/day divided into 4–6 doses

Thromboembolic Disorders
Adult: **PO** 325–650 mg 1–2 times/day

Kawasaki disease
80–100 mg/kg/day in divided doses q6h initially; then decrease to 3–5 mg/kg/day daily

STORAGE

Store at 15°–30° C (59°–86° F) in airtight container and dry environment unless otherwise directed by manufacturer. Store suppositories in a cool place or refrigerate but do not freeze.

ADMINISTRATION

Oral, Suppository
- Give with a full glass of water (240 mL), milk, food, or antacid to minimize gastric irritation.
- Enteric-coated tablets dissolve too quickly if administered with milk and should not be crushed or chewed.

ADVERSE EFFECTS Body as a Whole: Hypersensitivity (urticaria, <u>bronchospasm, anaphylactic shock</u> (<u>laryngeal edema</u>). **CNS:** Dizziness, confusion, drowsiness. **Special Senses:** Tinnitus, hearing loss. **GI:** *Nausea,* vomiting, diarrhea, anorexia, *heartburn, stomach pains,* ulceration, occult bleeding, GI bleeding. **Hematologic:** Thrombocytopenia, <u>hemolytic anemia</u>, prolonged bleeding time. **Skin:** Petechiae, easy bruising, rash. **Urogenital:** Impaired renal function. **Other:** Prolonged pregnancy and labor with increased bleeding.

DIAGNOSTIC TEST INTERFERENCE Bleeding time is prolonged 3–8 days (life of exposed platelets) following a single 325-mg (5 grains) dose of aspirin. Large doses of salicylates equivalent to 5 g or more of aspirin per day may cause prolonged ***prothrombin time*** by decreasing prothrombin production; interference with ***pregnancy tests*** (using mouse or rabbit); decreases in ***serum cholesterol, potassium, PBI, T_3 and T_4 concentrations,*** and an increase in ***T_3 resin uptake. Serum uric acid*** may increase when plasma salicylate levels are below 10 and decrease when above 15 mg/dL using colorimetric methods. **Urine 5-HIAA:** Aspirin may interfere with tests using fluorescent methods. **Urine ketones:** Salicylates interfere with Gerhardt test (reaction with ferric chloride produces a reddish color that persists after boiling). **Urine glucose:** Moderate to large doses of salicylates equivalent to an aspirin dosage ≥2.4 g/day may produce false-negative results with glucose oxidase methods (e.g., Clinistix, TesTape) and false-positive results with copper reduction methods (Benedict's solution, Clinitest). ***Urinary PSP excretion*** may be reduced by salicylates. Salicylates may cause ***urine VMA*** to be falsely elevated (by most tests), or reduced (by Pisano method). Salicylates may interfere with or cause false decreases in plasma theophylline levels using Schack and Waxler method. High plasma salicylate levels may cause abnormalities in ***liver function tests.***

INTERACTIONS Drug: Aminosalicylic acid increases risk of SALICYLATE toxicity. **Ammonium chloride** and other ACIDIFYING AGENTS decrease renal elimination and increase risk of SALICYLATE toxicity. ANTICOAGULANTS increase risk of bleeding. ORAL HYPOGLYCEMIC AGENTS increase hypoglycemic activity with aspirin doses >2 g/day. CARBONIC ANHYDRASE INHIBITORS enhance SALICYLATE toxicity. CORTICOSTEROIDS add to ulcerogenic effects. **Methotrexate** toxicity is increased. Low doses of SALICYLATES may antagonize uricosuric effects of **probenecid** and **sulfinpyrazone. Herbal: Feverfew, garlic, ginger, ginkgo** may increase bleeding potential.

PHARMACOKINETICS Absorption: 80–100% absorbed (depending on formulation), primarily in stomach and upper small intestine. Peak levels: 15 min to 2 h. **Distribution:** Widely distributed in most body tissues; crosses placenta. **Metabolism:** Aspirin is hydrolyzed to salicylate in GI mucosa, plasma, and erythrocytes; salicylate is metabolized in liver. **Elimination:** 50% of dose is eliminated in the urine in 2– 4 h (low doses) or 15–30 h (high doses). Excreted into breast milk. **Half-Life:** Aspirin 15–20 min; salicylate 2–18 h (dose dependent).

NURSING IMPLICATIONS

Assessment & Drug Effects

- Monitor for loss of tolerance to aspirin. Previous nonreaction to salicylates does not guarantee future safety. Some individuals develop an acute and specific intolerance to aspirin, although they may have taken it for years without incident. The reaction is nonimmunologic; symptoms usually occur 15 min to 3 h after ingestion: profuse rhinorrhea, erythema, nausea, vomiting, intestinal cramps, diarrhea.

- Monitor for salicylate toxicity. In adults, a sensation of fullness in the ears, tinnitus, and decreased or muffled hearing are the most frequent symptoms associated with chronic salicylate overdosage.
- Monitor children closely because salicylate toxicity is enhanced by the dehydration that frequently accompanies fever or illness. Children tend to manifest salicylate toxicity by hyperventilation, agitation, mental confusion or other behavioral changes, drowsiness, lethargy, sweating, and constipation.
- Monitor the diabetic child on aspirin carefully for indicated need of insulin adjustment. Children on high doses of aspirin are particularly prone to develop hypoglycemia.

Patient & Family Education

- Do not give aspirin to children or teenagers with symptoms of varicella (chickenpox) or influenza-like illnesses because of association of aspirin usage with Reye syndrome. Give acetaminophen or ibuprofen whenever possible to children instead of aspirin.
- Use enteric-coated tablets, extended-release tablets, buffered aspirin, or aspirin administered with an antacid to reduce GI disturbances.
- Take aspirin 1–2 day before menses when prescribed for dysmenorrhea. When experiencing heavy menstrual blood loss, take another analgesic, such as acetaminophen, instead of aspirin.
- Discontinue aspirin therapy about 1 wk before surgery to reduce risk of bleeding. Do not use aspirin-containing gum or gargles or chew aspirin products for at least 1 wk following oral surgery.
- Note: Chronic use of high-dose aspirin during the last 3 mo of pregnancy can prolong pregnancy and labor, increase maternal bleeding before and after delivery, and cause weight increase and hemorrhage in the neonate.
- Discontinue aspirin use with onset of ringing or buzzing in the ears, impaired hearing, dizziness, GI discomfort or bleeding, and report to prescriber.
- Do not use aspirin for self-medication of pain beyond 5 days without consulting a health care provider. Do not use aspirin longer than 3 days for fever (adults and children), never for fever over 38.9° C (102° F) or for recurrent fever without medical direction.
- Consult care provider before using aspirin for any fever accompanied by rash, severe headache, stiff neck, marked irritability, or confusion (all possible symptoms of meningitis).
- Avoid alcohol when taking large doses of aspirin.
- Observe and report signs of bleeding (e.g., petechiae, ecchymoses, bleeding gums, bloody or black stools, cloudy or bloody urine).
- Maintain adequate fluid intake for age when taking repeated doses of aspirin.
- Avoid other medications containing aspirin unless directed by prescriber, because of danger of overdosing (there are more than 500 OTC aspirin-containing compounds). Read labels carefully and check with pharmacist, physician, or nurse before taking OTC medications for common childhood illnesses.

■ Keep aspirin locked securely away; it is a common source of poisoning in children.
■ Do not breast feed while taking this drug.

ATENOLOL

(a-ten'oh-lole)
Apo-Atenolol ♣ , Tenormin
Classifications: AUTONOMIC NERVOUS SYSTEM AGENT; BETA-ADRENERGIC ANTAGONIST (SYMPATHOLYTIC, BLOCKING AGENT); ANTIHYPERTENSIVE
Prototype: Propranolol
Pregnancy Category: C

AVAILABILITY 25 mg, 50 mg, 100 mg tablets; 5 mg/10 mL vial

ACTIONS In therapeutic doses, atenolol selectively blocks beta$_1$-adrenergic receptors located chiefly in cardiac muscle. With large doses, preferential effect is lost and inhibition of beta$_2$-adrenergic receptors may lead to increased airway resistance, especially in patients with asthma or COPD. Mechanisms for antihypertensive action include central effect leading to decreased sympathetic outflow to periphery, reduction in renin activity with consequent suppression of the renin-angiotensin-aldosterone system, and competitive inhibition of catecholamine binding at beta-adrenergic receptor sites.
THERAPEUTIC EFFECTS Reduces rate and force of cardiac contractions (negative inotropic action); cardiac output is reduced, as well as systolic and diastolic BP. Atenolol decreases peripheral vascular resistance both at rest and with exercise.

USES Management of hypertension as a single agent or concomitantly with other antihypertensive agents, especially a diuretic, and in treatment of stable angina pectoris, MI.
UNLABELED USES Antiarrhythmic, to slow progression of congestive heart failure, mitral valve prolapse, adjunct in treatment of pheochromocytoma and of thyrotoxicosis; and for vascular headache prophylaxis.

CONTRAINDICATIONS Sinus bradycardia, greater than first-degree heart block, overt cardiac failure, cardiogenic shock. Safety during pregnancy (category C), lactation, or in children is not established.
CAUTIOUS USE Hypertensive patients with CHF controlled by digitalis and diuretics; asthma and COPD; diabetes mellitus; impaired renal function; hyperthyroidism.

ROUTE & DOSAGE

Hypertension, Angina
Child: **PO** 0.8–1.5 mg/kg/day (max 2 mg/kg/day)
Adult: **PO** 25–50 mg/day, may increase to 100 mg/day (max 200 mg/day)

Congestive Heart Failure
25–200 mg/day (Toprol XL formulation) Adjust dose in renal impairment.

STORAGE
Store in tightly closed, light-resistant container at 15°–30° C (59°–86° F) unless otherwise directed.

ADMINISTRATION

Oral
- Crush tablets, if necessary, before administration and give with fluid of patient's choice.

Intravenous

PREPARE **Direct:** Use undiluted or diluted in 10–50 mL of NS, D5W, D5/NS, D5/0.45NS, or 0.45NS.
ADMINISTER **Direct:** Give over 5 min. Do not exceed rate of 1 mg/min.

ADVERSE EFFECTS CNS: Dizziness, vertigo, light-headedness, syncope, fatigue or weakness, lethargy, drowsiness, insomnia, mental changes, depression. **CV:** *Bradycardia, hypotension, CHF,* cold extremities, leg pains, dysrhythmias. **GI:** Nausea, vomiting, diarrhea. **Respiratory:** Pulmonary edema, dyspnea, bronchospasm. **Other:** May mask symptoms of hypoglycemia; decreased sexual ability.

INTERACTIONS Drug: Atropine and other ANTICHOLINERGICS may increase atenolol absorption from GI tract; NSAIDS may decrease hypotensive effects; may mask symptoms of a hypoglycemic reaction induced by **insulin,** SULFONYLUREAS; may increase **lidocaine** levels and toxicity; pharmacologic and toxic effects of both atenolol and **verapamil** are increased. **Prazosin, terazocin** may increase severe hypotensive response to first dose of atenolol.

PHARMACOKINETICS Absorption: 50% of PO dose absorbed. **Peak:** 2–4 h PO; 5 min IV. **Duration:** 24 h. **Distribution:** Does not readily cross blood–brain barrier. **Metabolism:** No hepatic metabolism. **Elimination:** 40–50% excreted in urine; 50–60% excreted in feces. **Half-Life:** 6–7 h.

NURSING IMPLICATIONS

Assessment & Drug Effects
- Check apical pulse before giving oral drug, especially in patients receiving digitalis (both drugs slow AV conduction). If below 60 bpm (or other ordered parameter for child), withhold dose and consult physician.
- Monitor apical pulse, BP, respirations, and peripheral circulation throughout dosage adjustment period. Consult physician for acceptable parameters.

Patient & Family Education
- Adhere rigidly to dose regimen. Sudden discontinuation of drug can exacerbate angina and precipitate tachycardia or MI in patients with coronary artery disease, and thyroid storm in patients with hyperthyroidism.
- Make position changes slowly and in stages, particularly from recumbent to upright posture.

Common adverse effects in *italic;* life-threatening effects <u>underlined</u>; generic names in **bold;** drug classifications in SMALL CAPS; ♣ Canadian drug name; ❷ Prototype drug.

■ Do not breast feed while taking this drug without consulting physician.
■ Store this medication out of reach of children.

ATOMOXETINE

(a-to-mox′e-teen)
Strattera
Classifications: CENTRAL NERVOUS SYSTEM AGENT; PSYCHOTHERAPEUTIC; NOREPINEPHRINE REUPTAKE INHIBITOR
Pregnancy Category: C

AVAILABILITY 10 mg, 18 mg, 25 mg, 40 mg, 60 mg capsules

ACTIONS Exact mechanism of action is unknown, but is thought to be related to selective inhibition of the presynaptic norepinephrine transporter, resulting in norepinephrine reuptake inhibition.
THERAPEUTIC EFFECTS Improved attentiveness, ability to follow through on tasks with less distraction and forgetfulness, and diminished hyperactivity.

USES Treatment of attention deficit/hyperactivity disorder (ADHD) in adults and children.

CONTRAINDICATIONS Hypersensitive to atomoxetine or any of its constituents; concomitant use or use within 2 wk of MAOIs; narrow-angle glaucoma; pregnancy (category C).
CAUTIOUS USE Hypertension, tachycardia, cardiovascular or cerebrovascular disease; any condition that predisposes to hypotension; urinary retention or urinary hesitancy; concomitant use of CYP2D6 inhibitors (e.g., paroxetine, fluoxetine, quinidine), albuterol or other beta-2 agonists, vasopressor drugs; safety and efficacy in children <6 y and the older adult have not been established; lactation.

ROUTE & DOSAGE

ADHD

Child/Adolescent: **PO** *<70 kg,* start with 0.5 mg/kg/day. May increase after 3 days to target dose of 1.2 mg/kg/day. Administer once daily in morning or divide dose and give morning and late afternoon/early evening. Max dose is 1.4 mg/kg or 100 mg, whichever is less. *>70 kg,* max total daily dose is 100 mg
Adult: **PO** Start with 40 mg in morning. May increase after 3 days to target dose of 80 mg/day given either once in the morning or divided morning and late afternoon/early evening. May increase to max of 100 mg/day if needed

Hepatic Impairment

Child-Pugh Class B: Initial and target doses should be reduced to 50% of the normal dose
Child-Pugh Class C: Initial dose and target doses should be reduced to 25% of normal

Common adverse effects in *italic;* life-threatening effects <u>underlined;</u> generic names in **bold;** drug classifications in SMALL CAPS; ♣ Canadian drug name; ❷ Prototype drug.

137

STORAGE
Store at room temperature of 15°–30° C (59°–86° F).

ADMINISTRATION

Oral

- Note that total daily dose in children and adolescents is based on weight. Determine that ordered dose is appropriate for weight prior to administration of drug.
- Note manufacturer recommends dosage adjustments with concomitant administration of strong CYP2D6 inhibitors (e.g., paroxetine, fluoxetine, quinidine). Consult physician.

ADVERSE EFFECTS Body as a Whole: Flu-like syndrome, flushing, fatigue, fever, rigors. **CNS:** Dizziness, *headache,* somnolence, crying, tearfulness, irritability, mood swings, *insomnia,* depression, tremor, early morning awakenings, paresthesias, abnormal dreams, decreased libido, sleep disorder. **CV:** Increased blood pressure, sinus tachycardia, palpitations. **GI:** *Upper abdominal pain,* constipation, dyspepsia, *vomiting, decreased appetite,* anorexia, dry mouth, diarrhea, flatulence. **Endocrine:** Hot flushes. **Metabolic:** Weight loss. **Musculoskeletal:** Arthralgia, myalgia. **Respiratory:** *Cough,* rhinorrhea, nasal congestion, sinusitis. **Skin:** Dermatitis, pruritus, increased sweating. **Special Senses:** Mydriasis. **Urogenital:** Urinary hesitation/retention, dysmenorrhea, ejaculation dysfunction, impotence, delayed onset of menses, irregular menstruation, prostatitis.

INTERACTIONS Drug: Albuterol may potentiate cardiovascular effects of atomoxetine; **fluoxetine, paroxetine, quinidine** may increase atomoxetine levels and toxicity; MAOIS may precipitate a hypertensive crisis; may attenuate effects of ANTIHYPERTENSIVE AGENTS.

PHARMACOKINETICS Absorption: Well absorbed from GI tract. **Peak:** 1–2 h. **Metabolism:** Metabolized in liver by CYP2D6. **Elimination:** Primarily excreted in urine. **Half-Life:** 5.2 h.

NURSING IMPLICATIONS

Assessment & Drug Effects

- Evaluate for continuing therapeutic effectiveness especially with long-term use.
- Monitor cardiovascular status especially with preexisting hypertension.
- Monitor HR and BP at baseline, following a dose increase, and periodically while on therapy.
- Report increased aggression and irritability because these may indicate a need to discontinue the drug.

Patient & Family Education

- Report any of the following to physician: chest pains or palpitations, urinary retention or difficulty initiating voiding urine, appetite loss and weight loss, or insomnia.
- Make position changes slowly if you experience dizziness with arising from a lying or sitting position.

- Do not drive or engage in potentially hazardous activities until reaction to the drug is known.
- Do not breast feed while taking this drug without consulting prescriber.
- Store this medication out of reach of children.

ATOVAQUONE/PROGUANIL HYDROCHLORIDE

(a-to′-va-quone/pro′gua-nil)
Malarone, Malarone Pediatric
Classifications: ANTI-INFECTIVE; ANTIPROTOZOAL; ANTIMALARIAL
Prototype: Chloroquine HCl & Metronidazole
Pregnancy Category: C

AVAILABILITY Atovaquone 250 mg/proguanil HCl 100 mg (adult tablet), atovaquone 62.5 mg/proguanil HCl 25 mg tablets (pediatric tablet)

ACTIONS Combination of two antimalarial drugs. Atovaquone inhibits the electron transport system in the mitochondria of the malaria parasite, thus interfering with nucleic acid and ATP synthesis of the parasite. Proguanil interferes with DNA synthesis of the malaria parasite.
THERAPEUTIC EFFECTS Malarone is effective against strains of *Plasmodium* spp. and *P. falciparum* and *Pneumocystic carinii*.

USES Prevention and treatment of malaria due to *P. falciparum,* even in chloroquine-resistant areas; prevention and treatment of *P. carinii* pneumonia in susceptible children.

CONTRAINDICATIONS Known hypersensitivity to atovaquone or proguanil; pregnancy (category C); severe malaria.
CAUTIOUS USE Cerebral malaria, complicated malaria, pulmonary edema; renal failure; lactation; older adults. Use in children weighing <11 kg is not established.

ROUTE & DOSAGE

Prevention of Malaria

Child: **PO** *11–20 kg,* 1 pediatric tablet daily; *21–30 kg,* 2 pediatric tablets daily; *31–40 kg,* 3 pediatric tablets daily; *>40 kg* 1 adult tablet daily with food starting 1–2 days before travel to malarial area and continuing for 7 days after return
Adult: **PO** 1 tablet daily with food starting 1–2 days before travel to malarial area and continuing for 7 days after return

Treatment of Malaria

Child: **PO** *11–20 kg,* 1 adult tablet; *21–30 kg,* 2 adult tablets; *31–40 kg,* 3 adult tablets; *>40 kg,* 4 adult tablets as a single daily dose for 3 days
Adult: **PO** 4 tablets as a single daily dose for 3 days

STORAGE
Store at 15°–25° C (59°–77° F) in tightly closed containers.

ADMINISTRATION

Oral

▪ Give at the same time each day with food or a drink containing milk.
▪ Give a repeat dose if vomiting occurs within 1 h after dosing.

ADVERSE EFFECTS Body as a Whole: Fever, *myalgia,* back pain, asthenia, anorexia. **Digestive:** *Nausea, abdominal pain, diarrhea,* dyspepsia. **CNS:** *Headache.* **Respiratory:** Cough. **Skin:** Pruritus.

INTERACTIONS Drug: Rifampin, rifabutin, tetracycline may decrease serum levels; **metoclopramide** may decrease absorption.

PHARMACOKINETICS Absorption: Atovaquone (A), Poorly absorbed from GI tract, absorption is improved when taken with a fatty meal; **Proguanil (P),** Extensively absorbed. **Duration: A,** 6–23 wk after a 3-wk course of therapy. **Distribution: A,** Penetrates poorly into cerebrospinal fluid; >99.9% protein bound; **P,** 75% protein bound. **Metabolism: A,** Not metabolized; **P,** Metabolized by CYP2C19 to cycloguanil. **Elimination: A,** >94% excreted in feces over 21 days (enterohepatically cycled); **P,** Primarily excreted in urine. **Half-Life: A,** 2–3 days; **P,** 12–21 h.

NURSING IMPLICATIONS

Assessment & Drug Effects

▪ Lab tests: Monitor AST and ALT periodically, especially with long-term therapy.
▪ Monitor for S&S of parasitemia in patients receiving tetracycline and in those experiencing diarrhea or vomiting.
▪ Note: Only use metoclopramide to control vomiting if other antiemetics are not available.

Patient & Family Education

▪ Take this drug at the same time each day for maximum effectiveness. Take for entire course prescribed.
▪ Note: Absorption of this drug may be reduced with diarrhea and vomiting. Consult prescriber if either of these occurs.
▪ Do not breast feed while taking this drug without consulting physician.
▪ Store this medication out of reach of children.

ATRACURIUM BESYLATE

(a-tra-kyoor'ee-um)
Tracrium
Classifications: AUTONOMIC NERVOUS SYSTEM AGENT; SKELETAL MUSCLE RELAXANT, NONDEPOLARIZING; NEUROMUSCULAR BLOCKER
Prototype: Tubocurarine
Pregnancy Category: C

AVAILABILITY 10 mg/mL injection

ACTIONS Inhibits neuromuscular transmission by binding competitively with acetylcholine to muscle end plate receptors. Lacks analgesic action and has no apparent effect on pain threshold, consciousness, or cerebration. Given in general anesthesia only after unconsciousness has been induced by other drugs.

THERAPEUTIC EFFECTS Synthetic skeletal muscle relaxant pharmacologically similar to tubocurarine that produces shorter duration of neuromuscular blockade, exhibits minimal direct effects on cardiovascular system, and has less histamine-releasing action. Has minimal cumulative tendency with subsequent doses if recovery from the drug begins before dose is repeated.

USES Adjunct for general anesthesia to produce skeletal muscle relaxation during surgery; to facilitate endotracheal intubation. Especially useful for patients with severe renal or hepatic disease, limited cardiac reserve, and in patients with low or atypical pseudocholinesterase levels.

CONTRAINDICATIONS Myasthenia gravis. Safety during pregnancy (category C), lactation, or in children <2 y is not established; continuous IV infusion <2 yrs of age.

CAUTIOUS USE When appreciable histamine release would be hazardous (as in asthma or anaphylactoid reactions, significant cardiovascular disease), neuromuscular disease (e.g., Eaton-Lambert syndrome), carcinomatosis, electrolyte or acid–base imbalances, dehydration, impaired pulmonary function.

ROUTE & DOSAGE

Skeletal Muscle Relaxation

Child: **IV** *1 mo–2 y,* 0.3–0.4 mg/kg initial dose; further doses individualized.
Child/Adult: **IV** *≥2 y,* 0.4–0.5 mg/kg initial dose, then 0.08–0.1 mg/kg 20–45 min after the first dose if necessary, reduce doses if used with general anesthetics

Mechanical Ventilation

Adult: **IV** 5–9 mcg/kg/min by continuous infusion

STORAGE

Store at 2°–8° C (36°–46° F) to preserve potency unless otherwise directed. Avoid freezing.

ADMINISTRATION

Verify correct concentration and rate of infusion for infants and children with physician. Must be given only under direction of anesthesiologist.

Intravenous

PREPARE Direct: Give initial bolus dose undiluted. **Continuous:** Maintenance dose must be diluted with NS, D5W, or D5/NS. Do not mix in same syringe or administer through same needle as used for alkaline solutions (incompatible with alkaline solutions [e.g., barbiturates]).
ADMINISTER Direct: Give as bolus dose. **Continuous:** Give infusion.

ADVERSE EFFECTS CV: Bradycardia, tachycardia. **Respiratory:** <u>Respiratory depression and arrest</u>. **Other:** Increased salivation, <u>anaphylaxis</u>.

INTERACTIONS Drug: General anesthetics increase magnitude and duration of neuromuscular blocking action; aminoglycosides, **bacitracin, clindamycin, lidocaine, parenteral magnesium, polymyxin B, quinidine, quinine, trimethaphan, verapamil** increase neuromuscular blockade; diuretics may increase or decrease neuromuscular blockade; **lithium** prolongs duration of neuromuscular blockade; narcotic analgesics present possibility of additive respiratory depression; **succinylcholine** increases onset and depth of neuromuscular blockade; **phenytoin** may cause resistance to or reversal of neuromuscular blockade.

PHARMACOKINETICS Onset: 2 min. **Peak:** 3–5 min. **Duration:** 60–70 min. **Distribution:** Well distributed to tissues and extracellular fluids; crosses placenta; distribution into breast milk unknown. **Metabolism:** Rapid nonenzymatic degradation in bloodstream. **Elimination:** 70–90% excreted in urine in 5–7 h. **Half-Life:** 20 min.

NURSING IMPLICATIONS

Assessment & Drug Effects

- Lab tests: Baseline serum electrolytes, acid–base balance, and renal function as part of preanesthetic assessment.
- Note: Personnel and equipment required for endotracheal intubation, administration of oxygen under positive pressure, artificial respiration, and assisted or controlled ventilation must be immediately available.
- Evaluate degree of neuromuscular blockade and muscle paralysis to avoid risk of overdosage by qualified individual using peripheral nerve stimulator.
- Monitor BP, pulse, and respirations and evaluate patient's recovery from neuromuscular blocking (curare-like) effect as evidenced by ability to breathe naturally or to take deep breaths and cough, keep eyes open, lift head keeping mouth closed, adequacy of hand-grip strength. Notify physician if recovery is delayed.
- Note: Recovery from neuromuscular blockade usually begins 35–45 min after drug administration and is almost complete in about 1 h. Recovery time may be delayed in patients with cardiovascular disease or in edematous states.

ATROPINE SULFATE 🅟

(a′troe-peen)
Atropair ♣ , Atropisol, Isopto Atropine
Classifications: autonomic nervous system agent; anticholinergic (para-sympatholytic); antimuscarinic
Pregnancy Category: C

AVAILABILITY 0.4 mg tablets; 0.05 mg/mL, 0.1 mg/mL, 0.3 mg/mL, 0.4 mg/mL, 0.5 mg/mL, 0.8 mg/mL, 1 mg/mL injection

ACTIONS Acts by selectively blocking all muscarinic responses to acetylcholine (ACh), whether excitatory or inhibitory. Selective depression of

CNS relieves rigidity and tremor of Parkinson's syndrome. Antisecretory action (vagolytic effect) suppresses sweating, lacrimation, salivation, and secretions from nose, mouth, pharynx, and bronchi. Blocks vagal impulses to heart with resulting decrease in AV conduction time, increase in heart rate and cardiac output, and shortened PR interval.

THERAPEUTIC EFFECTS Atropine is a potent bronchodilator when bronchoconstriction has been induced by parasympathomimetics. Produces mydriasis (dilation of pupils) and cycloplegia (paralysis of accommodation) by blocking responses of iris sphincter muscle and ciliary muscle of lens to cholinergic stimulation.

USES Adjunct in symptomatic treatment of GI disorders (e.g., peptic ulcer, pylorospasm, GI hypermotility, irritable bowel syndrome) and spastic disorders of biliary tract. Relaxes upper GI tract and colon during hypotonic radiography. *Ophthalmic Use:* To produce mydriasis and cycloplegia before refraction and for treatment of anterior uveitis and iritis. *Preoperative Use:* To suppress salivation, perspiration, and respiratory tract secretions; to reduce incidence of laryngospasm, reflex bradycardia arrhythmia, and hypotension during general anesthesia. *Cardiac Uses:* For sinus bradycardia or asystole during CPR or that is induced by drugs or toxic substances (e.g., pilocarpine, beta-adrenergic blockers, organophosphate pesticides, and *Amanita* mushroom poisoning); for management of selected patients with symptomatic sinus bradycardia and associated hypotension and ventricular irritability; for diagnosis of sinus node dysfunction and in evaluation of coronary artery disease during atrial pacing; for management of chronic symptomatic sinus node dysfunction. *Other Uses:* Oral inhalation for short-term treatment and prevention of bronchospasms associated with asthma, bronchitis, and COPD and as drying agent in upper respiratory infection. Adjunctive therapy for hypermotility of GI tract.

CONTRAINDICATIONS Hypersensitivity to belladonna alkaloids; synechiae; angle-closure glaucoma; parotitis; obstructive uropathy, e.g., bladder neck obstruction caused by prostatic hypertrophy; intestinal atony, paralytic ileus, obstructive diseases of GI tract, severe ulcerative colitis, toxic megacolon; tachycardia secondary to cardiac insufficiency or thyrotoxicosis; acute hemorrhage; myasthenia gravis. Safety during pregnancy (category C) or lactation is not established.

CAUTIOUS USE Myocardial infarction, hypertension, hypotension; coronary artery disease, CHF, tachyarrhythmias; gastric ulcer, GI infections, hiatal hernia with reflux esophagitis; hyperthyroidism; chronic lung disease; hepatic or renal disease; older adults; debilitated patients; children <6 y of age; Down syndrome; blond haired/blue eyed, autonomic neuropathy, spastic paralysis, brain damage in children; patients exposed to high environmental temperatures; patients with fever.

ROUTE & DOSAGE

Preanesthesia

Child: **IV/IM/SC** *<5 kg,* 0.02 mg/kg; *>5 kg,* 0.01–0.02 mg/kg 30–60 min before surgery (max 0.4 mg/dose)
Adult: **IV/IM/SC** 0.2–1 mg 30–60 min before surgery

Arrhythmias

Child: **IV/IM** 0.01–0.03 mg/kg q15min for 1–2 doses (max 0.5 mg)
Adult: **IV/IM** 0.5–1 mg q1–2h prn (max 2 mg)

Organophosphate Antidote

Child: **IV/IM** 0.05 mg/kg q10–30min until muscarinic signs and symptoms subside
Adult: **IV/IM** 1–2 mg q5–60min until muscarinic signs and symptoms subside (may need up to 50 mg)

COPD

Child: **Inhalation** 0.03–0.05 mg/kg diluted with 3–5 mL saline, via nebulizer 3–4 times daily
Adult: **Inhalation** 0.025 mg/kg diluted with 3–5 mL saline, via nebulizer 3–4 times daily (max 2.5 mg/day)

Uveitis

Child/Adult: **Ophthalmic** 1–2 drops of solution or small amount of ointment in eye up to t.i.d.

Cycloplegia

Child: **Ophthalmic** 1–2 drops in eye b.i.d. for 1–3 days prior to procedure or a small amount of ointment in conjunctival sac t.i.d. for 1–3 days prior to procedure with last dose applied several hours before the procedure
Adult: **Ophthalmic** 1 drop of solution or small amount of ointment in eye 1 h before the procedure

STORAGE
Store at room temperature 15°–30° C (59°–86° F) in protected airtight, light-resistant containers unless otherwise directed by manufacturer.

ADMINISTRATION

Intravenous

PREPARE **Direct:** Give undiluted or diluted in up to 10 mL of sterile water.
ADMINISTER **Direct:** Give 1 mg or fraction thereof over 1 min directly into a Y-site.

ADVERSE EFFECTS CNS: Headache, ataxia, dizziness, excitement, irritability, convulsions, drowsiness, fatigue, weakness; mental depression, confusion, disorientation, hallucinations. **CV:** Hypertension or hypotension, ventricular tachycardia, palpitation, paradoxical bradycardia, AV dissociation, atrial or <u>ventricular fibrillation</u>. **GI:** Dry mouth with thirst, dysphagia, loss of taste; nausea, vomiting, constipation, delayed gastric emptying, antral stasis, paralytic ileus. **Urogenital:** Urinary hesitancy and retention, dysuria, impotence. **Skin:** Flushed, dry skin; anhidrosis, rash, urticaria, contact dermatitis, allergic conjunctivitis, fixed-drug eruption. **Special Senses:** Mydriasis, blurred vision, photophobia, increased intraocular pressure, cycloplegia, eye dryness, local redness.

DIAGNOSTIC TEST INTERFERENCE *Upper GI series:* Findings may require qualification because of anticholinergic effects of atropine (reduced gastric motility and delayed gastric emptying). *PSP excretion test:* Atropine may decrease urinary excretion of PSP (phenolsulfonphthalein).

INTERACTIONS Drug: Amantadine, ANTIHISTAMINES, TRICYCLIC ANTIDEPRESSANTS, **disopyramide, procainamide, quinidine** add to anticholinergic effects. **Levodopa** effects decreased. **Methotrimeptrazine** may precipitate extrapyramidal effects. Antipsychotic effects of PHENOTHIAZINES are decreased due to decreased absorption.

PHARMACOKINETICS Absorption: Well absorbed from all administration sites. **Peak Effect:** 30 min IM, 2–4 min IV, 1–2 h SC, 1.5–4 h inhalation, 30–40 min topical. **Duration:** Inhibition of salivation 4 h; mydriasis 7–14 days. **Distribution:** Distributed in most body tissues; crosses blood–brain barrier and placenta. **Metabolism:** Metabolized in liver. **Elimination:** 77–94% excreted in urine in 24 h. **Half-Life:** 2–3 h.

NURSING IMPLICATIONS

Assessment & Drug Effects
- Monitor vital signs. HR is a sensitive indicator of patient's response to atropine. Be alert to changes in quality, rate, and rhythm of HR and respiration and to changes in BP and temperature.
- Initial paradoxical bradycardia following IV atropine usually lasts only 1–2 min; it most likely occurs when IV is administered slowly (more than 1 min) or when small doses (less than 0.5 mg) are used. Postural hypotension occurs when patient ambulates too soon after parenteral administration.
- Note: Frequent and continued use of eye preparations, as well as overdosage, can have systemic effects. Some atropine deaths have resulted from systemic absorption following ocular administration in infants and children.
- Monitor I&O, especially after surgery (drug may contribute to urinary retention). Palpate lower abdomen for distention. Have patient void before giving atropine.
- Monitor CNS status. Side rails and supervision of activity may be indicated.
- Monitor infants and small children, for "atropine fever" (hyperpyrexia due to suppression of perspiration and heat loss), which increases the risk of heatstroke.
- Note: Intraocular tension and depth of anterior chamber should be determined before and during therapy with ophthalmic preparations to avoid glaucoma attacks (ophthalmic solutions and ointments are available in various strengths).
- Patients receiving atropine via inhalation sometimes manifest mild CNS stimulation with doses in excess of 5 mg and mental depression and other mental disturbances with larger doses.

Patient & Family Education
- Follow measures to relieve dry mouth: adequate hydration; small, frequent mouth rinses with tepid water; meticulous mouth and dental hygiene; chew gum or suck sugarless sourballs.
- Note: Drug causes drowsiness, sensitivity to light, blurring of near vision, and temporarily impairs ability to judge distance. Avoid driving and other activities requiring visual acuity and mental alertness.

- Discontinue ophthalmic preparations and notify physician if eye pain, conjunctivitis, palpitation, rapid pulse, or dizziness occurs.
- Do not breast feed while taking this drug without consulting physician.
- Store this medication out of reach of children.

AURANOFIN
(au-rane'eh-fin)
Ridaura
Classifications: GOLD COMPOUND; ANTI-INFLAMMATORY; ANTIRHEUMATIC
Prototype: Aurothioglucose
Pregnancy Category: C

AVAILABILITY 3 mg capsules

ACTIONS Strongly lipophilic and almost neutral in solution, properties that may facilitate transport of agent across cell membranes. Action appears to be immunomodulatory: serum immunoglobulin concentrations and rheumatoid factor titers are decreased; and anti-inflammatory: gold is taken up by macrophages with resulting inhibition of phagocytosis and lysosomal enzyme release.

THERAPEUTIC EFFECTS Auranofin is immunomodulatory and anti-inflammatory.

USES Management of active stage of classic or definite rheumatoid arthritis in adults who do not respond to or tolerate other antiarthritis agents (e.g., NSAIDS, other gold compounds).

UNLABELED USES Juvenile rheumatoid arthritis, active SLE, psoriatic arthritis.

CONTRAINDICATIONS History of gold-induced necrotizing enterocolitis, renal disease, exfoliative dermatitis or bone marrow aplasia; patient who has recently received radiation therapy, history of severe toxicity from previous exposure to gold or other heavy metals. Safety during pregnancy (category C), lactation, or by children is not established.

CAUTIOUS USE Inflammatory bowel disease, rash, liver disease, history of bone marrow depression; older adults; diabetes mellitus, CHF.

ROUTE & DOSAGE

Rheumatoid Arthritis
Child: **PO** Initially 0.1 mg/kg/day, may increase to 0.15 mg/kg/day in 1–2 divided doses (max 0.2 mg/kg/day)
Adult: **PO** 6 mg/day divided into 1–2 doses, may increase to 6–9 mg/day divided into 3 doses after 6 mo (max 9 mg/day)

STORAGE
- Store at 15°–30° C (59°–86° F); protect from light and moisture.
- Note: Expiration date is 4 y after date of manufacture.

Common adverse effects in *italic;* life-threatening effects <u>underlined</u>; generic names in **bold;** drug classifications in SMALL CAPS; ◆ Canadian drug name; ⊘ Prototype drug.

ADMINISTRATION

Oral

- Give capsule with food or fluid of patient's choice.

ADVERSE EFFECTS GI: *Diarrhea, abdominal cramping* and pain; *nausea,* vomiting, anorexia, dysphagia; *stomatitis,* glossitis, metallic taste; flatulence, constipation, GI bleeding, melena. **Hematologic:** Thrombocytopenia, leukopenia, eosinophilia, agranulocytosis, aplastic anemia. **Urogenital:** Proteinuria, hematuria, renal failure. **Skin:** *Rash, pruritus,* dermatitis, urticaria.

DIAGNOSTIC TEST INTERFERENCE Auranofin may enhance response to a *tuberculin skin test.*

PHARMACOKINETICS Absorption: 20% absorbed from small intestine. **Peak:** 2 h. **Distribution:** Highest concentrations in kidneys, spleen, lungs, adrenals, and liver; not known if crosses placenta; small amounts distributed into breast milk. **Elimination:** 60% of absorbed gold eliminated in urine, remainder in feces. **Half-Life:** 11–23 days.

NURSING IMPLICATIONS

Assessment & Drug Effects

- Monitor for therapeutic effectiveness, which develops slowly and is not usually apparent for 3–4 mo.
- Report any of following S&S promptly: Unexplained bleeding or bruising, metallic taste, sore mouth; pruritus, rash; diarrhea and melena; yellow skin and sclera; unexplained cough or dyspnea.
- Lab tests: Test for signs of possible impending gold toxicity including decreased Hgb; leukocytes <4000/mm^3; granulocytes <1500/mm^3; platelets <150,000/mm^3; proteinuria >500 mg/day. Also urinary protein and hepatic function.
- Note: Drug-induced thrombocytopenia is usually spontaneously reversible several weeks after drug is withdrawn.
- Continue medical surveillance and supportive therapy after drug is discontinued because adverse effects (such as difficulty in breathing, diarrhea and abdominal pain, fatigue, weakness, unexplained bleeding and bruising, metallic taste) may persist for many months.

Patient & Family Education

- Report adverse effects of therapy, especially abdominal cramping and pain; discontinuance of therapy may be necessary.
- Report metallic taste and pruritus with or without rash. These are among earliest symptoms of impending gold toxicity.
- Do not change dosage (dose or dose interval) by omission, increase, or decrease without first consulting prescriber.
- Use antidiarrheal OTC drug and high-fiber diet for drug-induced diarrhea.
- Avoid exposure to sunlight (especially between 10 a.m. and 4 p.m.) or to artificial ultraviolet light to prevent photosensitivity reaction.
- Rinse mouth with water frequently for symptomatic treatment of mild stomatitis. Avoid commercial mouth rinses; clean teeth with soft toothbrush and gentle brushing to avoid gingival trauma. Floss at least once daily.

- Do not breast feed while taking this drug without consulting physician.
- Store this medication out of reach of children.

AUROTHIOGLUCOSE ⓟ
(aur-oh-thye-oh-gloo'kose)
Gold thioglucose, Solganal
Classifications: GOLD COMPOUND; ANTI-INFLAMMATORY; ANTIRHEUMATIC
Pregnancy Category: C

AVAILABILITY 50 mg/mL injection

ACTIONS Mechanism of anti-inflammatory action not clearly understood. Gold uptake by macrophages with subsequent inhibition of migration and phagocytic action, thereby suppressing immune responsiveness, may be principal mechanism.
THERAPEUTIC EFFECTS Major clinical effect is suppression of joint inflammation in early arthritic disease. Has no effect on reparative process, but studies suggest that it may significantly slow or arrest disease progression.

USES Adjunctive treatment of both adult and juvenile active rheumatoid arthritis. Generally used when adequate trial with salicylates or other NSAIDS has not been satisfactory.
UNLABELED USES Psoriatic arthritis, Felty's syndrome, pemphigus, nondisseminated LE.

CONTRAINDICATIONS Gold allergy or history of severe toxicity from previous therapy with gold or other heavy metals; severe debilitation; uncontrolled diabetes mellitus; renal or hepatic insufficiency, history of hepatitis; uncontrolled CHF; marked hypertension; tuberculosis; severe anemia, hemorrhagic diathesis, agranulocytosis or other blood dyscrasias; disseminated LE, Sjögren's syndrome, recent radiation therapy; colitis; urticaria, eczema, history of exfoliative dermatitis. Safety during pregnancy (category C), lactation, or in children <6 y is not established.
CAUTIOUS USE Older adults; history of drug allergy or hypersensitivity; history of blood dyscrasias; history of renal or hepatic disease; compromised cerebral or cardiovascular circulation; presence of skin rash.

ROUTE & DOSAGE

Rheumatoid Arthritis
Child: **IM** 6–12 y, 0.25–1 mg/kg/wk (max 25 mg) for 20 wk **IM Maintenance Dose** 6–12 y, with improvement, 1 mg/kg (max 25 mg) q2–4wk
Adult: **IM** 10 mg first week, 25 mg second and third week, then 50 mg/wk to a cumulative dose of 1 g **IM Maintenance Dose** with improvement, 25–50 mg q2–3wk, then q3–4wk indefinitely or until adverse effects occur

STORAGE
Store at 15°–30° C (59°–86° F) in light-resistant containers unless otherwise directed. Protect from freezing and light.

ADMINISTRATION

Intramuscular

- Hold vial horizontally and shake vigorously to ensure uniform suspension. Heating vial to body temperature by placing in a warm-water bath facilitates drug withdrawal.
- Give drug by deep IM injection, in a site appropriate for age (see Part I). Use an 18- or 20-gauge, 1½-inch needle (for obese youth or adults a 2-inch needle may be preferable). Patient should be lying down when drug is administered.
- Have patients remain recumbent for 10 min after injection. Observe patient for 20–30 min after injection for hypersensitivity reactions.
- Note: Gold therapy is contraindicated following a severe reaction but may be attempted at reduced initial dosage schedule with careful monitoring after a mild reaction.

ADVERSE EFFECTS Body as a Whole: Hypersensitivity (<u>anaphylactic shock</u>, syncope, bradycardia, thickening of tongue, dysphagia, dyspnea), fever. **GI:** Nausea, vomiting, abdominal cramps, anorexia, metallic taste, diarrhea, hepatitis. **Hematologic:** Eosinophilia, <u>agranulocytosis</u>, thrombocytopenia, leukopenia, granulocytopenia, aplastic anemia. **Respiratory:** Pulmonary fibrosis, interstitial pneumonitis. **Skin:** *Pruritus, urticaria, erythema,* "gold dermatitis," fixed-drug eruptions, <u>exfoliative dermatitis</u> with alopecia and nail shedding; gingivitis, glossitis, <u>Stevens-Johnson syndrome</u>, photosensitivity reactions. **Urogenital:** Nephrotic syndrome, proteinuria, hematuria, vaginitis, nephrotic syndrome. **Other:** Immunologic destruction of synovial fluid, exacerbation of arthralgia (temporary), local irritation at injection site.

DIAGNOSTIC TEST INTERFERENCE Low *PBI* (by *chloric acid method*); test interference may persist for several weeks after gold therapy is discontinued.

INTERACTIONS ANTIMALARIALS, IMMUNOSUPPRESSANTS, **penicillamine, phenylbutazone** increase risk of blood dyscrasias.

PHARMACOKINETICS Absorption: Slowly and irregularly absorbed from IM site. **Peak:** 4–6 h. **Distribution:** Widely distributed, especially to synovial fluid; does not cross blood–brain barrier; crosses placenta. **Metabolism:** Unknown. **Elimination:** 50–90% of dose ultimately excreted in urine; 10–50% in feces; excreted into breast milk. **Half-Life:** 3–27 days.

NURSING IMPLICATIONS

Assessment & Drug Effects

- Monitor therapeutic effectiveness, which may not be apparent before 6–8 wk of gold therapy.
- Lab tests: Baseline renal and hepatic function tests, CBC, and urinalysis prior to initiation of therapy. Thereafter, perform urinalysis (for protein and sediment) before each injection. Determine CBC (including Hgb, RBC, WBC and differential, platelet counts) before every second injection throughout therapy.
- Withhold drug and notify physician of any of the following: Platelet count <100,000/mm^3, or leukocytes <4000/mm^3, granulocytes <1500/mm^3, eosinophils >5%, rapid fall in Hgb value, and presence of proteinuria or hematuria.

- Rule out pregnancy before gold treatment begins. Women of childbearing age should be warned about the potential hazards of becoming pregnant during therapy and counseled about the use of birth control.
- Note: During early treatment, some patients complain of exacerbation of joint pain after injection. It usually subsides after the first few injections.
- Monitor S&S of beginning gold toxicity. Toxicity generally involves skin and mucous membranes anywhere in body. Inspect skin carefully and examine mouth and throat. Report any of the following promptly: Itching that often precedes dermatitis and eosinophilia, bruising or bleeding, tenderness, metallic taste that frequently precedes sore mouth, tongue, or throat, gray-blue discoloration of skin and mucous membranes, diarrhea or loose stools, indigestion, unexplained malaise; signs of hepatotoxicity (yellow sclerae and skin, clay-colored stools, dark urine, pruritus).
- Note: Rapid improvement in joint pain and mobility also may signify that patient is approaching toxic tissue levels. Interruption of therapy, at least temporarily, may be indicated. Notify physician.

Patient & Family Education
- Review with health care provider and understand the list of possible adverse effects that should be reported. If therapy is interrupted at the onset of gold toxicity, serious reactions can be avoided.
- Note: Adverse reactions are most likely to occur during second and third month of therapy or when cumulative aurothioglucose dose is 300–500 mg. However, they may appear at any time during therapy or several months after treatment has been discontinued.
- Report any unusual color or odor to urine, or change in I&O ratio and pattern.
- Report unusual fatigue or weakness, malaise, chills, fever, sore throat; possible signs of bleeding (e.g., bleeding gums, nosebleeds, dark urine, black stools, petechiae, purpura, easy bruising). Report signs of hepatotoxicity (see Appendix D-1).
- Avoid contact with anyone who has a cold, recent vaccination, or has been exposed recently to a communicable disease.
- Report to physician need to increase the amount of aspirin or other prescribed NSAID for pain because this may indicate diminishing response to gold therapy.
- Minimize exposure to sunlight and artificial ultraviolet light because gray to blue pigmentation may occur on light-exposed skin areas.
- Use careful and thorough oral hygiene. Avoid overuse of mouthwashes, which contain alcohol; these enhance drying and irritation, and can change mouth flora.
- Do not breast feed while taking this drug without consulting physician.

AZELAIC ACID
(a′ze-laic)
Azelex, Finevin
Classifications: SKIN AND MUCOUS MEMBRANE AGENT; ANTIACNE
Prototype: Isotretinoin
Pregnancy Category: B

AVAILABILITY 20% cream

ACTIONS Azelaic acid is a naturally occurring dicarboxylic acid. The antimicrobial action may be attributable to inhibition of the microbial cellular protein synthesis. A normalization of keratinization may also contribute to its clinical effectiveness.
THERAPEUTIC EFFECTS Topical 20% azelaic acid possesses antimicrobial activity against *Propionibacterium acnes* and *Staphylococcus epidermidis*.

USES Mild to moderate inflammatory acne vulgaris.

CONTRAINDICATIONS Hypersensitivity to any component in the drug.
CAUTIOUS USE Dark complexion, pregnancy (category B), lactation. Safety and efficacy in children <12 y is not established.

ROUTE & DOSAGE

Acne Vulgaris
Child/Adult: **Topical** *>12 y,* apply thin film to clean and dry area b.i.d.

STORAGE
Store at 15°–30° C (59°–86° F).

ADMINISTRATION

Topical
- Wash and dry skin thoroughly prior to application of drug.
- Apply by thoroughly massaging a thin film of the cream into the affected area. Avoid occlusive dressing.
- Wash hands before and after application of cream.

ADVERSE EFFECTS Skin: Pruritus, burning, stinging, tingling, erythema, dryness, rash, peeling, irritation, contact dermatitis, vitiligo depigmentation, hypertrichosis. **Other:** Worsening of asthma.

PHARMACOKINETICS Absorption: Approximately 4% is absorbed through the skin. **Onset:** 4–8 wk. **Distribution:** Distributes into all tissues. **Metabolism:** Partially metabolized by beta oxidation in liver. **Elimination:** Excreted primarily in urine. **Half-Life:** 12 h.

NURSING IMPLICATIONS

Assessment & Drug Effects
- Assess for signs of hypopigmentation and report immediately.
- Monitor for sensitivity or severe irritation, which may warrant drug dosage reduction or discontinuation.

Patient & Family Education
- Learn proper application of cream and avoid contact with eyes or mucous membranes.
- Wash eyes with copious amounts of water if contact with medication occurs.

- Note: Transient pruritus, burning, and stinging are common; however, severe skin irritation or hypopigmentation should be reported.
- Do not breast feed while using this drug without consulting prescriber.
- Store this medication out of reach of children.

AZELASTINE HYDROCHLORIDE

(a-ze-las'teen)
Astelin, Optivar
Classifications: ANTIHISTAMINE; H_1-RECEPTOR ANTAGONIST; OCULAR ANTIHISTAMINE
Prototype: Diphenhydramine
Pregnancy Category: C

AVAILABILITY 137 mcg/spray nasal spray; 0.05% ophthalmic solution

ACTIONS First-generation antihistamine that is a potent histamine H_1-receptor antagonist.
THERAPEUTIC EFFECTS Effective in the symptomatic treatment of seasonal allergic rhinitis and as a nasal decongestant.

USES: Seasonal allergic rhinitis, itching associated with allergic conjunctivitis.

CONTRAINDICATIONS Hypersensitivity to azelastine; concurrent use of CNS depressants; pregnancy (category C), lactation, children <3 y.
CAUTIOUS USE Hepatic or renal disease; children <11 y; asthmatics.

ROUTE & DOSAGE

Allergic Rhinitis
Child: **Intranasal** *5–11 y,* 1 spray per nostril b.i.d.
Adult: **Intranasal** 2 sprays per nostril b.i.d.

STORAGE
Store the bottle upright at room temperature at 15°–30° C (59°–86° F). Should be discarded three months after priming.

ADMINISTRATION
Intranasal
- Prime delivery unit before first use (see manufacturer's instructions).
- Instruct patient to clear nasal passages prior to drug installation; then, tilt head forward slightly and sniff gently when drug is sprayed into each nostril.

ADVERSE EFFECTS Body as a Whole: Fatigue, dizziness. **GI:** Dry mouth, nausea. **Metabolic:** Weight gain. **CNS:** *Headache, somnolence.* **Respiratory:** Pharyngitis, *rhinitis,* paroxysmal sneezing, *cough,* asthma. **Special Senses:** *Bitter taste,* nasal burning, epistaxis, conjunctivitis.

INTERACTIONS Drug: Alcohol and CNS DEPRESSANTS may cause reduced alertness.

PHARMACOKINETICS Absorption: 40% absorbed from nasal inhalation. **Peak:** 2–3 h. **Metabolism:** Metabolized by CYP450 to active metabolites. **Elimination:** Excreted primarily in feces. **Half-Life:** 22 h.

NURSING IMPLICATIONS

Assessment & Drug Effects

- Monitor level of alertness especially with concurrent use of other CNS depressants.

Patient & Family Education

- Follow manufacturer's directions for priming the metered-dose spray unit before first use and after storage of >3 day.
- Tilt head forward while instilling spray. Avoid getting spray in eyes.
- Do not drive or engage in potentially hazardous activities until response to drug is known.
- Avoid concurrent use of CNS depressants, such as alcohol, while taking this drug.
- Discard spray unit and dispensing package bottle after 3 mo.
- Do not breast feed while using this drug.
- Store this medication out of reach of children.

AZITHROMYCIN

(a-zi-thro-mye'sin)
Zithromax
Classifications: ANTI-INFECTIVE; MACROLIDE ANTIBIOTIC
Prototype: Erythromycin
Pregnancy Category: B

AVAILABILITY 250 mg, 600 mg tablets; 100 mg/5 mL, 200 mg/5 mL, 1 g/packet oral suspension; 500 mg injection

ACTIONS A macrolide antibiotic that reversibly binds to the 50S ribosomal subunit of susceptible organisms and consequently inhibits protein synthesis.
THERAPEUTIC EFFECTS Effective for treatment of mild to moderate infections caused by pyogenic streptococci, *Streptococcus pneumoniae, Haemophilus influenzae,* and *Staphylococcus aureus.*

USES Pneumonia, lower respiratory tract infections, pharyngitis/tonsillitis, gonorrhea, nongonococcal urethritis, skin and skin structure infections due to susceptible organisms, otitis media, *Mycobacterium avium–intracellulare complex* infections.
UNLABELED USES Bronchitis, *Helicobacter pylori* gastritis.

CONTRAINDICATIONS Hypersensitivity to azithromycin, erythromycin, or any of the macrolide antibiotics.
CAUTIOUS USE Older adults or debilitated persons, hepatic or renal impairment, ventricular arrhythmias, pregnancy (category B), and lactation.

ROUTE & DOSAGE

Bacterial Infections

Child: **PO** ≥*6 mo,* 10 mg/kg on day 1, then 5 mg/kg for 4 more days (max 250 mg/day)
Adult: **PO** 500 mg on day 1, then 250 mg q24h for 4 more days **IV** 500 mg daily times at least 2 days, administer 1 mg/mL over 3 h or 2 mg/mL over 1 h

Otitis Media

Child: **PO** >*6 mo,* 30 mg/kg as a single dose *or* 10 mg/kg once daily (not to exceed 500 mg/day) for 3 days *or* 10 mg/kg as a single dose on day 1 followed by 5 mg/kg/day on days 2–5

Pharyngitis/Tonsillitis

Child: >*2 y,* 12 mg/kg/day × 5 days

Gonorrhea

Adult: **PO** 2 g as a single dose

Chancroid

Child: **PO** 20 mg/kg as single dose (max 1 g)
Adult: **PO** 1 g in a single dose

STORAGE

Store drug when diluted as directed for 24 h at or below 30° C (86° F) or for 7 days under 5° C (41° F).

ADMINISTRATION

Oral

- Tablets may be taken without regard to food.
- Do not give within 2 h of administration of an aluminum- or magnesium-containing antacid.

Intravenous

PREPARE **Intermittent:** Reconstitute 500-mg vial with 4.8 mL of sterile water for injection and shake until dissolved. Final concentration is 100 mg/mL. Solution must be further diluted to 1.0 or 2.0 mg/mL by adding 5 mL of the 100 mg/mL solution to 500 mL or 250 mL, respectively, of D5W, D5/NS, 0.45NS, or other compatible solution.
ADMINISTER **Intermittent:** Administer diluted solution over at least 60 min. Do not give a bolus dose.

ADVERSE EFFECTS CNS: Headache, dizziness. **GI:** Nausea, vomiting, diarrhea, abdominal pain; hepatotoxicity, mild elevations in liver function tests.

DIAGNOSTIC TEST INTERFERENCE Liver function tests: Reversible, asymptomatic elevations in *liver enzymes (AST, ALT, gamma glutamyl transferase, alkaline phosphatase)* have been reported in some patients treated with azithromycin.

INTERACTIONS Drug: ANTACIDS may decrease peak level of azithromycin. **Food:** Food will decrease the amount of azithromycin absorbed by 50%.

Common adverse effects in *italic;* life-threatening effects underlined; generic names in **bold;** drug classifications in SMALL CAPS; ✦ Canadian drug name; ❂ Prototype drug.

PHARMACOKINETICS Absorption: 37% of dose reaches the systemic circulation. **Onset:** 48 h. **Peak:** 2.5–4 h. **Distribution:** Extensively distributed to most tissues including sputum, blister, and vaginal secretions; tissue concentrations are often higher than serum concentrations. **Metabolism:** Metabolized in liver. **Elimination:** 5–12% of dose is excreted in urine; 50% eliminated in the bile. **Half-Life:** Increases with time after the dose due to slow elimination from tissue sites; ranges from 9.6–40 h.

NURSING IMPLICATIONS

Assessment & Drug Effects

- Monitor for and report loose stools or diarrhea because pseudomembranous colitis (see Appendix D-1) must be ruled out.
- Monitor PT and INR closely with concurrent warfarin use.

Patient & Family Education

- Take aluminum or magnesium antacids 2 h before or after drug.
- Report onset of loose stools or diarrhea.
- Do not breast feed while taking this drug without consulting prescriber.
- Store this medication out of reach of children.

AZTREONAM

(az-tree′oh-nam)

Azactam

Classifications: ANTI-INFECTIVE; BETA-LACTAM ANTIBIOTIC
Prototype: Imipenem-Cilastatin
Pregnancy Category: B

AVAILABILITY 500 mg, 1 g, 2 g vials

ACTIONS Differs structurally from other beta-lactam antibiotics (penicillins and cephalosporins) in having a monocyclic rather than a bicyclic nucleus. Acts by inhibiting synthesis of bacterial cell wall, primarily in aerobic, gram-negative bacteria.

THERAPEUTIC EFFECTS Highly resistant to beta-lactamases and does not readily induce their formation. Spectrum of activity limited to aerobic, gram-negative bacteria. Therapeutically active against *Haemophilus influenzae, Pseudomonas aeruginosa, Neisseria gonorrhoeae,* and against Enterobacteriaceae including most strains of *E. coli, Enterobacter, Klebsiella, Proteus, Providencia, Shigella, Salmonella,* and *Serratia.* There appears to be little cross-allergenicity with penicillins and cephalosporins.

USES Gram-negative infections of urinary tract, lower respiratory tract, skin and skin structures; and for intra-abdominal and gynecologic infections, septicemia, and as adjunctive therapy for surgical infections. Often used in combination with other antibiotics active against gram-positive and anaerobic bacteria in mixed infections.

CONTRAINDICATIONS Safety during pregnancy (category B), lactation, or on infants <9 mo is not established.

Common adverse effects in *italic;* life-threatening effects <u>underlined;</u> generic names in **bold;** drug classifications in SMALL CAPS; ◆ Canadian drug name; ⊘ Prototype drug.

155

CAUTIOUS USE History of hypersensitivity reaction to penicillin, cephalosporins, or to other drugs; impaired renal or hepatic function.

ROUTE & DOSAGE

Urinary Tract Infection
Adult: **IV/IM** 0.5–1 g q8–12h

Moderate to Severe Infections
Neonate: **IV/IM** *<7 day,* 60–90 mg/kg/day divided into doses q8–12h; *>7 days,* 60–120 mg/kg/day divided into doses q6–12h
Child: **IV/IM** *> 1 mo,* 90–120 mg/kg/day divided into doses q6–8h
Adult: **IV/IM** 1–2 g q6–8h (max 8 g/24 h)

Cystic Fibrosis
Child: **IV/IM** 50–200 mg/kg q6–8h (max 8 g/day)

STORAGE

Store powder for injection at <40° C (104° F), protected from light and moisture. Once reconstituted, is stable for 48 h at 15°–30° C (59°–86° F), or for 7 days when refrigerated at 2°–8° C (35°–46° F). If reconstituted with sodium chloride with benzyl alcohol or parabens, use immediately.

ADMINISTRATION

Intramuscular

- Reconstitute with at least 3 mL of diluent per gram of drug for IM injection. Immediately and vigorously shake vial to dissolve. Suitable diluents include sterile water for injection; bacteriostatic water for injection (with benzyl alcohol except for neonates and propyl parabens); NS 0.9% for injection.
- Give IM injections deeply into large muscle mass such as the lateral thigh (see Part I). Rotate injection sites.

Intravenous

- Verify correct IV concentration and rate of infusion/injection with physician before giving to neonates, infants, and children.

PREPARE **Direct:** Reconstitute a single dose with 6–10 mL of sterile water for injection. Immediately shake vial until solution is dissolved. Reconstituted solutions are colorless to light straw yellow and turn slightly pink on standing. **Intermittent:** Each gram of reconstituted aztreonam must be further diluted in at least 50 mL of D5W, NS, or other solution approved by manufacturer to yield a concentration not to exceed 20 mg/mL.

ADMINISTER **Direct:** Give over 3–5 min. **Intermittent:** Give over 20–60 min through Y-Site.

INCOMPATIBILITIES **Solution/Additive: Ampicillin, cephdrine, metronidazole, nafcillin.**

ADVERSE EFFECTS Body as a Whole: Hypersensitivity (urticaria, eosinophilia, <u>anaphylaxis</u>). **CNS:** Headache, dizziness, confusion, paresthesias, insomnia, seizures. **GI:** Nausea, *diarrhea,* vomiting, elevated

---

Common adverse effects in *italic;* life-threatening effects <u>underlined</u>; generic names in **bold;** drug classifications in SMALL CAPS; ♣ Canadian drug name; ☻ Prototype drug.

liver function tests. **Hematologic:** Eosinophilia. **Special Senses:** Tinnitus, nasal congestion, sneezing, diplopia. **Skin:** Rash, purpura, erythema multiforme, exfoliative dermatitis, diaphoresis; petechiae, pruritus. **Other:** Local reactions (phlebitis, thrombophlebitis [following IV], pain at injection sites), superinfections (gram-positive cocci), vaginal candidiasis.

DIAGNOSTIC TEST INTERFERENCE Aztreonam may cause transient elevations of *liver function tests,* increases in *PT* and *PTT,* minor changes in *Hgb,* and positive *Coombs' test.*

INTERACTIONS Drug: Imipenem-cilastatin, cefoxitin may be antagonistic; **probenecid** slows renal elimination of aztreonam.

PHARMACOKINETICS Peak: 1 h IM. **Distribution:** Widely distributed including synovial and blister fluid, bile, bronchial secretions, prostate, bone, and CSF; crosses placenta; distributed into breast milk in small amounts. **Metabolism:** Not extensively metabolized. **Elimination:** 60–70% excreted in urine within 24 h. **Half-Life:** 1.6–2.1 h.

NURSING IMPLICATIONS

Assessment & Drug Effects

- Lab tests: Obtain baseline C&S test prior to initiation of therapy. Start drug pending results.
- Baseline and periodic renal function tests, particularly in those with history of renal impairment.
- Inspect IV injection sites daily for signs of inflammation. Pain and phlebitis occur in a significant number of patients.

Patient & Family Education

- Determine previous hypersensitivity reactions to penicillins, cephalosporins, and other allergens prior to therapy.
- Monitor for S&S of opportunistic infections (diarrhea, rectal or vaginal itching or discharge, fever, cough) and promptly report onset to physician. Overgrowth of nonsusceptible organisms, particularly *staphylococci, streptococci,* and fungi, is a threat, especially in patients receiving prolonged or repeated therapy.
- Note: IV therapy may cause a change in taste sensation. Report interference with eating.
- Do not breast feed while taking this drug without consulting physician.

BACAMPICILLIN HYDROCHLORIDE

(ba-kam-pi-sill′in)
Penglobe ♣, Spectrobid
Classifications: ANTI-INFECTIVE; ANTIBIOTIC; AMINOPENICILLIN
Prototype: Ampicillin
Pregnancy Category: B

AVAILABILITY 400 mg tablets

Common adverse effects in *italic;* life-threatening effects underlined; generic names in **bold;** drug classifications in SMALL CAPS; ♣ Canadian drug name; ☻ Prototype drug.

157

B

ACTIONS Acid-stable, penicillinase-sensitive aminopenicillin that is rapidly hydrolyzed to ampicillin in body. Has broad spectrum of antimicrobial activity and exerts antibacterial action by inhibiting bacterial cell wall synthesis. More rapidly and completely absorbed from GI tract than ampicillin is, and serum concentrations attained are higher.
THERAPEUTIC EFFECTS Bacampicillin has a broad spectrum of antimicrobial activity against both gram-positive and gram-negative organisms.

USES Infections caused by susceptible microorganisms of upper and lower respiratory tract, urinary tract, skin and skin structures; acute uncomplicated gonorrhea.

CONTRAINDICATIONS Hypersensitivity to penicillins; pregnancy (category B); infectious mononucleosis or other viral diseases; children <25 kg.
CAUTIOUS USE History of allergy to cephalosporins; lactation.

ROUTE & DOSAGE

Moderate to Severe Infections
Child: **PO** 12.5–25 mg/kg q12h
Adult: **PO** 400–800 mg q12h

Gonorrhea
Adult: **PO** 1.6 g with 1 g probenecid for 1 dose

STORAGE
Store in tight container at 15°–30° C (59°–86° F) unless otherwise directed.

ADMINISTRATION
Oral
- Note: Tablets may be given without regard to food.
- Do not give concurrently with disulfiram (Antabuse).

ADVERSE EFFECTS Body as a Whole: Hypersensitivity (erythematous rash, anaphylaxis). **GI:** *Nausea,* vomiting, anorexia, *diarrhea.* **Hematologic:** Thrombocytopenia, eosinophilia, anemia. **Other:** Superinfections, fixed-drug eruption.

DIAGNOSTIC TEST INTERFERENCE High urine bacampicillin concentrations can result in false-positive ***urine glucose determinations with copper sulfate tests*** (Benedict's, Clinitest, Fehling's); ***glucose oxidase*** methods (Clinistix, TesTape) are not affected. ***Serum ALT*** and ***AST*** may increase.

INTERACTIONS Drug: Allopurinol increases incidence of rash; because ampicillin may interfere with ORAL CONTRACEPTIVE action, female patients should be advised to utilize nonhormonal contraception while on ANTIBIOTICS. **Food:** May decrease absorption of bacampicillin suspension; give 1 h before or 2 h after meals.

PHARMACOKINETICS Absorption: Rapidly and almost completely absorbed; hydrolyzed to ampicillin. **Distribution:** Most body tissues; crosses placenta; appears in breast milk. **Metabolism:** Metabolized in liver.

Common adverse effects in *italic;* life-threatening effects underlined; generic names in **bold;** drug classifications in SMALL CAPS; ♣ Canadian drug name; ☻ Prototype drug.

Elimination: 75% eliminated as ampicillin in urine within 8 h. **Half-Life:** 0.7–1.1 h.

NURSING IMPLICATIONS

Assessment & Drug Effects

- Determine previous hypersensitivity reactions to penicillins, cephalosporins, and other allergens prior to therapy.
- Lab tests: Baseline C&S tests prior to initiation of therapy; start drug pending results.
- Baseline and periodic checks of renal, hepatic, and hematopoietic status are advised during prolonged therapy, particularly in patients with history of impaired function of these systems, and in premature infants and neonates.

Patient & Family Education

- Report symptoms of an allergic hypersensitivity reaction immediately (see Appendix D-1).
- Report signs of superinfection.
- Take entire course of medication as prescribed.
- Do not breast feed while taking this drug without consulting physician.
- Store this medication out of reach of children.

BACITRACIN

(bass-i-tray′sin)
Baciguent, Bacitin
Classifications: ANTI-INFECTIVE; ANTIBIOTIC
Pregnancy Category: C

AVAILABILITY 50,000 unit vial; 500 units/g cream, powder, aerosol spray, 500 units/g ophthalmic ointment **Combination Products:** Available in topical forms with polymyxin B, neomycin, hydrocortisone, lidocaine

ACTIONS Polypeptide antibiotic derived from cultures of *Bacillus subtilis*. Precise mechanism of action not known. Appears to interfere with function of bacterial cell membrane by inhibiting cell wall synthesis. Spectrum of antibacterial activity similar to that of penicillin. Bactericidal or bacteriostatic depending on concentration and susceptibility of organism.

THERAPEUTIC EFFECTS Active against many gram-positive organisms including *Streptococci, Staphylococci, Pneumococci, Corynebacteria, Clostridia, Neisseria, Haemophilus influenzae,* and *Treponema pallidum*. Also active against *Gonococci* and *Meningococci;* ineffective against most other gram-negative organisms.

USES Parenteral therapy restricted to infants with *Staphylococcal* pneumonia and empyema due to susceptible organisms where adequate laboratory facilities and constant supervision are available. Used topically in treatment of superficial infections of skin.

Common adverse effects in *italic;* life-threatening effects <u>underlined</u>; generic names in **bold;** drug classifications in SMALL CAPS; ♣ Canadian drug name; ⊘ Prototype drug.

159

B

UNLABELED USES Orally for treatment of antibiotic-associated colitis. Has been used investigationally by various routes (intrathecal, intrapleural, intrasynovial) for serious infections.

CONTRAINDICATIONS Toxic reaction or renal dysfunction associated with bacitracin; impaired renal function; atopic individuals; pregnancy (category C).

CAUTIOUS USE Myasthenia gravis or other neuromuscular disease. Patients allergic to neomycin may be sensitive to bacitracin.

ROUTE & DOSAGE

Systemic Infections

Infant: **IM** <2.5 kg: up to 900 units/kg/24 h divided into doses given q8–12h; >2.5 kg: up to 1000 units/kg/24 h divided into doses given q8–12h (max treatment 12 days)
Adult: IM 10,000–25,000 units/6 h (max total daily dose 100,000 units)

Skin Infections

Adult: **Topical** Apply thin layer of ointment, powder or spray b.i.d. or t.i.d. and cover with dressing. May be dissolved in 0.9% sodium chloride or sterile water for injection and used as solution of 250–1000 units/mL for wet compress

Eye Infections

Apply 500 units/g ophthalmic ointment to eye daily, b.i.d., or t.i.d.

STORAGE

Dry bacitracin vials should be stored in refrigerator at 2°–8° C (36°–46° F). Store solution for a maximum of 1 wk if refrigerated. Inactivation occurs at room temperature. Store ointments in tightly closed containers at 15°–30° C (59°–86° F) unless otherwise directed.

ADMINISTRATION

Intramuscular

- Do not use parenteral bacitracin for longer than 12 days.
- Reconstitute with NS containing 2% procaine hydrochloride (prescribed). Do not reconstitute with diluents containing parabens because solution may precipitate or become cloudy.
- Alternate injection sites because injections are painful.

Topical

- Clean affected area prior to application. May be covered with a sterile bandage.

ADVERSE EFFECTS GI: Anorexia, nausea, vomiting, diarrhea, rectal itching and burning. **Hematologic:** Systemic use: Bone marrow depression, blood dyscrasias; eosinophilia. **Body as a Whole:** Hypersensitivity (erythema, anaphylaxis). **Urogenital:** Nephrotoxicity, dose related: Increased BUN, uremia, renal tubular and glomerular necrosis. **Special Senses:** Tinnitus. **Skin:** Redness, burning, itching. **Other:** Pain and inflammation at injection site, fever, superinfection, neuromuscular blockade with respiratory depression.

INTERACTIONS Drug: With AMINOGLYCOSIDES, possibility of additive nephrotoxic and neuromuscular blocking effects; with **tubocurarine** and other NONDEPOLARIZING SKELETAL MUSCLE RELAXANTS, possibility of additive neuromuscular blocking effects.

PHARMACOKINETICS Absorption: Poorly absorbed from intact or denuded skin or mucous membranes. **Peak:** 1–2 h IM. **Duration:** 6–8 h. **Distribution:** Widely distributed including peritoneal and ascitic fluids. **Elimination:** Slow renal excretion (10–40% in 24 h).

NURSING IMPLICATIONS

Assessment & Drug Effects

- Lab tests: Baseline C&S tests prior to initiation of therapy; start drug pending results.
- Determine BUN and nonprotein nitrogen (NPN); examine urine for albumin, casts, and cellular elements, before systemic therapy is started. Monitor renal function daily throughout therapy.
- Watch for signs of local allergic reaction (itching, burning, redness) with topical skin applications. Local reactions have preceded life-threatening anaphylactic episodes.
- Monitor I&O during parenteral therapy. Adequate urinary output is important to reduce possibility of renal toxicity. If fluid intake is inadequate or urinary output decreases, report to physician.
- Inspect urine for turbidity and hematuria, and watch for other S&S of urinary tract dysfunction. Report any changes in urination pattern (e.g., oliguria, urinary frequency, nocturia).
- Note: Prolonged use may result in overgrowth of nonsusceptible organisms, especially *Candida albicans.*

Patient & Family Education

- Report local allergic reactions with topical applications (e.g., itching, burning, redness).
- Store this medication out of reach of children.

BACLOFEN

(bak'loe-fen)
Lioresal, Lioresal DS
Classifications: AUTONOMIC NERVOUS SYSTEM AGENT; CENTRAL-ACTING SKELETAL MUSCLE RELAXANT
Prototype: Cyclobenzaprine
Pregnancy Category: C

AVAILABILITY 10 mg, 20 mg tablets; 500 mcg/mL, 2000 mcg/mL ampules for intrathecal injection and for use with compatible intrathecal pump

ACTIONS Centrally acting skeletal muscle relaxant. Precise mechanism of action not determined. Depresses monosynaptic and polysynaptic afferent reflex activity at spinal cord level.
THERAPEUTIC EFFECTS Reduces skeletal muscle spasm caused by upper motor neuron lesions.

B

USES To provide symptomatic relief of painful spasms in cerebral palsy, multiple sclerosis, and in the management of detrusor sphincter dyssynergia in spinal cord injury or disease.
UNLABELED USES Treatment of trigeminal neuralgia and of tardive dystonia associated with antipsychotic medications.

CONTRAINDICATIONS Safety during pregnancy (category C) lactation is not established.
CAUTIOUS USE Impaired renal and hepatic function; epilepsy; diabetes mellitus; stroke; psychiatric or brain disorders; older adults, children, especially intrathecal dosing.

ROUTE & DOSAGE

Muscle Spasm

Child: **PO** *2–7 y:* 10–15 mg/day divided into doses given q8h, may increase by 5–15 mg/day q3days (max 40 mg/day); *≥8 y:* 10–15 mg/day divided into doses given q8h, may increase by 5–15 mg/day q3days (max 60 mg/day)
Adult: **PO** 5 mg t.i.d., may increase by 5 mg/dose q3day prn (max 80 mg/day)
Child: **Intrathecal** Prior to infusion pump implantation, initiate trial dose of 25 mcg/mL bolus administered in intrathecal space. If response is positive, this becomes initial dose with pump. Daily dose can be increased slowly by 5–15% increments at 24 h intervals until condition improves. In children <12 y dose ranges from 24–1200 mcg daily, with an average dose of 274 mcg.
Adult: **Intrathecal** Prior to infusion pump implantation, initiate trial dose of 50 mcg/mL bolus administered in intrathecal space by barbotage over ≤1 min. Observe patient during next 4–8 h for significant decrease in muscle spasm. If response is less than desired, administer second bolus of 75 mcg/1.5 mL and observe 4–8 h. May repeat in 24 h with a 100 mcg/2 mL bolus if necessary. *Postimplant titration:* Use screening dose if response lasted >12 h or double screening dose if response lasted <12 h and administer over 24 h. After first 24 h, decrease dose by 10–30% q24h until desired response achieved. Maintenance doses range from 12–1500 mcg/day, with most patients maintained on 300–800 mcg/day

STORAGE

Store at 15°–30° C (59°–86° F) in tightly closed container unless otherwise directed.

ADMINISTRATION

Oral
▪ Give with food or milk to avoid GI distress.

Intrathecal
▪ Give by direct intrathecal injection (via lumbar puncture or catheter) over at least 1 min or longer. Must be administered by physician with expertise in neurologic treatment.

Common adverse effects in *italic;* life-threatening effects <u>underlined;</u> generic names in **bold;** drug classifications in SMALL CAPS; ♣ Canadian drug name; ❂ Prototype drug.

- Dilute *only* with sterile, preservative-free NS injection. Baclofen must be diluted to a concentration of 50 mcg/mL when preparing test doses.
- Intrathecal infusion pump: Do not abruptly discontinue because serious adverse effects may develop.

ADVERSE EFFECTS CNS: *Transient drowsiness,* vertigo, dizziness, weakness, fatigue, headache, confusion, insomnia; ataxia, loss of seizure control in epileptic patients; abrupt discontinuation of intrathecal administration may result in high fever, altered mental status, exaggerated rebound spasticity, and muscle rigidity that in rare cases has advanced to rhabdomyolysis, multiple organ-system failure, and death. **CV:** Hypotension. **Special Senses:** Tinnitus, nasal congestion; blurred vision, mydriasis, nystagmus, diplopia, strabismus, miosis. **GI:** Nausea, constipation, vomiting; mild increases in AST and alkaline phosphatase, jaundice. **Urogenital:** Urinary frequency.

DIAGNOSTIC TEST INTERFERENCE Possibility of increases in *blood glucose,* serum *alkaline phosphatase,* and *AST* levels.

INTERACTIONS Drug: Alcohol, CNS DEPRESSANTS, MAOIS, ANTIHISTAMINES compound CNS depression; baclofen may increase blood **glucose** levels, making it necessary to increase dosage of SULFONYLUREAS, **insulin.**

PHARMACOKINETICS Absorption: Readily absorbed from GI tract. **Peak:** 2–3 h. **Duration:** 8 h. **Distribution:** Minimal amounts cross blood–brain barrier; crosses placenta; distribution into breast milk unknown. **Metabolism:** 15% of dose metabolized in liver. **Elimination:** 70–85% excreted in urine within 72 h; some elimination in feces. **Half-Life:** 3–4 h.

NURSING IMPLICATIONS

Assessment & Drug Effects

- Supervise ambulation. Initially, the loss of spasticity induced by baclofen may affect patient's ability to stand or walk.
- Lab tests: Baseline and periodic BP, weight, blood sugar, hepatic function tests, and urine.
- Monitor for adverse neuropsychiatric or genitourinary symptoms that resemble those of the underlying disease. Assess them carefully and report to the physician.
- Observe carefully for side effects: mental confusion, depression, hallucinations.
- Monitor patients with epilepsy closely for possible loss of seizure control.

Patient & Family Education

- Note: CNS depressant effects will be additive to other CNS depressants, including alcohol.
- Monitor blood glucose for loss of glycemic control if diabetic.
- Do not drive or engage in other potentially hazardous activities until the response to drug is known.
- Report adverse reactions to physician. Most can be reduced by decreasing dosage. Incidence of CNS symptoms (drowsiness, dizziness, ataxia) is reportedly high in patients >40 y of age.

Common adverse effects in *italic;* life-threatening effects underlined; generic names in **bold;** drug classifications in SMALL CAPS; ♣ Canadian drug name; ☺ Prototype drug.

163

B

- Do not self-dose with OTC drugs without physician's approval.
- Do not stop this drug unless directed to do so by physician. Drug withdrawal needs to be accomplished gradually over a period of 2 wk or more. Abrupt withdrawal following prolonged administration may cause anxiety, agitated behavior, auditory and visual hallucinations, severe tachycardia, acute exacerbation of spasticity, and seizures.
- Do not breast feed while taking this drug without consulting physician.
- Store this medication out of reach of children.

BASILIXIMAB ☻

(bas-i-lix'i-mab)
Simulect
Classifications: IMMUNOSUPPRESSANT; MONOCLONAL ANTIBODY; INTERLEUKIN-2 RECEPTOR ANTIBODY
Pregnancy Category: B

AVAILABILITY 20 mg vials

ACTIONS Immunosuppressant agent that is an interleukin-2 receptor monoclonal antibody produced by recombinant DNA technology. Binds to and blocks interleukin-2R-alpha chain (CD-25 antibodies) on surface of activated T lymphocytes.
THERAPEUTIC EFFECTS Binding to CD-25 antibodies inhibits a critical pathway in the immune response of the lymphocytes involved in allograft rejection.

USES Prophylaxis of acute renal transplant rejection.

CONTRAINDICATIONS Hypersensitivity; serious infection or exposure to viral infections (e.g., chickenpox, herpes zoster); lactation.
CAUTIOUS USE History of untoward reactions to dacliximab or other monoclonal antibodies; pregnancy (category B).

ROUTE & DOSAGE

Prophylaxis for Transplant Rejection
Child: **IV** 2–15 y, 12 mg/m^2 (max 20 mg/dose) times 2 doses (1st dose 2 h before surgery, 2nd dose 4 days after transplant)
Adult: **IV** 20 mg times 2 doses (1st dose 2 h before surgery, 2nd dose 4 days after transplant)

STORAGE
If necessary the diluted solution may be stored at room temperature for 4 h or at 2°–8° C (36°–46° F) for 24 h. Discard after 24 h. Store undiluted drug at 2°–8° C (36°–46° F).

Common adverse effects in *italic;* life-threatening effects <u>underlined</u>; generic names in **bold**; drug classifications in SMALL CAPS; ♦ Canadian drug name; ☻ Prototype drug.

ADMINISTRATION

Intravenous

PREPARE IV **Infusion:** Add 5 mL sterile water for injection to a 20-mg vial, rock vial gently to dissolve then further dilute in an infusion bag to a volume of 50 mL of NS or D5W. The resulting solution has a concentration of 2.5 mg/mL. Invert IV bag to dissolve but do not shake. Discard if diluted solution is colored or has particulate matter. Use IV solution immediately.

ADMINISTER: Infuse the ordered dose of diluted drug over 20–30 min.

ADVERSE EFFECTS Body as a Whole: Pain, peripheral edema, edema, fever, viral infection, asthenia, arthralgia, acute hypersensitivity reactions with any dose. **CNS:** Headache, tremor, dizziness, insomnia, paresthesias, agitation, depression. **CV:** Hypertension, chest pain, hypotension, arrhythmias. **GI:** Constipation, nausea, diarrhea, abdominal pain, vomiting, dyspepsia, moniliasis, flatulence, GI hemorrhage, melena, esophagitis, erosive stomatitis. **Hematologic:** Anemia, thrombocytopenia, thrombosis, polycythemia. **Respiratory:** Dyspnea, URI, cough, rhinitis, pharyngitis, bronchospasm. **Skin:** Poor wound healing, acne. **Urogenital:** Dysuria, UTI, albuminuria, hematuria, oliguria, frequency, renal tubular necrosis, urinary retention. **Other:** Cataract, conjunctivitis. **Metabolic:** Hyperkalemia, hypokalemia, hyperglycemia, hyperuricemia, hypophosphatemia, hypocalcemia, increased weight, hypercholesterolemia, acidosis.

PHARMACOKINETICS Duration: 36 day. **Distribution:** Binds to interleukin-2R-alpha sites on lymphocytes. **Half-Life:** 7.2 ± 3.2 days in adults, 11.5 ± 6.3 days in children.

NURSING IMPLICATIONS

Assessment & Drug Effects

- Monitor carefully for and immediately report S&S of opportunistic infection or anaphylactoid reaction (see Appendix D-1).

Patient & Family Education

- Report any distressing adverse effects.
- Avoid vaccination for 2 wk following last dose of drug.
- Do not breast feed while taking this drug.

BCG (BACILLUS CALMETTE-GU'ERIN) VACCINE

(ba-cil'lus cal'met-te guer'in)

Tice, TheraCys

Classifications: VACCINE; ANTINEOPLASTIC; IMMUNOMODULATOR; BIOLOGICAL RESPONSE MODIFIER

Pregnancy Category: C

AVAILABILITY 50 mg, 81 mg, 120 mg powder for suspension

ACTIONS BCG vaccine is an immunization agent for tuberculosis (TB). It is an attenuated strain of the bacillus Calmette and Gu'erin strain of

BCG (BACILLUS CALMETTE-GU'ERIN) VACCINE

Mycobacterium bovis. BCG vaccine stimulates the reticuloendothelial system (RES) to produce macrophages that do not allow mycobacteria to multiply. BCG live is used intravesically as a biological response modifier for bladder cancer *in situ.* BCG live is thought to cause a local, chronic inflammatory response involving macrophage and leukocyte infiltration of the bladder. This local inflammatory response leads to destruction of superficial tumor cells.

THERAPEUTIC EFFECTS BCG is active immunotherapy, which stimulates the immune mechanism to reject the tumor in bladder cancer. It enhances the cytotoxicity of macrophages so that mycobacteria can not multiply.

USES To protect tuberculin skin test-negative infants and children, and groups with an excessive rate of new TB infections; carcinoma *in situ* of the bladder in adults (administration not described in this monograph for this use).

UNLABELED USES Malignant melanoma.

CONTRAINDICATIONS Impaired immune responses, immunosuppressive corticosteroid therapy, asymptomatic carriers with positive HIV serology; fever; UTI; lactation.

CAUTIOUS USE Hypersensitivity to BCG; pregnancy (category C).

ROUTE & DOSAGE

Prevention of Tuberculosis (Tice only)

Child: **Percutaneous** *<1 mo,* reduce adult dose by ¹/₂ (reconstitute with 2 mL), may need to revaccinate with full dose at 1 y; same as adult
Intradermal *<3 mo,* 0.05 mL; *>3 mo,* 0.1 mL
Adult: **Intradermal** 0.1 mL
Child/Adult: **Percutaneous** *>1 mo,* after reconstitution, 0.2–0.3 mL of vaccine is dropped onto the cleansed surface of the skin and administered using a multiple-puncture disk applied through the vaccine

---

STORAGE

Store dry BCG powder, reconstituted vaccine, and diluent refrigerated at 2°–8° C (36°–46° F). Use reconstituted solution within 2 h.

ADMINISTRATION

WARNING: Do not inject intravenously, subcutaneously, or intradermally.

Percutaneous

- Prepare solution: Add 1 mL sterile water for injection to 1 ampule of vaccine. Draw into syringe and expel back into ampule 3 times to mix.
- Administer drug by dropping 0.2–0.3 mL onto clean surface of skin; then use a sterile multiple-puncture disk to create percutaneous skin punctures.
- Instruct to keep vaccination site dry for 24 h; no dressing is needed.
- Important: Avoid contact with BCG vaccine during preparation and administration.

Intravesical Instillation

ADVERSE EFFECTS CNS: Intravesical administration: *malaise,* dizziness, headache, weakness. **Endocrine:** Hyperpyrexia. **GI:** Abdominal pain, anorexia, constipation, nausea, vomiting, diarrhea; hepatic dysfunction following intratumor injection, granulomatous hepatitis. **Hematologic:** Thrombocytopenia, eosinophilia, *anemia,* leukopenia, <u>disseminated intravascular coagulation</u>. **Respiratory:** Cough (rare), pulmonary granulomas, pulmonary infection. **Skin:** Abscess with recurrent discharge, red papule that scales or ulcerates in about 5–6 wk, dermatomyositis, granulomas at injection site 4–6 wk after inoculation, keloid formation, lupus vulgaris. **Body as a Whole:** Systemic BCG infection, *chills, flu-like syndrome,* <u>anaphylaxis</u> (rare), allergic reactions, lymphadenitis.

DIAGNOSTIC TEST INTERFERENCE Prior BCG vaccination may result in false-positive *tuberculin skin test (PPD).* Following BCG vaccination, tuberculin sensitivity may persist for months to years.

INTERACTIONS Drug: Concurrent antimycobacterial therapy **(aminosalicylic acid, capreomycin, cycloserine, ethambutol, ethionamide, isoniazid, pyrazinamide, rifabutin, rifampin, streptomycin)** that inhibits multiplication of BCG bacilli has the potential to antagonize or altogether negate the BCG vaccine-mediated immune response. **Cyclosporine** may reduce the immunologic response to BCG vaccine. **Cytomegalovirus immune globulin** and other live vaccines (measles/mumps/rubella, oral polio) may interfere with immune response to BCG. Previous vaccination with or other exposure to BCG may induce variable sensitivity to tuberculin. A greater booster effect following repeat tuberculin testing has been reported in individuals with prior BCG vaccination when compared with individuals without prior vaccination.

PHARMACOKINETICS Not studied.

NURSING IMPLICATIONS

Assessment & Drug Effects
- Monitor for S&S of systemic BCG infection: Fever, chills, severe malaise, or cough.
- Culture blood and urine, if systemic infection is suspected.
- Assess for regional lymph node enlargement and report fistula formation.

Patient & Family Education
- Review potential adverse effects.
- Keep vaccination site clean until local reaction has subsided. Report BCG administration to health care providers so TB tests are not performed (they will be positive). Chest radiographs are needed instead.
- Do not breast feed until cleared to do so by prescriber.

BECLOMETHASONE DIPROPIONATE

(be-kloe-meth'a-sone)

Beclovent, Beconase Nasal Inhaler. QVAR, QVAR Double Strength, Vancenase Nasal Inhaler, Vanceril, Vanceril D, Vancenase AQ

Classifications: HORMONE AND SYNTHETIC SUBSTITUTE; ADRENAL CORTICOSTEROID

Prototype: Hydrocortisone

Pregnancy Category: C

B

AVAILABILITY 42 mcg, 84 mcg metered-dose inhalers; QVAR 40 mcg, 80 mcg inhalers; 42 mcg nasal inhaler; 0.042%, 0.084% nasal spray. **See Appendix I-1.**

BELLADONNA TINCTURE
(bell-a-don′na)
Classifications: AUTONOMIC NERVOUS SYSTEM AGENT; ANTICHOLINERGIC (PARASYMPATHOLYTIC); ANTIMUSCARINIC, ANTISPASMODIC
Prototype: Atropine
Pregnancy Category: C

AVAILABILITY 27–33 mg/100 mL tincture

ACTIONS Reversibly blocks action of acetylcholine at parasympathetic neuroeffector sites.
THERAPEUTIC EFFECTS Belladonna inhibits smooth muscle contractions and suppresses secretions of secretory glands.

USES Adjunct in treatment of peptic ulcer disease, irritable bowel syndrome, and neurogenic bowel disturbances. Also has been used for dysmenorrhea, nocturnal enuresis, spasms of urinary tract, nausea and vomiting of pregnancy, vertigo, and for symptomatic relief of parkinsonism.

CONTRAINDICATIONS Hypersensitivity to anticholinergic drugs; obstructive uropathy, atony of urinary bladder; esophageal reflux, obstructive disease of GI tract, intestinal atony, paralytic ileus, severe ulcerative colitis, toxic megacolon; myasthenia gravis; narrow-angle glaucoma; unstable cardiovascular status in acute hemorrhages. Safety during pregnancy (category C), lactation, or in children is not established.
CAUTIOUS USE Autonomic neuropathy; heart disease, hypertension; patients >40 y (higher incidence of glaucoma).

ROUTE & DOSAGE

Antispasmodic
Child: **PO** 0.1 mL/kg/day in 3–4 divided doses (max 3.5 mL/day)
Adult: **PO** 0.6–1 mL t.i.d. or q.i.d.

STORAGE
Store at 15°–30° C (59°–86° F) in tightly covered, light-resistant containers, unless otherwise directed.

ADMINISTRATION
Oral
▪ Administer 30–60 min before meals and at bedtime.
▪ Space administration of antacid and belladonna preparations at least 2 h apart.

ADVERSE EFFECTS All: Dose related. **CNS:** Excitement (young children and older adults), confusion, delirium. **CV:** Rapid heart beat, tachycardia, palpitation. **Special Senses:** Blurred vision, mydriasis, photophobia. **GI:** *Dry mouth, constipation.* **Urogenital:** Urinary retention, urgency.

INTERACTIONS Drug: Amantadine, ANTIHISTAMINES, TRICYCLIC ANTIDEPRESSANTS, **quinidine, disopyramide, procainamide** have additive anticholinergic effects; **levodopa** effects decreased; **methotrimeprazine** may precipitate extrapyramidal effects; antipsychotic effects of PHENOTHIAZINES decreased (decreased absorption).

PHARMACOKINETICS Absorption: Readily absorbed from GI tract. **Onset:** 1–2 h. **Distribution:** Well distributed in body; crosses blood–brain barrier. **Elimination:** Excreted unchanged in urine.

NURSING IMPLICATIONS

Assessment & Drug Effects
- Monitor ambulation because drug may cause drowsiness and confusion.
- Monitor I&O and assess for urinary retention.

Patient & Family Education
- Note: Increase in fluid intake and bulk in diet may prevent or relieve constipation. Notify prescriber if constipation persists.
- Avoid hot baths, saunas, and strenuous work or exercise during hot and humid weather.
- Do not drive or engage in potentially hazardous activities until response to drug is known.
- Practice meticulous oral hygiene. Sugarless gum, lemon drops, and frequent sips of water may help dry mouth.
- Do not breast feed while taking this drug without consulting prescriber.
- Store this medication out of reach of children.

BENDROFLUMETHIAZIDE
(ben-droe-floo-meth-eye′a-zide)
Naturetin
Classifications: FLUID AND WATER BALANCE AGENT; THIAZIDE DIURETIC
Prototype: Hydrochlorothiazide
Pregnancy Category: C

AVAILABILITY 5 mg, 10 mg tablets

ACTIONS Thiazide diuretic chemically related to the sulfonamides. Similar to hydrochlorothiazide in pharmacologic action.
THERAPEUTIC EFFECTS Bendroflumethiazide decreases blood volume by increasing excretion of fluid and electrolytes. It has a hypotensive effect.

USES Management of edema associated with CHF, mild hypertension. **UNLABELED USES** Lithium-associated diabetes insipidus.

CONTRAINDICATIONS Anuria, hypersensitivity to thiazides, sulfonamides; pregnancy (category C), lactation.

Common adverse effects in *italic;* life-threatening effects underlined; generic names in **bold;** drug classifications in SMALL CAPS; ♣ Canadian drug name; ☻ Prototype drug.

169

B

CAUTIOUS USE Renal and hepatic disease; gout; diabetes mellitus.

ROUTE & DOSAGE

Hypertension
Child: **PO** 0.05–0.4 mg/kg/day in 1–2 divided doses
Adult: **PO** 2.5–20 mg/day in 1–2 divided doses

STORAGE
Store tablets in tightly closed container at 15°–30° C (59°–86° F) unless otherwise specified.

ADMINISTRATION

Oral
- Give drug early in a.m. after patient has eaten to reduce gastric irritation and prevent possibility of interrupted sleep due to diuresis. If 2 daily doses are ordered, administer second dose no later than 3 p.m.

ADVERSE EFFECTS CV: Orthostatic hypotension. **Metabolic:** Electrolyte imbalance, hypokalemia, hyperglycemia, impaired glucose tolerance, hyperuricemia. **Musculoskeletal:** Exacerbation of gout.

INTERACTIONS Drug: Cholestyramine, colestipol decrease absorption of the diuretic; **diazoxide** has additive effects; with **digoxin,** the hypokalemia may increase risk of **digitalis** toxicity; increases **lithium** levels and toxicity; may increase blood glucose levels, necessitating adjustment of hypoglycemic therapy (i.e., SULFONYLUREAS), **insulin.**

PHARMACOKINETICS Absorption: Readily absorbed from GI tract. **Onset:** 1–2 h. **Peak:** 6–12 h. **Duration:** 18–24 h. **Elimination:** Excreted unchanged in urine within 24 h.

NURSING IMPLICATIONS

Assessment & Drug Effects
- Monitor BP. Report a sudden fall in BP, which may initiate severe postural hypotension and potentially dangerous perfusion problems of the extremities. Antihypertensive effects are generally noted in 3–4 days; maximal effects may require 3–4 wk.
- Monitor I&O ratio and pattern, and weight, particularly during first phase of antihypertensive therapy.
- Lab tests: Periodic serum electrolytes. Report hypokalemia promptly.
- Report unexplained onset of joint pain and limitation of motion; may be due to hyperuricemia since thiazides interfere with uric acid excretion, although thiazides rarely precipitate acute gout.
- Monitor diabetics for loss of glycemic control.

Patient & Family Education
- Eat potassium-rich foods such as fruit juices, potatoes, cereals, skim milk, and bananas to prevent onset of hyperuricemia.
- Make position changes slowly and in stages to avoid dizziness or fainting.

- Report joint pain or limited joint movement.
- Avoid OTC drugs unless approved by prescriber.
- Do not breast feed while taking this drug.
- Store this medication out of reach of children.

BENZOCAINE

(ben_zoe-caine)

Americaine, Americaine Anesthetic Lubricant, Americaine-Otic, Anbesol, Benzocol, Chigger-Tox, Dermoplast, Foille, Hurricaine, Orabase with Benzocaine, Oracin, Orajel, Rhulicaine, Solarcaine, T-Caine, Unguentine

Classifications: CENTRAL NERVOUS SYSTEM AGENT; LOCAL ANESTHETIC (ESTER TYPE); ANTIPRURITIC
Prototype: Procaine
Pregnancy Category: C

AVAILABILITY 5% spray, cream, ointment; 6% cream; 8% lotion, 20% spray, ointment, gel, liquid. **Combination Products:** Available in combination topical products such as throat lozenges, gels, ointments, solutions

ACTIONS Produces surface anesthesia by inhibiting conduction of nerve impulses from sensory nerve endings. Probable action in certain OTC appetite suppressants is dulling taste for foods. Almost identical to procaine in chemical structure, but has prolonged duration of anesthetic action.
THERAPEUTIC EFFECTS Temporary relief of pain and discomfort.

USES Temporary relief of pain and discomfort in pruritic skin problems, minor burns and sunburn, minor wounds, and insect bites. Otic preparations are used to relieve pain and itching in acute congestive and serous otitis media, swimmer's ear, and otitis externa. Preparations are also available for toothache, minor sore throat pain, canker sores, hemorrhoids, rectal fissures, pruritus ani or vulvae, as male genital desensitizer to slow onset of ejaculation, and for use as anesthetic-lubricant for passage of catheters and endoscopic tubes.

CONTRAINDICATIONS Hypersensitivity to benzocaine or other PABA derivatives (e.g., sunscreen preparations), or to any of the components in the formulation; use of ear preparation in patients with perforated eardrum or ear discharge; applications to large areas; use in children <2 y. Safe use during pregnancy (category C) is not established.
CAUTIOUS USE History of drug sensitivity; denuded skin or severely traumatized mucosa; children <6 y.

ROUTE & DOSAGE

Anesthetic

Child: **Topical** Lowest concentration solutions.
Adult: **Topical** Lowest effective dose

Common adverse effects in *italic;* life-threatening effects <u>underlined</u>; generic names in **bold;** drug classifications in SMALL CAPS; ♣ Canadian drug name; ◑ Prototype drug.

171

B

STORAGE
Store at 15°–30° C (59°–86° F) in tight, light-resistant containers unless otherwise specified.

ADMINISTRATION

Topical
- Avoid contact of all preparations with eyes and be careful not to inhale mist when spray form is used.
- Do not use spray near open flame or cautery and do not expose to high temperatures. Hold can at least 12 inches (30 cm) away from affected area when spraying.
- Wash and neutralize chemical burns before benzocaine is applied.
- Clean and dry rectal area before administration of hemorrhoidal preparation. Usually administered morning and evening and after each bowel movement. Skin preparations may be administered t.i.d. or q.i.d.

ADVERSE EFFECTS Body as a Whole: Low toxicity; sensitization in susceptible individuals; allergic reactions, <u>anaphylaxis</u>. Methemoglobinemia reported in infants; also described in older children following prolonged use and large applications.

INTERACTION Drug: Benzocaine may antagonize antibacterial activity of SULFONAMIDES.

PHARMACOKINETICS Absorption: Poorly absorbed through intact skin; readily absorbed from mucous membranes. **Peak:** 1 min. **Duration:** 15–30 min. **Metabolism:** Metabolized by plasma cholinesterases and to a lesser extent by hepatic cholinesterases. **Elimination:** Metabolites excreted in urine.

NURSING IMPLICATIONS

Assessment & Drug Effects
- Assess swallowing when used on oral mucosa, because benzocaine may interfere with second (pharyngeal) stage of swallowing; hold food and liquids accordingly.
- Assess for sensitivity. Local anesthetics are potentially sensitizing to susceptible individuals when applied repeatedly or over extensive areas.
- Lozenge is dissolved slowly in mouth; avoid use in young children due to choking hazard.
- Otic solutions are instilled with 4–5 drops in external canal when tympanic membrane is intact q1–2h prn.

Patient & Family Education
- Use specific benzocaine preparation ONLY as prescribed or recommended by manufacturer. Generally the condition should improve within 2 days and medication should be stopped. Consult health care provider for conditions that continue more than 2 days.
- Discontinue medication if the condition persists, worsens, or if signs of sensitivity, irritation, or infection occur.
- Store this medication out of reach of children.

BENZONATATE 🅟

(ben-zoe′na-tate)
Tessalon
Classification: ANTITUSSIVE
Pregnancy Category: C

AVAILABILITY 100 mg capsules

ACTIONS Nonnarcotic antitussive chemically related to tetracaine. Antitussive activity reported to be somewhat less effective than that of codeine. Does not inhibit respiratory center at recommended doses.
THERAPEUTIC EFFECTS Decreases frequency and intensity of nonproductive cough.

USES Decreases frequency and intensity of nonproductive cough in acute and chronic respiratory conditions. Also used in bronchoscopy, thoracentesis, and other procedures when coughing must be avoided.

CONTRAINDICATIONS Safe use during pregnancy (category C) or lactation is not established.

ROUTE & DOSAGE

Antitussive
Child: **PO** <10 y, 8 mg/kg/day divided into 3–6 doses
Adult: **PO** 100 mg t.i.d. prn up to 600 mg/day

STORAGE
Store in airtight containers protected from light.

ADMINISTRATION
Oral
▪ Ensure that soft capsules called perles are swallowed whole.

ADVERSE EFFECTS Body as a Whole: Low incidence. **CNS:** Drowsiness, sedation headache, mild dizziness. **GI:** Constipation, nausea. **Skin:** Rash, pruritus.

PHARMACOKINETICS Onset: 15–20 min. **Duration:** 3–8 h.

NURSING IMPLICATIONS

Assessment & Drug Effects
▪ Auscultate lungs anteriorly and posteriorly at scheduled intervals.
▪ Observe character and frequency of coughing and volume and quality of sputum. Keep prescriber informed.

Patient & Family Education
▪ Do not chew, nor allow perle to dissolve in mouth; swallow whole. If perle dissolves in mouth, the mouth, tongue, and pharynx will be anesthetized. Also it is unpleasant to taste.

Common adverse effects in *italic;* life-threatening effects <u>underlined</u>; generic names in **bold;** drug classifications in SMALL CAPS; ♣ Canadian drug name; 🅟 Prototype drug.

173

B

- Do not breast feed while taking this drug without consulting prescriber.
- Store this medication out of reach of children.

BENZTHIAZIDE
(bens-thye′a-zide)
Aquatag, Exna, Hydrex, Marazide, Proaqua
Classifications: FLUID AND WATER BALANCE AGENT; THIAZIDE DIURETIC; ANTIHYPERTENSIVE
Prototype: Hydrochlorothiazide
Pregnancy Category: D

AVAILABILITY 50 mg tablets

ACTIONS Thiazide diuretic chemically related to sulfonamides. Similar to hydrochlorothiazide. Inhibits renal tubular reabsorption of sodium and chloride, resulting in excretion of sodium and water, accompanied by some loss of bicarbonate and potassium.
THERAPEUTIC EFFECTS Decreases blood volume resulting in a hypotensive effect.

USES Edema and adjunctively with other agents for treatment of mild hypertension.

CONTRAINDICATIONS Hypersensitivity to thiazides or sulfonamides; anuria; pregnancy (category D), lactation.
CAUTIOUS USE History of renal, hepatic, or pancreatic disease; history of gout; diabetes mellitus; hypercalcemia, hypokalemia.

ROUTE & DOSAGE

Edema
Child: **PO** 1–4 mg/kg/day divided into 3 doses
Adult: **PO** 25–200 mg/day or every other day

Hypertension
Adult: **PO** 25–100 mg/day after breakfast, may increase to 200 mg/day divided into 2–4 doses

STORAGE
Store tablets in tightly closed container at 15°–30° C (59°–86° F) unless otherwise directed.

ADMINISTRATION
Oral
- Give with food or milk to minimize gastric irritation unless otherwise directed by prescriber.
- Give as a single daily dose to promote diuresis, preferably early in the morning to prevent interrupted sleep.

ADVERSE EFFECTS Body as a Whole: Hypersensitivity (dermatitis, photosensitivity, urticaria). **CNS:** Headache, unusual fatigue. **CV:** Irregular

---

Common adverse effects in *italic*; life-threatening effects <u>underlined</u>; generic names in **bold**; drug classifications in SMALL CAPS; ♣ Canadian drug name; ☯ Prototype drug.

heartbeat, vasculitis, orthostatic hypotension, volume depletion. **GI:** Nausea, vomiting, anorexia, constipation, cramps, jaundice. **Metabolic:** Hyperglycemia, hypokalemia; hyperuricemia. **Hematologic:** (Rare) thrombocytopenia, agranulocytosis. **Other:** Increased thirst.

DIAGNOSTIC TEST INTERFERENCE *Serum PBI* levels may be decreased. Thiazides should be discontinued before *parathyroid function* tests because they tend to reduce *calcium* excretion.

INTERACTIONS Drug: Cholestyramine, colestipol decrease absorption of the diuretic; **diazoxide** has additive effects; with **digoxin**, hypokalemia may increase risk of **digitalis** toxicity; increases **lithium** levels and toxicity; may increase blood glucose levels, necessitating adjustment of dosage of SULFONYLUREAS, **insulin.**

PHARMACOKINETICS Absorption: Readily absorbed from GI tract. **Onset:** 2 h. **Peak:** 4–6 h. **Duration:** 12–18 h. **Distribution:** Crosses placenta; distributed into breast milk. **Elimination:** Excreted in urine within 24 h.

NURSING IMPLICATIONS

Assessment & Drug Effects

- Assess therapeutic effectiveness. Effects may be noted in 3 or 4 days; maximal effects usually require 3–4 wk.
- Assess patient carefully for signs of hypokalemia, (see Appendix D-1).
- Lab tests: Baseline and periodic blood counts, serum electrolytes, uric acid, blood sugar, NPN, BUN, and serum creatinine.
- Monitor I&O ratio and pattern.
- Monitor diabetics for loss of glycemic control.

Patient & Family Education

- Ingest potassium-rich foods such as fruit juices, bananas, and potatoes to prevent onset of hypokalemia.
- Weigh daily and report sudden weight gain to prescriber.
- Notify prescriber if nausea, vomiting, or diarrhea occurs in order to prevent dehydration.
- Avoid use of OTC drugs unless approved by prescriber.
- Notify physician of photosensitivity reaction (like an exaggerated sunburn). Thiazide-related photosensitivity is considered a photoallergy; it occurs 1½–2 wk after initial sun exposure.
- Do not breast feed while taking this drug.
- Store this medication out of reach of children.

BENZTROPINE MESYLATE

(benz'troe-peen)

Apo-Benzotropine ♣, Bensylate ♣, Cogentin, PMS Benzotropine ♣

Classifications: AUTONOMIC NERVOUS SYSTEM AGENT; ANTICHOLINERGIC (PARASYMPATHOLYTIC); ANTIPARKINSONISM AGENT

Prototype: Levodopa

Pregnancy Category: C

Common adverse effects in *italic;* life-threatening effects underlined; generic names in **bold;** drug classifications in SMALL CAPS; ♣ Canadian drug name; ⊘ Prototype drug.

175

B

AVAILABILITY 0.5 mg, 1 mg, 2 mg tablets; 1 mg/mL ampules

ACTIONS Synthetic centrally acting anticholinergic (antimuscarinic) agent. Acts by diminishing excess cholinergic effect associated with dopamine deficiency.
THERAPEUTIC EFFECTS Suppresses tremor and rigidity; does not alleviate tardive dyskinesia.

USES Symptomatic treatment of all forms of parkinsonism and to relieve extrapyramidal symptoms associated with neuroleptic drugs, e.g., haloperidol (Haldol), phenothiazines, thiothixene (Navane). Commonly used as supplement with trihexyphenidyl, carbidopa, or levodopa therapy.

CONTRAINDICATIONS Narrow-angle glaucoma; myasthenia gravis; obstructive diseases of GU and GI tracts; tendency to tachycardia; tardive dyskinesia, children <3 y. Safety during pregnancy (category C) or lactation is not established.
CAUTIOUS USE Children or debilitated patients, patients with poor mental outlook, mental disorders; hypertension; history of renal or hepatic disease.

ROUTE & DOSAGE

Extrapyramidal Reactions
Child: **PO/IM/IV** >3 y, 0.02–0.05 mg/kg, 1–2 times/day
Adult: **PO** 1–2 mg b.i.d. **IM/IV** 1–2 mg prn.

STORAGE
Store in tightly covered, light-resistant container at 15°–30° C (59°–86° F) unless otherwise directed.

ADMINISTRATION

Oral
- Give immediately after meals or with food to prevent gastric irritation. Tablet can be crushed and sprinkled on or mixed with food.
- Initiate and withdraw drug therapy gradually; effects are cumulative.

Intravenous

For IV administration to infants and children, verify correct IV concentration with physician.
PREPARE Direct: Give undiluted.
ADMINISTER Direct: Give 1 mg or a fraction thereof over 1 min.

ADVERSE EFFECTS CNS: *Sedation,* drowsiness, dizziness, paresthesias; agitation, irritability, restlessness, nervousness, insomnia, hallucinations, delirium, mental confusion, toxic psychosis, muscular weakness, ataxia, inability to move certain muscle groups. **CV:** Palpitation, tachycardia, flushing. **Special Senses:** Blurred vision, mydriasis, photophobia. **GI:** Nausea, vomiting, *constipation, dry mouth,* distention, <u>paralytic ileus</u>. **Urogenital:** Dysuria.

INTERACTIONS Drug: Alcohol, CNS DEPRESSANTS have additive sedation and depressant effects; **amantidine,** TRICYCLIC ANTIDEPRESSANTS, MAOIS,

PHENOTHIAZINES, **procainamide, quinidine** have additive anticholinergic effects and cause confusion, hallucinations, paralytic ileus.

PHARMACOKINETICS Onset: 15 min IM/IV; 1 h PO. **Duration:** 6–10 h.

NURSING IMPLICATIONS

Assessment & Drug Effects
- Assess therapeutic effectiveness. Clinical improvement may not be evident for 2–3 days after oral drug is started.
- Monitor I&O ratio and pattern. Advise patient to report difficulty in urination or infrequent voiding. Dosage reduction may be indicated.
- Closely monitor for appearance of S&S of onset of paralytic ileus including intermittent constipation, abdominal pain, diminution of bowel sounds on auscultation, and distention.
- Monitor for and report muscle weakness or inability to move certain muscle groups. Dosage reduction may be needed.
- Supervise ambulation and use bed side rails as necessary.
- Report immediately S&S of CNS depression or stimulation. These usually require interruption of drug therapy.

Patient & Family Education
- Do not drive or engage in potentially hazardous activities until response to drug is known. Seek help walking as necessary.
- Avoid alcohol and other CNS depressants because they may cause additive drowsiness. Do not take OTC cold, cough, or hay fever remedies unless approved by physician.
- Sugarless gum, hard candy, and rinsing mouth with tepid water will help dry mouth.
- Avoid doing manual labor or strenuous exercise in hot weather; diminished sweating may require dose adjustments because of possibility of heatstroke.
- Do not breast feed while taking this drug without consulting physician.
- Store this medication out of reach of children.

BERACTANT ⊙

(ber-ac'tant)
Survanta
Classifications: LUNG SURFACTANT
Pregnancy Category: Not applicable

AVAILABILITY 25 mg/mL suspension

ACTIONS Beractant is a sterile nonpyrogenic pulmonary surfactant. Endogenous pulmonary surfactant lowers surface tension on alveolar surfaces during respiration and stabilizes the alveoli against collapse at resting pressures. Deficiency of surfactant causes respiratory distress syndrome (RDS) in premature infants.
THERAPEUTIC EFFECTS Beractant lowers minimum surface tension and restores pulmonary compliance and oxygenation in premature infants.

Common adverse effects in *italic;* life-threatening effects underlined; generic names in **bold;** drug classifications in SMALL CAPS; ♣ Canadian drug name; ⊙ Prototype drug.

177

B

USES Prevention and treatment of RDS in premature infants, especially those weighing <1250 g.
UNLABELED USES Infants weighing <600 g or >1750 g; treatment of RDS in adults.

CONTRAINDICATIONS Nosocomial infections.

ROUTE & DOSAGE

Neonate: **Intratracheal** Instill mg/4 mL/kg/dose birth weight through endotracheal tube, may repeat no more frequently than q6h (max 4 doses in the first 48 h of life)

STORAGE

Store unopened vials inside carton to protect from light and refrigerated at 2°–8° C (36°–46° F) until ready to use.

ADMINISTRATION

Intratracheal

- Place refrigerated drug at room temperature for at least 20 min or warm in the hand for at least 8 min. Do not use artificial warming methods.
- Give to premature infants weighing less than 1250 g, or who have a surfactant deficiency, preferably within 15 min of birth.
- Give to infants requiring mechanical ventilation and with RDS confirmed by x-ray examination, within 8 h of birth.
- Suction infant before administration of beractant.
- Note: Drug color should be white to light brown. If drug has settled, swirl vial gently to suspend.
- Administer using a No. 5 French end-hole catheter inserted into the endotracheal tube. Divide dose into 4 equal amounts. Administer each separately: (1) downward with head turned to right, (2) downward with head turned to left, (3) upward with head turned to right, (4) upward with head turned to left
- Follow specific dosing procedure recommended by the manufacturer. Carefully read and follow exactly accompanying drug administration literature.
- Do not suction for 1 h after drug is administered unless signs of significant airway obstruction occur.
- Unopened vials warmed to room temperature will not lose potency if refrigerated within 8 h of warming. Drug should not be warmed and returned to refrigerator more than once.
- Note: Vials are for single use only. Discard unused drug in opened vials.

ADVERSE EFFECTS CV: *Transient bradycardia.* **Respiratory:** *Oxygen desaturation.* **Other:** Increased probability of post-treatment nosocomial sepsis in surfactant-treated infants was observed in controlled clinical trials but was not associated with increased mortality.

PHARMACOKINETICS Absorption: Absorbed from the alveolus into lung tissue, where it can be extensively catabolized and reutilized for further phospholipid synthesis and secretion. **Onset:** 0.5–4 h. **Peak:** 2 h. **Duration:** 48–72 h; may need multiple doses to sustain improvement.

Distribution: Not distributed to the systemic circulation. **Metabolism:** Surfactant is recycled and metabolized exclusively in the lungs. **Elimination:** Recycling may be a dominant metabolic pathway by which surfactant is taken up by type II pneumocytes and reused. **Half-Life:** 20–30 h.

NURSING IMPLICATIONS

Assessment & Drug Effects

- Monitor heart rate, color, chest expansion, facial expressions, oximeter, and endotracheal tube patency and position, during administration. Most adverse effects occur during dosing.
- Monitor postadministration and frequently with arterial or transcutaneous measurement of systemic oxygen and CO_2.
- Note: Crackles and moist breath sounds may occur transiently following drug administration. These do not necessarily indicate a need for suctioning.

BETAMETHASONE
(bay-ta-meth'a-sone)
Betnelan ♣, Celestone

BETAMETHASONE ACETATE AND BETAMETHASONE SODIUM PHOSPHATE
Celestone Soluspan

BETAMETHASONE BENZOATE
Beben ♣, Benisone, Uticort

BETAMETHASONE DIPROPIONATE
Alphatrex, Diprolene, Diprosone, Maxivate

BETAMETHASONE SODIUM PHOSPHATE (PH 8.5)
Betameth, Betnesol ♣, Celestone Phosphate, Celestone S, Cel-U-Jec, Selestoject

BETAMETHASONE VALERATE
Betacort, Betaderm ♣, Betatrex, Beta-Val, Betnovate ♣, Celestoderm ♣, Ectosone Lotion ♣, Luxiq, Metaderm ♣, Novobetamet ♣, Valisone, Valisone Scalp Lotion, Valnac, Psorion cream

Classifications: HORMONE AND SYNTHETIC SUBSTITUTE; ADRENAL CORTICOSTEROID; GLUCOCORTICOID; ANTI-INFLAMMATORY
Prototype: Hydrocortisone
Pregnancy Category: C

AVAILABILITY Betamethasone 0.6 mg tablets; 0.6 mg/5 mL syrup **Betamethasone Acetate and Betamethasone Sodium** 3 mg acetate, 3 mg sodium phosphate/mL suspension **Betamethasone Benzoate,**

Common adverse effects in *italic;* life-threatening effects <u>underlined</u>; generic names in **bold;** drug classifications in SMALL CAPS; ♣ Canadian drug name; ✪ Prototype drug.

179

B

Betamethasone Dipropionate, and Betamethasone Sodium Phosphate (PH 8.5) 4 mg/mL injection **Betamethasone Valerate** 0.1% ointment; 0.01%, 0.05%, 0.1% cream; 0.1% lotion; 1.2 mg/g foam
Combination Products: In combination with Clotrimazole as Lotrisone

ACTIONS Synthetic, long-acting glucocorticoid with minor mineralocorticoid properties but strong immunosuppressive, anti-inflammatory, and metabolic actions.
THERAPEUTIC EFFECTS Relieves anti-inflammatory manifestations and is an immunosuppressive agent.

USES Reduces serum calcium in hypercalcemia, suppresses undesirable inflammatory or immune responses, produces temporary remission in nonadrenal disease, and blocks ACTH production in diagnostic tests. Topical use provides relief of inflammatory manifestations of corticosteroid-responsive dermatoses.
UNLABELED USES Prevention of neonatal respiratory distress syndrome (hyaline membrane disease).

CONTRAINDICATIONS In patients with systemic fungal infections. Topical cream not recommended for children <12 y of age due to the high incidence of adrenal suppression. Pregnancy (category C), lactation, vaccines.
CAUTIOUS USE Ocular herpes simplex; concomitant use of aspirin; osteoporosis; diverticulitis, nonspecific ulcerative colitis, abscess or other pyrogenic infection, peptic ulcer disease; hypertension; renal insufficiency; myasthenia gravis.

ROUTE & DOSAGE

Anti-Inflammatory Agent
Child: **PO** 0.0175–0.25 mg/kg/day or 0.5–0.75 mg/m²/day divided into doses given q6–8h **IM** 0.0175–0.125 mg/kg/day or 0.5–0.75 mg/m²/day divided into doses given q6–8h
Adult: **PO** 0.6–7.2 mg/day **IM/IV** 0.5–9 mg/day as sodium phosphate

Respiratory Distress Syndrome Prophylaxis
Adult: **IM** 2 mL of sodium phosphate to mother once daily 2–3 days before delivery

STORAGE
Store in well-closed containers from 15°–30° C (59°–86° F)

ADMINISTRATION

Oral
- Give with food or milk to lessen stomach irritation.

Intra-Articular, Intramuscular, Intralesional
- Use Celestone Soluspan for intra-articular, IM, and intralesional injection. The preparation is not intended for IV use. Do not mix with diluents containing preservatives (e.g., parabens, phenol).
- Use 1% or 2% lidocaine hydrochloride if prescribed. Withdraw betamethasone mixture first, then lidocaine; shake syringe briefly.

Intravenous

PREPARE **Direct:** Give by direct IV undiluted or further diluted in D5W or NS.

ADMINISTER **Direct:** Give at a rate of 1 dose/min.

INCOMPATIBILITIES: **Solution/Additive: Amobarbital, ampicillin, bleomycin, colistimethate, dimenhydrinate, doxapram, doxorubicin, ephedrine, heparin, hydralazine, metaraminol, methicillin, nafcillin, pentobarbital, phenobarbital, prochlorperazine, promethazine, secobarbital,** TETRACYCLINES. **Y-Site: Ergotamine, phenytoin.**

ADVERSE EFFECTS Body as a Whole: Hypersensitivity or *anaphylactoid reactions;* aggravation or masking of infections; malaise, weight gain, obesity. Most adverse effects are dose and treatment duration dependent. **CNS:** Vertigo, headache, nystagmus, ataxia (rare), increased intracranial pressure with papilledema (usually after discontinuation of medication), mental disturbances, aggravation of preexisting psychiatric conditions, insomnia. **CV:** Hypertension; syncopal episodes, thrombophlebitis, thromboembolism or fat embolism, palpitation, tachycardia, necrotizing angiitis; CHF. **Endocrine:** Suppressed linear growth in children, decreased glucose tolerance; hyperglycemia, manifestations of latent diabetes mellitus; hypocorticism; amenorrhea and other menstrual difficulties. **Special Senses:** Posterior subcapsular cataracts (especially in children), glaucoma, exophthalmos, increased intraocular pressure with optic nerve damage, perforation of the globe, fungal infection of the cornea, decreased or blurred vision. **Metabolic:** Hypocalcemia; *sodium and fluid retention;* hypokalemia and hypokalemic alkalosis; negative nitrogen balance. **GI:** *Nausea,* increased appetite, ulcerative esophagitis, pancreatitis, abdominal distention, peptic ulcer with perforation and hemorrhage, melena; decreased serum concentration of vitamins A and C. **Hematologic:** Thrombocytopenia. **Musculoskeletal:** Osteoporosis, compression fractures, muscle wasting and weakness, tendon rupture, aseptic necrosis of femoral and humeral heads (all resulting from long-term use). **Skin:** Skin thinning and atrophy, *acne, impaired wound healing;* petechiae, ecchymosis, easy bruising; suppression of skin test reaction; hypopigmentation or hyperpigmentation, hirsutism, acneiform eruptions, subcutaneous fat atrophy; allergic dermatitis, urticaria, angioneurotic edema, increased sweating. **Urogenital:** Increased or decreased motility and number of sperm; urinary frequency and urgency, enuresis. **With Parenteral Therapy, IV Site:** Pain, irritation, necrosis, atrophy, sterile abscess; Charcot-like arthropathy following intra-articular use; burning and tingling in perineal area (after IV injection).

DIAGNOSTIC TEST INTERFERENCE May increase serum *cholesterol, blood glucose,* serum *sodium, uric acid* (in acute leukemia) and *calcium* (in bone metastasis). It may decrease serum *calcium, potassium, PBI, thyroxin (T_4), triiodothyronine (T_3) and reduce thyroid I-131* uptake. It increases *urine glucose* level and *calcium* excretion; decreases *urine 17-OHCS* and *17-KS* levels. May produce false-negative results with *nitroblue tetrazolium test* for systemic bacterial infection and may suppress reactions to skin tests.

INTERACTIONS Drug: BARBITURATES, **phenytoin, rifampin** may reduce pharmacologic effect of betamethasone by increasing its metabolism.

Common adverse effects in *italic*; life-threatening effects underlined; generic names in **bold**; drug classifications in SMALL CAPS; ♣ Canadian drug name; ❂ Prototype drug.

181

B

PHARMACOKINETICS Not studied.

NURSING IMPLICATIONS

Assessment & Drug Effects

- Assess therapeutic effectiveness. Response following intra-articular, intralesional, or intrasynovial administration occurs within a few hours and persists for 1–4 wk. Following IM administration response occurs in 2–3 h and persists for 3–7 days.

Patient & Family Education

- Monitor weight at least weekly.
- Discontinued slowly after systemic use of >1 wk. Abrupt withdrawal, especially following high doses or prolonged use, can cause dizziness, nausea, vomiting, fever, muscle and joint pain, weakness.
- Do not breast feed while taking this drug.
- Store this medication out of reach of children.

BETHANECHOL CHLORIDE ●

(be-than'e-kole)

Duvoid, Urabeth, Urecholine

Classifications: AUTONOMIC NERVOUS SYSTEM AGENT; DIRECT-ACTING CHOLINERGIC (PARASYMPATHOMIMETIC) AGENT

Pregnancy Category: C

AVAILABILITY 5 mg, 10 mg, 25 mg, 50 mg tablets; 5 mg/mL injection

ACTIONS Synthetic choline ester with effects similar to those of acetylcholine (ACh). Acts directly on postsynaptic receptors, and since it is not hydrolyzed by cholinesterase, its actions are more prolonged than those of ACh.

THERAPEUTIC EFFECTS Produces muscarinic effects primarily on GI tract and urinary bladder. Increases tone and peristaltic activity of esophagus, stomach, and intestine; contracts detrusor muscle of urinary bladder, usually enough to initiate micturition.

USES Acute postoperative and postpartum nonobstructive (functional) urinary retention, and for neurogenic atony of urinary bladder with retention.

UNLABELED USES In selected cases of adynamic ileus, gastric atony and retention, reflux esophagitis, congenital megacolon, familial dysautonomia; for prevention and treatment of bladder and salivary gland inhibition induced by tricyclic antidepressants, and for prophylaxis and treatment of phenothiazine-induced bladder dysfunction.

CONTRAINDICATIONS COPD; history of or active bronchial asthma; hyperthyroidism; recent urinary bladder surgery, cystitis, bacteriuria, urinary bladder neck or intestinal obstruction, peptic ulcer, recent GI surgery, peritonitis; marked vagotonia, pronounced vasomotor instability, AV conduction defects, severe bradycardia, hypotension or hypertension, coronary artery disease, recent MI; epilepsy, parkinsonism.

Safety during pregnancy (category C), lactation, or in children <8 y is not established.
CAUTIOUS USE Urinary retention; bacteriemia.

ROUTE & DOSAGE

Urinary Retention

Child: **PO** for gastroesophageal reflux: 0.1–0.2 mg/kg/dose or 0.6 mg/m^2/dose. Doses given 30 min–1 h before meals and at bedtime for a max of 4 doses/24 h **PO** for abdominal distention and urinary retention: 0.6 mg/kg/24 h divided into doses given q6–8h **SC** for abdominal distention and urinary retention: 0.12–0.2 mg/kg/24 h divided into doses given q6–8h
Adult: **PO** 10–50 mg b.i.d. to q.i.d. (max 120 mg/day) **SC** 2.5–5 mg t.i.d. or q.i.d. prn

STORAGE

Store at 15°–30° C (59°–86° F), unless otherwise directed.

ADMINISTRATION

Oral

- Give on an empty stomach (1 h before or 2 h after meals) to lessen possibility of nausea and vomiting, unless otherwise advised by prescriber.
- Determine minimum effective dose. Start with lowest dose and increase if needed.

Subcutaneous

- Determine minimum effective dose. Start with lowest dose and increase if needed.
- After inserting needle, aspirate carefully before injecting drug to avoid inadvertent entry into a blood vessel.
- Do NOT give by IM or IV; life-threatening symptoms of cholinergic stimulation can occur.
- Overdose management: Atropine sulfate 0.6–1.2 mg for adults administered IM, slow IV, or SC; and 0.01 mg/kg for infants and children repeated every 2 h, if necessary.

ADVERSE EFFECTS Body as a Whole: Dose-related. Increased sweating, malaise, headache, substernal pain or pressure, hypothermia. **CV:** Hypotension with dizziness, faintness, flushing, orthostatic hypotension (large doses); mild reflex tachycardia, atrial fibrillation (hyperthyroid patients), transient complete heart block. **Special Senses:** Blurred vision, miosis, lacrimation. **GI:** Nausea, vomiting, abdominal cramps, diarrhea, borborygmi, belching, salivation, fecal incontinence (large doses), urge to defecate (or urinate). **Respiratory:** Acute asthmatic attack, dyspnea (large doses).

DIAGNOSTIC TEST INTERFERENCE Bethanechol may cause increases in **serum amylase** and **serum lipase,** by stimulating pancreatic secretions, and may increase **AST, serum bilirubin,** and **BSP retention** by causing spasms in sphincter of Oddi.

B

INTERACTIONS Drug: Ambenonium, neostigmine, other CHOLINESTERASE INHIBITORS compound cholinergic effects and toxicity; **mecamylamine** may cause abdominal symptoms and hypotension; **atropine, epinephrine, procainamide, quinidine,** antagonize effects of bethanechol. Severe hypotension with ganglionic blockers like **trimethaphan.**

PHARMACOKINETICS Absorption: Well absorbed PO. **Onset:** 30 min PO; 5–15 min SC. **Peak:** 60–90 min PO; 15–30 min SC. **Duration:** 1–6 h PO; 2 h SC. **Distribution:** Does not cross blood–brain barrier. **Metabolism:** Unknown. **Elimination:** Unknown.

NURSING IMPLICATIONS

Assessment & Drug Effects

- Monitor BP and pulse. Observe patient for at least 1 h following SC administration. Report early signs of overdosage: Salivation, sweating, flushing, abdominal cramps, nausea.
- Monitor I&O. Observe and record patient's response to bethanechol and report any failure of the drug to relieve the particular condition for which it was prescribed.
- Monitor respiratory status. Promptly report dyspnea or any other indication of respiratory distress.
- Supervise ambulation as indicated by patient response to drug.

Patient & Family Education

- Make position changes slowly and in stages, particularly from lying down to standing.
- Do not stand still for prolonged periods; sit or lie down at first indication of faintness.
- Do not drive or engage in potentially hazardous activities until response to drug is known.
- Note: Drug may cause blurred vision; take appropriate precautions.
- Do not breast feed while taking this drug without consulting physician.
- Store this medication out of reach of children.

BIPERIDEN HYDROCHLORIDE

(bye-per'i-den)

Akineton

BIPERIDEN LACTATE

Akineton

Classifications: AUTONOMIC NERVOUS SYSTEM AGENT; ANTICHOLINERGIC (PARASYMPATHOLYTIC); ANTIPARKINSONISM AGENT
Prototype: Levodopa
Pregnancy Category: C

AVAILABILITY 2 mg tablets; 5 mg/mL injection

ACTIONS Synthetic tertiary amine, antimuscarinic. In common with other antiparkinsonism drugs has atropine-like (anticholinergic) action. Antiparkinsonism activity is thought to be caused by reducing central excitatory action of acetylcholine on cholinergic receptors in the extrapyramidal system.

THERAPEUTIC EFFECTS This action helps to establish some balance between cholinergic (excitatory) and dopaminergic (inhibitory) activity in the basal ganglia with the result of controlling the effect of extrapyramidal symptoms.

USES Adjunct in all forms of parkinsonism. Also used to control drug-induced parkinsonism (extrapyramidal symptoms) associated with reserpine and phenothiazine therapy.

CONTRAINDICATIONS Narrow-angle glaucoma; GI or GU obstruction, megacolon; tardive dyskinesia. Safety during pregnancy (category C), lactation, or in children is not established.

CAUTIOUS USE Older adults or debilitated patients; prostatic hypertrophy; glaucoma; cardiac arrhythmias; epilepsy; safety in children is not established.

ROUTE & DOSAGE

Child: **IM/IV** 0.04 mg/kg or 1.2 mg/m^2, may repeat q30min (max 8 mg/24 h)
Adult: **IM/IV** 2 mg injected slowly; may repeat q30min (max 8 mg/24h)

STORAGE
Store in tightly closed, light-resistant containers at 15°–30° C (59°–86° F) unless otherwise directed.

ADMINISTRATION
Intramuscular
- Give slowly, deep IM into a large muscle mass appropriate for age (see Part I).
- Monitor ambulation because incoordination may occur.

Intravenous

PREPARE **Direct:** Give undiluted.
ADMINISTER **Direct:** Infuse slowly at a rate of 2 mg or a fraction thereof over 1 min. Keep patient recumbent when receiving parenteral biperiden and for at least 15 min thereafter. Postural hypotension, disturbances of coordination, and temporary euphoria can occur following IV administration.

ADVERSE EFFECTS CNS: Drowsiness, dizziness, muscle weakness, lack of coordination, disorientation, euphoria, agitation, confusion. **CV:** Mild, transient postural hypotension (following IM), tachycardia. **Special Senses:** *Blurred vision,* photophobia. **GI:** *Dry mouth,* nausea, vomiting, constipation.

INTERACTIONS Drug: Alcohol and other CNS DEPRESSANTS increase sedation; **haloperidol,** PHENOTHIAZINES, OPIATES, TRICYCLIC ANTIDEPRESSANTS, **quinidine** increase risk of anticholinergic side effects.

PHARMACOKINETICS Unknown.

B

NURSING IMPLICATIONS

Assessment & Drug Effects

- Monitor BP and pulse after IV administration. Advise patient to make position changes slowly and in stages, particularly from recumbent to upright position.
- Monitor for and report immediately: Mental confusion, drowsiness, dizziness, agitation, hematuria, and decrease in urinary flow.
- Assess for and report blurred vision.
- Monitor I&O ratio and pattern.
- Note: Biperiden usually reduces muscle rigidity.

Patient & Family Education

- Do not drive or engage in potentially hazardous activities until response to drug is known.
- Note: Patients on prolonged therapy can develop tolerance; an increase in dosage may be required.
- Do not breast feed while taking this drug without consulting physician.

BISACODYL ⦿

(bis-a-koe′dill)

Apo-Bisacodyl ♣, Bisacolax, Bisco-Lax ♣, Dacodyl, Deficol, Dulcolax, Fleet Bisacodyl, Laxit ♣, Theralax

Classifications: GASTROINTESTINAL AGENT; STIMULANT LAXATIVE
Pregnancy Category: C

AVAILABILITY 5 mg tablets; 10 mg suppository

ACTIONS Expands intestinal fluid volume by increasing epithelial permeability.

THERAPEUTIC EFFECTS Induces peristaltic contractions by direct stimulation of sensory nerve endings in the colonic wall.

USES Temporary relief of acute constipation and for evacuation of colon before surgery, proctoscopic, sigmoidoscopic, and radiologic examinations. Also used to cleanse colon before delivery and to relieve constipation in patients with spinal cord damage.

CONTRAINDICATIONS Acute surgical abdomen, nausea, vomiting, abdominal cramps, intestinal obstruction, fecal impaction; use of rectal suppository in presence of anal or rectal fissures, ulcerated hemorrhoids, proctitis. Do NOT use in newborns.

CAUTIOUS USE Safety during pregnancy (category C), lactation, or in children is not established.

ROUTE & DOSAGE

Laxative

Child: **PO** ≥6 y, 5–10 mg prn **PR** ≥12 y, 10 mg; 2–11 y, 5–10 mg; <2 y, 5 mg
Adult: **PO** 5–15 mg prn (max 30 mg for special procedures) **PR** 10 mg prn

---

Common adverse effects in *italic*; life-threatening effects underlined; generic names in **bold**; drug classifications in SMALL CAPS; ♣ Canadian drug name; ⦿ Prototype drug.

STORAGE
Store tablets in tightly closed containers at temperatures not exceeding 30° C (86° F).

ADMINISTRATION

Oral

- Give in the evening or before breakfast because of action time required (approximately 6–10 h).
- Give enteric-coated tablets whole to avoid gastric irritation; do not cut or crush. Patient should not chew tablets. Preferably give with a full glass (240 mL) of water or other liquid or generous amount of water for age.
- Do not give within 1 h of antacids or milk. These substances may cause premature dissolution of enteric coating; early release of drug in stomach may result in gastric irritation and loss of cathartic action.

Rectal

- Suppository may be inserted at time bowel movement is desired. Usually effective in 15–60 min.
- Storage is same as tablets.

ADVERSE EFFECTS Systemic effects not reported. Mild cramping, nausea, diarrhea, fluid and electrolyte disturbances (especially potassium and calcium).

INTERACTIONS Drug: ANTACIDS will cause early dissolution of enteric-coated tablets, resulting in abdominal cramping.

PHARMACOKINETICS Absorption: 5–15% absorbed from GI tract. **Onset:** 6–8 h PO; 15–60 min PR. **Metabolism:** Metabolized in liver. **Elimination:** Excreted in urine, bile, and breast milk.

NURSING IMPLICATIONS

Assessment & Drug Effects

- Do not allow patient to chew or crush tablets.
- Do NOT use in newborn.
- Evaluate periodically patient's need for continued use of drug; bisacodyl usually produces 1 or 2 soft formed stools daily.
- Monitor patients receiving concomitant anticoagulants. Indiscriminate use of laxatives results in decreased absorption of vitamin K.

Patient & Family Education

- Add high-fiber foods slowly to regular diet to avoid gas and diarrhea. Ensure generous amount of daily fluid intake for age.
- Do not breast feed while taking this drug without consulting prescriber.
- Store this medication out of reach of children.

BISMUTH SUBSALICYLATE

(bis'muth)

Pepto-Bismol

Classifications: GASTROINTESTINAL AGENT; ANTIDIARRHEAL; SALICYLATE

Prototype: Diphenoxylate with atropine

Pregnancy Category: A

Common adverse effects in *italic;* life-threatening effects underlined; generic names in **bold;** drug classifications in SMALL CAPS; ♣ Canadian drug name; ⊘ Prototype drug.

187

B

AVAILABILITY 262 mg tablets/caplets; 130 mg/15 mL, 262 mg/15 mL, 524 mg/15 mL liquid

ACTIONS Hydrolyzed in GI tract to salicylate, which is believed to inhibit synthesis of prostaglandins responsible for GI hypermotility and inflammation.
THERAPEUTIC EFFECTS Effectiveness as an antidiarrheal also appears to be due to direct antimicrobial action and to an antisecretory effect on intestinal secretions exposed to toxins particularly of *Escherichia coli* and *Vibrio cholerae*.

USES Prophylaxis and treatment of traveler's diarrhea (turista) and for temporary relief of indigestion.
UNLABELED USES *Helicobacter pylori* associated with peptic ulcer disease.

CONTRAINDICATIONS Hypersensitivity to aspirin or other salicylates; concurrent use with aspirin; use for more than 2 day in presence of high fever or in children <3 y unless prescribed by physician; do not use with chickenpox or flu.
CAUTIOUS USE Diabetes and gout; concurrent use with salicylates and anticoagulants; pregnancy (category C), lactation.

ROUTE & DOSAGE

Diarrhea
Child: **PO** 3–6 y, 5 mL or ½ tab q30–60min prn (max 8 doses/day); 6–9 y, 10 mL or ⅔ tab q30–60min prn (max 8 doses/day); 9–12 y, 15 mL or 1 tab q30–60min prn (max 8 doses/day)
Adult: **PO** 30 mL or 2 tab q30–60min prn (max 8 doses/day)

Traveler's Diarrhea
Adult: **PO** 15–30 mL or 2–4 tab q.i.d. for 3 wk

Peptic Ulcer Disease
Child: **PO** <10 y, 15 mL q.i.d. for 6 wk
Adult: **PO** 2 tablets q.i.d. with 2 additional antibiotics for 10–14 days

STORAGE
Store at 15°–30° C (59°–86° F) unless otherwise directed.

ADMINISTRATION
Oral
- Ensure chewable tablets are chewed or crushed before being swallowed and followed with at least 8 oz water or other liquid.

ADVERSE EFFECTS GI: Temporary *darkening of stool* and tongue, metallic taste, bluish gum line; bleeding tendencies. With high doses: fecal impaction. **CNS:** Encephalopathy (disorientation, muscle twitching). **Hematologic:** Bleeding tendency. **Special Senses:** Tinnitus, hearing loss. **Urogenital:** Incontinence.

DIAGNOSTIC TEST INTERFERENCE Because bismuth subsalicylate is radiopaque, it may interfere with ***radiographic studies*** of GI tract.

Common adverse effects in *italic;* life-threatening effects <u>underlined</u>; generic names in **bold;** drug classifications in SMALL CAPS; ♣ Canadian drug name; ◐ Prototype drug.

B

INTERACTIONS Drug: Bismuth may decrease the absorption of TETRACY-CLINES, QUINOLONES **(ciprofloxacin, norfloxacin, ofloxacin).**

PHARMACOKINETICS Absorption: Undergoes chemical dissociation in GI tract to bismuth subcarbonate and sodium salicylate; bismuth is minimally absorbed, but the salicylate is readily absorbed (80%).

NURSING IMPLICATIONS

Assessment & Drug Effects

- Monitor bowel function; note that stools may darken and tongue may appear black. These are temporary effects and will disappear without treatment.
- Lab tests: *H. pylori* breath test when used for peptic ulcers. Do not give with chickenpox or flu-like symptoms. Do not give with other non-steroidal anti-inflammatory drugs so ask about OTC medicines. Ask for history of bleeding and do not administer in these cases.

Patient & Family Education

- Note: Bismuth contains salicylate. Use caution when taking aspirin and other salicylates. Many OTC medications for colds, fever, and pain contain salicylates.
- Consult prescriber if diarrhea is accompanied by fever or continues for more than 2 days.
- Note: Temporary grayish black discoloration of tongue and stool may occur.
- Do not breast feed while taking this drug without consulting prescriber.
- Store this medication out of reach of children.

BLEOMYCIN SULFATE

(blee-oh-mye′sin)
Blenoxane
Classifications: ANTINEOPLASTIC; ANTIBIOTIC
Prototype: Doxorubicin
Pregnancy Category: D

AVAILABILITY 15 units, 30 units powder for injection

ACTIONS A toxic drug with low therapeutic index; intensely cytotoxic. By unclear mechanism, blocks DNA, RNA, and protein synthesis. A cell cycle-phase nonspecific agent. Widely used in combination with other chemotherapeutic agents because it lacks significant myelosuppressive activity.

THERAPEUTIC EFFECTS This mixture of cytotoxic antibiotics from a strain of *Streptomyces verticillus* has strong affinity for skin and lung tumor cells, in contrast to its low affinity for cells in hematopoietic tissue.

USES As single agent or in combination with other chemotherapeutic agents, as adjunct to surgery and radiation therapy. Squamous cell carcinomas of head, neck, penis, cervix, and vulva; lymphomas (including

---

Common adverse effects in *italic;* life-threatening effects underlined; generic names in **bold;** drug classifications in SMALL CAPS; ♣ Canadian drug name; ⊘ Prototype drug.

reticular cell sarcoma, lymphosarcoma, Hodgkin's); testicular carcinoma; malignant pleural effusions.
UNLABELED USES *Mycosis fungoides* and *Verruca vulgaris* (common warts).

CONTRAINDICATIONS History of hypersensitivity or idiosyncrasy to bleomycin; women of childbearing age, pregnancy (category D), lactation.
CAUTIOUS USE Compromised hepatic, renal, or pulmonary function; previous cytotoxic drug or radiation therapy.

ROUTE & DOSAGE

Squamous Cell Carcinoma, Testicular Carcinoma
Child/Adult: **SC, IM, IV** 10–20 units/m^2 or 0.25–0.5 units/kg 1–2 times/wk (max 300–400 units)
Lymphomas
Child/Adult: **SC, IM, IV** 10–20 units/m^2 1–2 times/wk after a 1–2 units test dose times 2 doses
Hodgkin's Disease, Maintenance
Child/Adult: **SC, IM, IV** 1 units IM or IV/day or 5 units/wk

STORAGE
Store unopened ampules at 15°–30° C (59°–86° F) unless otherwise specified by manufacturer.

ADMINISTRATION
- Child: Must be given under care and direction of pediatric oncology specialist. Use recommended handling techniques for hazardous medications (see Part I).
- Note: Due to risk of anaphylactoid reaction, give lymphoma patients ≤2 units for first two doses. If no reaction, follow regular dosage schedule.

Subcutaneous/Intramuscular
- Reconstitute with sterile water, NS, or bacteriostatic water by adding 1–5 mL to the 15-units vial or 2–10 mL to the 30-units vial. Amount of diluent is determined by the total volume of solution that will be injected.
- Inject IM deeply into site appropriate for age (see Part I); change sites with each injection.

Intravenous
IV administration to infants and children: Verify correct IV concentration and rate of infusion with physician.

PREPARE **Intermittent:** Dilute each 15 U with at least 5 mL of sterile water or NS. May be further diluted in 50–100 mL of the chosen diluent. Do not dilute with any solution containing D5W.
ADMINISTER **Intermittent:** Give each 15 U or faction thereof over 10 min through Y-tube of free-flowing IV.
INCOMPATIBILITIES: **Solution/Additive: Aminophylline, ascorbic acid, carbenicillin,** CEPHALOSPORINS, **diazepam, hydrocortisone, methotrexate, mitomycin, nafcillin, penicillin G, terbutaline.**

ADVERSE EFFECTS Body as a Whole: Hypersensitivity (<u>anaphylactoid reaction</u>); *mild febrile reaction.* **CNS:** Headache, mental confusion. **GI:** Stomatitis, ulcerations of tongue and lips, anorexia, nausea, vomiting, diarrhea, weight loss. **Hematologic:** Thrombocytopenia, leukopenia. **Respiratory:** <u>Pulmonary toxicity</u> (dose and age-related); interstitial pneumonitis, pneumonia, or fibrosis. **Skin:** Diffuse alopecia (reversible), *hyperpigmentation, pruritic erythema,* vesiculation, acne, thickening of skin and nail beds, *patchy hyperkeratosis,* striae, peeling, bleeding. **Other:** Pain at tumor site; phlebitis; necrosis at injection site.

INTERACTIONS Drug: Other ANTINEOPLASTIC AGENTS increase bone marrow toxicity; decreases effects of **digoxin, phenytoin.**

PHARMACOKINETICS Distribution: Concentrates mainly in skin, lungs, kidneys, lymphocytes, and peritoneum. **Metabolism:** Unknown. **Elimination:** 60–70% recovered in urine as parent compound. **Half-Life:** 2 h.

NURSING IMPLICATIONS

Assessment & Drug Effects

- Start with a test dose. Monitor patient closely for at least 24 h (vital signs, auscultation of chest, careful observations). If there is no acute reaction (hypotension, hyperpyrexia, chills, confusion, wheezing, cardiopulmonary collapse), start regular dosage schedule. Anaphylactoid reaction can be fatal (see Appendix D-1). It may occur immediately or several hours after first or second dose, especially in lymphoma patients (10%).
- Therapeutic effectiveness: Favorable response, if any, is expected within 2 wk for treatment of Hodgkin's or testicular tumor, and within 3 wk for squamous cell cancers.
- Monitor vital signs. Febrile reaction (mild chills and fever) is relatively common in patients receiving bleomycin therapy. It usually occurs within the first few hours after administration of a large single dose and lasts about 4–12 h. Reaction tends to become less frequent with continued drug administration, but can recur at any time. Be alert for and report signs of infection such as respiratory infections, aching, rashes, gastrointestinal distress, etc. Assess immunization status prior to beginning therapy in order to be alert for diseases that pose risk.
- Monitor for and report any of the following: Unexplained bleeding or bruising; evidence of deterioration of renal function (changed I&O ratio and pattern, decreasing creatinine clearance, weight gain or edema); evidence of pulmonary toxicity (nonproductive cough, chest pain, dyspnea).
- Note: Stomatitis can be a dose limiting factor because oral ulcerations may interfere with adequate nutrient intake, leading to severe debilitation. Consult physician if an oral local anesthetic is indicated. Apply 10 min before meals to take effect so that patient can eat with less pain.
- Check weight at regular intervals under standard conditions. Weight loss and anorexia may persist a long time after therapy has been discontinued.

- Report symptoms of skin toxicity (hypoesthesia, urticaria, tender swollen hands) promptly. May develop in second or third week of treatment and after 150–200 units of bleomycin have been administered. Therapy may be discontinued.

Patient & Family Education
- Avoid OTC drugs during antineoplastic treatment period unless approved by physician.
- Report skin irritation, which may not develop for several weeks after therapy begins. Report signs of infections. Avoid exposure to persons with infectious diseases.
- Hyperpigmentation may occur in areas subject to friction and pressure, skin folds, nail cuticles, scars, and intramuscular sites.
- Do not breast feed while taking this drug.

BRETYLIUM TOSYLATE
(bre-til′ee-um)
Bretylate ♣, Bretylol
Classifications: CARDIOVASCULAR AGENT; ANTIARRHYTHMIC, CLASS III
Prototype: Amiodarone
Pregnancy Category: C

AVAILABILITY 2 mg/mL, 4 mg/mL, 50 mg/mL injection

ACTIONS Mechanism of action is complex and not fully understood. Suppresses ventricular fibrillation by direct action on the myocardium and ventricular tachycardia by adrenergic blockade. Shortly after administration, norepinephrine is released from adrenergic postganglionic nerve terminals, resulting in a moderate increase in BP, heart rate, and ventricular irritability. Subsequently (1–2 h), drug-induced release and reuptake of norepinephrine are blocked, leading to a state resembling surgical sympathectomy. Orthostatic hypotension commonly occurs as a result of peripheral adrenergic blockade; some degree of hypotension may occur even while patient is supine. In most patients, tolerance to this effect develops after several days.
THERAPEUTIC EFFECTS Suppresses arrhythmias with a reentry mechanism and decreases dispersion of ectopic foci. PR, QT, and QRS intervals are unchanged. Because onset of desired action is delayed, bretylium is not a first-line antiarrhythmic agent.

USES Short-term prophylaxis and treatment of ventricular fibrillation; life-threatening arrhythmias such as ventricular fibrillation not responsive to conventional therapy (e.g., lidocaine, procainamide, direct current [cardioversion]).

CONTRAINDICATIONS Contraindicated in arrhythmias caused by digoxin toxicity. Safety during pregnancy (category C), lactation, or in children is not established.
CAUTIOUS USE Digitalis-induced arrhythmias, patients with fixed cardiac output (e.g., severe aortic stenosis or severe pulmonary hypertension

Common adverse effects in *italic;* life-threatening effects <u>underlined</u>; generic names in **bold;** drug classifications in SMALL CAPS; ♣ Canadian drug name; ❷ Prototype drug.

because profound hypotension may result), sinus bradycardia, patients on digitalis maintenance, angina pectoris; impaired renal function.

ROUTE & DOSAGE

Ventricular Fibrillation

Child: **IV** 5 mg/kg, may repeat q10–20min (max 30 mg/kg) **IM** 2–5 mg/kg as single dose **Maintenance Dose IM, IV** 5 mg/kg/dose q6–8h
Adult: **IV** 5 mg/kg rapid IV injection, may increase to 10 mg/kg and repeat q15–30min (max 30 mg/kg/day); may also give by continuous infusion at 1–2 mg/min **IM** 5–10 mg/kg, may repeat in 1–2 h if arrhythmia persists, then 5–10 mg/kg q6–8h for maintenance

STORAGE

Store at 15°–30° C (59°–86° F) unless otherwise directed.

ADMINISTRATION

Limit use to patients in facilities adequately equipped and staffed for constant monitoring of ECG and BP and for cardiovascular/pulmonary resuscitation and cardioversion.

Intramuscular

- Administer no more than 5 mL in any one IM site, or administer smaller amounts as determined by recommended maximum for child's size.
- Keep a record of injection sites. Injection into same site can cause muscle atrophy, necrosis, and fibrosis.

Intravenous

- IV administration to infants and children: Verify correct IV concentration and rate of infusion/injection with physician.

PREPARE **Direct:** Give undiluted. **Intermittent:** Give diluted in 50 mL or more of NS or D5W.
ADMINISTER **Direct:** Give undiluted at a rate of 1 dose/15 sec.
Intermittent: Give diluted at a rate of 1–2 mg/min.
INCOMPATIBILITIES: **Solution/Additive: Dobutamine, nitroglycerin, phenytoin. Y-Site: Phenytoin.**

ADVERSE EFFECTS CV: Initial hypertension followed by supine and postural *hypotension* with dizziness, vertigo, light-headedness, faintness, syncope, transitory hypertension, bradycardia, increased frequency of PVCs, exacerbation of digitalis-induced arrhythmias. **GI:** *Nausea, vomiting* (particularly with rapid IV). **Respiratory:** Respiratory depression.

DIAGNOSTIC TEST INTERFERENCE *Urinary VMA, epinephrine,* and *norepinephrine* levels may be decreased during bretylium therapy.

INTERACTIONS Drug: Lidocaine, procainamide, propranolol, quinidine may antagonize antiarrhythmic effects and compound hypotension; ANTIHYPERTENSIVE AGENTS will add to hypotensive effects; increased sensitivity to digitalis and catecholamines.

PHARMACOKINETICS Onset: Minutes after IV; up to 6 h IM. **Peak:** 6–9 h. **Duration:** 6–24 h. **Distribution:** Does not cross blood–brain barrier; not

Common adverse effects in *italic;* life-threatening effects <u>underlined</u>; generic names in **bold**; drug classifications in SMALL CAPS; ♣ Canadian drug name; ☻ Prototype drug.

193

known if crosses placenta or distributed into breast milk. **Metabolism:** Not metabolized. **Elimination:** 70–80% excreted in urine in 24 h. **Half-Life:** 4–17 h.

NURSING IMPLICATIONS

Assessment & Drug Effects

- Anticipate vomiting. IV administration is associated with a high incidence of nausea and vomiting. These side effects can be minimized by slow administration of drug (≥10 min).
- Establish baseline readings and monitor BP and ECG when drug is administered. Observe for initial transient rise in BP, increased heart rate, PVCs and other arrhythmias, or worsening of existing arrhythmias, which may occur within a few minutes to 1 h after drug administration. Keep physician informed. Initial effect of hypertension is usually followed within 1 h by a fall in supine BP and by orthostatic hypotension.
- Use supine position until patient develops tolerance to hypotensive effect of bretylium (generally in several days). Hypotension can occur in the supine position, particularly in patients with severely compromised cardiac function. It may not readily respond to therapy (e.g., vasopressors, fluids); early reporting is essential.
- Raise or lower head of bed slowly; advise patient to make position changes slowly in order to prevent orthostatic hypotension.
- Monitor I&O, particularly in patients with impaired renal function.

Patient & Family Education

- Make position changes slowly. If allowed to be out of bed, dangle legs for a few minutes before standing, but do not stand still for prolonged periods. Males should sit on toilet to urinate.
- Do not breast feed while taking this drug without consulting physician.

BROMPHENIRAMINE MALEATE

(brome-fen-ir′a-meen)
Codimal-A, Conjec-B, Cophene-B, Dehist, Dimetane, Dimetane Extentabs, Nasahist B, Sinusol-B
Classifications: ANTIHISTAMINE (H₁-RECEPTOR ANTAGONIST)
Prototype: Diphenhydramine
Pregnancy Category: C

AVAILABILITY 10 mg/mL injection **Combination Products:** Ingredient in many oral combination products containing a decongestant, expectorant, and/or analgesic; available with phenylpropanolamine as Dimetapp or Bromanate

ACTIONS Antihistamine similar to diphenhydramine; shares properties of other antihistamines. Has less sedative effect than diphenhydramine. Competes with histamine for H₁-receptor sites on effector cells, thus blocking histamine-mediated responses.
THERAPEUTIC EFFECTS Effective against upper respiratory symptoms and allergic manifestations.

USES Symptomatic treatment of allergic manifestations. Also used in various cough mixtures and antihistamine-decongestant cold formulations.

CONTRAINDICATIONS Hypersensitivity to antihistamines; acute asthma; with MAOIS; pregnancy (category C), lactation; newborns.
CAUTIOUS USE Older adults; prostatic hypertrophy; narrow-angle glaucoma; cardiovascular or renal disease; hyperthyroidism.

ROUTE & DOSAGE

Allergy

Child: **PO** >12 y, 4–8 mg q6–8h *or* 8–12 mg of sustained release q8–12h (max 12 mg/24 h); *6–12 y,* 2–4 mg/dose q6–8h (max 12–16 mg/24 h), *<6 y,* 0.5 mg/kg/day divided into 3–4 doses (max 6–8 mg/24 h) **SC, IM, IV** 0.5 mg/kg/24 h divided into doses given q6–8h
Adult: **PO** 4–8 mg t.i.d. or q.i.d. *or* 8–12 mg of sustained release b.i.d. or t.i.d. **SC/IM/IV** 5–20 mg q6–12h (max 40 mg/24 h)

STORAGE
Store in tightly covered container at 15°–30° C (59°–86° F) unless otherwise directed. Elixir and parenteral form should be protected from light. Avoid freezing.

ADMINISTRATION
Oral
▪ Give with meals or a snack to prevent gastric irritation.

Subcutaneous/Intramuscular
▪ Give without further dilution or diluted to a 1:10 ratio with NS.

Intravenous
PREPARE Direct: Give undiluted or diluted with 10 mL D5W or NS.
ADMINISTER Direct: Give IV push slowly over 1 min to a recumbent patient.
INCOMPATIBILITIES: Solution/Additive: Radio-contrast media (diatrizoate, iothalamate).

ADVERSE EFFECTS Body as a Whole: Hypersensitivity reaction (urticaria, increased sweating, <u>agranulocytosis</u>). **CNS:** *Sedation,* drowsiness, dizziness, headache, disturbed coordination. **GI:** Dry mouth, throat, and nose, stomach upset, constipation. **Special Senses:** Ringing or buzzing in ears. **Skin:** Rash, photosensitivity.

DIAGNOSTIC TEST INTERFERENCE May cause false-negative *allergy skin tests.*

INTERACTIONS Drug: Alcohol and other CNS DEPRESSANTS add to sedation.

PHARMACOKINETICS Peak: 3–9 h. **Duration:** Up to 48 h. **Distribution:** Crosses placenta. **Elimination:** 40% excreted in urine within 72 h; 2% in feces. **Half-Life:** 12–34 h.

Common adverse effects in *italic;* life-threatening effects <u>underlined</u>; generic names in **bold;** drug classifications in SMALL CAPS; ♣ Canadian drug name; ❷ Prototype drug.

195

B

NURSING IMPLICATIONS

Assessment & Drug Effects

Discontinue 48 h before allergy testing.

- Drowsiness, sweating, transient hypotension, and syncope may follow IV administration; reaction to drug should be evaluated. Monitor and report results and side effects. Most symptoms respond to reduction in dosage.
- Lab tests: Periodic CBC in patients receiving long-term therapy.
- Be alert that when given in combination with phenylpropanolamine, additional cautions and teaching are needed.

Patient & Family Education

- Acute hypersensitivity reaction can occur within minutes to hours after drug ingestion. Reaction is manifested by high fever, chills, and possible development of ulcerations of mouth and throat, pneumonia, and prostration. Patient should seek medical attention immediately.
- Follow diligent mouth care. Sugarless gum, lemon drops, or frequent rinses with warm water may relieve dry mouth.
- Do not drive a car or other potentially hazardous activities until response to drug is known.
- Do not take alcoholic beverages or other CNS depressants (e.g., tranquilizers, sedatives, pain or sleeping medicines) without consulting physician.
- Do not breast feed while taking this drug.
- Store this medication out of reach of children.

BUDESONIDE

(bu-des'o-nide)

Entocort EC, Pulmicort Turbuhaler, Rhinocort, Rhinocort Aqua, Rhinocort Turbuhaler

Classifications: HORMONE AND SYNTHETIC SUBSTITUTE; ADRENAL CORTICOSTEROID; GLUCOCORTICOID; MINERALOCORTICOID

Prototype: Hydrocortisone

Pregnancy Category: B for inhaled, C for oral

AVAILABILITY 32 mcg/nasal aerosol; 200 mcg/metered oral inhalation; 3 mg capsule

ACTIONS Has potent glucocorticoid and weak mineralocorticoid activity. Its anti-inflammatory action on nasal mucosa is unknown.

THERAPEUTIC EFFECTS Glucocorticoids have a wide range of inhibitory activities against multiple cell types (e.g., neutrophils, macrophages) and mediators (e.g., histamine, cytokines) involved in allergic and nonallergic/irritant mediated inflammation; unapproved for but used in mild to moderate croup.

USES Treatment of allergic and perennial rhinitis, Crohn's disease; prophylaxis for asthma.

CONTRAINDICATIONS Hypersensitivity to budesonide, lactation.

Common adverse effects in *italic;* life-threatening effects <u>underlined</u>; generic names in **bold**; drug classifications in SMALL CAPS; ♣ Canadian drug name; ❷ Prototype drug.

CAUTIOUS USE Concomitant administration of systemic oral steroids; active or quiescent tuberculosis; infections of respiratory tract; in sun-treated fungal, bacterial, or systemic viral infections or ocular herpes simplex; recent nasal septal ulcers; recurrent epistaxis; nasal surgery or trauma; pregnancy (category C for oral; category B for inhaled). Safety and efficacy for children <6 y not established.

ROUTE & DOSAGE

Crohn's Disease
Adult: **PO** 9 mg once daily in morning for up to 8 wk, may taper to 6 mg daily for 2 wk prior to discontinuing. May repeat 8 wk course for recurring episodes of active Crohn's disease.

Croup (unapproved use)
Child: Nebulized mist with 2 mg

Asthma
Child: >6 y: One oral inhalation (200 mcg) b.i.d. and increase prn up to max 4 inhalations/day. Nasal inhalation 2 sprays in each nostril q.a.m. and g.h.s. or 4 sprays in each nostril q.a.m. Reduce to lowest effective dose to maintain control (max 8 sprays 250 mcg/day)
Adult: 1–2 inhalations b.i.d. (max 4 inhalations/day for someone with no prior steroid use or 8 mg/day for someone with prior inhaled or oral steroid use)

Asthma Prophylaxis, Rhinitis
See Appendix I-1

STORAGE
Store at 25° C (77° F); excursions permitted to 15°–30° C (59°–86° F).

ADMINISTRATION

Oral
- Ensure that capsules are swallowed whole and not chewed.
- Give only in the morning.
- Patients with moderate to severe liver disease should be monitored for increased S&S of hypercorticism. Reducing the dose of ENTOCORT EC capsules should be considered in these patients.
- Rinse mouth after oral inhalation.

ADVERSE EFFECTS Body as a Whole: Arthralgia, fatigue, fever, hyperkinesis, myalgia, asthenia, paresthesia, tremor. **CNS:** Dizziness, emotional lability, facial edema, nervousness, *headache,* agitation, confusion, insomnia, drowsiness. **CV:** Chest pain, hypertension, palpitations, sinus tachycardia. **GI:** Abdominal pain, dyspepsia, gastroenteritis, oral candidiasis, xerostomia, diarrhea, *nausea, vomiting,* cramps. **Hematologic:** Epistaxis. **Metabolic:** Hypokalemia, weight gain. **Respiratory:** Bronchospasms, *infections,* cough, rhinitis, sinusitis, dyspnea, hoarseness, wheezing. **Skin:** Eczema, pruritus, purpura, rash, alopecia. **Special Senses:** Contact dermatitis, reduced sense of smell, nasal pain. **Urogenital:** Intermenstrual bleeding, dysuria.

B

INTERACTIONS Drug: Ketoconazole may increase oral budesonide concentrations and toxicity; toxicity may also occur with **anastrozole** (high doses only), **clarithromycin, cyclosporine, danazol, delavirdine, diltiazem, erythromycin, fluconazole, fluoxetine, fluvoxamine, indinavir, isoniazid, INH, itraconazole, mibefradil, nefazodone, nelfinavir, nicardipine, norfloxacin, oxiconazole, quinidine, quinine, ritonavir, saquinavir, troleandomycin, verapamil,** and **zafirlukast. Food: Grapefruit juice** will significantly increase bioavailability of oral budesonide.

PHARMACOKINETICS Absorption: 20% of nasal inhalation dose, 6–13% of orally inhaled dose, and 9% of oral dose reach systemic circulation; PO form is absorbed from duodenum at pH >5.5; oral bioavailability increases 2.5 times in hepatic cirrhosis. **Onset:** 8–12 h inhaled, 2 wk oral. **Distribution:** 90% protein bound. **Metabolism:** 85% of absorbed dose undergoes first-pass metabolism to 2 inactive metabolites by CYP 3A4. **Elimination:** 60% excreted in urine, 40% in feces. **Half-Life:** 2–3.6 h.

NURSING IMPLICATIONS

Assessment & Drug Effects

- Monitor closely for signs and symptoms of hypercorticism if concomitant doses of ketoconazole or other CYP3A4 inhibitors (see DRUG INTERACTIONS) are being given.
- Monitor patients with moderate to severe liver disease for increased S&S of hypercorticism.
- Lab tests: Periodic serum potassium.

Patient & Family Education

- Notify the physician immediately for any of the following: Itching, skin rash, fever, swelling of face and neck, difficulty breathing, or if you develop signs and symptoms of infection.
- Do not drink grapefruit juice or eat grapefruit regularly.
- Avoid people with infections, especially those with chickenpox or measles if you have never had these conditions.
- Do not breast feed while taking this drug.
- Store this medication out of reach of children.

BUMETANIDE

(byoo-met′a-nide)
Bumex
Classifications: FLUID AND WATER BALANCE AGENT; LOOP DIURETIC
Prototype: Furosemide
Pregnancy Category: C

AVAILABILITY 0.5 mg, 1 mg, 2 mg tablets; 0.25 mg/mL injection

ACTIONS Sulfonamide derivative structurally related to furosemide and with similar pharmacologic effects. Diuretic activity is 40 times greater, however, and duration of action is shorter than that of furosemide. Causes both potassium and magnesium wastage.

THERAPEUTIC EFFECTS Inhibits sodium and chloride reabsorption by direct action on proximal ascending limb of the loop of Henle. Also appears to inhibit phosphate and bicarbonate reabsorption. Produces only mild hypotensive effects at usual diuretic doses.

USES Edema associated with CHF; hepatic or renal disease, including nephrotic syndrome. Has been used in management of postoperative and premenstrual edema, edema accompanying disseminated carcinoma, and mild hypertension. May be used concomitantly with a potassium-sparing diuretic.

CONTRAINDICATIONS Hypersensitivity to bumetanide or to other sulfonamides; anuria, markedly elevated BUN; hepatic coma; severe electrolyte deficiency; lactation. Avoid in neonates at risk for kernicterus due to displacement of bilirubin from albumin binding sites. Safety during pregnancy (category C) is not established.

CAUTIOUS USE Hepatic cirrhosis, as history of gout; history of hypersensitivity to furosemide, sulfonamides, with children.

ROUTE & DOSAGE

Edema

Neonates: **PO/IM/IV** 0.01–0.05 mg/kg q24–48h
Infant/Child: **PO/IM/IV** 0.015–0.1 mg/kg/dose given daily (max 10 mg/day)
Adult: **PO** 0.5–2 mg daily, may repeat at 4–5 h intervals if needed (max 10 mg/day) **IV/IM** 0.5–1 mg over 1–2 min, repeated q2–3h prn (max 10 mg/day)

STORAGE

Store in tight, light-resistant container at 15°–30° C (59°–86° F) unless otherwise directed.

ADMINISTRATION

Oral

- Give with food or milk to reduce risk of gastrointestinal irritation.
- Administered in the morning as a single dose, either daily or by intermittent schedule. For some patients, diuresis is reportedly more effective when administered in two divided doses, morning and evening.

Intramuscular

- Use undiluted solution for injection.

Intravenous

PREPARE Direct Continuous: Give direct IV undiluted or diluted for infusion with D5W, NS, RL.
ADMINISTER Direct: Give IV push at a rate of a single dose over 1–2 min. **Continuous:** Use diluted solution and give at prescribed rate.
INCOMPATIBILITIES: Solution/Additive: Dobutamine. Diluted infusion should be used within 24 h after preparation.

Common adverse effects in *italic;* life-threatening effects <u>underlined</u>; generic names in **bold;** drug classifications in SMALL CAPS; ♣ Canadian drug name; ☉ Prototype drug.

199

B

ADVERSE EFFECTS Body as a Whole: Sweating, hyperventilation, glycosuria. **CNS:** Dizziness, headache, weakness, fatigue. **CV:** Hypotension, ECG changes, chest pain, *hypovolemia.* **GI:** Nausea, vomiting, abdominal or stomach pain, GI distress, diarrhea, dry mouth. **Metabolic:** *Hypokalemia,* hyponatremia, hyperuricemia, hyperglycemia; *hypomagnesemia;* decreased calcium, chloride. **Musculoskeletal:** Muscle cramps, muscle pain, stiffness or tenderness; arthritic pain. **Special Senses:** Ear discomfort, ringing or buzzing in ears, impaired hearing.

INTERACTIONS Drug: AMINOGLYCOSIDES, **cisplatin** increase risk of ototoxicity; bumetanide increases risk of hypokalemia-induced **digoxin** toxicity; NONSTEROIDAL ANTI-INFLAMMATORY DRUGS (NSAID) may attenuate diuretic and hypotensive response; **probenecid** may antagonize diuretic activity; bumetanide may decrease renal elimination of **lithium.**

PHARMACOKINETICS Absorption: Readily absorbed from GI tract. **Onset:** 30–60 min PO; 40 min IV. **Peak:** 0.5–2 h. **Duration:** 4–6 h. **Distribution:** Distributed into breast milk. **Metabolism:** Partially metabolized in liver. **Elimination:** 80% excreted in urine in 48 h, 10–20% excreted in feces. **Half-Life:** 60–90 min.

NURSING IMPLICATIONS

Assessment & Drug Effects

Assess for allergies because allergy to sulfonamides may indicate allergy to bumetanide.

- Monitor I&O and report onset of oliguria or other changes in I&O ratio and pattern promptly.
- Monitor weight, BP, and pulse rate. Assess for hypovolemia by taking BP and pulse rate while patient is lying, sitting, and standing. Adminster oral doses with food.
- Lab tests: Serum electrolytes, blood studies, liver and kidney function tests, uric acid (particularly patients with history of gout), and blood glucose. Determine values initially and at regular intervals; measurements are especially important in patients receiving prolonged treatment, high doses, or who are on sodium restriction.
- Monitor for S&S of hypomagnesemia, hyponatremia, hypocalcemia, and hypokalemia (see Appendix D-1) especially in those receiving digitalis or who have CHF, hepatic cirrhosis, ascites, diarrhea, or potassium-depleting nephropathy.
- Monitor patients with hepatic disease carefully for fluid and electrolyte imbalances, which can precipitate encephalopathy (inappropriate behavior, altered mood, impaired judgment, confusion, drowsiness, coma).
- Question patient about hearing difficulty or ear discomfort. Patients at risk of ototoxic effects include those receiving the drug IV, especially at high doses, those with severely impaired renal function, and those receiving other potentially ototoxic or nephrotoxic drugs (see Appendix D-1).
- Monitor diabetics for loss of glycemic control.

Patient & Family Education

- Report symptoms of electrolyte imbalance to physician promptly (e.g., weakness, dizziness, fatigue, faintness, confusion, muscle cramps, headache, paresthesias).

Common adverse effects in *italic;* life-threatening effects <u>underlined;</u> generic names in **bold;** drug classifications in SMALL CAPS; ✦ Canadian drug name; ☻ Prototype drug.

- Eat potassium-rich foods such as fruit juices, potatoes, cereals, skim milk, and bananas while taking bumetanide.
- Report S&S of ototoxicity promptly to physician (see Appendix D-1). Parents should be alert for hearing problems in children.
- Monitor blood glucose for loss of glycemic control if diabetic.
- Do not breast feed while taking this drug.
- Store this medication out of reach of children.

BUPIVACAINE HYDROCHLORIDE

(byoo-piv′a-kane)
Marcaine, Sensorcaine
Classifications: CENTRAL NERVOUS SYSTEM AGENT; LOCAL ANESTHETIC (AMIDE-TYPE)
Prototype: Procaine
Pregnancy Category: C

AVAILABILITY 0.25%, 0.5%, 0.75% injection

ACTIONS Anesthetic of the amide type. Decreases sodium flux into nerve cell, inhibiting initial depolarization, and prevents propagation and conduction of the nerve impulse. Progression of anesthesia, related to diameter, myelination, and conduction velocity of affected fibers is manifested clinically as sequential loss of nerve function. May stimulate or depress the CNS or do both.

THERAPEUTIC EFFECTS Primary depressant effect is in medulla and higher centers affecting patient's reaction to pain, temperature, and touch, as well as proprioception and skeletal muscle tone.

USES Infiltration anesthesia; peripheral, sympathetic nerve, and epidural (including caudal) block anesthesia; 0.75% bupivacaine solution in dextrose is used for spinal anesthesia.

CONTRAINDICATIONS Known sensitivity to bupivacaine, local anesthetics, other amide-type anesthetics. Parabens, or metabisulfites; acidosis; heart block; severe hemorrhage; hypotension and shock; hypertension, cerebrospinal diseases; obstetrical paracervical anesthesia or spinal anesthesia in septicemia; topical or IV regional anesthesia; intercurrent use with chloroprocaine; history of malignant hyperthermia. Safety during pregnancy (category C) other than during labor, lactation, or children <12 y is not established.

CAUTIOUS USE Older adults or debilitated patient; hepatic or renal disease; known drug allergies and sensitivities; dysrhythmias; children >12 y; obstetrical delivery.

ROUTE & DOSAGE

Infiltration Anesthesia

Child: **Caudal block** 1–3.7 mg/kg; **Epidural block** 1.25 mg/kg
Adult: **IM Local infiltration, sympathetic block** 0.25% solution; **Lumbar epidural** 0.25%, 0.5%, 0.75% solutions; **Caudal block, peripheral nerve block** 0.25%, 0.5% solutions; **Retrobulbar block** 0.75% solution

---

Common adverse effects in *italic;* life-threatening effects underlined; generic names in **bold;** drug classifications in SMALL CAPS; ✦ Canadian drug name; ⊘ Prototype drug.

201

B

STORAGE
Store ampules at 15°–30° C (59°–86° F); protect from freezing. Solutions with epinephrine should be protected from light.

ADMINISTRATION

Intramuscular
- Inject slowly with frequent aspirations to avoid intravascular injection.

Intrathecal
- Do not use preparations containing preservatives for epidural or spinal anesthesia.
- Do not use multiple-dose vial for lumbar or caudal epidural block.

INCOMPATIBILITIES: **Solution/Additive: Sodium bicarbonate.**

ADVERSE EFFECTS Body as a Whole: Hypersensitivity (cutaneous lesions, urticaria, sneezing, diaphoresis, syncope, hyperthermia, angioneurotic edema [including <u>laryngeal edema</u>], <u>anaphylaxis, anaphylactoid reaction</u>). Seizures and cardiac arrest have been associated with inadvertent IV administration. **CNS:** Nervousness, unusual anxiety, excitement, dizziness, drowsiness, tremors, convulsions, unconsciousness, <u>respiratory arrest</u>. **Special Senses:** Pupillary constriction; blurred or double vision; tinnitus. **GI:** Nausea, vomiting. **Other:** Inflammation or sepsis at injection site, chills, pupillary constriction. **Associated with Epidural Anesthesia, Body as a Whole:** Total spinal block, persistent analgesia, paresthesia. **Urogenital:** Urinary retention, fecal incontinence, loss of perineal sensation and sexual function. **Other:** Slowing of labor, increased incidence of forceps delivery, cranial nerve palsies (with inadvertent intrathecal injection).

INTERACTIONS Drug: CNS DEPRESSANTS augment CNS depression; with **isoproterenol, ergonovine** there is persistent hypertension and a risk of CVA if bupivacaine used with **epinephrine.** MAOIS, TRICYCLIC ANTIDEPRESSANTS, PHENOTHIAZINES cause severe or prolonged hypotension or hypertension if bupivacaine used with **epinephrine.**

PHARMACOKINETICS Onset: 4–17 min for epidural, caudal, peripheral, or sympathetic block; within 1 min for spinal block. **Duration:** 3–5 h for epidural, caudal, peripheral, or sympathetic block; 1.25–2.5 h for spinal block. **Distribution:** Crosses placenta. **Metabolism:** Metabolized in liver. **Elimination:** 6% excreted unchanged in urine. **Half-Life:** 1.5–5.5 h in adults, 8.1 h in neonates.

NURSING IMPLICATIONS

Assessment & Drug Effects
- Monitor for signs of inadvertent intravascular injection, which can produce a transient "epinephrine response" (increased heart rate or systolic BP or both, circumoral pallor, palpitations, nervousness) within 45 sec in the unsedated patient and an increase by 20 bpm or more in heart rate for at least 15 sec in sedated patient.
- Vasoconstrictor-containing solution should be administered cautiously, if at all, to areas with end arteries (e.g., digits, penis) or to areas that

have a compromised blood supply; ischemia and gangrene can result. Inspect areas for evidence of reduced perfusion because of vasospasm: pale, cold, sensitive skin.

- Note: Systemic reactions (toxicity) are more apt to occur in children and may develop rapidly or be delayed for as long as 30 min after administration.
- Monitor for toxicity: CNS stimulation (unusual anxiety, excitement, restlessness) usually occurs first, followed by CNS depression (drowsiness, unconsciousness, respiratory arrest). However, because stimulation is apt to be transient or absent, drowsiness may be the first sign in some patients (especially children and older adults).
- Monitor BP and fetal heart rate continuously during labor because maternal hypotension may accompany regional anesthesia. Place mother on left side with legs elevated.
- Monitor cardiac and respiratory status continuously in patients receiving retrobulbar and dental blocks. Be cautious to avoid IV administration.
- Monitor for level of pain.

Patient & Family Education
- After spinal anesthesia, sensation to lower extremities may not return for 2.5–3.5 h.

BUPRENORPHINE HYDROCHLORIDE
(byoo-pre-nor′feen)
Buprenex, Subutex

BUPRENORPHINE HYDROCHLORIDE/NALOXONE HYDROCHLORIDE DIHYDRATE
Suboxone
Classifications: CENTRAL NERVOUS SYSTEM AGENT; ANALGESIC; NARCOTIC (OPIATE) AGONIST-ANTAGONIST
Prototype: Pentazocine
Pregnancy Category: C
Controlled Substance: Schedule III

AVAILABILITY 0.324 mg/mL injection; 2 mg, 8 mg sublingual tablets; 2 mg buprenorphine/0.5 mg naloxone, 8 mg buprenorphine/2 mg naloxone sublingual tablets

ACTIONS Opiate agonist-antagonist with agonist activity approximately 30 times that of morphine and antagonist activity equal to or up to 3 times greater than that of naloxone. Respiratory depression occurs infrequently probably due to drug's opiate antagonist activity. Psychologic and limited physical dependence develops infrequently; tolerance to drug rarely develops.
THERAPEUTIC EFFECTS Dose-related analgesia results from a high affinity of buprenorphine for mu opioid receptors and is an antagonist at the kappa-opiate receptors in the CNS. Naloxone is an antagonist at the mu-opioid receptor.

Common adverse effects in *italic;* life-threatening effects <u>underlined;</u> generic names in **bold;** drug classifications in SMALL CAPS; ◆ Canadian drug name; ● Prototype drug.

203

BUPRENORPHINE HYDROCHLORIDE

B

USES *Injectable* used principally for moderate to severe postoperative pain; also for pain associated with cancer and trigeminal neuralgia, accidental trauma, ureteral calculi, MI. *Sublingual tablets* used for treatment of opioid dependence.

UNLABELED USES *Injectable* to reverse fentanyl-induced anesthesia. *Sublingual tablets* may be used to ease cocaine withdrawal.

CONTRAINDICATIONS Known hypersensitivity to buprenorphine (both drug forms) or hypersensitivity to naloxone (Suboxone). Safety during pregnancy (category C), lactation, or in children <13 y is not established.

CAUTIOUS USE Patient with history of opiate use; compromised respiratory function (e.g., chronic obstructive pulmonary disease, cor pulmonale, decreased respiratory reserve, hypoxia, hypercapnia, or preexisting respiratory depression); concomitant use of other respiratory depressants; hypothyroidism, myxedema, Addison's disease; severe renal or hepatic impairment; debilitated patients; acute alcoholism, delirium tremens; prostatic hypertrophy, urethral stricture; comatose patient; patients with CNS depression, head injury or intracranial lesion; biliary tract dysfunction.

ROUTE & DOSAGE

Postoperative Pain
Child: **IV/IM** *2–12 y,* 2–6 mcg/kg q4–6h prn
Adult: **IV/IM** 0.3 mg q6h up to 0.6 mg q4h or 25–50 mcg/h by IV infusion

Opioid Dependence
Adult: **SL** Initiate with 8 mg daily Subutex on day 1 at least 4 h after last opioid dose, 16 mg daily Subutex on day 2, then switch to Suboxone for maintenance therapy at the same buprenorphine dose as day 2 (e.g., 16 mg daily). Adjust dose daily until opiate withdrawal effects are suppressed. Maintenance dose range: 4–24 mg/day buprenorphine

STORAGE
Store at 15°–30° C (59°–86° F); avoid freezing.

ADMINISTRATION

Sublingual
- Place SUBOXONE and SUBUTEX tablets under tongue until dissolved. For doses requiring more than 2 tablets, place all tablets at once under tongue, or if patient cannot accommodate all tablets, place 2 tablets at a time under tongue.
- Instruct to hold the tablets under tongue until dissolved; advise not to swallow.

Intramuscular
- Give undiluted, deep IM into a large muscle appropriate for age (see Part I).

Intravenous

PREPARE **Direct:** Give undiluted. Do not use if discolored or contains particulate matter.
ADMINISTER **Direct:** Give slowly at a rate of 0.3 mg over 2 min to the patient in a recumbent position.

ADVERSE EFFECTS CNS: *Sedation, drowsiness,* dizziness, vertigo, *headache,* amnesia, euphoria, asthenia, *insomnia, pain* (when used for withdrawal), *withdrawal symptoms.* **CV:** Hypotension, vasodilation. **Special Senses:** Miosis. **GI:** *Nausea,* vomiting, diarrhea, *constipation.* **Respiratory:** Respiratory depression, hyperventilation. **Skin:** Pruritus, injection site reactions, *sweating.*

INTERACTIONS Drug: Alcohol, OPIATES, other CNS DEPRESSANTS, BENZODI-AZEPINES augment CNS depression; **diazepam** may cause respiratory or cardiovascular collapse; AZOLE ANTIFUNGALS (e.g., **fluconazole**), MACROLIDE ANTIBIOTICS (e.g., **erythromycin**), and PROTEASE INHIBITORS (e.g., **saquinavir**) may increase buprenorphine levels.

PHARMACOKINETICS Absorption: Widely variable sublingual absorption. **Onset:** 10–30 min IM/IV. **Peak:** 1 h IM/IV; 2–6 h SL. **Duration:** 6–10 h. **Metabolism:** Metabolized extensively in liver by CYP3A4 to active metabolite norbuprenorphine. **Elimination:** 70% eliminated in feces and 30% in urine in 7 days. **Half-Life:** 2.2 h IM/IV; 37 h SL.

NURSING IMPLICATIONS

Assessment & Drug Effects

- Monitor respiratory status during therapy. Buprenorphine-induced respiratory depression is about equal to that produced by 10 mg morphine, but onset is slower, and if it occurs, it lasts longer.
- Note: Respiratory depression in the healthy adult plateaus or may even decrease in severity with doses of more than 1.2 mg because of antagonist activity of the drug.
- Use lower dosing of buprenorphine with a concurrent NSAID or other nonnarcotic analgesic due to additive analgesic effect.
- Monitor I&O ratio and pattern during buprenorphine therapy; urinary retention is a potential adverse effect.
- Lab tests: Baseline liver function, renal function, alkaline phosphatase, and PSA.
- Supervise ambulation; drowsiness occurs in 66% of patients taking this drug.

Patient & Family Education

- Do not drive or engage in other potentially hazardous activities until response to drug is known.
- Do not use alcohol or other CNS depressing drugs without consulting physician. An additive effect exists between buprenorphine hydrochloride and other CNS depressants including alcohol.
- Do not breast feed while taking this drug without consulting physician.
- Store this medication out of reach of children.

Common adverse effects in *italic;* life-threatening effects underlined; generic names in **bold;** drug classifications in SMALL CAPS; ♣ Canadian drug name; ✪ Prototype drug.

205

B

BUSPIRONE HYDROCHLORIDE
(byoo-spye'rone)
BuSpar
Classifications: CENTRAL NERVOUS SYSTEM AGENT; ANXIOLYTIC
Prototype: Lorazepam
Pregnancy Category: B

AVAILABILITY 5 mg, 10 mg, 15 mg tablets

ACTIONS First-generation agent in a new class of anxiolytics. Has chemical and pharmacologic properties unrelated to those of the benzodiazepines or other psychotherapeutic agents. Action is unclear, but appears to be focused mainly on the brain D_2-dopamine receptors. It has agonist effects on presynaptic dopamine receptors and also a high affinity for serotonin ($5-HT_{1A}$) receptors. Unlike other anxiolytics, it seems to cause less clinically significant impairment of cognitive and motor performance and produces minimal if any interaction with other CNS depressants, including alcohol.

THERAPEUTIC EFFECTS Antianxiety effect is due to its serotonin reuptake inhibition and agonist effects on dopamine receptors of the brain.

USES Management of anxiety disorders and for short-term treatment of generalized anxiety.

UNLABELED USES Adjuvant for nicotine withdrawal.

CONTRAINDICATIONS Concomitant use of alcohol and buspirone. Safety during pregnancy (category B), labor and delivery, lactation, or in children <18 y is not established.

CAUTIOUS USE Moderate to severe renal or hepatic impairment.

ROUTE & DOSAGE

Anxiety
Adult: **PO** 7.5–15 mg/day in divided doses, may increase by 5 mg/day q2–3 days as needed (max 60 mg/day)

STORAGE
Store at 15°–30° C (59°–86° F) in tightly closed container unless otherwise directed.

ADMINISTRATION

Oral
- Give with food to decrease nausea.
- Give 8 h before or after drinking grapefruit juice.

ADVERSE EFFECTS CNS: Numbness, paresthesia, tremors, *dizziness, headache,* nervousness, *drowsiness,* light-headedness, dream disturbances, decreased concentration, excitement, mood changes. **CV:** Tachycardia, palpitation. **Special Senses:** Blurred vision. **GI:** *Nausea,* vomiting, dry mouth, abdominal/gastric distress, diarrhea, constipation. **Urogenital:** Urinary frequency, hesitancy. **Musculoskeletal:** Arthralgias.

Common adverse effects in *italic;* life-threatening effects <u>underlined</u>; generic names in **bold**; drug classifications in SMALL CAPS; ✦ Canadian drug name; ❷ Prototype drug.

Respiratory: Hyperventilation, shortness of breath. **Skin:** Rash, edema, pruritus, flushing, easy bruising, hair loss, dry skin. **Other:** Fatigue, weakness.

DIAGNOSTIC TEST INTERFERENCE Buspirone may increase serum concentrations of *hepatic aminotransferases (ALT, AST)*.

INTERACTIONS Drug: May cause hypertension with MAOIS, **trazodone,** possible increase in liver transaminases; increased **haloperidol** serum levels.

PHARMACOKINETICS Absorption: Readily absorbed from GI tract but undergoes first-pass metabolism. **Onset:** 5–7 days. **Peak:** 1 h. **Metabolism:** Metabolized in liver. **Elimination:** 30–63% excreted in urine as metabolites within 24 h. **Half-Life:** 2–4 h.

NURSING IMPLICATIONS

Assessment & Drug Effects

- Monitor for therapeutic effectiveness. Desired response may begin within 7–10 day; however, optimal results take 3–4 wk. Reinforce the importance of continuing treatment to patient.
- Benzodiazepines or sedative-hypnotic drugs are withdrawn gradually before buspirone therapy is started. Observe patient for rebound symptoms, which may occur over varying time periods during first phase of treatment.
- Note: Buspirone may displace digoxin from its serum binding, increasing the potential for toxic serum levels of digoxin. If the two drugs must be given concomitantly, monitor cardiovascular parameters (BP, pulse) until dosage has been stabilized.
- Monitor for and report dystonia, motor restlessness, and involuntary repetitious movement of facial or cervical muscle.
- Observe for and report swollen ankles, decreased urinary output, changes in voiding pattern, jaundice, itching, nausea, or vomiting.

Patient & Family Education

- Take exactly as prescribed: Specifically, do not omit, skip, increase or decrease doses without advice of the prescriber.
- Report any of the following immediately: Involuntary, repetitive movements of face or neck; weakness, nervousness, nightmares, headache, or blurred vision; depression or thoughts of suicide.
- Do not use OTC drugs without advice of the prescriber while taking buspirone.
- Note: Adverse effects subside during continued therapy with or without dosage adjustment. Do not discontinue therapy.
- Do not drive or engage in other potentially hazardous activities until response to drug is known.
- Alert prescriber if you become pregnant; buspirone must be discontinued during pregnancy.
- Discuss limits of alcohol intake with prescriber; cautious use is generally advised.
- Note: It is important to understand the planned schedule for changes in doses and intervals to ensure low incidence of withdrawal or rebound symptoms when therapy is discontinued.
- Do not breast feed while taking this drug without consulting prescriber.
- Store this medication out of reach of children.

Common adverse effects in *italic;* life-threatening effects underlined; generic names in **bold;** drug classifications in SMALL CAPS; ✤ Canadian drug name; ◑ Prototype drug.

207

BUSULFAN
(byoo-sul′fan)
Busulfex, Myleran
Classifications: ANTINEOPLASTIC; ALKYLATING AGENT
Prototype: Cyclophosphamide
Pregnancy Category: D

AVAILABILITY 2 mg tablets; 6 mg/mL injection

ACTIONS Potent cytotoxic alkylating agent that may be mutagenic and carcinogenic. Cell-cycle nonspecific. Reduces total granulocyte mass but has little effect on lymphocytes and platelets except in large doses. May cause widespread epithelial cellular dysplasia severe enough to make it difficult to interpret exfoliative cytologic examinations from lung, breast, bladder, and uterine cervix.

THERAPEUTIC EFFECTS Causes cell death by acting predominantly on slowly proliferating stem cells by inducing cross linkage in DNA, thus blocking replication. Acquired resistance may develop, probably due to intracellular inactivation of busulfan.

USES Palliative treatment of chronic myelogenous (myeloid, granulocytic, myelocytic) leukemia for patients no longer responsive to radiation therapy or to previously tried antineoplastics. Does not appreciably extend survival time.

UNLABELED USES Polycythemia vera, severe thrombocytosis, as adjunct in treatment of myelofibrosis, allogenic bone transplantation in patients with acute nonlymphocytic leukemia.

CONTRAINDICATIONS Therapy-resistant chronic lymphocytic leukemia; lymphoblastic crisis of chronic myelogenous leukemia; bone marrow depression, immunizations (patient and household members), chickenpox (including recent exposure), herpetic infections. Safety during pregnancy (category D) or lactation is not established.

CAUTIOUS USE Persons of both genders in childbearing years; history of gout or urate renal stones; prior irradiation or chemotherapy.

ROUTE & DOSAGE

Chronic Myelogenous Leukemia
Child: **PO** 0.06–0.12 mg/kg/day or 1.8–4.6 mg/m²/day
Adult: **PO** 4–8 mg/day until maximal clinical and hematologic improvement, may use 1–4 mg/day if remission is shorter than 3 mo

Stem Cell Transplantation
Child: <12kg 1.1 mg/kg q6h × 4 days ≥12 kg 0.8 mg/kg q6h × 4 days
Adult: 0.8 mg/kg q6h × 4 days
(Stem cell transplant therapy given with cyclophosphamide and phenytoin)

STORAGE
Store in tightly capped, light-resistant container at 15°–30° C (59°–86° F), unless otherwise specified.

Common adverse effects in *italic;* life-threatening effects <u>underlined;</u> generic names in **bold;** drug classifications in SMALL CAPS; ♣ Canadian drug name; ⦿ Prototype drug.

ADMINISTRATION

Child: Given only under care and supervision of pediatric oncologist.

Oral

- Give at same time each day.
- Give on an empty stomach to minimize nausea and vomiting. Antiemetics routinely given.
- May be given with phenytoin prior to bone marrow transplant in order to prevent seizures caused by its effect of lowered seizure threshold.

IV

- Dilute injection solution with NS or D5W 10 times to achieve concentration of 0.5 mg/mL. Use 5-micro m nefron filter to withdraw drug. Do not mix with other drugs. Do not administer if any particulates are visualized in the preparation.

ADVERSE EFFECTS CNS: Decreases seizure threshold. **Hematologic:** Major toxic effects are related to bone marrow failure; agranulocytosis (rare), pancytopenia, thrombocytopenia, leukopenia, *anemia*. **Urogenital:** Flank pain, renal calculi, uric acid nephropathy, acute renal failure, gynecomastia, testicular atrophy, azoospermia, impotence, sterility in males, ovarian suppression, menstrual changes, amenorrhea (potentially irreversible), menopausal symptoms. **Respiratory:** Irreversible pulmonary fibrosis ("busulfan lung"). **Skin:** Alopecia, hyperpigmentation. **Other:** Endocardial fibrosis, dizziness, cholestatic jaundice, infections.

DIAGNOSTIC TEST INTERFERENCE Busulfan may decrease *urinary 17-OHCS* excretion, and may increase *blood and urine uric acid* levels. Drug-induced cellular dysplasia may interfere with interpretation of *cytologic studies.*

INTERACTIONS Drug: **Probenecid, sulfinpyrazone** may increase **uric acid** levels.

PHARMACOKINETICS Absorption: Readily absorbed from GI tract. **Peak:** 4 h. **Duration:** 4 h. **Metabolism:** Metabolized in liver. **Elimination:** 10–50% excreted in urine within 48 h.

NURSING IMPLICATIONS

Assessment & Drug Effects

- *Child:* Must be given under care and direction of pediatric oncology specialist. Use recommended handling techniques for hazardous medications (see Part I).
- *IV:* Initial pediatric doses are followed by therapeutic blood levels and dose adjustment as needed. Consult pharmacist and oncologist for blood collection methods.
- Be alert for and report signs of infection such as respiratory infections, aching, rashes, and gastrointestinal distress.
- Assess immunization status prior to beginning therapy in order to be alert for diseases that pose risk.
- Monitor for therapeutic effectiveness: Normal leukocyte count is usually achieved in about 2 mo.
- Monitor the following: Vital signs, weight, I&O ratio and pattern. Urge patient to increase fluid intake to 10–12 (8-oz) glasses daily (if allowed) to ensure adequate urinary output.

Common adverse effects in *italic;* life-threatening effects underlined; generic names in **bold;** drug classifications in SMALL CAPS; ♣ Canadian drug name; ◑ Prototype drug.

209

B

- Monitor for and report symptoms suggestive of superinfection (see Appendix D-1), particularly when patient develops leukopenia.
- Lab test: Baseline Hgb, Hct, WBC with differential, platelet count, liver function, kidney function, serum uric acid; repeat at least weekly.
- Avoid invasive procedures during periods of platelet count depression.

Patient & Family Education

- Report signs of infections. Avoid exposure to persons with infectious diseases. Report to physician any of the following: Easy bruising or bleeding, cloudy or pink urine, dark or black stools; sore mouth or throat, unusual fatigue, blurred vision, flank or joint pain, swelling of lower legs and feet; yellowing white of eye, dark urine, light-colored stools, abdominal discomfort, or itching (hepatotoxicity).
- Use contraceptive measures during busulfan therapy and for at least 3 mo after drug is withdrawn.
- Do not breast feed while taking this drug without consulting physician.
- Store this medication out of reach of children.

BUTABARBITAL SODIUM
(byoo-ta-bar′bi-tal)
Barbased, Butalan, Butisol Sodium, Sarisol No. 2
Classifications: CENTRAL NERVOUS SYSTEM AGENT; BARBITURATE; ANXIOLYTIC; SEDATIVE-HYPNOTIC
Prototype: Phenobarbital
Pregnancy Category: D
Controlled Substance: Schedule III

AVAILABILITY 15 mg, 30 mg, 50 mg, 100 mg tablets; 30 mg/5 mL elixir

ACTIONS Intermediate-acting barbiturate, similar to phenobarbital. Appears to act at thalamus level, where it interferes with transmission of impulses to the cerebral cortex.

THERAPEUTIC EFFECTS Preoperative sedative agent that also is an effective antianxiety agent.

USES Hypnotic in short-term treatment of simple insomnia, as sedative for relief of anxiety, and to provide sedation preoperatively.

CONTRAINDICATIONS Porphyria; uncontrolled pain; severe respiratory disease; history of addiction; pregnancy (category D); lactation.
CAUTIOUS USE Severe renal or hepatic impairment; acute abdominal conditions; older adults or debilitated patients. Safe use in children <12 y is not established.

ROUTE & DOSAGE

Daytime Sedation
Child: **PO** 7.5–30 mg t.i.d.
Adult: **PO** 15–30 mg t.i.d. or q.i.d.

Preoperative Sedation
Child: **PO** 2–6 mg/kg in 3 equally divided doses (max 100 mg)
Adult: **PO** 50–100 mg 60–90 min before surgery

Common adverse effects in *italic;* life-threatening effects underlined; generic names in **bold;** drug classifications in SMALL CAPS; ◆ Canadian drug name; ❷ Prototype drug.

Hypnotic
Adult: **PO** 50–100 mg at bedtime.

STORAGE
Store in tightly covered containers, preferably at 15°–30° C (59°–86° F), unless otherwise directed.

ADMINISTRATION

Oral
- Schedule slow withdrawal following long-term use to avoid precipitating withdrawal symptoms.

ADVERSE EFFECTS CNS: Drowsiness, *residual sedation* ("hangover"), headache. **GI:** Nausea, vomiting, constipation, diarrhea. **Skin:** Urticaria, skin rash. **Musculoskeletal:** Muscle or joint pain.

INTERACTIONS Drug: **Alcohol** and other CNS DEPRESSANTS add to CNS and respiratory depression; butabarbital increases the metabolism of ORAL ANTICOAGULANTS, BETA BLOCKERS, CORTICOSTEROIDS, **doxycycline, griseofulvin, quinidine,** THEOPHYLLINES, ORAL CONTRACEPTIVES, decreasing their effectiveness. **Herbal: Kava-kava, valerian** may potentiate sedation.

PHARMACOKINETICS Absorption: Readily absorbed from GI tract. **Onset:** 40–60 min. **Peak:** 3–4 h. **Duration:** 6–8 h. **Distribution:** Crosses placenta; distributed into breast milk. **Metabolism:** Metabolized in liver. **Elimination:** Excreted in urine primarily as metabolites. **Half-Life:** Average 100 h.

NURSING IMPLICATIONS

Assessment & Drug Effects
- Assess for adverse effects. Debilitated patients sometimes manifest excitement, confusion, or depression. Children also may react with paradoxical excitement. Use of side rails may be advisable. Report these reactions to prescriber.

Patient & Family Education
- Do not drive or engage in other potentially hazardous activities until response to drug is known.
- Do not drink alcoholic beverages while taking this drug. Other CNS depressants may produce additive drowsiness; do not take without approval of physician.
- Note: Prolonged use is not recommended because tolerance to drug occurs in about 14 days.
- Do not breast feed while taking this drug.
- Store this medication out of reach of children.

BUTENAFINE HYDROCHLORIDE
(bu-ten'a-feen)
Mentax
Classifications: ANTI-INFECTIVE; ANTIFUNGAL ANTIBIOTIC
Prototype: Fluconazole
Pregnancy Category: B

B

AVAILABILITY 1% cream

ACTIONS Exerts antifungal action by inhibiting sterol synthesis, which may enhance susceptibility of the fungal membrane to damage by butenafine.
THERAPEUTIC EFFECTS Antifungal effectiveness against interdigital *tinea pedis* (athlete's foot), *tinea corporis* (ringworm), and *tinea cruris* (jock itch).

USES Treatment of tinea pedis, tinea corporis, and tinea curis due to *Epidermophyton floccosum, Trichophyton mentagrophytes, Trichophyton rubrum.*

CONTRAINDICATIONS Hypersensitivity to butenafine.
CAUTIOUS USE Hypersensitivity to naftifine or tolnaftate; pregnancy (category B); lactation. Safety and efficacy in children <12 y are not established.

ROUTE & DOSAGE

Tinea Pedis
Child/Adult: **Topical** >12 y, Apply to affected area and surrounding skin b.i.d. for 7 days or daily for 4 wk
Tinea Corporis, Tinea Cruris
Child/Adult: **Topical** >12 y, Apply to affected area and surrounding skin once daily

STORAGE
Store at 5°–30° C (41°–86° F).

ADMINISTRATION

Topical
- Apply sufficient cream to cover affected skin and surrounding areas.
- Do not use occlusive dressing unless specifically directed to do so.

ADVERSE EFFECTS Skin: Burning/stinging at application site, contact dermatitis, erythema, irritation, itching.

NURSING IMPLICATIONS

Assessment & Drug Effects
- Note: 2–4 wk of therapy are usually required for effective treatment.

Patient & Family Education
- Discontinue medication and notify physician if irritation or sensitivity develops.
- Avoid contamination of toys and other objects.
- Avoid contact with mucous membranes.
- Wash hands thoroughly before and after application of cream.
- Do not breast feed while taking this drug without consulting physician.
- Store this medication out of reach of children.

CAFFEINE ⊘
(kaf-een')
Caffedrine, Dexitac, NoDoz, Quick Pep, S-250, Tirend, Vivarin

CAFFEINE CITRATE
Cafcit
Classifications: CENTRAL NERVOUS SYSTEM AGENT; RESPIRATORY AND CEREBRAL STIMULANT; XANTHINE
Prototype: Caffeine
Pregnancy Category: C

AVAILABILITY 100 mg, 150 mg, 200 mg tablets; 250 mg/mL solution; 20 mg/mL caffeine citrate injection

ACTIONS Chief action is thought to be related to inhibition of the enzyme phosphodiesterase, which results in higher concentrations of cyclic AMP. Releases epinephrine and norepinephrine from adrenal medulla, producing CNS stimulation. Small doses improve psychic and sensory awareness and reduce drowsiness and fatigue by stimulating cerebral cortex. Higher doses stimulate medullary, respiratory, vasomotor, and vagal centers. Produces smooth muscle relaxation (especially bronchi) and dilation of coronary, pulmonary, and systemic blood vessels by direct action on vascular musculature. Mild diuretic action may result from increase in renal blood flow and glomerular filtration rate and decrease in renal tubular reabsorption of sodium and water. Increases contractile force of heart and cardiac output by direct stimulation of myocardium. Also stimulates secretion of gastric acid and digestive enzymes.

THERAPEUTIC EFFECTS Effective in managing neonatal apnea, and as an adjuvant for pain control in headaches and following dural puncture. Relief of headache is perhaps due to mild cerebral vasoconstriction action and increased vascular tone. It acts as a bronchodilator in asthma and may improve psychomotor performance through CNS stimulation.

USES Orally as a mild CNS stimulant to aid in staying awake and restoring mental alertness, and as an adjunct in narcotic and nonnarcotic analgesia. Used parenterally as an emergency stimulant in acute circulatory failure, as a diuretic, and to relieve spinal puncture headache.

UNLABELED USES Topical treatment of atopic dermatitis; neonatal apnea.

CONTRAINDICATIONS Acute MI, symptomatic cardiac arrhythmias, palpitations; peptic ulcer; insomnia, panic attacks. Safe use during pregnancy (category C), in lactation, and in children not established.

CAUTIOUS USE Diabetes mellitus; hiatal hernia; hypertension with heart disease.

ROUTE & DOSAGE

Mental Stimulant
Adult: **PO** 100–200 mg q3–4h prn

Common adverse effects in *italic;* life-threatening effects <u>underlined</u>; generic names in **bold;** drug classifications in SMALL CAPS; ♣ Canadian drug name; ⊘ Prototype drug.

C

Circulatory Stimulant
Adult: **IM** 200–500 mg prn
Spinal Puncture Headaches
Adult: **IV** 500 mg over 1 h, may repeat times 1 dose
Neonatal Apnea
Neonate: **PO/IV** 10–20 mg/kg as a loading dose, followed by a maintenance dose of 5–10 mg/kg 24 h later administered once daily.
▪ Doses given in mg of caffeine citrate. To convert to mg of caffeine, divide citrate dose by 2.

STORAGE
▪ Store at 15°–30° C (59°–86° F). Discard injection solution with particulate matter or discoloration.
▪ Caffeine citrate injection stable in most IV solutions for 24 h.

ADMINISTRATION
Oral
▪ Give sustained-release oral preparations not less than 6 h before bedtime.
▪ Ensure that timed-release form of drug is not chewed or crushed. It must be swallowed whole.
Intramuscular
▪ Give deep IM into a large muscle appropriate for age (see Part I).
Intravenous
▪ Note: IV route (caffeine citrate) reserved for preparation emergency situations only.
PREPARE **Direct:** Give undiluted.
ADMINISTER **Direct:** Emergency situations: IV push at a rate of 250 mg or fraction thereof over 1 min. With neonates use caffeine without sodium benzoate and check with physician regarding preferred rate.

ADVERSE EFFECTS Body as a Whole: Weight loss, especially in premature infants. **CV:** Tingling of face, flushing, palpitation, tachycardia or bradycardia, ventricular ectopic beats. **GI:** Nausea, vomiting; epigastric discomfort, gastric irritation (oral form), diarrhea, hematemesis, kernicterus (neonates). **CNS:** *Nervousness, insomnia,* restlessness, irritability, confusion, agitation, fasciculations, delirium, twitching, tremors, clonic convulsions. **Respiratory:** Tachypnea. **Special Senses:** Scintillating scotomas, tinnitus. **Urogenital:** Increased neonate urination, diuresis.

DIAGNOSTIC TEST INTERFERENCE Caffeine reportedly may interfere with diagnosis of pheochromocytoma or neuroblastoma by increasing urinary excretion of ***catecholamines, VMA,*** and ***5-HIAA*** and may cause false-positive increases in ***serum urate*** (by ***Bittner method***).

INTERACTIONS Drug: Increases effects of **cimetidine;** increases cardiovascular stimulating effects of BETA-ADRENERGIC AGONISTS; possibly increases **theophylline** toxicity.

PHARMACOKINETICS Absorption: Rapidly absorbed. **Peak:** 15–45 min. **Distribution:** Widely distributed throughout body; crosses blood–brain barrier and placenta. **Metabolism:** Metabolized in liver. **Elimination:** Excreted in urine as metabolites; excreted in breast milk in small amounts. **Half-Life:** 3–5 h in adults, 36–144 h in neonates.

NURSING IMPLICATIONS

Assessment & Drug Effects

- ***Therapeutic level*** for neonatal apnea is 5–25 mg/L. Toxic level is 50 mg/L. Obtain sample for trough level 30 min prior to PO dose.
- Monitor vital signs closely because large doses may cause intensification rather than reversal of severe drug-induced depressions.
- Observe children closely following administration because they are more susceptible than adults to the CNS effects of caffeine.
- Lab tests: Monitor blood glucose and HbA$_{1c}$ levels in diabetics.

Patient & Family Education

- Caffeine in large amounts may impair glucose tolerance in diabetics.
- Do not consume large amounts of caffeine because headache, dizziness, anxiety, irritability, nervousness, and muscle tension may result from excessive use, as well as from abrupt withdrawal of coffee (or oral caffeine). Withdrawal symptoms usually occur 12–18 h following last coffee intake.
- Store this medication out of reach of children.

CALCITONIN (HUMAN)

(kal-si-toe′nin)
Cibacalcin

CALCITONIN (SALMON)

Calcimar, Miacalcin

Classifications: HORMONE AND SYNTHETIC SUBSTITUTE; BONE METABOLISM REGULATOR
Prototype: Etidronate
Pregnancy Category: C

AVAILABILITY 200 international units/mL injection; 200 international units/spray

ACTIONS Human calcitonin and salmon calcitonin are synthetic polypeptides. Pharmacologic actions are the same, but salmon calcitonin is considerably more potent and has a longer duration of action. Antibody formation occurs commonly with salmon calcitonin and only rarely with human calcitonin. Calcitonin opposes the effects of parathyroid hormone on bone and kidneys, reduces serum calcium by binding to a specific receptor site on osteoclast cell membrane, and alters transmembrane passage of calcium and phosphorus. Promotes renal excretion of calcium and phosphorus and causes transient sodium and water loss.

THERAPEUTIC EFFECTS Effective in osteoporosis due to inhibition of bone resorption. Effective in symptomatic hypercalcemia by rapidly lowering serum calcium.

USES Symptomatic Paget's disease of bone (osteitis deformans), postmenopausal osteoporosis, osteogenesis imperfecta. Orphan drug approval (calcitonin human): short-term adjunctive treatment of severe hypercalcemic emergencies.
UNLABELED USES Diagnosis and management of medullary carcinoma of thyroid; treatment of osteogenesis imperfecta.

CONTRAINDICATIONS Hypersensitivity to fish proteins, gelatin, or to synthetic calcitonin; history of allergy. Safe use in children, pregnancy (category C), and lactation not established.
CAUTIOUS USE Renal impairment; osteoporosis; pernicious anemia; Zollinger-Ellison syndrome.

ROUTE & DOSAGE

Paget's Disease
Adult: **SC** Human 0.5 mg/day *or* 2–3 times/wk *or* 0.25 mg/day up to 0.5 mg b.i.d. **SC/IM** Salmon 100 international units/day may decrease to 50–100 international units/day *or* every other day
Intranasal 1–2 sprays (200–400 units) daily

Hypercalcemia
Adult: **SC/IM** Salmon 4 international units/kg q12h, may increase to 8 units/kg q6h if needed

Osteogenesis Imperfecta
Child: **SC/IM** Salmon 2 units/kg/dose 3 times weekly with oral calcium supplements

STORAGE
Store (human) calcitonin at 25° C (77° F) or less, protected from light, unless otherwise specified by manufacturer. Store calcitonin (salmon) in refrigerator, preferably at 2°–8° C (36°–46° F) unless otherwise directed.

ADMINISTRATION
Allergy Test Dose
- An allergy skin test is usually done prior to initiation of therapy. For salmon protein, prepare 10 units/mL with NS and administer 0.1 ID. The appearance of more than mild erythema or wheal 15 min after intracutaneous injection indicates that the drug should not be given.

Intranasal
- Activate the pump prior to first use; hold bottle upright and depress white side arms 6 times.
- The nasal spray is administered in one nostril daily; alternate nostrils.

Subcutaneous
- Human calcitonin is administered only by SC injection; salmon calcitonin may be administered by SC or IM injection.

Common adverse effects in *italic;* life-threatening effects <u>underlined;</u> generic names in **bold;** drug classifications in SMALL CAPS; ♣ Canadian drug name; ❷ Prototype drug.

Intramuscular

- Use IM route when the volume to be injected is >2 mL. For appropriate IM site selection see Part I.
- Rotate injection sites.

ADVERSE EFFECTS Body as a Whole: Headache, eye pain, feverish sensation, hypersensitivity reactions, <u>anaphylaxis</u>. Reported for human calcitonin only: Urinary frequency, chills, chest pressure, weakness, paresthesias, tender palms and soles, dizziness, nasal congestion, shortness of breath. **GI:** *Transient nausea,* vomiting, anorexia, unusual taste sensation, abdominal pain, diarrhea. **Skin:** Inflammatory reactions at injection site, flushing of face or hands, pruritus of ear lobes, edema of feet, skin rashes. **Urogenital:** Nocturia, diuresis, abnormal urine sediment.

INTERACTIONS Drug: may decrease serum **lithium** levels.

PHARMACOKINETICS (salmon calcitonin). **Onset:** 15 min. **Peak:** 4 h. **Duration:** 8–24 h. **Distribution:** Does not cross placenta; distribution into breast milk unknown. **Metabolism:** Metabolized in kidneys. **Elimination:** Excreted in urine. **Half-Life:** 1.25 h (1 h for human calcitonin).

NURSING IMPLICATIONS

Assessment & Drug Effects

- Have on hand epinephrine 1:1000, antihistamines, and oxygen in the event of a reaction. Also have readily available parenteral calcium, particularly during early therapy. Hypocalcemic tetany is a theoretical possibility.
- Examine urine specimens periodically for sediment with long-term therapy.
- Lab tests: Monitor for hypocalcemia (see Signs & Symptoms, Appendix D-1). Theoretically, calcitonin can lead to hypocalcemic tetany. Latent tetany may be demonstrated by Chvostek's or Trousseau's signs and by **serum calcium values:** 7–8 mg/dL (latent tetany); below 7 mg/dL (manifest tetany).
- Examine nasal passages prior to treatment with the nasal spray and anytime nasal irritation occurs.
- Nasal ulceration and heavy bleeding are indications for drug discontinuation.

Patient & Family Education

- Use the SC route for self-administration. Instruct in administration technique.
- Watch for redness, warmth, or swelling at injection site and report to prescriber, because these may indicate an inflammatory reaction. The transient flushing that commonly occurs following injection of calcitonin, particularly during early therapy, may be minimized by administrating the drug at bedtime. Consult prescriber.
- Maintain your drug regimen even though symptoms have been ameliorated to prevent early relapses.
- Ensure that you feel comfortable using the nasal pump properly. Notify prescriber if significant nasal irritation occurs.
- Consult prescriber before using OTC preparations. Some supervitamins, hematinics, and antacids contain calcium and vitamin D (vitamin may antagonize calcitonin effects).
- Store this medication out of reach of children.

CALCITRIOL 🅿️

(kal-si-trye'ole)

Calcijex, Rocaltrol

Classifications: HORMONE AND SYNTHETIC SUBSTITUTE; VITAMIN D ANALOG

Pregnancy Category: C

AVAILABILITY 0.25 mcg, 0.5 mcg tablets; 1 mcg/mL oral solution; 1 mcg/mL, 2 mcg/mL injection

ACTIONS Synthetic form of an active metabolite of ergocalciferol (vitamin D_2). In the liver, cholecalciferol (vitamin D_3) and ergocalciferol (vitamin D_2) are enzymatically metabolized to calcifediol, an activated form of vitamin D_3. Calcifediol is biodegraded in the kidney to calcitriol, the most potent form of vitamin D_3. Patients with nonfunctioning kidneys are unable to synthesize sufficient calcitriol and therefore must receive it pharmacologically.

THERAPEUTIC EFFECTS By promoting intestinal absorption and renal retention of calcium, calcitriol elevates serum calcium levels, decreases elevated blood levels of phosphate and parathyroid hormone, and decreases subperiosteal bone resorption and mineralization defects in some patients.

USES Management of hypocalcemia in patients undergoing chronic renal dialysis and in patients with hypoparathyroidism or pseudohypoparathyroidism.

UNLABELED USES Selected patients with vitamin D-dependent rickets, familial hypophosphatemia (vitamin D-resistant rickets); management of hypocalcemia in premature infants.

CONTRAINDICATIONS Hypercalcemia or vitamin D toxicity; pregnancy (category C), lactation. Safe use in children not established.

CAUTIOUS USE Hyperphosphatemia, patients receiving digitalis glycosides.

ROUTE & DOSAGE

Hypocalcemia

Child: **PO** for renal failure: 0.01–0.05 mcg/kg/24h. Titrate by 0.005–0.01 mcg/kg/24h increments q4–8wk based on response. **IV route NOT preferred:** 0.01–0.05 mcg/kg 3 times/wk
Adult: **PO** 0.25 mcg/day, may be increased by 0.25 mcg/day q4–8wk for dialysis patients or q2–4wk for hypoparathyroid patients if necessary. **IV** 0.5 mcg 3 times/wk at the end of dialysis, may need up to 3 mcg 3 times/wk

STORAGE

Store away from moisture, light, and heat in tightly covered, light-resistant containers at 15°–30° C (59°–86° F). Avoid freezing. Will degrade upon exposure to light. Calcitriol injection does not contain preservative and unused portions should be discarded.

ADMINISTRATION

Oral

- Oral dose can be taken either with food or milk or on an empty stomach. Discuss with prescriber.
- When given for hypoparathyroidism, the dose is given in the morning.

Intravenous

PREPARE **Direct:** Give undiluted.
ADMINISTER **Direct:** Give IV push over 30–60 sec.

ADVERSE EFFECTS Body as a Whole: Muscle or bone pain. **CV:** Palpitation. **GI:** Anorexia, nausea, vomiting, dry mouth, thirst, constipation, abdominal cramps, metallic taste. **Metabolic:** Vitamin D intoxication, hypercalcemia, hypercalciuria, hyperphosphatemia. **CNS:** Headache, weakness, mental confusion. **Special Senses:** Blurred vision, photophobia. **Urogenital:** Increased urination.

INTERACTIONS Drug: THIAZIDE DIURETICS may cause hypercalcemia; calcifediol-induced hypercalcemia may precipitate digitalis arrhythmias in patients receiving DIGITALIS GLYCOSIDES.

PHARMACOKINETICS Absorption: Readily absorbed from GI tract. **Onset:** 2–6 h. **Peak:** 10–12 h. **Duration:** 3–5 days. **Metabolism:** Metabolized in liver. **Elimination:** Excreted mainly in feces. **Half-Life:** 3–6 h.

NURSING IMPLICATIONS

Assessment & Drug Effects

- Lab tests: Determine baseline and periodic levels of serum calcium, phosphorus, magnesium, alkaline phosphatase, creatinine; measure urinary calcium and phosphorous levels q24h.
- Effectiveness of therapy depends on an adequate daily intake of calcium and phosphate. The physician may prescribe a calcium supplement on an as-needed basis.
- Monitor for hypercalcemia (see Appendix D-1). During dosage adjustment period, monitor serum calcium levels particularly twice weekly to avoid hypercalcemia.
- If hypercalcemia develops, withhold calcitriol and calcium supplements and notify physician. Drugs may be reinitiated when serum calcium returns to normal.

Patient & Family Education

- Discontinue the drug if experiencing any symptoms of hypercalcemia (see Appendix D-1) and contact prescriber.
- Do not use any other source of vitamin D during therapy, since calcitriol is the most potent form of vitamin D_3. This will avoid the possibility of hypercalcemia.
- Consult prescriber before taking an OTC medication. (Many products contain calcium, vitamin D, phosphates, or magnesium, which can increase adverse effects of calcitriol.)
- Maintain an adequate daily fluid intake unless you have kidney problems, in which case consult your physician about fluids.

Common adverse effects in *italic;* life-threatening effects <u>underlined</u>; generic names in **bold;** drug classifications in SMALL CAPS; ♣ Canadian drug name; ❍ Prototype drug.

219

■ Do not breast feed while taking this drug.
■ Store this medication out of reach of children.

CALCIUM CHLORIDE

Calciject, Calcitrans, Solucalcine

Classifications: FLUID AND ELECTROLYTIC BALANCE AGENT; REPLACEMENT SOLUTION
Prototype: Calcium gluconate
Pregnancy Category: C

AVAILABILITY 10% injection

ACTIONS Actions similar to those of calcium gluconate. Ionizes more readily and thus is more potent than calcium gluconate and more irritating to tissues. Provides excess chloride ions that promote acidosis and temporary (1–2 day) diuresis secondary to excretion of sodium.

THERAPEUTIC EFFECTS Rapidly and effectively restores serum calcium levels in acute hypocalcemia of various origins and is an effective cardiac stabilizer under conditions of hyperkalemia or resuscitation.

USES Treatment of cardiac resuscitation when epinephrine fails to improve myocardial contractions; for treatment of acute hypocalcemia (as in tetany due to parathyroid deficiency, vitamin D deficiency, alkalosis, insect bites or stings, and during exchange transfusions), for treatment of hypermagnesemia, and for cardiac disturbances of hyperkalemia.

CONTRAINDICATIONS Ventricular fibrillation, hypercalcemia, digitalis toxicity, injection into myocardium or other tissue; pregnancy (category C). **CAUTIOUS USE** Digitalized patients; sarcoidosis, renal insufficiency, history of renal stone formation; cor pulmonale, respiratory acidosis, respiratory failure; lactation.

ROUTE & DOSAGE

All doses are in terms of *elemental calcium*: 1 g calcium chloride = 272 mg (13.6 mEq) elemental calcium

Hypocalcemia

Infant: **IV** <1 mEq/dose and then reassess
Child: **IV** 10–20 mg/kg; reassess condition and calcium level and repeat as needed; administered slowly
Adult: **IV** 0.5–1 g (7–14 mEq) at 1–3 day intervals as determined by patient response and serum calcium levels

Hypocalcemic Tetany

Neonate: **IV** 2.4 mEq/kg/day in divided doses
Child: **IV** 0.5–0.7 mEq/kg t.i.d. or q.i.d.
Adult: **IV** 4.5–16 mEq prn

CPR

Child: **IV** 20 mg/kg, may repeat in 10 min
Adult: **IV** 2.7–3.7 mEq×1

STORAGE
Store at room temperature of 15°–30° C (59°–86° F).

ADMINISTRATION
Intravenous

- IV administration to neonates, infants, and children: Verify correct IV concentration and rate of infusion with physician.

PREPARE **Direct:** May be given undiluted or diluted (preferred) with an equal volume of NS for injection. Solution should be warmed to body temperature before administration.

ADMINISTER **Direct:** Avoid rapid administration. Give at 0.5–1 mL/min or more slowly if irritation develops. Do not exceed 100 mg/min for IV push or 45–90 mg/kg/h for IV infusion; maximum concentration for infusion is 20 mg/mL. Avoid rapid administration. Use a small-bore needle and inject into a large vein to minimize venous irritation and undesirable reactions

INCOMPATIBILITIES: **Solution/Additive: Amphotericin B, chlophenir-amine, dobutamine. Y-Site: Amphotericin B cholesteryl complex, propofol, sodium bicarbonate**

ADVERSE EFFECTS Body as a Whole: Tingling sensation. With rapid IV, sensations of heat waves (peripheral vasodilation), fainting. **CV:** With rapid infusion, hypotension, bradycardia, cardiac arrhythmias, <u>cardiac arrest</u>. **Skin:** Pain and burning at IV site, severe venous thrombosis, necrosis and sloughing (with extravasation).

INTERACTIONS Drug: May enhance inotropic and toxic effects of **digoxin;** antagonizes the effects of **verapamil** and possibly other CAL-CIUM CHANNEL BLOCKERS.

PHARMACOKINETICS Distribution: Crosses placenta. **Elimination:** Primarily excreted in feces; small amounts excreted in urine, pancreatic juice, saliva, and breast milk.

NURSING IMPLICATIONS

Assessment & Drug Effects
- Monitor ECG and BP and observe patient closely during administration. IV injection may be accompanied by cutaneous burning sensation and peripheral vasodilation, with moderate fall in BP. Avoid extravasation, which may lead to necrosis; central line preferred. Do NOT administer SC or IM.
- Advise ambulatory patient to remain in bed for 15–30 min or more depending on response following injection.
- Observe digitalized patients closely because an increase in serum calcium increases risk of digitalis toxicity.
- Lab tests: Determine serum pH, calcium, and other electrolytes frequently as guides to dosage adjustments.

Patient & Family Education
- Remain in bed for 15–30 min or more following injection and depending on response.
- Symptoms of mild hypercalcemia, such as loss of appetite, nausea, vomiting, or constipation may occur. If hypercalcemia becomes

severe, call health care provider if feeling confused or extremely excited.

- Do not use other calcium supplements or eat foods high in calcium, like milk, cheese, yogurt, eggs, meats, and some cereals, during therapy.
- Do not breast feed while taking this drug without consulting physician.

CALCIUM GLUCEPTATE
(gloo-sep'tate)
Calcium Glucoheptonate, Glucalcium, Calcitrans
Classifications: FLUID AND ELECTROLYTIC BALANCE AGENT; REPLACEMENT SOLUTION
Prototype: Calcium gluconate
Pregnancy Category: C

AVAILABILITY 1.1 g/5 mL injection

ACTIONS Calcium is an essential element for regulating the excitation threshold of nerves and muscles, blood clotting mechanisms, cardiac function, maintenance of renal function, and body skeleton and teeth. Also plays a role in regulating neurotransmitters and hormones, and functional integrity of cell membranes and capillaries. Calcium gluceptate acts like digitalis on the heart, increasing cardiac muscle tone and force of systolic contractions (positive inotropic effect).

THERAPEUTIC EFFECTS Preferred for use when IM administration is required as in neonatal tetany. Rapidly and effectively restores serum calcium levels in acute hypocalcemia of various origins and is an effective cardiac stabilizer under conditions of hyperkalemia or resuscitation.

USES To correct hypocalcemia and following each 100 mL of exchange transfusion in newborns.

CONTRAINDICATIONS Ventricular fibrillation, hypercalcemia, digitalis toxicity, injection into myocardium or other tissue; pregnancy (category C). **CAUTIOUS USE** Digitalized patients; sarcoidosis, renal insufficiency, history of renal stone formation; cor pulmonale, respiratory acidosis, respiratory failure; lactation.

ROUTE & DOSAGE

All doses are in terms of *elemental calcium*: 1 g calcium gluceptate = 82 mg (4.1 mEq) elemental calcium

Hypocalcemia
Child: **IV** 200–500 mg/kg/day divided into doses given q6h.
IM 0.5–1.1 g/day in 2–5 mL (220 mg/mL)
Adult: **IV/IM** 500–1100 mg/dose

Cardiac Arrest
Child: **IV** 110 mg/dose q 10 min prn

Exchange Transfusions with Citrated Blood
Neonate: **IV** 0.5 mL after each 100 mL of blood exchanged

C

STORAGE
Store at 15°–30° C (59°–86° F). Check expiration dates.

ADMINISTRATION

Intramuscular

- IM injection may produce mild local reactions. Generally, this route is used only in adults when IV administration is not feasible.
- Recommended IM site for adults is the upper outer quadrant of the buttock and in infants (if prescribed) the midlateral thigh.

Intravenous

PREPARE **Direct:** May be given undiluted. Solution should be warmed to body temperature before administration.

ADMINISTER **Direct:** Give at a rate not to exceed 100 mg/min IV push or 150–300 mg/kg/h in maximum concentration of 55 mg/mL. Give more slowly if irritation develops. Avoid rapid administration.

- Patient may complain of a transient tingling sensation and metallic taste following IV administration.

ADVERSE EFFECTS Body as a Whole: Tingling sensation. With rapid IV, sensations of heat waves (peripheral vasodilation), fainting, **CV:** With rapid infusion, hypotension, bradycardia, cardiac arrhythmias, <u>cardiac arrest</u>. **Skin:** Pain and burning at IV site, severe venous thrombosis, necrosis and sloughing (with extravasation).

INTERACTIONS Drug: May enhance inotropic and toxic effects of **digoxin;** antagonizes the effects of **verapamil** and possibly other CALCIUM CHANNEL BLOCKERS.

PHARMACOKINETICS Duration: 2–3 h IV; 1–4 h IM. **Distribution:** Crosses placenta. **Elimination:** Primarily excreted in feces; small amounts excreted in urine, pancreatic juice, saliva, and breast milk.

NURSING IMPLICATIONS

See calcium gluconate for **NURSING IMPLICATIONS.**

CALCIUM GLUCONATE ℗

(gloo′koe-nate)
Kalcinate
Classifications: FLUID AND ELECTROLYTIC AND WATER BALANCE AGENT; REPLACEMENT SOLUTION
Pregnancy Category: B

AVAILABILITY 500 mg, 650 mg, 975 mg, 1 g tablets; 10% injection

ACTIONS Calcium is an essential element for regulating the excitation threshold of nerves and muscles, for blood clotting mechanisms, cardiac function (rhythm, tonicity, contractility), maintenance of renal function, for body skeleton and teeth. Also plays a role in regulating storage and release of neurotransmitters and hormones; regulating amino acid uptake and absorption of vitamin B_{12}, gastrin secretion, and in maintaining structural and functional integrity of cell membranes and

Common adverse effects in *italic;* life-threatening effects <u>underlined;</u> generic names in **bold;** drug classifications in SMALL CAPS; ♣ Canadian drug name; ℗ Prototype drug.

223

capillaries. Calcium gluconate acts like digitalis on the heart, increasing cardiac muscle tone and force of systolic contractions (positive inotropic effect).

THERAPEUTIC EFFECTS Rapidly and effectively restores serum calcium levels in acute hypocalcemia of various origins and effective cardiac stabilizer under conditions of hyperkalemia or resuscitation.

USES Negative calcium balance (as in neonatal tetany, hypoparathyroidism, vitamin D deficiency, alkalosis). Also to overcome cardiac toxicity of hyperkalemia, for cardiopulmonary resuscitation, to prevent hypocalcemia during transfusion of citrated blood. Also as antidote for magnesium sulfate, for acute symptoms of lead colic, to decrease capillary permeability in sensitivity reactions, and to relieve muscle cramps from insect bites or stings. Oral calcium may be used to maintain normal calcium balance during pregnancy, lactation, and childhood growth and to prevent primary osteoporosis. Also in osteoporosis, osteomalacia, chronic hypoparathyroidism, rickets, and as adjunct in treatment of myasthenia gravis and Eaton-Lambert syndrome.

UNLABELED USES To antagonize aminoglycoside-induced neuromuscular blockage, and as "calcium challenge" to diagnose Zollinger-Ellison syndrome and medullary thyroid carcinoma.

CONTRAINDICATIONS Ventricular fibrillation, metastatic bone disease, injection into myocardium; administration by SC or IM routes; renal calculi, hypercalcemia, predisposition to hypercalcemia (hyperparathyroidism, certain malignancies); pregnancy (category B).

CAUTIOUS USE Digitalized patients, renal or cardiac insufficiency, sarcoidosis, history of lithiasis, immobilized patients; lactation.

ROUTE & DOSAGE

All doses are in terms of *elemental calcium:* 1 g calcium gluconate = 90 mg (4.5 mEq, 9.3%) elemental calcium

Hypocalcemia

Neonate: **IV** 200–800 mg/kg/day divided into doses given q6h
Infant: **PO** 400–800 mg/kg/day divided into doses given q6h **IV** 200–500 mg/kg/day divided into doses given q6h
Child: **PO/IV** 200–500 mg/kg/day divided into doses given q6h
Adult: **PO/IV** 5–15 g/day divided into doses given q6h

Cardiac Arrest

Infant/Child: **IV** 100 mg/kg/dose (1 mL/kg/dose) q10 min
Adult: **IV** 500–800 mg/dose (5–8 mL/dose) q10 min (max 3 g/dose)

STORAGE
Store at 15°–30° C (59°–86° F). Check expiration dates.

ADMINISTRATION

Oral
- Ensure that chewable tablets are chewed or crushed before being swallowed with a liquid.
- Give with meals to enhance absorption.

Common adverse effects in *italic;* life-threatening effects <u>underlined</u>; generic names in **bold;** drug classifications in SMALL CAPS; ♣ Canadian drug name; ✪ Prototype drug.

Intravenous

PREPARE **Direct:** May be given undiluted. **Intermittent/Continuous:** May be diluted in 1000 mL of NS.

ADMINISTER **Direct:** Give direct IV at a rate of 0.5 mL or a fraction thereof over 1 min. Do not exceed 100 mg/min. **Intermittent/Continuous:** Give slowly, not to exceed 120–240 mg/kg/h (max concentration 50 mg/mL), through a small-bore needle into a large vein to avoid possibility of extravasation and resultant necrosis. With children, scalp veins and peripheral veins should be avoided. Avoid rapid infusion. High concentrations of calcium suddenly reaching the heart can cause fatal cardiac arrest. Do NOT administer IM or SC.

INCOMPATIBILITIES: **Solution/Additive: Amphotericin B, cefamandole, dobutamine, methylprednisolone, metoclopramide**. Many incompatibilities so check with pharmacy or manufacturer. **Y Site: Amphotericin B cholesteryl complex, fluconazole, indomethacin.**

- Injection should be stopped if patient complains of any discomfort.
- Patient should be advised to remain in bed for 15–30 min or more following injection, depending on response.

ADVERSE EFFECTS Body as a Whole: Tingling sensation. With rapid IV, sensations of heat waves (peripheral vasodilation), fainting. **GI:** PO preparation: Constipation, increased gastric acid secretion. **CV:** With rapid infusion, hypotension, bradycardia, cardiac arrhythmias, <u>cardiac arrest</u>. **Skin:** Pain and burning at IV site, severe venous thrombosis, necrosis and sloughing (with extravasation).

DIAGNOSTIC TEST INTERFERENCE IV calcium may cause false decreases in *serum and urine magnesium* (by *Titan yellow method)* and transient elevations of *plasma 11-OHCS* levels by *Glenn-Nelson technique.* Values usually return to control levels after 60 min; *urinary steroid values (17-OHCS)* may be decreased.

INTERACTIONS Drug: May enhance inotropic and toxic effects of **digoxin; magnesium** may compete for GI absorption; decreases absorption of TETRACYCLINES, QUINOLONES (**ciprofloxacin**); antagonizes the effects of **verapamil** and possibly other CALCIUM CHANNEL BLOCKERS (IV administration).

PHARMACOKINETICS Absorption: Approximately 1/3 of dose absorbed from small intestine. **Onset:** Immediately after IV. **Distribution:** Crosses placenta. **Elimination:** Primarily excreted in feces; small amounts excreted in urine, pancreatic juice, saliva, and breast milk.

NURSING IMPLICATIONS

Assessment & Drug Effects
- Assess for cutaneous burning sensations and peripheral vasodilation, with moderate fall in BP, during direct IV injection.
- Monitor ECG during IV administration to detect evidence of hypercalcemia: Decreased QT interval associated with inverted T wave.
- Observe IV site closely. Extravasation may result in tissue irritation and necrosis.

- Monitor for hypocalcemia and hypercalcemia (see Appendix D-1).
- Lab tests: Determine levels of calcium and phosphorus (tend to vary inversely) and magnesium frequently, during sustained therapy. Deficiencies in other ions, particularly magnesium, frequently coexist with calcium ion depletion.

Patient & Family Education

- Report S&S of hypercalcemia (see Appendix D-1) promptly to your care provider.
- Milk and milk products are the best sources of calcium (and phosphorus). Other good sources include dark green vegetables, soy beans, tofu, and canned fish with bones.
- Calcium absorption can be inhibited by zinc-rich foods: nuts, seeds, sprouts, legumes, soy products (tofu).
- Check with physician before self-medicating with a calcium supplement.
- Do not breast feed while taking this drug without consulting physician.
- Store this medication out of reach of children.

CALCIUM LACTATE

(lak'tate)
Cal-Lac, Calcimax, Calcium Unison, Ridactate
Classifications: FLUID AND ELECTROLYTIC BALANCE AGENT; REPLACEMENT SOLUTION
Prototype: Calcium gluconate
Pregnancy Category: B

AVAILABILITY 325 mg, 650 mg tablets

ACTIONS Oral calcium preparation reportedly well tolerated. Calcium is an essential element for regulating the excitation threshold of nerves and muscles, for blood clotting mechanisms, cardiac function, maintenance of renal function, for body skeleton and teeth. Also plays a role in regulating storage and release of neurotransmitters and hormones, and in maintaining structural and functional integrity of cell membranes and capillaries. It increases cardiac muscle tone and force of systolic contractions (positive inotropic effect).
THERAPEUTIC EFFECTS Rapidly and effectively restores serum calcium levels in mild hypocalcemia of various origins and effective for calcium maintenance therapy.

USES Mild hypocalcemia and maintenance calcium therapy.

CONTRAINDICATIONS Ventricular fibrillation, metastatic bone disease, injection into myocardium; administration by SC or IM routes; renal calculi, hypercalcemia, predisposition to hypercalcemia (hyperparathyroidism, certain malignancies); pregnancy (category B).
CAUTIOUS USE Digitalized patients, renal or cardiac insufficiency, sarcoidosis, history of lithiasis, immobilized patients; lactation.

Common adverse effects in *italic*; life-threatening effects underlined; generic names in **bold**; drug classifications in SMALL CAPS; ♦ Canadian drug name; ❂ Prototype drug.

ROUTE & DOSAGE

All doses are in terms of *elemental calcium:* 1 g calcium lactate = 130 mg (6.5 mEq, 13%) elemental calcium
Supplement for Mild Hypocalcemia
Child: **PO** 500 mg/kg/day divided into 3–4 doses (max 9 g/day)
Adult: **PO** 325 mg–1.3 g t.i.d. with meals

STORAGE
Store tightly closed at 15°–30° C (59°–86° F).

ADMINISTRATION
Oral

- Give with meals. Tablets or powder can be dissolved in hot water (if patient unable to swallow whole), then add cool water to make palatable.
- Calcium lactate may be administered with lactose (amount prescribed) to increase solubility.

ADVERSE EFFECTS GI: *Constipation* or laxative effect, acid rebound, nausea, eructation, *flatulence,* vomiting, fecal concretions. **Metabolic:** Hypercalcemia with alkalosis, metastatic calcinosis, hypercalciuria, hypomagnesemia, hypophosphatemia (when phosphate intake is low). **CNS:** Mood and mental changes. **Urogenital:** Polyuria, renal calculi.

INTERACTIONS Drug: May enhance inotropic and toxic effects of **digoxin; magnesium** may compete for GI absorption; decreases absorption of TETRACYCLINES, QUINOLONES **(ciprofloxacin).**

PHARMACOKINETICS Absorption: Approximately ⅓ of dose absorbed from small intestine. **Distribution:** Crosses placenta. **Elimination:** Primarily excreted in feces; small amounts excreted in urine, pancreatic juice, saliva, and breast milk.

NURSING IMPLICATIONS

Assessment & Drug Effects

- Monitor for hypercalcemia (see Signs & Symptoms, Appendix D-1).
- Lab tests: Check serum calcium levels periodically. Hypercalcemia can occur during prolonged administration particularly if patient is also taking vitamin D.
- Monitor increases in serum calcium in digitalized patients because this increases risk of digitalis toxicity.

Patient & Family Education

- Confer with prescriber regarding need for vitamin D supplementation.
- Calcium absorption can be inhibited by zinc-rich foods such as nuts, sprouts, legumes, and soy products.
- Take with meals; do not dissolve in milk.
- Do not breast feed while taking this drug without consulting physician.
- Store this medication out of reach of children.

Common adverse effects in *italic;* life-threatening effects underlined; generic names in **bold;** drug classifications in SMALL CAPS; ♣ Canadian drug name; ☻ Prototype drug.

227

CALCIUM POLYCARBOPHIL

(pol-ee-kar′boe-fil)
FiberCon, Mitrolan
Classifications: GASTROINTESTINAL AGENT; BULK LAXATIVE; ANTIDIARRHEAL
Prototype: Psyllium hydrophilic muciloid
Pregnancy Category: C

AVAILABILITY 500 mg, 625 mg tablets

ACTIONS Hydrophilic, bulk-producing laxative that restores normal moisture level and bulk content of intestinal tract. In constipation, retains free water in intestinal lumen, thereby indirectly opposing dehydrating forces of the bowel; in diarrhea, when intestinal mucosa is incapable of absorbing fluid, drug absorbs fecal fluid to form a gel. In both conditions, peristalsis is encouraged and a well-formed stool is produced.
THERAPEUTIC EFFECTS Relieves constipation or diarrhea associated with bowel disorders and acute nonspecific diarrhea.

USES Constipation or diarrhea associated with diverticulitis or irritable bowel syndrome; acute nonspecific diarrhea.

CONTRAINDICATIONS GI obstruction; narcotic-induced constipation; children <6 y.
CAUTIOUS USE Pregnancy (category C); lactation.

ROUTE & DOSAGE

Constipation or Diarrhea
Child: **PO** *<6 y, 500 mg 1–2 times/day (max 1.5 g/24 h); 6–12 y, 500 mg 1–3 times/day (max 3 g/24 h)*
Adult: **PO** *1 g q.i.d. as needed (max 6 g/24 h)*

STORAGE
Store tightly closed at 15°–30° C (59°–86° F).

ADMINISTRATION
Oral
- Administer with at least 180–240 mL (6–8 oz) water or other fluid of patient's choice when used as a laxative and with at least 60–90 mL (2–3 oz) of fluid when used as an antidiarrheal. Chewed tablets should not be swallowed dry.
- If diarrhea is severe, dose can be repeated every half hour up to maximum daily dose.

ADVERSE EFFECTS GI: *Flatulence,* abdominal fullness, <u>intestinal obstruction</u>; laxative dependence (long-term use).

PHARMACOKINETICS Absorption: Calcium polycarbophil is not absorbed from the intestine. Bowel movement usually occurs within 12–72 h. **Elimination:** Excreted in feces.

Common adverse effects in *italic;* life-threatening effects <u>underlined</u>; generic names in **bold**; drug classifications in SMALL CAPS; ♣ Canadian drug name; ☻ Prototype drug.

NURSING IMPLICATIONS

Assessment & Drug Effects

- Evaluate effectiveness of medication. If it is ineffective as an antidiarrheal, report to prescriber.
- Report rectal bleeding, very dark stools, or abdominal pain promptly.

Patient & Family Education

- A bowel movement is likely within 12–72 h.
- This is an OTC product. Take this drug exactly as ordered. Do not increase the dose if response is inadequate. Consult care provider. Do not use other laxatives while you are taking calcium polycarbophil.
- Do not breast feed while taking this drug without consulting physician.
- Store this medication out of reach of children.

CALFACTANT

(cal-fac′tant)

Infasurf

Classifications: LUNG SURFACTANT

Prototype: Beractant

Pregnancy Category: Not applicable

AVAILABILITY 35 mg/mL suspension

ACTIONS Pulmonary surfactant. Lowers the surface tension on alveolar surfaces during respiration and stabilizes the alveoli against collapse at resting pressure. Deficiency of surfactant causes respiratory disease syndrome (RDS) in premature infants.

THERAPEUTIC EFFECTS Effectively relieves and prevents RDS in neonates.

USE Prevention and treatment of RDS in infants at high risk for RDS.

CONTRAINDICATIONS Nosocomial infections.

ROUTE & DOSAGE

Prevention & Treatment of RDS

Infant: **Intratracheal** 3 mL/kg of birth weight administered through an endotracheal tube q12h for 3 doses

---

STORAGE

Refrigerate at 2°–8° C (36°–46° F).

ADMINISTRATION

Intratracheal

- Swirl vial to disperse suspension; do not dilute and DO NOT SHAKE. Visible flecks and foam may be present. Withdraw with 20-gauge or larger needle. Avoid excess foaming. Instill into the endotracheal tube, preferably within 30 min of birth. Divide into 2 portions and administer

---

the first while the infant is on one side and the other when moved to the other side. Administer each portion during ventilation over 20–30 breaths.

▪ Stop administration of calfactant if reflux into endotracheal tube occurs as indicated by cyanosis, bradycardia, or other signs of airway obstruction.

ADVERSE EFFECTS CV: *Bradycardia.* **Respiratory:** *Cyanosis, airway obstruction, reflux of surfactant* into endotracheal tube.

INTERACTIONS Drug: No clinically significant interactions established.

PHARMACOKINETICS Absorption: Absorbs rapidly to air; liquid interface of lung surface. No other human pharmacokinetic information available.

NURSING IMPLICATIONS

Assessment & Drug Effects
▪ Drug should be given under supervision of trained neonatologist.
▪ Monitor closely during and after administration; adjustments in oxygen therapy and ventilator pressures are usually needed. Suctioning may be required.

Patient & Family Education
▪ This drug will help baby to breathe properly and support normal respiratory function.

CAPSAICIN
(cap-say'i-sin)
Axsain, Capsaicin, Capsin, Capsacin-P, Dolorac, Zostrix, Zostrix-HP
Classifications: SKIN AND MUCOUS MEMBRANE AGENT: TOPICAL ANALGESIC

AVAILABILITY 0.025%, 0.075% lotion; 0.025%, 0.075%, 0.25% cream; 0.025%, 0.05% gel

ACTIONS Capsaicin is an alkaloid derived from plants and is the active ingredient in hot peppers. It is used as a topical analgesic. Capsaicin's precise mechanism is not fully understood. Substance P is thought to act as a principal neurotransmitter of pain sensations from the peripheral neurons to the CNS.
THERAPEUTIC EFFECTS It is thought that the drug renders skin and joints insensitive to pain by preventing the reaccumulation of substance P in peripheral sensory neurons. Thus capsaicin is an effective peripheral analgesic.

USES Temporary relief of pain from arthritis, neuralgias, diabetic neuropathy, and herpes zoster.
UNLABELED USES Phantom limb pain, psoriasis, intractable pruritus.

CONTRAINDICATIONS Hypersensitivity to capsaicin or any ingredient in the cream.
CAUTIOUS USE Patients on ACE inhibitors. Safety and efficacy in children <2 y have not been established.

ROUTE & DOSAGE

Analgesia

Child: >2 y, **Topical** Apply to affected area not more than 3–4 times/day
Adult: **Topical** Apply to affected area not more than 3–4 times/day

STORAGE

Stored at 15°–30° C (59°–86° F).

ADMINISTRATION

Topical

- Apply to affected areas only and avoid contact with eyes or broken or irritated skin.
- If applied with bare hand, wash immediately following application. An applicator or gloved hand may be used to apply cream.
- Avoid tight bandages over areas of application of the cream.

ADVERSE EFFECTS CNS: Concentration: Neurotoxicity, hyperalgesia. **Skin:** *Burning, stinging, redness,* itching. **Other:** Cough.

INTERACTIONS Drug: May increase incidence of cough with ACE INHIBITORS.

PHARMACOKINETICS Onset: Post-herpetic neuralgia: 2–6 wk.

NURSING IMPLICATIONS

Assessment & Drug Effects

- Monitor for significant pain relief, which may require 4–6 wk of application three or four times daily.
- Monitor for and report signs of skin breakdown because these generally indicate need for drug discontinuation.

Patient & Family Education

- Report local discomfort at site of application if discomfort is distressing or persists beyond the first 3–4 days of use.
- Use caution in handling contact lenses following application of cream. Wash hands thoroughly before touching lenses.
- Notify prescriber if symptoms do not improve or condition worsens within 14–28 days.
- Apply three or four times daily to maximize therapeutic effectiveness.
- Store this medication out of reach of children.

CAPTOPRIL ⊘

(kap′toe-pril)

Capoten

Classifications: CARDIOVASCULAR AGENT; ANGIOTENSIN-CONVERTING ENZYME INHIBITOR; ANTIHYPERTENSIVE

Pregnancy Category: C for first trimester and D for second and third trimesters

---

Common adverse effects in *italic;* life-threatening effects underlined; generic names in **bold;** drug classifications in SMALL CAPS; ♣ Canadian drug name; ⊘ Prototype drug.

231

AVAILABILITY 12.5 mg, 25 mg, 50 mg, 100 mg tablets

ACTIONS Lowers blood pressure by specific inhibition of the angiotensin-converting enzyme (ACE). This interrupts conversion sequences initiated by renin that lead to formation of angiotensin II, a potent endogenous vasoconstrictor. ACE inhibition alters hemodynamics without compensatory reflex tachycardia or changes in cardiac output (except in patient with CHF). Peripheral vascular resistance is lowered by vasodilation. Inhibition of ACE also leads to decreased circulating aldosterone. Reduced circulating aldosterone is associated with a potassium-sparing effect. In heart failure, captopril administration is followed by a fall in CVP and pulmonary wedge pressure; hypotensive action appears to be unrelated to plasma renin levels.

THERAPEUTIC EFFECTS Effective in stepped protocol management of hypertension to convert to normotensive range, and in congestive heart failure with resulting decreases in dyspnea and improved exercise tolerance.

USES Hypertension; in conjunction with digitalis and diuretics in CHF, diabetic nephropathy.

UNLABELED USE Idiopathic edema.

CONTRAINDICATIONS Pregnancy (category D) lactation. Safe use in children not established.

CAUTIOUS USE Impaired renal function, patient with solitary kidney; collagen-vascular diseases (scleroderma, SLE); patients receiving IMMUNOSUPPRESSANTS or other drugs that cause leukopenia or agranulocytosis; coronary or cerebrovascular disease; severe salt/volume depletion.

ROUTE & DOSAGE

Hypertension

Neonate: **PO** 0.1–0.4 mg/kg/day given in divided doses q6–8h
Infant: **PO** 0.15–0.3 mg/kg/dose given q8h, may titrate up to 6 mg/kg/day given in 1–4 divided doses
Child: **PO** 0.3–0.5 mg/kg/dose given q8h, may titrate up to max of 6 mg/kg/day given in 2–4 divided doses
Adult: **PO** 6.25–25 mg t.i.d., may increase gradually by 25 mg over 1 wk to 50 mg t.i.d. (max 450 mg/day)

STORAGE

Store in light-resistant containers at no more than 30° C (86° F) unless otherwise directed.

ADMINISTRATION

Oral

- Give Captopril 1 h before or 2 h after meals. Food reduces absorption by 30–40%.

ADVERSE EFFECTS Body as a Whole: Hypersensitivity reactions, serum sickness-like reaction, arthralgia, skin eruptions. **CV:** Slight increase in heart rate, first dose hypotension, dizziness, fainting. **GI:** Altered taste sensation (loss of taste perception, persistent salt or metallic taste); weight loss. **Hematologic:** Hyperkalemia, neutropenia, <u>agranulocytosis</u> (rare). **Respiratory:** *Cough.* **Skin:** *Maculopapular rash,* urticaria, pruritus, <u>angioedema</u>, photosensitivity. **Urogenital:** Azotemia, impaired renal function, nephrotic syndrome, membranous glomerulonephritis. **Other:** Positive antinuclear antibody (ANA) titers.

DIAGNOSTIC TEST INTERFERENCE In some patients, elevated ***urine protein levels*** may persist even after captopril has been discontinued. Possibility of transient elevations of ***BUN*** and ***serum creatinine,*** slight increase in ***serum potassium*** and ***serum prolactin,*** increases in ***liver enzymes,*** and false-positive ***urine acetone*** (using ***sodium nitroprusside reagent***). Captopril may decrease ***fasting blood sugar*** in the nondiabetic and cause hypoglycemia in the diabetic patient controlled with antidiabetic drug therapy.

INTERACTIONS Drug: NITRATES, DIURETICS, and ANTIHYPERTENSIVES enhance hypotensive effects. **Aspirin** and other NSAIDS may antagonize hypotensive effects. POTASSIUM-SPARING DIURETICS **(spironolactone, amiloride)** increase potassium levels. **Probenecid** decreases elimination and increases effects. **Food:** Food decreases absorption; take 30–60 min before meals.

PHARMACOKINETICS Absorption: 60–75% absorbed; food may decrease absorption 25–40%. **Onset:** 15 min. **Peak:** 1–2 h. **Duration:** 6–12 h. **Distribution:** Distributed to all tissues except CNS; crosses placenta. **Metabolism:** Some liver metabolism. **Elimination:** Excreted primarily in urine; excreted in breast milk.

NURSING IMPLICATIONS

Assessment & Drug Effects

- Monitor BP closely following the first dose. A sudden exaggerated hypotensive response may occur within 1–3 h of first dose, especially in those with high BP or on a diuretic and restricted salt intake.
- Advise bed rest and BP monitoring for the first 3 h after the initial dose.
- Monitor therapeutic effectiveness. At least 2 wk of therapy may be required before full therapeutic effects are achieved.
- Lab tests: Establish baseline urinary protein levels before initiation of therapy and check at monthly intervals for the first 8 mo of treatment and then periodically thereafter. Perform WBC and differential counts before therapy is begun and at approximately 2-wk intervals for the first 3 mo of therapy and then periodically thereafter.

Patient & Family Education

- Report to physician without delay the onset of unexplained fever, unusual fatigue, sore mouth or throat, easy bruising or bleeding (pathognomonic of agranulocytosis).
- Mild skin eruptions are most likely to appear during the first 4 wk of therapy and may be accompanied by fever and eosinophilia.
- Consult physician promptly if vomiting or diarrhea occur.
- Report darkening or crumbling of nail beds (reversible with dosage reduction).

- Taste impairment occurs in 5–10% of patients and generally reverses in 2–3 mo even with continued therapy.
- Use OTC medications only with approval of the physician. Inform surgeon or dentist that captopril is being taken. Alert diabetic patient that captopril may produce hypoglycemia. Monitor blood glucose and HbA$_{1c}$ closely during first few weeks of therapy.
- Do not breast feed while taking this drug.
- Store this medication out of reach of children.

CARBAMAZEPINE 🅟
(kar-ba-maz′e-peen)
Apo-Carbamazepine ♣ , Carbatrol, Epitol, Mazepine ♣ , PMSCarbamazepine ♣ , Tegretol, Tegretol XR
Classifications: CENTRAL NERVOUS SYSTEM AGENT; ANTICONVULSANT
Pregnancy Category: D

AVAILABILITY 100 mg chewable tablets; 200 mg tablets; 100 mg, 200 mg, 400 mg sustained-release tablets; 200 mg 300 mg sustained-release capsules; 100 mg/5 mL suspension

ACTIONS Structurally related to tricyclic antidepressants (TCAs) but lacks antidepressant properties. Anticonvulsant actions appear qualitatively similar to those of phenytoin. Like phenytoin, provides relief in trigeminal neuralgia by reducing synaptic transmission within trigeminal nucleus. Also has sedative, anticholinergic, antidepressant, and muscle relaxant (by inhibition of neuromuscular transmission) effects and slight analgesic actions.
THERAPEUTIC EFFECTS Effective anticonvulsant for a range of seizure disorders and as an adjuvant reduces depressive signs and symptoms and stabilizes mood. It is effective for pain and other symptoms associated with neurologic disorders.

USES Alone or concomitantly with other anticonvulsants in treatment of grand mal and psychomotor or temporal lobe epilepsy and mixed seizures in patients who have not responded satisfactorily to other agents. Also used for symptomatic treatment of trigeminal (tic douloureux) and glossopharyngeal neuralgias and for pain and paroxysmal symptoms associated with multiple sclerosis and other neurologic disorders.
UNLABELED USES Certain psychiatric disorders including prophylaxis and treatment of manic-depressive illness, treatment of schizoaffective illness, resistant schizophrenia, dyscontrol syndrome; for management of alcohol withdrawal, rage outbursts, and for antidiuretic effect in diabetes insipidus.

CONTRAINDICATIONS Hypersensitivity to carbamazepine and to TCAs; history of myelosuppression or hematologic reaction to other drugs; increased IOP; SLE; cardiac, hepatic, or renal disease; coronary artery disease; hypertension; MAO inhibitors; pregnancy (category D), lactation. Safe use in children <6 mo not established.

Common adverse effects in *italic;* life-threatening effects <u>underlined</u>; generic names in **bold**; drug classifications in SMALL CAPS; ♣ Canadian drug name; 🅟 Prototype drug.

CAUTIOUS USE History of cardiac disease.

ROUTE & DOSAGE

Epilepsy

Child: **PO** *<6 y,* 10–20 mg/kg/day given b.i.d. to q.i.d., may gradually increase weekly by 35 mg/kg/day, recommended max 35 mg/kg/day in 3–4 divided doses; *6–12 y,* 100 mg b.i.d., gradually increased to 400–800 mg/day in 3–4 divided doses (max 1 g/day); usual maintenance dose is 400–800 mg/24 h given b.i.d. to q.i.d.; *>12 y,* 200 mg b.i.d.; gradually increased by 200 mg/24 h at 1 wk intervals; give daily dose in 2–4 doses; usual maintenance dose is 800–1200 mg/24 h given b.i.d. to q.i.d.
Adult: **PO** 200 mg b.i.d., gradually increased to 800–1200 mg/day in 3–4 divided doses. Tegretol XR dosed b.i.d.

STORAGE

Store in tightly covered, light resistant container at a temperature not exceeding 30° C (86° F).

ADMINISTRATION

Oral

- Do not administer within 14 days of patient receiving a MAO inhibitor.
- Give with a meal to increase absorption.
- Ensure that chewable tablets are chewed or crushed before being swallowed with a liquid.
- Ensure that sustained-release form of drug is not chewed or crushed. It must be swallowed whole.
- Do not administer carbamazepine suspension simultaneously with other liquid medications because a precipitate may form in the stomach.

ADVERSE EFFECTS Body as a Whole: Myalgia, arthralgia, leg cramps, carbamazepine-induced SLE. **CV:** Edema, syncope, arrhythmias, <u>heart block</u>. **GI:** Nausea, vomiting, anorexia, abdominal pain, diarrhea, constipation, dry mouth and pharynx, abnormal liver function tests, hepatitis, cholestatic and hepatocellular jaundice, pancreatitis. **Endocrine:** Hypothyroidism, SIADH, hyponatremia. **Hematologic:** <u>Aplastic anemia</u>, *leukopenia* (transient), leukocytosis, <u>agranulocytosis</u>, eosinophilia, thrombocytopenia. **CNS:** Dizziness, vertigo, drowsiness, disturbances of coordination, ataxia, confusion, headache, fatigue, listlessness, speech difficulty, development of minor motor seizures, hyperreflexia, akathisia, involuntary movements, tremors, visual hallucinations, activation of latent psychosis, aggression; agitation, respiratory depression. **Skin:** Skin rashes, urticaria, petechiae, erythema multiforme, Stevens-Johnson syndrome, photosensitivity reactions, altered skin pigmentation, exfoliative dermatitis, alopecia. **Special Senses:** Abnormal hearing acuity, scotomas, conjunctivitis, blurred vision, transient diplopia, oculomotor disturbances, oscillopsia, nystagmus. **Urogenital:** Urinary frequency or retention, oliguria, impotence.

DIAGNOSTIC TEST INTERFERENCE False-negative ***pregnancy test*** results with tests involving ***human chorionic gonadotropin.***

INTERACTIONS Drug: Serum concentrations of other ANTICONVULSANTS may decrease because of increased metabolism; **verapamil, erythromycin, ketoconazole, nefazadone** may increase carbamazepine levels; decreases hypoprothrombinemic effects of ORAL ANTICOAGULANTS; increases metabolism of ESTROGENS, thus decreasing effectiveness of ORAL CONTRACEPTIVES. **Herbal: Ginkgo** may decrease anticonvulsant effectiveness.

PHARMACOKINETICS Absorption: Slowly absorbed from GI tract. **Peak:** 2–8 h. **Distribution:** Widely distributed; high concentrations in CSF; crosses placenta; distributed into breast milk. **Metabolism:** Metabolized in liver; can induce liver microsomal enzymes. **Elimination:** Excreted in urine and feces. **Half-Life:** 14–16 h (decreases with long-term use).

NURSING IMPLICATIONS

Assessment & Drug Effects

- Lab tests: Baseline and periodic CBCs including platelets, reticulocytes, serum electrolytes and serum iron, liver function tests, BUN, and complete urinalysis.
- ***Therapeutic blood level*** is 4–12 mg/L.
- Monitor for the following reactions, which commonly occur during early therapy: drowsiness, dizziness, light-headedness, ataxia, gastric upset. If these symptoms do not subside within a few days, dosage adjustments may be indicated.
- Withhold drug and notify physician if any of the following signs of myelosuppression occur: RBC <4 million/mm^3, Hct <32%, Hgb <11 g/dL, WBC <4000/mm^3, platelet count <100,000/mm^3, reticulocyte count <20,000/mm^3, serum iron >150 mg/dL.
- Monitor for toxicity, which can develop when serum concentrations are even slightly above the therapeutic range.
- Monitor I&O ratio and vital signs during period of dosage adjustment. Report oliguria, signs of fluid retention, changes in I&O ratio, and changes in BP or pulse patterns.
- Cardiac syncope may resemble epileptic seizures. Therefore, it is recommended that patients who experience an apparent increase in frequency of seizures or a change in their character should be checked by continuous ECG monitoring for 24 h.
- Doses higher than 600 mg/day may precipitate arrhythmias in patients with heart disease.
- Confusion and agitation may be aggravated; therefore, use of side rails and supervision of ambulation may be indicated.

Patient & Family Education

- Keep a record of any seizures and report to prescriber.
- Discontinue drug and notify physician immediately if early signs of toxicity or a possible hematologic problem appears (e.g., anorexia, fever, sore throat or mouth, malaise, unusual fatigue, tendency to bruise or bleed, petechiae, ecchymoses, bleeding gums, nose bleeds). Report rash immediately.
- Avoid hazardous tasks requiring mental alertness and physical coordination until reaction to drug is known, because dizziness, drowsiness, and ataxia are common adverse effects.

- Remain under close medical supervision throughout therapy.
- Avoid excessive sunlight, because photosensitivity reactions have been reported. Apply a sunscreen (if allowed) with SPF of 12 or above.
- Carbamazepine may cause breakthrough bleeding in females and may also affect the reliability of oral contraceptives.
- Be aware that abrupt withdrawal of any anticonvulsant drug may precipitate seizures or even status epilepticus.
- Do not breast feed while taking this drug.
- Store this medication out of reach of children.

CARBOPLATIN

(car-bo-pla′tin)
Paraplatin
Classifications: ANTINEOPLASTIC; ALKYLATING AGENT
Prototype: Cyclophosphamide
Pregnancy Category: D

AVAILABILITY 50 mg, 150 mg, 450 mg vials

ACTIONS Carboplatin is a platinum compound that is a chemotherapeutic agent. It produces interstrand DNA cross-linkages, thus interfering with DNA, RNA, and protein synthesis. Carboplatin is cell-cycle nonspecific, i.e., effective throughout the entire cell life cycle.
THERAPEUTIC EFFECTS Full or partial activity against a variety of cancers resulting in reduction or stabilization of tumor size and useful in patients with impaired renal function, patients unable to accommodate high-volume hydration, or patients at high risk for neurotoxicity and/or ototoxicity.

USES Monotherapy or combination therapy for ovarian cancer.
UNLABELED USES Combination therapy for breast, cervical, colon, endometrial, head and neck, and lung cancer; leukemia, lymphoma, and melanoma.

CONTRAINDICATIONS History of severe reactions to carboplatin or other platinum compounds, severe bone marrow depression; significant bleeding; impaired renal function; pregnancy (category D), and lactation.
CAUTIOUS USE Use with other nephrotoxic drugs.

ROUTE & DOSAGE

Ovarian Cancer

Adult: **IV** 360 mg/m^2 once q4wk, may be repeated when neutrophil count is at least 2000 mm^3 and platelet count is at least 100,000 mm^3. If neutrophil and platelet counts are lower, dose of carboplatin should be reduced by 50–75% of initial dose. Alternatively, 400 mg/m^2 as a 24-h infusion for 2 consecutive days can be used

Head and Neck and Small Cell Lung Cancer

Child: **IV** Up to 560 mg/m^2 once q4wk or up to 175 mg/m^2 q2wk. Other dosage regimens have been used for specific protocols

---

Common adverse effects in *italic;* life-threatening effects <u>underlined</u>; generic names in **bold;** drug classifications in SMALL CAPS; ✦ Canadian drug name; ⊘ Prototype drug.

237

Adult: **IV** 300–400 mg/m^2 q4wk

Important Note

Aluminum reacts with carboplatin to form an inactive precipitate; therefore, intravenous infusion sets and needles containing aluminum should not be used

STORAGE

Protect from light. Reconstituted solutions are stable for 8 h at room temperature; discard solutions 8 h after dilution.

ADMINISTRATION

Intravenous

- Child: Must be given under care and direction of pediatric oncology specialist. Use recommended handling techniques for hazardous medications (see Part I).

PREPARE IV **Infusion:** Do not use needles or IV sets containing aluminum. Immediately before use, reconstitute with either sterile water for injection or D5W or NS as follows: 50-mg vial plus 5 mL diluent; 150-mg vial plus 15 mL diluent; 450-mg vial plus 45 mL diluent. All dilutions yield 10 mg/mL. May be further diluted to 0.5 mg/mL with D5W or NS.

ADMINISTER IV **Infusion:** Give IV solution over 15 min or longer, depending on total amount of solution and patient tolerance. Lengthening duration of administration may decrease nausea and vomiting.

INCOMPATIBILITIES: **Solution/Additive: Sodium bicarbonate, fluorouracil, mesna. Y-Site: Amphotericin B cholesteryl complex**.

- Premedication with a parenteral antiemetic ½ h before and on a scheduled basis thereafter is normally used. ■ Do not repeat doses until the neutrophil count is at least 2000/mm^3 and platelet count at least 100,000/mm^3.

ADVERSE EFFECTS Body as a Whole: Hypersensitivity reactions. **GI:** *Mild to moderate nausea and vomiting, delayed nausea and vomiting >24 h after infusion,* anorexia, hypogeusia, dysgeusia, mucositis, diarrhea, constipation, elevated liver enzymes. **Hematologic:** <u>Thrombocytopenia, leukopenia, neutropenia, anemia</u>. **Metabolic:** *Mild hyponatremia, hypomagnesemia, hypocalcemia, and hypokalemia*. **CNS:** Peripheral neuropathy. **Skin:** Rash, alopecia. **Special Senses:** Tinnitus. **Urogenital:** Nephrotoxicity.

DIAGNOSTIC TEST INTERFERENCE Decreased *calcium levels;* mild increases in *liver function tests;* decreased levels of *magnesium, potassium,* and *sodium.*

INTERACTIONS Drug: AMINOGLYCOSIDES may increase the risk of ototoxicity and nephrotoxicity. May decrease **phenytoin** levels.

PHARMACOKINETICS Onset: 8 wk (2 cycles). **Duration:** 2–16 mo. **Distribution:** Highest concentration is seen in the liver, lung, kidney, skin, and tumors. Not bound to plasma proteins. **Metabolism:** Hydrolyzed in the serum. **Elimination:** Primarily eliminated by the kidneys; 60–80% excreted in urine within 24 h. **Half-Life:** 3 h.

NURSING IMPLICATIONS

Assessment & Drug Effects

- Monitor closely during first 15 min of infusion, because allergic reactions have occurred within minutes of carboplatin administration.
- Lab tests: Baseline and periodic CBC with differential, platelet count, Hgb and Hct. Monitor periodically kidney function with creatinine clearance tests and serum electrolytes.
- Be alert for and report signs of infection such as respiratory infections, aching, rashes, and gastrointestinal distress. Assess immunization status prior to beginning therapy in order to be alert for diseases that pose risk.
- Monitor results of peripheral blood counts. Median nadir occurs at day 21. Leukopenia, neutropenia, and thrombocytopenia are dose related and may produce dose-limiting toxicity.
- Monitor for peripheral neuropathy (e.g., paresthesias), ototoxicity, and visual disturbances.
- Monitor serum electrolyte studies, because carboplatin has been associated with decreases in sodium, potassium, calcium, and magnesium. Special precautions may be warranted for patients on diuretic therapy.

Patient & Family Education

- Learn about the range of potential adverse effects. Strategies for nausea prevention should receive special attention. Report signs of infections.
- During therapy there is risk for infection and hemorrhagic complications related to bone marrow suppression. Avoid unnecessary exposure to crowds or persons with infectious diseases. Report paresthesias (numbness, tingling), visual disturbances, or symptoms of ototoxicity (hearing loss and/or tinnitus).
- Do not breast feed while taking this drug.

CARISOPRODOL
(kar-eye-soe-proe′dole)
Rela, Soma
Classifications: AUTONOMIC NERVOUS SYSTEM AGENT; SKELETAL MUSCLE RELAXANT: CENTRAL-ACTING
Prototype: Cyclobenzaprine
Pregnancy Category: C

AVAILABILITY 350 mg tablets

ACTIONS Propanediol derivative carbamate with central depressant action pharmacologically related to meprobamate. Precise action mechanism of CNS depression is not clear. Skeletal muscle relaxant effect, unlike that of neuromuscular blocking agents, appears to be due to sedative action. Voluntary motor function is not lost, but there may be slight reduction in muscle tone leading to relief of pain and discomfort of muscle spasm.

THERAPEUTIC EFFECTS Effective spasmolytic and reduces pain associated with acute musculoskeletal disorders.

USES Skeletal muscle spasm, stiffness, and pain in a variety of musculoskeletal disorders and to relieve spasticity and rigidity in cerebral palsy.

CONTRAINDICATIONS Hypersensitivity to carisoprodol and related compounds (e.g., meprobamate, tybamate); acute intermittent porphyria; children <5 y; pregnancy (category C), lactation.

CAUTIOUS USE Impaired liver or kidney function, addiction-prone individuals.

ROUTE & DOSAGE

Muscle Spasm

Child: **PO** >5 y, 25 mg/kg/day divided into 4 doses
Adult: **PO** 350 mg t.i.d.

STORAGE

Store in tightly closed container at 15°–30° C (59°–86° F).

ADMINISTRATION

Oral

- Give with food, as needed, to reduce GI symptoms. Last dose should be taken at bedtime.

ADVERSE EFFECTS Body as a Whole: Eosinophilia, asthma, fever, anaphylactic shock. **CV:** Tachycardia, postural hypotension, facial flushing. **GI:** Nausea, vomiting, hiccups. **CNS:** *Drowsiness, dizziness,* vertigo, ataxia, tremor, headache, irritability, depressive reactions, syncope, insomnia. **Skin:** Skin rash, erythema multiforme, pruritus.

INTERACTIONS Drug: Alcohol, CNS DEPRESSANTS potentiate CNS effects.

PHARMACOKINETICS Onset: 30 min. **Duration:** 4–6 h. **Distribution:** Crosses placenta. **Metabolism:** Metabolized in liver. **Elimination:** Excreted by kidneys; excreted in breast milk (2–4 times the plasma concentrations). **Half-Life:** 8 h.

NURSING IMPLICATIONS

Assessment & Drug Effects

- Monitor for allergic or idiosyncratic reactions that generally occur from the first to the fourth dose in patients taking the drug for the first time. Symptoms usually subside after several hours; they are treated by supportive and symptomatic measures.

Patient & Family Education

- Avoid driving and other potentially hazardous activities until response to the drug has been evaluated. Drowsiness is a common side effect and may require reduction in dosage.
- Report to prescriber if symptoms of dizziness and faintness persist. Symptoms may be controlled by making position changes slowly and in stages.
- Do not take alcohol or other CNS depressants (effects may be additive) unless otherwise directed by prescriber.

- Discontinue drug and notify prescriber if skin rash, diplopia, dizziness, or other unusual signs or symptoms appear.
- Do not breast feed while taking this drug.
- Store this medication out of reach of children.

CARMUSTINE
(kar-mus′teen)
BCNU, BiCNU, Gliadel
Classifications: ANTINEOPLASTIC; ALKYLATING AGENT
Prototype: Cyclophosphamide
Pregnancy Category: D

AVAILABILITY 100 mg injection; 7.7 mg intracranial wafer

ACTIONS Highly lipid-soluble nitrosourea derivative with cell-cycle non-specific activity against rapidly proliferating cell populations. Produces cross-linkage of DNA strands, thereby blocking DNA, RNA, and protein synthesis. Major toxic effect is bone marrow suppression.
THERAPEUTIC EFFECTS Drug metabolites thought to be responsible for antineoplastic activities. Full or partial activity against a variety of cancers resulting in reduction or stabilization of tumor size and increased survival rates.

USES As single agent or in combination with other antineoplastics in treatment of Hodgkin's disease and other lymphomas, melanoma, primary and metastatic tumors of the brain, and GI tract malignancies.
UNLABELED USES Treatment of carcinomas of breast and lungs, Ewing's sarcoma, Burkitt's tumor, malignant melanoma, and topically for mycosis fungoides.

CONTRAINDICATIONS History of pulmonary function impairment; recent illness with or exposure to chickenpox or herpes zoster; infection, decreased circulating platelets, leukocytes, or erythrocytes; pregnancy (category D), lactation.
CAUTIOUS USE Hepatic and renal insufficiency; patient with previous cytotoxic medication, or radiation therapy, children <5 y.

ROUTE & DOSAGE

Previously Untreated Patients—Carcinoma
Child: **IV** 200–250 mg/m^2 q4–6wk as single dose. Doses adjusted based on hematologic parameters
Adult: **IV** 150–200 mg/m^2 q6wk in 1 dose *or* given over 2 days

Mycosis Fungoides
Adult: **Topical** 0.05–0.4% solution in 30% alcohol to paint entire body (60 mL) or ointment 1–2 times/day for 6–8 wk (10 mg/day) (must be specially compounded)
Intrancranial Wafer: Approximately 8 wafers placed in surgery with all chemotherapy withheld 4 wk prior to and 2 wk after surgery. Safety and efficacy of wafers not established in children

C

STORAGE

- Reconstituted solutions of carmustine are clear and colorless and may be stored at 2°–8° C (36°–46° F) for 24 h protected from light.
- Store unopened vials at 2°–8° C (36°–46° F), protected from light, unless otherwise directed by manufacturer.
- Signs of decomposition of carmustine in unopened vial: Liquefaction and appearance of oil film at bottom of vial. Discard drug in this condition.

ADMINISTRATION

Child: Must be given under care and direction of pediatric oncology specialist. Use recommended handling techniques for hazardous medications (see Part I).

- When administering IV to infants and children, verify correct IV concentration and rate of infusion with physician.

Intravenous

PREPARE IV **Infusion:** Wear disposable gloves; contact of drug with skin can cause burning, dermatitis, and hyperpigmentation. Add supplied diluent to the 100-mg vial. Further dilute with 27 mL of sterile water for injection to yield a concentration of 3.3 mg/mL. Each dose is then added to 100–500 mL of D5W or NS. If possible avoid using PVC IV tubing and bags.

ADMINISTER IV **Infusion:** Infuse a single dose over at least 1 h. Slow infusion over 1–2 h and adequate dilution will reduce pain of administration. Avoid starting infusion into dorsum of hand, wrist, or the antecubital veins; extravasation in these areas can damage underlying tendons and nerves leading to loss of mobility of entire limb.

INCOMPATIBILITIES: **Solution/Additive: Sodium bicarbonate. Y-Site: Allopurinol.** ■ Frequently check rate of flow and blood return; palpate injection site for extravasation. If there is any question about patency, line should be restarted.

ADVERSE EFFECTS Hematologic: Delayed <u>myelosuppression</u> (dose-related); thrombocytopenia. **CNS:** Dizziness, ataxia. **Respiratory:** <u>Pulmonary infiltration or fibrosis</u>. **Skin:** Skin flushing and burning pain at injection site, hyperpigmentation of skin (from contact). **Special Senses:** With high doses, eye infarctions, retinal hemorrhage, suffusion of conjunctiva. **GI:** Stomatitis, *nausea, vomiting*.

INTERACTIONS Drug: Cimetidine may potentiate neutropenia and thrombocytopenia.

PHARMACOKINETICS Distribution: Readily crosses blood–brain barrier; CSF concentrations 15–70% of plasma concentrations. **Metabolism:** Rapidly metabolized; metabolic fate not completely known. **Elimination:** 60–70% excreted in urine in 96 h; 6% excreted through lungs, 1% in feces; excreted in breast milk.

NURSING IMPLICATIONS

Assessment & Drug Effects

- Be alert for and report signs of infection such as respiratory infections, aching, rashes, and gastrointestinal distress. Assess immunization

status prior to beginning therapy in order to be alert for diseases that pose risk.
- Monitor for nausea and vomiting (dose related), which may occur within 2 h after drug administration and persist for up to 6 h. Prior administration of an antiemetic may help to decrease or prevent these adverse effects.
- Lab tests: Baseline CBC with differential and platelet count, repeat blood studies following infusion at weekly intervals for at least 6 wk. Baseline and periodic tests of hepatic and renal function.
- Platelet nadir usually occurs within 4–5 wk, and leukocyte nadir within 5–6 wk after therapy is terminated. Thrombocytopenia may be more severe than leukopenia; anemia is less severe.
- Check temperature daily. Avoid use of rectal thermometer to prevent injury to mucosa. An elevation of 0.6° F or more above usual temperature warrants reporting.
- Report symptoms of lung toxicity (cough, shortness of breath, fever) to the physician immediately.
- Be alert to signs of hepatic toxicity (jaundice, dark urine, pruritus, light-colored stools) and renal insufficiency (dysuria, oliguria, hematuria, swelling of lower legs and feet).

Patient & Family Education
- Report burning sensation immediately, because carmustine can cause burning discomfort even in the absence of extravasation. Infusion will be discontinued and restarted in another site. Ice application over the area may decrease the discomfort.
- Intense flushing of skin may occur during IV infusion. This usually disappears in 2–4 h.
- You will be highly susceptible to infection and to hemorrhagic disorders. Report signs of infection. Avoid exposure to crowds and those with infectious diseases. Be alert to hazardous periods that occur 4–6 wk after a dose of carmustine. If possible, avoid invasive procedures (e.g., IM injections, enemas, rectal temperatures) during this period.
- Report promptly the onset of sore throat, weakness, fever, chills, infection of any kind, or abnormal bleeding (ecchymosis, petechiae, epistaxis, bleeding gums, hematemesis, melena).
- Do not breast feed while taking this drug.

CEFACLOR
(sef′a-klor)
Ceclor, Ceclor CD
Classifications: ANTI-INFECTIVE; ANTIBIOTIC; SECOND-GENERATION CEPHALOSPORIN
Prototype: Cefonicid sodium
Pregnancy Category: B

AVAILABILITY 250 mg, 500 mg tablets; 250 mg, 500 mg capsules; 250 mg, 500 mg pulvules; 375 mg, 500 mg sustained-release tablets; 125 mg/5 mL, 187 mg/5 mL, 250 mg/5 mL, 375 mg/5 mL suspension

---

Common adverse effects in *italic*; life-threatening effects underlined; generic names in **bold**; drug classifications in SMALL CAPS; ♣ Canadian drug name; ❶ Prototype drug.

243

ACTIONS Semisynthetic, second-generation oral cephalosporin antibiotic similar to cefonicid. Possibly more active than other oral cephalosporins against gram-negative bacilli, especially beta-lactamase-producing *Haemophilus influenzae,* including ampicillin-resistant strains. Also active against *Escherichia coli, Proteus mirabilis, Klebsiella* sp. and certain gram-positive strains, e.g., *Streptococcus pneumoniae, S. pyogenes,* and *Staphylococcus aureus.* Preferentially binds to one or more of the penicillin-binding proteins (PBPs) located on cell walls of susceptible organisms. This inhibits third and final stage of bacterial cell wall synthesis, thus killing the bacterium.

THERAPEUTIC EFFECTS Effective in treating acute otitis media and acute sinusitis where the causative agent is resistant to other antibiotics. Useful in treating gonorrhea, respiratory and urinary tract infections. Partial cross-allergenicity between penicillins and cephalosporins has been reported.

USES Treatment of otitis media and infections of upper and lower respiratory tract, urinary tract, and skin and skin structures caused by ampicillin-resistant *H. influenzae;* acute uncomplicated UTI.

CONTRAINDICATIONS Hypersensitivity to cephalosporins and related antibiotics; pregnancy (category B), lactation. Safe use in infants <1 mo not established.

CAUTIOUS USE History of sensitivity to penicillins or other drug allergies; markedly impaired renal function.

ROUTE & DOSAGE

Mild to Moderate Infections

Child: **PO** 20–40 mg/kg/day divided into doses given q8h (max 2 g/day)
Adult: **PO** 250–500 mg q8h *or* Ceclor CD 250–500 mg q12h (max 4 g/day)

STORAGE

- Store tablets, capsules, and pulvules in tightly closed container at 15°–30° C (59°–86° F).
- After oral suspension is prepared, it should be kept refrigerated. Expiration date should appear on label. Discard unused portion after 14 days.

ADMINISTRATION

Oral

- Give sustained-release tablets with food to enhance absorption. Food does not affect absorption.
- Ensure that sustained-release tablets are not chewed or crushed. They must be swallowed whole.
- Shake suspension well before pouring.

ADVERSE EFFECTS Body as a Whole: Serum sickness-like reaction, eosinophilia, joint pain or swelling, fever, superinfections. **GI:** *Diarrhea;* nausea, vomiting, anorexia, <u>pseudomembranous colitis</u> (rare). **Skin:** Urticaria, pruritus, morbilliform eruptions.

DIAGNOSTIC TEST INTERFERENCE Cefaclor may produce positive *direct Coombs' test,* which can complicate *cross-matching procedures* and *hematologic studies.* False-positive *urine glucose* determinations may result with use of *copper sulfate reduction methods,* e.g., *Clinitest* or *Benedict's reagent,* but not with *glucose oxidase* (enzymatic) *tests* such as *Clinistix, Diastix, TesTape.*

INTERACTIONS Drug: Probenecid decreases renal excretion of cefaclor.

PHARMACOKINETICS Absorption: Well absorbed; acid stable. **Peak:** 30–60 min. **Elimination:** 60% of dose eliminated renally in 8 h; crosses placenta; excreted in breast milk. **Half-Life:** 0.5–1 h.

NURSING IMPLICATIONS

Assessment & Drug Effects

- Determine previous hypersensitivity to cephalosporins, penicillins, and other drug allergies, before therapy is initiated.
- Lab tests: Perform culture and sensitivity tests prior to and periodically during therapy.
- Diarrhea, the most frequent adverse effect, may be due to a pharmacologic effect or to associated change in intestinal flora. If it persists, interruption of therapy may be necessary.
- Monitor for manifestations of drug hypersensitivity (see Appendix D-1). Discontinue drug and promptly report them if they appear.
- Monitor for manifestations of superinfection (see Appendix D-1). Promptly report their appearance.

Patient & Family Education

- Report promptly any signs or symptoms of superinfection.
- Yogurt or buttermilk (if allowed) may serve as a prophylactic against intestinal superinfections by helping to maintain normal intestinal flora.
- Take the medication for the full course of therapy as directed by prescriber.
- Do not breast feed while taking this drug.
- Store this medication out of reach of children.

CEFADROXIL
(sef-a-drox'ill)
Duricef, Ultracef
Classifications: ANTI-INFECTIVE; ANTIBIOTIC; FIRST-GENERATION CEPHALOSPORIN
Prototype: Cefazolin
Pregnancy Category: B

AVAILABILITY 500 mg capsules; 1 g tablets; 125 mg/5 mL, 250 mg/5 mL, 500 mg/5 mL suspension

ACTIONS Semisynthetic, first-generation cephalosporin antibiotic with antibacterial spectrum similar to that of cefazolin. Bactericidal action (similar to that of penicillins): drug penetrates bacterial cell wall, resists beta-lactamases, and inactivates enzymes essential to cell wall synthesis. At equivalent doses, reportedly attains greater concentrations in serum and urine than other oral cephalosporins.

THERAPEUTIC EFFECTS Active against organisms that liberate cephalosporinase and penicillinase (beta-lactamases). According to clinical and laboratory evidence, partial cross-allergenicity exists between penicillins and cephalosporins. Effective in reducing signs and symptoms of urinary tract infections, bone and joint infections, skin and soft tissue infections, and pharyngitis.

USES Primarily in treatment of urinary tract infections caused by *Escherichia coli, Proteus mirabilis,* and *Klebsiella* sp.; infections of skin and skin structures caused by *Staphylococci* and *Streptococci;* and for treatment of *Group A beta-hemolytic streptococcal* pharyngitis and tonsillitis.

CONTRAINDICATIONS Hypersensitivity to cephalosporins and related antibiotics; pregnancy (category B), lactation.

CAUTIOUS USE Sensitivity to penicillins or other drug allergies; impaired renal function, history of colitis.

ROUTE & DOSAGE

Uncomplicated Urinary Tract Infection

Infant and Child: **PO** 30 mg/kg/day in 2 divided doses
Adult: **PO** 1–2 g/day in 1–2 divided doses

Skin and Skin Structure Infections, Streptococcal Pharyngitis, or Tonsillitis

Child: **PO** 30 mg/kg/day in 2 divided doses
Adult: **PO** 1 g/day in 1–2 divided doses

Adjustment for Renal Impairment Cl$_{cr}$ <25 mL/min

Child: **PO** 15 mg/kg q24h
Adult: **PO** 1 g q24h

STORAGE

Store in tight container unless otherwise directed. Oral suspensions are stable for 14 days under refrigeration at 2°–8° C (36°–46° F). Avoid freezing. Note expiration date on label; discard after 14 days.

ADMINISTRATION

Oral

- Give with food or milk to reduce nausea. If nausea persists, termination of therapy may be necessary.
- Follow direction for mixing oral suspension found on drug label. Reconstituted solution contains 125 mg or 250 mg cefadroxil per 5 mL suspension.
- Shake suspension well before use.

ADVERSE EFFECTS Body as a Whole: Hypersensitivity (rash, swollen eyelids [angioedema], pruritus, chills), superinfections. **GI:** Nausea, *diarrhea,* vomiting, heartburn, gastritis, bloating, abdominal cramps.

DIAGNOSTIC TEST INTERFERENCE False-positive *urine glucose* determinations using *copper sulfate reduction reagents,* such as *Clinitest* or *Benedict's reagent,* but not with *glucose oxidase tests,* e.g., *Clinistix, Diastix, TesTape. Cefadroxil-induced positive direct Coombs' test* may interfere with *cross-matching procedures* and *hematologic studies.*

INTERACTIONS Drug: Probenecid decreases renal excretion of cefadroxil.

PHARMACOKINETICS Absorption: Acid stable; rapidly absorbed from GI tract. **Peak:** 1 h. **Elimination:** 90% excreted unchanged in urine within 8 h; bacterial inhibitory levels persist 20–22 h; crosses placenta; excreted in breast milk. **Half-Life:** 1–12 h.

NURSING IMPLICATIONS

Assessment & Drug Effects
- Determine previous hypersensitivity to cephalosporins, penicillins, and other drug allergies, before therapy is initiated.
- Lab tests: Perform culture and sensitivity testing prior to and periodically during therapy.
- Lab tests: Perform baseline and periodic renal function studies in patients with renal function impairment, and monitor I&O ratio and pattern.
- Monitor for manifestations of drug hypersensitivity (see Appendix D-1). Discontinue drug and promptly report them if they appear.
- Monitor for manifestations of superinfection (see Signs & Symptoms, Appendix D-1). Promptly report their appearance.

Patient & Family Education
- Report promptly the onset of rash, urticaria, pruritus, or fever, because the possibility of an allergic reaction is high, if you are allergic to penicillin.
- Take medication for the full course of therapy as directed by your health care provider.
- Report promptly S&S of superinfections (see Appendix D-1).
- Do not breast feed while taking this drug.
- Store this medication out of reach of children.

CEFAMANDOLE NAFATE

(sef-a-man'dole)
Mandol
Classifications: ANTI-INFECTIVE; ANTIBIOTIC; SECOND-GENERATION CEPHALOSPORIN
Prototype: Cefonicid sodium
Pregnancy Category: B

AVAILABILITY 1 g, 2 g injection

ACTIONS Semisynthetic, second-generation cephalosporin antibiotic similar to other drugs of this class. Preferentially binds to one or more of the penicillin-binding proteins (PBP) located on cell walls of susceptible

---

organisms. This inhibits third and final stage of bacterial wall synthesis, thus killing the bacterium.

THERAPEUTIC EFFECTS Usually active against organisms susceptible to first-generation cephalosporins. In addition, it is active against the anaerobes *Clostridium* sp., *Peptococcus* sp., *Fusobacterium* sp.; and against some strains of *Providencia* sp., *Enterobacter, Serratia, Proteus, E. coli,* and *Klebsiella* resistant to first-generation cephalosporins. Inactive against *Enterococci,* methicillin-resistant *Staphylococci* (MRSA), *Listeria monocytogenes,* and *Pseudomonas.* Partial cross-allergenicity between penicillins and cephalosporins has been reported. Effective treatment for bone and joint infections, lower respiratory tract infections, peritonitis, urinary tract infections and surgical prophylaxis.

USES Serious infections of respiratory, genitourinary, and biliary tracts, skin and soft tissue, bones and joints, and in septicemia and peritonitis (caused by *E. coli* and other coliform microbes); also perioperative prophylaxis to reduce infections in patient undergoing potentially contaminated procedure.

CONTRAINDICATIONS Hypersensitivity to cephalosporins and related antibiotics; pregnancy (category B), lactation. Safe use in children between 1 and 6 mo not established.

CAUTIOUS USE History of sensitivity to penicillins or other drug allergies; renal function impairment; history of GI disease, particularly colitis.

ROUTE & DOSAGE

Moderate to Severe Infections
Child: **IV/IM** 50–100 mg/kg/day in 3–6 divided doses, up to 150 mg/kg/day (not to exceed adult doses)
Adult: **IV/IM** 500 mg–1 g q4–8h, up to 2 g q4h

Surgical Prophylaxis
Child: **IV/IM** 50–100 mg/kg 30–60 min before surgery, then q6h for 24 h
Adult: **IV/IM** 1–2 g 30–60 min before surgery, then q6h for 24 h

STORAGE
Protect from light. Reconstituted drug remains stable at room temperature for 24 h and when refrigerated at 5° C (41° F), for 96 h.

ADMINISTRATION

Intramuscular
- To each g of cefamandole add 3 mL of sterile water for injection or bacteriostatic water for injection, or NS, or D5W. Resulting solution contains 285 mg/mL. Administer IM deep into a large muscle mass appropriate for age such as gluteus maximus or vastus lateralis (see Part I).

Intravenous

PREPARE Direct: Reconstitute each g with 10 mL sterile water for injection, D5W, or NS. **Intermittent/Continuous:** May be further diluted in 100–1000 mL of D5W or NS.

ADMINISTER **Direct:** Give slowly over 3–5 min. **Intermittent/ Continuous:** The rate of infusion is determined by the amount of solution and status of patient.

INCOMPATIBILITIES: **Solution/Additive:** Ringer's lactate, calcium gluconate, calcium gluceptate, cimetidine, AMINOGLYCOSIDES, metronidazole, magnesium, ranitidine. **Y-Site:** AMINOGLYCOSIDES, **amiodarone, hetastarch.** ▪ Prolonged exposure to light causes cefamandole powder to discolor. Once reconstituted, cefamandole is no longer light sensitive. Solutions appear light yellow to amber. Do not use if otherwise colored or if a precipitate is present. ▪ After reconstitution, cefamandole may liberate CO_2. Do not store medication in syringes, because a buildup of pressure from CO_2 may force plunger out of barrel.

ADVERSE EFFECTS Body as a Whole: Drug fever, eosinophilia, pain, redness and induration, sterile abscess at injection site, superinfections. **GI:** Abdominal cramps, *diarrhea*, pseudomembranous colitis. **Hematologic:** Hypoprothrombinemia (vitamin K deficiency). **Skin:** Rash, urticaria.

DIAGNOSTIC TEST INTERFERENCE False-positive *urine glucose* determinations using *copper sulfate reduction methods,* e.g., *Clinitest* or *Benedict's reagent,* but not with *glucose oxidase* (enzymatic) *tests* such as *Clinistix, Diastix, TesTape.* Cefamandole-induced positive *direct Coombs' test* may interfere with *cross-matching procedures* and *hematologic studies.*

INTERACTIONS Drug: Probenecid decreases renal elimination of cefamandole; **alcohol** causes disulfiram reaction.

PHARMACOKINETICS Peak: 0.5–2 h IM; 10 min IV. **Distribution:** Poor CNS penetration even with inflamed meninges; extensive enterohepatic circulation; high concentrations in bile. **Metabolism:** Rapidly hydrolyzed in plasma to active metabolite. **Elimination:** 68–85% excreted unchanged in urine in 6–8 h. **Half-Life:** 30–120 min.

NURSING IMPLICATIONS

Assessment & Drug Effects

- Determine previous hypersensitivity to cephalosporins, penicillins, and other drugs, prior to initiating therapy.
- Lab tests: Perform C&S testing prior to and periodically during therapy. Cefamandole therapy may be instituted pending test results. Baseline and periodic studies of renal function and PT determinations should be performed.
- Monitor I&O rates and pattern: Particularly important in patients with impaired renal function or who are receiving high doses.
- Antibiotic-associated pseudomembranous enterocolitis (life threatening) is a superinfection caused by *Clostridia difficile* and may occur in 4–9 days or as long as 6 wk after cefamandole is discontinued (see Appendix D-1). Most likely to occur in the chronically ill patient, especially if undergoing abdominal surgery or if in an ICU.

Patient & Family Education

- Take medication for entire course as prescribed by health care provider.
- Check for fever in the presence of diarrhea and report fever and diarrhea to the prescriber.
- If you experience any signs or symptoms of hypersensitivity, discontinue the drug and consult with the prescriber.
- Avoid use of alcohol during and for 48–72 h after taking cefamandole. A drug-induced disulfiram-like reaction may follow alcohol intake.
- Report promptly any signs or symptoms of superinfection. Superinfections may occur, particularly during prolonged use of cephalosporins.
- Do not breast feed while taking this drug.

CEFAZOLIN SODIUM ⊙

(sef-a′zoe-lin)
Ancef, Kefzol, Zolicef
Classifications: ANTI-INFECTIVE; ANTIBIOTIC; FIRST-GENERATION CEPHALOSPORIN
Pregnancy Category: B

AVAILABILITY 250 mg, 500 mg, 1 g, injection

ACTIONS Semisynthetic, first-generation derivative of cephalosporin C; antibiotic activity similar to that of cefazolin. Activity against gram-negative organisms is limited. Bactericidal action: Preferentially binds to one or more of the penicillin-binding proteins (PBPs) located on cell walls of susceptible organisms. This inhibits third and final stage of bacterial cell wall synthesis, thus killing the bacterium.

THERAPEUTIC EFFECTS Effective treatment for bone and joint infections, biliary tract infections, enocarditis prophylaxis and treatment, respiratory tract and genital tract infections, septicemia and skin infections, and surgical prophylaxis.

USES Severe infections of urinary and biliary tracts, skin, soft tissue, and bone, and for bacteremia and endocarditis caused by susceptible organisms; also perioperative prophylaxis in patients undergoing procedures associated with high risk of infection, e.g., open heart surgery.

CONTRAINDICATIONS Hypersensitivity to any cephalosporin and related antibiotics; pregnancy (category B), lactation.
CAUTIOUS USE History of penicillin sensitivity, impaired renal function, patients on sodium restriction.

ROUTE & DOSAGE

Moderate to Severe Infections

Neonate: **IV** ≤*7 days,* 40 mg/kg/day divided into doses given q12h; *>7 day and <2000 g weight:* 40 mg/kg/day divided into doses given q8–12h; *>7 days and >2000 g weight:* 60 mg/kg/day divided into doses given q8–12h

Adjustment for Renal Impairment
Cl$_{cr}$ <35 mL/min: dose q12h

Child: **IV/IM** 25–100 mg/kg/day in 3–4 divided doses, up to 100 mg/kg/day (not to exceed 6 g/24 h)
Adult: **IV/IM** 250 mg–2 g q8h, up to 2 g q4h (max 12 g/day)
Surgical Prophylaxis
Child: **IV/IM** 25–50 mg/kg 30–60 min before surgery, then q8h for 24 h
Adult: **IV/IM** 1–2 g 30–60 min before surgery, then q8h for 24 h

STORAGE
Store powder at 15°–30° C (59°–86° F) and protect from light. Reconstituted solutions are stable for 24 h at room temperature and for 96 h refrigerated.

ADMINISTRATION
Intramuscular

- Preparation of IM solution: Reconstitute with sterile water for injection, bacteriostatic water for injection, or 0.9% sodium chloride injection.
- IM injections should be made deep into large muscle mass appropriate for age (see Part I). Pain on injection is usually minimal. Rotate injection sites.

Intravenous

- IV administration to neonates, infants, and children: Verify correct IV concentration and rate of infusion with physician.
PREPARE **Direct:** Dilute each 1 g with 10 mL of sterile water for injection. **Intermittent:** Further dilute with 50–100 mL of NS or D5W.
ADMINISTER **Direct/Intermittent:** Infuse 1 g over 5 min or longer as determined by the amount of solution. The risk of IV site reactions may be reduced by proper dilution of IV solution, use of small-bore IV needle in a large vein, and by rotating injection sites.
INCOMPATIBILITIES: **Solution/Additive:** AMINOGLYCOSIDES, **ascorbic acid, atracurium, bleomycin, cimetidine, hydromorphone, lidocaine, ranitidine, vitamin B complex with C. Y-Site: Amiodarone,** AMINOGLYCOSIDES, **amphotericin B cholesteryl complex, idarubicin, pentamidine, vinorelbine.**

ADVERSE EFFECTS Body as a Whole: <u>Anaphylaxis</u>, fever, eosinophilia, superinfections, seizure (high doses in patients with renal insufficiency). **GI:** *Diarrhea,* anorexia, abdominal cramps <u>pseudomembranous colitis</u>. **Skin:** Maculopapular rash, urticaria.

DIAGNOSTIC TEST INTERFERENCE Because of cefazolin effect on the ***direct Coombs' test,*** transfusion ***cross-matching procedures*** and ***hematologic studies*** may be complicated. False-positive ***urine glucose*** determinations are possible with use of ***copper sulfate tests*** (e.g., ***Clinitest*** or ***Benedict's reagent***) but not with ***glucose oxidase tests*** such as ***TesTape, Diastix,*** or ***Clinistix.***

INTERACTIONS Drug: Probenecid decreases renal elimination of cefazolin.

Common adverse effects in *italic;* life-threatening effects <u>underlined</u>; generic names in **bold;** drug classifications in SMALL CAPS; ✦ Canadian drug name; ❂ Prototype drug.

251

PHARMACOKINETICS Peak: 1–2 h IM; 5 min IV. **Distribution:** Poor CNS penetration even with inflamed meninges; high concentrations in bile and in diseased bone; crosses placenta. **Elimination:** 70% excreted unchanged in urine in 6 h; small amount excreted in breast milk. **Half-Life:** 90–130 min.

NURSING IMPLICATIONS

Assessment & Drug Effects

- Determine history of hypersensitivity to cephalosporins, penicillins, and other drugs, before therapy is initiated.
- Lab tests: Perform culture and sensitivity testing prior to and during therapy. Therapy may be initiated pending results.
- Monitor I&O rates and pattern: Be alert to changes in BUN, serum creatinine.
- If patient has had a reaction to penicillin, be alert to signs of hypersensitivity with use of cefazolin. Cross-allergenicity between cephalosporins and penicillin has been reported. Prompt attention should be given to onset of signs of hypersensitivity (see Appendix D-1).
- Promptly report the onset of diarrhea, which may or may not be dose related. It is seen especially in patients with history of drug-related GI disturbances. Pseudomembranous colitis, a potentially life-threatening condition, starts with diarrhea.

Patient & Family Education

- Report promptly any signs or symptoms of superinfection.
- Report signs of hemostatic defects: ecchymoses, petechiae, nosebleed.
- Do not breast feed while taking this drug.

CEFDINIR
(cef'di-nir)
Omnicef
Classifications: ANTI-INFECTIVE; THIRD-GENERATION CEPHALOSPORIN
Prototype: Cefotaxime sodium
Pregnancy Category: B

AVAILABILITY 300 mg capsules; 125 mg/5 mL suspension

ACTIONS Broad-spectrum semisynthetic third-generation cephalosporin antibiotic. Generally active against a wide variety of gram-positive and gram-negative bacteria.
THERAPEUTIC EFFECTS Effective against most *Enterobacteriaceae* and *Pseudomonas,* and most strains of *Staphylococci* and *Streptococci* including methicillin-resistant strains (MRSA). Effectively treats pneumonia, acute and chronic bronchitis, otitis media, sinusitis, vaginitis, and skin infections reducing or eliminating signs and symptoms of infection.

USES Community-acquired pneumonia, acute exacerbations of chronic bronchitis, acute maxillary sinusitis, pharyngitis, tonsillitis, uncomplicated skin infections, bacterial otitis media.

CONTRAINDICATIONS Hypersensitivity to cefdinir and other cephalosporins; pregnancy (category B)
CAUTIOUS USE Hypersensitivity to penicillins, penicillin derivatives; renal impairment; ulcerative colitis or antibiotic-induced colitis; bleeding disorders; lactation; GI disorders; liver or kidney disease. Safety and efficacy in neonates and infants <6 mo old not established.

ROUTE & DOSAGE

Community-Acquired Pneumonia, Skin Infections
Child 6 mo–12 y: **PO** 7 mg/kg q12h for 10 days
Adult: **PO** 300 mg q12h for 10 days

Chronic Bronchitis, Maxillary Sinusitis, Pharyngitis, Tonsillitis
Child 6 mo–12 y: **PO** 14 mg/kg q24h or 7 mg/kg q12h for 10 days
Adult: **PO** 600 mg q24h or 300 mg q12h for 10 days

STORAGE
Store reconstituted oral suspension in tightly closed container. Discard after 10 days.

ADMINISTRATION

Oral
- Do not give within 2 h of aluminum- or magnesium-containing antacids or iron supplements.
- Reconstitute oral suspension to 125 mg/mL by adding water (38-mL to 60-mL bottle or 63-mL to 100-mL bottle). Shake well before each use.
- Consult physician for dosage adjustment if creatinine clearance <30 mL/min and for patients on hemodialysis.

ADVERSE EFFECTS GI: *Diarrhea,* nausea, abdominal pain. **Metabolic:** Increased GGT, increased urine protein, hematuria. **CNS:** Headache. **Skin:** Rash, cutaneous moniliasis. **Urogenital:** Vaginal moniliasis, vaginitis.

DIAGNOSTIC TEST INTERFERENCE False positive for **ketones** or **glucose** in urine using **nitroprusside** or **Clinitest.**

INTERACTIONS Drug: ANTACIDS should be taken at least 2 h before or after cefdinir; **probenecid** prolongs cefdinir elimination; **iron** decreases absorption.

PHARMACOKINETICS Absorption: 16–25% bioavailability. **Peak:** 2–4 h. **Distribution:** 60–70% protein bound; penetrates sinus tissue, blister fluid, lung tissue, middle ear fluid. **Metabolism:** Not metabolized. **Elimination:** Excreted in urine. **Half-Life:** 1.6 h.

NURSING IMPLICATIONS

Assessment & Drug Effects
- Determine previous hypersensitivity to cephalosporins, penicillins, and other drug allergies, before therapy is initiated.
- Carefully monitor for and immediately report S&S of hypersensitivity, superinfection, or pseudomembranous colitis.

- Discontinue drug and notify physician if seizures associated with drug therapy occur.

Patient & Family Education
- Allow a minimum of 2 h between cefdinir and antacids containing aluminum or magnesium, or drugs containing iron.
- Immediately contact physician if a rash, diarrhea, or new infection (e.g., yeast infection) develops. Take entire course of medication as prescribed by health care provider.
- Drug may cause false positive for urine ketones or glucose. Consult package insert.
- Do not breast feed while taking this drug without consulting physician.
- Store this medication out of reach of children.

CEFIXIME
(ce-fix'ime)
Suprax
Classifications: ANTI-INFECTIVE; ANTIBIOTIC; THIRD-GENERATION CEPHALOSPORIN
Prototype: Cefotaxime sodium
Pregnancy Category: B

AVAILABILITY 200 mg, 400 mg tablets; 100 mg/5 mL suspension

ACTIONS A third-generation cephalosporin that is highly stable in the presence of beta-lactamases (penicillinases and cephalosporinases) and therefore has excellent activity against a wide range of gram-negative bacteria. It is bactericidal against susceptible bacteria. Cephalosporins inhibit mucopeptide synthesis in the bacterial cell wall.
THERAPEUTIC EFFECTS Effectively treats respiratory tract, urinary tract infection, otitis media and gonorrhea, reducing or eliminating signs and symptoms of infection.

USES Effective against *Streptococcus pyogenes, S. pneumoniae,* and gram-negative bacilli, including *Haemophilus influenzae, Branhamella catarrhalis,* and *Neisseria gonorrhoeae.* Little activity against *Staphylococci,* and no activity against *Pseudomonas aeruginosa;* also uncomplicated UTI, otitis media, pharyngitis, tonsillitis, and bronchitis.

CONTRAINDICATIONS Patients with known allergy to the cephalosporin group of antibiotics.
CAUTIOUS USE Allergy to penicillin, history of colitis, renal insufficiency, pregnancy (category B), lactation. Safety and effectiveness in infants <6 mo have not been established.

ROUTE & DOSAGE

Infection
Child: **PO** 8 mg/kg/day in 1–2 divided doses
Adult: **PO** 400 mg/day in 1–2 divided doses

Common adverse effects in *italic;* life-threatening effects <u>underlined;</u> generic names in **bold;** drug classifications in SMALL CAPS; ♣ Canadian drug name; ❶ Prototype drug.

STORAGE

After reconstitution, suspension may be kept for 14 days at room temperature or refrigerated. Store away from heat and light. Keep tightly closed and shake well before using.

ADMINISTRATION

Oral

- Do not substitute tablets for liquid in treatment of otitis media because of lack of bioequivalence.

ADVERSE EFFECTS GI: *Diarrhea,* loose stools, nausea, vomiting, dyspepsia, flatulence. **CNS:** Drug fever, headache, dizziness. **Skin:** Rash, pruritus, **Urogenital:** Vaginitis, genital pruritus.

INTERACTIONS Drug: AMINOGLYCOSIDES may increase risk of nephrotoxicity and have additive/synergistic effects. May decrease efficacy of ORAL CONTRACEPTIVES. **Probenecid** may increase levels.

PHARMACOKINETICS Absorption: 40–50% absorbed from GI tract. **Peak:** 2–6 h. **Distribution:** Distributed into breast milk. **Elimination:** 50% excreted in urine, 50% in bile. **Half-Life:** 3–4 h.

NURSING IMPLICATIONS

Assessment & Drug Effects

- Determine previous hypersensitivity reactions to cephalosporins, penicillins, and history of other allergies, particularly to drugs, prior to initiation of therapy.
- Lab tests: Perform culture and sensitivity tests prior to initiation of therapy and periodically during therapy. Therapy may be implemented pending test results.
- Discontinue if seizures associated with the drug therapy occur.
- Monitor for superinfections (see Appendix D-1) caused by overgrowth of nonsusceptible organisms, particularly during prolonged use.
- Monitor I&O rates and pattern.
- Carefully monitor anyone with a history of allergies, especially to drugs. Report manifestations of hypersensitivity.
- Promptly report loose stools or diarrhea, which may indicate pseudomembranous colitis (see Appendix D-1). Discontinuation of drug may be necessary.

Patient & Family Education

- Report loose stools or diarrhea during drug therapy and for several weeks after. This may indicate onset of pseudomembranous colitis.
- Take this antibiotic as prescribed by health care provider for the full course of treatment.
- Do not miss any doses and take the doses at evenly spaced times, day and night.
- Do not breast feed while taking this drug without consulting physician.
- Store this medication out of reach of children.

Common adverse effects in *italic;* life-threatening effects underlined; generic names in **bold;** drug classifications in SMALL CAPS; ♣ Canadian drug name; ⊘ Prototype drug.

255

CEFOPERAZONE SODIUM

(sef-oh-per′a-zone)
Cefobid
Classifications: ANTI-INFECTIVE; ANTIBIOTIC; THIRD-GENERATION CEPHALOSPORIN
Prototype: Cefotaxime sodium
Pregnancy Category: B

AVAILABILITY 1 g, 2 g injection

ACTIONS Semisynthetic third-generation cephalosporin antibiotic. Preferentially binds to one or more of the penicillin-binding proteins located on cell walls of susceptible organisms. This inhibits third and final stage of bacterial cell wall synthesis, thus killing the bacterium. Spectrum of activity is similar to that of cefotaxime.

THERAPEUTIC EFFECTS Generally active against a wide variety of gram-negative bacteria, including some strains of *Pseudomonas aeruginosa*. Also active against some organisms resistant to first- and second-generation cephalosporins and currently available aminoglycoside antibiotics and penicillins; e.g., *Escherichia coli, Klebsiella pneumoniae,* and *Serratia marcescens*. Other susceptible organisms include *Proteus mirabilis, Salmonella, Shigella, Haemophilus influenzae, Neisseria gonorrhoeae,* groups A and B *Streptococci, Staphylococcus aureus,* and some strains of *Pseudomonas* sp. Cefoperazone inhibits some strains of *Clostridium,* but *C. difficle* is resistant to the drug, as is *Listeria monocytogenes*. It has a broad antibacterial spectrum, including gram-positive bacteria and *Pseudomonas aeruginosa*. Effectively treats biliary tract infections, gynecologic infections and gonorrhea, intra-abdominal and soft tissue infections, respiratory tract infections, urinary tract infections, skin infections, septicemia, and surgical infections, reducing or eliminating signs and symptoms of infection.

USES Infections of skin and skin structures, urinary tract, respiratory tract; peritonitis and other intra-abdominal infections, pelvic inflammatory disease, endometritis and other infections of the female genital tract; bacterial septicemia.

UNLABELED USE Children <12 y.

CONTRAINDICATIONS Hypersensitivity to cephalosporins and related beta-lactam antibiotics; pregnancy (category B).

CAUTIOUS USE History of hypersensitivity to penicillins, history of allergy, particularly to drugs; hepatic disease, history of colitis or other GI disease, history of bleeding disorders; lactation.

ROUTE & DOSAGE

Moderate to Severe Infections

Child <12 y: **IV/IM** 100–200 mg/kg/day divided into doses q8–12h (max 12 g/24 h)
Adult: **IV/IM** 2–4 g/day in 2–4 divided doses (max 12 g/24 h in severe infection)

Common adverse effects in *italic;* life-threatening effects underlined; generic names in **bold;** drug classifications in SMALL CAPS; ✦ Canadian drug name; ☻ Prototype drug.

STORAGE

Store powder at 25° C (77° F) and protect from light. After reconstitution it is not necessary to protect from light. Solution stable at room temperature for 24 h. Refrigerated solution stable for 5 days, except if mixed with 10% dextrose. Store IV frozen solutions at −20° C (−4° F). After thawed, stable for 48 h at room temperature or 10 days refrigerated. Do not refreeze.

ADMINISTRATION

Intramuscular

- To prepare IM injections, appropriate diluents include sterile water for injection, bacteriostatic water for injection, and 0.5% lidocaine. See package insert for reconstitution procedure.
- Reconstitute for IM: Dilute each 1 g with 5 mL sterile water. Shake vigorously to dissolve. If concentrations of ≥250 mg/mL are needed for IM injection, 2% lidocaine should be added. See manufacturer's directions.
- Inject into large muscle mass appropriate for age (see Part I).

Intravenous

- IV administration to infants and children: Verify correct IV concentration and rate of infusion with physician. ▪ Rapid, direct (bolus) IV injections are not recommended.

PREPARE **Intermittent:** Dilute each 1 g with 5 mL sterile water. Shake vigorously to dissolve, then dilute in 50–100 mL of D5W or NS. **Continuous:** Further dilute in 500–1000 mL of the selected IV solution.

ADMINISTER **Intermittent:** Give over 15–30 min. **Continuous:** Give 500–1000 mL over 6–24 h.

INCOMPATIBILITIES **Solution/Additive:** AMINOGLYCOSIDES, doxapram. **Y-Site:** AMINOGLYCOSIDES, **amifostine, amphotericin B cholesteryl complex, cisatracurium, diltiazem, doxorubicin liposome, filgrastim, gemcitabine, hetastarch, labetalol, meperidine, ondansetron, pentamidine, perphenazine, promethazine, sargramostim, vinorelbine.**

ADVERSE EFFECTS Body as a Whole: Fever, eosinophilia, phlebitis (IV site), transient pain (IM site), superinfections. **GI:** Abdominal cramps, bloating, loose stools or *diarrhea*, pseudomembranous colitis, elevated liver function tests (AST, ALT, alkaline phosphatase). **Hematologic:** Abnormal PT/INR and PTT; hypoprothrombinemia. **Skin:** Skin rash, urticaria, pruritus. **Urogenital:** Transient increases in serum creatinine and BUN, oliguria.

DIAGNOSTIC TEST INTERFERENCE Cefoperazone can cause positive *direct Coombs' test,* which may interfer with *hematologic studies* and *cross-matching* procedures. False-positive results for *urine glucose* using *copper sulfate tests (Benedict's, Clinitest),* but not with *glucose enzymatic tests,* e.g., *Clinistix, TesTape, Diastix.* Also causes *prolonged prothrombin* twice during therapy.

INTERACTIONS Drug: Probenecid decreases renal elimination of cefoperazone; **alcohol** produces disulfiram reaction.

PHARMACOKINETICS Peak: 1–2 h IM; 15–20 min IV. **Distribution:** Low CNS penetration except with inflamed meninges; highest concentrations in bile; crosses placenta. **Elimination:** 70–75% excreted unchanged in bile in 6–12 h, small amount excreted in breast milk. **Half-Life:** 2 h.

NURSING IMPLICATIONS

Assessment & Drug Effects

- Determine hypersensitivity to cephalosporins, penicillins, and other drug allergies before therapy begins.
- Lab tests: Perform culture and sensitivity studies before initiation of therapy and during therapy, as indicated. Therapy may begin pending test results. Perform PTT and PT/INR before and during therapy.
- Observe for and question patient about signs of hemostatic defects: wound bleeding (e.g., surgical patient), nose bleeds, bleeding gums, bloody sputum, hematuria. Hypoprothrombinemia and vitamin K deficiency are possible complications of therapy and can result in significant blood loss in some patients. Patients at risk are those with poor nutritional states, malabsorption problems, patients on hyperalimentation regimens, and alcoholism. Vitamin K supplements may be prescribed for these patients, if indicated.
- Report the onset of loose stools or diarrhea. Most patients respond to replacement of fluids, electrolytes, and proteins. Discontinuation of drug may be required for some patients.
- Monitor *cefoperazone serum levels* (at steady state: 150 mg/mL) in patients with hepatic disease or biliary obstruction who are receiving over 4 g/day, patients with both hepatic and renal disease receiving over 1–2 g/day, and patients with renal impairment on high dose therapy.

Patient & Family Education

- Do not ingest alcohol within 72 h after drug administration because this will cause a disulfiram-like reaction (see Appendix D-1).
- Effects generally appear within 15–30 min after alcohol is taken and disappear spontaneously 1–2 h later.
- Report promptly any signs or symptoms of superinfection.
- Do not breast feed while taking this drug without consulting physician.

CEFOTAXIME SODIUM ⓟ

(sef-oh-taks'eem)

Claforan

Classifications: ANTI-INFECTIVE; BETA-LACTAM ANTIBIOTIC; THIRD-GENERATION CEPHALOSPORIN

Pregnancy Category: B

AVAILABILITY 500 mg, 1 g, 2 g injection

ACTIONS Broad-spectrum semisynthetic third-generation cephalosporin antibiotic. Preferentially binds to one or more of the penicillin-binding

proteins located on cell walls of susceptible organisms. This inhibits third and final stage of bacterial cell wall synthesis, thus killing the bacterium.
THERAPEUTIC EFFECTS Generally active against a wide variety of gram-negative bacteria including most of the Enterobacteriaceae. Also active against some organisms resistant to first- and second-generation cephalosporins and currently available aminoglycoside antibiotics and penicillins, e.g., *Escherichia coli, Klebsiella pneumoniae,* and *Serratia marcescens.* Other susceptible organisms: *Bacteroides fragilis, Morganella morganii, Proteus mirabilis, Salmonella, Shigella, Haemophilus influenzae, Neisseria gonorrhoeae,* groups A and B *Streptococci, Staphylococcus aureus, Bacteroides, Eubacterium, Peptostreptococcus,* and *Peptococcus.* Inhibits some strains of *Clostridium,* but *C. difficile* is resistant to the drug, as is *Listeria monocytogenes.* It is the drug of choice in the treatment of gram-negative adult bacillary meningitis, neonatal and childhood meningitis, and Enterobacteriaceae. Effectively treats bone and joint infections, CNS infections, gynecologic infections and gonorrhea, lower respiratory tract infections, intra-abdominal infections, skin and urinary tract infections, and is used for surgical prophylaxis to reduce or eliminate infection.

USES Serious infections of lower respiratory tract, skin and skin structures, bones and joints, CNS (including meningitis and ventriculitis), gynecologic and GU tract infections, including uncomplicated gonococcal infections caused by penicillinase-producing *Neisseria gonorrhoeae* (PPNG). Also used to treat bacteremia or septicemia, intra-abdominal infections, and for perioperative prophylaxis.
UNLABELED USES Currently recommended by CDC for treatment of disseminated gonococcal infections (gonococcal arthritis-dermatitis syndrome) and as drug of choice for gonococcal ophthalmia caused by PPNG in adults, children, and neonates.

CONTRAINDICATIONS Hypersensitivity to cephalosporins and other beta-lactam antibiotics; pregnancy (category B).
CAUTIOUS USE History of type I hypersensitivity reactions to penicillin; history of allergy to other beta-lactam; antibiotics; renal impairment; history of colitis or other GI disease; lactation.

ROUTE & DOSAGE

Moderate to Severe Infections
Child: **IV/IM** ≤1 wk, 50 mg/kg q12h; 1–4 wk, 50 mg/kg q8h; 1 mo–12 y, 100–200 mg/kg/day divided into doses q4–8h
Adult: **IV/IM** 1–2 g q8–12h, up to 2 g q4h (max 12 g/day)

Surgical Prophylaxis
Adult: **IV/IM** 1 g 30–90 min before surgery

STORAGE
Protect from excessive light. Reconstituted solutions may be stored in original containers for 24 h at room temperature; for 10 days under refrigeration at 5° C (41° F) or less; or for at least 13 wk in frozen state if frozen directly after reconstitution.

C

ADMINISTRATION

Intramuscular

- Add 3 mL sterile water for injection or bacteriostatic water for injection to vial containing 1 g drug, providing a solution of approximately 300 mg cefotaxime/mL.
- Administer IM injection deeply into large muscle mass appropriate for age (see Part I). Aspirate to avoid inadvertent injection into blood vessel. If IM dose is 2 g, divide dose and administer into 2 different sites.
- Risk of phlebitis may be reduced by use of a small needle in a large vein.

Intravenous

- IV administration to infants and children: Verify correct IV concentration and rate of infusion with prescriber. ■ Do not admix cefotaxime with sodium bicarbonate or any fluid with a pH >7.5.

PREPARE **Direct:** Add 10 mL diluent to vial with 1 or 2 g drug providing a solution containing 95 or 180 mg/mL, respectively. **Intermittent:** To 1 or 2 g drug add 50 or 100 mL D5W, NS, D5/NS, D5/0.45% NaCl, RL, or other compatible diluent. **Continuous:** Dilute in 500–1000 mL compatible IV solution.

ADMINISTER **Direct:** Give over 3–5 min. **Intermittent:** Give over 20–30 min, preferably via butterfly or scalp vein-type needles. **Continuous:** Infuse over 6–24 h.

INCOMPATIBILITIES: **Solution/Additive:** AMINOGLYCOSIDES, **amino-phylline, doxapram, sodium bicarbonate, vancomycin**. **Y-Site:** **Allopurinol,** AMINOGLYCOSIDES, **aminophylline, doxapram, filgrastim, fluconazole, gemcitabine, hetastarch, pentamidine, sodium bicarbonate, vancomycin.**

ADVERSE EFFECTS Body as a Whole: Fever, nocturnal perspiration, inflammatory reaction at IV site, phlebitis, thrombophlebitis; pain, induration, and tenderness at IM site, superinfections. **GI:** Nausea, vomiting, *diarrhea,* abdominal pain, colitis, <u>pseudomembranous colitis</u>, anorexia. **Metabolic:** Transient increases in serum AST, ALT, LDH, bilirubin, alkaline phosphatase concentrations. **Skin:** Rash, pruritus.

DIAGNOSTIC TEST INTERFERENCE May cause falsely elevated *serum* or *urine creatinine* values *(Jaffe reaction).* False-positive reactions for *urine glucose* have not been reported using *copper sulfate reduction methods,* e.g., *Benedict's, Clinitest;* however, since it has occurred with other cephalosporins, it may be advisable to use *glucose oxidase tests (Clinistix, TesTape, Diastix).* Positive *direct antiglobulin (Coombs') test* results may interfere with *hematologic studies* and *cross-matching* procedures.

INTERACTIONS Drug: Probenecid decreases renal elimination; **alcohol** produces disulfiram reaction.

PHARMACOKINETICS Peak: 30 min IM; 5 min IV. **Distribution:** CNS penetration except with inflamed meninges; also penetrates aqueous humor, ascitic and prostatic fluids; crosses placenta. **Metabolism:** Partially metabolized in liver to active metabolites. **Elimination:** 50–60% excreted unchanged in urine in 24 h; small amount excreted in breast milk. **Half-Life:** 1 h.

NURSING IMPLICATIONS

Assessment & Drug Effects

- Determine previous hypersensitivity reactions to cephalosporins and penicillins, and history of other allergies, particularly to drugs, before therapy is initiated.
- Lab tests: Perform culture and sensitivity tests before initiation of therapy and periodically during therapy if indicated. Therapy may be instituted pending test results. Serum creatinine, creatinine clearance, BUN should be evaluated at regular intervals during therapy and for several months after drug has been discontinued. Perform periodic hematologic studies (including PT and PTT) and evaluation of hepatic functions with high doses or prolonged therapy.
- Monitor I&O rates and patterns: Report change in I&O in patients with impaired renal function or with chronic UTI or who are receiving high dosages or an aminoglycoside concomitantly.
- Superinfection due to overgrowth of nonsusceptible organisms may occur, particularly with prolonged therapy.
- Report onset of diarrhea promptly. Check for fever. If diarrhea is mild, discontinuation of cefotaxime may be sufficient.
- If diarrhea is severe, suspect antibiotic-associated pseudomembranous colitis, a life-threatening superinfection (may occur in 4–9 days or as long as 6 wk after cephalosporin therapy is discontinued). Chronically ill or debilitated patients undergoing abdominal surgery or those in an intensive care unit are most vulnerable.

Patient & Family Education

- Report any early signs or symptoms of superinfection promptly. Superinfections caused by overgrowth of nonsusceptible organisms may occur, particularly during prolonged use.
- Report loose stools or diarrhea.
- Do not breast feed while taking this drug without consulting physician.

CEFOTETAN DISODIUM

(sef′oh-tee-tan)

Cefotan

Classifications: ANTI-INFECTIVE; ANTIBIOTIC; SECOND-GENERATION CEPHALOSPORIN

Prototype: Cefotaxime sodium

Pregnancy Category: B

AVAILABILITY 1 g, 2 g injection

ACTIONS Semisynthetic beta-lactam antibiotic, classified as a third-generation cephalosporin. Preferentially binds to one or more of the penicillin-binding proteins located on cell walls of susceptible organisms. This inhibits third and final stage of bacterial cell wall synthesis, thus killing the bacterium. Generally less active against susceptible *Staphylococci* than first-generation cephalosporins are but has broad

---

Common adverse effects in *italic;* life-threatening effects <u>underlined;</u> generic names in **bold;** drug classifications in SMALL CAPS; ✤ Canadian drug name; ☯ Prototype drug.

261

C

spectrum of activity against gram-negative bacteria when compared to first- and second-generation cephalosporins.

THERAPEUTIC EFFECTS Spectrum of activity is like that of cefotaxime including *Escherichia coli, Klebsiella* sp., *Enterobacter* sp., *Proteus* sp., *Streptococcus pneumoniae, Staphylococcus aureus,* penicillinase and non-penicillinase-producing *Haemophilus influenzae, Salmonella, Shigella, Neisseria gonorrhoeae,* and many anaerobes. Generally inactive against *Pseudomonas aeruginosa.* It is active against the Enterobacteriaceae and anaerobes, and shows moderate activity against gram-positive organisms. Effectively treats bone and joint infections, gynecologic and intra-abdominal infections, lower respiratory tract infections, skin infections, urinary tract infections, and is used for surgical prophylaxis, reducing or eliminating infection.

USES Infections caused by susceptible organisms in urinary tract, lower respiratory tract, skin and skin structures, bones and joints, gynecologic tract; also intra-abdominal infections, bacteremia, and perioperative prophylaxis.

CONTRAINDICATIONS Hypersensitivity to cephalosporins and related beta-lactam antibiotics; pregnancy (category B).
CAUTIOUS USE Lactation.

ROUTE & DOSAGE

Moderate to Severe Infections
Child: **IV/IM** 40–80 mg/kg/day divided into doses q12h
Adult: **IV/IM** 2–6 g/day divided into 2 doses (max 6 g/day)

Surgical Prophylaxis
Adult: **IV/IM** 1–2 g 30–60 min before surgery

STORAGE
Protect sterile powder from light; store at 22° C (71.6° F) or less; remains stable 24 mo after date of manufacture. May darken with age, but potency is unaffected. Reconstituted solutions: Stable for 24 h at 25° C (77° F); 96 h when refrigerated at 5° C (41° F); or at least 1 wk when frozen at −20° C (−4° F).

ADMINISTRATION

Intramuscular
- For IM reconstitution (follow manufacturer's directions for selection of diluent), add 2 mL diluent to 1 g vial; withdraw approximately 2.4 mL to yield 375 mg drug/mL.
- For IM administration, inject well into body of large muscle appropriate for age (see Part I).

Intravenous
- IV administration to infants and children: Verify correct IV concentration and rate of infusion with physician.

PREPARE **Direct:** Dilute each 1 g with 10 mL of sterile water for injection. **Intermittent:** Following reconstitution, dilute each 1 g with 50–100 mL of D5W or NS.

ADMINISTER Direct: Give over 3–5 min. **Intermittent:** Give a single dose over 30 min. For IV infusion, solution may be given for longer period of time through tubing system through which other IV solutions are being given.

INCOMPATIBILITIES: **Solution/Additive:** AMINOGLYCOSIDES, **doxapram,** HEPARIN, **promethazine,** TETRACYCLINES. **Y-Site:** AMINOGLYCOSIDES, **promethazine, vancomycin, vinorelbine.**

ADVERSE EFFECTS Body as a Whole: Fever, chills, injection site pain, inflammation, disulfiram-like reaction. **GI:** Nausea, vomiting, *diarrhea,* abdominal pain, antibiotic-associated colitis. **Hematologic:** Thrombocytopenia, prolongation of bleeding time or prothrombin time. **Skin:** Rash, pruritus.

DIAGNOSTIC TEST INTERFERENCE May cause falsely elevated *serum* or *urine creatinine* values *(Jaffe reaction).* False-positive reactions for *urine glucose* have not been reported using *copper sulfate reduction methods,* e.g., *Benedict's, Clinitest;* however, because it has occurred with other cephalosporins, it may be advisable to use *glucose oxidase tests (Clinistix, TesTape, Diastix).* Positive *direct antiglobulin (Coombs') test* results may interfere with *hematologic studies* and *cross-matching* procedures.

INTERACTIONS Drug: Probenecid decreases renal elimination of cefotetan; **alcohol** produces disulfiram reaction.

PHARMACOKINETICS Peak: 1.5–3 h IM. **Distribution:** Poor CNS penetration; widely distributed to body tissues and fluids, including bile, sputum, prostatic and peritoneal fluids; crosses placenta. **Elimination:** 51–81% excreted unchanged in urine; 20% excreted in bile; small amount excreted in breast milk. **Half-Life:** 180–270 min.

NURSING IMPLICATIONS

Assessment & Drug Effects
- Determine history of hypersensitivity to cephalosporins and penicillins, and other drug allergies, before therapy begins.
- Lab tests: Perform C&S studies before initiation of therapy and during therapy, as indicated. Therapy may begin pending test results. Perform periodic hematologic studies (including PT/INR and PTT) and evaluation of renal function, especially if cefotetan dose is high or if therapy is prolonged in order to recognize symptoms of nephrotoxicity and ototoxicity (see Appendix D-1).
- Report onset of loose stools or diarrhea. If diarrhea is severe, suspect pseudomembranous colitis (see Appendix D-1) caused by *Clostridium difficile.* Check temperature. Report fever and severe diarrhea to physician; drug should be discontinued.

Patient & Family Education
- Report promptly S&S of superinfection.
- Report loose stools or diarrhea.
- Do not breast feed while taking this drug without consulting physician.

C

CEFOXITIN SODIUM

(se-fox'i-tin)

Mefoxin

Classifications: ANTI-INFECTIVE; ANTIBIOTIC; SECOND-GENERATION CEPHALO-SPORIN

Prototype: Cefonicid sodium

Pregnancy Category: B

AVAILABILITY 1 g, 2 g injection

ACTIONS Semisynthetic, broad-spectrum beta-lactam antibiotic derivative of cephamycin C (produced by *Streptomyces lactamdurans*). Classified as second-generation cephalosporin; structurally and pharmacologically related to cephalosporins and penicillins. Antimicrobial spectrum of activity resembles that of cefonicid. Considerably less active than most cephalosporins against *Staphylococci*. Preferentially binds to one or more of the penicillin-binding proteins located on cell walls of susceptible organisms.

THERAPEUTIC EFFECTS It shows enhanced activity against a wide variety of gram-negative organisms and is effective for mixed aerobic-anaerobic infections. Effectively treats gynecologic, bone and joint and intra-abdominal infections, gonorrhea, skin and urinary tract infections, and is used for surgical prophylaxis, reducing or eliminating infection.

USES Infections caused by susceptible organisms in the lower respiratory tract, urinary tract, skin and skin structures, bones and joints; also intra-abdominal endocarditis, gynecological infections, septicemia, uncomplicated gonorrhea, and perioperative prophylaxis in prosthetic arthroplasty or cardiovascular surgery. May be cephalosporin of choice for mixed aerobic-anaerobic infections (e.g., *Bacteroides fragilis*).

CONTRAINDICATIONS Hypersensitivity to cephalosporins and related antibiotics; pregnancy (category B), lactation. Safe use in children <3 mo not established.

CAUTIOUS USE History of sensitivity to penicillin or other allergies, particularly to drugs; impaired renal function.

ROUTE & DOSAGE

Moderate to Severe Infections

Neonate: **IV/IM** 90–100 mg/kg/day divided into doses q8h
Child >3 mo: **IV/IM** 80–160 mg/kg/day divided into 4–6 doses (max 12 g/day)
Adult: **IV/IM** 4–12 g/24h divided into doses q6–8h

Surgical Prophylaxis

Child: **IV/IM** 30–40 mg/kg 30–60 min before surgery, then q6h for 24 h
Adult: **IV/IM** 2 g 30–60 min before surgery, then 2 g q6h for 24 h

Uncomplicated Gonorrhea

Adult: **IV/IM** 2 g given concurrently with 1 g probenecid PO

Common adverse effects in *italic;* life-threatening effects underlined; generic names in **bold;** drug classifications in SMALL CAPS; ✦ Canadian drug name; ⊘ Prototype drug.

C

STORAGE

- Reconstituted solution may become discolored (usually light yellow to amber) if exposed to high temperatures; however, potency is not affected. Solution may be cloudy immediately after reconstitution; let stand and it will clear.
- After reconstitution, solution is stable for 24 h at 25° C (77° F); 7 days when refrigerated at 4° C (39° F), or 30 wk when frozen at −20° C (−4° F).

ADMINISTRATION

Intramuscular

- Reconstitute each 1 g with 2 mL sterile water for injection or 0.5 or 1% lidocaine hydrochloride (without epinephrine), used to reduce discomfort of IM injection. After reconstitution for IM use, shake vial and allow solution to stand until it becomes clear.
- Administer IM injections deep into large muscle mass appropriate for age (see Part I). Aspirate before injecting drug. Rotate injection sites.

Intravenous

- IV administration to neonates, infants and children: Verify correct IV concentration and rate of infusion/injection with physician.

PREPARE **Direct:** Dilute each 1 g with 10 mL sterile water, D5W, or NS. **Intermittent:** Following reconstitution, dilute 1–2 g in 50–100 mL of D5W or NS.

ADMINISTER **Direct:** Give over 3–5 min. **Intermittent:** Give over 15 min or longer.

INCOMPATIBILITIES **Solution/Additive:** AMINOGLYCOSIDES, **ranitidine**. **Y-Site:** AMINOGLYCOSIDES, **filgrastim, hetastarch, pentamidine, vancomycin.**

ADVERSE EFFECTS Body as a Whole: Drug fever, eosinophilia, superinfections, local reactions: pain, tenderness, and induration (IM site), thrombophlebitis (IV site). **GI:** *Diarrhea*, <u>pseudomembranous colitis</u>. **Skin:** Rash, <u>exfoliative dermatitis</u>, pruritus, urticaria. **Urogenital:** Nephrotoxicity, interstitial nephritis.

DIAGNOSTIC TEST INTERFERENCE Cefoxitin causes false-positive (black-brown or green-brown color) ***urine glucose*** reaction with ***copper reduction reagents*** such as ***Benedict's*** or ***Clinitest,*** but not with ***enzymatic glucose oxidase reagents (Clinistix, TesTape).*** With high doses, falsely elevated ***Serum andurine creatinine*** (with ***Jaffee reaction***) reported. False-positive ***direct Coombs' test*** (may interfere with ***cross-matching procedures*** and ***hematologic studies***) has also been reported.

INTERACTIONS Drug: Probenecid decreases renal elimination of cefoxitin.

PHARMACOKINETICS Peak: 20–30 min IM; 5 min IV. **Distribution:** Poor CNS penetration even with inflamed meninges; widely distributed in body tissues including pleural, synovial, and ascitic fluid and bile; crosses placenta. **Elimination:** 85% excreted unchanged in urine in 6 h, small amount excreted in breast milk. **Half-Life:** 45–60 min.

Common adverse effects in *italic;* life-threatening effects <u>underlined</u>; generic names in **bold;** drug classifications in SMALL CAPS; ♣ Canadian drug name; ✪ Prototype drug.

265

C

NURSING IMPLICATIONS

Assessment & Drug Effects

- Determine previous hypersensitivity to cephalosporins, penicillins, and other drug allergies before therapy is initiated.
- Lab tests: Perform culture and sensitivity testing prior to and periodically during therapy. Periodic renal function tests.
- Inspect injection sites regularly. Report evidence of inflammation and patient's complaint of pain.
- Monitor I&O rates and pattern: Nephrotoxicity occurs most frequently in those with impaired renal function or who are receiving high doses of other nephrotoxic drugs.
- Be alert to S&S of superinfections.
- Report onset of diarrhea (may be dose related). If severe, pseudomembranous colitis (see Appendix D-1) must be ruled out.

Patient & Family Education

- Report promptly S&S of superinfection.
- Report watery or bloody loose stools or severe diarrhea.
- Report severe vomiting or stomach pain
- Report infusion site swelling, pain, or redness
- Do not breast feed while taking this drug.

CEFPODOXIME
(cef-po-dox′eem)
Vantin
Classifications: ANTI-INFECTIVE; ANTIBIOTIC; THIRD-GENERATION CEPHALOSPORIN
Prototype: Cefotaxime sodium
Pregnancy Category: B

AVAILABILITY 100 mg, 200 mg tablets; 50 mg/5 mL, 100 mg/5 mL suspension

ACTIONS Semisynthetic cephalosporin antibiotic with antibacterial activity resembling that of other third-generation cephalosporins. Stable in the presence of betalactamases. Highly active against gram-negative bacteria.

THERAPEUTIC EFFECTS Effective against most common pathogens causing upper and lower respiratory infections. Effectively treats gonorrhea, otitis media, upper and lower respiratory infections, and skin and urinary tract infections, reducing or eliminating infection.

USES Gonorrhea, otitis media, lower and upper respiratory tract infections, urinary tract infections.
UNLABELED USES Skin and soft tissue infections.

CONTRAINDICATIONS Hypersensitivity to cephalosporins and other beta-lactam antibiotics; pregnancy (category B).
CAUTIOUS USE Renal impairment, history of type I hypersensitivity reactions to penicillins; history of colitis or other GI disease; lactation.

Common adverse effects in *italic;* life-threatening effects <u>underlined</u>; generic names in **bold;** drug classifications in SMALL CAPS; ◆ Canadian drug name; ● Prototype drug.

ROUTE & DOSAGE

Respiratory Tract, Skin, and Soft Tissue Infections

Child: **PO** 10 mg/kg/day divided into doses q12h (max 400 mg/24h)
Adult: **PO** 200–800 mg/day divided into doses given q12h for 10 days

Urinary Tract Infections

Adult: **PO** 100 mg q12h

Gonorrhea

Adult: **PO** 200 mg as single dose

Otitis Media

Child 5 mo–12 y: **PO** 10 mg/kg/day divided into doses q12–24h

STORAGE

Store suspension for up to 14 days in a refrigerator at 2°–8° C (36°–46° F). Shake well before using.

ADMINISTRATION

Oral

- Give with food to enhance absorption.
- Give 1 h before or 2 h after an antacid.
- Consult physician regarding patients with renal impairment (i.e., creatinine clearance less than 30 mL/min); dosage intervals should be every 12 h.
- Patients on hemodialysis should be given usual dose 3 times weekly after hemodialysis.
- Preparation of oral suspension: To either the 50 mg/5 mL strength or the 100 mg/5 mL strength, add 25 mL of distilled water, then shake vigorously for 15 seconds. Next, to the 50 mg/5 mL strength add 33 mL, or to the 100 mg/5 mL strength add 32 mL, of distilled water, and shake for at least 3 minutes.

ADVERSE EFFECTS Body as a Whole: Eye itching, cough, epistaxis, fever, decreased appetite, malaise. **GI:** Diarrhea, nausea, vomiting, abdominal pain, soft stools, flatulance, pseudomembranous colitis (rare). **CNS:** (Rare) Headache, asthenia, dizziness, fatigue, anxiety, insomnia, flushing, nightmares, weakness. **Urogenital:** Vaginal candidiasis. **Skin:** Urticaria, rash, scaling, peeling.

INTERACTIONS Drug: ANTACIDS, **ranitidine** may decrease absorption. **Food:** Food may increase the absorption.

PHARMACOKINETICS Absorption: 40–50% absorbed from GI tract increased with food. **Onset:** Therapeutic effect in 3 days. **Distribution:** Distributes well into inflammatory, pulmonary, and pleural fluid, and tonsils. Some distribution into prostate. 40% bound to plasma proteins. Distributed into breast milk. **Elimination:** 80% excreted in urine. **Half-Life:** 2–3 h.

NURSING IMPLICATIONS

Assessment & Drug Effects

- Determine history of hypersensitivity reactions to cephalosporins and penicillins, and history of allergies, particularly to drugs, before therapy is initiated.

Common adverse effects in *italic;* life-threatening effects underlined; generic names in **bold;** drug classifications in SMALL CAPS; ♣ Canadian drug name; ☻ Prototype drug.

267

- Lab tests: Perform C&S tests before initiation of therapy and periodically during therapy, if indicated. Therapy may be instituted pending test results.
- Report onset of loose stools or diarrhea. Although pseudomembranous enterocolitis (see Appendix D-1) rarely occurs, this potentially life-threatening complication should be ruled out as the cause of diarrhea during and after antibiotic therapy.
- Monitor for manifestations of hypersensitivity. Discontinue drug and report S&S of hypersensitivity promptly.
- Monitor I&O rates and pattern: Especially important with high doses; report any significant changes.

Patient & Family Education
- Report any signs or symptoms of hypersensitivity immediately.
- Report loose stools, or diarrhea, especially if containing blood, mucus, or pus.
- Complete the full course of drug therapy as directed by health care provider even if symptoms improve.
- Do not breast feed while taking this drug without consulting prescriber.
- Store this medication out of reach of children.

CEFPROZIL
(cef′pro-zil)
Cefzil
Classifications: ANTI-INFECTIVE; ANTIBIOTIC; SECOND-GENERATION CEPHALOSPORIN
Prototype: Cefonicid sodium
Pregnancy Category: B

AVAILABILITY 250 mg, 500 mg tablets; 125 mg/5 mL, 250 mg/5 mL suspension

ACTION Semisynthetic, second-generation cephalosporin antibiotic with drug structure characterized by a beta-lactam ring; generally resistant to hydrolysis by betalactamases. Preferentially binds to proteins in cell walls of susceptible organisms, thus killing the bacteria. Also active against organisms susceptible to first-generation cephalosporin.
THERAPEUTIC EFFECTS Active against *Streptococcus pyogenes, S. pneumoniae, Haemophilus influenzae, Moraxella catarrhalis,* and *Staphylococcus aureus.* Effectively treats upper and lower respiratory tract infections, otitis media and sinusitis, and skin infections, eliminating or reducing infection.

USES Upper and lower respiratory tract infections, otitis media, skin infections.

CONTRAINDICATIONS Hypersensitivity to cephalosporin and related antibiotics; severely impaired renal or hepatic function; pregnancy (category B).
CAUTIOUS USE Lactation; patients with delayed reaction to penicillin or other drugs; GI disease, especially colitis.

ROUTE & DOSAGE

Mild to Moderate Infections
Adult: **PO** 500–1000 mg/day divided into doses q12–24 h for 10–14 days (max 1 g/24 h)

Otitis Media
Child 6 mo–12 y: **PO** 30 mg/kg/day divided into doses q12h

Pharyngitis/Tonsillitis
Child 2–12 y: 15 mg/kg/day divided into doses q12h

STORAGE
Store at 15°–30° C (59°–86° F) in tightly closed container. Refrigerate reconstituted suspension; discard after 14 days.

ADMINISTRATION

Oral
- Drug may be given without regard to meals.
- Consult prescriber for patients with impaired renal function. Dose is reduced by 50% when creatinine clearance is 0–30 mL/min.
- Administer after hemodialysis because drug is partially removed by dialysis.
- After reconstitution, oral suspension is refrigerated. Discard unused portion after 14 days.

ADVERSE EFFECTS Body as a Whole: Hypersensitivity reactions, superinfections. **GI:** Nausea, vomiting, diarrhea, abdominal pain. **Hematologic:** Eosinophilia. **CNS:** Headache. **Skin:** Rash, diaper rash. **Urogenital:** Genital pruritus, vaginal candidiasis.

DIAGNOSTIC TEST INTERFERENCE May cause a positive *direct Coombs' test;* false-negative results in the ferricyanide assay for *blood glucose;* false-positive reactions for *urine glucose* with *copper reduction tests* such as *Benedict's* or *Fehling's solution* or *Clinitest tablets;* increased *partial thromboplastin time,* indicating thrombocytosis, eosinophilia; minor elevations in *serum alanine aminotransferase (ALT), aspartate aminotransferase (AST),* and *bilirubin.*

INTERACTIONS Drug: Probenecid prolongs the elimination of cefprozil.

PHARMACOKINETICS Absorption: Readily absorbed from GI tract. **Peak:** 1–2 h. **Distribution:** Distributes into blister fluid at 50% of the serum level. **Elimination:** Primarily excreted by the kidneys. **Half-Life:** 1–2 h.

NURSING IMPLICATIONS

Assessment & Drug Effects
- Determine previous hypersensitivity to cephalosporins or penicillins before treatment.
- Withhold drug and notify physician if hypersensitivity occurs (e.g., rash, urticaria).

- Lab tests: Perform C&S tests before and periodically during therapy. Therapy may be initiated while results are pending.
- Monitor for and report diarrhea, because pseudomembranous colitis is a potential adverse effect.
- Monitor for and report signs of superinfection (see Appendix D-1).
- When given concurrently with other cephalosporins or aminoglycosides, monitor for signs of nephrotoxicity.

Patient & Family Education
- Complete the prescribed course of therapy, even if symptom free.
- Report rash or other signs of hypersensitivity immediately.
- Report signs of superinfection.
- Report loose stools and diarrhea even after completion of drug therapy.
- Do not breast feed while taking this drug without consulting physician.
- Store this medication out of reach of children.

CEFTAZIDIME
(sef′tay-zi-deem)
Fortaz, Tazicef, Tazidime
Classifications: ANTI-INFECTIVE; ANTIBIOTIC; THIRD-GENERATION CEPHALOSPORIN
Prototype: Cefotaxime sodium
Pregnancy Category: B

AVAILABILITY 500 mg, 1 g, 2 g injection

ACTIONS Semisynthetic, third-generation broad-spectrum cephalosporin antibiotic similar to cefotaxime but more active against *Pseudomonas aeruginosa* and less active against *Staphylococci* and *Bacteroides fragilis*. Preferentially binds to one or more of the penicillin-binding proteins located on cell walls of susceptible microbes; this inhibits third and final stage of bacterial cell wall synthesis, leading to cell death of the bacterium.
THERAPEUTIC EFFECTS Most strains of gonococci, meningococci, and *Haemophilus influenzae* are highly susceptible to ceftazidime; *Listeria monocytogenes* organisms are resistant. Emergence of resistance during treatment has been reported. May be used concomitantly with other antibiotics (e.g., aminoglycosides, vancomycin, clindamycin). It is effective against *Pseudomonas, Serratia,* and the Enterobacteriaceae. Effectively treats bone and joint infections, gynecologic and gram-negative infections, meningitis, intra-abdominal infections, septicemia and respiratory tract, urinary tract, and skin and soft tissue infections, by reducing or eliminating the infection.

USES To treat infections of cystic fibrosis, lower respiratory tract, skin and skin structures, urinary tract, bones and joints; also used to treat bacteremia, gynecologic, intra-abdominal and CNS infections (including meningitis).
UNLABELED USES Surgical prophylaxis.

CONTRAINDICATIONS Hypersensitivity to cephalosporins and related beta-lactam antibiotics; pregnancy (category B).
CAUTIOUS USE Lactation.

Common adverse effects in *italic;* life-threatening effects <u>underlined</u>; generic names in **bold;** drug classifications in SMALL CAPS; ♦ Canadian drug name; ❷ Prototype drug.

ROUTE & DOSAGE

Moderate to Severe Infections

Neonates: **IV/IM** ≥*7 days and >1200 g weight:* 150 mg/kg/24 h divided into doses and given q8h; ≥*7 days and <1200 g weight:* 100 mg/kg/24 h divided into doses and given q8h; *<7 days:* 100 mg/kg/24 h divided into doses q12h

Infant/Child: **IV/IM** 90–150 mg/kg/day divided into doses given q8h

Adult: **IV/IM** 1–2 g q8–12h, up to 2 g q6h

STORAGE

Store powder at 15°–30° C (59°–86° F) and protect from light. Reconstituted solution is stable 7 days when refrigerated at 4°–5° C (39°–41° F); for 18–24 h when stored at 15°–30° C (59°–86° F).

ADMINISTRATION

Intramuscular

- Reconstitute by adding 3 mL sterile water or bacteriostatic water for injection or 0.5% or 1% lidocaine HCl injection to 1-g vial to yield 280 mg/mL.
- Inject into large muscle mass appropriate for age of child (see Part I).

Intravenous

PREPARE **Direct:** Add 10 mL of sterile water for injection to 1 g to yield 280 mg/mL. **Intermittent:** Further dilute with 50–100 mL of D5W, NS, or RL.

ADMINISTER **Direct:** Give over 3–5 min. **Intermittent:** Give over 30–60 min. If given through a Y-type set, discontinue other solutions during infusion of ceftazidime.

INCOMPATIBILITIES **Solution/Additive:** AMINOGLYCOSIDES, **aminophylline, ranidine. Y-Site:** AMINOGLYCOSIDES, **amphotericin B cholesteryl complex, amsacrine, doxorubicin liposome, fluconazole, idarubicin, midazolam, pentamidine, sargramostim, vancomycin, warfarin.**

ADVERSE EFFECTS Body as a Whole: Fever, phlebitis, pain or inflammation at injection site, superinfections. **GI:** Nausea, vomiting, *diarrhea,* abdominal pain, metallic taste, drug-associated <u>pseudomembranous colitis</u>. **Skin:** Pruritus, rash, urticaria. **Urogenital:** Vaginitis, candidiasis.

DIAGNOSTIC TEST INTERFERENCE False-positive reactions for *urine glucose* have been reported using *copper sulfate* (e.g., *Benedict's solution, Clinitest*). *Glucose oxidase tests (Clinistix, TesTape)* are unaffected. May cause positive *direct antiglobulin (Coombs') test* results, which can interfere with *hematologic studies* and *transfusion cross-matching procedures.*

INTERACTIONS Drug: Probenecid decreases renal elimination of ceftazidine.

PHARMACOKINETICS Peak: 1 h after IM or IV. **Distribution:** CNS penetration with inflamed meninges; also penetrates bone, gallbladder, bile, endometrium, heart, skin, and ascitic and pleural fluids; crosses placenta.

Metabolism: Not metabolized. **Elimination:** 80–90% excreted unchanged in urine in 24 h; small amount excreted in breast milk. **Half-Life:** 25–60 min.

NURSING IMPLICATIONS

Assessment & Drug Effects

- Determine history of hypersensitivity to cephalosporins and penicillins, and other drug allergies, before therapy begins.
- Lab tests: Perform culture and sensitivity studies before initiation of therapy and during therapy as indicated. Therapy may begin pending test results.
- If administered concomitantly with another antibiotic, monitor renal function and report if symptoms of dysfunction appear (e.g., changes in I&O ratio and pattern, dysuria).
- Be alert to onset of rash, itching, and dyspnea. Check patient's temperature. If it is elevated, suspect onset of hypersensitivity reaction (see Appendix D-1).
- Monitor for superinfection (see Appendix D-1).
- If diarrhea occurs and is severe, suspect pseudomembranous colitis (caused by *Clostridium difficile*). Check temperature: Report fever and severe diarrhea to physician; drug should be discontinued.

Patient & Family Education

- Report loose stools or diarrhea promptly.
- Report any signs or symptoms of superinfection promptly.
- Do not breast feed while taking this drug without consulting physician.

CEFTIBUTEN
(sef-ti-bu′ten)
Cedax
Classifications: ANTI-INFECTIVE; BETA-LACTAM ANTIBIOTIC; THIRD–GENERATION CEPHALOSPORIN
Prototype: Cefotaxime sodium
Pregnancy Category: B

AVAILABILITY 400 mg capsules; 90 mg/5 mL, 180 mg/5 mL suspension

ACTIONS Ceftibuten is a broad-spectrum, third-generation beta-lactam antibiotic. Preferentially binds to one or more of the penicillin-binding proteins located in the cell wall of susceptible organisms. This inhibits third and final stage of bacterial cell wall synthesis, thus killing the bacterium. It is highly resistant to hydrolysis by most beta-lactamase bacteria. **THERAPEUTIC EFFECTS** It has antibacterial activity against both gram-negative and gram-positive bacteria, including *Haemophilus influenzae* (beta-lactamase-producing strains also), *Streptococcus pneumoniae,* and *S. pyogenes.* Effectively treats bronchitis, otitis media, pharyngitis and urinary tract infections, reducing or eliminating infection.

USES Acute bacterial exacerbations of chronic bronchitis caused by *H. influenzae, Moraxella catarrhalis,* or *S. pneumoniae;* acute bacterial

---

Common adverse effects in *italic;* life-threatening effects <u>underlined;</u> generic names in **bold;** drug classifications in SMALL CAPS; ◆ Canadian drug name; ❷ Prototype drug.

otitis media caused by *H. influenzae, M. catarrhalis,* or *S. pyogenes;* pharyngitis or tonsillitis caused by *S. pyogenes.*

CONTRAINDICATIONS Hypersensitivity to ceftibuten or cephalosporins.
CAUTIOUS USE Renal dysfunction, penicillin hypersensitivity, history of colitis or diabetes, pregnancy (category B), lactation. Safety and efficacy in infants <6 mo not established.

ROUTE & DOSAGE

Mild to Moderate Infections
Adult: **PO** 400 mg once daily for 10 days
Child 6 mo–12 y: **PO** 9 mg/kg/day in one dose (daily max 400 mg)
for 10 days

Adjustment for Renal Insufficiency (Adult Doses)
Cl_{cr} 30–49: 200 mg q24h; Cl_{cr} <30: 100 mg q24h

Adjustment for Renal Impairment (Child Doses)
Cl_{cr} 30–49 mL/min: 4.5 mg/kg/day; <30 mL/min: 2.25 mg/kg/day

STORAGE
Store capsules at 2°–25° C (36°–77° F); keep container tightly closed. Reconstituted oral suspension is stable for 14 days under refrigeration at 2°–8° C (36°–46° F).

ADMINISTRATION

Oral
- Give oral suspension 1 h before or 2 h after a meal.
- Children weighing more than 45 kg may receive adult daily dose.
- Hemodialysis patients should receive drug at the end of dialysis.

ADVERSE EFFECTS Body as a Whole: Dyspnea, dysuria, fatigue, vaginitis, moniliasis, urticaria, pruritus, rash, paresthesia, taste perversion. **GI:** Nausea, vomiting, diarrhea, dyspepsia, abdominal pain, anorexia, constipation, dry mouth, eructation, flatulence. **CNS:** Headache, dizziness, nasal congestion, somnolence.

INTERACTIONS Drug: AMINOGLYCOSIDES may increase risk of nephrotoxicity and have additive/synergistic effects. May decrease efficacy of ORAL CONTRACEPTIVES. **Probenecid** may increase levels.

PHARMACOKINETICS Absorption: Rapidly absorbed from GI tract. **Peak:** Approx 2–3 h. **Distribution:** Bronchial mucosa levels are approx 37% of plasma levels, middle ear levels approx 50% of plasma levels. **Elimination:** Excreted primarily in urine. **Half-Life:** 1.5–2.5 h.

NURSING IMPLICATIONS

Assessment & Drug Effects
- Determine history of hypersensitivity reactions to cephalosporins, penicillins, or other drugs, before therapy is initiated. Monitor for S&S of hypersensitivity; report their appearance promptly and discontinue drug.

Common adverse effects in *italic;* life-threatening effects underlined; generic names in **bold;** drug classifications in SMALL CAPS; ♣ Canadian drug name; ● Prototype drug.

273

C

- Lab tests: Perform culture and sensitivity tests before initiation of therapy. Dosage may be started pending test results.
- Monitor for S&S of superinfection or pseudomembranous colitis (see Appendix D-1); immediately report either to physician.
- Closely monitor patients with renal impairment; if seizures develop discontinue drug and notify physician.

Patient & Family Education
- If on dialysis treatment, take this drug after dialysis.
- Report any S&S of hypersensitivity, superinfection, and pseudomembranous colitis promptly.
- Do not breast feed while taking this drug without consulting physician.
- Store this medication out of reach of children.

CEFTIZOXIME SODIUM
(sef-ti-zox'eem)
Cefizox
Classifications: ANTI-INFECTIVE; ANTIBIOTIC; THIRD-GENERATION CEPHALOSPORIN
Prototype: Cefotaxime sodium
Pregnancy Category: B

AVAILABILITY 500 mg, 1 g, 2 g injection

ACTIONS Semisynthetic third-generation cephalosporin antibiotic. Preferentially binds to one or more of the penicillin-binding proteins located on cell walls of susceptible organisms. This inhibits third and final stage of bacterial cell wall synthesis, thus killing the bacterium. Spectrum of activity similar to that of cefotaxime. Generally resistant to inactivation by beta-lactamases that act principally as cephalosporinases and penicillinases.

THERAPEUTIC EFFECTS *Clostridium difficile,* enterococci including *Streptococcus faecalis,* and most strains of *Listeria monocytogenes* are resistant to ceftizoxime. Incompatible with the aminoglycoside antibiotics. Evidence of partial cross-allergenicity among cephalosporins and other beta-lactamase antibiotics has been reported. It is used for gram-negative bacillary meningitis and drug-resistant Enterobacteriaceae. Effectively treats endocarditis, bone and joint infections, gonorrhea and gynecologic infections including pelvic inflammatory disease (PID), *E. coli* infections, *Haemophilus influenzae* infections, intra-abdominal infections, meningitis, osteomyelitis, lower respiratory tract infections, *Serratia* sp. infections, septicemia and skin infections, urinary tract infections, and is used for surgical prophylaxis, reducing or eliminating infection.

USES Infections caused by susceptible organisms in lower respiratory tract, skin and skin structures, urinary tract, bones and joints; also used to treat intra-abdominal infections, PID, uncomplicated gonorrhea, meningitis *(Haemophilus influenzae, Streptococcus pneumoniae),* and for surgical prophylaxis.

UNLABELED USES Meningitis caused by *Neisseria meningitidis* and *Escherichia coli.*

Common adverse effects in *italic;* life-threatening effects <u>underlined</u>; generic names in **bold;** drug classifications in SMALL CAPS; ◆ Canadian drug name; ☺ Prototype drug.

C

CONTRAINDICATIONS Hypersensitivity to cephalosporins and other beta-lactam antibiotics; pregnancy (category B).
CAUTIOUS USE Lactation.

ROUTE & DOSAGE

Moderate to Severe Infections

Child: **IV/IM** ≥6 mo, 150–200 mg/kg/24 h divided into doses q6–8h
Adult: **IV/IM** 2–12 g/24 h divided into doses q8–12h

STORAGE

Store powder at 15°–30° C (59°–86° F) and protect from light. Reconstituted solution stable at room temperature for 24 h or refrigerated for 96 h.

ADMINISTRATION

Intramuscular

- Reconstitute as follows with sterile water for injection: add 1.5 mL to 500 mg to yield 280 mg/mL; add 3 mL to 1 g or 6 mL to 2 g to yield 270 mg/mL.
- Give deep IM into a large muscle appropriate for age (see Part I). Give no more than 1 g into a single injection site.

Intravenous

PREPARE Direct: Reconstitute each 1 g with 10 mL sterile water. Shake well. **Intermittent:** Further dilute in 50–100 mL D5W, NS, D5/NS, D5/0.45% NaCl, RL, or other compatible IV solution.
ADMINISTER Direct: Give over 3–5 min. **Intermittent:** Give over 30 min.
INCOMPATIBILITIES: Solution/Additive: AMINOGLYCOSIDES. **Y-Site:** AMINO-GLYCOSIDES, **filgrastim.**

ADVERSE EFFECTS Body as a Whole: Fever, phlebitis, vaginitis, pain and induration at injection site, paresthesia. **GI:** Nausea, vomiting, diarrhea, pseudomembranous colitis. **Skin:** Rash, pruritus.

DIAGNOSTIC TEST INTERFERENCE Ceftizoxime causes false-positive *direct Coombs' test* (may interfere with *cross-matching procedures* and *hematologic studies*).

INTERACTIONS Drug: Probenecid decreases renal elimination of ceftizoxime.

PHARMACOKINETICS Peak: 1 h after IM or IV. **Distribution:** Crosses placenta. **Metabolism:** Not metabolized. **Elimination:** 80–90% excreted unchanged in urine in 24 h; small amount excreted in breast milk. **Half-Life:** 25–60 min.

NURSING IMPLICATIONS

Assessment & Drug Effects

- Determine history of hypersensitivity reactions to cephalosporins, penicillin, or other drugs before therapy is instituted. Report to physician history of allergy, particularly to drugs.

- Lab tests: Perform culture and sensitivity tests before initiation of therapy and periodically during therapy if indicated. Therapy may be instituted pending test results.
- Be alert to symptoms of hypersensitivity reaction. Serious reactions may require emergency measures.

Patient & Family Education
- Report loose stools or diarrhea promptly.
- Report any signs or symptoms of hypersensitivity promptly.
- Do not breast feed while taking this drug without consulting physician.

CEFTRIAXONE SODIUM

(sef-try-ax'one)
Rocephin
Classifications: ANTI-INFECTIVE; ANTIBIOTIC; THIRD-GENERATION CEPHALOSPORIN
Prototype: Cefotaxime sodium
Pregnancy Category: B

AVAILABILITY 250 mg, 500 mg, 1 g, 2 g injection

ACTIONS Semisynthetic third-generation cephalosporin antibiotic. Preferentially binds to one or more of the penicillin-binding proteins located on cell walls of susceptible organisms. This inhibits third and final stage of bacterial cell wall synthesis, thus killing the bacterium.
THERAPEUTIC EFFECTS Spectrum of activity similar to that of cefotaxime including most Enterobacteriaceae, most gram-positive aerobic cocci, *Neisseria meningitidis,* and most strains of penicillinase-producing and non-penicillinase-producing *Neisseria gonorrhoeae.* Has some activity against *Treponema pallidum* but none against most strains of *Clostridia.* Effectively treats bone and joint infections, gonorrhea and intra-abdominal infections, meningitis and lower respiratory tract infections, otitis media, pelvic inflammatory disease, *Proteus* infections, septicemia, skin and soft tissue infections, urinary tract infections, and is used for surgical prophylaxis, reducing or eliminating infection.

USES Infections caused by susceptible organisms in lower respiratory tract, skin and skin structures, urinary tract, bones and joints; also intra-abdominal infections, pelvic inflammatory disease, uncomplicated gonorrhea, meningitis, and surgical prophylaxis.

CONTRAINDICATIONS Hypersensitivity to cephalosporins and related antibiotics; neonates with hyperbilirubinemia; pregnancy (category B).
CAUTIOUS USE Lactation.

ROUTE & DOSAGE

Moderate to Severe Infections
Child: **IV/IM** 50–75 mg/kg/day in 2 divided doses (max 2 g/day)
Adult: **IV/IM** 1–4 g/24 h given q12–24h (max 4 g/day)

Common adverse effects in *italic;* life-threatening effects <u>underlined;</u> generic names in **bold;** drug classifications in SMALL CAPS; ♣ Canadian drug name; ◑ Prototype drug.

C

Meningitis
Child: **IV/IM** 75 mg/kg loading dose, then 100 mg/kg/day divided
into 2 doses (max 4 g/day)
Adult: **IV/IM** 2 g q12h

Surgical Prophylaxis
Adult: **IV/IM** 1 g 30–120 min before surgery

Uncomplicated Gonorrhea
Child: IM 125 mg as single dose
Adult: IM 250 mg as single dose

STORAGE
Protect sterile powder from light. Store at 15°–25° C (59°–77° F). Reconstituted solutions stability depends on diluent and concentration of solution; see manufacturer's instructions.

ADMINISTRATION
Intramuscular
- Reconstitute the 1-g or 2-g vial by adding 2.1 mL or 4.2 mL, respectively,
of sterile water for injection. Can reconstitute with 1% lidocaine (without epinephrine) to reduce pain of injection. Yields 3.50 mg/mL. See
manufacturer's directions for other dilutions.
- Give deep IM into a large muscle appropriate for age (see Part I).

Intravenous
- IV administration to infants and children: Verify correct IV concentration and rate of infusion with physician.

PREPARE **Intermittent:** Reconstitute each 250 mg with 2.4 mL of sterile
water, D5W, NS, or D5/NS to yield 100 mg/mL. Further dilute with
50–100 mL of the selected IV solution.

ADMINISTER **Intermittent:** Give over 30 min.

INCOMPATIBILITIES **Solution/Additive:** AMINOGLYCOSIDES, **aminophylline, clindamycin, lidocaine, metronidazole, theophylline.**
Y-Site: AMINOGLYCOSIDES, **amphotericin B cholesteryl complex,
amsacrine, fluconazole, filgrastim, labetalol, pentamidine,
vancomycin, vinorelbine.**

ADVERSE EFFECTS Body as a Whole: Pruritus, fever, chills, pain, induration at IM injection site; phlebitis (IV site). **GI:** *Diarrhea,* abdominal
cramps, <u>pseudomembranous colitis</u>, biliary sludge. **Urogenital:** Genital
pruritus; moniliasis.

DIAGNOSTIC TEST INTERFERENCE Causes prolonged *PT/INR* during
therapy.

INTERACTIONS Drug: Probenecid decreases renal elimination of ceftriaxone; **alcohol** produces disulfiram reaction.

PHARMACOKINETICS Peak: 1.5–4 h after IM; immediately after IV infusion.
Distribution: Widely distributed in body tissues and fluids; good CNS penetration, especially with inflamed meninges; crosses placenta. **Metabolism:**

Not metabolized. **Elimination:** 33–65% excreted unchanged in urine; also excreted in bile; small amount excreted in breast milk. **Half-Life:** 5–10 h.

NURSING IMPLICATIONS

Assessment & Drug Effects

- Determine history of hypersensitivity reactions to cephalosporins and penicillins and history of other allergies, particularly to drugs, before therapy is initiated.
- Lab tests: Perform culture and sensitivity tests before initiation of therapy and periodically during therapy. Dosage may be started pending test results. Periodic coagulation studies (PT and INR) should be done.
- Inspect injection sites for induration and inflammation. Rotate sites. Note IV injection sites for signs of phlebitis (redness, swelling, pain).
- Monitor for manifestations of hypersensitivity. Report their appearance promptly and discontinue drug.
- Watch for and report these signs: petechiae, ecchymotic areas, epistaxis, or any unexplained bleeding. Ceftriaxone appears to alter vitamin K-producing gut bacteria; therefore, hypoprothrombinemic bleeding may occur.
- Check for fever if diarrhea occurs: Report both promptly. The incidence of antibiotic-produced pseudomembranous colitis (see Appendix D-1) is higher than with most cephalosporins. Most vulnerable patients: chronically ill or debilitated older adult patients undergoing abdominal surgery.

Patient & Family Education

- Report any signs of bleeding.
- Report loose stools or diarrhea promptly.
- Do not breast feed while taking this drug without consulting physician.

CEFUROXIME SODIUM
(se-fyoor-ox′eem)
Kefurox, Zinacef

CEFUROXIME AXETIL
Ceftin
Classifications: ANTI-INFECTIVE; ANTIBIOTIC; SECOND-GENERATION CEPHALO-SPORIN
Prototype: Cefonicid sodium
Pregnancy Category: B

AVAILABILITY 125 mg, 250 mg, 500 mg tablets; 125 mg/5 mL, 250 mg/5 mL suspension; 750 mg, 1.5 g injection

ACTIONS Semisynthetic second-generation cephalosporin antibiotic with structure similar to that of the penicillins. Resistance against beta-lactamase-producing strains exceeds that of first-generation cephalosporins. Antimicrobial spectrum of activity resembles that of cefonicid. Preferentially binds to one or more of the penicillin binding proteins located on cell walls of susceptible organisms. This inhibits third and final stage of bacterial cell wall synthesis, thus killing the bacterium. Partial cross-allergenicity between other beta-lactam antibiotics and cephalosporins has been reported.

THERAPEUTIC EFFECTS It is effective for the treatment of penicillinase-producing *Neisseria gonorrhoea* (PPNG). Effectively treats bone and joint infections, bronchitis, meningitis, gonorrhea, otitis media, pharyngitis/tonsillitis, sinusitis, lower respiratory tract infections, skin and soft tissue infections, urinary tract infections, and is used for surgical prophylaxis, reducing or eliminating infection.

USES Infections caused by susceptible organisms in the lower respiratory tract, urinary tract, skin, and skin structures; also used for treatment of meningitis, gonorrhea, and otitis media and for perioperative prophylaxis (e.g., open-heart surgery), early Lyme disease.

CONTRAINDICATIONS Hypersensitivity to cephalosporins and related antibiotics; pregnancy (category B), lactation.
CAUTIOUS USE History of allergy, particularly to drugs; penicillin sensitivity; renal insufficiency; history of colitis or other GI disease; potent diuretics.

ROUTE & DOSAGE

Moderate to Severe Infections

Neonate: **IM/IV** 20–60 mg/kg/day divided into doses q12h
Child 3 mo–12 y: **PO** 10–20 mg/kg (125–250 mg) q12h (max 1 g/24 h). **IV/IM** 75–100 mg/kg/day divided into doses q8h (max 6 g/day)
Adult: **PO** 250–500 mg q12h **IV/IM** 750 mg–1.5 g q6–8h

Bacterial Meningitis

Child: **IV/IM** 75–150 mg/kg/day divided into doses q6–8h; reduced to 75–100 mg/kg/day upon improvement
Adult: **IV/IM** 3 g q8h

Surgical Prophylaxis

Adult: **IV/IM** 1.5 g 30–60 min before surgery, then 750 mg q8h for 24 h

STORAGE

Store tablets and powder at 15°–30° C (59°–86° F) and protect from light. Powder and solutions may range in color from light yellow to amber without adversely affecting product potency. After reconstitution, store suspension at 2°–30° C (36°–86° F). Discard after 10 days. Reconstituted parenteral solution stable at room temperature for 24 h or refrigerated for 48 h.

ADMINISTRATION

Oral

- Cefuroxime tablets and oral suspension are not substitutable on a mg-for-mg basis.
- The oral suspension is for infants and children 3 mo to 12 y. Each teaspoon (5 mL) contains the equivalent of 125 mg cefuroxime. Shake oral suspension well before each use.

Intramuscular

- Shake IM suspension gently before administration. IM injections should be made deeply into large muscle mass appropriate for age (see Part I). Rotate injection sites.

[C]

Intravenous

- IV administration to neonates, infants and children: Verify correct IV concentration and rate of infusion/injection with physician.

PREPARE **Direct:** Dilute each 750 mg with 9 mL sterile water, D5W, or NS. **Intermittent:** Further dilute in 50–100 mL of compatible solution. **Continuous:** May be added to 1000 mL of IV compatible solution.

ADMINISTER **Direct:** Give slowly over 3–5 min. **Intermittent:** Give over 30 min. **Continuous:** Give over 6–24 h.

INCOMPATIBILITIES **Solution/Additive:** AMINOGLYCOSIDES, **doxapram, ranitidine, sodium bicarbonate. Y-Site:** AMINOGLYCOSIDES, **filgrastim, fluconazole, midazolam, sodium bicarbonate, vancomycin, vinorelbine.**

ADVERSE EFFECTS Body as a Whole: Thrombophlebitis (IV site); pain, burning, cellulitis (IM site); superinfections, positive Coombs' test. **GI:** *Diarrhea,* nausea, antibiotic-associated colitis. **Skin:** Rash, pruritus, urticaria. **Urogenital:** Increased serum creatinine and BUN, decreased creatinine clearance.

DIAGNOSTIC TEST INTERFERENCE Cefuroxime causes false-positive (black-brown or green-brown color) *urine glucose* reaction with *copper reduction reagents,* e.g., *Benedict's* or *Clinitest,* but not with *enzymatic glucose oxidase reagents,* e.g., *Clinistix, TesTape.* False-positive *direct Coombs' test* (may interfere with *cross-matching procedures* and *hematologic studies*) has been reported.

INTERACTIONS Drug: Probenecid decreases renal elimination of cefuroxime, thus prolonging its action.

PHARMACOKINETICS Absorption: Axetil salt well absorbed from GI tract; hydrolyzed to active drug in GI mucosa. **Peak:** PO 2 h; IM 30 min. **Distribution:** Widely distributed in body tissues and fluids; adequate CNS penetration with inflamed meninges; crosses placenta. **Elimination:** 66–100% excreted in urine in 24 h; excreted in breast milk. **Half-Life:** 1–2 h.

NURSING IMPLICATIONS

Assessment & Drug Effects

- Determine history of hypersensitivity reactions to cephalosporins, penicillins, and history of allergies, particularly to drugs, before therapy is initiated.
- Lab tests: Perform culture and sensitivity tests before initiation of therapy and periodically during therapy if indicated. Therapy may be instituted pending test results. Monitor periodically BUN and creatinine clearance.
- Inspect IM and IV injection sites frequently for signs of phlebitis.
- Report onset of loose stools or diarrhea. Although pseudomembranous colitis (see Appendix D-1) rarely occurs, this potentially life-threatening complication should be ruled out as the cause of diarrhea during and after antibiotic therapy.

- Monitor for manifestations of hypersensitivity. Discontinue drug and report their appearance promptly.
- Monitor I&O rates and pattern, especially in severely ill patients receiving high doses. Report any significant changes.

Patient & Family Education
- Report loose stools or diarrhea promptly.
- Report any signs or symptoms of hypersensitivity.
- Do not breast feed while taking this drug.
- Store this medication out of reach of children.

CEPHALEXIN
(sef-a-lex′in)
Cefanex, Ceporex_A, Keflet, Keflex, Keftab, Novolexin_A
Classifications: ANTI-INFECTIVE; ANTIBIOTIC; FIRST-GENERATION CEPHALOSPORIN
Prototype: Cefazolin
Pregnancy Category: B

AVAILABILITY 250 mg, 500 mg capsules; 250 mg, 500 mg, 1 g tablets; 125 mg/5 mL, 250 mg/5 mL suspension

ACTIONS Semisynthetic derivative of cephalosporin C. Broad-spectrum, first-generation cephalosporin antibiotic with anti-infective activity similar to that of cefazolin but reportedly less potent. Preferentially binds to one or more of the penicillin-binding proteins located on cell walls of susceptible organisms. This inhibits third and final stage of bacterial cell wall synthesis, thus killing the bacterium. Ineffective against many gram-negative or anaerobic organisms. Cross-allergenicity between cephalosporins and penicillins has been reported.
THERAPEUTIC EFFECTS Active against many gram-positive aerobic cocci and much less active against gram-negative bacteria. Effectively treats osteomyelitis, otitis media, streptococcal pharyngitis, prostate and respiratory infections, skin and urinary tract infections, eliminating or reducing infection.

USES To treat infections caused by susceptible pathogens in respiratory and urinary tracts, middle ear, skin, soft tissue, and bone.

CONTRAINDICATIONS Hypersensitivity to cephalosporins and related antibiotics; pregnancy (category B), lactation. Safe use in infants <1 mo not established.
CAUTIOUS USE History of hypersensitivity to penicillin or other drug allergy; severely impaired renal function.

ROUTE & DOSAGE

Mild to Moderate Infection
Child: **PO** 25–100 mg/kg/day in 4 divided doses
Adult: **PO** 250–500 mg q6h

Skin and Skin Structure Infections
Adult: **PO** 500 mg q12h
Otitis Media
Child: **PO** 75–100 mg/kg/day in 4 divided doses

STORAGE
Store tablets and capsules tightly covered at 15°–30° C (59°–86° F). Refrigerated suspension stable for 14 days if refrigerated; discard after that date.

ADMINISTRATION
Oral
- Label should indicate expiration date. Shake suspension well before pouring.

ADVERSE EFFECTS Body as a Whole: Angioedema, <u>anaphylaxis</u>, superinfections. **GI:** *Diarrhea* (generally mild), nausea, vomiting, anorexia, abdominal pain. **CNS:** Dizziness, headache, fatigue. **Skin:** Rash, urticaria.

DIAGNOSTIC TEST INTERFERENCE False-positive ***urine glucose*** determinations using ***copper sulfate reagents,*** e.g., *Clinitest, Benedict's reagent,* but not with ***glucose oxidase (enzymatic) tests,*** e.g., *Tes-Tape, Diastix, Clinistix.* Positive ***direct Coombs' test*** may complicate transfusion ***cross-matching procedures*** and ***hematologic studies.***

INTERACTIONS Drug: Probenecid decreases renal elimination of cephalexin.

PHARMACOKINETICS Absorption: Rapidly absorbed from GI tract; stable in stomach acid. **Peak:** 1 h. **Distribution:** widely distributed in body fluids with highest concentration in kidney; crosses placenta. **Elimination:** 80–100% eliminated unchanged in urine in 8 h; excreted in breast milk. **Half-Life:** 38–70 min.

NURSING IMPLICATIONS
Assessment & Drug Effects
- Determine history of hypersensitivity reactions to cephalosporins and penicillin and history of other drug allergies before therapy is initiated.
- Lab tests: Evaluate renal and hepatic function periodically in patients receiving prolonged therapy.
- Monitor for manifestations of hypersensitivity. Discontinue drug and report their appearance promptly.

Patient & Family Education
- Take medication for the full course of therapy as directed by health care provider. Refrigerate solution and shake well before giving dose.
- Keep physician informed if adverse reactions appear.
- Be alert to S&S of superinfections. These symptoms should be reported promptly and appropriate therapy instituted.
- Do not breast feed while taking this drug.
- Store this medication out of reach of children.

CEPHAPIRIN SODIUM
(sef-a-pye'rin)
Cefadyl
Classifications: ANTI-INFECTIVE; ANTIBIOTIC; FIRST-GENERATION CEPHALOSPORIN
Prototype: Cefazolin
Pregnancy Category: B

AVAILABILITY 1 g injection

ACTIONS Semisynthetic, first-generation, broad-spectrum cephalosporin antibiotic similar to cefazolin. Reported to cause less tissue irritation and to be less nephrotoxic than cefazolin. Preferentially binds to one or more of the penicillin-binding proteins (PBP) located on cell walls of susceptible organisms. This inhibits third and final stage of bacterial cell wall synthesis, thus killing the bacterium. Cross-allergenicity between cephalosporins and penicillins has been reported.

THERAPEUTIC EFFECTS Effectively treats osteomyelitis, respiratory tract infections, skin infections, urinary tract infections, *Streptococcal* infections, infective endocarditis, septicemia, and is used for preoperative prophylaxis, reducing or eliminating infection.

USES Serious infections of respiratory and urinary tracts, skin and soft tissue, and for osteomyelitis, septicemia, and endocarditis caused by susceptible pathogens, e.g., group A *beta-hemolytic streptococci,* penicillinase- and non-penicillinase-producing *Staphylococcus aureus, Streptococcus pneumoniae, viridans streptococci, Haemophilus influenzae, Escherichia coli, Proteus mirabilis,* and *Klebsiella* sp.; also to prevent postoperative infection when infection at operative site is a risk.

CONTRAINDICATIONS Hypersensitivity to cephalosporins and related antibiotics; pregnancy (category B), lactation. Safe use in children <3 mo not established.

CAUTIOUS USE History of sensitivity to penicillins and other allergies, particularly to drugs; sodium restriction, impaired renal function.

ROUTE & DOSAGE

Mild to Moderate Infection
Child: **IM/IV** 40–80 mg/kg/day divided into 4 doses
Adult: **IM/IV** 500 mg–1 g q4–6h up to 12 g/day

Perioperative Prophylaxis
Adult: **IM/IV** 1–2 g 30–60 min before surgery, 1–2 g during surgery, then 1–2 g q6h for 24 h

Adjustment for Renal Impairment
Cl_{cr} <5 mg/dL: **IM/IV** 7.5–15 mg/kg q12h

STORAGE
After reconstitution, depending on diluent and amount used, solutions retain potency for 12–48 h at room temperature or for 10 days if

refrigerated at 4° C. See package insert for specific information. Solutions may become slightly yellow, but this does not affect potency.

ADMINISTRATION

Intramuscular

- Reconstitute the 500-mg and 1-g vials with 1 or 2 mL sterile water for injection or bacteriostatic water for injection, respectively. Resulting solutions will contain 500 mg of cephapirin per 1.2 mL.
- IM injections should be made deep into large muscle mass appropriate for age of child (see Part I). Rotate injection sites.

Intravenous

PREPARE **Direct:** Reconstitute 1-g or 2-g vial with at least 10 mL bacteriostatic water for injection, D5W, or NS. **Intermittent:** Further dilute with 50–100 mL of D5W or NS.

ADMINISTER **Direct:** Give over 5 min. **Intermittent:** Give over 30 min

INCOMPATIBILITIES **Solution/Additive:** AMINOGLYCOSIDES, **aminophylline, ascorbic acid, epinephrine, norepinephrine, mannitol, phenytoin,** TETRACYCLINES, **thiopental.** **Y-Site:** AMINOGLYCOSIDES, TETRACYCLINES, **thiopental, phenytoin.**

ADVERSE EFFECTS Body as a Whole: Rash, urticaria, drug fever, eosinophilia, serum sickness-like reactions, <u>anaphylaxis</u>. **GI:** Nausea, vomiting, *diarrhea,* abdominal cramps. **Other:** Needle site reactions (infrequent).

DIAGNOSTIC TEST INTERFERENCE False-positive *urine glucose* determinations, using *copper sulfate reduction methods,* e.g., *Clinitest* or *Benedict's reagent,* but not with *glucose oxidase (enzymatic) tests,* e.g., *Clinistix, Diastix, TesTape.* Positive *Coombs' test* may **complicate cross-matching procedures** and **hematologic studies.**

INTERACTIONS Drug: **Probenecid** decreases renal elimination of cephapirin.

PHARMACOKINETICS Peak: 30 min after IM; 5 min after IV. **Distribution:** Widely distributed in body fluids with highest concentration in kidney; crosses placenta. **Metabolism:** Partially metabolized in liver and kidneys. **Elimination:** 60–85% eliminated unchanged in urine in 6 h; excreted in breast milk. **Half-Life:** 36–54 min.

NURSING IMPLICATIONS

Assessment & Drug Effects

- Determine history of previous hypersensitivity to cephalosporins, penicillins, and other allergies, particularly to drugs, before therapy begins.
- Lab tests: Perform culture and sensitivity testing before treatment is begun. Therapy may be initiated before results are obtained. Monitor periodically renal function.
- Advise patient to report changes in I&O ratio and pattern or evidence of blood or pus in urine.
- Monitor for manifestations of hypersensitivity. Discontinue drug and report their appearance promptly.

Common adverse effects in *italic;* life-threatening effects <u>underlined</u>; generic names in **bold;** drug classifications in SMALL CAPS; ♣ Canadian drug name; ❷ Prototype drug.

Patient & Family Education
- Report promptly any S&S of superinfections.
- Report S&S of hypersensitivity.
- Do not breast feed while taking this drug.

CEPHRADINE
(sef'ra-deen)
Anspor, Velosef
Classifications: ANTI-INFECTIVE; ANTIBIOTIC; FIRST-GENERATION CEPHALOSPORIN
Prototype: Cefazolin
Pregnancy Category: B

AVAILABILITY 250 mg, 500 mg capsules; 125 mg/5 mL, 250 mg/5 mL suspension; 250 mg, 500 mg, 1 g, 2 g injection

ACTIONS Semisynthetic acid-stable, first-generation, broad-spectrum cephalosporin similar to cefazolin. Preferentially binds to one or more of the penicillin-binding proteins located on cell walls of susceptible organisms. This inhibits third and final stage of bacterial cell wall synthesis, thus killing the bacterium. Cross-allergenicity between cephalosporins and penicillins has been reported.

THERAPEUTIC EFFECTS Active against many gram-positive aerobic cocci and much less active against gram-negative bacteria. Effectively treats bone infections, otitis media, respiratory tract infections, septicemia and skin infections, and urinary tract infections, reducing or eliminating infection.

USES Serious infections of respiratory and urinary tracts, skin and soft tissues, and for otitis media caused by susceptible pathogens; for perioperative prophylaxis, in cesarean section (intraoperative and postoperative); in septicemia (due to *Streptococcus pneumoniae, Staphylococcus aureus, Proteus mirabilis,* and *Escherichia coli*). Also used to treat urinary tract infections due to *Klebsiella* sp. and enterococci *(Streptococcus faecalis)*.

CONTRAINDICATIONS Hypersensitivity to cephalosporins and related antibiotics; pregnancy (category B), lactation. Safe use in children <9 mo not established.

CAUTIOUS USE History of penicillin or other allergies, particularly to drugs; impaired renal function, sodium restriction (parenteral cephradine).

ROUTE & DOSAGE

Mild to Moderate Infection

Child: **PO** 25–50 mg/kg/day divided into 2–4 doses (maximum dose 4 g/day). **IM/IV** 50 to 100 mg/kg/day divided into 4 doses (maximum dose 8 g/day)
Adult: **PO** 250–500 mg q6h or 500 mg–1 g q12h up to 4 g/day. **IM/IV** 2–4 g/day divided into 4 doses (max 8 g/day)

Perioperative Prophylaxis
Adult: **PO** 1 g 30–60 min before surgery; 1 g during surgery; then 1 g q4–6h for 24 h

STORAGE
Store at 15°–30° C (59°–86° F) in tightly closed, light-resistant containers. Reconstituted oral suspension may be stored at room temperature up to 7 days or in refrigerator for up to 14 days. After reconstitution, IM or IV solutions should be used within 2 h if kept at room temperature or 24 h if refrigerated. Protect from concentrated light or direct sunlight.

ADMINISTRATION
Oral
- Oral cephradine may be given without regard to meals (acid stable); however, the presence of food may delay absorption.

Intramuscular
- Inject deep into large muscle mass appropriate for age of child to minimize pain and induration of IM site (see Part I).

Intravenous

PREPARE **Direct:** Dilute each 500 mg with 5 mL sterile water for injection. **Intermittent:** Further dilute in 10–20 mL of D5W or NS. Do not mix with RL.
ADMINISTER **Direct:** Give over 3–5 min. **Intermittent:** Give over 30–60 min.
INCOMPATIBILITIES: **Solution/Additive:** AMINOGLYCOSIDES, TPN SOLUTIONS, other ANTIBIOTICS. **Y-Site:** AMINOGLYCOSIDES, TPN SOLUTIONS, other ANTIBIOTICS. ▪ The risk of thrombophlebitis may be reduced by proper dilution of IV fluid, use of small IV needles and large veins, and by alternating injection sites.

ADVERSE EFFECTS Body as a Whole: Joint pains, eosinophilia, tightness in chest, pain, induration and tissue sloughing (IM injection site); thrombophlebitis (IV site); paresthesias, superinfections. **GI:** *Diarrhea* or loose stools, abdominal pain, heartburn. **CNS:** Dizziness. **Skin:** Urticaria, rash, pruritus.

DIAGNOSTIC TEST INTERFERENCE Cephradine causes false-positive (black-brown or green-brown color) ***urine glucose*** reaction with ***copper reduction reagents,*** (e.g., as ***Benedict's*** or ***Clinitest***), but not with ***enzymatic glucose oxidase reagents,*** e.g., Clinistix, TesTape. False-positive ***direct Coombs' test*** (may interfere with ***crossmatching procedures*** and ***hematologic studies***) has also been reported.

INTERACTIONS Drug: Probenecid decreases renal elimination of cephradine.

PHARMACOKINETICS Absorption: Well absorbed from GI tract. **Peak:** 1 h after PO; 1–2 h after IM; 5 min after IV. **Distribution:** Widely distributed in body fluids, with highest concentration in kidney; crosses placenta. **Elimination:** 80–90% eliminated unchanged in urine in 6 h; excreted in breast milk. **Half-Life:** 1–2 h.

Common adverse effects in *italic;* life-threatening effects <u>underlined;</u> generic names in **bold;** drug classifications in SMALL CAPS; ✦ Canadian drug name; ❷ Prototype drug.

NURSING IMPLICATIONS

Assessment & Drug Effects

- Determine history of previous hypersensitivity to cephalosporins, penicillins, and other drug allergies before therapy is initiated.
- Inspect IV insertion site frequently for thrombophlebitis.
- Lab tests: Perform culture and sensitivity tests and renal function studies before and periodically during drug therapy.
- Consult physician if patient's creatinine clearance is below normal. Recommended dosage schedule in patients with reduced renal function is lowered based on creatinine clearance determinations and severity of infection.
- Pseudomembranous enterocolitis, a potentially life-threatening superinfection caused by *Clostridium difficile,* may occur during or after cephalosporin therapy. If diarrhea occurs, check for fever. Report diarrhea and fever promptly.
- Monitor for signs of superinfection. Report their appearance promptly.

Patient & Family Education

- Take this medication for the full course of therapy as directed by your health care provider. Therapy is usually continued for at least 48–72 h after you become asymptomatic.
- Superinfections caused by overgrowth of nonsusceptible organisms may occur. Report early signs and symptoms promptly.
- Report loose stools or diarrhea promptly.
- Do not breast feed while taking this drug.
- Store this medication out of reach of children.

CETIRIZINE

(ce-tir′i-zeen)
Reactine ♣ , Zyrtec
Classifications: ANTIHISTAMINE; H₁-RECEPTOR ANTAGONIST; NONSEDATING
Prototype: Loratidine
Pregnancy Category: B

AVAILABILITY 5 mg, 10 mg tablets; 5 mg/5 mL syrup

ACTIONS Cetirizine is a potent H₁-receptor antagonist and thus an antihistamine without significant anticholinergic or CNS activity. Low lipophilicity combined with its H₁-receptor selectivity probably accounts for its relative lack of anticholinergic and sedative properties.

THERAPEUTIC EFFECTS Effectively treats allergic rhinitis, and chronic urticaria by eliminating or reducing the local and systemic effects of histamine release.

USES Seasonal and perennial allergic rhinitis and chronic idiopathic urticaria.

CONTRAINDICATIONS Hypersensitivity to H₁-receptor antihistamines; lactation, children <2 y.

CAUTIOUS USE Moderate to severe renal impairment, pregnancy (category B), children.

ROUTE & DOSAGE

Allergic Rhinitis
Child: **PO** *2 to 5 y:* 2.5 mg daily. (max 5 mg/day); ≥6 y: 5–10 mg daily.
Adult: **PO** 5–10 mg daily.

Chronic Urticaria
Adult: **PO** 10 mg daily or b.i.d.

STORAGE
Store tightly covered at room temperature.

ADMINISTRATION

Oral
- Consult prescriber about dosage if significant adverse effects appear. As elimination half-life is prolonged in the debilitated, dosage adjustments may be warranted.

ADVERSE EFFECTS GI: Constipation, diarrhea, dry mouth. **CNS:** *Drowsiness, sedation, headache,* depression.

INTERACTIONS Drug: Theophylline may decrease cetirizine clearance leading to toxicity.

PHARMACOKINETICS Absorption: Readily absorbed from GI tract. **Peak:** 1 h. **Distribution:** 93% protein bound; minimal CNS concentrations. **Metabolism:** Minimal. **Elimination:** 60% excreted unchanged in urine within 24 h, 5% excreted in feces. **Half-Life:** 7.4 h.

NURSING IMPLICATIONS

Assessment & Drug Effects
- Monitor for drug interactions. As the drug is highly protein bound, the potential for interactions with other protein-bound drugs exists.
- Monitor for sedation.

Patient & Family Education
- Do not use in combination with OTC antihistamines.
- Do not engage driving or other hazardous activities, before experiencing your responses to the drug.
- Do not breast feed while taking this drug without consulting physician.
- Store this medication out of reach of children.

CHARCOAL, ACTIVATED (LIQUID ANTIDOTE)
Actidose, Charcoaid, Charcocaps, Charcodote, Insta-Char
Classifications: ANTIDOTE; ADSORBENT
Pregnancy Category: C

Common adverse effects in *italic;* life-threatening effects <u>underlined;</u> generic names in **bold;** drug classifications in SMALL CAPS; ✦ Canadian drug name; ☻ Prototype drug.

AVAILABILITY 208 mg/mL, 15 g, 30 g 50 mg liquid/suspension

ACTIONS Residue from destructive distillation of organic materials treated to reduce particle size, which increases surface area and adsorptive power. Activated charcoal (carbon) is a chemically inert, odorless, tasteless, fine black powder with wide spectrum of adsorptive activity. Acts by binding (adsorbing) toxic substances, thereby inhibiting their GI absorption, enterohepatic circulation, and thus bioavailability.

THERAPEUTIC EFFECTS Recent studies indicate that administration by "gastric dialysis" (repetitive doses) effectively increases clearance of drugs already absorbed into the systemic circulation. Action appears to result from increased rate of drug diffusion from plasma into GI tract where it is adsorbed by activated charcoal. Effectively adsorbs toxins in the gut preventing their systemic absorption and impact.

USES General-purpose emergency antidote in the treatment of poisonings by most drugs and chemicals: acetaminophen, aspirin, atropine, barbiturates, digitalis glycosides, phenytoin, propoxyphene, strychnine, tricyclic antidepressants, among many others. Gastric dialysis (repetitive doses) in uremia to adsorb various waste products from GI tract; severe acute poisoning. Has been used to adsorb intestinal gases in treatment of dyspepsia, flatulence, and distention (value in these conditions not established). Sometimes used topically as a deodorant for foul-smelling wounds and ulcers.

CONTRAINDICATIONS Reportedly not effective for poisonings by cyanide, mineral acids, caustic alkalis, organic solvents, iron, ethanol, methanol.

CAUTIOUS USE Pregnancy (category C); lactation.

ROUTE & DOSAGE

Acute Poisonings
Infant <1 y: **PO** 1 g/kg
Child 1–12 y: **PO** 1–2 g/kg or 15–30 g in at least 6–8 oz of water
Adult: **PO** 30–100 g in at least 180–240 mL (6–8 oz) of water or 1 g/kg

Gastric Dialysis
Adult: **PO** 20–40 g q6h for 1 or 2 days

GI Disturbances
Adult: **PO** 520–975 mg p.c. up to 5 g/day

STORAGE
Store at 15°–30° C (59°–86° F) in tightly closed glass or metal containers.

ADMINISTRATION

Oral
- Activated charcoal tablets or capsules are less adsorptive and thus less effective than powder or liquid form; therefore, they are not recommended in treatment of acute poisoning.

- Drug is most effective when administered as soon as possible after acute poisoning (preferably within 30 min).
- Sorbital may be added to stimulate catharsis.
- In an emergency, dose may be approximated by stirring sufficient activated charcoal into tap water to make a slurry the consistency of soup (about 20–30 g in at least 240 mL of water).
- Activated charcoal can be swallowed or given through a nasogastric tube. If administered too rapidly, patient may vomit.
- If necessary, palatability may be improved by adding a small amount of concentrated fruit juice or chocolate powder to the slurry. Reportedly, these agents do not appreciably alter adsorptive activity.

ADVERSE EFFECTS GI: Vomiting (rapid ingestion of high doses), constipation, diarrhea (from sorbitol).

INTERACTIONS Drug: May decrease absorption of all other oral medications—administer at least 2 h apart.

PHARMACOKINETICS Absorption: Not absorbed. **Elimination:** Excreted in feces.

NURSING IMPLICATIONS

Assessment & Drug Effects
- Record appearance, color, consistency, frequency, and relative amount of stools. Inform patient that activated charcoal will color feces black.

Patient & Family Education
- Call Poison Control Center before using. Review prevention of poisonings and what to do if they occur at each health promotion visit during childhood.
- Do not breast feed while taking this drug without consulting physician.
- Store this medication out of reach of children.

CHLORAL HYDRATE
(klor′al hye′drate)
Aquachloral Supprettes, Noctec, Novochlorhydrate ◆
Classifications: CENTRAL NERVOUS SYSTEM AGENT; ANXIOLYTIC, SEDATIVE-HYPNOTIC
Prototype: Secobarbital
Pregnancy Category: C
Controlled Substance: Schedule IV

AVAILABILITY 500 mg capsules; 250 mg/5 mL, 500 mg/5 mL syrup; 324 mg, 500 mg, 648 mg suppositories

ACTIONS Produces "physiologic sleep" by mild cerebral depression with little effect on respirations or BP and little or no hangover.
THERAPEUTIC EFFECTS Chloral hydrate is a sedative-hypnotic that does not affect sleep physiology (e.g., REM sleep) in low doses. Has little or no analgesic action.

USES Short-term management of insomnia, for general sedation prior to procedures, for sedation before and after surgery, to reduce anxiety associated with drug withdrawal, and alone or with paraldehyde to prevent or suppress alcohol withdrawal symptoms.

CONTRAINDICATIONS Known hypersensitivity to chloral hydrate or chloral derivatives; severe hepatic, renal, or cardiac disease; rectal dosage form in patients with proctitis; oral use in patients with esophagitis, gastritis, gastric or duodenal ulcers; pregnancy (category C), lactation. **CAUTIOUS USE** History of intermittent porphyria, asthma, history of or proneness to drug dependence, depression, suicidal tendencies.

ROUTE & DOSAGE

Sedative
Child: **PO/PR** 25–50 mg/kg/day, divided q6–8h (max 500 mg/dose)
Adult: **PO/PR** 250 mg t.i.d. p.c.

Hypnotic
Child: **PO/PR** 50 mg/kg 15–30 min before bedtime or 30 min before surgery (max 1 g)
Adult: **PO/PR** 500 mg–1 g 15–30 min before bedtime or 30 min before surgery (max 2 g/24h)

Sedation for Procedures
Child: **PO/PR** 25–100 mg/kg/dose (max 1 g/dose for infants and 2 g/dose for children)

EEG Premedication
Child: **PO/PR** 20–25 mg/kg 30–60 min prior to procedure

STORAGE
Store at 15°–30° C (59°–86° F) in tightly covered, light-resistant containers.

ADMINISTRATION

Oral
- Dilute liquid preparations in chilled fluids to minimize unpleasant taste.
- Watch to see that drug is not cheeked and hoarded.

Rectal
- Moisten suppository with a water-based lubricant, such as K-Y jelly, prior to insertion.

ADVERSE EFFECTS Body as a Whole: <u>Angioedema</u>, eosinophilia, breath odor, leukopenia, ketonuria, renal and hepatic damage, <u>sudden death</u>. **CV:** Arrhythmias, <u>cardiac arrest</u>. **GI:** *Nausea, vomiting, diarrhea,* severe gastritis. **CNS:** Dizziness, motor incoordination, headache. **Skin:** Purpura, urticaria, erythematous rash, eczema, erythema multiforme, fixed drug eruptions. **Special Senses:** Conjunctivitis.

DIAGNOSTIC TEST INTERFERENCE False-positive results for *urine glucose* with *Benedict's solutions,* and possibly with *Clinitest* but not with *glucose oxidase methods* (e.g., *Clinistix, Diastix, TesTape*). Possible interference with fluorometric test for *urine catecholamines* (if chloral hydrate is administered within 48 h of test) and **urinary 17-OHCS** determinations (by modification of **Reddy, Jenkins, Thorn procedure**).

INTERACTIONS Drug: Alcohol, BARBITURATES, **paraldehyde,** other CNS DEPRESSANTS potentiate CNS depression; tachycardia may also occur with **alcohol;** increases anticoagulant effect of ORAL ANTICOAGULANTS; **furosemide** IV can produce flushing, diaphoresis, BP changes.

PHARMACOKINETICS Absorption: Readily absorbed from oral or rectal administration. **Onset:** 30–60 min. **Peak:** 1–3 h. **Duration:** 4–8 h. **Distribution:** Well distributed to all tissues; 70–80% protein bound; crosses placenta. **Metabolism:** Metabolized in liver to the active metabolite trichloroethanol. **Elimination:** Excreted primarily by kidneys, with a small amount excreted in feces via bile. **Half-Life:** 8–11 h.

NURSING IMPLICATIONS

Assessment & Drug Effects

- Chloral hydrate is not intended for relief of pain. When used in the presence of pain, it may cause excitement and delirium.
- Do not exceed 2 weeks of use.
- Monitor for signs of respiratory depression. Chloral hydrate may depress muscles needed for breathing.
- Do not discontinue abruptly following prolonged use. Sudden withdrawal from dependent patients may produce delirium, mania, or convulsions.
- Monitor for S&S of allergic skin reactions, which may occur within several hours or as long as 10 days after drug administration.
- Evaluate patient's response to chloral hydrate and continued need for the drug.

Patient & Family Education

- Do not ambulate without assistance until response to drug is known.
- Avoid concomitant use of alcoholic beverages.
- Avoid driving and other potentially hazardous activities while under the influence of chloral hydrate.
- Do not breast feed while taking this drug.
- Store this medication out of reach of children.

CHLORAMBUCIL

(klor-am'byoo-sil)

Leukeran

Classifications: ANTINEOPLASTIC; ALKYLATING AGENT
Prototype: Cyclophosphamide
Pregnancy Category: D

AVAILABILITY 2 mg tablets

ACTIONS Potent aromatic derivative of the alkylating agent nitrogen mustard, which is slowest acting and least toxic of the nitrogen mustards. A cell-cycle nonspecific drug (kills both resting and dividing cells), it causes cytotoxic cross-linkage in DNA, thus preventing synthesis of DNA, RNA, and proteins. Myelosuppression in therapeutic doses is moderate and rapidly reversible.

THERAPEUTIC EFFECTS Lymphocytic effect is marked, thus it is effective in treatment of various lymphomas.

USES As single agent or in combination with other antineoplastics in treatment of chronic lymphocytic leukemia, malignant lymphomas including lymphosarcoma, Hodgkin's disease, and giant follicular lymphoma, and in treatment of carcinoma of the ovary, breast, and testes.
UNLABELED USES Nonneoplastic conditions: vasculitis complicating rheumatoid arthritis, autoimmune hemolytic anemias associated with cold agglutinins, lupus glomerulonephritis, idiopathic nephrotic syndrome, polycythemia vera, macroglobulinemia.

CONTRAINDICATIONS Hypersensitivity to chlorambucil or to other alkylating agents; administration within 4 wk of a full course of radiation or chemotherapy; full dosage if bone marrow is infiltrated with lymphomatous tissue or is hypoplastic; smallpox and other vaccines; pregnancy (category D), lactation.
CAUTIOUS USE Excessive or prolonged dosage, pneumococcus vaccination, history of seizures or head trauma.

ROUTE & DOSAGE

Malignant Diseases (Lymphomas, Hodgkin's Disease, etc.)
Child: **PO** 0.1–0.2 mg/kg/day in single or divided doses
Adult: **PO** 0.1–0.2 mg/kg/day (usual dose 4–10 mg/day)

STORAGE
Store in tightly closed, light-resistant container.

ADMINISTRATION
Child: Must be given under care and direction of pediatric oncology specialist. Use recommended handling techniques for hazardous medications (see Part I).

Oral
- Control nausea and vomiting by giving entire daily dose at one time, 1 h before breakfast or 2 h after evening meal, or at bedtime. Consult physician.
- With confirmation of bone marrow depression (low platelet and neutrophil counts or peripheral lymphocytosis), it is recommended that dosage not exceed 0.1 mg/kg.

ADVERSE EFFECTS Body as a Whole: Drug fever, skin rashes, papilledema, alopecia, peripheral neuropathy, sterile cystitis, pulmonary complications, seizures (high doses). **GI:** Low incidence of gastric discomfort, <u>hepatotoxicity</u>. **Hematologic:** <u>Bone marrow depression</u>: *leukopenia,* thrombocytopenia, anemia. **Metabolic:** Sterility, hyperuricemia.

INTERACTIONS Drug: May have to adjust dose of **allopurinol, colchicine** because of chlorambucil-associated hyperuricemia.

PHARMACOKINETICS Absorption: Rapidly and completely absorbed from GI tract. **Peak:** 1 h. **Distribution:** Extensively bound to plasma and tissue proteins; crosses placenta. **Metabolism:** Extensively metabolized in liver. **Elimination:** 60% eliminated in urine as metabolites within 24 h. **Half-Life:** 1.5–2.5 h.

NURSING IMPLICATIONS

Assessment & Drug Effects

- Lab tests: CBC, Hgb, total and differential leukocyte counts, and serum uric acid initially and at least once weekly during treatment.
- Assess immunization status prior to beginning therapy in order to be alert for diseases that pose risk.
- Leukopenia usually develops after the third week of treatment; it may continue for up to 10 days after last dose, then rapidly return to normal.
- Avoid or reduce to minimum injections and other invasive procedures (e.g., rectal temperatures, enemas) when platelet count is low because of danger of bleeding.
- Monitor for S&S of skin rashes, which are rare, but appear to show a consistent pattern: pustular eruption on mouth, chin, cheeks; urticarial erythema on trunk that spreads to legs. The rash occurs early in treatment period and lasts about 10 days after last dose.
- Assess immunization status prior to beginning therapy in order to be alert for diseases that pose risk.

Patient & Family Education

- Keep appointments with physician. During treatment it is dangerous to go longer than 2 wk without a clinical examination and blood studies.
- Avoid contact with crowds and those with infectious diseases.
- Notify physician if the following symptoms occur: Unusual bleeding or bruising, sores on lips or in mouth; flank, stomach, or joint pain; fever, chills, or other signs of infection, sore throat, cough, dyspnea.
- Report immediately the onset of cutaneous reaction.
- Drink generous amount of fluid daily for age and size and report to physician if urine output decreases below normal amounts.
- Report to physician immediately if pregnant, because there is a potential hazard to the fetus.
- Do not breast feed while taking this drug.
- Store this medication out of reach of children.

CHLORAMPHENICOL

(klor-am-fen′i-kole)

Chlorofair, Chloromycetin, Chloroptic, Chloroptic S.O.P., Fenicol, Isopto Fenicol, Novochlorocap ✚, Ophthochlor, Pentamycetin ✚

CHLORAMPHENICOL SODIUM SUCCINATE

Chloromycetin Sodium Succinate

Classifications: ANTI-INFECTIVE; ANTIBIOTIC
Pregnancy Category: C

AVAILABILITY 250 mg capsules; 100 mg/mL injection; 5 mg/mL ophth solution; 10 mg/g ointment; 0.5% otic solution.

ACTIONS Synthetic broad-spectrum antibiotic formerly derived from *Streptomyces venezuelae*. Principally bacteriostatic but may be bactericidal in certain species (e.g., *Haemophilus influenzae*) or when given in higher concentrations. Believed to act by binding to the 50S ribosome of bacteria and thus interfering with protein synthesis.

THERAPEUTIC EFFECTS Effective against a wide variety of gram-negative and gram-positive bacteria and most anaerobic microorganisms.

USES Severe infections when other antibiotics are ineffective or are contraindicated. Particularly effective against *Salmonella typhi* and other *Salmonella* sp., *Streptococcus pneumoniae, Neisseria,* meningeal infections caused by *H. influenzae,* and infections involving *Bacteroides fragilis* and other anaerobic organisms, *Rickettsia rickettsii* (cause of Rocky Mountain spotted fever) and other rickettsiae, the lymphogranuloma-psittacosis group *(Chlamydia),* and *Mycoplasma.* Also used in cystic fibrosis anti-infective regimens and topically for infections of skin, eyes, and external auditory canal.

CONTRAINDICATIONS History of hypersensitivity or toxic reaction to chloramphenicol; treatment of minor infections, prophylactic use; typhoid carrier state, history or family history of drug-induced bone marrow depression, concomitant therapy with drugs that produce bone marrow depression; pregnancy (category C); lactation.

CAUTIOUS USE Impaired hepatic or renal function, premature and full-term infants, children; intermittent porphyria; patients with G6PD deficiency; patient or family history of drug-induced bone marrow depression.

ROUTE & DOSAGE

Serious Infections

Neonate: **IV** 25–50 mg/kg/day in divided doses q12–24 h
Infant/Child: **PO/IV** 50–75 mg/kg/day divided into doses q6h (max 4 g/day)
Adult: **PO/IV** 50 mg/kg/day divided into 4 doses. **Topical** 1–2 drops of ophthalmic solution q3–6h or small strip of ophthalmic ointment in lower conjunctival sac q3–6h or 2–3 drops of otic solution in ear t.i.d.

Meningitis

Child/Adult: **IV** 75–100 mg/kg/day divided q6h

STORAGE

- Do not use cloudy solutions.
- Store topical ophthalmic, otic, and skin preparations, PO forms, and unopened ampules at room temperature and protected from light unless otherwise directed by manufacturer.

ADMINISTRATION

Oral

- Give preferably with a full glass of water (or generous amount of water appropriate for younger child) on an empty stomach, at least 1 h before or 2 h after a meal, to achieve optimum blood levels.

Ophthalmic

- Apply light pressure to lacrimal duct after instillation for 1–2 min to prevent drainage into nasopharynx and systemic absorption. This is an extremely important step to decrease absorption. Several cases of aplastic anemia have been associated with use of ophthalmic preparations.

Intravenous

- IV administration to neonates, infants, children: Verify correct IV concentration and rate of infusion with physician.

PREPARE **Direct:** Dilute each 1 g with 10 mL of sterile water or D5W. **Intermittent:** Further dilute in 50–100 mL of D5W. **Continuous:** Dilute with additional D5W for a longer infusion time.

ADMINISTER **Direct:** Give slowly over a period of at least 1 min. **Intermittent:** Give over 30–60 min. **Continuous:** Infuse over 4–6h.

INCOMPATIBILITIES **Solutions/Additives: Chlorpromazine, glycopyrrolate, metoclopramide, polymyxin B, prochlorperazine, promethazine,** TETRACYCLINES, **vancomycin. Y-Site: Fluconazole.** ■ Solution for infusion may form crystals or a second layer when stored at low temperatures. Solution can be clarified by shaking vial.

ADVERSE EFFECTS Body as a Whole: Hypersensitivity, <u>angioedema</u>, dyspnea, fever, <u>anaphylaxis</u>, superinfections, Gray syndrome. **GI:** Nausea, vomiting, diarrhea, perianal irritation, enterocolitis, glossitis, stomatitis, unpleasant taste, xerostomia. **Hematologic:** <u>Bone marrow depression</u> (dose-related and reversible): reticulocytosis, leukopenia, granulocytopenia, thrombocytopenia, increased plasma iron, reduced Hgb, hypoplastic anemia, hypoprothrombinemia. Non-dose-related and irreversible <u>pancytopenia</u>, <u>agranulocytosis</u>, <u>aplastic anemia</u>, paroxysmal nocturnal hemoglobinuria, leukemia. **CNS:** Neurotoxicity: headache, mental depression, confusion, delirium, digital paresthesias, peripheral neuritis. **Skin:** Urticaria, contact dermatitis, maculopapular and vesicular rashes, fixed-drug eruptions. **Special Senses:** Visual disturbances, optic neuritis, optic nerve atrophy, contact conjunctivitis.

DIAGNOSTIC TEST INTERFERENCE Possibility of false-positive results for *urine glucose* by *copper reduction methods* (e.g., *Benedict's solution, Clinitest*). Chloramphenicol may interfere with *17-OHCS* (urinary steroid) determinations (modification of *Reddy, Jenkins, Thorn procedure* not affected), with *urobilinogen excretion,* and with responses to *tetanus toxoid* and possibly other active immunizing agents.

INTERACTIONS Drug: The metabolism of **chlorpropamide, dicumarol, phenytoin, tolbutamide** may be decreased, prolonging their activity. **Phenobarbital** decreases chloramphenicol levels. The response to **iron** preparations, **folic acid,** and **vitamin B$_{12}$** may be delayed.

PHARMACOKINETICS Absorption: Rapidly absorbed from GI tract. **Peak:** 1–3 h PO; 1 h IV. **Distribution:** Widely distributed to most body tissues including saliva and ascitic, pleural and synovial fluid; concentrates in liver and kidneys; penetrates CNS; crosses placenta. **Metabolism:** Primarily inactivated in liver. **Elimination:** Much longer in neonates; metabolite and free drug excreted in urine; excreted in breast milk. **Half-Life:** 1.5 to 4.1 h.

NURSING IMPLICATIONS

Assessment & Drug Effects

- Lab tests: Perform bacterial culture and susceptibility tests prior to first dose and periodically thereafter. Baseline CBC, platelets, serum iron, and reticulocyte cell counts before initiation of therapy, at 48-h intervals during therapy, and periodically. Monitor chloramphenicol blood levels weekly or more frequently with hepatic dysfunction and in patients receiving therapy for longer than 2 wk. ***Desired concentrations:*** Therapeutic level 15–20 mg/L for meningitis, 10–20 mg/L for other infections. Trough: 5–15 mg/L for meningitis, 5–10 mg/L for other infections.

- Measure IV peak 30 min after end of infusion, PO peak 2 h after PO dose; measure IV+PO trough 30 min before next scheduled dose.
- Monitor blood studies. Chloramphenicol should be discontinued upon appearance of leukopenia, reticulocytopenia, thrombocytopenia, or anemia.
- Non-dose-related irreversible bone marrow depression may appear weeks or months after drug therapy is terminated. The potential for this side effect is greatest in patients with impaired hepatic or renal function, infants, children, and premenopausal women.
- Observe the patient closely, because blood studies are not always reliable predictors of irreversible bone marrow depression.
- Check temperature at least q4h. Usually chloramphenicol is discontinued if temperature remains normal for 48 h.
- Monitor I&O ratio or pattern: Report any appreciable change.
- More frequent determinations of serum glucose are recommended in patients receiving oral antidiabetic agents.
- Monitor for S&S of Gray syndrome, which has occurred 2–9 days after initiation of high-dose chloramphenicol therapy in premature infants and neonates and in children ≤2 y. Report early signs: abdominal distention, failure to feed, pallor, changes in vital signs. Early detection and prompt termination of therapy can interrupt a potentially fatal course.

Patient & Family Education
- A bitter taste may occur 15–20 sec after IV injection; it usually lasts only 2–3 min.
- Report immediately sore throat, fever, fatigue, petechiae, nose bleeds, bleeding gums, or other unusual bleeding or bruising, or any other suspicious sign or symptom. Drug therapy should be discontinued if abnormal bleeding occurs.
- Watch for S&S of superinfection.
- Follow dosage and duration of therapy as prescribed by health care provider.
- Avoid prolonged or frequent intermittent use of topical preparations because systemic absorption and toxicity can occur.
- Withhold medication and check with physician immediately if signs of hypersensitivity reaction, irritation, superinfection, or other adverse reactions appear.
- Do not breast feed while taking this drug.
- Store this medication out of reach of children.

CHLORDIAZEPOXIDE HYDROCHLORIDE

(klor-dye-az-e-pox′ide)
Libritabs, Librium, Lipoxide, Medilium ♣, Novopoxide ♣, Sereen, Solium ♣
Classifications: CENTRAL NERVOUS SYSTEM AGENT; ANXIOLYTIC; SEDATIVE-HYPNOTIC; BENZODIAZEPINE
Prototype: Lorazepam
Pregnancy Category: D
Controlled Substance: Schedule IV

CHLORDIAZEPOXIDE HYDROCHLORIDE

AVAILABILITY 5 mg, 10 mg, 25 mg capsules; 10 mg, 25 mg tablets; 100 mg/amp injection
Combination Products: Limbitrol (in combination with amitriptyline)

ACTIONS Benzodiazepine derivative. Acts on the limbic, thalamic, and hypothalamic areas of the CNS. Has long-acting hypnotic properties. Causes mild suppression of REM sleep and of deeper phases, particularly stage 4, while increasing total sleep time.
THERAPEUTIC EFFECTS Produces mild anxiolytic (reduces anxiety), sedative, anticonvulsant, and skeletal muscle relaxant effects.

USES Relief of various anxiety and tension states, preoperative apprehension and anxiety, and for management of alcohol withdrawal.
UNLABELED USES Essential, familial, and senile action tremors.

CONTRAINDICATIONS Hypersensitivity to chlordiazepoxide and other benzodiazepines; narrow-angle glaucoma, prostatic hypertrophy, shock, comatose states, primary depressive disorder or psychoses, pregnancy (category D), lactation, oral use in children <6 y, parenteral use in children <12 y, acute alcohol intoxication.
CAUTIOUS USE Anxiety states associated with impending depression, history of impaired hepatic or renal function; addiction-prone individuals, blood dyscrasias; children; hyperkinesis.

ROUTE & DOSAGE

Mild Anxiety, Preoperative Anxiety
Child: **PO** 5 mg b.i.d. to q.i.d.; may be increased to 10 mg t.i.d.
Adult: **PO** 5–10 mg t.i.d. or q.i.d. **IM/IV** 50–100 mg 1 h before surgery

Severe Anxiety and Tension
Adult: **PO** 20–25 mg t.i.d. or q.i.d. **IM/IV** 50–100 mg, then 25–50 mg t.i.d. or q.i.d.

Alcohol Withdrawal Syndrome
Adult: **PO** 50–100 mg prn up to 300 mg/day. **IM/IV** 50–100 mg, may repeat in 2–3 h if necessary

STORAGE
Store in tight, light-resistant containers at room temperature unless otherwise specified by manufacturer. The special diluent supplied by manufacturer for IM preparation should be kept refrigerated, preferably at 2°–8° C (36°–46° F) until ready for use.

ADMINISTRATION
Oral
- Give with or immediately after meals or with milk to reduce GI distress. If an antacid is prescribed, it should be taken at least 1 h before or after chlordiazepoxide to prevent delay in drug absorption.
- Supervise drug ingestion to prevent "cheeking" pills, a maneuver that leads to hoarding or omission of drug.

Intramuscular
- Prepare parenteral solution immediately before use; discard unused portion. Drug is unstable in light and when in solution.

- Use special diluent provided by manufacturer to make the IM solution. Add diluent carefully to avoid bubble formation; gently agitate until solution is clear. Resulting solution: 50 mg/mL. Discard diluent if it is not clear.
- Inject into muscle mass appropriate for age (see Part I).

Intravenous

PREPARE **Direct:** Dilute each 100-mg ampule of dry powder with 5 mL sterile water for injection or NS. Agitate gently until dissolved. DO NOT use supplied diluent, which is for IM injection only.

ADMINISTER **Direct:** Give at a rate of 100 mg or a fraction thereof over at least 1 min.

INCOMPATIBILITIES **Y-Site: Cefepime.**

ADVERSE EFFECTS Body as a Whole: Edema, pain in injection site, jaundice, hiccups, <u>respiratory depression</u>. **CV:** Orthostatic hypotension, tachycardia, changes in ECG patterns seen with rapid IV administration. **GI:** Nausea, dry mouth, vomiting, constipation, increased appetite. **CNS:** *Drowsiness,* dizziness, *lethargy,* changes in EEG pattern; vivid dreams, nightmares, headache, vertigo, syncope, tinnitus, confusion, hallucinations, paradoxical rage, depression, delirium, ataxia. **Skin:** Photosensitivity, skin rash. **Urogenital:** Urinary frequency.

DIAGNOSTIC TEST INTERFERENCE Chlordiazepoxide increases ***serum bilirubin, AST*** and ***ALT;*** decreases ***radioactive iodine uptake;*** and may falsely increase readings for ***urinary 17-OHCS*** (modified ***Glenn-Nelson*** technique).

INTERACTIONS Drug: Alcohol, CNS DEPRESSANTS, ANTICONVULSANTS potentiate CNS depression; **cimetidine** increases **chlordiazepoxide** plasma levels, thus increasing toxicity; may decrease antiparkinson effects of **levodopa;** may increase **phenytoin** levels; smoking decreases sedative and antianxiety effects. **Herbal: Kava-kava, valerian** may potentiate sedation.

PHARMACOKINETICS Absorption: Well absorbed from GI tract; slow erratic absorption from IM. **Peak:** 1–4 h PO; 15–30 min IM; 3–30 min IV. **Distribution:** Widely distributed throughout body; crosses placenta. **Metabolism:** Metabolized in liver to long-acting active metabolite. **Elimination:** Slowly excreted in urine (may last several days); excreted in breast milk. **Half-Life:** 5–30 h.

NURSING IMPLICATIONS

Assessment & Drug Effects

- Monitor for signs and symptoms of orthostatic hypotension and tachycardia, which occur more frequently with parenteral administration. Patient should stay recumbent 2–3 h after IM or IV injection; observe closely and monitor vital signs.
- Check BP and pulse before giving benzodiazepine in early part of therapy. If blood pressure falls 20 mm Hg or more or if pulse rate is above 120 bpm or level set for children by prescriber, delay medication and consult physician.
- Lab tests: Periodic blood cell counts and liver function tests are recommended during prolonged therapy.

- Monitor for signs and symptoms of agranulocytosis: sore throat or mouth, upper respiratory infection, fever, and malaise. Total and differential WBC counts should be ordered immediately, and protective isolation instituted.
- Monitor I&O until drug dosage is stabilized. Report changes in I&O ratio and dysuria. Cumulative (overdosage) effects can result in renal dysfunction.
- Monitor for S&S of paradoxic reactions—excitement, stimulation, disturbed sleep patterns, acute rage—which may occur during first few weeks of therapy in psychiatric patients and in hyperactive and aggressive children receiving chlordiazepoxide. Withhold drug and report to physician.
- If given in combination product with amitriptyline (Limbitrol), can increase risk of suicidal thinking and behavior in children and adolescents with major depressive disorder, obsessive compulsive disorder, and other psychiatric disorders. Observe closely for worsening of condition, suicidality, and behavior changes. Instruct family and caregivers to monitor for these symptoms and discuss with prescriber. A MedGuide describing risks and stating whether the drug is approved for the child'/adolescent' condition should be provided for all families when antidepressants are prescribed.
- Assess patient's sleep pattern. If dreams or nightmares interfere with rest, notify physician. A change in the dosing schedule, dose, or an alternate drug may be prescribed.
- Supervise ambulation and other activities. Observe for signs of developing physical or psychologic dependency such as requests for change in drug regimen (dose and dose interval), diminishing favorable response (e.g., disturbed sleep pattern, increase in psychomotor activity), withdrawal symptoms. Investigate the symptoms of ataxia, vertigo, slurred speech; the patient may be taking more than the prescribed dose.
- Abrupt discontinuation of drug in patients receiving high doses for long periods (≥4 mo) has precipitated withdrawal symptoms, but not for at least 5–7 days because of slow elimination.

Patient & Family Education

- Take drug specifically as prescribed: do not skip, increase, or decrease doses, change intervals, or terminate therapy without physician's advice and do not lend or offer any of drug to another person.
- Do not take OTC drugs unless prescribed.
- Long-term use of this drug may cause xerostomia. Good oral hygiene can alleviate the discomfort.
- Avoid activities requiring mental alertness until reaction to the drug has been evaluated.
- Avoid drinking alcoholic beverages. When combined with chlordiazepoxide, effects of both are potentiated.
- If pregnant during therapy or intending to become pregnant, communicate with physician about continuing therapy.
- Avoid excessive sunlight. Photosensitivity has been reported. Use sunscreen lotion (SPF 12 or above) if allowed.
- Do not breast feed while taking this drug.
- Store this medication out of reach of children.

CHLOROQUINE HYDROCHLORIDE ℗

(klor'oh-kwin)

Aralen Hydrochloride

CHLOROQUINE PHOSPHATE

Aralen Phosphate

Classifications: ANTI-INFECTIVE; ANTIMALARIAL

Pregnancy Category: C

AVAILABILITY Hydrochloride: 250 mg, 500 mg tablets; 5 mg, 50 mg/mL ampule; **Phosphate:** 250 mg, 500 mg tablets

ACTIONS Antimalarial activity is believed to be based on its ability to form complexes with DNA of parasite, thereby inhibiting replication and transcription to RNA and nucleic acid synthesis. Highly active against asexual erythrocytic forms of the four species of *Plasmodium: P. vivax, P. malariae, P. ovale,* and most strains of *P. falciparum.* Action mechanism is unknown. **THERAPEUTIC EFFECTS** Acts as a suppressive agent in patient with *P. vivax* or *P. malariae* malaria; terminates acute attacks and increases intervals between treatment and relapse of malaria. Abolishes the acute attack of *P. falciparum* malaria but does not prevent the infection. Chloroquine-resistant strains have been reported. Also acts as a tissue amebicide, has anti-inflammatory, antihistamine, and antiserotonic properties.

USES Suppression and treatment of malaria caused by *P. malariae, P. ovale, P. vivax,* and susceptible forms of *P. falciparum,* and in the treatment of extraintestinal amebiasis. Concomitant therapy with primaquine is necessary for radical cure of *P. vivax* and *P. malariae* malarias.

UNLABELED USES Discoid and systemic lupus erythematosus, porphyria cutanea tarda, solar urticaria, polymorphous light eruptions, and in rheumatoid arthritis (as second-line therapy).

CONTRAINDICATIONS Hypersensitivity to 4-aminoquinolines, psoriasis; porphyria, renal disease, 4-aminoquinoline-induced retinal or visual field changes; long-term therapy in children; pregnancy (category C), lactation. Safe use in women of childbearing potential not established.

CAUTIOUS USE Impaired hepatic function, alcoholism, eczema, patients with G6PD deficiency, infants and children, hematologic, GI, and neurologic disorders.

ROUTE & DOSAGE

Doses are expressed in terms of chloroquine base: 500 mg tablet = 300 mg base; 50 mg injection = 40 mg base

Acute Malaria

Child: **PO** 10 mg base/kg, then 5 mg base/kg at 6, 24, and 48 h. **IM** 5 mg base/kg q12h

Adult: **PO** 600 mg base followed by 300 mg base at 6, 24, and 48 h. **IM** 200 mg base q6h prn, not to exceed 800 mg base/24 h

Malaria Suppression

Child: **PO** 5 mg base/kg the same day each week starting 2 wk before

Common adverse effects in *italic;* life-threatening effects <u>underlined;</u> generic names in **bold;** drug classifications in SMALL CAPS; ♣ Canadian drug name; ℗ Prototype drug.

301

exposure and continuing for 4–6 wk after leaving the area of exposure (max 300 mg base/wk)

Adult: **PO** 300 mg base the same day each week starting 2 wk before exposure and continuing for 4–6 wk after leaving the area of exposure (max 300 mg base/wk)

Extraintestinal Amebiasis

Child: **PO** 10 mg base/kg/day for 2–3 wk
Adult: **PO** 600 mg base/day for 2 days, then 300 mg base/day for 2–3 wk

Rheumatoid Arthritis, SLE

Adult: **PO** 150 mg base/day with evening meal

STORAGE

Store tablets and ampules preferably at 15°–30° C (59°–86° F), unless otherwise directed by manufacturer. Store tablets in tightly closed container.

ADMINISTRATION

Oral

- Give immediately before or after meals to minimize GI distress.
- Monitor child's dose closely. Children are extremely susceptible to overdosage.

Intramuscular

- IM administration should generally be reserved for those who cannot take the oral form.
- Give undiluted, deep IM into a large muscle appropriate for age (see Part I).

ADVERSE EFFECTS Body as a Whole: Slight weight loss, myalgia, lymphedema of upper limbs. **CV:** Hypotension; ECG changes. **GI:** *Diarrhea,* abdominal cramps, *nausea,* vomiting, anorexia. **Hematologic:** Hemolytic anemia in patients with G6PD deficiency. **CNS:** Mild transient headache, fatigue, irritability, confusion, nightmares, skeletal muscle weakness, paresthesias, reduced reflexes, vertigo. **Skin:** Bleaching of scalp, eyebrows, body hair, and freckles, pruritus, patchy alopecia (reversible). **Special Senses:** (Usually reversible) Blurred vision, disturbances of accommodation, night blindness, scotomas, visual field defects, photophobia, corneal edema, opacity or deposits, ototoxicity (rare).

INTERACTIONS Drug: Aluminum- and **magnesium**-containing ANTACIDS and LAXATIVES decrease chloroquine absorption, so separate administration by at least 4 h; chloroquine may interfere with response to **rabies vaccine.**

PHARMACOKINETICS Absorption: Rapidly and almost completely absorbed. **Peak:** 1–2 h. **Distribution:** Widely distributed; concentrates in lungs, liver, erythrocytes, eyes, skin, and kidneys; crosses placenta. **Metabolism:** Partially metabolized in liver to active metabolites. **Elimination:** Eliminated in urine; excreted in breast milk. **Half-Life:** 70–120 h.

NURSING IMPLICATIONS

Assessment & Drug Effects

- Lab tests: CBC and ECG are advised before initiation of therapy and periodically thereafter in patients on long-term therapy. A test for G6PD deficiency is recommended for American blacks and individuals of Mediterranean ancestry before therapy.

- Monitor for changes in vision. Retinopathy (generally irreversible) can be progressive even after termination of therapy. Patient may be asymptomatic or complain of night blindness, scotomas, visual field changes, blurred vision, or difficulty in focusing. Chloroquine should be discontinued immediately.
- Question patients on long-term therapy regularly about skeletal muscle weakness. Periodic tests should be made of muscle strength and deep tendon reflexes. Positive signs are indications to terminate therapy.

Patient & Family Education
- Report promptly visual or hearing disturbances, muscle weakness, or loss of balance, symptoms of blood dyscrasia (fever, sore mouth or throat, unexplained fatigue, easy bruising or bleeding).
- Use of dark glasses in sunlight or bright light may provide comfort (because of photophobia) and reduce risk of ocular damage. When drug is taken after exposure but no disease has occurred, families need to understand the concept and need for period of prophylaxis.
- Avoid driving or other potentially hazardous activities until reaction to drug is known.
- May cause rusty yellow or brown discoloration of urine.
- Do not breast feed while taking this drug.
- Store this medication out of reach of children.

CHLOROTHIAZIDE
(klor-oh-thye′a-zide)
Diachlor, Diuril, SK-Chlorothiazide

CHLOROTHIAZIDE SODIUM
Sodium Diuril
Classifications: ELECTROLYTE AND WATER BALANCE AGENT; THIAZIDE DIURETIC; ANTIHYPERTENSIVE
Prototype: Hydrochlorothiazide
Pregnancy Category: C

AVAILABILITY 250 mg, 500 mg tablets; 250 mg/5 mL suspension; 500 mg injection

ACTIONS Thiazide diuretic chemically related to sulfonamides. Primary action is production of diuresis by direct action on the distal convoluted tubules. Inhibits reabsorption of sodium, potassium, and chloride ions. Promotes renal excretion of sodium (and water), bicarbonate, and potassium; decreases renal calcium excretion and supports uric acid excretion.
THERAPEUTIC EFFECTS Antihypertensive mechanism is unclear but correlates with contraction of extracellular and intravascular fluid volumes and direct vasodilatory effect on vascular wall. This initially reduces cardiac output with subsequent decrease in peripheral resistance through autoregulatory mechanisms.

USES Adjunctively to manage edema associated with CHF, hepatic cirrhosis, renal dysfunction, corticosteroid, or estrogen therapy. Used alone

---

Common adverse effects in *italic*; life-threatening effects underlined; generic names in **bold**; drug classifications in SMALL CAPS; ◆ Canadian drug name; ❷ Prototype drug.

303

as step 1 agent in stepped care approach, or in combination with other agents for treatment of hypertension.

UNLABELED USES To reduce polyuria of central and nephrogenic diabetes insipidus, to prevent calcium-containing renal stones, and to treat renal tubular acidosis.

CONTRAINDICATIONS Hypersensitivity to thiazide or sulfonamides; anuria; hypokalemia; IV use in infants and children; pregnancy (category C).

CAUTIOUS USE History of sulfa allergy; impaired renal or hepatic function or gout; lactation; hypercalcemia, diabetes mellitus, debilitated patients, pancreatitis, sympathectomy, jaundiced children.

ROUTE & DOSAGE

Hypertension, Edema
Adult: **PO** 250 mg–1 g/day divided into 1–2 doses **IV** 250 mg–1 g/day divided into 1–2 doses

Edema
Child: **PO** <6 mo, 20–40 mg/kg/day given in 1 or 2 doses; >6 mo, 20 mg/kg/day divided into 2 doses **IV** <6 mo, 2–4 mg/kg/day divided into 2 doses; >6 mo, 4 mg/kg/day

STORAGE
Store tablets, oral solutions, and parenteral dosage forms at 15°–30° C (59°–86° F) unless otherwise directed by manufacturer. Unused reconstituted IV solutions may be stored at room temperature up to 24 h. Use only clear solutions.

ADMINISTRATION

Oral
- Give with or after food to prevent gastric irritation. Extent of absorption appears to be increased by taking it with food.
- Schedule daily doses to avoid nocturia and interrupted sleep.

Intravenous
- Reserve for emergency or when patient unable to take oral medication.
- IV administration to infants and children: Verify correct IV concentration and rate of infusion with physician.

***PREPARE* Intermittent:** Reconstitute the 500-mg vial with at least 18 mL sterile water for injection. May be further diluted with D5W or NS.

***ADMINISTER* Intermittent:** Give at a rate of 0.5 g over 5 min.

***INCOMPATIBILITIES* Solution/Additive: Amikacin, chlorpromazine, hydralazine, insulin, levorphanol, morphine, norepinephrine, polymyxin B, procaine, prochlorperazine, promazine, promethazine, streptomycin, triflupromazine, vancomycin.**

ADVERSE EFFECTS Body as a Whole: Fever, respiratory distress, anaphylactic reaction. **CV:** Irregular heart beat, weak pulse, orthostatic hypotension. **GI:** Vomiting, acute pancreatitis, diarrhea. **Hematologic:** Agranulocytosis (rare), aplastic anemia (rare), asymptomatic hyperuricemia, hyperglycemia, glycosuria, SIADH secretion. **Metabolic:** *Hypokalemia,*

hypercalcemia, hyponatremia, hypochloremic alkalosis, elevated cholesterol and triglyceride levels. **CNS:** Unusual fatigue, dizziness, mental
changes, vertigo, headache. **Skin:** Urticaria, photosensitivity, skin rash.

DIAGNOSTIC TEST INTERFERENCE Chlorothiazide (thiazides) may cause:
marked increases in *serum amylase* values, decrease in *PBI* determinations; increase in excretion of *PSP;* increase in *BSP retention;* false-
negative *phentolamine* and *tyramine* tests; interference with *urine
steroid* determinations, and possibly the *histamine test* for pheochromocytoma. Thiazides should be discontinued at least 3 day before
bentiromide test (thiazides can invalidate test) and before *parathyroid
function tests* because they tend to decrease calcium excretion.

INTERACTIONS Drug: Amphotericin B, CORTICOSTEROIDS increase hypokalemic effects of chlorothiazide; the hypoglycemic effects of SULFONYL-
UREAS and **insulin** may be antagonized; **cholestyramine, colestipol**
decrease thiazide absorption; intensifies hypoglycemic and hypotensive
effects of **diazoxide;** increased potassium and magnesium loss may
cause **digoxin** toxicity; decreases **lithium** excretion, increasing its toxicity; increases risk of NSAID-induced renal failure and may attenuate diuresis.

PHARMACOKINETICS Absorption: Incompletely absorbed PO. **Onset:** 2 h
PO; 15 min IV. **Peak:** 3–6 h PO; 30 min IV. **Duration:** 6–12 h PO; 2 h IV.
Distribution: Distributed throughout extracellular tissue; concentrates in
kidney; crosses placenta. **Metabolism:** Does not appear to be metabolized.
Elimination: Excreted in urine and breast milk. **Half-Life:** 45–120 min.

NURSING IMPLICATIONS

Assessment & Drug Effects

- Monitor for therapeutic effect. Antihypertensive action of a thiazide diuretic requires several days before effects are observed; usually optimum therapeutic effect is not established for 3–4 wk.
- Lab tests: Baseline and periodic determinations are indicated for blood
  count, serum electrolytes, CO_2, BUN, creatinine, uric acid, and blood
  glucose.
- Monitor for hyperglycemia. Thiazide therapy can cause hyperglycemia
  and glycosuria in diabetic and diabetic-prone individuals. Dosage adjustment of hypoglycemic drugs may be required.
- Asymptomatic hyperuricemia can be produced because of interference
  with uric acid excretion.
- Establish baseline weight before initiation of therapy. Weigh patient at
  the same time each a.m. under standard conditions. Report rapid or
  gradual weight gain. Tell patient to report signs of edema (hands, ankles, pretibial areas).
- Monitor BP closely during early drug therapy.
- Inspect skin and mucous membranes daily for evidence of petechiae in
  patients receiving large doses and those on prolonged therapy.
- Monitor I&O rates and patterns: Excessive diuresis or oliguria may
  cause electrolyte imbalance and necessitate prompt dosage adjustment.
- Monitor patients on digitalis therapy for S&S of hypokalemia. Even
  moderate reduction in serum potassium can precipitate digitalis intoxication in these patients.

Common adverse effects in *italic;* life-threatening effects <u>underlined</u>; generic names
in **bold;** drug classifications in SMALL CAPS; ♣ Canadian drug name; ⊘ Prototype drug.

305

C

- Thiazide preparations are extremely irritating to the tissues, and great care must be taken to avoid extravasation. If infiltration occurs, stop medication, remove needle, and apply ice if area is small.

Patient & Family Education

- Urination will occur in greater amounts and with more frequency than usual, and there will be an unusual sense of tiredness. With continued therapy, diuretic action decreases; hypotensive effects usually are maintained, and sense of tiredness diminishes.
- If orthostatic hypotension is a troublesome symptom consult physician for measures that will help tolerate the effect and to prevent falling.
- Report to physician any illness accompanied by prolonged vomiting or diarrhea.
- Avoid drinking large quantities of coffee or other caffeine drinks. Caffeine is a CNS stimulant with diuretic effects.
- Report S&S of hypokalemia, hypercalcemia, or hyperglycemia.
- Hypokalemia may be prevented if the daily diet contains potassium rich foods. Banana, orange juice, potato are examples of potassium rich foods. Collaborate with dietitian and other care providers.
- Report photosensitivity reaction to physician if it occurs. Thiazide-related photosensitivity is considered a photoallergy (radiation changes drug structure and makes it allergenic for some individuals). It occurs 1½–2 wk after initial sun exposure.
- Do not breast feed while taking this drug without consulting physician.
- Store this medication out of reach of children.

CHLORPHENIRAMINE MALEATE

(klor-fen-eer'a-meen)
Aller-Chlor, Chlo-Amine, Chlorate, Chlor-Pro, Chlorspan, Chlortab, Chlor-Trimeton, Chlor-Tripolon ♣, Novopheniram ♣, Pfeiffer Allergy, Phenetron, Telachlor, Teldrin, Trymegan
Classifications: ANTIHISTAMINE (H₁-RECEPTOR ANTAGONIST)
Prototype: Diphenhydramine
Pregnancy Category: B first and second trimester; category D in third trimester

---

AVAILABILITY 2 mg, 4 mg tablets; 8 mg, 12 mg sustained-release tablets; 2 mg/5 mL syrup

ACTIONS Antihistamine that competes with histamine for H₁-receptor sites on effector cells, thus it prevents histamine action that promotes capillary permeability and edema formation and constrictive action on respiratory, gastrointestinal, and vascular smooth muscles. It generally produces less drowsiness than other antihistamines, but adverse effects involving CNS stimulation may be more common.
THERAPEUTIC EFFECTS Has effective antihistamine reaction resulting in decreasing allergic symptomatology.

USES Symptomatic relief of various uncomplicated allergic conditions; to prevent transfusion and drug reactions in susceptible patients, and as adjunct to epinephrine and other standard measures in anaphylactic reactions.

CONTRAINDICATIONS Hypersensitivity to antihistamines of similar structure; lower respiratory tract symptoms, narrow-angle glaucoma, obstructive prostatic hypertrophy or other bladder neck obstruction, GI obstruction or stenosis; pregnancy (category B in first and second trimester, and category D in third trimester), lactation; premature and newborn infants; during or within 14 days of MAOI therapy.

CAUTIOUS USE Convulsive disorders, increased intraocular pressure, hyperthyroidism, cardiovascular disease, hypertension, diabetes mellitus, history of bronchial asthma, older adult patients, patients with G6PD deficiency.

ROUTE & DOSAGE

Symptomatic Allergy Relief
Child: **PO** *2–6 y,* 1 mg q4–6h; *6–12 y,* 2 mg q4–6h (max 12 mg/day)
Adult: **PO** 2–4 mg t.i.d. or q.i.d. *or* 8–12 mg b.i.d. or t.i.d. (max 24 mg/day)

Allergic Reactions to Blood
Adult: **SC/IV/IM** 10–20 mg (max 40 mg/day)

STORAGE
Store at 15°–30° C (59°–86° F). Protect syrup and injection forms from light to prevent discoloration; keep tightly closed.

ADMINISTRATION

Oral
- Give on an empty stomach for fastest response.
- Sustained-release tablets should be swallowed whole and not crushed or chewed.
- Ensure that chewable tablets are chewed or crushed before being swallowed with a liquid.

Subcutaneous/Intramuscular/Intravenous
- The 100 mg/mL preparation is intended for IM or SC use only. It should not be administered IV because it contains preservatives. The 10 mg/mL injection can be given IV, IM, or SC. It contains no preservatives.

Intravenous
PREPARE **Direct:** Give undiluted.
ADMINISTER **Direct:** Give 10 mg or fraction thereof over at least 1 min.
- If patient manifests any reaction after parenteral administration, drug should be discontinued. (Exception: Patient may experience transitory stinging sensation that rarely lasts longer than a few minutes.)

ADVERSE EFFECTS Body as a Whole: Sensation of chest tightness. **CV:** Palpitation, tachycardia, mild hypotension or hypertension. **GI:** Epigastric distress, anorexia, nausea, vomiting, constipation, or diarrhea. **CNS:** *Drowsiness,* sedation, headache, dizziness, vertigo, fatigue, disturbed coordination, tremors, euphoria, nervousness, restlessness, insomnia. **Special Senses:** *Dryness of mouth,* nose, and throat, tinnitus, vertigo, acute labyrinthitis, thickened bronchial secretions, blurred vision, diplopia. **Urogenital:** Urinary frequency or retention, dysuria.

DIAGNOSTIC TEST INTERFERENCE Antihistamines should be discontinued 4 days before *skin testing* procedures for allergy because they may obscure otherwise positive reactions.

INTERACTIONS Drug: Alcohol (ethanol) and other CNS DEPRESSANTS produce additive sedation and CNS depression.

PHARMACOKINETICS Absorption: Well absorbed from GI tract; about 45% of dose reaches systemic circulation intact. **Onset:** Within 6 h. **Peak:** 2–6 h. **Distribution:** Highest concentrations in lung, heart, kidney, brain, small intestine, and spleen. **Half-Life:** 12–43 h.

NURSING IMPLICATIONS

Assessment & Drug Effects

- Monitor for CNS depression and sedation, especially when chlorpheniramine is given in combination with other CNS depressants.
- Monitor BP in hypertensive patients because chlorpheniramine may elevate BP.

Patient & Family Education

- Avoid driving a car and other potentially hazardous activities until drug response has been determined.
- Avoid alcohol intake. Antihistamines have additive effects with alcohol.
- Report any of the following: Palpitations or tinnitus.
- Consult prescriber before taking additional OTC drugs for allergy relief.
- Do not breast feed while taking this drug.
- Store this medication out of reach of children.

CHLORPROMAZINE ⊘
(klor-proe′ma-zeen)

CHLORPROMAZINE HYDROCHLORIDE

Chlorpromanyl ✦, Largactil ✦, Novochlorpromazine ✦, Ormazine, Promapar, Promaz, Sonazine, Thorazine, Thor-Prom
Classifications: CENTRAL NERVOUS SYSTEM AGENT; PSYCHOTHERAPEUTIC; ANTIPSYCHOTIC; PHENOTHIAZINE; ANTIEMETIC
Pregnancy Category: C

AVAILABILITY 10 mg, 25 mg, 50 mg, 100 mg, 200 mg tablets; 30 mg, 75 mg, 150 mg sustained-release capsules; 10 mg/5 mL syrup; 30 mg/mL, 100 mg/mL oral concentrate; 25 mg, 100 mg suppositories; 25 mg/mL injection

ACTIONS Phenothiazine derivative with actions at all levels of CNS with a mechanism that produces strong antipsychotic effects. Actions on hypothalamus and reticular formation produce strong sedation, hypotension, and depressed temperature regulation. Has strong alpha-adrenergic blocking action and weak anticholinergic effects. Directly depresses the heart; may increase coronary blood flow. Exerts quinidine-like antiarrhythmic action. Antiemetic effect due to suppression of the chemoreceptor trigger zone (CTZ). Inhibitory effect on dopamine reuptake may be the basis for moderate extrapyramidal symptoms. Antipsychotic drugs

---

Common adverse effects in *italic;* life-threatening effects <u>underlined;</u> generic names in **bold;** drug classifications in SMALL CAPS; ✦ Canadian drug name; ⊘ Prototype drug.

are sometimes called neuroleptics because they tend to reduce initiative and interest in the environment, decrease displays of emotions or affect, suppress spontaneous movements and complex behavior, and decrease psychotic symptoms. Spinal reflexes and unconditioned nociceptive-avoidance behaviors remain intact.

THERAPEUTIC EFFECTS Mechanism that produces strong antipsychotic effects is unclear, but thought to be related to blockade of postsynaptic dopamine receptors in the brain. Also has antiemetic effects due to its action on the CTZ.

USES To control manic phase of manic-depressive illness, for symptomatic management of psychotic disorders, including schizophrenia, in management of severe nausea and vomiting, to control excessive anxiety and agitation before surgery, and for treatment of severe behavior problems in children, e.g., attention deficit disorder. Also used for treatment of acute intermittent porphyria, intractable hiccups, and as adjunct in treatment of tetanus.

CONTRAINDICATIONS Hypersensitivity to phenothiazine derivatives; withdrawal states from alcohol; comatose states, brain damage, bone marrow depression, Reye's syndrome; children <6 mo; pregnancy (category C), lactation.
CAUTIOUS USE Agitated states accompanied by depression, seizure disorders, respiratory impairment due to infection or COPD; glaucoma, diabetes, hypertensive disease, peptic ulcer, prostatic hypertrophy; thyroid, cardiovascular, and hepatic disorders; patients exposed to extreme heat or organophosphate insecticides; previously detected breast cancer.

ROUTE & DOSAGE

Psychotic Disorders, Agitation
Child: **PO** >6 mo, 0.55 mg/kg q4–6h prn up to 500 mg/day **PR** >6 mo, 1.1 mg/kg q6–8h **IM/IV** >6 mo, 0.55 mg/kg q6–8h
Adult: **PO** 25–100 mg t.i.d. or q.i.d., may need up to 1000 mg/day **IM/IV** 25–50 mg up to 600 mg q4–6h

Nausea and Vomiting
Child: **PO** >6 mo, 0.55 mg/kg q4–6h prn up to 500 mg/day **PR** >6 mo, 1.1 mg/kg q6–8h **IM/IV** >6 mo, 0.55 mg/kg q6–8h
Adult: **PO** 10–25 mg q4–6h prn **PR** 50–100 mg q6–8h **IM/IV** 25–50 mg q3–4h prn

Intractable Hiccups
Adult: **PO/IM/IV** 25–50 mg t.i.d. or q.i.d.

STORAGE
Store all forms at 15°–30° C (59°–86° F) and protect from light. Avoid freezing.

ADMINISTRATION
Oral
- Give with food or a full glass of fluid to minimize GI distress.
- Ensure that oral drug is swallowed and not hoarded. Suicide attempt is

C

a constant possibility in depressed patients, particularly when they are improving.

- Mix chlorpromazine concentrate just before administration in at least ½ glass juice, milk, water, coffee, tea, carbonated beverage, or with semi-solid food.
- Ensure that sustained-release form of drug is not chewed or crushed. It must be swallowed whole.

Intramuscular/Intravenous

- Avoid parenteral drug contact with skin, eyes, and clothing because of its potential for causing contact dermatitis.
- Keep patient recumbent for at least ½ h after parenteral administration. Observe closely. Report hypotensive reactions.

Intramuscular

- Inject IM preparations slowly and deep into large muscle mass appropriate for age of child (see Part I). Avoid SC injection; it may cause tissue irritation and nodule formation. If irritation is a problem, consult prescriber about diluting medication with normal saline or 2% procaine. Rotate injection sites.

Intravenous

PREPARE **Direct:** Dilute 25 mg with 24 mL of NS to yield 1 mg/mL. **Continuous:** May be further diluted in up to 1000 mL of NS.

ADMINISTER **Direct:** Administer 1 mg or fraction thereof over 1 min for adults and over 2 min for children. **Continuous:** Give slowly at a rate not to exceed 1 mg/min. Lemon yellow color of parenteral preparation does not alter potency; if otherwise colored or markedly discolored, solution should be discarded.

INCOMPATIBILITIES **Solution/Additive: Aminophylline, amphotericin B, ampicillin, chloramphenicol, chlorothiazide, cimetidine, dimenhydrinate, furosemide, heparin, methohexital, penicillin G, pentobarbital, phenobarbital, thiopental. Y-Site: Allopurinol, amifostine, aminophylline, amphotericin B; cholesteryl complex, aztreonam, cefepime, chloramphenicol, chlorothiazide, etoposide, fludarabine, melphalan, methotrexate, paclitaxel, piperacillin/tazobactam, remifentanil, sargramostim.**

ADVERSE EFFECTS Body as a Whole: Idiopathic edema, muscle necrosis (following IM), SLE-like syndrome, <u>sudden unexplained death</u>. **CV:** Orthostatic hypotension, palpitation, tachycardia, ECG changes (usually reversible): prolonged QT and PR intervals, blunting of T waves, ST depression. **GI:** Dry mouth; constipation, <u>adynamicileus</u>, cholestatic jaundice, aggravation of peptic ulcer, dyspepsia, increased appetite. **Hematologic:** <u>Agranulocytosis</u>, thrombocytopenic purpura, <u>pancytopenia</u> (rare). **Metabolic:** Weight gain, hypoglycemia, hyperglycemia, glycosuria (high doses), enlargement of parotid glands. **CNS:** *Sedation, drowsiness,* dizziness, restlessness, <u>neuroleptic malignant syndrome</u>, tardive dyskinesias, tumor, syncope, headache, weakness, insomnia, reduced REM sleep, bizarre dreams, cerebral edema, convulsive seizures, <u>hypothermia,</u> inability to sweat, depressed cough reflex, *extrapyramidal symptoms,* EEG changes. **Respiratory:** <u>Laryngospasm</u>. **Skin:** Fixed-drug eruption, urticaria, reduced perspiration, contact

Common adverse effects in *italic;* life-threatening effects <u>underlined</u>; generic names in **bold;** drug classifications in SMALL CAPS; ♣ Canadian drug name; ✪ Prototype drug.

dermatitis, exfoliative dermatitis, photosensitivity, eczema, anaphylactoid reactions, hypersensitivity vasculitis; hirsutism (long term therapy). **Special Senses:** Blurred vision, lenticular opacities, mydriasis, photophobia. **Urogenital:** Anovulation, infertility, pseudopregnancy, menstrual irregularity, gynecomastia, galactorrhea, priapism, inhibition of ejaculation, reduced libido, urinary retention and frequency.

DIAGNOSTIC TEST INTERFERENCE Chlorpromazine (phenothiazines) may increase *cephalin flocculation,* and possibly other *liver function tests;* also may increase *PBI.* False-positive result may occur for *amylase, 5-hydroxyindoleacetic acid, porphobilinogens, urobilinogen (Ehrlich's reagent),* and *urine bilirubin (Bili-Labstix).* False-positive or false-negative *pregnancy test* results possibly caused by a metabolite of phenothiazines, which discolors urine depending on test used.

INTERACTIONS Drug: Alcohol, CNS DEPRESSANTS increase CNS depression; ANTACIDS, ANTIDIARRHEALS decrease absorption—space administration 2 h before or after administration of chlorpromazine; **phenobarbital** increases metabolism of phenothiazine; GENERAL ANESTHETICS increase excitation and hypotension; antagonizes antihypertensive action of **guanethidine; phenylpropanolamine** poses possibility of sudden death; TRICYCLIC ANTIDEPRESSANTS intensify hypotensive and anticholinergic effects; ANTICONVULSANTS decrease seizure threshold—may need to increase anticonvulsant dose. **Herbal: Kava-kava** increases risk and severity of dystonic reaction.

PHARMACOKINETICS Absorption: Rapid absorption with considerable first pass metabolism in liver; rapid absorption after IM. **Onset:** 30–60 min. **Peak:** 2–4 h PO; 15–20 min IM. **Duration:** 4–6 h. **Distribution:** Widely distributed; accumulates in brain; crosses placenta. **Metabolism:** Metabolized in liver. **Elimination:** Excreted in urine as metabolites; excreted in breast milk. **Half-Life:** Biphasic 2 and 30 h.

NURSING IMPLICATIONS

Assessment & Drug Effects

- Establish baseline BP (in standing and recumbent positions), and pulse, before initiating treatment.
- Monitor BP frequently. Hypotensive reactions, dizziness, and sedation are common during early therapy, particularly in patients on high doses and with parenteral doses. Patients usually develop tolerance to these adverse effects; however, lower doses or longer intervals between doses may be required.
- Lab tests: Periodic CBC with differential, liver function tests, urinalysis, and blood glucose.
- Monitor cardiac status with baseline ECG in patients with preexisting cardiovascular disease.
- Be alert for signs of neuroleptic malignant syndrome. Report immediately.
- Observe and record smoking since it increases metabolism of phenothiazines, resulting in shortened half-life and more rapid clearance of drug. Higher dosage in smokers may be required. Advise patient to stop or at least reduce smoking, if possible.

- Monitor I&O ratio and pattern: Urinary retention due to mental depression and compromised renal function may occur. If serum creatinine becomes elevated, therapy should be discontinued.
- Monitor for antiemetic effect of chlorpromazine, which may obscure signs of overdosage of other drugs or other causes of nausea and vomiting.
- Be alert to complaints of diminished visual acuity, reduced night vision, photophobia, and a perceived brownish discoloration of objects. Patient may be more comfortable with dark glasses.
- Monitor diabetics or prediabetics on long-term, high-dose therapy for reduced glucose tolerance and loss of diabetes control.
- Ocular examinations (and EEG recommended before and periodically during prolonged therapy.

Patient & Family Education
- Take medication as prescribed and keep appointments for follow-up evaluation of dosage regimen. Improvement may not be experienced until 7 or 8 wk into therapy.
- Do not alter dosing regimen, and do not give the drug to another person.
- May cause pink to red-brown discoloration of urine.
- Wear protective clothing and sunscreen lotion with SPF above 12 when outdoors, even on dark days. Photosensitivity associated with chlorpromazine therapy is a phototoxic reaction. Severity of response depends on amount of exposure and drug dose. Exposed skin areas have appearance of an exaggerated sunburn. If reaction occurs, report to physician.
- Practice meticulous oral hygiene. Oral candidiasis occurs frequently in patients receiving phenothiazines.
- Report extrapyramidal symptoms that occur most often in patients on high dosage, the pediatric patient with severe dehydration and acute infection, and females.
- Avoid driving a car or undertaking activities requiring precision and mental alertness until drug response is known.
- Do not abruptly stop this drug. Abrupt withdrawal of drug or deliberate dose skipping, especially after prolonged therapy with large doses, can cause onset of extrapyramidal symptoms and severe GI disturbances. When drug is to be discontinued, dosage must be tapered off gradually over a period of several weeks.
- Do not breast feed while taking this drug.
- Store this medication out of reach of children.

CHLORTHALIDONE
(klor-thal_i-done)
Hygroton, Hylidone, Novothalidone ♣, Thalitone, Uridon ♣
Classifications: ELECTROLYTE AND WATER BALANCE AGENT; THIAZIDE DIURETIC
Prototype: Hydrochlorothiazide
Pregnancy Category: B

Common adverse effects in *italic;* life-threatening effects underlined; generic names in **bold;** drug classifications in SMALL CAPS; ♣ Canadian drug name; ◑ Prototype drug.

AVAILABILITY 15 mg, 25 mg, 50 mg, 100 mg tablets

ACTIONS Sulfonamide derivative. Differs chemically from thiazides but shares similar actions. Increases excretion of sodium and chloride by inhibiting their reabsorption in the cortical diluting segment of the ascending loop of Henle. Reportedly, in some individuals, it causes elevations in total cholesterol, LDL cholesterol, and triglycerides.
THERAPEUTIC EFFECTS Antihypertensive effect is correlated to the decrease in extracellular and intracellular volumes. Decreased volume results in reduced cardiac output with subsequent decrease in peripheral resistance.

USES Edema associated with CHF, renal decompensation, hepatic cirrhosis, corticosteroid and estrogen therapy; as sole agent or with other antihypertensives to treat hypertension.

CONTRAINDICATIONS Hypersensitivity to sulfonamide derivatives; anuria, hypokalemia; pregnancy (category B), lactation. Safe use in children not established.
CAUTIOUS USE History of renal and hepatic disease, gout, SLE, diabetes mellitus.

ROUTE & DOSAGE

Hypertension
Child: **PO** 2 mg/kg 3 times/wk
Adult: **PO** 12.5–25 mg/day, may be increased to 100 mg/day if needed
Edema
Adult: **PO** 50–100 mg/day, may be increased to 200 mg/day if needed

STORAGE
Store tablets in tightly closed container at 15°–30° C (59°–86° F).

ADMINISTRATION
Oral
- Administer as single dose in a.m. to reduce potential for interrupted sleep because of diuresis.
- Consult physician when chlorthalidone is used as a diuretic; an intermittent dose schedule may reduce incidence of adverse reactions.

ADVERSE EFFECTS CV: Orthostatic hypotension. **GI:** Anorexia, nausea, vomiting, diarrhea, constipation, cramping, jaundice. **Hematologic:** <u>Agranulocytosis</u>, thrombocytopenia, <u>aplastic anemia</u>. **CNS:** Dizziness, vertigo, paresthesias, headache. **Metabolic:** *Hypokalemia,* hyponatremia, hypochloremia, hypercalcemia, glycosuria, hyperglycemia, exacerbation of gout. **Skin:** Rash, urticaria, photosensitivity, vasculitis. **Urogenital:** Impotence.

INTERACTIONS Drug: Increased risk of **digoxin** toxicity because of hypokalemia; CORTICOSTEROIDS, **amphotericin B** increase hypokalemia; decreases **lithium** elimination; may antagonize the hypoglycemic effects

---

of SULFONYLUREAS; NSAIDS may attenuate diuretic effects; **cholestyramine** decreases thiazide absorption.

PHARMACOKINETICS Absorption: Readily absorbed from GI tract. **Onset:** 2 h. **Peak:** 3–6 h. **Duration:** 24–72 h. **Distribution:** Crosses placenta; appears in breast milk. **Elimination:** 30–60% excreted in urine in 24 h. **Half-Life:** 54 h.

NURSING IMPLICATIONS

Assessment & Drug Effects

- Establish baseline BP measurements and check at regular intervals during period of dosage adjustment when chlorthalidone is used for hypertension.
- Be alert to signs of hypokalemia.
- Lab tests: Baseline and periodic: serum electrolytes (particularly K, Mg, Ca), serum uric acid, creatinine, BUN, and uric acid and blood glucose (especially in patients with diabetes).
- Monitor lithium and digoxin levels closely when either of these drugs is used concurrently.

Patient & Family Education

- Maintain adequate potassium intake, monitor weight, and make a daily estimate of I&O ratio.
- Do not breast feed while taking this drug.
- Store this medication out of reach of children.

CHLORZOXAZONE

(klor-zox′a-zone)
Paraflex, Parafon Forte
Classifications: AUTONOMIC NERVOUS SYSTEM AGENT; CENTRALLY ACTING SKELETAL MUSCLE RELAXANT
Prototype: Cyclobenzaprine
Pregnancy Category: C

AVAILABILITY 250 mg, 500 mg tablets

ACTIONS Centrally acting skeletal muscle relaxant. Acts indirectly by depressing nerve transmission through polysynaptic pathways in spinal cord, subcortical centers, and brain stem; also possibly has a sedative effect.
THERAPEUTIC EFFECTS Effectively controls muscle spasms and pain associated with musculoskeletal conditions. Not effective for spastic or dyskinetic CNS disorders, e.g., cerebral palsy.

USE Symptomatic treatment of muscle spasm and pain associated with various musculoskeletal conditions.

CONTRAINDICATIONS Impaired liver function; pregnancy (category C), lactation.
CAUTIOUS USE Patients with known allergies or history of drug allergies; history of liver disease.

ROUTE & DOSAGE

Skeletal Muscle Relaxant
Child: **PO** 20 mg/kg/day divided into 3–4 doses
Adult: **PO** 250–500 mg t.i.d. or q.i.d. (max 3 g/day)

STORAGE

Store in tightly closed container at 15°–30° C (59°–86° F).

ADMINISTRATION

Oral

- Give with food or meals to prevent gastric distress. If necessary, tablet may be crushed and mixed with food or liquid, e.g., milk, fruit juice.

ADVERSE EFFECTS GI: Anorexia, heartburn, nausea, vomiting, constipation, diarrhea, abdominal pain, hepatotoxicity: jaundice, liver damage. **CNS:** *Drowsiness, dizziness,* light-headedness, headache, malaise, overstimulation. **Skin:** Erythema, rash, pruritus, urticaria, petechiae, ecchymoses.

INTERACTIONS Drug: Alcohol, CNS DEPRESSANTS add to CNS depression.

PHARMACOKINETICS Absorption: Readily absorbed from GI tract. **Onset:** 1 h. **Peak:** 1–4 h. **Duration:** 3–4 h. **Distribution:** Not known if crosses placenta or distributed into breast milk. **Metabolism:** Metabolized in liver. **Elimination:** Excreted in urine. **Half-Life:** 66 min.

NURSING IMPLICATIONS

Assessment & Drug Effects

- Monitor ambulation during early drug therapy; some patients may require supervision.
- Lab tests: Periodic liver function tests are advised in patients receiving long-term therapy even if sporadic.
- Note: Since chlorzoxazone metabolite may discolor urine, dark urine cannot be a reliable sign of a hepatotoxic reaction.

Patient & Family Education

- Avoid activities requiring mental alertness, judgment, and physical coordination until reaction to drug is known, because sedation, drowsiness, and dizziness may occur.
- Drug may discolor urine orange to purplish red, but this is of no clinical significance.
- Discontinue drug and notify physician if signs of hypersensitivity or of liver dysfunction appear (abdominal discomfort, yellow sclerae or skin, pruritus, malaise, nausea, vomiting).
- Check with physician before taking an OTC depressant (e.g., antihistamine, sedative, alcohol) because effects may be additive.
- Do not breast feed while using this drug.
- Store this medication out of reach of children.

Common adverse effects in *italic;* life-threatening effects <u>underlined</u>; generic names in **bold;** drug classifications in SMALL CAPS; ♣ Canadian drug name; ● Prototype drug.

315

CHOLESTYRAMINE RESIN Pr
(koe-less-tear′a-meen)
LoCHOLEST, Questran, Questran Light, Prevalyte
Classifications: CARDIOVASCULAR AGENT; ANTILIPEMIC; BILE ACID SEQUESTRANT
Pregnancy Category: C

AVAILABILITY 4 g powder for suspension; 1 g tablet

ACTIONS Anion-exchange resin used for its cholesterol-lowering effect. Adsorbs and combines with intestinal bile acids in exchange for chloride ions to form an insoluble, nonabsorbable complex that is excreted in the feces. As a result, bile salts are continually (but not entirely) prevented from reentry into the enterohepatic circulation, thus, increasing fecal loss of bile acids. This leads to lowered serum total cholesterol by decreasing low density lipoprotein (LDL) cholesterol.

THERAPEUTIC EFFECTS The resin anion-exchange agent increases fecal loss of bile acids, which leads to lowered serum total cholesterol by decreasing LDL cholesterol, and reducing bile acid deposit in dermal tissues (decreasing pruritis). Serum triglyceride levels may increase or remain unchanged.

USES As adjunct to diet therapy in management of patients with primary hypercholesterolemia (type IIa hyperlipedemia) with a significant risk of atherosclerotic heart disease and MI; for relief of pruritus secondary to partial biliary stasis.

UNLABELED USES To control diarrhea caused by excess bile acids in colon; for hyperoxaluria.

CONTRAINDICATIONS Complete biliary obstruction, hypersensitivity to bile acid sequestrants; pregnancy (category C), lactation. Safe use in children ≤6 y not established.

CAUTIOUS USE Bleeding disorders; hemorrhoids; impaired GI function, peptic ulcer, malabsorption states (e.g., steatorrhea); phenylketonuria (Questran Light only).

ROUTE & DOSAGE

Hypercholesterolemia
Child: **PO** 240 mg/kg/day divided into 3 doses
Adult: **PO** 4 g b.i.d. to q.i.d. a.c. and at bedtime, may need up to 24 g/day

STORAGE
Store in tightly closed container at 15°–30° C (59°–86° F).

ADMINISTRATION

Oral
- Place contents of one packet or one level scoopful on surface of at least 120 to 180 mL (4–6 oz) of water or other preferred liquid. Permit drug to hydrate by standing without stirring 1–2 min, twirling glass

occasionally, then stir until suspension is uniform. Rinse glass with small amount of liquid and have patient drink remainder to ensure entire dose is taken. Administer before meals.

- Always dissolve cholestyramine powder before administration; it is irritating to mucous membranes and may cause esophageal impaction if administered dry.

ADVERSE EFFECTS GI: *Constipation,* fecal impaction, hemorrhoids, abdominal pain and distension, flatulence, bloating sensation, belching, nausea, vomiting, heartburn, anorexia, diarrhea, steatorrhea. **Endocrine:** Increased libido. **Metabolic:** Weight loss or gain, iron, calcium, vitamin A, D, and K deficiencies (from poor absorption); hypoprothrombinemia, hyperchloremic acidosis, decreased erythrocyte folate levels, **Skin:** Rash, irritations of skin, tongue, and perianal areas. **Special Senses:** Arcus juvenilis, uveitis.

DIAGNOSTIC TEST INTERFERENCE Cholestyramine therapy may be accompanied by increased *serum AST, phosphorus, chloride,* and *alkaline phosphatase* levels; decreased *serum calcium, sodium,* and *potassium* levels.

INTERACTIONS Drug: Decreases the absorption of ORAL ANTICOAGULANTS, **digoxin,** TETRACYCLINES, **penicillins, phenobarbital,** THYROID HORMONES, THIAZIDE DIURETICS, IRON SALTS, FAT-SOLUBLE VITAMINS (A, D, E, K) from the GI tract—administer cholestyramine 4 h before or 2 h after these drugs.

PHARMACOKINETICS Absorption: Not absorbed from GI tract. **Elimination:** Excreted in feces as insoluble complex.

NURSING IMPLICATIONS

Assessment & Drug Effects

- Administer 4 h before or 2 h after vitamins A, D, E and K if they are given orally.
- Monitor therapeutic effect. Serum cholesterol levels are reduced within 24–48 h after treatment starts and may continue to decline for a year. After withdrawal of cholestyramine, cholesterol levels usually return to baseline level in about 2 to 4 wk.
- Be alert to early symptoms of hypoprothrombinemia (petechiae, ecchymoses, abnormal bleeding from mucous membranes, tarry stools) and report their occurrence promptly. Long-term use of cholestyramine resin can increase bleeding tendency.
- Preexisting constipation may be worsened especially in those taking >24 g/day.
- Consult prescriber regarding supplemental vitamins A and D and folic acid that may be required by patient on long-term therapy.
- Lab tests: Periodic CBC, platelet count, serum electrolytes, and lipid profile.

Patient & Family Education

- Report constipation immediately. High-bulk diet with adequate fluid intake is an essential adjunct to cholestyramine treatment and generally resolves the problems of constipation and bloating sensation.

- Do not omit doses. Sudden withdrawal can promote uninhibited absorption of other drugs taken concomitantly, leading to toxicity or overdosage.
- GI adverse effects usually subside after the first month of drug therapy.
- The following symptoms may be drug-induced and should be reported promptly: severe gastric distress with nausea and vomiting, unusual weight loss, black stools, severe hemorrhoids (GI bleeding), sudden back pain.
- Do not breast feed while using this drug.
- Store this medication out of reach of children.

CHOLINE MAGNESIUM TRISALICYLATE
(cho'leen mag-ne'si-um tri-sal'ici-late)
Trilisate
Classifications: CENTRAL NERVOUS SYSTEM AGENT; ANALGESIC, SALICYLATE; ANTIPYRETIC
Prototype: Aspirin
Pregnancy Category: C

AVAILABILITY 500 mg, 750 mg, 1000 mg tablets; 500 mg/5 mL liquid

ACTIONS Trilisate is a nonsteroidal, anti-inflammatory preparation combining choline salicylate and magnesium salicylate. Mode of action is by inhibiting prostaglandin synthesis.
THERAPEUTIC EFFECTS Trilisate has anti-inflammatory, analgesic and antipyretic action. Platelet aggregation is not affected.

USES Osteoarthritis, rheumatoid arthritis, and other arthrides. Preferable to aspirin for patients with GI bleeding.

CONTRAINDICATIONS Hypersensitivity to nonacetylated salicylates; children <6 y; children and teenagers with chickenpox, influenza, or flu symptoms because of the potential for Reye's syndrome; pregnancy (category C); contraindicated in late pregnancy, near term, or in labor and delivery.
CAUTIOUS USE Chronic renal and hepatic failure, peptic ulcer; patients on coumadin or heparin; lactation; older adults.

ROUTE & DOSAGE

Arthritis
Adult: **PO** 1.5–2.5 g/day divided into 2–3 doses (max 4.5 g/day)
Mild to Moderate Pain, Fever
Child: **PO** 30–60 mg/kg/day divided into 3–4 doses
Adult: **PO** 2–3 g/day divided into 2 doses

STORAGE
Store at 15°–30° C (59°–86° F).

ADMINISTRATION

Oral

■ Give with food to reduce gastric upset. Do not give with antacids.

ADVERSE EFFECTS GI: Vomiting, diarrhea. **CNS:** Headache, vertigo, confusion, drowsiness. **Special Senses:** Tinnitus.

INTERACTIONS Drug: Aminosalicylic acid increases risk of salicylate toxicity; **ammonium chloride** and other **acidifying agents** decrease its renal elimination, increasing risk of salicylate toxicity; ANTICOAGULANTS increase risk of bleeding; CARBONIC ANHYDRASE INHIBITORS enhance salicylate toxicity; CORTICOSTEROIDS compound ulcerogenic effects; increases **methotrexate** toxicity; low doses of salicylates may antagonize uricosuric effects of **probenecid, sulfinpyrazone.**

PHARMACOKINETICS Absorption: Readily absorbed from small intestine. **Onset:** 30 min. **Peak:** 1–3 h. **Metabolism:** Metabolized in liver. **Elimination:** Excreted in urine. **Half-Life:** 2–3 h.

NURSING IMPLICATIONS

Assessment & Drug Effects

■ As with other NSAIDS, the antipyretic and anti-inflammatory effects may mask usual S&S of infection or other diseases.
■ Assess for GI discomfort; nausea, gastric irritation, indigestion, diarrhea, and constipation are frequent complaints.
■ Monitor for S&S of bleeding. Closely monitor PT if used concurrently with warfarin.

Patient & Family Education

■ Avoid taking aspirin, NSAIDs, or acetaminophen concurrently with drug.
■ Avoid dangerous activities until reaction to drug is determined, due to possible CNS effects (e.g., vertigo, drowsiness).
■ Report tinnitus or persistent gastric irritation and epigastric pain.
■ Report any unexplained bruising or bleeding to physician.
■ Hypoglycemic effects may be enhanced for those with type 2 diabetes taking an oral hypoglycemic agent (OHA).
■ Do not give to children or teenagers with chickenpox, influenza, or flu symptoms because of association with Reye syndrome.
■ Do not breast feed while taking this drug without consulting physician.
■ Store this medication out of reach of children.

CHOLINE SALICYLATE

(koe′leen)

Arthropan

Classifications: CENTRAL NERVOUS SYSTEM AGENT; ANALGESIC, SALICYLATE; ANTIPYRETIC

Prototype: Aspirin

Pregnancy Category: C

AVAILABILITY 870 mg/5 mL liquid

ACTIONS Choline salt of salicylic acid available commercially as a liquid preparation that is a nonsteroidal anti-inflammatory agent. Mode of action is by inhibiting prostaglandin synthesis.

THERAPEUTIC EFFECTS Reported to be less potent than aspirin as an analgesic, anti-inflammatory, and antipyretic, and produces less gastric irritation and bleeding. Unlike aspirin, believed to have no appreciable effect on platelet function.

USES Analgesic and anti-inflammatory in rheumatoid arthritis, rheumatic fever, osteoarthritis, and other conditions for which oral salicylates are usually recommended. May be indicated for patients who have difficulty swallowing tablets or capsules or as an alternative preparation for patients who show gastric intolerance to aspirin or who should avoid sodium-containing salicylates.

CONTRAINDICATIONS Salicylate hypersensitivity; children <12 y; children and teenagers with chickenpox, influenza, or flu symptoms because of the potential for Reye's syndrome; pregnancy (category C); contraindicated in late pregnancy, near term, or in labor and delivery.

CAUTIOUS USE Chronic renal and hepatic failure, peptic ulcer; patients on coumadin or heparin; lactation; older adults.

ROUTE & DOSAGE

Analgesic, Antipyretic
Child: **PO** 2–11 y, 2 g (11.5 mL)/m^2 in 4–6 divided doses
Adult: **PO** 435–870 mg (2.5–5 mL) q4h

Arthritis
Child: **PO** 107–134 mg (0.6–0.8 mL)/kg/day in 4–6 divided doses
Adult: **PO** 4.8–7.2 g (28–41 mL)/day in 4–6 divided doses

STORAGE
Store in tightly capped container at 15°–30° C (59°–86° F). Protect from freezing.

ADMINISTRATION

Oral

- May be mixed with or followed by fruit juice, a carbonated beverage, or water. Do not administer with an antacid.
- If patient requires an antacid, administer choline salicylate before meals and the antacid 2 h after meals.

ADVERSE EFFECTS GI: *Nausea,* vomiting, hepatotoxicity. **CNS:** Dizziness, sweating, mental confusion, hyperventilation. **Special Senses:** Tinnitus, deafness.

DIAGNOSTIC TEST INTERFERENCE As for aspirin with the exception of *5-HIAA,* which is not affected by choline salicylate.

INTERACTIONS Drug: Aminosalicylate increases risk of salicylate toxicity; increases risk of bleeding with ORAL ANTICOAGULANTS; SULFONYLUREAS pose increased risk of hypoglycemia with large doses of salicylates; CARBONIC ANHYDRASE INHIBITORS cause metabolic acidosis that may increase salicylate toxicity; CORTICOSTEROIDS add to ulcerogenic effects; may increase **methotrexate** levels; small doses of salicylates may blunt uricosuric effects of **probenecid, sulfinpyrazone.**

PHARMACOKINETICS Absorption: Readily absorbed from GI tract. **Peak:** 10–30 min. **Distribution:** Widely distributed in most body tissues; crosses placenta; distributed in breast milk. **Elimination:** Excreted in urine. **Half-Life:** 2–3 h.

NURSING IMPLICATIONS

Assessment & Drug Effects

■ Monitor effectiveness of drug in relieving pain in arthritic joints.
■ Assess for signs of bleeding, especially in patients on anticoagulant therapy.

Patient & Family Education

■ Report any of the following to physician: Tinnitus, persistent gastric irritation, epigastric pain, unexplained bruising or bleeding.
■ This drug is available OTC. Do not exceed recommended dosage and keep medicine out of the reach of children.
■ Avoid concurrent use of other drugs containing aspirin or salicylates unless otherwise advised by prescriber.
■ Do not breast feed without consulting prescriber.
■ Store this medication out of reach of children.

CHORIONIC GONADOTROPIN

(go-nad'oh-troe-pin)
Antuitrin, A.P.L., Chorex, Chorigon, Choron 10, Corgonject-5, Follutein, Glukor, Gonic, HCG, Pregnyl, Profasi HP
Classifications: HORMONE & SYNTHETIC SUBSTITUTE
Pregnancy Category: X

AVAILABILITY 5,000 units, 10,000 units, 20,000 units in vials

ACTIONS Human chorionic gonadotropin (HCG) is a polypeptide hormone produced by the placenta and extracted from urine during first trimester of pregnancy. Actions nearly identical to those of pituitary luteinizing hormone (LH). Promotes production of gonadal steroid hormones by stimulating interstitial cells of the testes to produce androgen, and the corpus luteum of the ovary to produce progesterone.
THERAPEUTIC EFFECTS Administration of HCG to women of childbearing age with normal functioning ovaries causes maturation of the ovarian follicle and triggers ovulation. When given during normal pregnancy, it maintains corpus luteum after LH decreases, supports continuing secretion of estrogen and progesterone, and prevents ovulation.

USES Prepubertal cryptorchidism not due to anatomic obstruction and male hypogonadism secondary to pituitary deficiency. Also used in

---

Common adverse effects in *italic;* life-threatening effects underlined; generic names in **bold;** drug classifications in SMALL CAPS; ♣ Canadian drug name; ✪ Prototype drug.

C

conjunction with menotropins to induce ovulation and pregnancy in infertile women in whom the cause of anovulation is secondary; ovulation usually occurs within 18 h. To stimulate spermatogenesis in males with hypogonadism.

UNLABELED USES Corpus luteum dysfunction.

CONTRAINDICATIONS Known hypersensitivity to HCG, hypogonadism of testicular origin, hypertrophy or tumor of pituitary, prostatic carcinoma or other androgen-dependent neoplasms, precocious puberty; children <4 y. Pregnancy (category X).

CAUTIOUS USE Epilepsy, migraine, asthma, cardiac or renal disease; lactation.

ROUTE & DOSAGE

Prepubertal Cryptorchidism

Child: **IM** 4000 units 3 times/wk for 3 wk *or* 5000 units every other day for 4 doses, *or* 500–1000 units 3 times/wk for 4–6 wk

STORAGE

Store powder for injection at 15°–30° C (59°–86° F). Following reconstitution solution is stable for 30–90 days, depending on manufacturer, when refrigerated; thereafter potency decreases.

ADMINISTRATION

- Reconstitute only with diluent supplied by manufacturer.
- Inject it into appropriate muscle mass for age (see Part I).

ADVERSE EFFECTS Body as a Whole: Edema, pain at injection site, arterial thromboembolism. **Endocrine:** Gynecomastia, precocious puberty, increased urinary steroid excretion, ectopic pregnancy (incidence low). When used with menotropins (human menopausal gonadotropin): Ovarian hyperstimulation (ascites with or without pain, pleural effusion, ruptured ovarian cysts with resultant hemoperitoneum, multiple births). **CNS:** Headache, irritability, restlessness, depression, fatigue.

DIAGNOSTIC TEST INTERFERENCE *Pregnancy tests:* Possibility of false results.

INTERACTIONS Drug: No clinically significant drug interactions established. **Herbal: Black cohosh** may antagonize fertility effects.

PHARMACOKINETICS Onset: 2 h. **Peak:** 6 h. **Distribution:** Testes in males, ovaries in females. **Elimination:** 10–12% excreted in urine within 24 h. **Half-Life:** 23 h.

NURSING IMPLICATIONS

Assessment & Drug Effects

- Assess prepubescent males for development of secondary sex characteristics.

Patient & Family Education

- Treatment for prepubertal cryptorchidism is usually started between 4 and 9 y. HCG can help predict whether orchidopexy will be needed in the future.
- Report to physician if the following appear: Axillary, facial, pubic hair; penile growth; acne; deepening of voice. Induction of androgen secretion by HCG may induce precocious puberty in patient treated for cryptorchidism.
- Observe for signs of fluid retention. A weight chart should be maintained for a biweekly record. Report to health care provider if weight gain is associated with edema.

CIMETIDINE ⊕
(sye-met′i-deen)
Novocimetine ♣ , Peptol ♣ , Tagamet, Tagamet HB
Classifications: GASTROINTESTINAL AGENT; ANTISECRETORY (H₂-RECEPTOR ANTAGONIST)
Pregnancy Category: B

AVAILABILITY 100 mg, 200 mg, 400 mg, 800 mg tablets; 300 mg/5 mL liquid; 150 mg/mL injection

ACTIONS Enzyme inhibitor structurally similar to histamine. Belongs to the antihistamine group with high selectivity for histamine H_2-receptors on parietal cells of the stomach (minimal effect on H_1 receptors). By reversible competitive inhibition of histamine at the H_2-receptor sites, it suppresses all phases of daytime and nocturnal basal gastric acid secretion in the stomach. Indirectly reduces pepsin secretion; it is not a cholinergic. Has no effect on lower esophageal sphincter pressure, gastric motility or emptying, biliary or pancreatic secretion.
THERAPEUTIC EFFECTS Cimetidine blocks the H_2 receptor on the parietal cells of the stomach, thus decreasing gastric acid secretion, raises the pH of the stomach and, thereby, reduces pepsin secretion.

USES Short-term treatment of active duodenal ulcer and prevention of ulcer recurrence (at reduced dosage) after it is healed. Also used for short-term treatment of active benign gastric ulcer, pathologic hypersecretory conditions such as Zollinger-Ellison syndrome, and heartburn.
UNLABELED USES Prophylaxis of stress-induced ulcers, upper GI bleeding, and aspiration pneumonitis; gastroesophageal reflux; chronic urticaria; acetaminophen toxicity.

CONTRAINDICATIONS Known hypersensitivity to cimetidine or other H_2-receptor antagonists; lactation, pregnancy (category B). Safe use in children <16 y not established.
CAUTIOUS USE Critically ill; impaired renal or hepatic function; organic brain syndrome; gastric ulcers; immunocompromised patients.

ROUTE & DOSAGE

Duodenal Ulcer

Neonate: **PO/IM/IV** 5–10 mg/kg/day divided into doses q8–12h
Infant: **PO/IM/IV** 10–20 mg/kg/day divided into doses q6–12h
Child: **PO/IM/IV** 20–40 mg/kg/day divided into 4 doses
Adult: **PO** 300 mg q.i.d. *or* 400 mg b.i.d. *or* 800 mg at bedtime
IM/IV 300 mg q6–8h

Duodenal Ulcer, Maintenance Therapy

Adult: **PO** 400 mg at bedtime

Gastric Ulcer

Adult: **PO** 300 mg q.i.d. with meals and at bedtime **IM/IV** 300 mg q6–8h

Heartburn

Adult: **PO** 200 mg 2–4 times/day

Pathologic Hypersecretory Disease

Adult: **PO** 300 mg q.i.d. with meals and at bedtime, may increase up to 2400 mg/day **IM/IV** 300 mg q6–8h, may increase up to 2400 mg/day

Adjustment for Renal Impairment

Cl_{cr} 20–40 mL/min: dose q8h
Cl_{cr} <20 mL/min: dose q12h

STORAGE

Store all forms at 15°–30° C (59°–86° F) protected from light. Parenteral solutions are stable for 48 h at room temperature when added to commonly used IV solutions for dilution. Follow manufacturer's directions.

ADMINISTRATION

Oral

- Give 1 h before or 2 h after an antacid.

Intravenous

- IV administration to neonates, infants and children: Verify correct IV concentration and rate of infusion/injection with physician.

PREPARE **Direct:** Dilute 300 mg in 18 mL D5W or NS to yield 300 mg/ 20 mL. **Intermittent:** Dilute 300 mg in 50 mL D5W or NS. **Continuous:** Further dilute in up to 1000 mL of selected IV solution.

ADMINISTER **Direct:** Give 300 mg or fraction thereof over last 5 min. **Intermittent:** Give over 15–20 min. **Continuous:** Give a loading dose of 150 mg at the intermittent infusion rate; then give continuous infusion equally spaced over 24 h.

INCOMPATIBILITIES **Solution/Additive: Amphotericin B, atropine, cefamandole, cefazolin, chlorpromazine, pentobarbital, secobarbital. Y-Site: Allopurinol, amphotericin B cholesteryl complex, amsacrine, cefepime, indomethacin, warfarin.**

ADVERSE EFFECTS Body as a Whole: Fever. **CV:** (Rare) <u>Cardiac arrhythmias and cardiac arrest</u> after rapid IV bolus dose. **GI:** Mild transient diarrhea; severe diarrhea, constipation, abdominal discomfort. **Hematologic:** Increased prothrombin time; neutropenia (rare), thrombocytopenia (rare), <u>aplastic anemia</u>. **Metabolic:** Slight increase in serum uric acid, BUN, creatinine; transient pain at IM site; hypospermia. **Musculoskeletal:** Exacerbation of joint symptoms in patients with preexisting arthritis. **CNS:** Drowsiness, dizziness, light-headedness, depression, headache, reversible confusional states, paranoid psychosis. **Skin:** Rash, Stevens-Johnson syndrome, reversible alopecia. **Urogenital:** Gynecomastia and breast soreness, galactorrhea, reversible impotence.

DIAGNOSTIC TEST INTERFERENCE Cimetidine may cause false-positive *hemoccult test for gastric bleeding* if test is performed within 15 min of oral cimetidine administration.

INTERACTIONS Drug: Cimetidine decreases the hepatic metabolism of **warfarin, phenobarbital, phenytoin, diazepam, propranolol, lidocaine, theophylline,** thus increasing their activity and toxicity; ANTACIDS may decrease absorption of cimetidine.

PHARMACOKINETICS Absorption: 70% of oral dose absorbed from GI tract. **Peak:** 1–1.5 h. **Distribution:** Widely distributed; crosses blood–brain barrier and placenta. **Metabolism:** Metabolized in liver. **Elimination:** Most of drug excreted in urine in 24 h; excreted in breast milk. **Half-Life:** 2 h.

NURSING IMPLICATIONS

Assessment & Drug Effects

- Ulcer healing may occur within the first 2 wk of therapy but generally requires at least 4 wk in most individuals. Short-term (i.e., 8-wk) therapy of active duodenal ulcer does not prevent ulcer recurrence when drug is discontinued.
- Monitor pulse of patient during first few days of drug regimen. Bradycardia after PO as well as IV administration should be reported. Pulse usually returns to normal within 24 h after drug discontinuation.
- Monitor I&O ratio and pattern.
- Report loss of bowel sounds, absence of bowel movement or flatus, vomiting, crampy pain, abdominal distention. Adynamic ileus has been reported in patients receiving cimetidine to prevent and treat stress ulcers.
- Lab tests: Periodic evaluations of blood count and renal and hepatic function are advised during therapy.
- Be alert to onset of confusion. Symptoms occur within 2–3 days after first dose. Report immediately; drug should be withdrawn. Symptoms usually resolve within 3–4 days after therapy is discontinued.
- Check BP and report an elevation to the prescriber, if patient complains of severe headache.
- Cimetidine impairs absorption of protein-bound vitamin B_{12}; therefore, patient who takes cimetidine in divided doses to continuously suppress acid gastric secretion is at risk for vitamin B_{12} deficiency (no risk for patient who takes drug at bedtime to suppress nocturnal acid production).

Patient & Family Education

- Cimetidine must be taken exactly as prescribed. Sudden discontinuation of therapy reportedly has caused perforation of chronic peptic ulcer.
- Seek advice about self-medication with any OTC drug.

C

- Report breast tenderness or enlargement. Mild bilateral gynecomastia and breast soreness may occur after ≥ 1 mo of therapy. It may disappear spontaneously or remain throughout therapy.
- Report recurrence of gastric pain or bleeding (black, tarry stools or "coffee-grounds" vomitus) immediately and notify prescriber if diarrhea continues more than 1 day.
- Avoid driving and other potentially hazardous activities until reaction to drug is known.
- Duodenal or gastric ulcer is a chronic, recurrent condition that requires long-term maintenance drug therapy.
- Maintenance therapy at reduced dosage after healing of active duodenal ulcer appears to limit recurrence, particularly if other therapeutic measures are taken such as avoiding smoking and reducing stress.
- Do not breast feed while taking this drug.
- Store this medication out of reach of children.

CIPROFLOXACIN HYDROCHLORIDE ⓟ
(ci-pro-flox′a-cin)
Cipro, Cipro IV, Cipro XR

CIPROFLOXACIN OPHTHALMIC

Ciloxan

Classifications: ANTI-INFECTIVE; QUINOLONE ANTIBIOTIC
Pregnancy Category: C

AVAILABILITY 100 mg, 250 mg, 500 mg, 750 mg tablets; 500 mg extended-release tablets; 50 mg/mL, 100 mg/mL suspension; 200 mg, 400 mg injection; 3.5 mg/mL ophthalmic solution

ACTIONS Synthetic quinolone that is a broad-spectrum bactericidal agent. Inhibits DNA-gyrase, an enzyme necessary for bacterial DNA replication and some aspects of transcription, repair, recombination, and transposition.

THERAPEUTIC EFFECTS Effective against many gram-positive and gram-negative organisms including *Citrobacter diversus, Enterobacter cloacae, Enterobacter aerogenes, Escherichia coli, Haemophilus influenzae, Klebsiella pneumoniae, Neisseria gonorrhoeae, Proteus mirabilis, P. vulgaris, Pseudomonas aeruginosa, Serratia marcescens, Staphylococcus aureus, S. pyogenes, Shigella,* and *Salmonella.* Less active against gram-positive than gram-negative bacteria, although active against many gram-positive aerobic bacteria, including penicillinase-producing, non-penicillinase-producing, and methicillin-resistant *Staphylococci.* However, many strains of *Streptococci* are relatively resistant to the drug. Inactive against most anaerobic bacteria. Resistant to some strains of methicillin-resistant *Staphylococcus aureus* (MRSA).

USES UTIs, lower respiratory tract infections, skin and skin structure infections, bone and joint infections, GI infection or infectious diarrhea, chronic bacterial prostatitis, nosocomial pneumonia, acute sinusitis; post-exposure prophylaxis for anthrax. **Ophthalmic:** Corneal ulcers, bacterial conjunctivitis caused by *Staphylococci, Streptococci,* and *P. aeruginosa.*

CONTRAINDICATIONS Known hypersensitivity to ciprofloxacin or other quinolones, pregnant women (category C), lactation.
CAUTIOUS USE Known or suspected CNS disorders (i.e., severe cerebral arteriosclerosis or seizure disorders), patients receiving theophylline derivatives or caffeine, severe renal impairment and crystalluria during ciprofloxacin therapy, and patients on coumarin therapy. This and other quinolones have caused arthropathy in developing animals, and safety in children under 18 y is not proven. Has been used in children when no other agent is available. Use with extreme caution.

ROUTE & DOSAGE

Uncomplicated UTI
Adult: **PO** 250 mg q12h or 500 mg XR daily for 3 days **IV** 200 mg q12h, infused over 60 min

Complicated UTI
Adult: **PO** 1000 mg XR daily for 7–14 days **IV** 400 mg q12h, infused over 60 min

Acute Sinusitis
Adult: **PO** 500 mg b.i.d. for 10 days

Moderate to Severe Systemic Infection
Child: **PO** 20–30 mg/kg/day divided into 2 doses (max 1.5 g/day) **IV** 10–20 g/kg/day divided into 2 doses (max 800 mg/day)
Adult: **PO** 500–750 mg q12h **IV** 200–400 mg q12h, infused over 60 min

Renal Impairment
Cl_{cr} 30–50 mL/min: **PO** 250–500 mg q12h, **IV** no change in dose; <30 mL/min: **PO** 250–500 mg q 18 h, **IV** 200–400 mg q 18–24h

Cystic Fibrosis
Child: **PO** 40 mg/kg/day divided into 2 doses (max 2 g/day) **IV** 30 mg/kg/day divided into 3 doses (max 1.2 g/day)

Bacterial Conjunctivitis
Adult: **Ophthalmic** 1–2 drops in conjunctival sac q2h while awake for 2 days, then 1–2 drops q4h while awake for the next 5 days.
Ointment: ½-inch ribbon into conjunctival sac t.i.d. times 2 days, then b.i.d. times 5 days

Corneal Ulcers
Adult: **Ophthalmic** 2 drops q15min for 6 h, 2 drops q30min for the next 18 h, then 2 drops q1h for 24 h, then 2 drops q4h for 14 days

STORAGE
Store in tightly closed containers at a temperature of <30° C (<86° F). Reconstituted IV solution is stable for 14 days refrigerated.

ADMINISTRATION
- For patients with renal impairment, oral and IV doses are lowered according to creatinine clearance.

Oral

- Do not give an antacid within 4 h of the oral ciprofloxacin dose.

Intravenous

PREPARE **Intermittent:** Dilute in NS or D5W to a final concentration of 0.5–2 mg/mL. Typical dilutions are 200 mg in 100–250 mL and 400 mg in 250–500 mL.

ADMINISTER **Intermittent:** Give slowly over 60 min. Avoid rapid infusion and use of a small vein.

INCOMPATIBILITIES **Solution/Additive: Aminophylline, clindamycin, heparin. Y-Site: Aminophylline, ampicillin, ampicillin/sulbactam, cefepime, dexamethasone, furosemide, heparin, hydrocortisone, phenytoin, propofol, sodium bicarbonate, theophylline, warfarin.**

- Discontinue other IV infusion while infusing ciprofloxacin or infuse through another site.

ADVERSE EFFECTS GI: Nausea, vomiting, diarrhea, cramps, gas. **Metabolic:** Transient increases in liver transaminases, alkaline phosphatase, lactic dehydrogenase, and eosinophilia count. **Musculoskeletal:** Tendon rupture. **CNS:** Headache, vertigo, malaise, seizures (especially with rapid IV infusion). **Skin:** Rash, phlebitis, pain, burning, pruritus, and erythema at infusion site. **Special Senses:** *Local burning and discomfort, crystalline precipitate on superficial portion of cornea,* lid margin crusting, scales, foreign body sensation, itching, and conjunctival hyperemia.

DIAGNOSTIC TEST INTERFERENCE Ciprofloxacin does not interfere with *urinary glucose* determinations using *cupric sulfate solution* or with *glucose ovadase tests;* may cause false positive on *opiate screening tests.*

INTERACTIONS Drug: May increase **theophylline** levels 15–30%; ANTACIDS, **sulcralfate, iron** decrease absorption of ciprofloxacin; may increase PT for patients on **warfarin.**

PHARMACOKINETICS Absorption: 60–80% absorbed from GI tract. **Ophthalmic:** Minimal absorption through cornea or conjuctiva. **Onset:** Topical 0.5–2 h. **Duration:** Topical 12 h. **Peak:** 1–2 h. **Distribution:** Widely distributed including prostate, lung, and bone; crosses placenta; distributed into breast milk. **Elimination:** Excreted primarily in urine with some biliary excretion. **Half-Life:** 3.5–4 h.

NURSING IMPLICATIONS

Assessment & Drug Effects

- Lab tests: Culture and sensitivity tests should be done prior to initial dose. Treatment may be implemented pending results.
- Monitor urine pH; it should be less than 6.8, especially in those receiving high doses of ciprofloxacin, to reduce the risk of crystalluria.
- Monitor I&O ratio and patterns; patients should be well hydrated; assess for signs and symptoms of crystalluria.
- Monitor plasma theophylline concentrations, because drug may interfere with half-life.

- Administration with theophylline derivatives or caffeine can cause CNS stimulation.
- Assess for signs and symptoms of GI irritation (e.g., nausea, diarrhea, vomiting, abdominal discomfort) in clients receiving high dosages.
- Monitor PT and INR in patients receiving coumarin therapy.
- Assess for signs and symptoms of superinfections (see Appendix D-1).

Patient & Family Education
- Fluid intake of 2–3 L/day is advised for adults, if not contraindicated; give generous amounts appropriate for age of child.
- Report sudden, unexplained joint pain.
- Restrict caffeine due to the effects (e.g., nervousness, insomnia, anxiety, tachycardia).
- Report possible toxicity. If taking theophylline derivatives, there is potential for adverse effects.
- Report nausea, diarrhea, vomiting, and abdominal pain or discomfort.
- Use caution with hazardous activities until reaction to drug is known. Drug may cause light-headedness.
- Do not breast feed while taking this drug
- Store this medication out of reach of children.

CISATRACURIUM BESYLATE

(cis-a-tra-kyoo-ri′um)
Nimbex
Classifications: AUTONOMIC NERVOUS SYSTEM AGENT; SKELETAL MUSCLE RELAXANT, NONDEPOLARIZING
Prototype: Tubocurarine chloride
Pregnancy Category: B

AVAILABILITY 2 mg/mL, 10 mg/mL injection

ACTIONS Cisatracurium is a neuromuscular blocking agent with intermediate onset and duration of action compared with similar agents. It binds competitively to cholinergic receptors on motor end plate of neurons, antagonizing the action of acetylcholine.
THERAPEUTIC EFFECTS Antagonism of acetylcholine blocks neuromuscular transmission of nerve impulses. This action can be reversed or antagonized by acetylcholinesterase inhibitors (e.g., neostigmine).

USES Adjunct to general anesthesia to facilitate tracheal intubation and provide skeletal muscle relaxation during surgery or mechanical ventilation.

CONTRAINDICATIONS Hypersensitivity to cisatracurium or other related agents; rapid-sequence endotracheal intubation. Not studied in children <2 y.
CAUTIOUS USE History of hemiparesis, electrolyte imbalances, burn patients, neuromuscular diseases (e.g., myasthenia gravis), older adults, renal function impairment, pregnancy (category B), lactation.

ROUTE & DOSAGE

Intubation

Child ≥2 y: **IV** 0.1 mg/kg given over 5–10 sec
Adult: **IV** 0.15 or 0.20 mg/kg

Maintenance

Child ≥2 y: **IV** 1–2 mcg/kg/min
Adult: **IV** 0.03 mg/kg q20min prn *or* 1–2 mcg/kg/min

Mechanical Ventilation in ICU

Adult: **IV** 3 mcg/kg/min (can range from 0.5–10.2 mcg/kg/min)

STORAGE

Refrigerate vials at 2°–8° C (36°–46° F). Protect from light. Diluted solutions may be stored refrigerated or at room temperature for 24 h.

ADMINISTRATION

- Administer carefully adjusted, individualized doses using a peripheral nerve stimulator to evaluate neuromuscular function.
- Give only by or under supervision of expert clinician familiar with the drug's actions and potential complications.
- Have immediately available personnel and facilities for resuscitation and life support and an antagonist of cisatracurium.
- Refer to manufacturer's guidelines for preparation and administration. Note that 10-mL multiple-dose vials contain benzyl alcohol and should not be used with neonates.

Intravenous

PREPARE **Direct:** Give undiluted. **IV Infusion:** Dilute 10 mg in 95 mL or 40 mg in 80 mL of compatible IV fluid to prepare 0.1 mg/mL or 0.4 mg/mL, respectively, IV solution. Compatible IV fluids include D5W, NS, D5/NS, and D5/RL. **ICU IV Infusion:** Dilute the contents of the 200 mg vial (i.e., 10 mg/mL) in 1000 mL or 500 mL of compatible IV fluid to prepare 0.2 mg/mL or 0.4 g/mL, respectively, IV solutions.

ADMINISTER **Direct:** Give a single dose over 5–10 sec **IV Infusion:** Adjust the rate based on patient's weight.

INCOMPATIBILITIES **Solution/Additive: Ketorolac, propofol, sodium bicarbonate. Y-Site: Amphotericin B, amphotericin B cholesteryl complex, cefoperazone, cefuroxime, diazepam, sodium bicarbonate.**

ADVERSE EFFECTS CV: Bradycardia, hypotension, flushing. **Respiratory:** Bronchospasm. **Skin:** Rash.

PHARMACOKINETICS Onset: Varies with dose from 1.5 to 3.3 min (higher the dose, faster the onset). **Peak:** Varies with dose from 1.5 to 3.3 min (higher the dose, faster to peak). **Duration:** Varies with dose from 46 to 121 min (higher dose, longer recovery time). **Metabolism:** Undergoes Hoffman elimination (pH- and temperature-dependent degradation) and hydrolysis by plasma esterases. **Elimination:** Excreted in urine. **Half-Life:** 22 min.

NURSING IMPLICATIONS

Assessment & Drug Effects

- Perform neuromuscular monitoring only on nonparetic limbs.
- Monitor for bradycardia, hypotension, and bronchospasms; monitor ICU patients for spontaneous seizures.
- Antagonists should not be given when complete neuromuscular block is present.

CISPLATIN (cis-DDP, cis-PLATINUM II)

(sis′pla-tin)
Abiplatin ♣, Platinol
Classifications: ANTINEOPLASTIC; ALKYLATING AGENT
Prototype: Cyclophosphamide
Pregnancy Category: D

AVAILABILITY 1 mg/mL injection

ACTIONS A heavy metal complex with platinum as central atom surrounded by 2 chloride atoms and 2 ammonia molecules in the cis chemical position. Biochemical properties similar to those of bifunctional alkylating agents. Produces interstrand and intrastrand cross-linkage in DNA of rapidly dividing cells, thus preventing DNA, RNA, and protein synthesis.
THERAPEUTIC EFFECTS Cell-cycle nonspecific, i.e., effective throughout the entire cell life cycle. Carcinogenicity has not been fully studied, but other compounds with similar action mechanisms and mutogenicity have been studied.

USES Established combination therapy (cisplatin, vinblastine, bleomycin) in patient with metastatic testicular tumors and with doxorubicin for metastatic ovarian tumors following appropriate surgical or radiation therapy.
UNLABELED USES Carcinoma of endometrium, bladder, head, and neck; childhood cancers of osteogenic sarcoma, neuroblastoma, recurrent brain tumor.

CONTRAINDICATIONS History of hypersensitivity to cisplatin or other platinum-containing compounds; impaired renal function; myelosuppression; impaired hearing; history of gout and urate renal stones; hypomagnesia; concurrent administration with loop diuretics; Raynard syndrome; pregnancy (category D), lactation. Safe use in children not established although some experimental regimens have been used.
CAUTIOUS USE Previous cytotoxic drug or radiation therapy with other ototoxic and nephrotoxic drugs; hyperuricemia. Electrolyte imbalances, hepatic impairment; history of circulatory disorders.

ROUTE & DOSAGE

Testicular Neoplasms
Adult: **IV** 20 mg/m^2/day for 5 days q3–4wk for 3 courses

Ovarian Neoplasms

Adult: **IV** *Combination therapy:* 50 mg/m^2 once q3–4wk;
Single agent: 100 mg/m^2 once q3–4wk

Osteogenic Sarcoma and Neuroblastoma

Child: **IV** 90 mg/m^2 once q3wk *or* 30 mg/m^2 once every week

Recurrent Brain Tumor

Child: **IV** 60 mg/m^2 once daily for 2 consecutive days q3–4wk

---

STORAGE

Store at 15°–30° C (59°–86° F). Do not refrigerate. Protect from light. Once vial is opened, solution is stable for 28 days protected from light or 7 days in fluorescent light.

ADMINISTRATION

- Administer only under supervision of a qualified pediatric oncology specialist experienced in the use of antineoplastics.
- Usually a parenteral antiemetic agent is administered ½ h before cisplatin therapy is instituted and given on a scheduled basis throughout day and night as long as necessary.
- Before the initial dose is given, hydration is started with 1–2 L IV infusion fluid to reduce risk of nephrotoxicity and ototoxicity.

Intravenous

PREPARE **IV Infusion:** Use disposable gloves when preparing cisplatin solutions. If drug accidentally contacts skin or mucosa, wash immediately and thoroughly with soap and water. Do not use any equipment containing aluminum. Withdraw required dose and dilute in 2 L D5W 5% dextrose in ½ or ⅓ normal saline containing 37.5 g mannitol.
ADMINISTER **IV Infusion:** Give 2 L over 6–8 h
INCOMPATIBILITIES **Solution/Additive: 5% dextrose, fluorouracil, mesna, metoclopramide, sodium bicarbonate, thiotepa. Y-Site: Amifostine, amphotericin B, cholesteryl, cefepime, piperacillin/ tazobactam, thiotepa, TPN.**

- Hydration and forced diuresis are continued for at least 24 h after drug administration to ensure adequate urinary output.

ADVERSE EFFECTS Body as a Whole: <u>Anaphylactic-like reactions</u>. **CV:** Cardiac abnormalities. **GI:** *Marked nausea, vomiting*, anorexia, stomatitis, xerostomia, diarrhea, constipation. **Hematologic:** Myelosuppression (25–30% patients): leukopenia, thrombocytopenia; hemolytic anemia, hemolysis. **Metabolic:** Hypocalcemia, *hypomagnesemia*, hyperuricemia, elevated AST, SIADH. **CNS:** Seizures, headache; peripheral neuropathies (may be irreversible): paresthesia, unsteady gait, clumsiness of hands and feet, exacerbation of neuropathy with exercise, loss of taste. **Special Senses:** Ototoxicity (may be irreversible): tinnitus, hearing loss, deafness, vertigo, blurred vision, changes in ability to see colors (optic neuritis, papilledema). **Urogenital:** Nephrotoxicity.

INTERACTIONS Drug: AMINOGLYCOSIDES, **amphotericin B, vancomycin,** other **nephrotoxic drugs** increase nephrotoxicity and acute

---

Common adverse effects in *italic;* life-threatening effects <u>underlined</u>; generic names in **bold;** drug classifications in SMALL CAPS; ✦ Canadian drug name; ⬤ Prototype drug.

renal failure—try to separate by at least 1–2 wk; AMINOGLYCOSIDES, **furosemide** increase risk of ototoxicity.

PHARMACOKINETICS Peak: Immediately after end of infusion. **Distribution:** Widely distributed in body fluids and tissues; concentrated in kidneys, liver, and prostate; accumulated in tissues. **Metabolism:** Not completely known. **Elimination:** 15–50% of dose excreted in urine within 24–48 h. **Half-Life:** 73–290 h.

NURSING IMPLICATIONS

Assessment & Drug Effects

- Obtain baseline ECG and cardiac monitoring during induction therapy because of possible myocarditis or focal irritability.
- Lab tests: The following tests should be done *before* initiating every course of therapy and repeated each week during treatment period: serum uric acid, serum creatinine, BUN, urinary creatinine clearance. CBC and platelet counts are done weekly for 2 wk after each course of treatment. Monitor periodically serum electrolytes and liver function tests.
- A repeat course of therapy should not be given until (1) serum creatinine is below 1.5 mg/dL; (2) BUN is below 25 mg/dL; (3) platelets >100,000/mm^3; (4) WBC >4000/mm^3; (5) audiometric test is within normal limits.
- Monitor urine output and specific gravity for 4 consecutive hours before treatment and for 24 h after therapy. Report if output is less than 100 mL/h or if specific gravity is more than 1.030. A urine output of less than 75 mL/h necessitates medical intervention to avert a renal emergency.
- Audiometric testing should be performed before the first dose and before each subsequent dose. Ototoxicity (reported in 31% of patients) may occur after a single dose of 50 mg/m^2. Children who receive repeated doses are especially susceptible.
- Monitor for anaphylactoid reactions (particularly in patient previously exposed to cisplatin), which may occur within minutes of drug administration.
- Monitor closely for dose-related adverse reactions. Drug action is cumulative; therefore, severity of most adverse effects increases with repeated doses.
- Nephrotoxicity (reported in 28–36% of patients receiving a single dose of 50 mg/m^2) usually occurs within 2 wk after drug administration and becomes more severe and prolonged with repeated courses of cisplatin.
- Suspect ototoxicity if patient manifests tinnitus or difficulty hearing in the high frequency range.
- Intractable nausea and vomiting severe enough to warrant discontinuation of drug usually begin 1–4 h after treatment and may last 24 h or persist for up to 1 wk after treatment is ended.
- Monitor and report abnormal electrolyte levels: sodium >145 or <135 mEq/L, and potassium >5 or <3.5 mEq/L.
- Monitor results of blood studies. The nadirs in platelet and leukocyte counts occur between day 18 and 23 (range: 7.5–45) with most patients recovering in 13–62 days. A decrease in Hgb (more than 2 g/dL decrease from baseline) occurs at approximately the same time and with the same frequency.

- Check BP, mental status, pupils, and fundi every hour during therapy. Hydration and mannitol may increase the danger of elevated intracranial pressure (ICP).
- Neurologic examinations at regular intervals should include tests of muscle strength, Romberg, vibratory and position sense, tests of sensation.
- Monitor and report abnormal bowel elimination pattern. Constipation and the possibility of fecal impaction may be caused by neurotoxicity; diarrhea is a possible response to GI irritation.
- Inspect oral membranes for xerostomia (white patches and ulcerations) and tongue for signs of fungal overgrowth (black, furry appearance).
- Institute infection precautions promptly if a temperature increase of 0.6° F over the previous reading is noted.
- Be alert for and report signs of infection such as respiratory infections, aching, rashes, and gastrointestinal distress. Assess immunization status prior to beginning therapy in order to be alert for diseases that pose risk.
- Weigh the patient under standard conditions every day. A gradual ascending weight profile occurring over a period of several days should be reported.

Patient & Family Education

- Continue maintenance of adequate hydration (at least 3000 mL/24 h oral fluid if physician agrees) and report promptly: Reduced urinary output, flank pain, anorexia, nausea, vomiting, dry mucosae, itching skin, urine odor on breath, fluid retention, and weight gain.
- Avoid rapid changes in position to minimize risk of dizziness or falling.
- Tingling, numbness, and tremors of extremities, loss of position sense and taste, and constipation are early signs of neurotoxicity. Report their occurrence promptly to prevent irreversibility. Pain with heel walking and difficulty in getting out of bed or chair are late indicators of nerve damage.
- Report tinnitus or any hearing impairment.
- Report promptly evidence of unexplained bleeding and easy bruising.
- Report unusual fatigue, fever, sore mouth and throat, abnormal body discharges. Report signs of infections.
- Avoid exposure to persons with infectious diseases.
- Do not breast feed while taking this drug.

CLARITHROMYCIN

(clar'i-thro-my-sin)
Biaxin Filmtabs, Biaxin XL
Classifications: ANTI-INFECTIVE; MACROLIDE ANTIBIOTIC
Prototype: Erythromycin
Pregnancy Category: C

AVAILABILITY 250 mg, 500 mg tablets; 500 mg sustained-release tablets; 125 mg/5 mL, 250 mg/5 mL suspension

ACTIONS A semisynthetic macrolide antibiotic that binds to the 50S ribosomal subunit of susceptible bacterial organisms and thus inhibits protein synthesis of the bacteria.

THERAPEUTIC EFFECTS Active against both aerobic and anaerobic gram-positive and gram-negative organisms including *Streptococcus pyogenes, S. pneumoniae, Haemophilus influenzae, Moraxella catarrhalis, Mycoplasma pneumoniae*, and *Staphylococcus aureus*.

USES Treatment of upper respiratory, lower respiratory infections; acute maxillary sinusitis; otitis media; and skin and soft tissue infections caused by clinically significant aerobic and anaerobic gram-negative and gram-positive organisms, including *S. aureus, H. influenzae, S. pneumoniae, M. catarrhalis, S. pyogenes, M. pneumoniae*. Prevention and treatment of *Mycobacterium avium complex* (MAC) infections in patients with HIV. Used in combination for *H. pylori*.

CONTRAINDICATIONS Hypersensitivity to clarithromycin, erythromycin, or any other macrolide antibiotics; patients receiving cisapride, astemizole, or pimozide; suspected or potential bacteremias; acute porphyria; severe hepatic or biliary disease; pregnancy (category C). Safety and efficacy in children <6 y not established.

CAUTIOUS USE Renal impairment, older adults, and lactation.

ROUTE & DOSAGE

Mild to Moderate Infections
Child: **PO** 7.5 mg/kg q12h
Adult: **PO** 250–500 mg b.i.d. or 500 mg XL daily for 10–14 days

Mycobacterial Infections
Child: **PO** 7.5 mg/kg q12h
Adult: **PO** 500 mg q12h

***H. pylori* Infections**
Adult: **PO** 500 mg b.i.d. to t.i.d.

Renal Impairment
Cl_{cr} <30 mL/min, decrease dose by ½ or double the dosing interval

STORAGE

Store all forms at 15°–30° C (59°–86° F). Shake suspension well before use. Reconstituted suspension stable at room temperature for 14 days.

ADMINISTRATION

Oral
- Ensure that sustained-release form of drug is not chewed or crushed. It must be swallowed whole.

ADVERSE EFFECTS GI: Diarrhea, abdominal discomfort, nausea, abnormal taste, dyspepsia. **Hematologic:** Eosinophilia. **CNS:** Headache. **Skin:** Rash, urticaria.

DIAGNOSTIC TEST INTERFERENCE May increase *serum AST* and *ALT* levels.

INTERACTIONS Drug: May increase **theophylline** levels; drugs known to interact with **erythromycin** (i.e., **digoxin, carbamazepine, triazolam, warfarin, ergotamine**) should be monitored carefully for increased levels and toxicity; **pimozide** may increase risk of arrhythmias.

Common adverse effects in *italic;* life-threatening effects underlined; generic names in **bold;** drug classifications in SMALL CAPS; ♣ Canadian drug name; ☻ Prototype drug.

335

PHARMACOKINETICS Absorption: Readily absorbed from GI tract; 50% reaches the systemic circulation. **Peak:** 2–4 h. **Distribution:** Widely distributes into most body tissue (excluding CNS); high pulmonary tissue concentrations. **Metabolism:** Partially metabolized in the liver; active 14-OH metabolite acts synergistically with the parent compound against *H. influenzae.* **Elimination:** 20% excreted unchanged in urine; 10–15% of 14-OH metabolite excreted in urine. **Half-Life:** 3–5 h.

NURSING IMPLICATIONS

Assessment & Drug Effects

- Inquire about previous hypersensitivity to other macrolides (e.g., erythromycin) before treatment.
- Withhold drug and notify physician, if hypersensitivity occurs (e.g., rash, urticaria).
- Monitor for and report loose stools or diarrhea, because pseudomembranous colitis must be ruled out.
- When clarithromycin is given concurrently with anticoagulants, digoxin, or theophylline, blood levels of these drugs may be elevated. Monitor appropriate serum levels and assess for S&S of drug toxicity.

Patient & Family Education

- Complete prescribed course of therapy.
- Report rash or other signs of hypersensitivity immediately.
- Report loose stools or diarrhea even after completion of drug therapy.
- Do not breast feed without consulting physician.
- Store this medication out of reach of children.

CLEMASTINE FUMARATE

(klem′as-teen)
Tavist, Tavist-1
Classifications: ANTIHISTAMINE (H₁-RECEPTOR ANTAGONIST)
Prototype: Diphenhydramine
Pregnancy Category: B

AVAILABILITY 1.34 mg, 2.68 mg tablets; 0.67 mg/5 mL syrup

ACTIONS An antihistamine (H_1-receptor antagonist) that competes for H_1-receptor sites on effector cells, thus blocking histamine release. Has greater selectivity for preripheral H_1 receptors and, consequently, produces little sedation. Has prominent antipruritic activity and low incidence of unpleasant adverse effects.

THERAPEUTIC EFFECTS Effective in controlling various allergic reactions, e.g., nasal congestion, sneezing, itching.

USES Symptomatic relief of allergic rhinitis (sneezing, rhinorrhea, pruritus) and mild uncomplicated allergic skin manifestations such as urticaria and angioedema.

CONTRAINDICATIONS Hypersensitivity to clemastine or to other antihistamines of similar chemical structure; lower respiratory tract symptoms,

including acute asthma; concomitant MAOI therapy. Pregnancy (category B), lactation. Safe use in children <6 y not established.
CAUTIOUS USE History of bronchial asthma, increased intraocular pressure, GI or GU obstruction, hyperthyroidism, cardiovascular disease, hypertension, older adults.

ROUTE & DOSAGE

Allergic Rhinitis
Child: **PO** <6 y, 0.05 mg/kg/day divided into 2 doses (max 1 mg/day); >6 y, 0.67 mg b.i.d., may increase up to 3 mg/day
Adult: **PO** 1.34 mg b.i.d., may increase up to 8.04 mg/day

Allergic Urticaria
Child: **PO** 1 mg b.i.d., may increase up to 4 mg/day
Adult: **PO** 2.68 mg b.i.d. or t.i.d., may increase up to 8.04 mg/day

STORAGE
Store at 15°–30° C (59°–86° F).

ADMINISTRATION

Oral
- Drug may be administered with food, water, or milk to reduce possibility of gastric irritation.

ADVERSE EFFECTS Body as a Whole: <u>Anaphylaxis</u>, excess perspiration, chills. **CV:** Hypotension, palpitation, tachycardia, extrasystoles. **GI:** *Dry mouth,* epigastric distress, anorexia, nausea, vomiting, diarrhea, constipation. **Hematologic:** Hemolytic anemia, thrombocytopenia, <u>agranulocytosis</u>. **CNS:** Sedation, *transient drowsiness,* dry nose and throat, headache, dizziness, weakness, fatigue, disturbed coordination; confusion, restlessness, nervousness, hysteria, convulsions, tremors, irritability, euphoria, insomnia, paresthesias, neuritis. **Respiratory:** Dry nose and throat, thickening of bronchial secretions, tightness of chest, wheezing, nasal stuffiness. **Skin:** Urticaria, rash, photosensitivity. **Special Senses:** Vertigo, tinnitus, acute labyrinthitis, blurred vision, diplopia. **Urogenital:** Difficult urination, urinary retention, early menses.

INTERACTIONS Drug: Alcohol and other CNS DEPRESSANTS increase sedation; MAOIS may prolong and intensify anticholinergic effects.

PHARMACOKINETICS Absorption: Readily absorbed from GI tract. **Peak:** 5–7 h. **Duration:** 10–12 h. **Distribution:** Distributed into breast milk. **Metabolism:** Metabolized in liver. **Elimination:** Excreted chiefly in urine.

NURSING IMPLICATIONS

Assessment & Drug Effects
- Monitor for drowsiness, poor coordination, or dizziness, especially in the debilitated person. Supervision of ambulation may be warranted.
- Assess for symptomatic relief with use of the medication.
- Lab tests: Periodic hematological studies with long-term use.

Common adverse effects in *italic;* life-threatening effects <u>underlined</u>; generic names in **bold;** drug classifications in SMALL CAPS; ♣ Canadian drug name; ✪ Prototype drug.

337

Patient & Family Education

- Check with physician before taking alcohol or other CNS depressants, since effects may be additive.
- Clemastine may cause lethargy and drowsiness; therefore, necessary safety precautions should be taken.
- Avoid driving and other potentially hazardous activities until response to the drug has been established.
- Take frequent sips of water or suck sugarless hard candy to relieve dry mouth.
- Do not breast feed while taking this drug.
- Store this medication out of reach of children.

CLINDAMYCIN HYDROCHLORIDE ℗

(klin-da-mye′sin)
Cleocin, Dalacin C ◆

CLINDAMYCIN PALMITATE HYDROCHLORIDE

Cleocin Pediatric

CLINDAMYCIN PHOSPHATE

Cleocin Phosphate, Cleocin T, Dalacin C, Cleocin Vaginal Ovules or Cream
Classifications: ANTI-INFECTIVE; ANTIBIOTIC
Pregnancy Category: B

AVAILABILITY 75 mg, 150 mg, 300 mg capsules; 75 mg/5 mL oral suspension; 150 mg/mL injection; 2% vaginal cream; 100 mg suppositories; 10 mg gel, lotion

ACTIONS Semisynthetic derivative of lincomycin with which it shares neuromuscular blocking properties and other actions. Reported to have a greater degree of antibacterial activity *in vitro,* better absorption, and lower incidence of GI adverse effects than lincomycin. Suppresses protein synthesis by binding to 50S subunits of bacterial ribosomes, and therefore inhibits other antibiotics (e.g., erythromycin) that act at this site.
THERAPEUTIC EFFECTS Particularly effective against susceptible strains of anaerobic streptococci, *Bacteroides* (especially *B. fragilis*), *Fusobacterium, Actinomyces israelii, Peptococcus,* and *Clostridium* sp. Also effective against aerobic gram-positive cocci, including *Staphylococcus aureus, S. epidermidis,* Streptococci (except *S. faecalis*), and *Pneumococci.*

USES Serious infections when less toxic alternatives are inappropriate. Topical applications are used in treatment of acne vulgaris. Vaginal applications are used in treatment of bacterial vaginosis in nonpregnant women.
UNLABELED USES In combination with pyrimethamine for toxoplasmosis in patients with AIDS.

CONTRAINDICATIONS History of hypersensitivity to clindamycin or lincomycin; history of regional enteritis, ulcerative colitis, or antibiotic-associated colitis. Pregnancy (category B), lactation. Not recommended for infants <1 mo.

CAUTIOUS USE History of GI disease, renal or hepatic disease; atopic individuals (history of eczema, asthma, hay fever); older patients >60 y.

ROUTE & DOSAGE

Moderate to Severe Infections

Neonate: **IM/IV** *<7 day,* 10–15 mg/kg/day divided into doses q8–12h; *>7 day,* 10–20 mg/kg/day divided into doses q6–12h
Child: **PO** 10–30 mg/kg/day q6–8h. **IM/IV** 25–40 mg/kg/day q6–8h
Adult: **PO** 150–450 mg q6h **IM/IV** 300–900 mg q6–8h (max 2700 mg/day)

Acne Vulgaris

Adult: **Topical** Apply to affected areas b.i.d.

Bacterial Vaginosis

Adult: **Topical** Insert 1 suppository intravaginally at bedtime for 3 days, or insert 1 applicator full of cream intravaginally at bedtime for 7 days

STORAGE

Store all forms at 15°–30° C (59°–86° F). Note expiration date of oral solution; retains potency for 14 days at room temperature. Do not refrigerate, because chilling causes thickening and thus makes pouring it difficult.

ADMINISTRATION

- Determine history of any previous sensitivities to drugs or other allergens prior to administration.

Oral

- Administer clindamycin capsules with a 240-mL (8-oz) glass of water or generous amount of fluid for age to prevent esophagitis.

Intramuscular

- Deep IM injection is recommended into muscle appropriate for age (see Part I). Rotate injection sites and observe daily for evidence of inflammatory reaction. Single IM doses should not exceed 600 mg.

Intravenous

- IV administration to neonates, infants and children: Verify correct IV concentration and rate of infusion with physician.

PREPARE **Intermittent:** Each 18 mg must be diluted with at least 1 mL of D5W, NS, D5/0.45% NaCl, or other compatible solution. Final concentration should never exceed 18 mg/mL.
ADMINISTER **Intermittent:** Never give a bolus dose. Do not give >1200 mg in a single 1-h infusion. Infusion rate should not exceed 30 mg/min.
INCOMPATIBILITIES **Solution/Additive: Aminophylline, ceftriaxone, ciprofloxacin, fluconazole, ranitidine, tobramycin. Y-Site: Allopurinol, filgrastim, fluconazole, idarubicin.**

ADVERSE EFFECTS Body as a Whole: Fever, serum sickness, sensitization, swelling of face (following topical use), generalized myalgia,

---

Common adverse effects in *italic;* life-threatening effects <u>underlined;</u> generic names in **bold;** drug classifications in SMALL CAPS; ♣ Canadian drug name; ● Prototype drug.

339

superinfections, proctitis, vaginitis, pain, induration, sterile abscess (following IM injections); thrombophlebitis (IV infusion). **CV:** Hypotension (following IM), <u>cardiac arrest</u> (rapid IV). **GI:** *Diarrhea,* abdominal pain, flatulence, bloating, *nausea, vomiting,* <u>pseudomembranous colitis</u>; esophageal irritation, loss of taste, medicinal taste (high IV doses), jaundice, abnormal liver function tests. **Hematologic:** Leukopenia, eosinophilia, <u>agranulocytosis</u>, thrombocytopenia. **Skin:** *Skin rashes,* urticaria, pruritus, dryness, contact dermatitis, gram-negative folliculitis, irritation, oily skin.

DIAGNOSTIC TEST INTERFERENCE Clindamycin may cause increases in *serum alkaline phosphatase, bilirubin, creatine phosphokinase (CPK)* from muscle irritation following IM injection; *AST, ALT.*

INTERACTIONS Drug: Chloramphenicol, erythromycin possibly are mutually antagonistic to clindamycin; neuromuscular blocking action enhanced by NEUROMUSCULAR BLOCKING AGENTS **(atracurium, tubocurarine, pancuronium).**

PHARMACOKINETICS Absorption: Approximately 90% absorbed from GI tract; 10% of topical application is absorbed through skin. **Peak:** 45–60 min PO; 3 h IM. **Duration:** 6 h PO; 8–12 h IM. **Distribution:** Widely distributed except for CNS; crosses placenta; distributed into breast milk. **Metabolism:** Metabolized in liver. **Elimination:** Excreted in urine and feces. **Half-Life:** 2–3 h.

NURSING IMPLICATIONS

Assessment & Drug Effects
- Lab tests: Culture and sensitivity testing should be performed initially and periodically during therapy. Periodic CBC with differential and platelet count.
- Monitor BP and pulse in patients receiving drug parenterally. Hypotension has occurred following IM injection. Advise patient to remain recumbent following drug administration until BP has stabilized. Severe diarrhea and colitis, including pseudomembranous colitis, have been associated with oral (highest incidence), parenteral, and topical clindamycin. Report immediately the onset of watery diarrhea, with or without fever; passage of tarry or bloody stools, pus, intestinal tissue, or mucus; abdominal cramps, or ileus. Symptoms may appear within a few days to 2 wk after therapy is begun or up to several weeks following cessation of therapy.
- Closely observe patients for development of colitis.
- Be alert to signs of superinfection.
- Be alert for signs of anaphylactoid reactions, which require immediate attention.

Patient & Family Education
- Take drug for the full course of therapy as prescribed.
- Report loose stools or diarrhea promptly.
- Stop drug therapy if significant diarrhea develops (more than 5 loose stools daily) and notify physician.
- Do not self-medicate with antidiarrheal preparations. Antiperistaltic agents may prolong and worsen diarrhea by delaying removal of toxins from colon.

- If using topical preparation for acne, discontinue other acne preparations unless otherwise directed by physician. Keep medication away from eyes.
- Because 10% absorption of topical medication is possible, report the onset of systemic reactions to physician.
- Do not breast feed while taking this drug.
- Store this medication out of reach of children.

CLOFAZIMINE
(kloe-fa′zi-meen)
Lamprene
Classifications: ANTI-INFECTIVE; ANTILEPROSY AGENT
Prototype: Dapsone
Pregnancy Category: C

AVAILABILITY 50 mg capsules

ACTIONS Exerts a slow bactericidal effect on *Mycobacterium leprae* (Hansen's bacillus). Binds preferentially to DNA of all mycobacteria and inhibits their growth. Its anti-inflammatory action (precise mechanism unknown) controls erythema nodosum leprosum reactions. Bacterial killing is not detectable in biopsy tissue from leprosy patient until 50 days after start of therapy.

THERAPEUTIC EFFECTS Exerts a slow bactericidal effect on *M. leprae* (Hansen's bacillus) and has anti-inflammatory activity. Clofazimine is not effective against all forms of leprosy. Does not show cross-resistance with rifampin or dapsone. Has no clinically useful activity against microorganisms other than mycobacteria.

USES Chiefly in multi-infective therapy of multibacillary leprosy (with dapsone, rifampin, ethionamide) to prevent development of drug resistance. Also in lepromatous leprosy, including dapsone-resistant lepromatous leprosy and leprosy complicated by erythema nodosum leprosum (lepra) reaction.

UNLABELED USES *Mycobacterium avium-intracellulare complex* infections in patients with AIDS.

CONTRAINDICATIONS Pregnancy (category C), lactation, children <12 y.
CAUTIOUS USE Patients with GI problems.

ROUTE & DOSAGE

Dapsone-resistant Leprosy
Child: **PO** 1 mg/kg/day in combination with dapsone and rifampin
Adult: **PO** 100 mg/day in combination with 1 or more antileprosy drugs for 3 y, then 100 mg/day as monotherapy

Erythema Nodosum Leprosum
Adult: **PO** 100–300 mg/day for up to 3 mo; taper dose to 100 mg/day as soon as possible

C

Mycobacterium avium-intracellulare

Child: **PO** 1–2 mg/kg/day (max 100 mg/day)
Adult: **PO** 100 mg 1–3 times/day

STORAGE

Store capsules at 15°–30° C (59°–86° F); protect from moisture.

ADMINISTRATION

Oral

- Drug should be taken with meals or milk to reduce gastric irritation.
- Doses of more than 100 mg/day are given for as short a period of time as possible and should be administered under close medical supervision.

ADVERSE EFFECTS GI: *Abdominal/epigastric pain* (dose-related), *nausea, vomiting, diarrhea,* bowel obstruction, hepatitis, jaundice, enlarged liver. **Hematologic:** Eosinophilia. **Metabolic:** Hypokalemia; elevated albumin, serum bilirubin, and AST. **CNS:** Drowsiness, fatigue, headache, giddiness, dizziness, neuralgia, taste disorder. **Skin:** *Pink-brown skin discoloration, ichthyosis, dryness,* rash, pruritus, phototoxicity, erythema nodosum leprosum (lepra) reaction. **Special Senses:** *Conjunctival and corneal discoloration,* dryness, burning, itching, irritation.

INTERACTIONS Drug: Isoniazid may decrease clofazimine concentrations in skin. **Food:** Food will increase absorption.

PHARMACOKINETICS Absorption: Slowly absorbed from GI tract; approximately 50% absorbed. **Peak:** 4–12 h. **Distribution:** Distributed predominantly to fatty tissues and reticuloendothelial system; crosses placenta; distributed into breast milk. **Elimination:** Primarily eliminated in feces through bile. **Half-Life:** 70 days.

NURSING IMPLICATIONS

Assessment & Drug Effects

- Assess for serious adverse effects (e.g., pain in bones and joints, GI bleeding, diminished vision). Reactions are usually reversible but may require months or years to diminish.
- Lab tests: Periodic WBC with differential, serum electrolytes, serum albumin, and liver function tests.
- Drug-induced reddish-brown discoloration of skin, cornea, conjunctiva, and body fluids (including tears, sweat, sputum, urine, and feces) occurs in 75–90% of patients within a few weeks of treatment. Skin discoloration may take months or years to disappear after drug is discontinued.
- Monitor for the onset of tender, erythematous nodules with lymphadenopathy, joint swelling, epistaxis, iritis, which suggests a type 2 leprosy reactional state. Dosage may be increased to 200 mg/day. After reactive episode is controlled, dosage is tapered to 100 mg/day as soon as possible. Patient should remain under medical surveillance during the episode.

Patient & Family Education

- Adhere strictly to established drug regimen. No drug dosage should be omitted, increased, or decreased without advice of health care provider.
- Report promptly bone and joint pain; GI bleeding, colicky abdominal pain, nausea, vomiting, diarrhea; diminished vision.
- Minimize use of soap, avoid applying it directly to dry skin, and thoroughly rinse it off.
- When dizziness, drowsiness, or visual impairment adverse effects are experienced, do not drive or work with hazardous equipment. These symptoms are generally dose related. Discuss with care provider.
- Do not breast feed while taking this drug.
- Store this medication out of reach of children.

CLOMIPRAMINE HYDROCHLORIDE

(clo-mi'pra-meen)
Anafranil
Classifications: CENTRAL NERVOUS SYSTEM AGENT; PSYCHOTHERAPEUTIC; TRICYCLIC ANTIDEPRESSANT
Prototype: Imipramine
Pregnancy Category: C

AVAILABILITY 25 mg, 50 mg, 75 mg capsules

ACTIONS Inhibits the reuptake of norepinephrine and serotonin at the presynaptic neuron. Elevates serum levels of these two amines.
THERAPEUTIC EFFECTS The basis of its antidepressant effects is thought to be due to the elevated serum levels of norepinephrine and serotonin. Exhibits anticholinergic, antihistaminic, hypotensive, sedative, mild analgesic, and peripheral vasodilator effects.

USES Obsessive-compulsive disorder (OCD).
UNLABELED USES Panic disorder, anxiety, agoraphobia.

CONTRAINDICATIONS Hypersensitivity to other tricyclic compounds; acute recovery period after MI, children <10 y, pregnancy (category C), lactation.
CAUTIOUS USE History of convulsive disorders, children and adolescents, prostatic hypertrophy, urinary retention, cardiovascular, hepatic, GI, or blood disorders.

ROUTE & DOSAGE

Obsessive-Compulsive Disorder
Child: **PO** *10–18 y*, 100–200 mg/day given in divided doses, start at 50 mg/day and titrate upward as needed
Adult: **PO** 75–300 mg/day given in divided doses

Depression
Adult: **PO** 50–150 mg/day in single or divided doses

STORAGE
Store at 15°–30° C (59°–86° F).

ADMINISTRATION

Oral

- Give in divided doses with meals to reduce GI adverse effects.
- Following titration to the full dose, drug may be given as a single dose at bedtime to reduce daytime sedation.

ADVERSE EFFECTS Body as a Whole: Diaphoresis. **CV:** Hypotension, tachycardia. **GI:** Constipation, *dry mouth.* **Endocrine:** Galactorrhea, hyperprolactinemia, amenorrhea, *weight gain.* **Hematologic:** Leukopenia, <u>agranulocytosis</u>, thrombocytopenia, anemia. **CNS:** Mania, *tremor,* dizziness, hyperthermia, <u>neuroleptic malignant syndrome</u>, seizures (especially with abrupt withdrawal). **Urogenital:** Delayed ejaculation, anorgasmia.

DIAGNOSTIC TEST INTERFERENCE Clomipramine appears to elevate serum ***prolactin*** levels. ***Serum AST and ALT*** are elevated. Serum levels of ***triiodothyronine (T_3) and free triiodothyronine (FT_3)*** have been significantly reduced from baseline. ***Thyroxine-binding globulin (TBG)*** levels were increased from baseline, whereas ***thyroxine (T_4), free thyroxine (FT_4),*** and reverse T_3 were unchanged.

INTERACTIONS Drug: MAOIS may precipitate hyperpyrexic crisis, tachycardia, or seizures; ANTIHYPERTENSIVE AGENTS potentiate orthostatic hypotension; CNS DEPRESSANTS, **alcohol** add to CNS depression; **norepinephrine** and other SYMPATHOMIMETICS may increase cardiac toxicity; **cimetidine** decreases hepatic metabolism, thus increasing imipramine levels; **methylphenidate** inhibits metabolism of **imipramine** and thus may increase its toxicity. **Herbal: Ginkgo** may decrease seizure threshold; **St. John's wort** may cause serotonin syndrome.

PHARMOCOKINETICS Absorption: Rapidly absorbed from GI tract; 20–78% reaches systemic circulation. **Onset:** Depression: approx 2 wk; OCD: approx 4–10 wk. **Peak:** 2–6 h. **Distribution:** Widely distributed including the CSF; crosses placenta. **Metabolism:** Extensive first-pass metabolism in the liver; active metabolite is desmethylclomipramine. **Elimination:** 50–60% excreted in urine, 24–32% in feces. **Half-Life:** 20–30 h.

NURSING IMPLICATIONS

Assessment & Drug Effects

- Monitor for seizures, especially in those with predisposing factors such as alcoholism, brain injury, or concurrent therapy with other drugs that lower seizure threshold.
- Lab tests: Periodic CBC with differential, platelet count, and Hct and Hgb. Monitor liver functions, especially with long-term therapy.
- Monitor for and report signs of neuroleptic malignant syndrome.
- Monitor for sedation and vertigo, especially at the beginning of therapy and following dosage increases. Supervision of ambulation may be indicated.
- Notify physician of fever and complaints of sore throat because these may indicate need to rule out adverse hematologic changes.
- Antidepressants increase risk of suicidal thinking and behavior in children and adolescents with major depressive disorder, obsessive

compulsive disorder, and other psychiatric disorders. Observe closely for worsening of condition, suicidality, and behavior changes. Instruct family and caregivers to monitor for these symptoms and discuss with prescriber. A MedGuide describing risks and stating whether the drug is approved for the child's/adolescent's condition should be provided for all families when antidepressants are prescribed.

Patient & Family Education
- Do not take OTC drugs or discontinue therapy without consent of prescriber. Abrupt discontinuation may cause nausea, headache, malaise, or seizures.
- Report worsening of condition, suicidal thoughts and behavior changes to prescriber immediately.
- Can cause impotence or ejaculation failure in males. Advise them to report this problem to physician.
- Report promptly a sore throat accompanied by fever.
- Use caution with ambulation until response to drug is known.
- Moderate alcohol intake because it may potentiate adverse drug effects.
- Do not breast feed while taking this drug.
- Store this medication out of reach of children.

CLONAZEPAM

(kloe-na′zi-pam)
Klonopin, Rivotril ♣
Classifications: CENTRAL NERVOUS SYSTEM AGENT; ANTICONVULSANT; BENZODIAZEPINE
Prototype: Diazepam
Pregnancy Category: C
Controlled Substance: Schedule IV

AVAILABILITY 0.5 mg, 1 mg, 2 mg tablets

ACTIONS BENZODIAZEPINE derivative with strong anticonvulsant activity and several other pharmacologic properties characteristic of the drug class.
THERAPEUTIC EFFECTS Suppresses spike and wave discharge in absence seizures (petit mal) and decreases amplitude, frequency, duration, and spread of discharge in minor motor seizures.

USES Alone or with other drugs in absence, myoclonic, and akinetic seizures, Lennox-Gastaut syndrome, absence seizures refractory to succinimides or valproic acid, and for infantile spasms and restless legs.
UNLABELED USES Panic disorder, complex partial seizure pattern and generalized tonic-clonic convulsions.

CONTRAINDICATIONS Hypersensitivity to benzodiazepines; liver disease; acute narrow-angle glaucoma; pregnancy (category C), lactation.
CAUTIOUS USE Renal disease; COPD; drug-controlled open-angle glaucoma; addiction-prone individuals; children (because of unknown consequences of long-term use on growth and development); patient with mixed seizure disorders.

Common adverse effects in *italic;* life-threatening effects underlined; generic names in **bold;** drug classifications in SMALL CAPS; ♣ Canadian drug name; ♥ Prototype drug.

345

ROUTE & DOSAGE

Seizures

Child: **PO** <10 y, 0.01–0.03 mg/kg/day (not to exceed 0.05 mg/kg/day) divided into 3 doses; may increase by 0.25–0.5 mg q3days until seizures are controlled or until intolerable adverse effects occur (max recommended dose 0.2 mg/kg/day)
Adult: **PO** 1.5 mg/day divided into 3 doses, increased by 0.5–1 mg q3days until seizures are controlled or until intolerable adverse effects occur (max recommended dose 20 mg/day)

Panic Disorders

Adult: **PO** 1–2 mg/day given in divided doses (max 4 mg/day)

STORAGE

Store in tightly closed container protected from light at 15°–30° C (59°–86° F).

ADMINISTRATION

Oral

- Give largest dose at bedtime if daily dose cannot be equally divided.
- If clonazepam is to replace a different anticonvulsant, verify whether or not the prior drug should be gradually tapered.

ADVERSE EFFECTS CV: Palpitations. **GI:** Dry mouth, sore gums, anorexia, coated tongue, increased salivation, increased appetite, nausea, constipation, diarrhea. **Hematologic:** Anemia, leukopenia, thrombocytopenia, eosinophilia. **CNS:** *Drowsiness, sedation, ataxia,* insomnia, aphonia, choreiform movements, coma, dysarthria, "glassy-eyed" appearance, headache, hemiparesis, hypotonia, slurred speech, tremor, vertigo, confusion, depression, hallucinations, aggressive behavior problems, hysteria, suicide attempt. **Respiratory:** Chest congestion, respiratory depression, rhinorrhea, dyspnea, hypersecretion in upper respiratory passages. **Skin:** Hirsutism, hair loss, skin rash, ankle and facial edema. **Special Senses:** Diplopia, nystagmus, abnormal eye movements. **Urogenital:** Increased libido, dysuria, enuresis, nocturia, urinary retention.

DIAGNOSTIC TEST INTERFERENCE Clonazepam causes transient elevations of *serum transaminase* and *alkaline phosphatase.*

INTERACTIONS Drug: Alcohol and other CNS DEPRESSANTS increase sedation and CNS depression; may increase **phenytoin** levels. **Herbal: Kava-kava, valerian** may potentiate sedation.

PHARMACOKINETICS Absorption: Readily absorbed from GI tract. **Onset:** 60 min. **Peak:** 1–2 h. **Duration:** Up to 12 h in adults; 6–8 h in children. **Distribution:** Crosses placenta; distributed into breast milk. **Metabolism:** Metabolized in liver. **Elimination:** Excreted in urine primarily as metabolites. **Half-Life:** 18–40 h.

NURSING IMPLICATIONS

Assessment & Drug Effects

- Monitor I&O ratio and patterns: Excess accumulation of metabolites because of impaired excretion leads to toxicity.

- Assess carefully for signs of overdosage or drug interaction, i.e., increased depressant adverse effects, if multiple anticonvulsants are being given.
- Lab testes: Periodic liver function tests, platelet counts, blood counts, and renal function tests.
- Watch patient to see that he or she does not cheek the tablet. Both psychological and physical dependence may occur in the patient on long-term, high-dose therapy. Limit availability of large amounts of drug in the addiction-prone individual.
- Monitor for S&S of overdose, including somnolence, confusion, irritability, sweating, muscle and abdominal cramps, diminished reflexes, coma.

Patient & Family Education

- Report loss of seizure control promptly. Anticonvulsant activity is often lost after 3 mo of therapy; dosage adjustment may reestablish efficacy.
- Do not abruptly discontinue this drug. Abrupt withdrawal can precipitate seizures. Other withdrawal symptoms include convulsion, tremor, abdominal and muscle cramps, vomiting, sweating.
- Take drug as prescribed and do not alter dosing regimen without consulting health care provider.
- Do not self-medicate with OTC drugs before consulting the physician.
- Do not drive a car or engage in other activities requiring mental alertness and physical coordination until reaction to the drug is known. Drowsiness occurs in approximately 50% of patients.
- Carry identification (e.g., Medic Alert) bearing information about medication in use and the diagnosis. Report medication to dentists and all other health care providers.
- Do not breast feed while taking this drug.
- Store this medication out of reach of children.

CLONIDINE HYDROCHLORIDE

(kloe'ni-deen)

Catapres, Catapres-TTS, Dixaril ♣ , Duraclon

Classifications: CARDIOVASCULAR AGENT; CENTRAL-ACTING ANTIHYPERTENSIVE; ANALGESIC

Prototype: Methyldopa

Pregnancy Category: C

AVAILABILITY 0.1 mg, 0.2 mg, 0.3 mg tablets; 0.1 mg/24 h, 0.2 mg/24 h, 0.3 mg/24 h transdermal patch; 100 mcg/mL, 500 mcg/mL injection

ACTIONS Centrally acting antiadrenergic derivative. Stimulates alpha$_2$-adrenergic receptors in CNS to inhibit sympathetic vasomotor centers. Central actions reduce plasma concentrations of norepinephrine. Decreases systolic and diastolic BP and heart rate. Orthostatic effects tend to be mild and occur infrequently. Also inhibits renin release from kidneys.

THERAPEUTIC EFFECTS Decreases systolic and diastolic BP and heart rate. Orthostatic effects tend to be mild and occur infrequently. Reportedly minimizes or eliminates many of the common clinical S&S associated with withdrawal of heroin, methadone, or other opiates.

CLONIDINE HYDROCHLORIDE

USES Step 2 drug in stepped-care approach to treatment of hypertension, either alone or with diuretic or other antihypertensive agents. Epidural administration as adjunct therapy for severe pain.
UNLABELED USES Prophylaxis for migraine; treatment of dysmenorrhea, menopausal flushing, diarrhea, paroxysmal localized hyperhidroses; alcohol, smoking, opiate, and benzodiazepine withdrawal; in the clonidine suppression test for diagnosis of pheochromocytoma; Gilles de la Tourette syndrome; attention deficit disorder with hyperactivity (ADHD) in children.

CONTRAINDICATIONS Pregnancy (category C), lactation. Use of clonidine patch in polyarteritis nodosa, scleroderma, SLE.
CAUTIOUS USE Severe coronary insufficiency, recent MI, sinus node dysfunction, cerebrovascular disease; chronic renal failure; Raynaud's disease, thromboangiitis obliterans; history of mental depression.

ROUTE & DOSAGE

Hypertension

Child: **PO** 5–10 mcg/kg/day, divided into doses q8–12h, may increase to 5–25 mcg/kg/day divided into doses q6h (max 0.9 mg/day)
Adult: **PO** 0.1 mg b.i.d. or t.i.d., may increase by 0.1–0.2 mg/day until desired response is achieved (max 2.4 mg/day) **Transdermal** 0.1 mg patch once q7day; may increase by 0.1 mg q1–2wk

Severe Pain

Child: **Epidural** Start infusion at 0.5 mcg/kg/h and titrate to response
Adult: **Epidural** Start infusion at 30 mcg/h and titrate to response. Use rates >40 mcg/h with caution

ADHD

Child: **PO** 5 mcg/kg/day divided into 4 doses (average dose, 0.15–0.2 mg/day). **Transdermal** 0.2–0.3 mg/day applied q5–7days

STORAGE
Store in tightly closed container at 15°–30° C (59°–86° F).

ADMINISTRATION
- Give last PO dose immediately before patient retires to ensure overnight BP control and to minimize daytime drowsiness.
- Oral dosage is increased gradually over a period of weeks so as not to lower BP abruptly (especially important in the older adult). Follow-up visits should be scheduled every 2–4 wk until BP stabilizes, then every 2–4 mo.
- Apply transdermal patch to dry skin, free of hair and rash. Avoid irritated, abraded, or scarred skin. Recommended areas for applying transdermal patch are upper outer arm and anterior chest. Less drug is absorbed from thighs. Rotate application sites and keep a record.
- During change from PO clonidine to transdermal system, PO clonidine should be maintained for at least 24 h after patch is applied.
- Do not abruptly discontinue drug. It should be withdrawn over a period of 2–4 days. Abrupt withdrawal resembles sympathetic stimulation and may result in restlessness and headache 2–3 h after a missed dose and a hypertensive crisis within 8–18 h.

ADVERSE EFFECTS CV: *Hypotension (epidural),* postural hypotension (mild), peripheral edema, ECG changes, tachycardia, bradycardia, flushing, rapid increase in BP with abrupt withdrawal. **GI:** *Dry mouth, constipation,* abdominal pain, pseudo-obstruction of large bowel, altered taste, nausea, vomiting, hepatitis, hyperbilirubinemia, weight gain (sodium retention). **CNS:** *Drowsiness, sedation,* dizziness, headache, fatigue, weakness, sluggishness, dyspnea, vivid dreams, nightmares, insomnia, behavior changes, agitation, hallucination, nervousness, restlessness, anxiety, mental depression. **Skin:** Rash, pruritus, thinning of hair, exacerbation of psoriasis; with transdermal patch: hyperpigmentation, recurrent herpes simplex, skin irritation, contact dermatitis, mild erythema. **Special Senses:** Dry eyes. **Urogenital:** Impotence, loss of libido.

DIAGNOSTIC TEST INTERFERENCE Possibility of decreased urinary excretion of *aldosterone, catecholamines,* and *VMA* (however, sudden withdrawal of clonidine may cause increases in these values); transient increases in *blood glucose;* weakly positive *direct antiglobulin (Coombs') tests.*

INTERACTIONS Drug: Alcohol and other CNS DEPRESSANTS add to CNS depression; TRICYCLIC ANTIDEPRESSANTS may reduce antihypertensive effects. OPIATE ANALGESICS increase hypotension with epidural clonidine. Increased risk of bradycardia or AV block when epidural clonidine is used with **digoxin,** CALCIUM CHANNEL BLOCKERS, or BETA-BLOCKERS.

PHARMACOKINETICS Absorption: Readily absorbed from GI tract. **Onset:** 30–60 min PO; 1–3 days transdermal. **Peak:** 2–4 h PO; 2–3 days transdermal. **Duration:** 8 h PO; 7 days transdermal. **Distribution:** Widely distributed; crosses blood–brain barrier; not known if crosses placenta or distributed into breast milk. **Metabolism:** Metabolized in liver. **Elimination:** 80% excreted in urine, 20% in feces. **Half-Life:** 6–20 h.

NURSING IMPLICATIONS

Assessment & Drug Effects

- Monitor BR closely. Determine positional changes (supine, sitting, standing).
- With epidural administration, frequently monitor BP and HR. Hypotension is a common side effect that may require intervention.
- Monitor BP closely whenever a drug is added to or withdrawn from therapeutic regimen.
- Monitor I&O during period of dosage adjustment. Report change in I&O ratio or change in voiding pattern.
- Determine weight daily. Patients not receiving a concomitant diuretic agent may gain weight, particularly during first 3 or 4 days of therapy, because of marked sodium and water retention.
- Supervise closely patients with history of mental depression, because they may be subject to further depressive episodes.

Patient & Family Education

- Although postural hypotension occurs infrequently, make position changes slowly and in stages, particularly from recumbent to upright position, and dangle and move legs a few minutes before standing. Lie down immediately if faintness or dizziness occurs.

- Avoid potentially hazardous activities until reaction to drug has been determined due to possible sedative effects.
- Do not omit doses or stop the drug without consulting your health care provider.
- Do not take OTC medications, alcohol, or other CNS depressants without prior discussion with care provider.
- Examine site when transdermal patch is removed and report to physician if erythema, rash, irritation, or hyperpigmentation occurs.
- If transdermal patch loosens, tape it in place with adhesive. The patch should never be cut or trimmed.
- Do not breast feed while taking this drug.
- Store this medication out of reach of children.

CLORAZEPATE DIPOTASSIUM

(klor-az′e-pate)

Novoclopate ♣, Tranxene, Tranxene-SD

Classifications: CENTRAL NERVOUS SYSTEM AGENT; ANXIOLYTIC; SEDATIVE-HYPNOTIC; ANTICONVULSANT; BENZODIAZEPINE

Prototype: Lorazepam

Pregnancy Category: D

Controlled Substance: Schedule IV

AVAILABILITY 3.75 mg, 7.5 mg, 15 mg capsules and tablets; 11.25 mg, 22.5 mg long-acting tablets

ACTIONS Anxiolytic qualitatively similar to lorazepam. It has depressant effects on the CNS, thus controlling anxiety associated with stress.

THERAPEUTIC EFFECTS Effective in controlling anxiety and withdrawal symptoms of alcohol.

USES Management of anxiety disorders, short-term relief of anxiety symptoms, as adjunct in management of partial seizures, and symptomatic relief of acute alcohol withdrawal.

CONTRAINDICATIONS Hypersensitivity to clorazepate and other benzodiazepines; acute narrow-angle glaucoma; depressive neuroses, psychotic reactions, drug abusers. Safe use during pregnancy (category D), lactation, and in children <9 y not established.

CAUTIOUS USE Debilitated patients; hepatic disease; kidney disease.

ROUTE & DOSAGE

Anxiety

Adult: **PO** 15 mg/day at bedtime, may increase to 15–60 mg/day given in divided doses (max 60 mg/day)

Acute Alcohol Withdrawal

Adult: **PO** 30 mg followed by 30–60 mg in divided doses (max 90 mg/day), taper by 15 mg/day over 4 days to 7.5–15 mg/day until stable

Common adverse effects in *italic;* life-threatening effects <u>underlined;</u> generic names in **bold;** drug classifications in SMALL CAPS; ♣ Canadian drug name; ❷ Prototype drug.

Partial Seizures
Child: 9–12 y, **PO** 3.75–7.5 mg b.i.d., may increase by no more than 3.75 mg/wk (max 60 mg/day)
Adult: **PO** 7.5 mg t.i.d.

STORAGE
Store in light-resistant container at 15°–30° C (59°–86° F).

ADMINISTRATION

Oral

- Give with food to minimize gastric distress. Give antacid no less than 1 h before or 1 h after drug ingestion.
- Ensure that long-acting form of drug is not chewed or crushed. It must be swallowed whole.
- Taper drug dose gradually over several days when drug is to be discontinued. Abrupt termination may lead to memory impairment, severe GI symptoms, muscle pain, restlessness, irritability, fatigue, insomnia.

ADVERSE EFFECTS Body as a Whole: Allergic reactions. **CV:** Hypotension. **GI:** GI disturbances, abnormal liver function tests, xerostomia. **Hematologic:** Decreased Hct, blood dyscrasias. **CNS:** *Drowsiness,* ataxia, dizziness, headache, paradoxical excitement, mental confusion, insomnia. **Special Senses:** Diplopia, blurred vision.

INTERACTIONS Drug: Alcohol and other CNS DEPRESSANTS compound CNS depression; clorazepate increases effects of **cimetidine, disulfiram,** causing excessive sedation. **Herbal: Ginkgo** may decrease anticonvulsant effectiveness.

PHARMACOKINETICS Absorption: Decarboxylated in stomach; absorbed as active metabolite, desmethyldiazepam. **Peak:** 1 h. **Duration:** 24 h. **Distribution:** Crosses placenta; distributed into breast milk. **Metabolism:** Metabolized in liver to oxazepam. **Elimination:** Excreted primarily in urine. **Half-Life:** 30–200 h.

NURSING IMPLICATIONS

Assessment & Drug Effects

- Drowsiness, a common side effect, is more likely to occur at initiation of therapy and with dose increments on successive days.
- Lab tests: Periodic blood counts and tests of liver and kidney function should be performed throughout therapy.
- Monitor patient with history of cardiovascular disease in early therapy for drug-induced responses. If systolic BP drops more than 20 mm Hg or if there is a sudden increase in pulse rate, withhold drug and notify prescriber.

Patient & Family Education

- Take drug as prescribed and do not change dose or abruptly stop taking the drug without instructions from health care provider.

Common adverse effects in *italic;* life-threatening effects <u>underlined</u>; generic names in **bold;** drug classifications in SMALL CAPS; ♣ Canadian drug name; ☻ Prototype drug.

351

- Do not self-dose with OTC drugs (cold remedies, sleep medications, antacids) without consulting prescriber.
- Avoid driving and other potentially hazardous activities until reaction to drug is known.
- Do not use alcohol and other CNS depressants while on clorazepate therapy.
- If a woman becomes pregnant during therapy or intends to become pregnant, communicate with prescriber about the desirability of discontinuing the drug.
- Do not breast feed while taking this drug.
- Store this medication out of reach of children.

CLOTRIMAZOLE

(kloe-trim'a-zole)

Canesten ♣, Gyne-Lotrimin, Gyne-Lotrimin-3, Lotrimin, Mycelex, Mycelex-G

Classifications: ANTI-INFECTIVE; ANTIBIOTIC; ANTIFUNGAL

Prototype: Fluconazole

Pregnancy Category: B (topical); category C (oral)

AVAILABILITY 1% cream, solution, lotion; 10 mg troches; 100 mg, 200 mg, 500 mg vaginal tablets; 1% vaginal cream

ACTIONS Has broad-spectrum fungicidal activity. Acts by altering fungal cell membrane permeability, permitting loss of phosphorous compounds, potassium, and other essential intracellular constituents with consequent loss of ability to replicate.

THERAPEUTIC EFFECTS Active against *Trichophyton rubrum, T. mentagrophytes, Epidermophyton floccosum, Microsporum canis, Malassezia furfur,* and *Candida* sp., including *Candida albicans.* Natural or acquired fungal resistance to clotrimazole is rare.

USES Dermal infections including tinea pedis, tinea cruris, tinea corporis, tinea versicolor; also vulvovaginal and oropharyngeal candidiasis.

UNLABELED USE Trichomoniasis.

CONTRAINDICATIONS Ophthalmic uses; systemic mycoses. Safe use during pregnancy (category C for oral troches, category B for topical preparations), lactation, and in children <3 y not established.

CAUTIOUS USE Hepatic impairment.

ROUTE & DOSAGE

Dermal Infections

Adult: **Topical** Apply small amount onto affected areas b.i.d. a.m. and p.m.

Vulvovaginal Infections

Adult: **Intravaginal** Insert 1 applicator full or one 100 mg vaginal tablet into vagina at bedtime for 7 days, or one 500 mg vaginal tablet at bedtime for 1 dose

Oropharyngeal Candidiasis
Child/Adult: **PO** 1 troche (lozenge) 5 times/day q3h for 14 days

STORAGE
Store cream and solution formulations at 15°–30° C (59°–86° F); do not store troches or vaginal tablets above 35° C (95° F).

ADMINISTRATION
- Instruct patient taking the oral lozenge to allow it to dissolve slowly in mouth over 15–30 min for maximum effectiveness. Before using, evaluate the child's ability to follow directions for use of lozenge.
- Apply skin cream and solution preparations sparingly. Protect hands with latex gloves when applying medication.
- Avoid contact of clotrimazole preparations with the eyes.
- Do not use occlusive dressings unless directed by physician to do so.
- Consult health care provider about skin cleansing procedure before applying medication. Regardless of procedure used, dry skin thoroughly.

ADVERSE EFFECTS GI: Abnormal liver function tests; occasional nausea and vomiting (with oral troche). **Skin:** Stinging, erythema, edema, vesication, desquamation, pruritus, urticaria, skin fissures. **Urogenital:** Mild burning sensation, lower abdominal cramps, bloating, cystitis, urethritis, mild urinary frequency, vulval erythema and itching, pain and vaginal soreness during intercourse.

INTERACTIONS Drug: Intravaginal preparations may inactivate SPERMI-CIDES.

PHARMACOKINETICS Absorption: Minimal systemic absorption; minimally absorbed topically. **Peak:** High saliva concentrations <3 h; high vaginal concentrations in 8–24 h. **Metabolism:** Metabolized in liver. **Elimination:** Eliminated as metabolite in bile.

NURSING IMPLICATIONS

Assessment & Drug Effects
- Evaluate effectiveness of treatment. Report any signs of skin irritation with dermal preparations.
- Anticipate signs of clinical improvement within the first week of drug use.

Patient & Family Education
- Use clotrimazole as directed and for the length of time prescribed.
- Generally, clinical improvement is apparent during first week of therapy. Report to health care provider if condition worsens or if signs of irritation or sensitivity develop, or if no improvement is noted after 4 wk of therapy.
- If receiving the drug vaginally, sexual partner may experience burning and irritation of penis or urethritis; refrain from sexual intercourse during therapy or have sexual partner wear a condom.
- Do not breast feed while taking this drug.
- Store this medication out of reach of children.

Common adverse effects in *italic;* life-threatening effects <u>underlined;</u> generic names in **bold;** drug classifications in SMALL CAPS; ✦ Canadian drug name; ☻ Prototype drug.

353

C

CLOXACILLIN, SODIUM
(klox-a-sill'in)
Apo-Cloxi ♣ , Cloxapen, Cloxilean, Novocloxin ♣ , Orbenin, Tegopen
Classifications: ANTI-INFECTIVE; ANTIBIOTIC; NATURAL PENICILLIN; BETA-LACTAM
Prototype: Penicillin G
Pregnancy Category: B

AVAILABILITY 250 mg, 500 mg capsules; 125 mg/5 mL oral suspension

ACTIONS Semisynthetic, acid-stable, penicillinase-resistant, isoxazolyl penicillin. Effective against most gram-positive bacteria.
THERAPEUTIC EFFECTS In common with other isoxazolyl penicillins (dicloxacillin, oxacillin), highly active against most penicillinase-producing staphylococci, less potent than penicillin G against penicillin-sensitive microorganisms, and generally ineffective against gram-negative bacteria and methicillin-resistant staphylococci (MRSA).

USES Primarily in infections caused by penicillinase-producing staphylococci and penicillin-resistant staphylococci. May be used to initiate therapy in suspected staphylococcal infections pending culture and susceptibility test results. As with other penicillins, serum concentrations are enhanced by concurrent use of probenecid.

CONTRAINDICATIONS Sensitivity to penicillins; pregnancy (category B), lactation. Safe use in neonates not established.
CAUTIOUS USE History of or suspected atopy or allergy (asthma, eczema, hives, hay fever), renal or hepatic function impairment, history of allergy to cephalosporins.

ROUTE & DOSAGE

Mild to Moderate Infections
Child: **PO** <20 kg: 12.5–25 mg/kg q6h (max 4 g/day)
Adult: **PO** 250–500 mg q6h

STORAGE
Store capsules at 15°–30° C (59°–86° F). Reconstituted suspension stable for 14 days if refrigerated, and 3 days at room temperature.

ADMINISTRATION
Oral
- Give on an empty stomach (at least 1 h before or 2 h after meals) unless otherwise advised by prescriber. Food reduces rate and extent of drug absorption.
- After reconstitution PO solution retains potency for 14 days if refrigerated (shake well before pouring).

ADVERSE EFFECTS Body as a Whole: Wheezing, sneezing, chills, drug fever, anaphylaxis, superinfections. **GI:** *Nausea,* vomiting, flatulence,

diarrhea. **Hematologic:** Eosinophilia, leukopenia, <u>agranulocytosis</u>.
Metabolic: Elevated AST, ALT; jaundice (possibly of allergic etiology).
Skin: Pruritus, urticaria, rash.

INTERACTIONS Drug: Probenecid decreases cloxacillin elimination.

PHARMACOKINETICS Absorption: 37–60% absorbed from GI tract. **Peak:**
0.5–2 h. **Duration:** 4–6 h. **Distribution:** Distributed throughout body with
highest concentrations in liver, kidney, spleen, bone, bile, and pleural
fluid; low CSF penetration; crosses placenta; distributed into breast milk.
Metabolism: Metabolized in liver. **Elimination:** Excreted primarily in urine
with some elimination through bile. **Half-Life:** 30–60 min.

NURSING IMPLICATIONS

Assessment & Drug Effects

- Determine previous exposure and sensitivity to penicillins and cephalosporins and other allergic reactions of any kind before treatment is initiated.
- Monitor for S&S of anaphylactoid reaction or other S&S of hypersensitivity reaction as with other penicillins.
- Lab tests: Periodic assessments of renal, hepatic, and hematopoietic
function are advised in patients on long-term therapy.

Patient & Family Education

- Take medication around the clock, do not miss a dose, and continue
taking the medication until it is finished.
- Report to health care provider the onset of hypersensitivity reaction and
superinfections.
- Check with care provider if GI adverse effects (nausea, vomiting, diar-
rhea) appear.
- Do not breast feed while taking this drug.
- Store this medication out of reach of children.

CODEINE

(koe'deen)

CODEINE PHOSPHATE

Paveral ◆

CODEINE SULFATE

Classifications: CENTRAL NERVOUS SYSTEM AGENT; NARCOTIC (OPIATE)
AGONIST ANALGESIC; ANTITUSSIVE
Prototype: Morphine
Pregnancy Category: C
Controlled Substance: Schedule II

AVAILABILITY 15 mg, 30 mg, 60 mg tablets; 15 mg/5 mL oral solution; 30
mg, 60 mg injection

C

ACTIONS Opium derivative similar to morphine. In equianalgesic doses, parenteral codeine produces degree of respiratory depression similar to that of morphine. In contrast to morphine, orally administered codeine is about 60% as potent as the parenteral form. Histamine-releasing action appears to be more potent than that of morphine and may result in hypotension, flushing, and rarely bronchoconstriction.
THERAPEUTIC EFFECTS Analgesic potency is about one-sixth that of morphine; antitussive activity is also a little less than that of morphine.

USES Symptomatic relief of mild to moderately severe pain when control cannot be obtained by nonnarcotic analgesics and to suppress hyperactive or nonproductive cough.

CONTRAINDICATIONS Hypersensitivity to codeine or other morphine derivatives; acute asthma, COPD; increased intracranial pressure, head injury, acute alcoholism, hepatic or renal dysfunction, hypothyroidism. Pregnancy (category C), lactation. Safe use in neonates not established.
CAUTIOUS USE Very young children; those with history of drug abuse.

ROUTE & DOSAGE

Analgesic
Child: **PO/IM/SC** 0.5–1 mg/kg q4–6h prn. (max 60 mg/dose)
Adult: **PO/IM/SC** 15–60 mg q.i.d.

Antitussive
Child: **PO** 2–6 y, 2.5–5 mg q4–6h (max 30 mg/24 h); 6–12 y, 5–10 mg q4–6h (max 60 mg/24 h)
Adult: **PO** 10–20 mg q4–6h prn (max 120 mg/24h)

STORAGE
Preserve in tightly covered, light-resistant containers at 15°–30° C (59°–86° F). Do not freeze injection solution.

ADMINISTRATION
Oral
- Administer PO codeine with milk or other food to reduce possibility of GI distress.

Subcutaneous/Intramuscular
- Give parenterally to achieve greatest effectiveness. An oral dose is about 60% as effective as an equal parenteral dose.

ADVERSE EFFECTS Body as a Whole: Shortness of breath, anaphylactoid reaction. **CV:** Palpitation, hypotension, orthostatic hypotension, bradycardia, tachycardia, <u>circulatory collapse</u>. **GI:** *Nausea,* vomiting, *constipation.* **CNS:** *Dizziness,* light-headedness, *drowsiness,* sedation, lethargy, euphoria, agitation; restlessness, exhilaration, convulsions, narcosis, respiratory depression. **Skin:** Diffuse erythema, rash, urticaria, *pruritus,* excessive perspiration, facial flushing, fixed-drug eruption. **Special Senses:** Miosis. **Urogenital:** Urinary retention.

INTERACTIONS Drug: Alcohol and other CNS DEPRESSANTS augment CNS depressant effects. **Herbal: St. John's wort** may cause increased sedation.

PHARMACOKINETICS Absorption: Readily absorbed from GI tract. **Onset:** 15–30 min. **Peak:** 1–1.5 h. **Duration:** 4–6 h. **Distribution:** Crosses placenta; distributed into breast milk. **Metabolism:** Metabolized in liver. **Elimination:** Excreted in urine. **Half-Life:** 2.5–4 h.

NURSING IMPLICATIONS

Assessment & Drug Effects

- Record relief of pain and duration of analgesia.
- Evaluate effectiveness as cough suppressant. Treatment of cough is directed toward decreasing frequency and intensity of cough without abolishing cough reflex, need to remove bronchial secretions.
- Although codeine has less abuse liability than morphine, dependence is a major unwanted effect.
- Supervision of ambulation and use other safety precautions as warranted because drug may cause dizziness and light-headedness.
- Monitor for nausea, a common side effect. Report nausea accompanied by vomiting. Change to another analgesic may be warranted.

Patient & Family Education

- Make position changes slowly and in stages particularly from recumbent to upright posture. Lie down immediately if light-headedness or dizziness occurs.
- Lie down when feeling nauseated and notify prescriber if this symptom persists. Nausea appears to be aggravated by ambulation.
- Codeine may impair ability to perform tasks requiring mental alertness, so avoid driving and other potentially hazardous activities.
- Do not take alcohol or other CNS depressants unless approved by prescriber.
- Hyperactive cough may be lessened by avoiding irritants such as smoking, dust, fumes, and other air pollutants. Humidification of ambient air may provide some relief.
- Do not breast feed while taking this drug.
- Store this medication out of reach of children.

COLFOSCERIL PALMITATE

(col-fos'ce-ril)
Exosurf Neonatal
Classification: LUNG SURFACTANT
Prototype: Beractant
Pregnancy Category: Not applicable

AVAILABILITY 108 mg powder for injection

ACTIONS Synthetic lung surfactant. Endogenous pulmonary surfactant lowers surface tension on alveolar surfaces during respiration and stabilizes the alveoli against collapse at resting pressures.

Common adverse effects in *italic;* life-threatening effects underlined; generic names in **bold;** drug classifications in SMALL CAPS; ✤ Canadian drug name; ❷ Prototype drug.

357

THERAPEUTIC EFFECTS Deficiency of surfactant causes respiratory distress syndrome (RDS) in premature infants. Colfosceril lowers minimum surface tension on alveolar surfaces and restores pulmonary compliance and oxygenation in premature infants.

USES Prophylactic treatment of infants with birth weights <1350 g who are at risk of developing RDS. Prophylactic therapy of infants with birth weights >1350 g who show evidence of pulmonary immaturity.
UNLABELED USES Rescue treatment of infants with established RDS; RDS in adults.

CONTRAINDICATIONS Infants who have major congenital abnormalities or who are suspected of having congenital infections.

ROUTE & DOSAGE

Prophylaxis

Infant: **Intratracheal** 3 doses of 5 mL/kg are recommended, with the first dose being given as soon as possible after birth and repeat doses 12 and 24 h later to infants who remain on mechanical ventilation

Rescue Therapy

Infant: **Intratracheal** 2 doses of 5 mL/kg are recommended, the first dose being initiated as soon as the diagnosis of RDS is confirmed and the second 12 h later in infants remaining on mechanical ventilation

STORAGE
Store at 15°–30° C (59°–86° F) in a dry place. Reconstituted solution is stable for 12 h.

ADMINISTRATION

Intratracheal

- Reconstitute immediately before use if possible. Use only supplied diluent for reconstitution.
- Reconstitute as follows: (1) Withdraw diluent with 18- or 19-gauge needle attached to 10- to 12-mL syringe; (2) inject into vial by allowing vacuum to draw diluent in; (3) do not withdraw needle and aspirate as much of solution as possible back into syringe; (4) maintain vacuum and quickly release plunger. Repeat steps 3 and 4 three or four times to ensure adequate mixing.
- Reconstituted drug is a milky white suspension. Gently shake if needed to resuspend it.
- Withdraw entire ordered dose into syringe while maintaining vacuum in vial.
- Before administration of drug, ensure that endotracheal tube tip is in the trachea.
- Before administration of drug, the infant should be suctioned. If possible, avoid suctioning for 2 h after drug administration.
- Drug is administered without interrupting mechanical ventilation. Use side port on the endotracheal tube adaptor.
- Administer dose in halves, each half over 1–2 min. Give first half dose with head in midline position; then turn head and torso to the right.

Wait 30 sec; then return to midline position for second half dose. Give each dose in short bursts timed with inspiration. After second half dose, turn head and torso to left for 30 sec; then return to midline.
- Slow or stop drug administration and adjust ventilator rate or F$_{IO2}$ if any of the following occur: Heart rate decreases, infant becomes dusky or agitated, or O$_2$ saturation drops.

INCOMPATIBILITIES Solution/Additive: Do not mix any antibiotics with surfactant; this may inactivate surfactant.

ADVERSE EFFECTS CV: Bradycardia, tachycardia. **Respiratory:** Decreased oxygen saturation, mucous plugging, apnea, pulmonary hemorrhage.

INTERACTIONS Drug: No clinically significant interactions established.

PHARMACOKINETICS Absorption: Absorbed from the alveolus into lung tissue. **Duration:** At least 7 days. **Distribution:** Distributes uniformly to all lobes of the lung, distal airways, and alveolar spaces. **Metabolism:** Recycled and metabolized exclusively in the lungs. **Half-Life:** 20–36 h.

NURSING IMPLICATIONS

Assessment & Drug Effects
- During administration of drug, continuous ECG and transcutaneous monitoring are required. Also monitor chest expansion and facial expression.
- Monitor pulmonary function during administration. Rapid changes may require immediate adjustment of peak inspiratory pressure, ventilator rate, or F$_{IO2}$.
- Monitor continuously for 30 min following administration. Frequent arterial blood gas sampling is required to prevent hyperoxia and hypocarbia.

COLISTIMETHATE SODIUM
(koe-lis-ti-meth′ate)
Coly-Mycin M
Classifications: URINARY TRACT ANTI-INFECTIVE; ANTIBIOTIC
Prototype: Trimethoprim
Pregnancy Category: B

AVAILABILITY 150 mg injection

ACTIONS Polymyxin antibiotic and parenteral form of colistin. Similar to polymyxin B in structure and actions but about one-third to one-fifth as potent. Antibacterial activity and overall toxicity are less, but nephrotoxic potential is almost identical with that of polymyxin B. Believed to act by affecting phospholipid component in bacterial cytoplasmic membranes with resulting damage and leakage of essential intracellular components.

THERAPEUTIC EFFECTS Bactericidal against most gram-negative organisms including *Pseudomonas aeruginosa, Escherichia coli, Enterobacter*

---

aerogenes, Haemophilus sp., *Klebsiella pneumoniae, Brucella, Salmo-nella, Shigella, Bordetella, Pasteurella,* and *Vibrio.* Not effective against *Proteus* or *Neisseria* species. Complete cross-resistance and cross-sensitivity to polymyxin B reported but not to broad-spectrum antibiotics.

USES Particularly for severe, acute and chronic UTIs caused by susceptible strains of gram-negative organisms resistant to other antibiotics. Has been used with carbenicillin for *Pseudomonas* sepsis in children with acute leukopenia.

CONTRAINDICATIONS Hypersensitivity to polypeptide antibiotics; concomitant use of drugs that potentiate neuromuscular blocking effect (aminoglycoside antibiotics, other polymyxins, anticholinesterases, curariform muscle relaxants, ether, sodium citrate); nephrotoxic and ototoxic drugs; pregnancy (category B).
CAUTIOUS USE Impaired renal function; myasthenia gravis; older adult patients, infants; lactation.

ROUTE & DOSAGE

Urinary Tract Infections
Child/Adult: **IM/IV** 2.5–5 mg/kg/day divided into 2–4 doses (max 5 mg/kg/day)
Renal Impairment
Cl_{cr} 1.3–1.5 mg/dL: 2.5–3.8 mg/kg/day divided into 2 doses; Cl_{cr} 1.6–2.5 mg/dL: 2.5 mg/kg/day in a single dose or divided into 2 doses; Cl_{cr} 2.6–4 mg/dL: 1.5 mg/kg q36h

STORAGE
Reconstituted solution may be stored in refrigerator at 2°–8° C (36°–46° F) or at controlled room temperature of 15°–30° C (59°–86° F). Use within 7 days. Store unopened vials at controlled room temperature.

ADMINISTRATION
Intramuscular
- Reconstitute each 150-mg vial with 2 mL of sterile water for injection to yield a concentration of 75 mg/mL. Swirl vial gently during reconstitution to avoid bubble formation. IM injection should be made deep into upper outer quadrant of buttock. Patients commonly experience pain at injection site. Rotate sites.

Intravenous
PREPARE **Direct/Intermittent:** Prepare first half of total daily dose as directed for IM then further dilute with 20 mL sterile water for injection. Prepare second half of total daily dose by diluting further in 50 mL or more of D5W, NS, D5/NS, RL, or other compatible solution. IV infusion solution should be freshly prepared and used within 24 h.
ADMINISTER **Direct/Intermittent:** First half of total daily dose: Give slowly over 3–5 min. Second half of total daily dose: Starting 1–2 h after

Common adverse effects in *italic;* life-threatening effects <u>underlined;</u> generic names in **bold;** drug classifications in SMALL CAPS; ✦ Canadian drug name; ✪ Prototype drug.

the first half dose has been given, infuse the second half dose over the next 22–23 h.

INCOMPATIBILITIES **Solution/Additive: Carbenicillin, cephalothin, erythromycin, hydrocortisone, kanamycin.**

ADVERSE EFFECTS Body as a Whole: Drug fever, pain at IM site. **GI:** GI disturbances. **CNS:** Circumoral, lingual, and peripheral paresthesias; visual and speech disturbances, neuromuscular blockade (generalized muscle weakness, dyspnea, respiratory depression or paralysis), seizures, psychosis. **Respiratory:** Respiratory arrest after IM injection. **Skin:** Pruritus, urticaria, dermatoses. **Special Senses:** Ototoxicity. **Urogenital:** Nephrotoxicity.

INTERACTIONS Drug: Tubocurarine, pancuronium, atracurium, AMINOGLYCOSIDES may compound and prolong respiratory depression; AMINOGLYCOSIDES, **amphotericin B, vancomycin** augment nephrotoxicity.

PHARMACOKINETICS Peak: 1–2 h IM. **Duration:** 8–12 h. **Distribution:** Widely distributed in most tissues except CNS; crosses placenta; distributed into breast milk in low concentrations. **Metabolism:** Metabolized in liver. **Elimination:** 66–75% excreted in urine within 24 h. **Half-Life:** 2–3 h.

NURSING IMPLICATIONS

Assessment & Drug Effects

- Lab tests: Culture and sensitivity tests should be performed initially and periodically during therapy to determine responsiveness of causative organisms. Baseline renal function tests should be performed prior to therapy; frequent monitoring of renal function and urine drug levels is advisable during therapy. Impaired renal function increases the possibility of nephrotoxicity, apnea, and neuromuscular blockade.
- Report restlessness or dyspnea promptly. Respiratory arrest has been reported after IM administration.
- Monitor I&O ratio and patterns: Decrease in urine output or change in I&O ratio and rising BUN, serum creatinine, and serum drug levels (without dosage increase) are indications of renal toxicity. If they occur, withhold drug and report to prescriber.
- Close monitoring of infants is essential. They are particularly prone to renal toxicity.
- Be alert to neurologic symptoms: Changes in speech and hearing, visual changes, drowsiness, dizziness, ataxia, and transient paresthesias should be reported.
- Monitor closely postoperative patients who have received curariform muscle relaxants, ether, or sodium citrate for signs of neuromuscular blockade (delayed recovery, muscle weakness, depressed respiration).

Patient & Family Education

- Avoid operating a vehicle or other potentially hazardous activities while on drug therapy because of the possibility of transient neurologic disturbances.
- Do not breast feed without consulting the prescriber.

CORTICOTROPIN
(kor-ti-koe-troe′pin)
ACTH, Acthar

CORTICOTROPIN REPOSITORY

ACTH Gel, Acthron, Cortigel, Cortrophin-Gel, Cotropic Gel, H. P. Acthar Gel

Classifications: HORMONE AND SYNTHETIC SUBSTITUTE; ADRENAL CORTICOSTEROID

Prototype: Prednisone

Pregnancy Category: C

AVAILABILITY 25 unit, 40 unit vials for injection **Repository** 40 units/mL, 80 units/mL

ACTIONS Adrenocorticotropic hormone (ACTH) extracted from pituitary of domestic animals (usually pigs). Stimulates functioning adrenal cortex to produce and secrete corticosterone, cortisol (hydrocortisone), several weak androgens, and limited amounts of aldosterone.

THERAPEUTIC EFFECTS Therapeutic effects appear more rapidly than do those of prednisone. Suppresses further release of corticotropin by negative-feedback mechanism. Chronic administration of exogenous corticosteroids decreases ACTH store and causes structural changes in pituitary. Lack of ACTH stimulation can lead to adrenal cortex atrophy.

USES Diagnostic test of adrenocortical function and adjunctively to treat adrenal insufficiency secondary to inadequate corticotropin secretion. Used to treat infantile spasms.

CONTRAINDICATIONS Ocular herpes simplex; recent surgery; CHF; scleroderma; osteoporosis; systemic fungoid infections; hypertension; sensitivity to porcine proteins; conditions accompanied by primary adrenocortical insufficiency or hyperfunction; pregnancy (category C), lactation.

CAUTIOUS USE Patients with latent tuberculosis or those reacting to tuberculin; hypothyroiditis, impaired hepatic function.

ROUTE & DOSAGE

Diagnostic Test

Adult: **IV** 10–25 units in 500 mL D5W infused over 8 h

Therapeutic

Child: **IM/IV/SC** 1.6 units/kg/day in repository gel for infantile spasms, divided into doses given q6–8h; repository 0.8 units/kg/day divided into doses given q12h

Adult: **IM/SC** 40–80 units/day, dose and frequency individualized; **Repository** 40–80 units q24–72h

STORAGE

Reconstituted injection solution is stable for 24 h or 7 days, depending on product, when stored at 2°–8° C (36°–46° F). Store repository at 2°–15° C (36°–59° F). Store corticotropin zinc hydroxide at 15°–30° C (59°–86° F).

ADMINISTRATION

Subcutaneous/Intramuscular

- Dosage is individualized. Changes in dosage regimen are gradual and only after full drug effects have become apparent.
- Corticotropin repository is only for SC and IM use. Do not use IV.
- Shake corticotropin zinc hydroxide bottle well before injecting drug deep into appropriate muscle for age.

Intravenous

- IV administration to infants and children: Verify correct IV concentration and rate of infusion with physician.

PREPARE Continuous: Use only the vial labeled for IV use. Dilute powder with 2 mL sterile water or NS for injection; desired dose is withdrawn from vial and further diluted with 500 mL of D5W.

ADMINISTER Continuous: Give over 8 h.

INCOMPATIBILITIES Solution/Additive: Aminophylline, sodium bicarbonate.

- Administration of the hormone at high dosage levels is tapered rather than withdrawn suddenly. A 2–5 day period of adrenocortical hypofunction follows discontinuation of corticotropin.

ADVERSE EFFECTS Body as a Whole: May impair growth, loss of muscle mass, hypersensitivity, activation of latent tuberculosis, vertebral compression fracture. **GI:** Nausea, vomiting, abdominal distention, peptic ulcer with perforation and hemorrhage. **Endocrine:** Hirsutism, amenorrhea, osteoporosis, cushingoid state, activation of latent diabetes mellitus. **Metabolic:** Sodium and water retention; potassium and calcium loss, negative nitrogen balance, hyperglycemia. **CNS:** Euphoria, insomnia, headache, convulsions, papilledema, mood swings, depression. **Skin:** Acne, impaired wound healing, fragile skin, petechiae, ecchymosis. **Special Senses:** Cataract, glaucoma.

INTERACTIONS Drug: Aspirin, NSAIDS increase potential for hypoprothrombinemia; BARBITURATES, **phenytoin, rifampin** decrease effects of corticotropin; ESTROGENS may increase corticotropin binding and effects; **amphotericin B,** THIAZIDE AND LOOP DIURETICS increase potassium loss.

PHARMACOKINETICS Absorption: Readily absorbed from IM site. **Onset:** 6 h. **Duration:** 2–4 h IV/IM; 12–24 h repository. **Distribution:** Concentrated in many tissues; not known if crosses placenta or distributed into breast milk. **Metabolism:** Metabolized in liver. **Elimination:** Excreted in urine. **Half-Life:** <20 min.

C

NURSING IMPLICATIONS

Assessment & Drug Effects

- Before giving corticotropin to patient with suspected sensitivity to porcine proteins, hypersensitivity skin testing should be performed.
- Observe patient closely for 15 min for hypersensitivity reactions during IV administration or immediately after SC or IM injections (urticaria, pruritus, dizziness, nausea, vomiting, anaphylactic shock). Epinephrine 1:1000 should be readily available for emergency treatment.
- Prolonged use of corticotropin increases risk of hypersensitivity reaction.
- Adrenal response to corticotropin is measured against a baseline plasma cortisol level 1 h before the 8-h test. Another plasma level is determined after at least 1 h of the infusion.
- Corticotropin may suppress S&S of chronic disease.
- New infections can appear during treatment. Because of decreased resistance and inability to localize the infection, it may be severe. Report immediately.
- Monitor carefully growth and development of a child receiving this drug.

Patient & Family Education

- Corticotropin administration increases requirements for insulin and oral antidiabetic agents. If you have diabetes mellitus, monitor blood glucose closely until response to the drug is stabilized.
- Monitor weight and report a steady gain, especially if accompanied by edema. Also promptly report headache, muscle weakness, abdominal pain.
- Do not self-medicate with OTC drugs without consulting physician.
- Eye examinations should be done before initiation of expected long-term therapy and periodically during treatment. Report to physician if blurred vision occurs.
- Dietary salt restriction and potassium supplementation may be necessary to minimize edema caused by overstimulation of the adrenal cortex by corticotropin.
- Do not receive live vaccine immunizations while receiving corticotropin.
- Do not breast feed while taking this drug.
- Keep this medication out of reach of children.

CORTISONE ACETATE
(kor'ti-sone)
Cortistan, Cortone
Classifications: HORMONE AND SYNTHETIC SUBSTITUTE; SYNTHETIC ADRENAL CORTICOSTEROID; GLUCOCORTICOID
Prototype: Prednisone
Pregnancy Category: D

AVAILABILITY 5 mg, 10 mg, 25 mg tablets; 50 mg/mL injection

ACTIONS Short-acting synthetic steroid with prominent glucocorticoid activity and mineralocorticoid effects approximately equal to those of

prednisone (cortisol). Because therapeutic activity of cortisone results from its conversion in body to cortisol, its effects simulate those of hydrocortisone. Metabolic effects include promotion of protein, carbohydrate, and fat metabolism and interference with linear growth in children.
THERAPEUTIC EFFECTS Mineralocorticoid actions include promotion of sodium retention and potassium excretion. May foster development of osteoporosis. Has anti-inflammatory and immunosuppressive actions.

USES Replacement therapy for primary or secondary adrenocortical insufficiency and inflammatory and allergic disorders.

CONTRAINDICATIONS Hypersensitivity to glucocorticoids; psychoses; viral or bacterial diseases of skin; Cushing's syndrome, immunologic procedures; pregnancy (category D), lactation. Safe use in children not established.
CAUTIOUS USE Diabetes mellitus; hypertension, CHF; active or arrested tuberculosis; active or latent peptic ulcer.

ROUTE & DOSAGE

Replacement or Inflammatory Disorders

Child: **PO** 2.5–10 mg/kg/day divided into doses q6–8h; **IM** 1–5 mg/kg/day divided into doses q12–24h
Adult: **PO/IM** 20–300 mg/day divided into 1 or more doses; reduced periodically by 10–25 mg/day to lowest effective dose

STORAGE

Store at 15°–30° C (59°–86° F) in tightly closed container. Protect from heat and freezing.

ADMINISTRATION

Oral

- Administer cortisone (usually in a.m.) with food or fluid of patient's choice to reduce gastric irritation.
- Sodium chloride and a mineralocorticoid are usually given with cortisone as part of replacement therapy.

Intramuscular

- Parenteral cortisone is a suspension (25 mg/mL) and therefore should not be used IV. Shake bottle well before withdrawing dose.
- Give deep IM into a large muscle mass appropriate for age. (see Part I)
- Drug must be gradually tapered rather than withdrawn abruptly.

ADVERSE EFFECTS Body as a Whole: Impaired growth. **CV:** CHF, hypertension, *edema.* **GI:** *Nausea,* peptic ulcer, pancreatitis. **Endocrine:** Hyperglycemia. **Hematologic:** Thrombocytopenia. **Musculoskeletal:** *Compression fracture,* osteoporosis, muscle weakness. **CNS:** Euphoria, insomnia, vertigo, nystagmus. **Skin:** Impaired wound healing, petechiae, ecchymosis, acne. **Special Senses:** *Cataracts,* glaucoma, blurred vision.

INTERACTIONS Drug: BARBITURATES, **phenytoin, rifampin** decrease effects of cortisone.

PHARMACOKINETICS Absorption: Readily absorbed from GI tract. **Onset:** Rapid PO; 24–48 h IM. **Peak:** 2 h PO; 24–48 h IM. **Duration:** 1.25–1.5 days. **Distribution:** Concentrated in many tissues; crosses placenta; distributed into breast milk. **Metabolism:** Metabolized in liver. **Elimination:** Excreted in urine. **Half-Life:** 0.5 h; HPA suppression: 8–12 h.

NURSING IMPLICATIONS

Assessment & Drug Effects

- Monitor for S&S of Cushing's syndrome, especially in those on long-term therapy.
- Lab tests: Periodic blood glucose and CBC with platelet count.
- Cortisone may mask some signs of infection, and new infections may appear. Monitor growth and development regularly.
- Be alert to clinical indications of infection: Malaise, anorexia, depression, and evidence of delayed healing. (Classic signs of inflammation are suppressed by cortisone.)
- Report ecchymotic areas, unexplained bleeding, and easy bruising.

Patient & Family Education

- Take drug exactly as prescribed. Do not alter dose intervals or stop therapy abruptly.
- Monitor weight and report a steady gain especially if it is accompanied by signs of fluid retention (e.g., edema of ankles or hands).
- Report changes in visual acuity, including blurring, promptly.
- Inform care providers, including dentist that cortisone is being taken. Carry identification card or jewelry that states drug being taken and health care provider's name.
- Do not breast feed while taking this drug.
- Keep this medication out of reach of children.

COSYNTROPIN

(koe-sin-troe′pin)
Cortrosyn
Classification: DIAGNOSTIC AGENT
Prototype: Prednisone
Pregnancy Category: C

AVAILABILITY 0.25 mg injection

ACTIONS Synthetic polypeptide resembling corticotropin (ACTH) in relation to the first 24 of the 39 amino acids in naturally occurring ACTH. Has less immunologic activity and is associated with less risk of sensitivity than corticotropin.

THERAPEUTIC EFFECTS In patient with normal adrenocortical function, stimulates adrenal cortex to secrete corticosterone, cortisol (hydrocortisone), several weak androgenic substances, and limited amounts of aldosterone.

USES Diagnostic tool to differentiate primary adrenal from secondary (pituitary) adrenocortical insufficiency.

UNLABELED USE In individuals with normal adrenocortical function for the long-term treatment of chronic inflammatory or degenerative disorders responsive to glucocorticoids.

CONTRAINDICATIONS History of allergic disorders; scleroderma, osteoporosis; systemic fungal infections, ocular herpes simplex; recent surgery; history of or presence of peptic ulcer; CHF; hypertension; adrenocortical insufficiency and adrenocortical hyperfunction; pregnancy (category C), lactation; immunizations, tuberculosis, infections. **CAUTIOUS USE** Multiple sclerosis, acute gouty arthritis, mental disturbances, diabetes, abscess, pyrogenic infections, diverticulitis, renal insufficiency, myasthenia gravis, children.

ROUTE & DOSAGE

Rapid Screening Test
Neonate: **IM/IV** 0.015 mg/kg
Child <2 y: **IM** 0.125 mg injected over 2 min **IV** 0.125 mg at 0.04 mg/h over 6 h
Child >2 y/Adult: **IM/IV** 0.25 mg injected over 2 min

STORAGE
Reconstituted solutions remain stable 24 h at room temperature or 21 days at 2°–8° C (36°–46° F).

ADMINISTRATION
Intramuscular
- Reconstitute cosyntropin powder by adding 1.1 mL NS (diluent provided by manufacturer) to vial labeled 0.25 mg to provide solution containing 0.25 mg/mL.
- Inject deep IM into a large muscle mass appropriate for age. (see Part I)

Intravenous
- IV administration to neonates, infants and children: Verify correct IV concentration and rate of infusion/injection with physician.
PREPARE Direct: Reconstitute as for IM. **IV Infusion:** Further dilute in 250–500 mL of D5W or NS.
ADMINISTER Direct: Give over 2 min. **IV Infusion:** Give at an approximate rate of 40 mcg/h over 4–6 h.
- Cosyntropin should not be added to blood or to plasma infusions.

ADVERSE EFFECTS Body as a Whole: Mild fever. **GI:** Chronic pancreatitis. **Skin:** Pruritus.

DIAGNOSTIC TEST INTERFERENCE Cortisone, hydrocortisone, estrogen, spironolactone, elevated **bilirubin,** and presence of **free hgb** in plasma may interfere with **plasma cortisol** determinations.

INTERACTIONS Drug: Cortisone, hydrocortisone can exhibit abnormally high baseline values of cortisol and a decreased response to cosyntropin test.

PHARMACOKINETICS Absorption: Plasma cortisol levels double in 15–30 min. **Peak:** 1 h. **Duration:** 2–4 h. **Distribution:** Unknown; does not cross placenta. **Metabolism:** Unknown.

NURSING IMPLICATIONS

Assessment & Drug Effects

- Normal 17-KS levels in men are 10–25 mg/24 h; in women <50 y, 5–15 mg/24 h.
- Normal 17-OHCS levels in men are 5–12 mg/24 h; in women, 3–10 mg/24 h; in children 8–12 y, <4.5 mg/24 h; in younger children, 1.5 mg/24 h. Levels may be slightly higher in obese or muscular individuals.
- See prednisone for further information.

CROMOLYN SODIUM ⓟ

(kroe'moe-lin)

Disodium Cromoglycate, Crolom, DSCG, Fivent ♣ , Intal, Nasalcrom, Opticrom, Rynacrom ♣ , Vistacrom ♣ , Gastrocrom

Classification: MAST CELL STABILIZER
Pregnancy Category: B

AVAILABILITY 20 mg/2 mL solution for nebulization; 800 mcg spray; 40 mg/mL nasal solution; 4% ophthalmic solution; 100 mg/5 mL oral concentrate ampules

ACTIONS Synthetic asthma-prophylactic agent with unique action. Inhibits release of bronchoconstrictors—histamine and SRS-A (slow reacting substance of anaphylaxis) from sensitized pulmonary mast cells, thereby suppressing an allergic response. Has no intrinsic bronchodilator, antihistaminic, or vasoconstrictor properties, thus only of value when taken prophylactically.

THERAPEUTIC EFFECTS Particularly effective for IgE-mediated or "extrinsic asthma" precipitated by exposure to specific allergen, e.g., pollens, dust, animal dander by inhibiting the release of brochoconstrictor substances.

USES Primarily for prophylaxis of mild to moderate seasonal and perennial bronchial asthma and allergic rhinitis. Also used for prevention of exercise-related bronchospasm, prevention of acute bronchospasm induced by known pollutants or antigens, and for prevention and treatment of allergic rhinitis. Orally for systemic mastocytosis. **Ophthalmic use:** Allergic ocular disorders, conjunctivitis, vernal keratoconjunctivitis.

UNLABELED USES Orally for prophylaxis of GI and systemic reactions to food allergy.

CONTRAINDICATIONS Use of aerosol (because of fluorocarbon propellants) in patients with coronary artery disease or history of arrhythmias; dyspnea, acute asthma, status asthmaticus; patients unable to coordinate

---

actions or follow instructions, pregnancy (category B), lactation. Safe use in children <6 y not determined; use of capsule not recommended for children.
CAUTIOUS USE Renal or hepatic dysfunction.

ROUTE & DOSAGE

Allergies

Child: **Inhalation** >6 y, Metered dose inhaler or capsule: Same as for adult; >6 y, nasal solution: same as for adult
Adult: **Inhalation** Metered dose inhaler or capsule: 1 spray or 1 capsule inhaled q.i.d.; nasal solution: 1 spray in each nostril 3–6 times/day at regular intervals

Mastocytosis

Child: **PO** *2–12 y,* 1 ampule q.i.d. 30 min a.c. and at bedtime
Adult: **PO** 2 ampules q.i.d. 30 min a.c. and at bedtime

STORAGE

Protect from moisture and heat. Store in tightly closed, light-resistant container at 15°–30° C (59°–86° F).

ADMINISTRATION

- Patients should receive detailed instructions for loading and administering the spinhaler or nasalmatic device. See manufacturer's instructions. Therapeutic effect is dependent on proper inhalation technique.
- Advise child to clear as much mucus as possible before inhalation treatments. Then exhale as completely as possible before placing inhaler mouthpiece between lips, tilt head backward and inhale rapidly and deeply with steady, even breaths. Remove inhaler from mouth, hold breath for a few seconds, then exhale into the air. Repeat until entire dose is taken.
- Caution child not to exhale into inhaler because moisture from breath will interfere with its proper operation. Also inform child that capsule is intended for inhalation only and is ineffective if swallowed. Periodically observe the child's technique and correct as needed.

ADVERSE EFFECTS Body as a Whole: Peripheral eosinophilia, <u>angioedema</u>, <u>bronchospasm</u>, <u>anaphylaxis</u> (rare). **GI:** Swelling of parotid glands, dry mouth, slightly bitter after-taste, *nausea,* vomiting, esophagitis. **CNS:** Headache, dizziness, peripheral neuritis. **Skin:** Erythema, urticaria, rash, contact dermatitis. **Special Senses:** *Sneezing, nasal stinging and burning,* dryness and *irritation of throat and trachea; cough;* nasal congestion, itchy, puffy eyes, lacrimation, *transient ocular burning, stinging.*

INTERACTIONS Drug: No clinically significant interactions established.

PHARMACOKINETICS Absorption: Approximately 8% of dose absorbed from lungs. **Onset:** 1 wk with regular use. **Peak:** 15 min. **Duration:** 4–6 h; may last as long as 2–3 wk. **Elimination:** Excreted in bile and urine in equal amounts. **Half-Life:** 80 min.

NURSING IMPLICATIONS

Assessment & Drug Effects

- Withhold drug and notify physician if any of the following occur: Angioedema or bronchospasm.
- Monitor for exacerbation of asthmatic symptoms including breathlessness and cough that may occur in patients receiving cromolyn during corticosteroid withdrawal.
- For patients with asthma, therapeutic effects may be noted within a few days but generally not until after 1–2 wk of therapy.

Patient & Family Education

- Throat irritation, cough, and hoarseness can be minimized by gargling with water, drinking a few swallows of water, or by sucking on a lozenge after each treatment.
- Talk to your physician about what to do in the event of an acute asthmatic attack. Cromolyn is of no value in acute asthma.
- Cromolyn does not eliminate the continued need for therapy with bronchodilators, expectorants, antibiotics, or corticosteroids, but the amount and frequency of use of these medications may be appreciably reduced.
- Report any unusual signs or symptoms. Hypersensitivity reactions can be severe and life threatening. Drug should be discontinued if an allergic reaction occurs.
- Treatment with cromolyn 15 min before doing protracted exercises reportedly blunts the effects of vigorous exercise as well as cold air.
- Ophthalmic use: Do not wear soft contact lenses during therapy with ophthalmic drug. They may be worn within a few hours after therapy is discontinued.
- Learn the proper technique for instillation of ophthalmic drops.
- Do not breast feed while taking this drug.
- Keep this medication out of reach of children.

CROTAMITON
(kroe-tam′i-tonn)
Eurax
Classifications: SKIN AND MUCOUS MEMBRANE AGENT; SCABICIDE; ANTIPRURITIC
Prototype: Lindane
Pregnancy Category: C

AVAILABILITY 10% cream, lotion

ACTIONS Scabicidal and antipruritic agent. Available in an emollient lotion base or in a vanishing cream.

THERAPEUTIC EFFECTS By unknown mechanisms, drug eradicates *Sarcoptes scabiei* and effectively relieves itching.

USES Treatment of scabies and for symptomatic treatment of pruritus.

CONTRAINDICATIONS Application to acutely inflamed skin, raw or weeping surfaces, eyes, or mouth; history of previous sensitivity to crotamiton; pregnancy (category C).

Common adverse effects in *italic;* life-threatening effects underlined; generic names in **bold;** drug classifications in SMALL CAPS; ♣ Canadian drug name; ☻ Prototype drug.

ROUTE & DOSAGE

Scabies

Child/Adult: **Topical** Apply a thin layer of cream from neck to toes; apply a second layer 24 h later. Bathe 48 h after last application to remove drug

STORAGE

Store in tightly closed containers at 15°–30° C (59°–86° F). Do not freeze.

ADMINISTRATION

Topical

- Shake container well before use of solution.
- The skin must be thoroughly dry before applying medication.
- If drug accidentally contacts eyes, thoroughly flush out medication with water.
- Pruritus treatment: Massage medication gently into affected areas until it is completely absorbed. Repeat as needed (usually effective for 6–10 h).

ADVERSE EFFECTS Skin: Skin irritation (particularly with prolonged use), rash, erythema, sensation of warmth, allergic sensitization.

INTERACTIONS Drug: No clinically significant interactions established.

NURSING IMPLICATIONS

Assessment & Drug Effects

- Monitor for and report significant skin irritation or allergic sensitization.

Patient & Family Education

- Review package insert before treatment begins.
- Discontinue medication and report to health care provider if irritation or sensitization develops.
- Store this medication out of reach of children.

CYANOCOBALAMIN

(sye-an-oh-koe-bal-a′-min)
Anacobin ♣, Bedoz ♣, Betalin 12, Cobex, Crystamine, Crysti-12, Cyanabin, Cyanoject, Kaybovite, Nascobal, Redisol, Rubesol, Rubion ♣, Rubramin PC
Classifications: HORMONE AND SYNTHETIC SUBSTITUTE; VITAMIN B$_{12}$
Pregnancy Category: A; C (parenteral)

AVAILABILITY 25 mcg, 50 mcg, 100 mcg, 250 mcg tablets; 400 mcg/unit, 500 mcg/0.1 mL nasal gel

ACTIONS Vitamin B$_{12}$ is a cobalt-containing B complex vitamin produced by *Streptomyces griseus*. Essential for normal growth, cell reproduction, maturation of RBCs, nucleoprotein synthesis, maintenance of nervous

Common adverse effects in *italic;* life-threatening effects <u>underlined;</u> generic names in **bold;** drug classifications in SMALL CAPS; ♣ Canadian drug name; ◐ Prototype drug.

371

system (myelin synthesis), and believed to be involved in protein and carbohydrate metabolism. Also acts as coenzyme in various biologic reactions. Vitamin B_{12} deficiency results in megaloblastic anemia, dysfunction of spinal cord with paralysis, GI lesions.

THERAPEUTIC EFFECTS Therapeutically effective for treatment of vitamin B_{12} deficiency and pernicious anemia.

USES Vitamin B_{12} deficiency due to malabsorption syndrome as in pernicious (Addison's) anemia, sprue; GI pathology, dysfunction, or surgery; fish tapeworm infestation, and gluten enteropathy. Also used in B_{12} deficiency caused by increased physiologic requirements or inadequate dietary intake, and in vitamin B_{12} absorption (Schilling) test.

UNLABELED USES To prevent and treat toxicity associated with sodium nitroprusside.

CONTRAINDICATIONS History of sensitivity to vitamin B_{12}, other cobalamins, or cobalt; early Leber's disease (hereditary optic nerve atrophy), indiscriminate use in folic acid deficiency. Safe use during pregnancy (category A, category C [parenteral or when above RDA]), lactation, and in children not established.

CAUTIOUS USE Heart disease, anemia, pulmonary disease.

ROUTE & DOSAGE

Vitamin B_{12} Deficiency
Child: **IM/Deep SC** 100 mcg/day for 10–15 days, then 60 mcg/mo
Adult: **IM/Deep SC** 30 mcg/day for 5–10 days, then 100–200 mcg/mo

Pernicious Anemia
Child: **IM** 30–50 mcg/day for 2 wk to total of 1000 mcg, then 100 mcg/mo
Adult: **IM/Deep SC** 100–1000 mcg/day for 2–3 wk, then 100–1000 mcg q2–4wk **Intranasal** One pump of gel in one nostril once weekly

Diagnosis of Megaloblastic Anemia
Adult: **IM/Deep SC** 1 mcg/day for 10 days while maintaining a low folate and vitamin B_{12} diet

Schilling Test
Adult: **IM/Deep SC** 1000 mcg times 1 dose

Nutritional Supplement
Child: **PO** <1 y, 0.3 mcg/day, ≥1 y, 1 mcg/day
Adult: **PO** 1–25 mcg/day

STORAGE
Preserve in light-resistant containers at room temperature preferably at 15°–30° C (59°–86° F) unless otherwise directed by manufacturer.

ADMINISTRATION

Oral
- PO preparations may be mixed with fruit juices. However, administer promptly because ascorbic acid affects the stability of vitamin B_{12}.
- Administration of oral vitamin B_{12} with meals increases its absorption.

Subcutaneous/Intramuscular

- Give deep SC by slightly tenting the skin at the injection site.
- IM may be given into any normal IM injection site.

ADVERSE EFFECTS Body as a Whole: Feeling of swelling of body, <u>anaphylactic shock, sudden death</u>. **CV:** Peripheral vascular thrombosis, pulmonary edema, CHF. **GI:** Mild transient diarrhea. **Hematologic:** Unmasking of polycythemia vera (with correction of vitamin B$_{12}$ deficiency). **Metabolic:** Hypokalemia. **Skin:** Itching, rash, flushing. **Special Senses:** Severe optic nerve atrophy (patients with Leber's disease).

DIAGNOSTIC TEST INTERFERENCE Most antibiotics, methotrexate, and pyrimethamine may produce invalid diagnostic *blood assays for vitamin B$_{12}$*. Possibility of false positive test for *intrinsic factor antibodies.*

INTERACTIONS Drug: Alcohol, aminosalicylic acid, neomycin, colchicine may decrease absorption of oral cyanocobalamin; **chloramphenicol** may interfere with therapeutic response to cyanocobalamin.

PHARMACOKINETICS Absorption: Intestinal absorption requires presence of intrinsic factor in terminal ileum. **Distribution:** Widely distributed; principally stored in liver, kidneys, and adrenals; crosses placenta, excreted in breast milk. **Metabolism:** Converted in tissues to active coenzymes; enterohepatically cycled. **Elimination:** 50–95% of doses ≥100 mcg are excreted in urine in 48 h. **Half-Life:** 6 days (400 days in liver).

NURSING IMPLICATIONS

Assessment & Drug Effects

- Lab tests: Before initiation of therapy, reticulocyte and erythrocyte counts, Hgb, Hct, vitamin B$_{12}$, and serum folate levels should be determined; then repeated between 5 and 7 days after start of therapy and at regular intervals during therapy. Monitor potassium levels during the first 48 h. Conversion to normal erythropoiesis increases erythrocyte potassium requirement and can result in severe hypokalemia and sudden death.
- Obtain a careful history of sensitivities. Sensitization to cyanocobalamin can take as long as 8 y to develop.
- Monitor vital signs in patients with cardiac disease and in those receiving parenteral cyanocobalamin, and be alert to symptoms of pulmonary edema, which generally occur early in therapy.
- Therapeutic response to drug therapy is usually dramatic, occurring within 48 h. Effectiveness is measured by laboratory values and improvement in manifestations of vitamin B$_{12}$ deficiency.
- Characteristically, reticulocyte concentration rises in 3–4 days, peaks in 5–8 days, and then gradually declines as erythrocyte count and Hgb rise to normal levels (in 4–6 wk).
- Obtain a complete diet and drug history and inquire into alcohol drinking patterns for all patients receiving cyanocobalamin to identify and correct poor habits.

Patient & Family Education

- Notify physician of any intercurrent disease or infection. Increased dosage may be required.
- To prevent irreversible neurologic damage resulting from pernicious anemia, drug therapy must be continued throughout life.
- Rich food sources of B_{12} are nutrient-added breakfast cereals, vitamin B_{12}-fortified soy milk, organ meats, clams, oysters, egg yolk, crab, salmon, sardines, muscle meat, milk, and dairy products.
- Do not breast feed while taking this drug.
- Store this medication out of reach of children.

CYCLIZINE HYDROCHLORIDE

(sye′kli-zeen)
Marezine, Marzine ◆

CYCLIZINE LACTATE

Marezine Lactate, Marzine

Classifications: ANTIHISTAMINE (H_1-RECEPTOR ANTAGONIST); ANTIVERTIGO AGENT; ANTIEMETIC
Prototype: Meclizine
Pregnancy Category: B

AVAILABILITY 50 mg tablets; 50 mg/mL injection

ACTIONS Piperazine antihistamine (H_1-receptor blocking agent) structurally and pharmacologically related to other cyclizine compounds (e.g., buclizine, hydroxyzine, meclizine). In common with these agents, it exhibits CNS depression and anticholinergic, antispasmodic, local anesthetic, and antihistaminic activity. Mechanism of action is not known.

THERAPEUTIC EFFECTS Has prominent depressant action on labyrinthine excitability and on conduction in vestibular-cerebellar pathways, thus producing marked antimotion and antiemetic effects.

USES Chiefly for prevention and treatment of motion sickness and post-operative nausea and vomiting.

CONTRAINDICATIONS Pregnancy (category B), lactation, children <6 y.
CAUTIOUS USE Narrow-angle glaucoma; prostatic hypertrophy; obstructive disease of GU or GI tracts; postoperative patients.

ROUTE & DOSAGE

Motion Sickness

Child: **PO** 6–12 y, 25 mg q4–6h prn (max 75 mg/day) **IM** 6–12 y, 1 mg/kg t.i.d. prn (max 75 mg/day)
Adult: **PO** 50 mg 30 min before travel, then q4–6h prn (max 200 mg/day) **IM** 50 mg q4–6h prn

Postoperative Vomiting

Adult: **IM** 50 mg 15–30 min before end of operation, may repeat q4–6h (t.i.d.) prn during first few days after surgery

Common adverse effects in *italic;* life-threatening effects <u>underlined</u>; generic names in **bold**; drug classifications in SMALL CAPS; ◆ Canadian drug name; ✪ Prototype drug.

STORAGE

- Store tablets in tightly closed, light-resistant container at 15°–30° C (59°–86° F). Store parenteral form at 5°–10° C (41°–50° F). When parenteral solution is stored at room temperature for prolonged periods, it may become slightly yellow, but this does not indicate loss of potency.

ADMINISTRATION

Oral

- Give dose 30 min prior to any activity likely to cause motion sickness.

Intramuscular

- Aspirate needle carefully before injecting IM. Anaphylactic reactions following inadvertent IV injection have been reported.
- For prophylaxis of postoperative nausea and vomiting, drug usually prescribed with preoperative medication or is administered 20–30 min before expected termination of surgery.

ADVERSE EFFECTS CV: Hypotension, palpitation, tachycardia. **GI:** Anorexia, nausea, vomiting, diarrhea, or constipation, cholestatic jaundice. **CNS:** *Drowsiness,* excitement, euphoria, auditory and visual hallucinations, hyperexcitability alternating with drowsiness, convulsions, respiratory paralysis (rare). **Skin:** Urticaria, rash. **Special Senses:** *Dry mouth,* nose, and throat; blurred vision, diplopia; tinnitus. **Other:** Pain at IM injection site.

DIAGNOSTIC TEST INTERFERENCE Because cyclizine is an antihistamine, inform patient that ***skin testing*** procedures should not be scheduled for about 4 days after drug is discontinued or false-negative reactions may result.

INTERACTIONS Drug: Alcohol, BARBITURATES, CNS DEPRESSANTS (e.g., HYPNOTICS, SEDATIVES, and ANXIOLYTICS) may compound effects of cyclizine.

PHARMACOKINETICS Onset: Rapid. **Duration:** 4–6 h. **Metabolism:** Unknown.

NURSING IMPLICATIONS

Assessment & Drug Effects

- Monitor postoperative patient's vital signs closely, because cyclizine can cause hypotension.
- Monitor for and report signs of CNS stimulation (e.g., hyperexcitability, euphoria). Dose reduction or discontinuation of drug may be indicated.

Patient & Family Education

- Take cyclizine with food or a glass of milk or water to minimize GI irritation.
- Do not drive a car or engage in other potentially hazardous activities until reaction to the drug is known. Adverse effects include drowsiness and dizziness.
- Alcohol, barbiturates, narcotic analgesic, and other CNS depressants may compound sedative action.
- Do not breast feed while taking this drug.
- Store this medication out of reach of children.

CYCLOBENZAPRINE HYDROCHLORIDE ⊕
(sye-kloe-ben′za-preen)
Cycoflex, Flexeril
Classifications: AUTONOMIC NERVOUS SYSTEM AGENT; SKELETAL MUSCLE RELAXANT, CENTRAL ACTING
Pregnancy Category: B

AVAILABILITY 10 mg tablets

ACTIONS Structurally and pharmacologically related to tricyclic antidepressants. Relieves skeletal muscle spasm of local origin without interfering with muscle function. Believed to act primarily within CNS at brain stem; some action at spinal cord level is also probable. Depresses tonic somatic motor activity, although both gamma and alpha motor neurons are affected.

THERAPEUTIC EFFECTS In common with other tricyclic compounds, it increases circulating norepinephrine by blocking its synaptic reuptake, thus producing its antidepressant effect. Also has sedative effects and potent central and peripheral anticholinergic activity.

USES Short-term adjunct to rest and physical therapy for relief of muscle spasm associated with acute musculoskeletal conditions. Not effective in treatment of spasticity associated with cerebral palsy or cerebral or cord disease.

CONTRAINDICATIONS Acute recovery phase of MI, patients with cardiac arrhythmias, heart block or conduction disturbances, CHF, hyperthyroidism. Use for periods longer than 2 or 3 wk not recommended by manufacturer. Pregnancy (category B), lactation. Safe use in children <15 y not established.

CAUTIOUS USE Patients receiving anticholinergic medications; prostatic hypertrophy, history of urinary retention, angle-closure glaucoma; increased IOP, seizures; cardiovascular disease; hepatic impairment; older adults, debilitated patients; history of psychiatric illness.

ROUTE & DOSAGE

Muscle Spasm
Adult: **PO** 20–40 mg/day in 2–4 divided doses (max 60 mg/day). Should not be administered to child <15 y of age

STORAGE
Store in tightly closed container, preferably at 15°–30° C (59°–86° F) unless otherwise directed by manufacturer.

ADMINISTRATION
Oral
- Do not administer drug if patient is receiving an MAO INHIBITOR (e.g., furazolidone, isocarboxazid, pargyline, tranylcypromine).
- Cyclobenzaprine is intended for short-term (2–3 wk) use.

Common adverse effects in *italic;* life-threatening effects <u>underlined</u>; generic names in **bold**; drug classifications in SMALL CAPS; ♣ Canadian drug name; ⊕ Prototype drug.

ADVERSE EFFECTS Body as a Whole: <u>Edema of tongue</u> and face, sweating, myalgia, hepatitis, alopecia. Shares toxic potential of tricyclic antidepressants. **CV:** Tachycardia, syncope, palpitation, vasodilation, chest pain, orthostatic hypotension, dyspnea; with high doses, possibility of severe arrhythmias. **GI:** *Dry mouth,* indigestion, unpleasant taste, coated tongue, tongue discoloration, vomiting, anorexia, abdominal pain, flatulence, diarrhea, paralytic ileus. **CNS:** *Drowsiness, dizziness,* weakness, fatigue, asthenia, paresthesias, tremors, muscle twitching, insomnia, euphoria, disorientation, mania, ataxia. **Skin:** Pruritus, urticaria, skin rash. **Urogenital:** Increased or decreased libido, impotence.

INTERACTIONS Drug: Alcohol, BARBITURATES, other CNS DEPRESSANTS enhance CNS depression; potentiates anticholinergic effects of **phenothiazine** and other ANTICHOLINERGICS; MAO INHIBITORS may precipitate hypertensive crisis—use with extreme caution.

PHARMACOKINETICS Absorption: Well absorbed from GI tract with some first-pass elimination in liver. **Onset:** 1 h. **Peak:** 3–8 h. **Duration:** 12–24 h. **Distribution:** Highly protein bound (93%). **Metabolism:** Metabolized in liver to inactive metabolites. **Elimination:** Slowly excreted in urine with some elimination in feces; may be excreted in breast milk. **Half-Life:** 1–3 days.

NURSING IMPLICATIONS

Assessment & Drug Effects

- Supervision of ambulation may be indicated because of risk of drowsiness and dizziness.
- Withhold drug and notify physician if signs of hypersensitivity (e.g., pruritus, urticaria, rash) appear.

Patient & Family Education

- Avoid driving and other potentially hazardous activities until reaction to drug is known. Adverse effects include drowsiness and dizziness.
- Avoid alcohol and other CNS DEPRESSANTS (unless otherwise directed by physician) because cyclobenzaprine enhances their effects.
- Dry mouth may be relieved by increasing total fluid intake (if not contraindicated).
- Keep prescriber informed of therapeutic effectiveness. Spasmolytic effect usually begins within 1 or 2 days and may be manifested by lessening of pain and tenderness, increase in range of motion, and ability to perform ADL.
- Do not breast feed while taking this drug.
- Store this medication out of reach of children.

CYCLOPENTOLATE HYDROCHLORIDE ℗

(sye-kloe-pen′toe-late)

Ak-Pentolate, Cyclogyl, Pentalair

Classifications: EYE PREPARATION; CYCLOPLEGIC; MYDRIATIC

Pregnancy Category: C

Common adverse effects in *italic;* life-threatening effects <u>underlined</u>; generic names in **bold;** drug classifications in SMALL CAPS; ♣ Canadian drug name; ℗ Prototype drug.

377

AVAILABILITY 0.5%, 1%, 2% ophthalmic solution **Combination Products:** Available in combination with phenylephrine in ophthalmic solution

ACTIONS Tertiary amine antimuscarinic compound with systemic side effects and CNS toxicity, similar to those of atropine. Acts by blocking response of iris sphincter muscle and muscle of accommodation in the ciliary body to cholinergic stimulation.

THERAPEUTIC EFFECTS Results in dilation and paralysis ☯ accommodation of the eyes. It binds to melanin in pupil; thus highly pigmented eyes may be less responsive to cycloplegic and mydriatic actions of the drug.

USES Induction of cycloplegia or mydriasis for ophthalmic diagnostic procedures.

CONTRAINDICATIONS Narrow-angle glaucoma, excessively increased intraocular pressure; pregnancy (category C), lactation.

CAUTIOUS USE Children with brain damage, Down syndrome, cerebral palsy, blue-eyed individuals.

ROUTE & DOSAGE

Cycloplegia or Mydriasis

Neonate/Infant: Cyclopentolate with phenylephrine is recommended due to decreased amounts of cyclopentolate in this product.

Child: **Topical** 1 drop of 0.5–1% solution in eye 40–50 min before procedure, followed by 1 drop in 5 min; may need 2% solution in patients with darkly pigmented eyes

Adult: **Topical** 1 drop of 1% solution in eye 40–50 min before procedure, followed by 1 drop in 5 min; may need 2% solution in patients with darkly pigmented eyes

ADMINISTRATION

Topical

- Clarify with prescriber which strength (1% or 2%) should be used.
- Ask child or youth to remove soft contact lenses prior to installation of drops.

ADVERSE EFFECTS Body as a Whole: Flushing, fever. **CNS:** Drowsiness dysarthria, disorientation, ataxia, hallucinations, hyperkinesis, psychosis, seizures. **CV:** Sinus tachycardia, hypotension. **GI:** Dry mouth, abdominal distention in infants. **Skin:** Rash, contact urticaria. **Special Senses:** Burning, stinging, transient increases in intraocular pressure, irritation, punctate keratitis, blurred vision, hyperemia, synechiae, conjunctivitis, photophobia. **Urogenital:** Urinary retention.

INTERACTIONS Drug: May interfere with the ocular antihypertensive effects of **carbachol, pilocarpine, physostigmine.**

PHARMACOKINETICS Peak: 15–60 min. **Duration:** 24 h.

Common adverse effects in *italic;* life-threatening effects <u>underlined</u>; generic names in **bold;** drug classifications in SMALL CAPS; ♣ Canadian drug name; ☯ Prototype drug.

NURSING IMPLICATIONS

Assessment & Drug Effects
- Monitor cardiac status especially with preexisting heart disease.

Patient & Family Education
- Do not touch the dropper to any surface, including your skin or eyes.
- Exercise caution when driving or engaging in other potentially hazardous activities because cyclopentolate ophthalmic may cause blurred vision. If you experience blurred vision, avoid these activities.
- Protect your eyes when in bright light. Cyclopentolate ophthalmic solution may cause increased light sensitivity.
- Do not wear soft contact lenses when the eye drops are being used.
- Report immediately any of the following: Difficulty breathing, swelling of your lips, tongue, or face or hives; palpitations; unusual behavior.
- Do not breast feed while using this drug.
- Keep this medication out of reach of children.

CYCLOPHOSPHAMIDE ⊘
(sye-kloe-foss′fa-mide)
Cytoxan, Neosar, Procytox ✦
Classifications: ANTINEOPLASTIC; ALKYLATING AGENT
Pregnancy Category: C

AVAILABILITY 25 mg, 50 mg tablets; 100 mg, 200 mg, 500 mg, 1 g, 2 g vials

ACTIONS Cell-cycle nonspecific alkylating agent chemically related to the nitrogen mustards. Action mechanism unknown but thought to be the result of cross-linkage of DNA strands, thereby blocking synthesis of DNA, RNA, and protein. Associated with increased risk of secondary malignancies that may be detected several years after cyclophosphamide has been discontinued.
THERAPEUTIC EFFECTS Has pronounced immunosuppressive activity and is a highly toxic drug; thus therapeutic effects are usually accompanied by some evidence of toxicity.

USES As single agent or in combination with other chemotherapeutic agents in treatment of malignant lymphoma, multiple myeloma, leukemias, mycosis fungoides (advanced disease), neuroblastoma, adenocarcinoma of ovary, carcinoma of breast, or malignant neoplasms of lung. Useful in conditioning regimens for bone marrow transplantation.
UNLABELED USES To prevent rejection in homotransplantation; to treat severe rheumatoid arthritis, multiple sclerosis, systemic lupus erythematosus, Wegener's granulomatosis, nephrotic syndrome.

CONTRAINDICATIONS Men and women in childbearing years; serious infections (including chickenpox, herpes zoster); live virus vaccines; myelosuppression; pregnancy (category C), lactation.
CAUTIOUS USE History of radiation or cytotoxic drug therapy; hepatic and renal impairment, recent history of steroid therapy; bone marrow

---

infiltration with tumor cells; history of urate calculi and gout; patients with leukopenia, thrombocytopenia.

ROUTE & DOSAGE

Neoplasm

Child: **PO Initial:** 2–8 mg/kg or 60–250 mg/m^2 **Maintenance:** 2–5 mg/kg *or* 50–150 mg/m^2 twice weekly **IV Initial:** 2–8 mg/kg *or* 60–250 mg/m^2

Adult: **PO Initial:** 1–5 mg/kg/day **Maintenance:** 1–5 mg/kg q7–10 days **IV Initial:** 40–50 mg/kg in divided doses over 2–5 days up to 100 mg/kg **Maintenance:** 10–15 mg/kg q7–10 days *or* 3–5 mg twice weekly

Rhematoid Arthritis

Child/Adult: **PO** 1.5–2.5 mg/kg/day in combination with other agents **IV** 0.5–1 g/m^2 monthly for 6 mo then q2–3mo in combination with other agents

STORAGE

Store cyclophosphamide PO solution in refrigerator at 2°–8° C (36°–46° F). Use within 14 days.

ADMINISTRATION

Oral

- Child: Must be given under care and direction of pediatric oncology specialist. Use recommended handling techniques for hazardous medications (see Part I).
- Administer PO drug on empty stomach. If nausea and vomiting are severe, however, it may be taken with food. An antiemetic medication may be prescribed to be given before the drug.

Intravenous

IV PREPARE **Direct:** Add 5 mL sterile water for injection or bacteriostatic water for injection (paraben-preserved only) to each 100 mg and shake gently to dissolve. **Intermittent:** May be further diluted with 100–250 mL D5W, NS, D5/NS, RL, or other compatible solution.
ADMINISTER **Direct/Intermittent:** Give each 100 mg or fraction thereof over 10–15 min.
INCOMPATIBILITIES **Y-Site: Amphotericin B, cholesteryl complex.**

ADVERSE EFFECTS Body as a Whole: Transient dizziness, fatigue, facial flushing, diaphoresis, drug fever, <u>anaphylaxis</u>, secondary neoplasia. **GI:** *Nausea, vomiting,* mucositis, *anorexia,* hepatotoxicity, diarrhea. **Hematologic:** <u>Leukopenia</u>, *neutropenia,* acute myeloid leukemia, anemia, thrombophlebitis, interference with normal healing. **Metabolic:** Severe hyperkalemia, SIADH, hyponatremia, weight gain (but without edema) or weight loss, hyperuricemia. **Respiratory:** <u>Pulmonary emboli</u> and edema, pneumonitis, <u>interstitial pulmonary fibrosis</u>. **Skin:** *Alopecia* (reversible), transverse ridging of nails, pigmentation of nail beds and skin (reversible), nonspecific dermatitis <u>toxic epidermal necrolysis</u>,

Stevens-Johnson syndrome. **Urogenital:** Sterile hemorrhagic and non-hemorrhagic cystitis, bladder fibrosis, nephrotoxicity.

DIAGNOSTIC TEST INTERFERENCE Cyclophosphamide suppresses positive reactions to *Candida, mumps, trichophytons,* and *tuberculin PPD skin tests. Papanicolaou (PAP)* smear may be falsely positive.

INTERACTIONS Drug: Succinylcholine, prolonged neuromuscular blocking activity; **doxorubicin** may increase cardiac toxicity.

PHARMACOKINETICS Absorption: Readily absorbed from GI tract. **Peak:** 1 h PO. **Distribution:** Widely distributed, including brain, breast milk; crosses placenta. **Metabolism:** Metabolized in liver. **Elimination:** Excreted in urine as active metabolites and unchanged drug. **Half-Life:** 4–6 h.

NURSING IMPLICATIONS

Assessment & Drug Effects

- Lab tests: Total and differential leukocyte count, platelet count, and Hct are determined initially and at least 2 times per week during maintenance period. Baseline and periodic determinations of liver and kidney function and serum electrolytes also should be made. Microscopic urine examinations are recommended after large IV doses.
- Thrombocytopenia is rare, but if it occurs (count of 100,000/mm^3 or lower), assess for signs of unexplained bleeding or easy bruising. If platelet count indicates thrombocytopenia (≤100,000/mm^3), drug will be discontinued.
- Marked leukopenia is the most serious side effect. It can be fatal. Nadir may occur in 2–8 days after first dose but may be as late as 1 mo after a series of several daily doses. Leukopenia usually reverses 7–10 days after therapy is discontinued.
- During severe leukopenic period, protect patient from infection and trauma and from visitors and medical personnel who have colds or other infections.
- Report onset of unexplained chills, sore throat, tachycardia. Monitor temperature carefully and report an elevation immediately. The development of fever in a neutropenic patient (granulocyte count <1000) is a medical emergency because sepsis can develop quickly in these patients.
- Observe and report character of wound drainage. During period of neutropenia, purulent drainage may become serosanguineous because there are not enough WBCs to create pus. Because of suppressed immune mechanisms, wound healing may be prolonged or incomplete.
- Be alert for and report additional signs of infection such as respiratory infections, aching, rashes, and gastrointestinal distress.
- Assess immunization status prior to beginning therapy in order to be alert for diseases that pose risk.
- Monitor I&O ratio and patterns: Because the drug is a chemical irritant, PO and IV fluid intake is generally increased to help prevent renal irritation and hemorrhagic cystitis. Have patient void frequently, especially after each dose and just before retiring to bed.

- Watch for symptoms of water intoxication or dilutional hyponatremia; patients are usually well hydrated as part of the therapy.
- Promptly report hematuria or dysuria. Drug schedule is usually interrupted and fluids are forced.
- Record body weight at least twice weekly (basis for dose determination). Alert physician to sudden change or slow, steady weight gain or loss over a period of time that appears inconsistent with caloric intake.
- Diarrhea may signal onset of hyperkalemia, particularly if accompanied by colicky pain, nausea, bradycardia, and skeletal muscle weakness. These symptoms warrant prompt reporting to physician.
- Monitor for hyperuricemia, which occurs commonly during early treatment period in patients with leukemias or lymphoma. Report edema of lower legs and feet; joint, flank, or stomach pain.
- Protect patient from potential sources of infection. Cyclophosphamide makes the patient particularly susceptible to varicella-zoster infections (chickenpox, herpes zoster).
- Report any sign of overgrowth with opportunistic organisms, especially in patient receiving corticosteroids or who has recently been on steroid therapy.
- Report fever, dyspnea, and nonproductive cough. Pulmonary toxicity is not common, but the already debilitated patient is particularly susceptible.

Patient & Family Education

- Adhere to dosage regimen and do not omit, increase, decrease, or delay doses. If for any reason drug cannot be taken, notify physician.
- Be alert for and report additional signs of infection such as respiratory infections, aching, rashes, and gastrointestinal distress.
- Alopecia occurs in about 33% of patients on cyclophosphamide therapy. Hair loss may be noted 3 wk after therapy begins; regrowth (often differs in texture and color) usually starts 5–6 wk after drug is withdrawn and may occur while on maintenance doses.
- Use adequate means of contraception during and for at least 4 mo after termination of drug treatment. Breast feeding should be discontinued before cyclophosphamide therapy is initiated.
- Amenorrhea may last up to 1 y after cessation of therapy in 10–30% of women.
- Do not breast feed while taking this drug.
- Store this medication out of reach of children.

CYCLOSPORINE 🅟

(sye′kloe-spor-een)
Gengraf, Neoral, Sandimmune
Classification: IMMUNOSUPPRESSANT
Pregnancy Category: C

AVAILABILITY Sandimmune: 25 mg, 50 mg, 100 mg capsules; 100 mg/mL oral solution; **Gengraf, Neoral:** (microemulsion) 25 mg, 100 mg capsules; 100 mg/mL oral solution; 50 mg/mL injection

ACTIONS Immunosuppressant agent derived from extract of a soil fungus. Action in reducing transplant rejection appears to be due to selective and reversible inhibition of helper T-lymphocytes (which normally stimulate antibody production).

THERAPEUTIC EFFECTS This creates an imbalance in favor of suppressor T-lymphocytes (which inhibit antibody production); thus immune response is subdued. Unlike other immunosuppressive agents, it does not cause clinically significant bone marrow suppression.

USES In conjunction with adrenal corticosteroids to prevent organ rejection after kidney, liver, and heart transplants (allografts). Has had limited use in pancreas, bone marrow, and heart/lung transplantations. Also used for treatment of chronic transplant rejection in patients previously treated with other immunosuppressants; rheumatoid arthritis, severe psoriasis.

UNLABELED USES Sjögren's syndrome, to prevent rejection of heart-lung and pancreatic transplants, ulcerative colitis.

CONTRAINDICATIONS Hypersensitivity to cyclosporine or to ingredients in commercially available formulations, e.g., Cremophor (polyoxyl 35 castor oil); recent contact with or bout of chickenpox, herpes zoster; administration of live virus vaccines to patient or family members; RA patients with abnormal renal function, uncontrolled hypertension, or malignancies; pregnancy (category C), lactation.

CAUTIOUS USE Renal, hepatic, pancreatic, or bowel dysfunction; hyperkalemia; hypertension; infection; malabsorption problems (e.g., liver transplant patients).

ROUTE & DOSAGE

Prevention of Organ Rejection

Child: **PO** Same as for adult **IV** Same as for adult
Adult: **PO** 14–18 mg/kg beginning 4–12 h before transplantation and continued for 1–2 wk after surgery, then gradual reduction by 5%/wk (max dose of microemulsion, 10 mg/kg/day) **Maintenance:** 5–10 mg/kg/day **IV** 5–6 mg/kg beginning 4–12 h before transplantation (administer over 2–6 h); give same daily dose until patient can take oral form

Rheumatoid Arthritis (Neoral)

Adult: **PO** 2.5 mg/kg/day divided into 2 doses, may increase by 0.5–0.75 mg/kg/day q4wk to a max of 4 mg/kg/day

Severe Psoriasis (Neoral)

Adult: **PO** 1.25 mg/kg b.i.d. If significant improvement has not occurred after 4 wk, may increase dose by 0.5 mg/kg/day every 2 wk to max of 4 mg/kg/day

STORAGE

Store preferably at 15°–30° C (59°–86° F) in well-closed containers. Do not refrigerate. Protect ampules from light.

Common adverse effects in *italic;* life-threatening effects <u>underlined</u>; generic names in **bold;** drug classifications in SMALL CAPS; ♣ Canadian drug name; ❂ Prototype drug.

C

ADMINISTRATION

Oral

- Do not dilute oral solution with grapefruit juice. Dilute with orange or apple juice, stir well, then administer immediately.
- Neoral (microemulsion) and Sandimmune are not bioequivalent and cannot be used interchangeably without physician supervision.

Intravenous

PREPARE IV infusion: Dilute each 1 mL immediately before administration in 20–100 mL of D5W or NS.

ADMINISTER IV Infusion: Give by slow infusion over approximately 2–6 h. Rapid IV can result in nephrotoxicity.

INCOMPATIBILITIES Solution/Additive: Magnesium Sulfate. Y-Site: Amphotericin B cholesteryl complex, TPN.

ADVERSE EFFECTS Body as a Whole: Lymphoma, gynecomastia, chest pain, leg cramps, edema, fever, chills, infection, toxic states, weight loss, increased risk of skin malignancies in psoriasis patients previously treated with methotrexate, psoralens, or UV light therapy. (Rash, fever, chills may be due to castor oil vehicle in injectable products and neoral oral product. May necessitate the need to use oral Sandimmune.) **CV:** *Hypertension,* MI (rare). **GI:** Gingival hyperplasia, diarrhea, nausea, *vomiting,* abdominal discomfort, anorexia, gastritis, constipation. **Hematologic:** Leukopenia, anemia, thrombocytopenia, *hypermagnesemia, hyperkalemia,* hyperuricemia, *decreased serum bicarbonate,* hyperglycemia. **CNS:** *Tremor,* convulsions, headache, paresthesias, hyperesthesia, flushing, night sweats, insomnia, visual hallucinations, confusion, anxiety, flat affect, depression, lethargy, weakness, paraparesis, ataxia, amnesia. **Skin:** *Hirsutism,* acne, oily skin, flushing. **Special Senses:** Sinusitis, tinnitus, hearing loss, sore throat. **Urogenital:** Urinary retention, frequency, *nephrotoxicity (oliguria).*

DIAGNOSTIC TEST INTERFERENCE *Hyperlipidemia* and abnormalities in *electrophoresis* reported; believed to be due to polyoxyl 35 castor oil (Cremophor) in IV cyclosporine.

INTERACTIONS Drug: AMINOGLYCOSIDES, **danazol, diltiazem, doxycycline, erythromycin, ketoconazole, methylprednisolone, metoclopramide, nicardipine,** NSAIDS, **prednisolone, verapamil** may increase cyclosporine levels; **carbamazepine, isoniazid, octreotide, phenobarbital, phenytoin, rifampin** may decrease cyclosporine levels; **acyclovir,** AMINOGLYCOSIDES, **amphotericin B, cimetidine, cotrimoxazole, erythromycin, ketoconazole, melphalan, ranitidine, trimethoprim** may increase risk of nephrotoxicity; POTASSIUM-SPARING DIURETICS, ACE INHIBITORS **(captopril, enalapril)** may potentiate hyperkalemia. **Herbal: St. John's wort** may decrease cyclosporine levels.

PHARMACOKINETICS Absorption: Variably and incompletely absorbed (30%). Microemulsion formulation (Neoral) has less variability in absorption and may produce significantly higher serum levels compared with the standard formulation. **Peak:** 3–4 h. **Distribution:** Widely distributed; 33–47% distributed to plasma; 41–50% to RBCs; crosses placenta;

Common adverse effects in *italic;* life-threatening effects underlined; generic names in **bold;** drug classifications in SMALL CAPS; ♣ Canadian drug name; ⊘ Prototype drug.

distributed into breast milk. **Metabolism:** Extensively metabolized in liver, including significant first-pass metabolism; considerable entero-hepatic circulation. **Elimination:** Primarily eliminated in bile and feces; 6% excreted in urine. **Half-Life:** 19–27 h.

NURSING IMPLICATIONS

Assessment & Drug Effects

- Observe patients receiving the drug parenterally for at least 30 min con-tinuously after start of IV infusion and at frequent intervals thereafter to detect allergic or other adverse reactions.
- Hypersensitivity reactions have been associated with Cremophor emul-sifying agent in the parenteral formulation but not with the PO solution, which does not contain this ingredient.
- Monitor I&O ratio and pattern: Nephrotoxicity has been reported in about one-third of transplant patients. It has occurred in mild forms as late as 2–3 mo after transplantation. In severe form, it can be irre-versible, and therefore early recognition is critical.
- Record immunization status before therapy. Be alert for infectious diseases.
- Monitor vital signs. Be alert to indicators of local or systemic infection that can be fungal, viral, or bacterial. Also report significant rise in BP.
- Lab tests: Baseline and periodic tests are advised for (1) renal function (BUN, serum creatinine), (2) liver function (AST, ALT, serum amylase, bilirubin, and alkaline phosphatase), and (3) serum potassium.
- Lab tests: In psoriasis patients, CBC, BUN, uric acid, potassium, lipids, and magnesium should be monitored biweekly during first 3 mo.
- Periodic tests should be made of neurologic function. Neurotoxic ef-fects generally occur over 13–195 days after initiation of cyclosporine therapy. Signs and symptoms are reportedly fully reversible with dosage reduction or discontinuation of drug.
- Monitor blood or plasma drug concentrations at regular intervals, par-ticularly in patients receiving the drug orally for prolonged periods, as drug absorption is erratic.

Patient & Family Education

- Use the specially calibrated pipette provided to measure dose.
- Take medication with meals to reduce nausea or GI irritation.
- Enhance palatability of oral solution by mixing it with milk, chocolate milk, or orange juice, preferably at room temperature. Mix in a glass rather than a plastic container. Stir well, drink immediately, and rinse glass with small quantity of diluent to ensure getting entire dose.
- Take medication at same time each day to maintain therapeutic blood levels.
- Keep scheduled follow-up appointments. Report signs of infections. Avoid exposure to persons with infectious diseases.
- If possible, see a dentist before start of cyclosporine treatment, and practice good oral hygiene. Inspect mouth daily for white patches, sores, swollen gums.
- Hirsutism is reversible with discontinuation of drug.
- Do not breast feed while taking this drug.
- Store this medication out of reach of children.

Common adverse effects in *italic;* life-threatening effects underlined; generic names in **bold;** drug classifications in SMALL CAPS; ✦ Canadian drug name; ❍ Prototype drug.

385

CYPROHEPTADINE HYDROCHLORIDE
(si-proe-hep′ta-deen)
Periactin, Vimicon ♣
Classifications: ANTIHISTAMINE, H₁-RECEPTOR ANTAGONIST; ANTIPRURITIC
Prototype: Diphenhydramine
Pregnancy Category: B

AVAILABILITY 4 mg tablets

ACTIONS Potent piperidine antihistamine with pharmacologic actions similar to those of azatadine. Acts by competing with histamine for H_1-receptor sites on effector cells, thus preventing histamine mediated responses.

THERAPEUTIC EFFECTS Produces mild central depression and moderate anticholinergic effects; lacks antiemetic action. Has significant antipruritic, local anesthetic, and antiserotonin activity.

USES Symptomatic relief of various allergic conditions, including hay fever, vasomotor rhinitis, allergic conjunctivitis, urticaria caused by cold sensitivity, and pruritus of allergic dermatoses. Effective in treatment of anaphylactoid reactions as adjunct to epinephrine and other standard measures after acute symptoms have been controlled.

UNLABELED USES Cushing's disease, carcinoid syndrome, vascular headaches, appetite stimulant.

CONTRAINDICATIONS Hypersensitivity to cyproheptadine or other H_1-receptor antagonist antihistamines; acute asthma attack. Safe use during pregnancy (category B), lactation, and in children <2 y not established.

CAUTIOUS USE Older adult and debilitated patients; patients predisposed to urinary retention; glaucoma; asthma; hyperthyroidism; cardiovascular disease, hypertension; GI or GU tract obstruction.

ROUTE & DOSAGE

Allergies
Child: **PO** 0.25 mg/kg/day in 3–4 divided doses (max 12 mg/day for 2–6 y, 16 mg/day for 6–12 y)
Adult: **PO** 4 mg t.i.d. or q.i.d. (4–20 mg/day), max 0.5 mg/kg/day

STORAGE
Store in tightly covered container at 15°–30° C (59°–86° F) unless otherwise directed.

ADMINISTRATION
Oral
▪ GI adverse effects may be minimized by administering drug with food or milk.

ADVERSE EFFECTS GI: *Dry mouth,* nausea, vomiting, epigastric distress, appetite stimulation, weight gain, transient decrease in fasting blood sugar level, increased serum amylase level, cholestatic jaundice. **CNS:** *Drowsiness,* dizziness, faintness, headache, tremulousness, fatigue, disturbed coordination. **Respiratory:** Thickened bronchial secretions. **Skin:** Skin rash. **Special Senses:** Dry nose and throat. **Urogenital:** Urinary frequency, retention, and difficult urination.

DIAGNOSTIC TEST INTERFERENCE As a general rule, antihistamines are discontinued about 4 days before *skin testing procedures* are to be performed because they may produce false-negative results.

INTERACTIONS Drug: Alcohol and CNS DEPRESSANTS add to CNS depression; TRICYCLIC ANTIDEPRESSANTS and other ANTICHOLINERGICS have additive anticholinergic effects; may inhibit pressor effects of **epinephrine.**

PHARMACOKINETICS Absorption: Readily absorbed from GI tract. **Duration:** 6–9 h. **Distribution:** Distribution into breast milk not known. **Metabolism:** Metabolized in liver. **Elimination:** Excreted in urine.

NURSING IMPLICATIONS

Assessment & Drug Effects
- Monitor level of alertness. In some patients, the sedative effect disappears spontaneously after 3–4 days of drug administration.
- Because drug may cause dizziness, supervision of ambulation and other safety precautions may be warranted.

Patient & Family Education
- Avoid activities requiring mental alertness and physical coordination, such as driving a car, until reaction to the drug is known.
- Drug causes sedation, dizziness, and hypotension. Report these symptoms. Children are more apt to manifest CNS stimulation, e.g., confusion, agitation, tremors, hallucinations. Reduction in dosage may be indicated.
- Cyproheptadine may increase and prolong the effects of alcohol, barbiturates, narcotic analgesics, anxiolytics, and other CNS depressants.
- Monitor weight and keep physician informed of any significant weight gain.
- Maintain sufficient fluid intake to help to relieve dry mouth and also reduce risk of cholestatic jaundice.
- Do not breast feed while taking this drug.

CYTARABINE

(sye-tare'a-been)
ARA-C, Cytosar-U, Cytosine Arabinoside, DepoCyt, Tarabine
Classifications: ANTINEOPLASTIC; ANTIMETABOLITE; IMMUNOSUPPRESSANT
Prototype: Fluorouracil
Pregnancy Category: D

AVAILABILITY 10 mg/mL liposomal, 20 mg/mL, 100 mg, 500 mg, 1g, 2 g injection

C

ACTIONS Pyrimidine analog with cell-phase specificity affecting rapidly dividing cells in S phase (DNA synthesis). In certain conditions prevents development of cell from G_1 to S phase. Interferes with DNA and RNA synthesis.

THERAPEUTIC EFFECTS Antineoplastic agent that has strong myelosuppressant activity. Immunosuppressant properties are exhibited by obliterated cell-mediated immune responses, such as delayed hypersensitivity skin reactions.

USES To induce and maintain remission in acute myelocytic leukemia, acute lymphocytic leukemia, and meningeal leukemia and for treatment of lymphomas. Used in combination with other antineoplastics in established chemotherapeutic protocols.

CONTRAINDICATIONS History of drug-induced myelosuppression; immunization procedures; pregnancy (category D) particularly during first trimester, lactation. Safe use in infants not established.

CAUTIOUS USE Impaired renal or hepatic function, gout, drug-induced myelosuppression.

ROUTE & DOSAGE

Leukemias

Child/Adult: **IV** 200 mg/m² by continuous infusion over 24 h **SC** 1 mg/kg 1–2 times/wk **Intrathecal** 5–75 mg once q4days or once a day for 4 days

STORAGE

Store cytarabine in refrigerator until reconstituted. Reconstituted solutions may be stored at 15°–30° C (59°–86° F) for 48 h. Discard solutions with a slight haze.

ADMINISTRATION

- Child: Must be given under care and direction of pediatric oncology specialist. Use recommended handling techniques for hazardous medications (see Part I).

Intrathecal

- For intrathecal injection, reconstitute with an isotonic, buffered diluent without preservatives. Follow manufacturer's recommendations.

Intravenous

PREPARE Direct: Reconstitute with bacteriostatic water for injection (without benzyl alcohol for neonates) as follows: Add 5 mL to the 100-mg vial to yield 20 mg/mL; add 10 mL to the 500-mg vial to yield 50 mg/mL. **IV Infusion:** May be further diluted with 100 mL or more of D5W or NS.

ADMINISTER Direct: Give at a rate of 100 mg or a fraction thereof over 3 min. **IV Infusion:** Give over 30 min or longer depending on the total volume of IV solution to be infused.

INCOMPATIBILITIES Solution/Additive: Fluorouracil, gentamicin, heparin, insulin, nafcillin, oxacillin, penicillin G. Y-Site: Allopurinol, ganciclovir, TPN.

Common adverse effects in *italic;* life-threatening effects underlined; generic names in **bold;** drug classifications in SMALL CAPS; ✦ Canadian drug name; ⊘ Prototype drug.

ADVERSE EFFECTS Body as a Whole: Weight loss, sore throat, fever, thrombophlebitis and pain at injection site; pericarditis, bleeding (any site), pneumonia. Potentially carcinogenic and mutagenic. **GI:** *Nausea, vomiting,* diarrhea, stomatitis, oral or anal inflammation or ulceration, esophagitis, anorexia, <u>hemorrhage</u>, hepatotoxicity, jaundice. **Hematologic:** *Leukopenia, thrombocytopenia,* anemia, megaloblastosis, myelosuppression (reversible); transient hyperuricemia. **CNS:** Headache, <u>neurotoxicity</u>; peripheral neuropathy, brachial plexus neuropathy, personality change, neuritis, vertigo, lethargy, somnolence, confusion. **Skin:** Rash, erythema, freckling, cellulitis, skin ulcerations, pruritus, urticaria, bulla formation, desquamation. **Special Senses:** Conjunctivitis, keratitis, photophobia. **Urogenital:** Renal dysfunction, urinary retention.

INTERACTIONS Drug: GI toxicity may decrease **digoxin** absorption; decreases AMINOGLYCOSIDES activity against *Klebsiella pneumoniae*.

PHARMACOKINETICS Peak: 20–60 min SC. **Distribution:** Crosses blood–brain barrier in moderate amounts; crosses placenta. **Metabolism:** Metabolized primarily in liver. **Elimination:** 80% excreted in urine in 24 h. **Half-Life:** 1–3 h.

NURSING IMPLICATIONS

Assessment & Drug Effects

- Inspect patient's mouth before the administration of each dose. Record nausea and vomiting, which are common. Antiemetics are used early to prevent problems. Toxicity necessitating dosage alterations almost always occurs. Report adverse reactions immediately.
- Lab tests: Hct and platelet counts and total and differential leukocyte counts should be evaluated daily during initial therapy. Serum uric acid and hepatic function tests should be performed at regular intervals throughout treatment period.
- Be alert for and report signs of infection such as respiratory infections, aching, rashes, and gastrointestinal distress.
- Assess immunization status prior to beginning therapy in order to be alert for diseases that pose risk.
- Hyperuricemia due to rapid destruction of neoplastic cells may accompany cytarabine therapy. A regimen that includes a uricosuric agent such as allopurinol, urine alkalinization, and adequate hydration may be started. To reduce potential for urate stone formation, fluids are forced in excess of 2 L, if tolerated. Consult physician.
- Monitor I&O ratio and pattern.
- Monitor body temperature. Be alert to the most subtle signs of infection, especially low-grade fever, and report promptly.
- When platelet count falls below 50,000/mm^3 and polymorphonuclear leukocytes to below 1000/mm^3, therapy may be suspended. WBC nadir is usually reached in 5–7 days after therapy has been stopped. Therapy is restarted with appearance of bone marrow recovery and when preceding cell counts are reached.
- Provide good oral hygiene to diminish adverse effects and chance of superinfection. Stomatitis and cheilosis usually appear 5–10 days into the therapy.

Common adverse effects in *italic;* life-threatening effects <u>underlined</u>; generic names in **bold;** drug classifications in SMALL CAPS; ♣ Canadian drug name; ❂ Prototype drug.

D

Patient & Family Education

- Report promptly protracted vomiting or signs of nephrotoxicity (see Appendix D-1).
- Flu-like syndrome occurs usually within 6–12 wk after drug administration and may recur with successive therapy. Report chills, fever, achy joints and muscles. Report signs of infections. Avoid exposure to persons with infectious diseases.
- Report any signs and symptoms of superinfection (see Appendix D-1).
- Do not breast feed while taking this drug.

DACARBAZINE

(da-kar'ba-zeen)
DTIC, DTIC-Dome, Imidazole Carboxamide
Classifications: ANTINEOPLASTIC; ALKYLATING AGENT
Prototype: Cyclophosphamide
Pregnancy Category: C

AVAILABILITY 10 mg/mL injection

ACTIONS Cytotoxic agent with alkylating properties, which is cell-cycle nonspecific. Interferes with purine metabolism and with RNA and protein synthesis in rapidly proliferating cells.
THERAPEUTIC EFFECTS Has minimal immunosuppressive activity; reportedly carcinogenic, mutagenic, and teratogenic.

USES As single agent or in combination with other antineoplastics in treatment of metastatic malignant melanoma, refractory Hodgkin's disease, various sarcomas, and neuroblastoma.
UNLABELED USES Soft-tissue metastatic sarcoma and malignant glucagonoma.

CONTRAINDICATIONS Hypersensitivity to dacarbazine; lactation. Safe use during pregnancy (category C) is not established.

ROUTE & DOSAGE

Malignant Melanoma
Adult: **IV** 2–4.5 mg/kg/day for 10 days repeated at 4-wk intervals
Hodgkin's Disease
Child: **IV** 200–470 mg/m^2/day over 5 days q21–28days
Adult: **IV** 2–4.5 mg/kg/day for 10 days repeated at 4-wk intervals or 150 mg/m^2/day for 5 days repeated at 4-wk intervals

STORAGE
Store reconstituted solution up to 72 h at 4° C (39° F) or at room temperature 15°–30° C (59°–86° F) for up to 8 h. Store diluted reconstituted solution for 24 h at 4° C (39° F) or at room temperature for up to 8 h. Protect from light. Change from ivory to pink color indicates decomposition.

D

ADMINISTRATION

Intravenous

- Child: Must be given under care and direction of pediatric oncology specialist. Use recommended handling techniques for hazardous medications (see Part I). ■ IV administration to infants and children: Verify correct IV concentration and rate of infusion with physician.
  - Wear gloves when handling this drug. If solution gets into the eyes, wash them with soap and water immediately, then irrigate with water or isotonic saline.

***PREPARE* Direct:** Reconstitute drug with sterile water for injection to make a solution containing 10 mg/mL dacarbazine (pH 3.0–4.0) by adding 9.9 mL to 100 mg or 19.8 mL to 200 mg. **IV Infusion:** Dilute further in 50 mL of D5W or NS.

***ADMINISTER* Direct:** Give by direct IV over 1 min. **IV Infusion:** Infuse IV over 30 min. If possible, avoid using antecubital vein or veins on dorsum of hand or wrist where extravasation could lead to loss of mobility of entire limb. Avoid veins in extremity with compromised venous or lymphatic drainage and veins near joint spaces.

***INCOMPATIBILITIES:* Solution/Additive: Heparin, hydrocortisone sodium succinate.** ■ Administer dacarbazine only to patients under close supervision because close observation and frequent laboratory studies are required during and after therapy. ■ IV extravasation: Monitor injection site frequently (instruct patient to do so, if able). Give prompt attention to patient's complaint of swelling, stinging, and burning sensation around injection site. Extravasation can occur painlessly and without visual signs. Danger areas for extravasation are dorsum of hand or ankle (especially if peripheral arteriosclerosis is present), joint spaces, and previously irradiated areas. If extravasation is suspected, infusion should be stopped immediately and restarted in another vein. Report to the physician. Prompt institution of local treatment is IMPERATIVE.

ADVERSE EFFECTS Body as a Whole: Hypersensitivity (erythematosus, urticarial rashes, hepatotoxicity, photosensitivity); facial paresthesia and flushing, flu-like syndrome, myalgia, malaise, anaphylaxis. **CNS:** Confusion, headache, seizures, blurred vision. **GI:** *Anorexia, nausea, vomiting.* **Hematologic:** <u>Severe leukopenia and thrombocytopenia</u>, mild anemia. **Skin:** Alopecia. **Other:** *Pain along injected vein.*

PHARMACOKINETICS Distribution: Localizes primarily in liver. **Metabolism:** Extensively metabolized in liver. **Elimination:** 35–50% excreted in urine in 6 h. **Half-Life:** 5 h.

NURSING IMPLICATIONS

Assessment & Drug Effects

- Monitor IV site carefully for extravasation; if suspected, discontinue IV immediately and notify physician.
- Note: Skin damage by dacarbazine can lead to deep necrosis requiring surgical debridement, skin grafting, and even amputation. The very

D

young, comatose, and debilitated patients are especially at risk. Other risk factors include establishing an IV line in a vein previously punctured several times and the use of nonplastic catheters.

- Lab tests: Monitor for hematopoietic toxicity that usually appears about 4 wk after first dose. Generally, a leukocyte count of <3000/mm^3 and a platelet count of <100,000/mm^3 require suspension or cessation of therapy.
- Avoid, if possible, all tests and treatments during platelet nadir requiring needle punctures (e.g., IM). Observe carefully and report evidence of unexplained bleeding.
- Monitor for severe nausea and vomiting (>90% of patients) that begin within 1 h after drug administration and may last for as long as 12 h. Food may be withheld for several hours before the dose is given and treatment may be accompanied by use of an antiemetic.
- Be alert for and report signs of infection such as respiratory infections, aching, rashes, and gastrointestinal distress.
- Assess immunization status prior to beginning therapy in order to be alert for diseases that pose risk.
- Check patient's mouth for ulcerative stomatitis prior to the administration of each dose.
- Monitor I&O ratio and pattern and daily temperature. Renal impairment extends the half-life and increases danger of toxicity. Report symptoms of renal dysfunction and even a slight elevation of temperature.

Patient & Family Education
- Learn about all potential adverse drug effects.
- Report flu-like syndrome that may occur during or even a week after treatment is terminated and last 7–21 days. Symptoms frequently recur with successive treatments. Report signs of infections. Avoid exposure to persons with infectious diseases and be alert for signs of infection.
- Avoid prolonged exposure to sunlight or to ultraviolet light during treatment period and for at least 2 wk after last dose. Protect exposed skin with sunscreen lotion (SPF 15) and avoid exposure in midday.
- Report promptly the onset of blurred vision or paresthesia.
- Do not breast feed while taking this drug.

DACTINOMYCIN
(dak-ti-noe-mye′sin)
Actinomycin-D, Cosmegen
Classifications: ANTINEOPLASTIC; ANTIBIOTIC
Prototype: Doxorubicin
Pregnancy Category: C

AVAILABILITY 0.5 mg injection

ACTIONS Potent cytotoxic antibiotic derived from mixture of actinomycins produced by *Streptomyces parvulus*. Toxic properties preclude its use as antibiotic. Complexes with DNA, thereby inhibiting DNA, RNA, and protein synthesis. Causes delayed myelosuppression. Potentiates effects of x-ray therapy; the converse also appears likely.

THERAPEUTIC EFFECTS Drug has antineoplastic properties that result from inhibiting DNA and RNA synthesis.

USES As single agent or in combination with other antineoplastics or radiation to treat Wilms' tumor, rhabdomyosarcoma, carcinoma of testes and uterus, Ewing's sarcoma, and sarcoma botryoides.
UNLABELED USES Malignant melanoma, trophoblastic tumors, Kaposi's sarcoma, osteogenic sarcoma, among others.

CONTRAINDICATIONS Chickenpox, herpes zoster, and other viral infections; pregnancy (category C), lactation, infants <6 mo.
CAUTIOUS USE Previous therapy with antineoplastics or radiation within 3–6 wk, bone marrow depression; infections; history of gout; impairment of kidney or liver function; obesity.

ROUTE & DOSAGE

Neoplasms

Child: **IV** 15 mcg/kg/day (max 500 mcg) for 5 days or 2.5 mg/m^2 over 7 days, may repeat at 2–4 wk intervals if tolerated
Adult: **IV** 500 mcg/day for 5 days max, may repeat at 2–4 wk intervals if tolerated; if patient is obese or edematous, give 400–600 mcg/m^2/day to relate dosage to lean body mass. Monitor for symptoms of toxicity from overdosage

Isolation Perfusion

Adult: **IV** 50 mcg/kg for lower extremity or pelvis; 35 mcg/kg for upper extremity
Do not exceed 15 mcg/kg or 400–600 mcg/m^2 as daily dose for 5 days in either adults or children.

STORAGE
Store drug at 15°–30° C (59°–86° F) unless otherwise directed. Protect from heat and light.

ADMINISTRATION

Intravenous

- Child: Must be given under care and direction of pediatric oncology specialist. Use recommended handling techniques for hazardous medications (see Part I). ■ Use gloves and eye shield when preparing solution. If skin is contaminated, rinse with running water for 10 min; then rinse with buffered phosphate solution. If solution gets into the eyes, wash with water immediately; then irrigate with water or isotonic saline for 10 min.
PREPARE **Direct:** Reconstitute 0.5-mg vial by adding 1.1 mL sterile water (without preservative) for injection; the resulting solution will contain approximately 0.5 mg/mL. **IV Infusion:** Further dilute in 50 mL of D5W or NS for infusion.
ADMINISTER **Direct:** Use two-needle technique for direct IV: Withdraw calculated dose from vial with one needle, change to new needle to

give directly into vein without using an infusion. Give over 2–3 min. Or give directly into an infusing solution of D5W or NS, or into tubing or side arm of a running IV infusion. **IV Infusion:** Give diluted solution as a single dose over 15–30 min.

ADVERSE EFFECTS GI: *Nausea, vomiting,* anorexia, abdominal pain, diarrhea, proctitis, GI ulceration, *stomatitis,* cheilitis, glossitis, dysphagia, hepatitis. **Hematologic:** Anemia (including aplastic anemia), agranulocytosis, *leukopenia, thrombocytopenia,* pancytopenia, reticulopenia. **Skin:** Acne, desquamation, hyperpigmentation and reactivation of erythema especially over previously irradiated areas, *alopecia* (reversible). **Other:** Malaise, fatigue, lethargy, fever, myalgia, anaphylaxis, gonadal suppression, hypocalcemia, hyperuricemia, thrombophlebitis; *necrosis, sloughing, and contractures at site of extravasation;* hepatitis, hepatomegaly.

INTERACTIONS Drug: Elevated **uric acid** level produced by dactinomycin may necessitate dose adjustment of ANTIGOUT AGENTS; effects of both dactinomycin and other MYELOSUPPRESSANTS are potentiated; effects of both **radiation** and dactinomycin are potentiated, and dactinomycin may reactivate erythema from previous radiation therapy; **vitamin K** effects (antihemorrhagic) decreased, leading to prolonged clotting time and potential hemorrhage. Disrupts serum level testing of various antibiotics.

PHARMACOKINETICS Distribution: Concentrated in liver, spleen, kidneys, and bone marrow; does not cross blood–brain barrier; crosses placenta; distribution into breast milk not known. **Elimination:** 50% excreted unchanged in bile and 10% in urine; only 30% excreted in urine over 9 days. **Half-Life:** 36 h.

NURSING IMPLICATIONS

Assessment & Drug Effects

- Observe injection site frequently; if extravasation occurs, stop infusion immediately. Restart infusion in another vein. Report to physician. Institute prompt local treatment to prevent thrombophlebitis and necrosis.
- Monitor for severe toxic effects that occur with high frequency. Effects usually appear 2–4 days after a course of therapy is stopped and may reach maximal severity 1–2 wk following discontinuation of therapy.
- Use antiemetic drugs to control nausea and vomiting, which often occur a few hours after drug administration. Vomiting may be severe enough to require intermittent therapy. Observe patient daily for signs of drug toxicity.
- Lab tests: Frequent renal, hepatic, and bone marrow function tests are advised. Perform WBC counts daily, and platelet counts every 3 days to detect hematopoietic depression.
- Monitor temperature and inspect oral membranes daily for stomatitis.
- Monitor for stomatitis, diarrhea, and severe hematopoietic depression. These may require prompt interruption of therapy until drug toxicity subsides.
- Be alert for and report signs of infection such as respiratory infections, aching, rashes, and gastrointestinal distress.

- Assess immunization status prior to beginning therapy in order to be alert for diseases that pose risk.
- Report onset of unexplained bleeding, jaundice, and wheezing. Also, be alert to signs of agranulocytosis (see Appendix D-1). Report to physician. Antibiotic therapy, protective isolation, and discontinuation of the antineoplastic are indicated.
- Observe and report symptoms of hyperuricemia (see Appendix D-1). Urge patient to increase fluid intake up to 3000 mL/day if adolescent or generous amount of fluid for age of child.

Patient & Family Education
- Note: Infertility is a possible, irreversible adverse effect of this drug.
- Learn preventive measures to minimize nausea and vomiting.
- Report signs of infections. Avoid exposure to persons with infectious diseases.
- Note: Alopecia (hair loss) is an anticipated reversible adverse effect of this drug. Seek appropriate supportive guidance.
- Do not breast feed while taking this drug.

DANTROLENE SODIUM
(dan'troe-leen)
Dantrium
Classifications: AUTONOMIC NERVOUS SYSTEM AGENT; CENTRAL-ACTING SKELETAL MUSCLE RELAXANT
Prototype: Cyclobenzaprine
Pregnancy Category: C

AVAILABILITY 25 mg, 50 mg, 100 mg capsules; 20 mg vial

ACTIONS Hydantoin derivative, structurally related to phenytoin, with peripheral skeletal muscle relaxant action. Directly relaxes the spastic muscle by interfering with calcium ion release from sarcoplasmic reticulum. Clinical doses produce about a 50% decrease in contractility of skeletal muscles but no effect on smooth or cardiac muscles.
THERAPEUTIC EFFECTS Relief of spasticity may be accompanied by muscle weakness sufficient to affect overall functional capacity of the patient.

USES Orally for the symptomatic treatment of skeletal muscle spasms secondary to spinal cord injury, stroke, cerebral palsy, multiple sclerosis. Used intravenously for the management of malignant hyperthermia. Oral dantrolene has been used prophylactically (2 or 3 days before anesthesia) for patients with a history of malignant hyperthermia or with a family history of the disorder.
UNLABELED USES Neuroleptic malignant syndrome, exercise-induced muscle pain, and flexor spasms.

CONTRAINDICATIONS Active hepatic disease; when spasticity is necessary to sustain upright posture and balance in locomotion or to maintain increased body function; spasticity due to rheumatic disorders. Safe use

---

during pregnancy (category C), lactation, or in children <5 y is not established. Because long-term administration in children under 5 y is not established, the benefits to the child must be carefully weighed against possible side effects that can occur years after therapy.

CAUTIOUS USE Impaired cardiac or pulmonary function.

ROUTE & DOSAGE

Relief of Spasticity

Child: **PO** 0.5 mg/kg b.i.d., increase to 0.5 mg/kg t.i.d. or q.i.d., may increase by 0.5 mg/kg up to 3 mg/kg b.i.d. to q.i.d. (max 100 mg q.i.d.)
Adult: **PO** 25 mg once/day, increase to 25 mg b.i.d. to q.i.d., may increase q4–7days up to 100 mg b.i.d. to q.i.d.

Malignant Hyperthermia

Child/Adult: **IV** 1 mg/kg rapid direct IV push repeated prn up to a total of 10 mg/kg **PO** May be necessary to continue orally with 1–2 mg/kg q.i.d. for 1–3 days to prevent recurrence

STORAGE

Store both PO and parenteral forms at 15°–30° C (59°–86° F) unless otherwise directed.

- Store capsules in tightly closed, light-resistant container. Contents of vial (for IV use) must be protected from direct light and used within 6 h after reconstitution, because it does not contain a preservative.

ADMINISTRATION

Oral

- Prepare oral suspension for a single dose, when necessary, by emptying contents of capsule(s) into fruit juice or other liquid. Shake suspension well before pouring. Avoid contamination, keep refrigerated, and use within several days, because it does not contain a preservative.

Intravenous

PREPARE Direct: Dilute each 20 mg with 60 mL sterile water without preservatives. Shake until clear.
ADMINISTER Direct: Give by rapid direct IV push. Avoid extravasation; solution has a high pH and therefore is extremely irritating to tissue. Ensure IV patency prior to IV push.

ADVERSE EFFECTS Body as a Whole: Hypersensitivity (pruritus, urticaria, eczematoid skin eruption, photosensitivity, eosinophilic pleural effusion). **CNS:** Drowsiness, *muscle weakness,* dizziness, light-headedness, unusual fatigue, speech disturbances, headache, confusion, nervousness, mental depression, insomnia, euphoria, seizures. **CV:** Tachycardia, erratic BP. **Special Senses:** Blurred vision, diplopia, photophobia. **GI:** *Diarrhea,* constipation, nausea, vomiting, anorexia, swallowing difficulty, alterations of taste, gastric irritation, abdominal cramps, GI bleeding; hepatitis, jaundice, hepatomegaly, <u>hepatic necrosis</u> (all related to prolonged use of high doses). **Urogenital:** Crystalluria with pain or burning with urination, urinary frequency, urinary retention, nocturia, enuresis, difficult erection.

INTERACTIONS Drug: Alcohol and other CNS DEPRESSANTS compound CNS depression; **estrogens** increase risk of hepatotoxicity; **verapamil** and other CALCIUM CHANNEL BLOCKERS increase risk of ventricular fibrillation and cardiovascular collapse with IV dantrolene.

PHARMACOKINETICS Absorption: About 35% slowly and incompletely absorbed from GI tract. **Peak:** 5 h. **Distribution:** Crosses placenta. **Metabolism:** Metabolized in liver. **Elimination:** excreted in urine chiefly as metabolites. **Half-Life:** 8.7 h.

NURSING IMPLICATIONS

Assessment & Drug Effects

- Monitor for therapeutic effectiveness. Improvement may not be apparent until 1 wk or more of drug therapy.
- Monitor vital signs during IV infusion. Also monitor ECG, CVP, and serum potassium.
- Supervise ambulation and other activities until patient's reaction to drug is known. Relief of spasticity may be accompanied by some loss of strength.
- Note: Most common adverse effects are generally transient, lasting up to 14 days after initiation of therapy. Keep physician informed.
- Perform periodic developmental testing on child to identify enhanced or impaired developmental progression of expected tasks.
- Monitor patients with impaired cardiac or pulmonary function closely for cardiovascular or respiratory symptoms such as tachycardia, BP changes, feeling of suffocation.
- Monitor for and report symptoms of allergy and allergic pleural effusion: Shortness of breath, pleuritic pain, dry cough.
- Alert physician if improvement is not evident within 45 days. Drug may be discontinued because of the possibility of hepatotoxicity (see Appendix D-1).
- Lab tests: Perform baseline and regularly scheduled hepatic function tests (alkaline phosphatase, AST, ALT, total bilirubin), blood cell counts, and renal function tests.
- Monitor bowel function. Persistent diarrhea may necessitate drug withdrawal. Severe constipation with abdominal distention and signs of intestinal obstruction have been reported.

Patient & Family Education

- Record child's acquisition of developmental tasks.
- Report promptly the onset of jaundice: yellow skin or sclerae; dark urine, clay-colored stools, itching, abdominal discomfort. Hepatotoxicity frequently occurs between 3rd and 12th month of therapy.
- Do not drive or engage in other potentially hazardous activities until response to drug is known.
- Do not use OTC medications, alcoholic beverages, or other CNS depressants unless otherwise advised by prescriber. Liver toxicity occurs more commonly when other drugs are taken concurrently.

- Do not breast feed while taking this drug without consulting prescriber.
- Store this medication out of reach of children.

D

DAPSONE ℗

(dap'sone)

Avlosulfon ✤, DDS

Classifications: ANTI-INFECTIVE; ANTILEPROSY (SULFONE) AGENT

Pregnancy Category: C

AVAILABILITY 25 mg, 100 mg tablets

ACTIONS Sulfone derivative chemically related to sulfonamides, with bacteriostatic and bactericidal activity similar to that group. Interferes with bacterial cell growth by competitive inhibition of folic acid synthesis by susceptible organisms.

THERAPEUTIC EFFECTS Spectrum of activity includes *Mycobacterium leprae* (Hansen's bacillus), *M. tuberculosis,* and limited activity against *Pneumocystis carinii* and *Plasmodium.* Drug is effective against dapsone-sensitive multibacillary (borderline, borderline lepromatous, or lepromatous) leprosy, and dapsone-sensitive paucibacillary (indeterminate, tuberculoid, or borderline tuberculoid) leprosy. Resistant strains of initially susceptible *M. leprae* develop slowly in a stepwise fashion over periods of 5–24 y.

USES Drug of choice for treatment of all forms of leprosy (unless organism is shown to be dapsone resistant). Used in dapsone-sensitive multibacillary leprosy (with clofazimine and rifampin) and in dapsone-sensitive paucibacillary leprosy (with rifampin, clofazimine, or ethionamide). Also used prophylactically in contacts of patients with all forms of leprosy except tuberculoid and indeterminate leprosy. Used for treatment of dermatitis herpetiformis.

UNLABELED USES Chemoprophylaxis of malaria (with pyrimethamine), systemic and discoid lupus erythematosus, pemphigus vulgaris, dermatosis (especially those associated with bullous eruptions, mucocutaneous lesion, inflammation or pustules); rheumatoid arthritis, allergic vasculitis; treatment of initial episodes of *P. carinii* pneumonia (with trimethoprim) in limited number of adults with AIDS.

CONTRAINDICATIONS Hypersensitivity to sulfones or its derivatives; advanced renal amyloidosis, anemia, methemoglobin reductase deficiency. Safe use during pregnancy (category C) or lactation is not established.

CAUTIOUS USE Chronic renal, hepatic, pulmonary, or cardiovascular disease, refractory anemias, albuminuria, G6PD deficiency.

ROUTE & DOSAGE

Tuberculoid and Indeterminate-Type Leprosy

Adult: **PO** 100 mg/day (with 6 mo of rifampin 600 mg/day) for a minimum of 3 y

Lepromatous and Borderline Lepromatous Leprosy

Child: **PO** 1–2 mg/kg/day once daily in combination therapy (max 100 mg/day)
Adult: **PO** 100 mg/day for ≥10 y

Dermatitis Herpetiformis

Adult: **PO** 50 mg/day, may be increased to 300 mg/day if necessary (max 500 mg/day)

Prophylaxis for Close Contacts of Patient with Multibacillary Leprosy

Child: **PO** *<6 mo,* 6 mg 3 times/wk; *6–23 mo,* 12 mg 3 times/wk; *2–5 y,* 25 mg 3 times/wk; *6–12 y,* 25 mg/day
Adult: **PO** 50 mg/day

P. carinii Pneumonia Prophylaxis

Child: **PO** 2 mg/kg once daily (max 100 mg/day)
Adult: **PO** 50 mg b.i.d. or 100 mg daily

STORAGE
Store in tightly covered, light resistant containers at 15°–30° C (59°–86° F). Drug discoloration apparently does not indicate a chemical change.

ADMINISTRATION

Oral

- Give with food to reduce possibility of GI distress. Tablets are sometimes crushed and given in syrup to children; effectiveness of this practice has not been measured.

ADVERSE EFFECTS Body as a Whole: Hypersensitivity (cutaneous reactions); erythema multiforme, exfoliative dermatitis, <u>toxic epidermal necrolysis</u> [rare], allergic rhinitis, urticaria, fever, infectous mononucleosis-like syndrome. **CNS:** Headache, nervousness, insomnia, vertigo; paresthesia, *muscle weakness.* **CV:** Tachycardia. **GI:** Anorexia, nausea, vomiting, abdominal pain; <u>toxic hepatitis,</u> cholestatic jaundice (reversible with discontinuation of drug therapy); increased ALT, AST, LDH; hyperbilirubinemia. **Hematologic:** In patient with or without G6PD deficiency, *dose-related hemolysis,* Heinz body formation, *methemoglobinemia with cyanosis,* hemolytic anemia; <u>aplastic anemia</u> (rare), <u>agranulocytosis.</u> **Skin:** Drug induced lupus erythematosus, phototoxicity. **Special Senses:** Blurred vision, tinnitus. **Other:** Male infertility; sulfone syndrome (fever, malaise, exfoliative dermatitis, hepatic necrosis with jaundice, lymphadenopathy, methemoglobinemia, anemia).

INTERACTIONS Drug: Activated charcoal decreases dapsone absorption and enterohepatic circulation; **pyrimethamine, trimethoprim** increase risk of adverse hematologic reactions; **rifampin** decreases dapsone levels 7- to 10-fold. **Didanosine** may decrease drug activity against <u>P. carinii.</u>

PHARMACOKINETICS Absorption: Rapidly and nearly completely absorbed from GI tract. **Peak:** 2–8 h. **Distribution:** Distributed to all body tissues; high concentrations in kidney, liver, muscle, and skin; crosses placenta; distributed into breast milk. **Metabolism:** Metabolized in liver. **Elimination:** 70–85% excreted in urine; remainder excreted in feces; traces of drug may be found in body for 3 wk after discontinuation of repeated doses. **Half-Life:** 20–30 h.

NURSING IMPLICATIONS

Assessment & Drug Effects

- Monitor for therapeutic effectiveness that may not appear for leprosy until after 3–6 mo of therapy. Skin lesions respond well; recovery from nerve involvement is usually limited.
- Lab tests: Perform baseline then weekly CBC during the first month of therapy, at monthly intervals for at least 6 mo, and semiannually thereafter.
- Determine periodic dapsone blood levels.
- Perform liver function tests in patients who complain of malaise, fever, chills, anorexia, nausea, vomiting, and have jaundice. Dapsone therapy is usually suspended until etiology is identified.
- Monitor severity of anemia. Nearly all patients demonstrate hemolysis. Manufacturer states that Hgb level is generally decreased by 1–2 g/dL; reticulocytes increase by 2–12%; RBC life span is shortened; and methemoglobinemia occurs in most patients receiving dapsone.
- Monitor temperature during first few weeks of therapy. If fever is frequent or severe, leprosy reactional state should be ruled out. Reduction of or interruption of therapy may be sufficient for improvement.
- Report cyanotic appearance or mucous membranes with brownish hue to physician as possible methemoglobinemia.

Patient & Family Education

- Report symptoms of leprosy that do not improve within 3 mo or get worse.
- Report the appearance of a rash with bullous lesions around elbows and other joints promptly. Drug-induced or worsening skin lesions require withdrawal of dapsone.
- Report symptoms of peripheral neuropathy with motor loss (muscle weakness) promptly.
- Do not breast feed while taking this drug without consulting physician.
- Store this medication out of reach of children.

DAUNORUBICIN HYDROCHLORIDE

(daw-noe-roo'bi-sin)
Cerubidine

DAUNORUBICIN CITRATED LIPOSOMAL

DaunoXome
Classifications: ANTINEOPLASTIC; ANTIBIOTIC
Prototype: Doxorubicin HCl
Pregnancy Category: D

AVAILABILITY Daunorubicin HCl 10 mg, 20 mg, 50 mg, 100 mg, 150 mg lyophilized vials; 2 mg/mL injection **Daunorubicin Citrated Liposomal** 2 mg/mL (equivalent to 50 mg daunorubicin base) injection

ACTIONS Cytotoxic and antimitotic glycoside antibiotic; cell-cycle specific for S-phase of cell division. Toxic properties preclude its use as an antibiotic. Mechanism of action unclear but may be due to rapid intercalating of DNA molecule resulting in inhibition of DNA, RNA, and protein synthesis. **THERAPEUTIC EFFECTS** A potent bone marrow suppressant with immunosuppressive properties as well as antineoplastic properties. Interferes with DNA and RNA synthesis. Induces cardiac toxicity and may be mutagenic and carcinogenic (development of secondary carcinomas).

USES To induce remission in acute nonlymphocytic leukemia (myelogenous, monocytic, erythroid) in adults.
UNLABELED USES Solid tumors of childhood and non-Hodgkin's lymphoma.

CONTRAINDICATIONS Severe myelosuppression; immunizations (patient, family), and preexisting cardiac disease unless risk–benefit is evaluated; lactation; uncontrolled systemic infection. Safe use during pregnancy (category D) is not established.
CAUTIOUS USE History of gout, urate calculi, hepatic or renal function impairment; older adult patients with inadequate bone reserve due to age or previous cytotoxic drug therapy, tumor cell infiltration of bone marrow, patient who has received potentially cardiotoxic drugs or related antineoplastics.

ROUTE & DOSAGE

Neoplasms

Child: **IV** As combination therapy, <2 y, calculated on body weight (mg/kg) rather than body surface area; ≥2 y, 25–45 mg/m^2; max cumulative dose lower in children than adults to prevent cardiotoxicity (max total cumulative dose, 400–450 mg/m^2)
Adult: **IV** As a single agent, 30–60 mg/m^2/day for 3–5 days q3–4wk (max total cumulative dose, 500–600 mg/m^2); as combination therapy, 30–45 mg/m^2/day on days 1, 2, 3 of first course and days 1 and 2 of subsequent courses

Kaposi's Sarcoma (DaunoXome)

Adult: **IV** 40 mg/m^2 over 1 h, repeat q2wk (for serum bilirubin >3 mg/dL or S$_{cr}$ >3 mg/dL, administer half normal dose)

STORAGE
Store reconstituted solution at room temperature (15°–30° C; 59°–86° F) for 24 h and under refrigeration at 2°–8° C (36°–46° F) for 48 h. Protect from light.

ADMINISTRATION
Intravenous

- Child: Must be given under care and direction of pediatric oncology specialist. Use recommended handling techniques for hazardous medications (see Part I). ▪ Use gloves during preparation for infusion to prevent skin contact with this drug. If contact occurs, decontaminate skin with copious amounts of water with soap.

D

PREPARE **Direct:** Reconstitute 20 mg vial with 4 mL sterile water for injection. The concentration of the solution will be 5 mg/mL. ▪ Withdraw dose into syringe containing 10–15 mL normal saline. **IV Infusion:** Dilute further in 100 mL NS as required.

ADMINISTER **Direct:** Inject over approximately 3 min into the tubing or side arm of a rapidly flowing IV infusion of D5W or NS. **Infusion:** Give a single dose over 30 min.

Specific to DaunoXome

PREPARE **IV Infusion:** Each vial of DaunoXome contains the equivalent of 50 mg daunorubicin base. Dilute with enough D5W to produce a concentration of 1 mg/1 mL.

ADMINISTER **IV Infusion:** Give DaunoXome over 60 min. Do not use a filter with DaunoXome.

INCOMPATIBILITIES: **Solution/Additive: Dexamethasone, heparin.**
▪ Avoid extravasation because it can cause severe tissue necrosis.

ADVERSE EFFECTS Body as a Whole: Fever. **CNS:** Amnesia, anxiety, ataxia, confusion, hallucinations, emotional lability, tremors. **CV:** Pericarditis, myocarditis, arrhythmias, peripheral edema, CHF, hypertension, tachycardia. **GI:** *Acute nausea and vomiting* (mild), anorexia, *stomatitis,* mucositis, diarrhea (occasionally) hemorrhage. **Urogenital:** Dysuria, nocturia, polyuria, dry skin. **Hematologic:** <u>Bone marrow depression,</u> *thrombocytopenia, leukopenia,* anemia. **Skin:** Generalized *alopecia* (reversible), transverse pigmentation of nails, severe cellulitis or tissue necrosis at site of drug extravasation. **Endocrine:** Hyperuricemia, gonadal suppression.

PHARMACOKINETICS Distribution: Highest concentrations in spleen, kidneys, liver, lungs, and heart; does not cross blood–brain barrier; crosses placenta; distribution into breast milk not known. **Metabolism:** Metabolized in liver to active metabolite. **Elimination:** 25% excreted in urine, 40% in bile. **Half-Life:** 18.5–26.7 h.

NURSING IMPLICATIONS

Assessment & Drug Effects

▪ Monitor for therapeutic effectiveness. A profound suppression of bone marrow is required to induce a complete remission. Nadirs for thrombocytes and leukocytes are usually reached in 10–14 days.
▪ Monitor serum bilirubin; drug dose needs to be reduced when bilirubin is >1.2 mg/dL.
▪ Lab tests: Preform Hct, platelet count, total and differential leukocyte count, serum uric acid, chest x-ray, and cardiac, hepatic, and renal function tests prior to and periodically during therapy.
▪ Monitor BP, temperature, pulse, and respiratory function during treatment.
▪ Be alert for and report signs of infection such as respiratory infections, aching, rashes, and gastrointestinal distress.
▪ Assess immunization status prior to beginning therapy in order to be alert for diseases that pose risk.
▪ Monitor for S&S of acute CHF. It can occur suddenly, especially when total dosage exceeds 550 mg/m^2, or in patients with compromised heart function because of previous radiation therapy to heart area.

- Report immediately: Breathlessness, orthopnea, change in pulse and BP parameters. Early clinical diagnosis of drug-induced CHF is essential for successful treatment.
- Report promptly S&S of superinfections including elevation of temperature, chills, upper respiratory tract infection, tachycardia, overgrowth with opportunistic organisms because myelosuppression imposes risk of superimposed infection (see Appendix D-1).
- Protect patient from contact with persons with infections. The most hazardous period is during nadirs of thrombocytes and leukocytes.
- Control nausea and vomiting (usually mild) by antiemetic therapy.
- Inspect oral membranes daily. Mucositis may occur 3–7 days after drug is administered.

Patient & Family Education
- Loss of hair is probable; recovery is usual in 6–10 wk.
- A transient effect of the drug is to turn urine red on the day of infusion.
- Report signs of infections. Avoid exposure to persons with infectious diseases.
- Use barrier contraceptives during treatment because this drug is teratogic. Tell your physician immediately if you become pregnant during therapy.
- Do not breast feed while taking this drug.

DEFEROXAMINE MESYLATE

(de-fer-ox′a-meen)
Desferal
Classifications: CHELATING AGENT; ANTIDOTE
Pregnancy Category: C

AVAILABILITY 500 mg vials

ACTIONS Chelating agent isolated from *Streptomyces pilosus* with specific affinity for ferric ion and low affinity for calcium.
THERAPEUTIC EFFECTS Binds ferric ions to form a stable watersoluble chelate readily excreted by kidneys. Main effect is removal of iron from ferritin, hemosiderin, and transferrin.

USES Adjunct in treatment of acute iron intoxication. Has been used in management of hemochromatosis and hemosiderosis secondary to increased iron storage as from multiple transfusions used in treatment of congenital anemias, e.g., thalassemia (Cooley's or Mediterranean anemia), sickle cell anemia, and other chronic anemias.
UNLABELED USES To promote aluminum excretion in aluminum-associated dialysis encephalopathy and aluminum accumulation in bones of patients in renal failure.

CONTRAINDICATIONS Severe renal disease, anuria, pyelonephritis; pregnancy (category C), and children <3 y of age. For all children the benefits of therapy must be weighed against possible long-term effects of drug on bone development and growth.
CAUTIOUS USE History of pyelonephritis; lactation.

ROUTE & DOSAGE

Acute Iron Intoxication

Child: **IM/IV** 20 mg/kg or 600 mg/m^2 followed by 10 mg/kg or 300 mg/m^2 at 4 h intervals for 2 doses, subsequent doses of 10 mg/kg q4–12h may be given if necessary (max 6 g/24 h), infuse at ≤15 mg/kg/h
Adult: **IM/IV** 1 g followed by 500 mg at 4 h intervals for 2 doses, subsequent doses of 500 mg q4–12h may be given if necessary (max 6 g/24 h), infuse at ≤15 mg/kg/h

Chronic Iron Overload

Child/Adult: **IM** 500 mg–1 g/day **IV** 2 g with each unit of blood transfused, infuse at ≤15 mg/kg/h **SC** 1–2 g/day (20–40 mg/kg/day) infused over 8–24 h (max for a child, 6 g/day or 2 g/dose)

STORAGE

Store at 15°–30° C (59°–86° F) for not longer than 1 wk. Protect from light.

ADMINISTRATION

Subcutaneous/Intramuscular

- Reconstitute by adding 2 mL sterile water for injection to 500-mg vial to yield 250 mg/mL. Dissolve drug completely before it is withdrawn from vial.
- Administer SC dose over 8–24 h using portable minipump devices; rate not to exceed 20–40 mg/kg in 8–24 h.
- Use IM route for all patients not in shock; preferred route for acute intoxication.

Intravenous

For infants and children: Verify correct IV concentration and rate with physician. Must be given slowly; see rate below.
PREPARE **IV Infusion:** Reconstitute by adding 5 mL sterile water for injection to 500-mg vial to yield 100 mg/mL. ▪ After drug is completely dissolved, withdraw prescribed amount from vial and add to NS, D5W, or RL solution.
ADMINISTER **IV Infusion:** Give initial dose at a rate not to exceed 15 mg/kg/h. ▪ Give subsequent doses at a rate not to exceed 125 mg/h. ▪ Do not infuse IV rapidly; such infusion is associated with the occurrence of more adverse effects.

ADVERSE EFFECTS Body as a Whole: Hypersensitivity (generalized itching, cutaneous wheal formation, rash, fever, <u>anaphylactoid reaction</u>); impaired growth in children on long-term therapy; decreased ascorbic acid levels. **CV:** *Hypotension,* tachycardia, cardiac failure when treatment accompanied by high ascorbic acid doses. **Respiratory:** Adult respiratory distress syndrome. **Special Senses:** Decreased hearing; blurred vision, decreased visual acuity and visual fields, color vision abnormalities, night blindness, retinal pigmentary degeneration. **GI:** Abdominal discomfort, diarrhea. **Urogenital:** Dysuria, exacerbation of pyelonephritis, orange-rose discoloration of urine. **Other:** *Pain and induration at injection site.*

DIAGNOSTC TEST INTERFERENCE Interferes with gallium scintography; discontinue drug 48 h before procedure.

INTERACTIONS Drug: Causes ascorbic acid deficiency; treatment with **ascorbic acid** common. However high doses of **ascorbic acid** increases risk of cardiac failure. Loss of consciousness when given with **prochlorperazine.**

PHARMACOKINETICS Distribution: Widely distributed in body tissues. **Metabolism:** Forms nontoxic complex with iron. **Elimination:** Excreted primarily in urine; some excreted in feces.

NURSING IMPLICATIONS

Assessment & Drug Effects

- Monitor vital signs, particularly BP and respiratory effort.
- Lab tests: Perform baseline kidney function tests prior to drug administration.
- Monitor injection site. If pain and induration occur, move infusion to another site.
- Monitor I&O ratio and pattern. Report any change. Observe stools for blood (iron intoxication frequently causes necrosis of GI tract).
- Note: Periodic ophthalmoscopic (slit lamp) examinations and audiometry are advised for patients on prolonged or high-dose therapy for chronic iron overload.
- Measure the child on each health care visit and plot growth on grids. Report change in height channels. Growth generally improves but may be impaired by long-term therapy.
- Iron overload increases chance of infection so be alert for symptoms of infection.

Patient & Family Education

- Deferoxamine chelate makes urine turn a reddish color.
- Report blurred vision or any other visual abnormality.
- Be sure child has regular health care visits for monitoring of growth and sensory function.
- Report signs of infection or unusual symptoms promptly.
- Because ascorbic acid is frequently given during therapy, ask family about other sources of vitamin C intake such as multivitamins. High doses of ascorbic acid can be associated with cardiac failure.
- Do not breast feed while taking this drug without consulting physician.

DELAVIRDINE MESYLATE

(del-a-vir′deen)
Rescriptor
Classifications: ANTI-INFECTIVE; ANTIVIRAL; NONNUCLEOSIDE REVERSE TRANSCRIPTASE INHIBITOR
Prototype: Nevirapine
Pregnancy Category: C

D

AVAILABILITY 100 mg tablets

ACTIONS Nonnucleoside reverse transcriptase inhibitor (NNRTI) of HIV-1 binds directly to reverse transcriptase (RT) and blocks RNA- and DNA-dependent DNA polymerase activities.
THERAPEUTIC EFFECTS Thus, it prevents replication of the HIV-1 virus. HIV-2 RT and human DNA polymerases such as polymerases alpha, gamma, and delta are not inhibited by delavirdine. Resistant strains appear rapidly.

USES Treatment of HIV infection in combination with other antiretroviral agents.

CONTRAINDICATIONS Hypersensitivity to delavirdine; lactation.
CAUTIOUS USE Impaired liver function, pregnancy (category C). Safety and efficiency in children ≤16 y have not been established.

ROUTE & DOSAGE

HIV Infection
Adult: **PO** 400 mg t.i.d. for those over 16 y

STORAGE
Store at 20°–25° C (68°–77° F) and protect from high humidity in a tightly closed container.

ADMINISTRATION
Oral
- Disperse in water by adding a single dose to at least 3 oz of water, let stand for a few minutes, then stir to create a uniform suspension just prior to administration.
- Give drug to patients with achlorhydria with an acid beverage such as orange or cranberry juice.

ADVERSE EFFECTS Body as a Whole: Headache, fatigue, allergic reaction, chills, edema, arthralgia. **CNS:** Abnormal coordination, agitation, amnesia, anxiety, confusion, dizziness. **CV:** Chest pain, bradycardia, palpitations, postural hypotension, tachycardia. **GI:** Nausea, vomiting, diarrhea, increased LFTs, abdominal cramps, anorexia, aphthous stomatitis. **Hematologic:** Neutropenia. **Respiratory:** Bronchitis, cough, dyspnea. **Skin:** *Rash,* pruritus.

INTERACTIONS Drug: ANTACIDS, H$_2$-RECEPTOR ANTAGONISTS decrease absorption; **didanosine** and **delavirdine** should be taken 1 h apart to avoid decreased delavirdine levels; **clarithromycin, fluoxetine, ketoconazole** may increase delavirdine levels; **carbamazepine, phenobarbital, phenytoin, rifabutin, rifampin** may decrease delavirdine levels; delavirdine may increase levels of **clarithromycin, astemizole, indinavir, saquinavir, dapsone, rifabutin, alprazolam, midazolam, triazolam,** DIHYDROPYRIDINE, CALCIUM CHANNEL BLOCKERS (e.g., **nifedipine, nicardipine,** etc.), **cisapride, quinidine, warfarin. Herbal:** St. John's **wort** may decrease antiretroviral activity.

PHARMACOKINETICS Absorption: Rapidly absorbed from GI tract, 80% reaches systemic circulation. **Peak:** 1 h. **Distribution:** 98% protein bound. **Metabolism:** Metabolized in the liver by the CYP3A enzymes. **Elimination:** Approximately 51% excreted in urine, 44% in feces. **Half-Life:** 2–11 h.

NURSING IMPLICATIONS

Assessment & Drug Effects

- Therapeutic effectiveness: Indicated by decreased viral load.
- Monitor for and immediately report appearance of a rash, generally within 1–3 wk of starting therapy; rash is usually diffuse, maculopapular, erythematous, and pruritic.

Patient & Family Education

- Take this drug exactly as prescribed. Missed doses increase risk of drug resistance.
- Do not take antacids and delavirdine at the same time; separate by at least 1 h.
- Report all prescription and nonprescription drugs used to physician because of multiple drug interactions.
- Discontinue medication and notify physician if rash is accompanied by any of the following: Fever, blistering, oral lesions, conjunctivitis, swelling, muscle or joint pain.
- Be alert for signs of infection and report promptly.
- Keep regular health care appointments to monitor condition.
- Do not breast feed while taking this drug.
- Store this medication out of reach of children.

DEMECLOCYCLINE HYDROCHLORIDE

(dem-e-kloe-sye′kleen)
Declomycin
Classifications: ANTI-INFECTIVE; ANTIBIOTIC; TETRACYCLINE
Prototype: Tetracycline
Pregnancy Category: D

AVAILABILITY 150 mg capsules; 150 mg, 300 mg tablets

ACTIONS Broad-spectrum, tetracycline antibiotic isolated from mutant strain of *Streptomyces aureofaciens*. Similar to tetracycline but is absorbed more readily, excreted much more slowly.
THERAPEUTIC EFFECTS Drug has longer duration of effective blood levels than tetracycline; therefore intervals between doses can be longer. Primarily bacteriostatic in action.

USES Similar to those of tetracycline.
UNLABELED USES Treatment of chronic SIADH (syndrome of inappropriate [excessive] antidiuretic hormone) secretion.

Common adverse effects in *italic;* life-threatening effects <u>underlined</u>; generic names in **bold;** drug classifications in SMALL CAPS; ♣ Canadian drug name; ⊘ Prototype drug.

407

D

CONTRAINDICATIONS Hypersensitivity to any of the tetracyclines; cirrhosis, common bile duct obstruction; period of tooth development (last half of pregnancy [category D], lactation, children <8 y causes permanent yellow discoloration of teeth, enamel hypoplasia, and retarded bone growth).

CAUTIOUS USE Impaired renal or hepatic function; nephrogenic insipidus; use of capsule or tablet formulations in patients with esophageal compression or obstruction.

ROUTE & DOSAGE

Anti-Infective

Child: **PO** *>8 y,* 6.6–13.2 mg/kg/day divided into 2–3 doses; alternatively 300 mg/m^2 may be given in 2–3 divided doses
Adult: **PO** 150 mg q6h or 300 mg q12h (max 2.4 g/day)

Gonorrhea

Adult: **PO** 600 mg followed by 300 mg q12h for 4 days

SIADH

Adult: **PO** 600–1200 mg/day in 3–4 divided doses

STORAGE

Store in tight, light-resistant containers, preferably at 15°–30° C (59°–86° F) unless otherwise directed.

ADMINISTRATION

Oral

- Give not less than 1 h before or 2 h after meals. Foods rich in iron (e.g., red meat or dark green vegetables) or calcium (e.g., milk products) impair absorption.
- Concomitant therapy: Do not give antacids with tetracyclines.
- Check expiration date before giving drug. Renal damage and death have resulted from use of outdated tetracyclines.
- Request prescriber order to give with light meal if gastric distress is a problem. Absorption may be reduced; keep meal dairy free. Tetracyclines form toxic products when outdated or exposed to light, heat, or humidity.

ADVERSE EFFECTS Body as a Whole: Hypersensitivity (*photosensitivity,* <u>pericarditis, anaphylaxis</u> [rare]). **GI:** *Nausea,* vomiting, *diarrhea,* esophageal irritation or ulceration, enterocolitis, abdominal cramps, anorexia. **Urogenital:** Diabetes insipidus, azotemia, hyperphosphatemia. **Skin:** Pruritus, erythematous eruptions, exfoliative dermatitis.

DIAGNOSTIC TEST INTERFERENCE Like other tetracyclines, demeclocycline may cause false increases in ***urine catecholamines*** (**fluorometric** methods); false decreases in ***urine urobilinogen;*** and false-negative ***urine glucose*** with **glucose oxidase** methods (e.g., **Clinistix, TesTape**).

Common adverse effects in *italic;* life-threatening effects <u>underlined</u>; generic names in **bold;** drug classifications in SMALL CAPS; ♣ Canadian drug name; ❷ Prototype drug.

INTERACTIONS Drug: ANTACIDS, IRON PREPARATION, **calcium, magnesium, zinc, kaolin-pectin, sodium bicarbonate** can significantly decrease demeclocycline absorption; effects of **desmopressin** and demeclocycline antagonized; increases **digoxin** absorption, increasing risk of **digoxin** toxicity; **methoxyflurane** increases risk of renal failure. **Food:** Dairy products significantly decrease demeclocycline absorption; food may decrease drug absorption also.

D

PHARMACOKINETICS Absorption: 60–80% absorbed from GI tract. **Peak:** 3–4 h. **Distribution:** Concentrated in liver; crosses placenta; distributed into breast milk. **Metabolism:** Metabolized in liver; enterohepatic circulation. **Elimination:** 40–50% excreted in urine and 31% in feces in 48 h. **Half-Life:** 10–17 h.

NURSING IMPLICATIONS

Assessment & Drug Effects

- Lab tests: C&S prior to initial therapy and periodically during prolonged therapy. With prolonged therapy, add periodic evaluations of serum drug levels, electrolytes, and renal, hepatic, and hematopoietic systems.
- Monitor I&O ratio and pattern and record weights in patients with impaired kidney or liver function, or on prolonged or high dose therapy. Some patients develop diabetes insipidus-like syndrome (SIADH).
- CDC (www.cdc.gov) states that tetracycline alone is not adequate treatment for gonorrhea.

Patient & Family Education

- Do not use antacids while taking this drug.
- Take drug on an empty stomach to enhance absorption. Because esophageal irritation and ulceration have been reported, take each dose with a full glass (240 mL) of water; and avoid taking drug within 1 h of lying down or bedtime.
- Notify prescriber if gastric distress is a problem; a snack or light meal free of dairy products may be added to the regimen.
- Report symptoms of any infections; this is VERY important (see Appendix D-1).
- Demeclocycline-induced phototoxic reaction can be unusually severe. Avoid sunlight as much as possible and use sunscreen.
- Do not breast feed while taking this drug.
- Store this medication out of reach of children.

DESIPRAMINE HYDROCHLORIDE

(dess-ip′ra-meen)
Norpramin, Pertofrane
Classifications: CENTRAL NERVOUS SYSTEM AGENT; PSYCHOTHERAPEUTIC; TRICYCLIC ANTIDEPRESSANT
Prototype: Imipramine
Pregnancy Category: C

AVAILABILITY 10 mg, 25 mg, 50 mg, 75 mg, 100 mg, 150 mg tablets

---

D

ACTIONS Dibenzoxazepine tricyclic antidepressant (TCA) and secondary amine. Desipramine is the active metabolite of imipramine and has similar pharmacologic actions. Unlike imipramine, onset of action is more rapid, and it has lower potential for producing sedative and anticholinergic effects and orthostatic hypotension.

THERAPEUTIC EFFECTS In common with other TCAs, antidepressant activity appears to be related to inhibition of reuptake of norepinephrine and serotonin in the CNS. Restoration of the levels of these neurotransmitters is a proposed mechanism of antidepressant action.

USES Endogenous depression and various depression syndromes.
UNLABELED USES Attention deficit disorder in children >6 y and adolescents; to prevent depression in cocaine withdrawal.

CONTRAINDICATIONS Hypersensitivity to tricyclic compounds; recent MI. Safe use during pregnancy (category C) and lactation not established. Because of sudden collapse and death in children, the manufacturer does not recommend use in children <12 years of age.
CAUTIOUS USE Urinary retention, prostatic hypertrophy; narrow-angle glaucoma; epilepsy; alcoholism; adolescents, older adults; thyroid; cardiovascular, renal, and hepatic disease; suicidal tendency; ECT; elective surgery.

ROUTE & DOSAGE

Antidepressant

Child: **PO** *6–12 y,* 1–3 mg/kg/day in divided doses (max 5 mg/kg/day)
Adolescent: **PO** 25–50 mg/day (max 150 mg/day) in divided doses
Adult: **PO** 75–100 mg/day at bedtime or in divided doses, may gradually increase to 150–300 mg/day if needed in hospitalized patients

STORAGE
Store drug in tightly closed container at 15°–30° C (59°–86° F) unless otherwise specified.

ADMINISTRATION
Oral
- Give drug with or immediately after food to reduce possibility of gastric irritation.
- Give maintenance dose at bedtime to minimize daytime sedation.

ADVERSE EFFECTS Body as a Whole: Hypersensitivity (rash, urticaria, photosensitivity). **CNS:** *Drowsiness,* dizziness, weakness, fatigue, headache, insomnia, confusional states, depressive reaction, paresthesias, ataxia; collapse and sudden death in children. **CV:** *Postural hypotension,* hypotension, palpitation, tachycardia, ECG changes, flushing, heart block. **Special Senses:** Tinnitus, parotid swelling; blurred vision, disturbances in accommodation, mydriasis, increased IOP. **GI:** *Dry mouth, constipation,* bad taste, diarrhea, nausea. **Urogenital:** *Urinary retention,* frequency, delayed micturition, nocturia; impaired sexual function, galactorrhea. **Hematologic:** Bone marrow depression and agranulocytosis (rare). **Other:** Sweating, craving for sweets, weight gain or loss, SIADH secretion, hyperpyrexia, eosinophilic pneumonia.

INTERACTIONS Drug: May somewhat decrease response TO ANTIHYPERTEN-SIVES; CNS DEPRESSANTS, **alcohol,** HYPNOTICS, BARBITURATES, SEDATIVES potentiate CNS depression; may increase hypoprothombinemic effect of ORAL ANTICOAGULANTS; **ethchlorvynol** may cause transient delirium; **levodopa,** SYMPATHOMIMETICS (e.g., **epinephrine, norepinephrine**) pose possibility of sympathetic hyperactivity with hypertension and hyperpyrexia; MAO IN-HIBITORS pose possibility of severe reactions, toxic psychosis, cardiovascular instability; **methylphenidate** increases plasma TCA levels; THYROID AGENTS may increase possibility of arrhythmias; **cimetidine** may increase plasma TCA levels. **Herbal: Ginkgo** may decrease seizure threshold; **St. John's wort** may cause **serotonin** syndrome.

PHARMACOKINETICS Absorption: Rapidly absorbed from GI tract and injection sites. **Peak:** 4–6 h. **Distribution:** Crosses placenta. **Metabolism:** Metabolized in liver. **Elimination:** Primarily excreted in urine. **Half-Life:** 7–60 h.

NURSING IMPLICATIONS

Assessment & Drug Effects

- Monitor for therapeutic effectiveness: Usually not realized until after at least 2 wk of therapy.
- Monitor BP and pulse rate during early phase of therapy, particularly in child, debilitated, or cardiovascular patients. If BP rises or falls more than 20 mm Hg or if there is a sudden increase in pulse rate or change in rhythm, withhold drug and inform physician.
- Antidepressants increase risk of suicidal thinking and behavior in children and adolescents with major depressive disorder, obsessive compulsive disorder, and other psychiatric disorders. Observe closely for worsening of condition, suicidality, and behavior changes. Instruct family and caregivers to monitor for these symptoms and discuss with prescriber. A MedGuide describing risks and stating whether the drug is approved for the child's/adolescent's condition should be provided for all families when antidepressants are prescribed.
- Note: Drowsiness, dizziness, and orthostatic hypotension are signs of impending toxicity in patient on long-term, high-dosage therapy. Prolonged QT or QRS intervals indicate possible toxicity. Report to prescriber.
- Observe patient with history of glaucoma. Report symptoms that may signal acute attack: Severe headache, eye pain, dilated pupils, halos of light, nausea, vomiting.
- Monitor bowel elimination pattern and I&O ratio. Severe constipation and urinary retention are potential problems of TCA therapy.
- Note: Norpramin tablets may contain tartrazine, which can cause allergic-type reactions including bronchial asthma in susceptible individuals. Such individuals are frequently also sensitive to aspirin.

Patient & Family Education

- Make all position changes slowly and in stages, particularly from recumbent to standing position.
- Do not drive or engage in other potentially hazardous activities until reaction to drug is known.
- Monitor children and adolescents closely. Report behavior changes and suicidal thoughts immediately to prescriber.

D

- Take medication exactly as prescribed; do not change dose or dose intervals.
- Note: Patients who receive high doses for prolonged periods may experience withdrawal symptoms including headache, nausea, musculoskeletal pain, and weakness if drug is discontinued abruptly.
- Do not take OTC drugs unless physician has approved their use.
- Stop, or at least limit, smoking because it may increase the metabolism of desipramine, thereby diminishing its therapeutic action.
- Do not breast feed while taking this drug without consulting physician.
- Store this medication out of reach of children.

DESMOPRESSIN ACETATE

(des-moe-pres′sin)

DDAVP, Stimate

Classifications: HORMONES AND SYNTHETIC SUBSTITUTES; PITUITARY (ANTIDIURETIC) HORMONE

Prototype: Vasopressin

Pregnancy Category: B

AVAILABILITY 0.1 mg, 0.2 mg, tablets; 0.1 mg/mL, 1.5 mg/mL nasal solution; 4 mcg/mL, 15 mcg/mL injection

ACTIONS Synthetic analog of the natural human posterior pituitary (antidiuretic) hormone, arginine vasopressin. Has more specific and longer duration of action than antidiuretic hormone and lower incidence of allergic reactions. Also, oxytocic and vasopressor actions are not apparent at therapeutic dosages. Unlike vasopressin, it does not stimulate release of adrenocorticotropic hormone nor does it increase plasma cortisol, growth hormone, prolactin, or luteinizing hormone levels.

THERAPEUTIC EFFECTS Reduces urine volume and osmolality in patients with central diabetes insipidus by increasing reabsorption of water by kidney collecting tubules. Produces a dose-related increase in factor VIII (antihemophilic factor) and von Willebrand's factor.

USES To control and prevent symptoms and complications of central (neurohypophyseal) diabetes insipidus, and to relieve temporary polyuria and polydipsia associated with trauma or surgery in the pituitary region.

UNLABELED USES To increase factor VIII activity in selected patients with mild to moderate hemophilia A and in type I von Willebrand's disease or uremia, and to control enuresis in children.

CONTRAINDICATIONS Nephrogenic diabetes insipidus, type II B von Willebrand's disease. Safe use during pregnancy (category B) or lactation is not established.

CAUTIOUS USE Coronary artery insufficiency, hypertensive cardiovascular disease.

ROUTE & DOSAGE

Diabetes Insipidus

Child: **Intranasal** *3 mo–12 y*, 0.05–0.3 mL (5–30 mcg of 0.1 mg/mL nasal solution) in 1–2 divided doses; ½ dose into each nostril **IV/SC** 0.3 mcg/kg infused over 15–30 min **PO** 0.05 mg titrated to response *Adult:* **Intranasal** 0.1–0.4 mL (10–40 mcg of 0.1 mg/mL nasal solution) in 1–3 divided doses **IV/SC** 2–4 mcg in 2 divided doses; ½ dose into each nostril **PO** 0.2–0.4 mg/day

D

Enuresis

Child: **PO** ≥6 y, 0.2 mg at bedtime, may titrate up to 0.6 mg at bedtime. *Child/Adult >6 y:* **Intranasal** 5–40 mcg at bedtime; ½ dose into each nostril

Hemophilia A and Von Willebrand's Disease

Child/Adult: **Intranasal** 2–4 mcg/kg/dose
Child/Adult: **IV/SC** *>3 mo,* 0.3 mcg/kg 30 min preop, may repeat in 48 h if needed

STORAGE

Store parenteral and nasal solution in refrigerator preferably at 4° C (39.2° F) unless otherwise directed. Avoid freezing. Nasal spray can be stored at room temperature. Discard solutions that are discolored or contain particulate matter.

ADMINISTRATION

Oral

- Note that 0.2 mg PO is equivalent to 10 mcg (0.1 mL of 0.1 mg/mL nasal solution) intranasal.

Intranasal

- Follow manufacturer's instructions for proper technique with nasal spray. Each dose is divided to administer ½ into each nostril.
- Give initial dose in the evening, and observe antidiuretic effect. Dose is increased each evening until uninterrupted sleep is obtained. If daily urine volume is more than 2 L for adult (over 12 years) after nocturia is controlled, morning dose is started and adjusted daily until urine volume does not exceed 1.5–2 L/24 h. Check expected fluid volumes for younger children with prescriber.

Intravenous

***PREPARE* Direct:** Give undiluted for diabetes insipidus. **IV Infusion:** Dilute 0.3 mcg/kg in 10 mL of NS (children ≤10 kg) or 50 mL of NS (children >10 kg and adults) for von Willebrand's disease (type I).
***ADMINISTER* Direct:** Give direct IV over 30 sec for diabetes insipidus. **IV Infusion:** Give over 15–30 min for von Willebrand's disease (type I).

ADVERSE EFFECTS All: Dose related hyponatremia, water intoxication. **CNS:** *Transient headache, drowsiness, listlessness.* **Special Senses:** Nasal congestion, rhinitis, nasal irritation. **GI:** Nausea, heartburn, mild abdominal cramps. **Other:** Vulval pain, shortness of breath, slight rise in BP, facial flushing, pain and swelling at injection site.

INTERACTIONS Drug: Demeclocycline, lithium, other VASOPRESSORS may decrease antidiuretic response; **carbamazepine, chlorpropamide, clofibrate** may prolong antidiuretic response.

PHARMACOKINETICS Absorption: 10–20% absorbed through nasal mucosa. **Onset:** 15–60 min. **Peak:** 1–5 h. **Duration:** 5–21 h. **Distribution:** Small amount crosses blood–brain barrier; distributed into breast milk. **Half-Life:** 76 min.

D

NURSING IMPLICATIONS

Assessment & Drug Effects

- Monitor I&O ratio and pattern (intervals). Fluid intake must be carefully controlled, particularly in the very young to avoid water retention and sodium depletion.
- Weigh patient daily and observe for edema. Severe water retention may require reduction in dosage and use of a diuretic.
- Monitor BP during dosage-regulating period and whenever drug is administered parenterally.
- Monitor urine and plasma osmolality. An increase in urine osmolality and a decrease in plasma osmolality indicate effectiveness of treatment in diabetes insipidus.

Patient & Family Education

- Report upper respiratory tract infection or nasal congestion.
- Follow manufacturer's instructions for insertion to ensure delivery of drug high into nasal cavity and not down throat. A flexible calibrated plastic tube is provided.
- Have family keep a log of bed wetting when drug is used for treatment of enuresis. Inform family carefully of recommended fluid intake and output.
- Do not breast feed while taking this drug without consulting prescriber.
- Store this medication out of reach of children.

DEXAMETHASONE

(dex-a-meth'a-sone)

Aeroseb-Dex, Decaderm, Decadron, Decaspray, Deronil ♣, Dexameth, Dexamethasone Intensol, Dexasone, Dexone, Hexadrol, Maxidex, Mymethasone, Oradexon ♣

DEXAMETHASONE ACETATE

Dalalone D.P., Dalalone-LA, Decadron-LA, Decaject-LA, Dexacen LA-8, Dexasone-LA, Dexo-LA, Dexon LA, Dexone LA, Solurex-LA

DEXAMETHASONE SODIUM PHOSPHATE

AK-Dex, Alba Dex, Dalalone, Decadrol, Decadron Phosphate, Decaject, Dex-4, Dexacen-4, Dexasone, Dexon, Dexone, Hexadrol Phosphate, Maxidex Ophthalmic, Savacort-D, Solurex
Available in combination with neomycin as NeoDecadron, AK-Neo-Dex, NeoDecadron Ocumeter, Neo-Dex-ide

Classifications: HORMONES AND SYNTHETIC SUBSTITUTES, ADRENAL CORTICOSTEROID; GLUCOCORTICOID; STEROID
Prototype: Prednisone
Pregnancy Category: C

Common adverse effects in *italic;* life-threatening effects <u>underlined</u>; generic names in **bold**; drug classifications in SMALL CAPS; ♣ Canadian drug name; ☀ Prototype drug.

AVAILABILITY Dexamethasone 0.25 mg, 0.5 mg, 0.75 mg, 1 mg, 1.5 mg, 2 mg, 4 mg, 6 mg tablets; 0.5 mg/5 mL, 0.5 mg/0.5 mg oral solution; 0.01%, 0.04% topical aerosol **Dexamethasone Acetate** 8 mg/mL, 16 mg/mL injection suspension **Dexamethasone Sodium Phosphate** 4 mg/mL, 10 mg/mL, 20 mg/mL, 24 mg/mL injection; 0.1% cream; 0.1% ophthalmic solution, suspension; 0.05% ophthalmic ointment.

D

Combination Products: Available in combination with neomycin and polymyxin B as AK-Trol, Dexacidin, Dexasporin, Maxitrol, Ocu-Trol, Dex-Ide, Maxitrol; in combination with tobramycine as TobraDex, Decadron Phosphate Turbinaire, AK-Dex, Decadron phosphate Ocumeter

ACTIONS Long-acting synthetic adrenocorticoid with intense anti-inflammatory (glucocorticoid) activity and minimal mineralocorticoid activity. **Anti-Inflammatory Action:** Prevents accumulation of inflammatory cells at sites of infection; inhibits phagocytosis, lysosomal enzyme release, and synthesis of selected chemical mediators of inflammation; reduces capillary dilation and permeability. **Immunosuppression:** Not clearly understood, but may be due to prevention or suppression of delayed hypersensitivity immune reaction.

THERAPEUTIC EFFECTS Drug has anti-inflammatory and immunosuppression properties.

USES Adrenal insufficiency concomitantly with a mineralocorticoid; inflammatory conditions, allergic states, collagen diseases, hematologic disorders, cerebral edema, and addisonian shock. Also palliative treatment of neoplastic disease, as adjunctive short-term therapy in acute rheumatic disorders and GI diseases, and as a diagnostic test for Cushing's syndrome and for differential diagnosis of adrenal hyperplasia and adrenal adenoma.

UNLABELED USES As an antiemetic in cancer chemotherapy; as a diagnostic test for endogenous depression; and to prevent hyaline membrane disease in premature infants.

CONTRAINDICATIONS Systemic fungal infection, acute infections, active or resting tuberculosis, vaccinia, varicella, administration of live virus vaccines (to patient, family members), latent or active amebiasis. **Ophthalmic use:** Primary open-angle glaucoma, eye infections, superficial ocular herpes simplex, keratitis and tuberculosis of eye. Safe use during pregnancy (category C), lactation, or in children is not established.

CAUTIOUS USE Stromal herpes simplex, keratitis, GI ulceration, renal disease, diabetes mellitus, hypothyroidism, myasthenia gravis, CHF, cirrhosis, psychic disorders, seizures.

ROUTE & DOSAGE

Allergies, Inflammation, Neoplasias

Child: **PO/IV/IM** 0.08–0.3 mg/kg/day divided into doses q6–12h
Adult: **PO** 0.25–4 mg b.i.d. to q.i.d. **IM** 8–16 mg q1–3wk or 0.8–1.6 mg intralesional q1–3wk

Cerebral Edema

Child: **PO/IV/IM** 1–2 mg/kg loading dose, then 1–1.5 mg/kg/day divided into doses q4–6h (max 16 mg/day)

Adult: **IV** 10 mg followed by 4 mg q4h, reduce dose after 2–4 days
then taper over 5–7 days

Meningitis

Child >6 wk: **IV** 0.6 mg/kg/24 h divided into doses given q6h for
10 days

Croup

Child: **IM, IV** 0.6 mg/kg/dose one time

Airway Edema

Child: **PO/IM/IV** 0.5–2 mg/kg/24 h divided into doses q6h; begun
24 h before extubation and continue for 4–6 doses after extubation

Antiemetic

Child: **IV** 10 mg/m^2/dose (max 20 mg) for initial dose, then
5 mg/m^2/dose q6h

Shock

Adult: **IV** 1–6 mg/kg as a single dose or 40 mg repeated q2–6h
if needed

Dexamethasone Suppression Test

Adult: **PO** 0.5 mg q6h for 48 h

Inflammation

Child/Adult: **Ophthalmic/Topical/Inhalation/Intranasal
See Appendix I-1**

STORAGE

Store at 15°–30° C (59°–86° F) unless otherwise directed. Do not store or
expose aerosol to temperature above 48.9° C (120° F); do not puncture or
discard into a fire or an incinerator.

ADMINISTRATION

Oral

- Give the once-daily dose in morning with food or liquid of patient's
  choice.
- Taper dosage over a period of time before discontinuing because
  adrenal suppression can occur with prolonged use.

Intramuscular

- Give IM injection deep into a large muscle mass appropriate for age (e.g.,
  gluteus maximus for older children and vastus lateralis for younger). (see
  Part I) Avoid SC injection: Atrophy and sterile abscesses may occur.
- Use repository form, dexamethasone acetate, for IM or local injection
  only. The white suspension settles on standing; mild shaking will resuspend drug.

Intravenous

PREPARE **Direct:** Give undiluted. **Intermittent:** Dilute in D5W or NS for
infusion.
ADMINISTER **Direct:** Give direct IV push over 30 sec or less. **Intermittent:**
Set rate as prescribed or according to amount of solution to infuse.

INCOMPATIBILITIES: **Solution/Additive:** Daunorubicin, doxapram, doxorubicin, glycopyrrolate, metaraminol, vancomycin.

ADVERSE EFFECTS *Aerosol Therapy: Nasal irritation,* dryness, epistaxis, rebound congestion, bronchial asthma, anosomia, perforation of nasal septum. *Systemic Absorption*—**CNS:** Euphoria, insomnia, convulsions, increased ICP, vertigo, headache, psychic disturbances. **CV:** CHF, hypertension, *edema.* **Endocrine:** Menstrual irregularities, *hyperglycemia;* cushingoid state; growth suppression in children; hirsutism. **Special Senses:** *Posterior subcapsular cataract,* increased IOP, glaucoma, exophthalmos. **GI:** Peptic ulcer with possible perforation, abdominal distention, nausea, increased appetite, heartburn, dyspepsia, pancreatitis, bowel perforation, *oral candidiasis.* **Musculoskeletal:** Muscle weakness, loss of muscle mass, vertebral compression fracture, pathologic fracture of long bones, tendon rupture. **Skin:** Acne, *impaired wound healing,* petechiae, ecchymoses, diaphoresis, allergic dermatitis, hypo- or hyperpigmentation, SC and cutaneous atrophy, burning and tingling in perineal area (following IV injection).

DIAGNOSTIC TEST INTERFERENCE *Dexamethasone suppression test for endogenous depression:* False-positive results may be caused by **alcohol, glutethimide, meprobamate;** false-negative results may be caused by high doses of benzodiazepines (e.g., **chlordiazepoxide** and **cyproheptadine**), long-term glucocorticoid treatment, **indomethacin, ephedrine,** estrogens or hepatic enzyme-inducing agents **(phenytoin)** may also cause false-positive results in *test for Cushing's syndrome.*

INTERACTIONS Drug: BARBITURATES, **phenytoin, rifampin** increase steroid metabolism—dosage of dexamethasone may need to be increased; **amphotericin B,** DIURETICS compound potassium loss; **ambenonium, neostigmine, pyridostigmine** may cause severe muscle weakness in patients with myasthenia gravis; may inhibit antibody response to VACCINES, TOXOIDS.

PHARMACOKINETICS Absorption: Readily absorbed from GI tract. **Onset:** Rapid onset. **Peak:** 1–2 h PO; 8 h IM. **Duration:** 2.75 days PO; 6 days IM; 1–3 wk intralesional, intra-articular. **Distribution:** Crosses placenta; distributed into breast milk. **Elimination:** Hypothalamus-pituitary axis suppression: 36–54 h. **Half-Life:** 3–4.5 h.

NURSING IMPLICATIONS

Assessment & Drug Effects

- Monitor and report S&S of Cushing's syndrome (see Appendix D-1) or other systemic adverse effects.
- Monitor neonates born to a mother who has been receiving a corticosteroid during pregnancy for symptoms of hypoadrenocorticism.
- Take careful history of immunization status because drug can cause immunosuppression, and exposure to susceptible diseases must be minimized.
- Monitor for S&S of a hypersensitivity reaction (see Appendix D-1). The acetate and sodium phosphate formulations may contain bisulfites,

parabens, or both; these inactive ingredients are allergenic to some individuals.

Patient & Family Education

- Take drug exactly as prescribed.
- Report lack of response to medication or malaise, orthostatic hypotension, muscular weakness and pain, nausea, vomiting, anorexia, hypoglycemic reactions (see Appendix D-1), or mental depression to physician. These symptoms may signal hypoadrenocorticism.
- Report exposure to communicable diseases. Inform health care provider of drug before any treatments such as immunizations or dental care.
- Report changes in appearance and easy bruising to physician. These symptoms may signal hyperadrenocorticism.
- Note: Hiccups that occur for several hours following each dose may be a complication of high-dose oral dexamethasone.
- Keep appointments for checkups; make sure electrolytes and BP are evaluated during therapy at regular intervals.
- Add potassium-rich foods to diet; report signs of hypokalemia (see Appendix D-1). Concomitant potassium-depleting diuretic can enhance dexamethasone-induced potassium loss.
- Note: Dexamethasone dose regimen may need to be altered during stress (e.g., surgery, infections, emotional stress, illness, acute bronchial attacks, trauma). Consult prescriber if change in living or working environment is anticipated.
- Discontinue drug gradually under the guidance of the prescriber. Do not stop taking without instructions. Report conditions that cause the drug not to be taken (nausea and vomiting).
- Note: It is important to prevent exposure to infection, trauma, and sudden changes in environmental factors, as much as possible, because drug is an immunosuppressor.
- Do not breast feed while taking this drug without consulting physician.
- Store this medication out of reach of children.

DEXCHLORPHENIRAMINE MALEATE

(dex-klor-fen-eer′a-meen)
Dexchlor, Poladex T. D., Polaramine, Polargen
Classifications: ANTIHISTAMINE (H₁-RECEPTOR ANTAGONIST)
Prototype: Diphenhydramine
Pregnancy Category: B

AVAILABILITY 2 mg tablets; 4 mg, 6 mg sustained-release tablets; 2 mg/5 mL syrup

ACTIONS Competes for H₁-receptor sites on cells thus blocking histamine release.

THERAPEUTIC EFFECTS H₁-receptor antagonist and antihistamine. In common with other antihistamines, has anticholinergic properties and produces mild to moderate drowsiness and sedation.

USES Perennial and seasonal allergic rhinitis, other manifestations of allergy, and vasomotor rhinitis. Also as adjunct to epinephrine in treatment of anaphylactic reactions.

CONTRAINDICATIONS Hypersensitivity to antihistamines of similar class; acute asthmatic attack, lower respiratory tract symptoms, newborns, premature infants. Safe use during pregnancy (category B) or lactation is not established. Not for use in newborns. Safety for those under 2 y not established. Safety of 4-mg sustained-release tablets not established in those under 6 y, or 6-mg tablets in those under 12 y.

CAUTIOUS USE Increased intraocular pressure; asthma; hyperthyroidism; renal and cardiovascular disease.

ROUTE & DOSAGE

Allergic Rhinitis

Child: **PO** 2–5 y, 0.5 mg q4–6h (max 3 mg/24 h); *6–11 y,* 1 mg q4–6h (max 6 mg/24 h) or 4 mg of sustained-release tablets at bedtime
Adult: **PO** 2 mg q4–6h or 4–6 mg of sustained-release tablets at bedtime or q8–10h during the day

STORAGE

Store at 15°–30° C (59°–86° F) unless otherwise directed.

ADMINISTRATION

Oral

- Ensure that sustained-release form of drug is not chewed or crushed. It must be swallowed whole.
- Give regular tablet whole or crushed and taken with fluid or mixed with food.
- Give medication with food, water, or milk to lessen GI distress.

ADVERSE EFFECTS CNS: *Drowsiness,* dizziness, weakness, headache, excitation, neuritis, disturbed coordination, insomnia, euphoria, paresthesias; paradoxical excitement in young children. **Special Senses:** Vertigo, tinnitus, acute labyrinthitis; blurred vision. **CV:** Palpitation, tachycardia, hypotension, extrasystoles. **GI:** Nausea, vomiting, anorexia, *dry mouth,* constipation, diarrhea. **Urogenital:** Difficulty in urinating, *urinary retention,* urinary frequency, early menses. **Hematologic:** Agranulocytosis (rare), hemolytic or hypoplastic anemia. **Skin:** Skin eruptions, photosensitivity.

DIAGNOSTIC TEST INTERFERENCE In common with other antihistamines, dexchlorpheniramine may interfere with ***skin tests for allergy;*** discontinue dexchlorpheniramine at least 72 h before tests.

INTERACTIONS Drug: Alcohol and other CNS DEPRESSANTS, MAO INHIBITORS compound CNS depression.

PHARMACOKINETICS Absorption: Readily absorbed from GI tract. **Onset:** 15–30 min. **Peak:** 3 h. **Distribution:** Small amounts distributed into breast milk. **Metabolism:** Metabolized in liver. **Elimination:** Excreted in urine within 24 h.

D

NURSING IMPLICATIONS

Assessment & Drug Effects

- Supervise ambulation and take safety precautions, especially in the very young.
- Monitor I&O and assess for difficulty voiding (e.g., frequency or retention).

Patient & Family Education

- Swallow timed or sustained-release tablet whole. Do not break, crush, or chew.
- Any child should be under the care of a health care professional when taking this medication. Do not self-medicate young children with this drug.
- Do not drive or engage in other potentially hazardous activities until reaction to drug is known.
- Ask prescriber about the use of alcohol, tranquilizers, sedatives, or other CNS depressants because the effects of dexchlorpheniramine will be additive.
- Discontinue dexchlorpheniramine about 4 days before skin tests for allergies, because it can make test results inaccurate.
- Do not breast feed while taking this drug without consulting physician.
- Store this medication out of reach of children.

DEXMETHYLPHENIDATE

(dex-meth-ill-fen′i-date)
Focalin
Classifications: CENTRAL NERVOUS SYSTEM AGENT; CEREBRAL STIMULANT
Prototype: Amphetamine
Pregnancy Category: C
Controlled Substance: Schedule II

AVAILABILITY 2.5 mg, 5 mg, 10 mg tablets

ACTIONS Thought to block the reuptake of norepinephrine and dopamine into the presynaptic neurons and, thereby, increasing release of these substances into the synapse. The mode of action in controlling the symptoms of attention deficit hyperactivity disorder (ADHD) by Focalin is not fully understood.

THERAPEUTIC EFFECTS Focalin is used for control of ADHD syndrome in conjunction with other measures (psychological, educational, and social). The use of stimulants is contraindicated in patients who exhibit ADHD symptoms secondary to environmental factors, and/or other primary psychiatric disorders including psychosis.

USES Attention deficit hyperactivity disorder.

CONTRAINDICATIONS Hypersensitivity to dexmethylphenidate or methylphenidate; severe agitation, anxiety, or tension; glaucoma; motor tics other than Tourette's syndrome; concurrent or recent MAOI therapy; children <6 y; seizures; pregnancy (category C).

CAUTIOUS USE Moderate to severe hepatic insufficiency; Tourette's syndrome; depression; emotional instability; alcoholism or drug dependence; history of seizure disorders; psychotic symptomatology; hypertension or other cardiovascular disease; hyperthyroidism; lactation.

ROUTE & DOSAGE

Attention Deficit Hyperactivity Disorder

Child/Adult: PO >6 y, 2.5 mg b.i.d., may increase by 2.5 mg–5 mg/ day at weekly intervals to max of 20 mg/day. If converting from methylphenidate, start with ½ of methylphenidate dose

STORAGE
Store at 15°–30° C (59°–86° F).

ADMINISTRATION

Oral
- Do not administer with or within 14 days following discontinuation of a MAO inhibitor.
- Give b.i.d. doses at least 4 h apart.

ADVERSE EFFECTS Body as a Whole: Fever, allergic reactions. **CNS:** Dizziness, insomnia, nervousness, tics, abnormal thinking, hallucinations, emotional lability, CNS overstimulation or sympathomimetic effects (angina, anxiety, agitation, biting, blurred vision, delirium, diaphoresis, flushing or pallor, hallucinations, hyperthermia, labile blood pressure and heart rate (hypotension or hypertension), mydriasis, palpitations, paranoia, purposeless movements, psychosis, sinus tachycardia, tachypnea, or tremor). **CV:** Hypertension, tachycardia. **GI:** *Abdominal pain,* decreased appetite, nausea, vomiting.

INTERACTIONS Drug: Additive stimulant effects with other STIMULANTS (including **amphetamine, caffeine**); increased vasopressor effects with **dopamine, epinephrine, norepinephrine, phenylpropanolamine, pseudoephedrine;** MAO INHIBITORS may cause hypertensive crisis; antagonizes hypotensive effects of **bretylium, guanethidine;** may inhibit metabolism and increase serum levels of **fosphenytoin, phenobarbital, phenytoin, primidone, warfarin,** TRICYCLIC ANTIDEPRESSANTS.

PHARMACOKINETICS Absorption: Well absorbed. **Peak:** 1–1.5 h. **Metabolism:** De-esterified in liver. No interaction with CYP450 system. **Elimination:** Primarily excreted in urine. **Half-Life:** 2.2 h.

NURSING IMPLICATIONS

Assessment & Drug Effects
- Withhold drug and notify prescriber if patient has a seizure. Monitor closely for loss of seizure control with a prior history of seizures.

D

- Monitor BP in all patients receiving this drug. Monitor cardiac status and report palpitations or other signs of arrhythmias.
- Monitor for potential abuse and dependence on this drug. Careful supervision is needed during drug withdrawal because severe depression may occur.
- Monitor child behavior at school, home, and other settings.
- Lab tests: Periodic CBC, differential, platelet counts, and LFTs during prolonged therapy.
- Concurrent drugs: Monitor patients on BP-lowering drugs for loss of BP control. Monitor plasma levels of oral anticoagulants and anticonvulsants; doses of these drugs may need to be decreased.

Patient & Family Education

- Withhold drug and report immediately any of the following signs of overdose: Vomiting, agitation, tremors, muscle twitching, convulsions, confusion, hallucinations, delirium, sweating, flushing, headache, or high temperature.
- Note that drug is usually discontinued if improvement is not observed after appropriate dosage adjustment over 1 mo.
- Keep log of child behavior at school, home, and other settings.
- Drug has high potential for abuse. Keep locked and secure.
- Do not breast feed while taking this drug without consulting prescriber.

DEXRAZOXANE
(dex-ra-zox'ane)
Zinecard
Classifications: CHELATING AGENT; CARDIOPROTECTIVE FOR DOXORUBICIN
Pregnancy Category: C

AVAILABILITY 250 mg, 500 mg vials for injection

ACTIONS Drug is a derivative of EDTA that readily penetrates cell membranes. The mechanism by which dexrazoxane exerts its cardioprotective activity is not fully understood.

THERAPEUTIC EFFECTS Dexrazoxane is converted intracellularly to a chelating agent that interferes with iron-mediated free radical generation thought to be partially responsible for one form of cardiomyopathy.

USES Reduction of the incidence and severity of cardiomyopathy associated with doxorubicin in women with metastatic breast cancer who have received a cumulative doxorubicin dose of 300 mg/m^2.

CONTRAINDICATIONS Chemotherapy regimens that do not contain anthracycline, lactation.
CAUTIOUS USE Myelosuppresion, pregnancy (category C). Safety and efficacy in children have not been established.

ROUTE & DOSAGE

Cardiomyopathy

Child/Adult: **IV** 10 parts dexrazoxane to 1 part doxorubicin or 500 mg/m^2 for every 50 mg/m^2 of doxorubicin, repeated q3wk

Common adverse effects in *italic;* life-threatening effects <u>underlined;</u> generic names in **bold;** drug classifications in SMALL CAPS; ♣ Canadian drug name; ✪ Prototype drug.

STORAGE
Store reconstituted solutions for 6 h at 15°–30° C (59°–86° F).

ADMINISTRATION

Intravenous

D

- Wear gloves when handling dexrazoxane. Immediately wash with soap and water if drug contacts skin or mucosa. ■ Doxorubicin dose MUST be started within 30 min of beginning dexrazoxane.

PREPARE **Direct:** Reconstitute by adding 25 or 50 mL of 0.167 M sodium lactate injection (provided by manufacturer) to the 250- or 500-mg vial, respectively, to produce a 10 mg/mL solution. **IV Infusion:** Further dilute with NS or D5W in an IV bag to a concentration of 1.3–5.0 mg/mL for infusion.

ADMINISTER **Direct:** Give slow IV push. **IV Infusion:** Give over 10 min.

ADVERSE EFFECTS All: Adverse effects of dexrazoxane are difficult to distinguish from those of the chemotherapeutic agents. Pain at injection site, leukopenia, granulocytopenia, and thrombocytopenia appear to occur more frequently with the addition of dexrazoxane than with placebo.

PHARMACOKINETICS Distribution: Not bound to plasma proteins. **Metabolism:** Metabolized in liver. **Elimination:** 42% excreted in urine. **Half-Life:** 2–2.5 h.

NURSING IMPLICATIONS

Assessment & Drug Effects

- Monitor cardiac function. Drug does not eliminate risk of doxorubicin cardiotoxicity.
- Lab tests: Monitor hepatic, renal, and hematopoietic status throughout course of therapy.
- Note: Adverse effects are likely due to concurrent cytotoxic drugs rather than dexrazoxane.

Patient & Family Education

- Report any of the following to physician: Worsening shortness of breath, swelling extremities, or chest pains.
- Do not breast feed while taking this drug.

DEXTRAN 40

(dex'tran)

Gentran 40, Hyskon, 10% LMD, Rheomacrodex

Classifications: BLOOD DERIVATIVE; PLASMA VOLUME EXPANDER; REPLACEMENT SOLUTION

Prototype: Albumin

Pregnancy Category: C

AVAILABILITY 10% solution in D5W or NS

D

ACTIONS Low-molecular-weight polysaccharide. As a hypertonic colloidal solution, produces immediate and short-lived expansion of plasma volume by increasing colloidal osmotic pressure and drawing fluid from interstitial to intravascular space. Reduces possibility of deep venous thrombosis and pulmonary embolism, primarily by inhibiting venous stasis and platelet adhesiveness.

THERAPEUTIC EFFECTS Cardiovascular response to volume expansion includes increased BP, pulse pressure, CVP, cardiac output, venous return to heart, and urinary output.

USES Adjunctively to expand plasma volume and provide fluid replacement in treatment of shock or impending shock caused by hemorrhage, burns, surgery, or other trauma. Also used in prophylaxis and therapy of venous thrombosis and pulmonary embolism. Used as priming fluid or as additive to other primers during extracorporeal circulation.

CONTRAINDICATIONS Hypersensitivity to dextrans, renal failure, hypervolemic conditions, severe CHF, thrombocytopenia, significant anemia, hypofibrinogenemia or other marked hemostatic defects including those caused by drugs (e.g., heparin, warfarin); pregnancy (category C), lactation.

CAUTIOUS USE Active hemorrhage; severe dehydration; chronic liver disease; impaired renal function; patients susceptible to pulmonary edema or CHF.

ROUTE & DOSAGE

Shock

Child: **IV** Total dose ≤20 mL/kg in first 24 h and then ≤10 mL/kg/day (max 5 days total)
Adult: **IV** 500 mL administered rapidly (over 15–30 min), additional doses may be given more slowly up to 20 mL/kg in the first 24 h (doses up to 10 mL/kg/day may be given for an additional 4 days if needed)

Prophylaxis for Thromboembolic Complications

Adult: **IV** 500–1000 mL (10 mL/kg) on the day of operation followed by 500 mL/day for 2–3 days, may continue with 500 mL q2–3days for up to 2 wk if necessary

Priming for Extracorporeal Circulation

Adult: **IV** 10–20 mL/kg added to perfusion circuit

STORAGE

Store at a constant temperature, preferably 25° C (77° F). Once opened, discard unused portion because dextran contains no preservative.

ADMINISTRATION

Intravenous

If blood is to be administered, draw a cross-match specimen before dextran infusion.
PREPARE **IV Infusion:** Use only if seal is intact, vacuum is detectable, and solution is absolutely clear.

D

ADMINISTRATION IV Infusion: Specific flow rate should be prescribed by physician. For emergency treatment of shock in adults give first 500 mL rapidly (e.g., 20–40 mL/min); give remaining portion of the daily dose over 8–24 h or at the rate prescribed.

ADVERSE EFFECTS Body as a Whole: Hypersensitivity (mild to generalized urticaria, pruritus, <u>anaphylactic shock</u> [rare], angioedema, dyspnea). **Other:** Renal tubular vacuolization (osmotic nephrosis), stasis, and blocking; oliguria, <u>renal failure</u>; increased AST and ALT, interference with platelet function, prolonged bleeding and coagulation times.

DIAGNOSTIC TEST INTERFERENCE When blood samples are drawn for study, notify laboratory that patient has received dextran. *Blood glucose:* False increases (utilizing *ortho-toluidine methods* or *sulfuric* or *acetic acid* hydrolysis). *Urinary protein:* False increases (utilizing *Lowry method*). *Bilirubin assays:* False increases when alcohol is used. *Total protein assays:* False increases using *biuret reagent*. *Rh testing, blood typing* and *cross-matching* procedures: Dextran may interfere with results (by inducing rouleaux formation) when *proteolytic enzyme techniques* are used (*saline agglutination* and *indirect antiglobulin methods* reportedly not affected).

PHARMACOKINETICS Onset: Volume expansion within minutes of infusion. **Duration:** 12 h. **Metabolism:** Degraded to glucose and metabolized to CO_2 and water over a period of a few weeks. **Elimination:** 75% excreted in urine within 24 h; small amount excreted in feces.

NURSING IMPLICATIONS

Assessment & Drug Effects

- Evaluate patient's state of hydration before dextran therapy begins. Record hourly intake and output and current weight. Administration to severely dehydrated patients can result in renal failure.
- Lab tests: Baseline Hct prior to and after initiation of dextran (dextran usually lowers Hct). Notify physician if Hct is depressed below 30% by volume.
- Monitor vital signs and observe patient closely for at least the first 30 min of infusion. Hypersensitivity reaction is most likely to occur during the first few minutes of administration. Terminate therapy at the first sign of a hypersensitivity reaction (see Appendix D-1).
- Monitor CVP as an estimate of blood volume status and a guide for determining dosage. Normal CVP: 5–10 cm H_2O.
- Observe for S&S of circulatory overload (see Appendix D-1).
- Note: When sodium restriction is indicated, know that 500 mL of dextran 40 in 0.9% normal saline contains 77 mEq of both sodium and chloride.
- Monitor I&O ratio and check urine specific gravity every 30 min as therapy begins and then at regular intervals. Low urine specific gravity may signify failure of renal dextran clearance and is an indication to discontinue therapy.

D

- Report oliguria, anuria, or lack of improvement in urinary output (dextran usually causes an increase in urinary output). Discontinue dextran at first sign of renal dysfunction. Weigh daily.
- High doses are associated with transient prolongation of bleeding time and interference with normal blood coagulation.

Patient & Family Education

- Report immediately S&S of bleeding: Easy bruising, blood in urine or dark tarry stool.
- Do not breast feed while taking this drug.

DEXTROAMPHETAMINE SULFATE

(dex-troe-am-fet′a-meen)

Dexampex, Dexedrine, Oxydess II ♣, Spancap No. 1

Classifications: CENTRAL NERVOUS SYSTEM AGENT; RESPIRATORY AND CEREBRAL STIMULANT; AMPHETAMINE; ANOREXIANT

Prototype: Amphetamine

Pregnancy Category: C

Controlled Substance: Schedule II

AVAILABILITY 5 mg, 10 mg tablets; 5 mg, 10 mg, 15 mg sustained-release capsules

ACTIONS Dextrorotatory isomer of amphetamine. Anorexigenic action is thought to result from CNS stimulation and possibly from loss of acuity of smell and taste.

THERAPEUTIC EFFECTS On a weight basis, has less pronounced effect on cardiovascular and peripheral nervous systems and is a more potent appetite suppressant than amphetamine. CNS stimulating effect approximately twice that of racemic amphetamine. In hyperkinetic children, amphetamines reduce motor restlessness by an unknown mechanism.

USES Adjunct in short-term treatment of exogenous obesity, narcolepsy, and attention deficit disorder with hyperactivity in children (also called minimal brain dysfunction or hyperkinetic syndrome).

UNLABELED USES Adjunct in epilepsy to control ataxia and drowsiness induced by barbiturates; to combat sedative effects of trimethadione in absence seizures.

CONTRAINDICATIONS Hypersensitivity to sympathomimetic amines, glaucoma, agitated states, psychoses (especially in children), advanced arteriosclerosis, symptomatic heart disease, moderate to severe hypertension, hyperthyroidism, history of drug abuse, during or within 14 days of MAO INHIBITOR therapy, as anorexiant in children <12 y, for attention deficit disorder in children <3 y, lactation.

CAUTIOUS USE Pregnancy (category C). Safety and efficacy in children <3 y have not been established.

ROUTE & DOSAGE

Narcolepsy

Child: **PO** *6–12 y,* 5 mg/day in 1–3 doses, may increase by 5 mg/day at weekly intervals (max 60 mg/day); *>12 y,* 10 mg/day in 1–3 doses, may increase by 10 mg/day at weekly intervals (max 60 mg/day)
Adult: **PO** 5–20 mg 1–3 times/day at 4–6 h intervals

Attention Deficit Disorder

Child: **PO** *3–5 y,* 2.5 mg 1–2 times/day given every morning, may increase by 2.5 mg at weekly intervals; *≥6 y,* 5 mg 1–2 times/day given every morning, may increase by 5 mg at weekly intervals (max 40 mg/day)

STORAGE

Store in tightly closed containers at 15°–30° C (59°–86° F) unless otherwise directed.

ADMINISTRATION

Oral

- Ensure that sustained-release capsule is not chewed or crushed. It MUST be swallowed whole.
- Give 30–60 min before meals for treatment of obesity. Give long-acting form in the morning.
- Give last dose no later than 6 h before patient retires (10–14 h before bedtime for sustained-release form) to avoid insomnia.

ADVERSE EFFECTS CNS: Nervousness, *restlessness,* hyperactivity, *insomnia,* euphoria, dizziness, headache; ***with prolonged use***—severe depression, psychotic reactions; paradoxical reactions in children. **CV:** Palpitation, tachycardia, elevated BP. **GI:** Dry mouth, unpleasant taste, anorexia, weight loss, diarrhea, constipation, abdominal pain. **Other:** Slowed growth, unusual fatigue, increased intraocular pressure, marked dystonia of head, neck, and extremities; sweating.

DIAGNOSTIC TEST INTERFERENCE Dextroamphetamine may cause significant elevations in ***plasma corticosteroids*** (evening levels are highest) and increases in ***urinary epinephrine*** excretion (during first 3 h after drug administration).

INTERACTIONS Drug: Acetazolamide, sodium bicarbonate decrease dextroamphetamine elimination; **ammonium chloride, ascorbic acid** increase dextroamphetamine elimination; effects of both BARBITURATES and dextroamphetamine may be antagonized; **furazolidone** may increase BP effects of AMPHETAMINES—interaction may persist for several weeks after discontinuing **furazolidone;** large doses of antacids decrease urinary excretion; antagonizes antihypertensive effects of **guanethidine, guanadrel;** MAO INHIBITORS, **selegiline** can cause hypertensive crisis (fatalities reported)—do not administer AMPHETAMINES during or within 14 days of these drugs; PHENOTHIAZINES may inhibit mood-elevating effects of AMPHETAMINES; TRICYCLIC ANTIDEPRESSANTS enhance dextroamphetamine effects because of increased **norepi-nephrine** release; BETA-ADRENERGIC AGONISTS increase cardiovascular adverse effects.

PHARMACOKINETICS Absorption: Rapid. **Peak:** 1–5 h. **Duration:** Up to 10 h. **Distribution:** All tissues especially the CNS. **Metabolism:** Metabolized in liver. **Elimination:** Renal elimination; excreted in breast milk. **Half-Life:** 10–30 h.

NURSING IMPLICATIONS

Assessment & Drug Effects

- Not recommended in children under 5 y because diagnosis of ADHD is difficult in young children.
- Monitor growth rate closely in children.
- Interrupt therapy or reduce dosage periodically to assess effectiveness in behavior disorders.
- Note: Tolerance to anorexic effects may develop after a few weeks, however, tolerance does not appear to develop when dextroamphetamine is used to treat narcolepsy.

Patient & Family Education

- Swallow sustained-release capsule whole with a liquid; do not chew or crush.
- Give early in day for treatment of ADHD and avoid medication in afternoon and evening. Ensure that child has health supervision visits for monitoring of growth and of behavioral symptoms. Record child's behavior at school, home, and other settings. Record sleep patterns and report to prescriber.
- Do not drive or engage in other potentially hazardous activities until response to drug is known.
- Taper drug gradually following long-term use to avoid extreme fatigue, mental depression, and prolonged sleep pattern.
- Keep medication securely stored because a high risk for abuse is present.
- Do not breast feed while taking this drug.

DEXTROMETHORPHAN HYDROBROMIDE

(dex-troe-meth-or-fan)

Balminil DM ✦ , Benylin DM, Cremacoat 1, Delsym, DM Cough, Hold, Koffex ✦ , Mediquell, Neo-DM ✦ , Ornex DM ✦ , Pedia Care, Pertussin 8 Hour Cough Formula, Robidex ✦ , Robitussin DM, Romilar CF, Romilar Children's Cough, Sedatuss ✦ , Sucrets Cough Control

Classifications: ANTITUSSIVE
Prototype: Benzonatate
Pregnancy Category: C

AVAILABILITY 30 mg capsules; 2.5 mg, 5 mg, 7.5 mg, 15 mg lozenges; 10 mg/15 mL, 3.5 mg/5 mL, 7.5 mg/5 mL, 15 mg/5 mL liquid; 15 mg/15 mL, 10 mg/5 mL syrup. **Combination Products:** Available in many OTC cold

---

Common adverse effects in *italic;* life-threatening effects <u>underlined;</u> generic names in **bold;** drug classifications in SMALL CAPS; ✦ Canadian drug name; ❷ Prototype drug.

and cough preparations, such as with acetaminophen, chlorphenir-amine, pseudoephedrine, and guaifenesin.

ACTIONS Nonnarcotic derivative of levorphanol. Chemically related to morphine but without central hypnotic or analgesic effect or capacity to cause tolerance or addiction. Antitussive activity comparable to that of codeine but is less likely than codeine to cause constipation, drowsiness, or GI disturbances.
THERAPEUTIC EFFECTS Controls cough spasms by depressing cough center in medulla. Temporarily relieves coughing spasm.

USE Temporary relief of cough spasms in nonproductive coughs due to colds, pertussis, and influenza.

CONTRAINDICATIONS Asthma, productive cough, persistent or chronic cough; hepatic function impairment; patients on MAO inhibitors; pregnancy (category C).
CAUTIOUS USE Chronic pulmonary disease; children <2y.

ROUTE & DOSAGE

Cough

Child: **PO** 2–6 y, 2.5–5 mg q4h or 7.5 mg q6–8h (max 30 mg/day) or 15 mg sustained action liquid b.i.d.; 6–12 y, 5–10 mg q4h or 15 mg q6–8h (max 60 mg/day) or 30 mg sustained action liquid b.i.d.
Adult: **PO** 10–20 mg q4h or 30 mg q6–8h (max 120 mg/day) or 60 mg of sustained action liquid b.i.d.

STORAGE
Store between 15°–30° C (59°–86° F). Liquid solutions should be tightly covered and in light resistant containers.

ADMINISTRATION
Oral
- Do not give lozenges to children <6 y or those unable to follow directions due to choking hazard.
- Ensure that extended-release form of drug is not chewed or crushed. It MUST be swallowed whole.
- Note: Although soothing local effect of the syrup may be enhanced if given undiluted, depression of cough center depends only on systemic absorption of drug.

ADVERSE EFFECTS CNS: Dizziness, drowsiness, CNS depression with very large doses; excitability, especially in children. **GI:** GI upset, constipation, abdominal discomfort.

INTERACTIONS Drug: High risk of excitation, hypotension, and hyper-pyrexia with MAO INHIBITORS.

PHARMACOKINETICS Absorption: Readily absorbed from GI tract. **Onset:** 15–30 min. **Duration:** 3–6 h. **Metabolism:** Metabolized in liver. **Elimination:** Excreted in urine.

Common adverse effects in *italic;* life-threatening effects <u>underlined;</u> generic names in **bold;** drug classifications in SMALL CAPS; ♣ Canadian drug name; ✪ Prototype drug.

429

NURSING IMPLICATIONS

Assessment & Drug Effects
- Monitor for dizziness and drowsiness, especially when concurrent therapy with CNS depressant is used.
- Monitor S&S of respiratory distress; take vital signs; be aware of signs of infection particulary in young children.

Patient & Family Education
- Avoid self-medication of young children with OTC preparations, especially when using combination drug forms. Consult with health care provider about child's symptoms and recommended treatment.
- Avoid irritants such as smoking, dust, fumes, and other air pollutants to lesson unnecessary cough. Humidify ambient air to provide some relief.
- Note: Treatment aims to decrease the frequency and intensity of cough without completely eliminating protective cough reflex.
- While dextromethorphan is available OTC, any cough persisting longer than 1 wk–10 days needs to be medically diagnosed.
- Store this medication out of reach of children.

DEXTROTHYROXINE SODIUM
(dex-troe-thye-rox′een)
Choloxin
Classifications: CARDIOVASCULAR DRUG; ANTILIPEMIC; LIPID-LOWERING AGENT
Pregnancy Category: C

AVAILABILITY 2 mg, 4 mg tablets

ACTIONS Sodium salt and dextrorotatory isomer of thyroxine. Reduces serum cholesterol and LDL levels in hyperlipidemia; triglycerides and beta-lipoproteins may also be lowered from previously elevated levels, but effect is variable.

THERAPEUTIC EFFECTS By an unclear mechanism, liver is stimulated to increase catabolism and excretion of cholesterol and its degradation products via the biliary route into feces. Greatest decrease in serum cholesterol occurs in patients with highest baseline concentrations, with maximum therapeutic effects in 1 or 2 mo.

USES Adjunct to other medications in the treatment of primary hypercholesterolemia (type IIa hyperlipidemia), particularly euthyroid patients with significant risk but no evidence of coronary artery disease.

CONTRAINDICATIONS Euthyroids with one or more of the following: known organic heart disease including angina pectoris, arrhythmias, decompensated or borderline compensated cardiac states; history of MI or CHF; rheumatic heart disease; hypertension; advanced liver or kidney disease; history of iodism; pregnancy (category C), lactation; 2 wk prior to elective surgery.

CAUTIOUS USE Hypothyroid patients with concomitant coronary artery disease; women of childbearing age with familial hypercholesterolemia; diabetes mellitus; liver and kidney impairment; children, older adults.

ROUTE & DOSAGE

D

Euthyroid Hyperlipidemia

Child: **PO** 0.05 mg/kg/day, increased by not more than 0.05 mg/kg every month if needed (max 4 mg/day)
Adult: **PO** 1–2 mg/day, increased by 1 or 2 mg every month if needed (max 8 mg/day)

STORAGE

Store medication in light- and moisture-proof container at 15°–30° C (59°–86° F) unless otherwise specified.

ADMINISTRATION

Oral

■ Give at any time without respect to meals.

ADVERSE EFFECTS All: Mainly due to increased metabolism. **CNS:** Insomnia, nervousness, dizziness, psychic changes, paresthesias. **CV:** Angina pectoris, palpitation, cardiac arrhythmia, ECG evidence of ischemic myocardial changes, increase in heart size; MI (relationship not conclusive), worsening of peripheral vascular disease. **Special Senses:** Tinnitus, hoarseness; visual disturbances, exophthalmos, retinopathy, lid lag. **GI:** Nausea, constipation, diarrhea, bitter taste, weight loss. **Other:** Acneiform rash, pruritus, coryza, conjunctivitis, stomatitis, brassy taste, laryngitis, bronchitis.

INTERACTIONS Drug: Cholestyramine, colestipol decrease absorption of dextrothyroxine; compounds thyroid effects of other THYROID PREPARATIONS; increases risk of hypoprothrombinemia associated with **warfarin; digoxin** may enhance myocardial stimulation; may increase blood **glucose,** requiring adjustment of **insulin** and SULFONYLUREAS.

PHARMACOKINETICS Absorption: About 25% absorbed from GI tract. **Distribution:** Crosses placenta; distribution into breast milk not known. **Metabolism:** Metabolized in liver. **Elimination:** Excreted in urine and feces. **Half-Life:** 18 h.

NURSING IMPLICATIONS

Assessment & Drug Effects

■ Monitor for therapeutic effectiveness. Initial decrease in cholesterol levels may not occur until 2 wk–1 mo after initiation of therapy. Maximum decrease usually occurs during second or third month of therapy.
■ Lab test: Determine & evaluate serum lipids initially and at periodic intervals during therapy. Patient should follow a normal diet for several days prior to the test.
■ Observe patients with cardiac disease closely, particularly during early therapy and at frequent intervals throughout the treatment period.

D

- Note: Hypothyroid patients with organic heart disease have a high incidence of adverse effects.
- Report immediately new S&S of cardiac disease or increased decompensation in the borderline compensated patient. Dose adjustment may be indicated.
- Concomitant drugs: Carefully monitor coagulation studies with warfarin.
- Monitor diabetics for loss of glycemic control.

Patient & Family Education
- Note: Serum lipids generally return to pretreatment levels within 6 wk–3 mo after drug is withdrawn. Instruct family in diet that reduces lipid levels.
- Report chest pain, palpitations, sweating, diarrhea, headache, or skin rash to physician.
- Report to physician immediately any of the following: Acne-type rash, itching, conjunctivitis, inflamed mouth, significant nasal discharge, brassy taste, laryngitis, or bronchitis.
- Do not take OTC medications without care provider's approval.
- Inform care provider or dentist in an emergency situation that you are taking dextrothyroxine before any surgery is performed.
- Do not breast feed while taking this drug.
- Store this medication out of reach of children.

DIAZEPAM ℗
(dye-az-e-pam)
Apo-Diazepam ♣, Diastat, Diazemuls ♣, E-Pam ♣, Meval ♣, Novodipam ♣, Valium, Valrelease, Vivol ♣

DIAZEPAM EMULSIFIED
Dizac
Classifications: CENTRAL NERVOUS SYSTEM AGENT; BENZODIAZEPINE ANTICONVULSANT; ANXIOLYTIC
Pregnancy Category: D

AVAILABILITY 2 mg, 5 mg, 10 mg tablets; 1 mg/mL, 5 mg/mL, 5 mg/5 mL oral solution; 5 mg/mL injection; 2.5 mg, 5 mg, 10 mg, 15 mg, 20 mg rectal gel

ACTIONS Psychotherapeutic agent related to chlordiazepoxide; reportedly superior in antianxiety and anticonvulsant activity, with somewhat shorter duration of action. Like chlordiazepoxide, it appears to act at both limbic and subcortical levels of CNS.
THERAPEUTIC EFFECTS Shortens REM and stage 4 sleep but increases total sleep time. Antianxiety and anticonvulsant agent.

USES Management of status epilepticus. Management of anxiety disorders, for short-term relief of anxiety symptoms, to allay anxiety and tension prior to surgery, cardioversion and endoscopic procedures, as an amnesic, and treatment for restless legs. Also used to alleviate acute withdrawal symptoms of alcoholism, voiding problems in older adults, and adjunctively for relief of skeletal muscle spasm associated with cerebral palsy, paraplegia, athetosis, stiffman syndrome, tetanus.

CONTRAINDICATIONS *Injectable form:* Shock, coma, acute alcohol intoxication, depressed vital signs, obstetrical patients, infants <30 days of age. *Tablet form:* Infants <6 mo of age, acute narrow-angle glaucoma, untreated open-angle glaucoma; during or within 14 days of MAO INHIBITOR therapy. Safe use during pregnancy (category D) and lactation is not established.

CAUTIOUS USE Epilepsy, psychoses, mental depression; myasthenia gravis; impaired hepatic or renal function; drug abuse, addiction prone individuals. Injectable diazepam used with extreme caution in older adults, the very ill, and patients with COPD.

ROUTE & DOSAGE

Status Epilepticus

Neonate/Child: **IV** 0.3–0.75 mg/kg/dose q15–30min times 2–3 doses; *>1 mo,* 0.2–0.5 mg/kg/dose q15–30min (max *<5 y,* 5 mg *>5 y* 10 mg); *>5 y,* 1 mg slowly q2–5min up to 10 mg, repeat if needed q2–4h (max 10 mg)
Adult: **IV/IM** 5–10 mg, repeat if needed at 10–15 min intervals up to 30 mg, then repeat if needed q2–4h (max 30 mg)

Anxiety, Muscle Spasm, Convulsions, Alcohol Withdrawal

Child: **IV** 0.04–0.2 mg/kg/dose q2–4h (max 0.5 mg/kg in 8 h)
PO *>6 mo,* 1–2.5 mg b.i.d. or t.i.d.; 0.12–0.8 mg/kg/day or 3.5–24 mg/m²/day divided into 3–4 doses
Adult: **PO** 2–10 mg b.i.d. to q.i.d. or 15–30 mg/day sustained-release
IV/IM 2–10 mg, repeat if needed in 3–4 h

Epilepsy

Child: **PO** 6–15 mg/day

STORAGE

Store in tight, light-resistant containers at 15°–30° C (59°–86° F), unless otherwise specified by manufacturer. Store Dizac emulsion at 2°–8° C (36°–46° F). Do not freeze.

ADMINISTRATION

Note: Dizac emulsion is administered by IV only.

Oral

- Ensure that sustained-release form is not chewed or crushed. It MUST be swallowed whole. Give other tablets crushed with fluid or mixed with food if necessary.
- Supervise oral ingestion to ensure drug is swallowed.
- Avoid abrupt discontinuation of diazepam. Taper doses to termination.

Common adverse effects in *italic;* life-threatening effects <u>underlined</u>; generic names in **bold;** drug classifications in SMALL CAPS; ♣ Canadian drug name; ⊘ Prototype drug.

433

Intramuscular

- Give deep into large muscle mass appropriate for age. Inject slowly. Rotate injection sites.
- Do NOT give emulsion form (Dizac) as IM or SC. It is for IV use only.

Intravenous

PREPARE **Direct:** Do not dilute or mix with any other drug.

ADMINISTER **Direct:** Give direct IV by injecting drug slowly, taking at least 1 min for each 5 mg (1 mL) given to adults and taking at least 3 min to inject 0.25 mg/kg body weight of children. Do not exceed rate of 2 mg/min. ▪ If injection cannot be made directly into vein, inject slowly through infusion tubing as close as possible to vein insertion. ▪ The emulsion form is incompatible with filters with pore sizes <5 microns or via polyvinyl chloride (PVC) infusion sets. Rate of administration for emulsion form should not exceed 5 mg/min. ▪ Avoid small veins and take extreme care to avoid intra-arterial administration or extravasation.

INCOMPATIBILITIES **Solution/Additive: Bleomycin, benzquinamide, dobutamine, doxapram, doxorubicin, fluorouracil, glycopyrrolate, heparin, nalbuphone, sufentanil.** Emulsion also incompatible with **morphine. Y-Site: Furosemide, heparin, potassium chloride, vitamin B complex with C.** Emulsion also incompatible with **morphine.** Do not mix emulsion with any other drugs. Do not administer through **PVC** infusion sets.

ADVERSE EFFECTS Body as a Whole: Throat and chest pain. **CNS:** *Drowsiness,* fatigue, ataxia, confusion, paradoxic rage, dizziness, vertigo, amnesia, vivid dreams, headache, slurred speech, tremor; EEG changes, tardive dyskinesia. **CV:** Hypotension, tachycardia, edema, <u>cardiovascular collapse</u>. **Special Senses:** Blurred vision, diplopia, nystagmus. **GI:** Xerostomia, nausea, constipation, hepatic dysfunction. **Urogenital:** Incontinence, urinary retention, gynecomastia (prolonged use), menstrual irregularities, ovulation failure. **Respiratory:** Apnea, hiccups, coughing, <u>laryngospasm</u>. **Other:** Pain, venous thrombosis, phlebitis at injection site.

INTERACTIONS Drug: Alcohol, CNS DEPRESSANTS, ANTICONVULSANTS potentiate CNS depression; **cimetidine** increases diazepam plasma levels, increases toxicity; may decrease antiparkinson effects of **levodopa;** may increase **phenytoin** levels; smoking decreases sedative and antianxiety effects. **Herbal: Kava kava, valerian** may potentiate sedation.

PHARMACOKINETICS Absorption: Readily absorbed from GI tract; erratic IM absorption. **Onset:** 30–60 min PO; 15–30 min IM; 1–5 min IV. **Peak:** 1–2 h PO. **Duration:** 15 min–1 h IV; up to 3 h PO. **Distribution:** Crosses blood–brain barrier and placenta; distributed into breast milk. **Metabolism:** Metabolized in liver to active metabolites. **Elimination:** Excreted primarily in urine. **Half-Life:** 20–50 h.

NURSING IMPLICATIONS

Assessment & Drug Effects

- Take history of other medications and herbal products.
- Monitor for adverse reactions. Most are dose related. Physician will rely on accurate observation and reports of patient response to the drug to determine lowest effective maintenance dose.

- Emergency treatment is followed by long-lasting anticonvulsants. Observe for desired and adverse effects of all drugs.
- Monitor for therapeutic effectiveness. Maximum effect may require 1–2 wk; patient tolerance to therapeutic effects may develop after 4 wk of treatment.
- Observe necessary preventive precautions for suicidal tendencies that may be present in anxiety states accompanied by depression.
- Observe patient closely and monitor vital signs when diazepam is given parenterally; hypotension, muscular weakness, tachycardia, and respiratory depression may occur.
- Lab tests: Periodic CBC and liver function tests during prolonged therapy.
- Supervise ambulation. Adverse reactions such as drowsiness and ataxia are more likely to occur in debilitated patients or those receiving larger doses. Dosage adjustment may be necessary.
- Monitor I&O ratio, including urinary and bowel elimination.
- Note: Smoking increases metabolism of diazepam; lowering clinical effectiveness. Heavy smokers may need a higher dose than the non-smoker.
- Note: Psychic and physical dependence may occur in patients on long-term high dosage therapy, in those with histories of alcohol or drug addiction, or in those who self-medicate.

Patient & Family Education

- Report use of this drug to all health care professionals. Monitor and report any seizure activity. Instruct school and other settings in emergency treatment of seizures.
- Avoid alcohol and other CNS depressants during therapy unless otherwise advised by prescriber. Concomitant use of these agents can cause severe drowsiness, respiratory depression, and apnea.
- Do not drive or engage in other potentially hazardous activities or those requiring mental precision until reaction to drug is known.
- Tell physician if you become or intend to become pregnant during therapy; drug may need to be discontinued.
- Take drug as prescribed; do not change dose or dose intervals.
- Check with physician before taking any OTC drugs.
- Do not breast feed while taking this drug without consulting physician.
- Store this medication out of reach of children.

DIAZOXIDE

(dye-az-ox′ide)

Hyperstat I. V., Proglycem

Classifications: CARDIOVASCULAR AGENT; ANTIHYPERTENSIVE; VASODILATOR; SULFONYLUREA

Prototype: Hydralazine

Pregnancy Category: C

AVAILABILITY 50 mg capsules; 50 mg/mL suspension; 15 mg/mL injection

D

ACTIONS Rapid-acting thiazide nondiuretic hypotensive and hyperglycemic agent. In contrast to thiazide diuretics, causes sodium and water retention and decreases urinary output, probably because it increases proximal tubular reabsorption of sodium and decreases glomerular filtration rate. Hypotensive effect may be accompanied by marked reflex increase in heart rate, cardiac output, and stroke volume; thus cerebral and coronary blood flow are usually maintained.
THERAPEUTIC EFFECTS Reduces peripheral vascular resistance and BP by direct vasodilatory effect on peripheral arteriolar smooth muscles, perhaps by direct competition for calcium receptor sites.

USES Intravenously for emergency lowering of BP in hospitalized patients with malignant hypertension, particularly when associated with renal impairment. Not effective in pheochromocytoma. Commonly used with a diuretic such as furosemide (Lasix) to counteract diazoxide-induced sodium and water retention. Orally in treatment of various diagnosed hypoglycemic states due to hyperinsulinism when other medical treatment or surgical management has been unsuccessful or is not feasible.

CONTRAINDICATIONS Hypersensitivity to diazoxide or to other thiazides; cerebral bleeding, eclampsia; aortic coarctation; AV shunt, significant coronary artery disease. Safe use during pregnancy (category C) or lactation is not established. Use of oral diazoxide for functional hypoglycemia or in presence of increased bilirubin in newborns.
CAUTIOUS USE Diabetes mellitus; impaired cerebral or cardiac circulation; impaired renal function; patients taking corticosteroids or estrogen–progestogen combinations; hyperuricemia, history of gout, uremia.

ROUTE & DOSAGE

Severe Hypertension
Child/Adult: **IV** 1–3 mg/kg up to 150 mg, repeat at 5–15 min intervals if necessary
Hypoglycemia
Infants/Neonates: **PO** 8–15 mg/kg/day divided into doses given q8–12h
Child/Adult: **PO** 3–8 mg/kg/day divided into doses given q8–12h

STORAGE
Do not give darkened solutions. Store capsules, oral suspension, and injectables at 2°–30° C (36°–86° F) unless otherwise directed. Protect from light, heat, and freezing.

ADMINISTRATION
Intravenous
Note: Give any prescribed diuretic 30–60 min prior to IV diazoxide. Keep patient recumbent 8–10 h because of possible additive hypotensive effect.
PREPARE **Direct:** Give undiluted.
ADMINISTER **Direct:** Give IV by rapid direct injection over 10–30 sec. Keep patient recumbent while receiving IV and for at least 30 min following

Common adverse effects in *italic;* life-threatening effects underlined; generic names in **bold;** drug classifications in SMALL CAPS; ✦ Canadian drug name; ◯ Prototype drug.

administration. ■ Check IV injection site frequently. Solution is strongly alkaline. Extravasation of medication into tissues can cause severe inflammatory reaction. Administered drug by peripheral vein ONLY.

ADVERSE EFFECTS CNS: headache, weakness, malaise, *dizziness,* polyneuritis, sleepiness, insomnia, euphoria, anxiety, extrapyramidal signs. **CV:** Palpitations, atrial and ventricular arrhythmias, flushing, shock; *orthostatic hypotension*, CHF, transient hypertension. **Special Senses:** Tinnitus, momentary hearing loss; burred vision, transient cataracts, subconjunctival hemorrhage, ring scotoma, diplopia, lacrimation, papilledema. **GI:** *Nausea, vomiting,* abdominal discomfort, diarrhea, constipation, ileus, anorexia, transient loss of taste, impaired hepatic function. **Hematologic:** Transient neutropenia, eosinophilia, decreased Hgb/Hct, decreased IgG. **Body as a Whole:** Hypersensitivity (rash, fever, leukopenia); chest and back pain, muscle cramps. **Urogenital:** Decreased urinary output, nephrotic syndrome (reversible), hematuria, increased nocturia, proteinuria, azotemia; inhibition of labor. **Skin:** Pruritus, flushing, monilial dermatitis, herpes, hirsutism; loss of scalp hair, sweating, sensation of warmth, burning, or itching. **Endocrine:** Advance in bone age (children), *hyperglycemia, sodium and water retention, edema,* hyperuricemia, glycosuria, enlargement of breast lump, galactorrhea; decreased immunoglobulinemia, hirsutism.

DIAGNOSTIC TEST INTERFERENCE Diazoxide can cause false-negative response to *glucagon.*

INTERACTIONS Drug: SULFONYLUREAS antagonize effects; THIAZIDE DIURETICS may intensify hyperglycemia and antihypertensive effects; **phenytoin** increases risk of hyperglycemia, and diazoxide may increase **phenytoin** metabolism, causing loss of seizure control.

PHARMACOKINETICS Onset: 30–60 sec IV; 1 h PO. **Peak:** 5 min IV. **Duration:** 2–12 or more hours IV; 8 h PO. **Distribution:** Crosses blood–brain barrier and placenta. **Metabolism:** Partially metabolized in the liver. **Elimination:** Excreted in urine. **Half-Life:** 21–45 h.

NURSING IMPLICATIONS

Assessment & Drug Effects

■ Monitor for therapeutic effectiveness. Discontinue if not effective in 2 or 3 wk.
■ Lab tests: Initial blood glucose, serum electrolytes, and CBC and at regular intervals in patients receiving multiple doses.
■ Monitor BP q5min for the first 15–30 min or until stabilized, then hourly for balance of drug effect.
■ Notify physician immediately if BP continues to fall 30 min or more after IV drug administration. Cause other than drug effect is probable.
■ Monitor pulse: Tachycardia has occurred immediately following IV; palpitation and bradycardia have also been reported.
■ Report promptly any change in I&O ratio.
■ Observe patient closely for S&S of CHF (see Appendix D-1).
■ Monitor diabetics carefully for loss of glycemic control.

D

- Evaluate serum electrolyte levels at regular intervals, particularly in patients with impaired renal function; hypokalemia potentiates hyperglycemic effect of diazoxide.
- Note: In contrast to IV diazoxide, oral administration usually does not produce marked effects on BP. However, do make periodic measurements of BP and vital signs.
- Monitor signs and symptoms for up to 7 days for both oral and parenteral forms; essential because of long half-life of diazoxide.

Patient & Family Education
- Note: Drug may cause hyperglycemia and glycosuria in diabetic and diabetic-prone individuals. Closely monitor blood and urine glucose; report any abnormalities to prescriber.
- Report palpitations, chest pain, dizziness, fainting, or severe headache.
- Note: Lanugo-type hirsutism occurs frequently, commonly in children and women. It is reversible with discontinuation of drug.
- Do not breast feed while taking this drug without consulting prescriber.
- Store this medication out of reach of children.

DIBUCAINE
(dye'byoo-kane)
Nupercainal
Classifications: CENTRAL NERVOUS SYSTEM AGENT; ANESTHETIC, LOCAL (AMIDE-TYPE)
Prototype: Procaine
Pregnancy Category: C

AVAILABILITY 1% ointment; 0.5% cream

ACTIONS Long-acting anesthetic of the amide type and reportedly one of the most potent and most toxic. Appears to inhibit initiation and conduction of nerve impulses by reducing permeability of nerve cell membrane to sodium ions.

THERAPEUTIC EFFECTS Relief of pain and itching due to inhibiting conduction of nerve impulses.

USES Fast, temporary relief of pain and itching due to hemorrhoids and other anorectal disorders, nonpoisonous insect bites, sunburn, minor burns, cuts, and scratches.

CONTRAINDICATIONS Hypersensitivity to amide-type anesthetics, pregnancy (category C), children <1 y.
CAUTIOUS USE Lactation, children <12 y.

ROUTE & DOSAGE

Itching Due to Insect Bites or Hemorrhoids
Child: **Topical** Apply skin cream or ointment to affected area as needed (max 1/4 oz [7g]/24 h)

Adult: **Topical** Apply skin cream or ointment to affected area as needed (max 1 oz [28 g]/24 h); insert rectal ointment morning and evening and after each bowel movement

D

STORAGE
Store at 15°–30° C (59°–86° F) in tight, light-resistant containers.

ADMINISTRATION

Topical
■ Apply cream preparation after bathing or swimming (water soluble).

ADVERSE EFFECTS Skin: Irritation, contact dermatitis; rectal bleeding (suppository).

PHARMACOKINETICS Absorption: Poorly absorbed from intact skin; readily absorbed from mucous membranes or abraded skin. **Onset:** 15 min. **Duration:** 2–4 h.

NURSING IMPLICATIONS

Patient & Family Education
■ Use OTC preparations as directed. Always review package instructions.
■ Consult health care provider before using this or any skin preparation with young children due to increased potential for absorption.
■ Discontinue if irritation or rectal bleeding (following use of rectal preparations) develops and consult physician.
■ Hemorrhoids can be caused or worsened by constipation, excessive straining at stool, excessive standing, sitting, and coughing.
■ Physician may prescribe sitz baths 3–4 times/day to reduce the swelling and pain of hemorrhoids.
■ Note: Medication is intended for temporary relief of mild to moderate itching or pain. Seek medical advice for continuing discomfort, pain, bleeding, or sensation of rectal pressure.
■ Do not breast feed while taking this drug without consulting prescriber.
■ Store this medication out of reach of children.

DICLOFENAC SODIUM
(di-klo'fen-ak)
Voltaren, Voltaren-XR, Solaraze

DICLOFENAC POTASSIUM
Cataflam
Classifications: CENTRAL NERVOUS SYSTEM AGENT; ANALGESIC; ANTIPYRETIC; NSAID
Prototype: Ibuprofen
Pregnancy Category: B

D

AVAILABILITY Diclofenac Sodium 25 mg, 50 mg, 75 mg tablets; 100 mg sustained-release tablets; 0.1% ophthalmic solution; 3% gel. **Diclofenac Potassium** 50 mg tablets

ACTIONS Although its exact mechanism of action has not been fully elucidated, it appears to be a potent inhibitor of cyclooxygenase, thereby decreasing the synthesis of prostaglandins.
THERAPEUTIC EFFECTS Nonsteroidal anti-inflammatory drug (NSAID) with analgesic and antipyretic activity.

USES Analgesic and antipyretic effects in symptomatic treatment of rheumatoid arthritis, osteoarthritis, and ankylosing spondylitis. Has been used in some children age 3–16 y for juvenile rheumatoid arthritis, but optimal doses and uses are not clearly established. Used in acute soft-tissue injuries including sprains and strains; dysmenorrhea; headache, migraine, and dental, minor surgical, and postpartum pain; and renal or biliary colic. **Ophthalmic:** Cataract surgery; photophobia associated with refractive surgery. **Topical:** Treatment of actinic keratosis.

CONTRAINDICATIONS Hypersensitivity to diclofenac, patients in whom asthma, urticaria, angioedema, bronchospasm, severe rhinitis, shock, or other sensitivity reaction is precipitated by aspirin or other NSAIDs, pregnancy (category B), lactation.
CAUTIOUS USE Children; patients receiving anticoagulant therapy; history of GI disease; GU tract problems such as dysuria, cystitis, hematuria, nephritis, nephrotic syndrome, patients who must restrict their sodium intake; impaired hepatic function; SLE; heart failure; hypertension.

ROUTE & DOSAGE

Rheumatoid Arthritis
Child: **PO** 2–3 mg/kg/dose with doses given b.i.d. or t.i.d. for juvenile rheumatoid arthritis
Adult: **PO** 150–200 mg/day in 3–4 divided doses

STORAGE
Store at 15°–30° C (59°–86° F) away from heat and direct light.

ADMINISTRATION
Oral
- Ensure that sustained-release or enteric-coated forms of drug are not chewed or crushed. MUST be swallowed whole.
- Should be given with food or milk to decrease the risk of gastric irritation.
- Schedule administration 30 min before physical therapy or planned exercise to keep discomfort at a minimum.
- Discontinue therapy about 1 wk before surgery to reduce risk of bleeding.
- Use with caution in anyone who must restrict sodium intake.

Common adverse effects in *italic;* life-threatening effects underlined; generic names in **bold;** drug classifications in SMALL CAPS; ♣ Canadian drug name; ⦾ Prototype drug.

ADVERSE EFFECTS CNS: Dizziness, headache, drowsiness. **Special Senses:** Tinnitus. **Skin:** Rash, pruritus. **GI:** *Dyspepsia,* nausea, vomiting, abdominal pain, bleeding cramps, constipation, diarrhea, indigestion, abdominal distension, flatulence, peptic ulcer; liver enzymes, transaminases increased, liver test abnormalities. **CV:** Fluid retention, hypertension, CHF. **Respiratory:** Asthma. **Body as a Whole:** Back, leg, or joint pain. **Endocrine:** Hyperglycemia. **Hematologic:** Prolonged bleeding time; inhibits platelet aggregation.

DIAGNOSTIC TEST INTERFERENCE Liver function test values may be increased. Liver function test abnormalities may return to normal despite continued use; however, if significant abnormalities occur, clinical signs and symptoms consistent with liver disease develop, or systemic manifestations such as eosinophilia or rash occur, the medication should be discontinued. Serum uric acid concentrations may be decreased because of increased renal clearance.

INTERACTIONS Drug: Increases **cyclosporine**-induced nephrotoxicity; increases **methotrexate** levels (increases toxicity); may decrease BP-lowering effects of DIURETICS; may increase levels and toxicity of **lithium;** may increase **digoxin** levels. **Herbal: Feverfew, garlic, ginger, ginkgo** may increase risk of bleeding.

PHARMACOKINETICS Absorption: Readily absorbed from GI tract; 50–60% reaches systemic circulation. **Peak:** 2–3 h. **Distribution:** Widely distributed including synovial fluid and into breast milk. **Metabolism:** Extensively metabolized in liver. **Elimination:** 50–70% excreted in urine, 30–35% in feces. **Half-Life:** 1.2–2 h.

NURSING IMPLICATIONS

Assessment & Drug Effects

- Monitor for therapeutic effectiveness. Up to 3 wk may be needed for beneficial effects with rheumatoid arthritis.
- Lab tests: Periodic liver function, serum uric acid concentrations, Hct, PT/INR, and blood glucose.
- Observe and report signs of bleeding (e.g., petechiae, ecchymoses, bleeding gums, bloody or black stools, cloudy or bloody urine).
- Monitor BP for hypertension and blood sugar for hyperglycemia.
- Monitor diabetics closely for loss of diabetic control.
- Monitor for increased serum sodium and potassium in patients receiving potassium-sparing diuretics.
- Monitor weight and report gains greater than 1 kg (2 lb)/24 h.
- Monitor for S&S of GI irritation and ulceration.

Patient & Family Education

Oral Form

- Do not lie down for 15–30 min after taking medicine to decrease esophageal irritation.
- Discontinue use with onset of ringing or buzzing in the ears, impaired hearing, dizziness, GI discomfort, or bleeding and notify

prescriber. Watch for black-colored stools, nosebleeds, and bleeding gums.

- Do not take aspirin or other OTC analgesics without permission of the prescriber.
- Inform all health care providers (dental and other health care) about use of this drug.
- Avoid alcohol or other CNS depressants.
- Do not drive or engage in other potentially hazardous activities until reaction to drug is known.
- Note: Diabetics need to monitor blood glucose carefully for loss of glycemic control.
- Do not breast feed while taking this drug.
- Store this medication out of reach of children.

DICLOXACILLIN SODIUM
(dye-klox-a-sill'in)
Dycill, Dynapen, Pathocil
Classifications: ANTI-INFECTIVE; ANTIBIOTIC; SEMISYNTHETIC PENICILLIN
Prototype: Penicillin G potassium
Pregnancy Category: B

AVAILABILITY 125 mg, 250 mg, 500 mg capsules; 62.5 mg/5 mL suspension

ACTIONS Semisynthetic, acid-stable, penicillinase-resistant isoxazolyl penicillin. Action is bactericidal. Inhibits biosynthesis of bacterial cell wall during stage of active multiplication.

THERAPEUTIC EFFECTS Reportedly the most active of the isoxazolyl penicillins (cloxacillin, oxacillin) against penicillinase-producing *Staphylococci*. Generally ineffective against methicillin-resistant *Staphylococci* and gram-negative bacteria.

USES Primarily in systemic infections caused by penicillinase-producing *Staphylococci* and penicillin-resistant *Staphylococci*.

CONTRAINDICATIONS Hypersensitivity to penicillins. Safe use during pregnancy (category B) or in neonates is not established.

CAUTIOUS USE History of or suspected atopy or allergy (asthma, eczema, hives, hay fever); history of hypersensitivity to cephalosporins; lactation; renal or hepatic impairment. Experience using this drug with neonates and infants is very limited.

ROUTE & DOSAGE

Mild to Moderate Infections
Child: **PO** <40 kg, 12.5–25 mg/kg/day divided into doses given q6h (max 4 g/day)
Adult: **PO** 125–500 mg q6h (max 4 g/day)

Severe Infections
Child: **PO** *<40 kg,* 50–100 mg/kg/day divided into doses given q6h
Adult: **PO** 125–500 mg q6h (max 4 g/day)

STORAGE
Store reconstituted oral suspensions for 7 days at room temperature (15°–30° C; 59°–86° F) or 14 days under refrigeration at 2°–8° C (36°–46° F). Date and label container. Store capsules at room temperature in tightly covered containers unless otherwise directed.

ADMINISTRATION

Oral
- Give on an empty stomach at least 1 h before or 2 h after meals. Food reduces drug absorption.
- Reconstitute powder for oral suspension by shaking container to loosen powder. Add water according to label starting with half of the amount, then shake vigorously. Add remaining half and shake again vigorously. Shake well before each use.

ADVERSE EFFECTS Body as a Whole: Hypersensitivity (pruritus, urticaria, rash, wheezing, sneezing, <u>anaphylaxis</u>; eosinophilia). **GI:** Nausea, vomiting, flatulence, *diarrhea,* abdominal pain. **Other:** Transient elevations of ALT, superinfections.

INTERACTION Drug: Probenecid decreases dicloxacillin elimination.

PHARMACOKINETICS Absorption: 35–76% absorbed from GI tract. **Peak:** 0.5–2 h. **Duration:** 4–6 h. **Distribution:** Distributed throughout body with highest concentrations in liver and kidney; low CSF penetration; crosses placenta; distributed into breast milk. **Metabolism:** Metabolized in liver. **Elimination:** Excreted primarily in urine with some elimination through bile. **Half-Life:** 30–60 min.

NURSING IMPLICATIONS

Assessment & Drug Effects
- Note: Take care to establish previous exposure and sensitivity to penicillins and cephalosporins as well as other allergic reactions of any kind before initiating therapy.
- Obtain C&S prior to initiation of therapy to determine susceptibility of causative organism. Therapy may begin pending test results.
- Lab tests: Baseline blood cultures, WBC, and differential counts and at least weekly for patients on prolonged therapy. Periodic ALT and AST determinations, urinalysis, BUN, and creatinine are also advised for these patients.

Patient & Family Education
- Take medication around the clock. Do not miss a dose and continue taking medication until it is all gone, unless otherwise directed by prescriber.

Common adverse effects in *italic;* life-threatening effects <u>underlined</u>; generic names in **bold;** drug classifications in SMALL CAPS; ♣ Canadian drug name; ☯ Prototype drug.

443

D

- Check with prescriber if GI side effects appear.
- Watch for and report the signs of hypersensitivity reactions and super-infections (see Appendix D-1).
- Do not breast feed while taking this drug without consulting physician.
- Store this medication out of reach of children.

DIDANOSINE (DDI)

(di-dan'o-sine)
Videx, Videx EC
Classifications: ANTI-INFECTIVE; ANTIRETROVIRAL AGENT; NUCLEOSIDE REVERSE TRANSCRIPTASE INHIBITOR
Prototype: Zidovudine
Pregnancy Category: B

AVAILABILITY 25 mg, 50 mg, 100 mg, 150 mg, 200 mg tablets; 125 mg, 200 mg, 250 mg, 400 mg delayed-release capsules; 100 mg, 167 mg, 250 mg, 2 g, 4 g powder for oral solution

ACTIONS DDI interferes with the HIV RNA-dependent DNA polymerase (reverse transcriptase), thus preventing replication of the virus.
THERAPEUTIC EFFECTS Synthetic purine nucleotide that inhibits replication of HIV.

USES Advanced HIV infection in patients who are intolerant to zidovudine (AZT) or who demonstrate significant clinical or immunologic deterioration during zidovudine therapy.

CONTRAINDICATIONS Hypersensitivity to any of the components in the formulation, pregnancy (category B), lactation.
CAUTIOUS USE Individuals with peripheral vascular disease, history of neuropathy, chronic pancreatitis, renal impairment, or any liver impairment. Safety and efficacy of delayed-release capsules have not been established in children; other dosage forms are well tested in children.

ROUTE & DOSAGE

Neonates/Infants: PO 100 mg/m^2/day divided into doses given q12h
Child <13 y: **PO** 180 mg/m^2/day divided into doses given q12h, may increase daily dose to 300 mg/m^2 as needed
Adult: **PO** <60 kg, tablets, 250 mg daily or 125 mg b.i.d. (take 2 tablets at each dose to ensure adequate buffering); <60 kg, powder, 167 mg b.i.d.; ≥60 kg, tablets, 400 mg daily or 200 mg b.i.d.; ≥60 kg, powder, 250 mg b.i.d.

Note: Children in early puberty (Tanner stages I–II) are dosed as children; those in Tanner stages III–IV are dosed as child or adult with close monitoring; and those in Tanner stage V are dosed as adults.

Alternative child dosing:

BSA (m²)	Chewable Tablet	Powder
<0.4	25 mg q12h	31 mg q12h
0.5–0.7	50 mg q12h	62 mg q12h
0.8–1	75 mg q12h	94 mg q12h
1.1–1.4	100 mg q12h	125 mg q12h

STORAGE

Store tablets in tightly covered containers at room temperature 15°–30° C (59°–86° F). Store reconstituted liquid in a tightly closed flint-glass or plastic container in refrigerator for up to 30 days.

ADMINISTRATION

Oral

- Give drug on an empty stomach. Food should not be consumed within 15–30 min of drug administration.
- Give with water. Do NOT give with fruit juice or any other acid-containing liquid.
- If the child is receiving other medications, care regarding administration schedule is needed. Give 1 h before indinavir, 2 h before or after delavirdine, ritonavir, fluoroquinolones, ketaconazole, itraconazole, tetracyclines, dapsone. Give at least two tablets to provide adequate buffering. For example, for a 50-mg dose, give two 25-mg tablets.
- Chewable tablets must be thoroughly chewed or crushed and dispersed in at least 30 mL (1 oz) of water and immediately swallowed.
- Mix powder for oral solution (buffered) with at least 120 mL (4 oz) of water, stir until dissolved (requires 2–3 min), and immediately swallowed.
- Note: Powder for oral solution (pediatric) is prepared by pharmacist to yield a concentration of 10 mg/mL. Shake solution thoroughly before administration.
- Dosage reduction may be indicated in those with renal or hepatic impairment.
- Store reconstituted liquid in a tightly closed container in refrigerator for up to 30 days.

ADVERSE EFFECTS CV: Palpitations, thrombophlebitis, arrhythmias, *vasodilation.* **CNS:** *Headache, dizziness, nervousness, insomnia, peripheral neuropathy,* lethargy, poor coordination, seizures. **Special Senses:** Retinal depigmentation, photophobia, blurred vision, optic neuritis, diplopia, blindness. **GI:** *Abdominal pain, nausea, vomiting, diarrhea,* constipation, stomatitis, dry mouth, <u>pancreatitis</u>, increased liver enzymes. **Hematologic:** Increased WBC, neutrophil, lymphocyte, and platelet counts; increased Hgb, thrombocytopenia, ecchymosis, hemorrhage, petechiae. **Metabolic:** Hypocalcemia, hypokalemia, hypomagnesemia, hyperuricemia (asymptomatic), *hypertriglyceridemia.* **Musculoskeletal:** Muscle atrophy, myalgia, arthritis, decreased strength. **Respiratory:** *Asthma, cough, dyspnea, epistaxis, rhinitis, rhinorrhea,* hypoventilation, pharyngitis, rhonchi or rales, sinusitis, congestion. **Skin:** Rash, impetigo, eczema, *pruritus, sweating,* erythema.

Common adverse effects in *italic;* life-threatening effects <u>underlined</u>; generic names in **bold;** drug classifications in SMALL CAPS; ♣ Canadian drug name; ⊘ Prototype drug.

INTERACTIONS Drug: ALUMINUM- and MAGNESIUM-CONTAINING ANTACIDS may increase the aluminum- and magnesium-associated adverse effects of tablets. The effectiveness of **dapsone** in prophylaxis of *Pneumocystis carinii* pneumonia may be reduced by concomitant didanosine. Concomitant administration with **delaviridine** may decrease absorption of both drugs. May cause additive neuropathy with **zalcitabine** (ddC). **Food:** Absorption is significantly decreased by food. Take on an empty stomach.

PHARMACOKINETICS Absorption: Rapidly absorbed from GI tract when administered to fasting patient with antacids; 23–40% reaches systemic circulation. **Peak:** 0.6–1 h. **Distribution:** Distributed primarily to body water; 21% reaches CSF; crosses placenta. **Elimination:** 36% excreted in urine. **Half-Life:** 0.8–1.5 h.

NURSING IMPLICATIONS

Assessment & Drug Effects
- Monitor for S&S of pancreatitis (e.g., abdominal pain, nausea, vomiting, elevated serum amylase). Report immediately to physician and withhold drug until ruled out.
- Monitor for S&S of peripheral neuropathy (e.g., numbness, tingling, burning, pain in hands or feet). Report to physician; dose reduction may be indicated.
- Monitor patients with renal impairment for drug toxicity and hypermagnesemia manifested by muscle weakness and confusion.

Patient & Family Education
- Report immediately to physician any of the following: Abdominal pain, nausea, or vomiting.
- Do not breast feed while taking this drug.
- Store this medication out of reach of children.

DIGOXIN 🅟
(di-jox′in)
Lanoxicaps, Lanoxin
Classifications: CARDIOVASCULAR AGENT; CARDIAC GLYCOSIDE; ANTIARRHYTHMIC
Pregnancy Category: A

AVAILABILITY 0.05 mg, 0.1 mg, 0.2 mg capsules; 0.125 mg, 0.25 mg, 0.5 mg tablets; 0.05 mg/mL elixir; 0.25 mg/mL, 0.1 mg/mL injection

ACTIONS Widely used cardiac glycoside of *Digitalis lanata*. Acts by increasing the force and velocity of myocardial systolic contraction (positive inotropic effect). It also decreases conduction velocity through the atrioventricular node. Action is more prompt and less prolonged than that of digitalis and digitoxin.

THERAPEUTIC EFFECTS Increases the contractility of the heart muscle (positive inotropic effect).

USES Rapid digitalization and for maintenance therapy in CHF, atrial fibrillation, atrial flutter, paroxysmal atrial tachycardia.

CONTRAINDICATIONS Digitalis hypersensitivity, ventricular fibrillation, ventricular tachycardia unless due to CHF. Full digitalizing dose not given if patient has received digoxin during previous week or if slowly excreted cardiotonic glycoside has been given during previous 2 wk.

CAUTIOUS USE Renal insufficiency, hypokalemia, advanced heart disease, acute MI, incomplete AV block, cor pulmonale; hypothyroidism; lung disease; pregnancy (category A), lactation, premature and immature infants, children, older adults, or debilitated patients.

ROUTE & DOSAGE

Digitalizing Dose

Child:

Age	PO Dose (mcg/kg)	IM/IV Dose (mcg/kg)
Premature	20	15
Full-term newborn	30	20
<2 y	40–50	30–40
2–10 y	30–40	20–30
>10 y and <100 kg	10–15	8–12

Adult: **PO** 10–15 mcg/kg (1 mg) in divided doses over 24–48 h
IV 10–15 mcg/kg (1 mg) in divided doses over 24 h

Maintenance Dose

Child:

Age	PO Dose (mcg/kg/day)	IM/IV Dose (mcg/kg/day)
Premature	5	3–4
Full-term newborn	8–10	6–8
<2 y	10–12	7.5–9
2–10 y	8–10	6–8
>10 y and <100 kg	2.5–5	2–3

Note: Adjust doses downward in renal failure.

Adult: **PO/IV** 0.1–0.375 mg/day

STORAGE

Store tablets, elixir, and injection solution at 15°–30° C (59°– 86° F).

D

ADMINISTRATION

Oral

- Give without regard to food. Administration after food may slightly delay rate of absorption, but total amount absorbed is not affected.
- Crush and mix tablet with fluid or food if patient cannot swallow it whole, or obtain new order for elixir form.

Intravenous

One-half of digitalizing dose is given at once, then ¼ of digitalizing dose q 8–18 hr for 2 doses. For children under 10 y, daily dose is given in divided doses b.i.d.; for those >10 y, it is given daily.

***PREPARE* Direct:** Give undiluted or diluted in 4 mL of sterile water, D5W, or NS (less diluent may cause precipitation).

***ADMINISTER* Direct:** Give each dose over at least 5 min.

***INCOMPATIBILITIES* Solution/Additive: Dobutamine, doxapram.**

- Monitor IV site frequently. Infiltration of parenteral drug into subcutaneous tissue can cause local irritation and sloughing.

ADVERSE EFFECTS CNS: Fatigue, muscle weakness, headache, facial neuralgia, mental depression, paresthesias, hallucinations, confusion, drowsiness, agitation, dizziness. **CV:** Arrhythmias, hypotension, <u>AV block</u>. **Special Senses:** Visual disturbances. **GI:** Anorexia, *nausea,* vomiting, diarrhea. **Other:** Diaphoresis, recurrent malaise, dysphagia.

INTERACTIONS Drug: ANTACIDS, **cholestyramine, colestipol** decrease digoxin absorption; DIURETICS, CORTICOSTEROIDS, **amphotericin B,** LAXATIVES, **sodium polystyrene sulfonate** may cause hypokalemia, increasing the risk of digoxin toxicity; **calcium IV** may increase risk of arrhythmias if administered together with digoxin; **amiodarone, flecainide, quinidine, verapamil** significantly increase digoxin levels, and digoxin dose should be decreased by 50%; **erythromycin** may increase digoxin levels; **succinylcholine** may potentiate arrhythmogenic effects; **nefazodone** may increase digoxin levels. **Herbal: Ginseng** increase digoxin toxicity; **ma-huang, ephedra** may induce arrhythmias.

PHARMACOKINETICS Absorption: Absorption: 70% PO tablets; 90% PO liquid and capsules. **Onset:** 1–2 h PO; 5–30 min IV. **Peak:** 6–8 h PO; 1–5 h IV. **Duration:** 3–4 days in fully digitalized patient. **Distribution:** Widely distributed; tissue levels significantly higher than plasma levels; crosses placenta. **Metabolism:** Approximately 14% in liver. **Elimination:** 80–90% excreted by kidneys; may appear in breast milk. **Half-Life:** Premature, 61–170 h; full-term newborn, 35–45 h; infants, 18–25 h; children, 35 h.

NURSING IMPLICATIONS

Assessment & Drug Effects

- Be familiar with patient's baseline data (e.g., quality of peripheral pulses, blood pressure, clinical symptoms, serum electrolytes, creatinine clearance) as a foundation for making assessments.
- Lab tests: Baseline and periodic serum digoxin, potassium, magnesium, and calcium. Notify physician of abnormal values. Draw blood samples for determining plasma digoxin levels at least 6 h after daily dose and preferably just before next scheduled daily dose; should be taken

5–6 days after continuous dosing with the medication. ***Therapeutic range*** of serum digoxin is 0.8–2 ng/mL; toxic levels are >2 ng/mL.

- Take apical pulse for 1 full min noting rate, rhythm, and quality before administering. If changes are noted, withhold digoxin, take rhythm strip if patient is on ECG monitor, notify physician promptly. Take EKG 6 h after dose.
- Withhold medication and notify physician if apical pulse falls below ordered parameters (e.g., <50 or 60/min in adults and <60 to 100/min in children depending on age).
- Monitor for S&S of drug toxicity: In children, cardiac arrhythmias are usually reliable signs of early toxicity. Early indicators in adults (anorexia, nausea, vomiting, diarrhea, visual disturbances) are rarely initial signs in children.
- Monitor I&O ratio during digitalization, particularly in patients with impaired renal function. Also monitor for edema daily and auscultate chest for rales.
- Monitor serum digoxin levels closely during concurrent antibiotic–digoxin therapy, which can precipitate toxicity because of altered intestinal flora.
- Observe patients closely when being transferred from one preparation (tablet, elixir, or parenteral) to another; when tablet is replaced by elixir potential for toxicity increases since ≥30% of drug is absorbed.

Patient & Family Education

- Report to physician if pulse falls below determined lower level or rises above upper level.
- Suspect toxicity and report to physician if any of the following occur: Anorexia, nausea, vomiting, diarrhea, or visual disturbances. Report upset stomach or inability to take drug immediately.
- Weigh each day under standard conditions. Report weight gain >1 kg (2 lb)/day for older children or any increase for young children.
- Take digoxin PRECISELY as prescribed; do not skip or double a dose or change dose intervals, and take it at same time each day.
- Do not administer OTC medications to the child, especially those for coughs, colds, allergy, GI upset, or obesity, without prior approval of physician.
- Continue with brand originally prescribed unless otherwise directed by physician.
- Keep drug locked and out of reach of children. It has high risk for toxicity during accidental ingestion. Consider that visits to grandparents and other may provide access to this drug; evaluate the environment to ensure child safety.
- Do not breast feed while taking this drug without consulting physician.

DIGOXIN IMMUNE FAB (OVINE)

(di-jox′in)

Digibind, DigiFab

Classifications: ANTIDOTE
Pregnancy Category: C

AVAILABILITY 38 mg, 40 mg vial

ACTIONS Purified fragments of antibodies specific for digoxin (but also effective for digitoxin) produced in sheep immunized with digoxin–albumin conjugate. Use of fragments of antidigoxin antibodies (Fab) instead of whole antibody molecules permits more extensive and faster distribution to serum and toxic cellular sites.

THERAPEUTIC EFFECTS FAB acts by selectively complexing with circulating digoxin or digitoxin, thereby preventing drug from binding at receptor sites; the complex is then eliminated in urine.

USES Treatment of potentially life-threatening digoxin or digitoxin intoxication in carefully selected patients.

CONTRAINDICATIONS Hypersensitivity to sheep products; renal or cardiac failure. Safe use during pregnancy (category C) or lactation is not established.

CAUTIOUS USE Prior treatment with sheep antibodies or ovine Fab fragments; history of allergies; impaired renal function.

ROUTE & DOSAGE

Serious Digoxin Toxicity Secondary to Overdose

Child/Adult: **IV** Dosages vary according to amount of digoxin to be neutralized; dosages are based on total body load or steady-state serum digoxin concentrations (see package insert); some patients may require a second dose after several hours.
Total body digoxin load (TBL) = serum digoxin level (ng/mL) $\times 5.6 \times$ wt in kg divided by 1000; alternatively TBL = mg digoxin ingested $\times 0.8$
Dose of immune fab in # vials = TBL divided by 0.5

STORAGE

Use reconstituted solutions promptly or refrigerate at 2°–8° C (36°–46° F) for up to 4 h.

ADMINISTRATION

Intravenous

***PREPARE* Direct:** Reconstitute by dissolving 38 mg (1 vial) in 4 mL of sterile water for injection; mix gently (solution will contain 9.5 mg/mL). **IV Infusion:** Dilute further with any volume of NS compatible with cardiac status.

***ADMINISTER* Direct:** Give undiluted bolus only if cardiac arrest is imminent. **IV Infusion:** Give IV infusion over 15–30 min, through a 0.22-micron membrane filter. ■ For administration to infants: Reconstitute for direct IV and administer with a tuberculin syringe. For small doses (e.g., 2 mg or less), dilute the reconstituted 40-mg vial with 36 mL of NS to yield 1 mg/mL. Closely monitor for fluid overload.

ADVERSE EFFECTS Adverse reactions associated with use of digoxin immune Fab are related primarily to the effects of **digitalis** withdrawal on the heart (see Nursing Implications). Allergic reactions have been reported rarely. Hypokalemia.

DIAGNOSTIC TEST INTERFERENCE Digoxin immune Fab may interfere with *serum digoxin* determinations by immunoassay tests.

INTERACTIONS Drug: Not established.

PHARMACOKINETICS Onset: <1 min after IV administration. **Elimination:** Excreted in urine over 5–7 days. **Half-Life:** 14–20 h.

NURSING IMPLICATIONS

Assessment & Drug Effects

- Perform skin testing for allergy prior to administration of immune Fab, particularly in patients with history of allergy or who have had previous therapy with immune Fab.
- Keep emergency equipment and drugs immediately available before skin testing is done or first dose is given and until patient is out of danger.
- Monitor for therapeutic effectiveness: Reflected in improvement in cardiac rhythm abnormalities, mental orientation and other neurologic symptoms, and GI and visual disturbances. S&S of reversal of digitalis toxicity occurs in 15–60 min in adults and usually within minutes in children.
- Baseline and frequent vital signs and EGG during administration.
- Lab tests: Baseline and periodic serum potassium and serum digoxin; serum digoxin or digitoxin concentration (this measurement will not be accurate for at least 5–7 days after therapy begins because of test interference by immune Fab).
- Note: Serum potassium is particularly critical during first several hours following administration of immune Fab. Monitor closely.
- Monitor closely: Cardiac status may deteriorate as inotropic action of digitalis is withdrawn by action of immune Fab. CHF, arrhythmias, increase in heart rate, and hypokalemia can occur.
- Make sure serum digoxin levels and ECG readings are obtained for at least 2–3 wk.

Patient & Family Education

- If digitalis poisoning was a result of inaccurate administration or child poisoning, complete a thorough history and teaching to avoid future problems. Refer to home health care nurse for home visit.
- Do not breast feed while taking this drug without consulting physician.

DIHYDROTACHYSTEROL

(dye-hye-droe-tak-iss'ter-ole)
DHT, DHT Intensol, Hytakerol
Classifications: VITAMIN D; REGULATOR OF SERUM CALCIUM
Pregnancy Category: A

AVAILABILITY 0.125 mg, 0.2 mg, 0.4 mg tablets; 0.2 mg/mL oral solution; 0.125 mg capsules 1 mg = 120,000 international units vitamin D_2

Common adverse effects in *italic;* life-threatening effects underlined; generic names in **bold;** drug classifications in SMALL CAPS; ♣ Canadian drug name; ● Prototype drug.

451

ACTIONS Oil-soluble reduction product of ergocalciferol (vitamin D₂) with pharmacologic actions similar to those of both ergocalciferol and parathyroid hormone. In comparison with ergocalciferol, dihydrotachysterol promotes less intestinal absorption of calcium but almost equal phosphate diuresis.

THERAPEUTIC EFFECTS Acts like parathyroid hormone in ability to raise serum calcium concentrations rapidly; also reported to increase intestinal absorption of sodium, potassium, and magnesium.

USES Hypocalcemia associated with hypoparathyroidism, both postoperative and idiopathic, and in pseudohypoparathyroidism. Also for prophylaxis of hypocalcemic tetany following thyroid surgery.

UNLABELED USES Vitamin D-resistant rickets (familial hypophosphatemia), osteoporosis, and renal osteodystrophy.

CONTRAINDICATIONS Sensitivity to vitamin D; hypercalcemia and hypocalcemia associated with renal insufficiency and hyperphosphatemia; hypervitaminosis D. Safe use during pregnancy (category A), lactation, or in children in amounts exceeding RDA is not established. Pregnancy category changes to D if used in doses above RDA.

CAUTIOUS USE Renal stones, renal failure, heart disease.

ROUTE & DOSAGE

Hypoparathyroidism, Pseudohypoparathyroidism
Neonate: **PO** 0.05–0.1 mg/day
Infant/Child: **PO** 1–5 mg/day for 4 days, then 0.5–1.5 mg/day
Adult: **PO** 0.75–2.5 mg/day for several days, then 0.2–1 mg/day (may need 1.5 mg/day)

Rickets
Child: **PO** 0.5 mg one time *or* 13–50 mcg/day daily until healed

Thyroidectomy-Induced Hypocalcemia
Adult: **PO** 0.25 mg/day

Renal Osteodystrophy
Child: **PO** 0.1–0.5 mg/day
Adult: **PO** 0.1–0.6 mg/day

STORAGE
Store in tightly closed, light-resistant containers at 15°–30° C (59°–86° F) unless otherwise directed.

ADMINISTRATION

Oral
▪ Withhold drug if signs and symptoms of hypercalcemia appear (see Appendix D-1) and report to physician.

ADVERSE EFFECTS Body as a Whole: Hypervitaminosis A **CNS:** Drowsiness, headache, weakness, vertigo, ataxia, atonia, mental depression. **Endocrine:** Hypercalcemia. **GI:** Anorexia, nausea, vomiting, metallic taste, dry mouth, thirst, diarrhea, constipation, abdominal pain. **Urogenital:** Nocturia, polyuria, renal calculi. **Special Senses:** Tinnitus.

INTERACTIONS Drug: Not established.

PHARMACOKINETICS Absorption: Readily absorbed from small intestines. **Peak:** 2 wk. **Duration:** 2 wk. **Distribution:** Distributed in breast milk. **Metabolism:** Metabolized in liver to active metabolite. **Elimination:** Excreted primarily in bile and feces.

D

NURSING IMPLICATIONS

Assessment & Drug Effects

- Lab tests: Serum and urinary calcium levels at least weekly during first month of therapy until they are stabilized, then monthly thereafter.
- Supplement with 10–15 g of oral calcium lactate or gluconate daily; adequate calcium intake is necessary for clinical response to therapy.
- Restrict dietary phosphate or administer calcium carbonate supplements with meals, or both, to bind intestinal phosphates and improve calcium balance in patients with hyperphosphatemia.
- Monitor hypoparathyroid patients receiving thiazide diuretics closely; they are prone to develop hypercalcemia.

Patient & Family Education

- Teach the family to recognize S&S of hypercalcemia (see Appendix D-1).
- Do not breast feed while taking this drug without consulting prescriber.
- Store this medication out of reach of children.

DILTIAZEM

(dil-tye′a-zem)
Cardizem, Cardizem CD, Cardizem LA, Cardizem SR, Cardizem Lyo-Ject, Cartia XT Dilacor XR, Tiamate, Tiazac, Taztia XT

DILTIAZEM IV

Cardizem IV
Classifications: CARDIOVASCULAR AGENT; CALCIUM CHANNEL BLOCKING AGENT; ANTIHYPERTENSIVE
Prototype: Verapamil
Pregnancy Category: C

AVAILABILITY 30 mg, 60 mg, 90 mg, 120 mg tablets; 120 mg, 180 mg, 240 mg sustained-release tablets; 60 mg, 90 mg, 120 mg, 180 mg, 240 mg, 300 mg, 360 mg sustained-release capsules; 120 mg, 180 mg, 240 mg, 300 mg, 360 mg, 420 mg extended-release tablets; 25 mg, 50 mg vials

ACTIONS Slow channel blocker with pharmacologic actions similar to those of verapamil. Inhibits calcium ion influx through slow channels into cell of myocardial and arterial smooth muscle (both coronary and peripheral blood vessels). As a result, intracellular calcium remains at subthreshold levels insufficient to stimulate cell excitation and contraction. Slows SA and AV node conduction (antiarrhythmic effect) without affecting normal arterial action potential or intraventricular conduction.

Common adverse effects in *italic;* life-threatening effects <u>underlined;</u> generic names in **bold;** drug classifications in SMALL CAPS; ♣ Canadian drug name; ❂ Prototype drug.

453

D

THERAPEUTIC EFFECTS Dilates coronary arteries and arterioles and inhibits coronary artery spasm; thus myocardial oxygen delivery is increased (antianginal effect). By vasodilation of peripheral arterioles drug decreases total peripheral vascular resistance and reduces arterial BP at rest (antihypertensive effect).

USES Vasospastic angina (Prinzmetal's variant or at rest angina), chronic stable (classic effort-associated) angina, essential hypertension. **IV form:** Atrial fibrillation, atrial flutter, supraventricular tachycardia.
UNLABELED USES Prevention of reinfarction in non-Q-wave MI.

CONTRAINDICATIONS Known hypersensitivity to drug; sick sinus syndrome (unless pacemaker is in place and functioning); second- or third-degree AV block; severe hypotension (systolic <90 mm Hg or diastolic <60 mm Hg); patients undergoing intracranial surgery; bleeding aneurysms. Safe use during pregnancy (category C), lactation, or in children is not established.
CAUTIOUS USE CHF (especially if patient is also receiving beta-blocker), conduction abnormalities; renal or hepatic impairment; older adults.

ROUTE & DOSAGE

Child: **PO** 1.5–2 mg/kg/day divided into doses given t.i.d. or q.i.d. (max 3.5 mg/kg/day)
Adolescent: **PO** immediate release: 30–120 mg/dose with doses t.i.d. or q.i.d. (usual range: 180–360 mg/day); extended release: 120–300 mg/day given in 1 dose for Cardizem CD, Dilacor XR, Tiazac, and given in 2 doses for Cardizem SR
Adult: **PO** 60–120 mg sustained-release b.i.d. (usual range: 240–360 mg/day). Cardizem LA 120–360 mg at bedtime (max 540 mg/day)

STORAGE
Store at 15°–30° C (59°–86° F).

ADMINISTRATION

Oral

- Do not crush sustained-release capsules or tablets. They must be swallowed whole.
- Withhold if systolic BP is <90 mm Hg or diastolic is <60 mm Hg.
- Give before meals and at bedtime.

Intravenous

PREPARE **Direct:** Give undiluted. **Continuous:** For IV infusion, add to a volume of D5W, NS, or D5/0.45% NaCl that can be administered in 24 h or less.
ADMINISTER **Direct:** Give as a bolus dose over 2 min. A second bolus may be given after 15 min. **Continuous:** Give at a rate 5–15 mg/h. Infusion duration longer than 24 h and infusion rate >15 mg/h are not recommended.
INCOMPATIBILITIES **Solution/Additive: Furosemide. Y-Site: Furosemide.**

Common adverse effects in *italic;* life-threatening effects underlined; generic names in **bold**; drug classifications in SMALL CAPS; ♣ Canadian drug name; ❷ Prototype drug.

ADVERSE EFFECTS CNS: *Headache,* fatigue, dizziness, asthenia, drowsiness, nervousness, insomnia, confusion, tremor, gait abnormality. **CV:** Edema, arrhythmias, angina, second- or third-degree AV block, bradycardia, CHF, flushing, hypotension, syncope, palpitations. **GI:** Nausea, constipation, anorexia, vomiting, diarrhea, impaired taste, weight increase. **Skin:** Rash.

INTERACTIONS Drug: BETA-BLOCKERS, **digoxin** may have additive effects on AV node conduction prolongation; may increase **digoxin** or **quinidine** levels; **cimetidine** may increase diltiazem levels, thus increasing effects; may increase **benzodiazepines, beta-blockers, carbamazepine, cyclosporine, fentanyl** levels.

PHARMACOKINETICS Absorption: Approximately 80% absorbed from GI tract, with 40% reaching systemic circulation. **Peak:** 2–3 h; 6–11 h sustained release; 11–18 h Cardizem LA. **Distribution:** Distributed into breast milk. **Metabolism:** Metabolized in liver. **Elimination:** Excreted primarily in urine with some elimination in feces. **Half-Life:** 3.5–9 h PO; 2 h IV.

NURSING IMPLICATIONS

Assessment & Drug Effects
- Check BP and ECG before initiation of therapy and monitor particularly during dosage adjustment period.
- Lab tests: Do baseline and periodic liver and renal function tests.
- Monitor for and report S&S of CHF.
- Monitor for headache. An analgesic may be required.
- Supervise ambulation as indicated.

Patient & Family Education
- Make position changes slowly and in stages; light-headedness and dizziness (hypotension) are possible.
- Do not drive or engage in other potentially hazardous activities until reaction to drug is known.
- Keep follow-up appointments and prescriber informed.
- Do not breast feed while taking this drug without consulting prescriber.
- Store this medication out of reach of children.

DIMENHYDRINATE
(dye-men-hye′dri-nate)
Apo-Dimenhydrinate ♦, Calm-X, Dimenhydrinate Injection, Dimentabs, Dinate, Dommanate, Dramanate, Dramamine, Dramilin, Dramocen, Dramoject, Dymenate, Gravol ♦, Hydrate, Marmine, Motion-Aid, Nauseatol ♦, Novodimenate ♦, PMS Dimenhydrinate ♦, Travamine ♦, Travel Aid, Travel Eze, Wehamine
Classifications: ANTIHISTAMINE (H₁-RECEPTOR ANTAGONIST); ANTIEMETIC; ANTIVERTIGO AGENT
Prototype: Diphenhydramine
Pregnancy Category: B

D

AVAILABILITY 50 mg tablets; 50 mg/mL injection; 15.62 mg/5 mL, 12.5 mg/4 mL, 12.5 mg/5 mL liquid

ACTIONS H_1-receptor antagonist and salt of diphenhydramine, with which it shares similar properties.
THERAPEUTIC EFFECTS Precise mode of antinauseant action not known, but thought to involve ability to inhibit cholinergic stimulation in vestibular and associated neural pathways.

USES Chiefly in prevention and treatment of motion sickness. Also has been used in management of vertigo, nausea, and vomiting associated with radiation sickness, labyrinthitis, Ménière's syndrome, stapedectomy, anesthesia, and various medications.

CONTRAINDICATIONS Narrow-angle glaucoma, vomiting of unknown origin. Safe use during pregnancy (category B), lactation, or in children <2 y is not established.
CAUTIOUS USE Convulsive disorders, when taken with ototoxic agents or in history of seizures.

ROUTE & DOSAGE

Motion Sickness

Child: **PO/IM/IV** *2–12 y,* 5 mg/kg/day divided into doses q6h (max PO doses 2–5 y: 75 mg/day; 6–12 y: 150 mg/day)
Adult: **PO** 50–100 mg q4–6h (max 400 mg/24 h) **IV/IM** 50 mg as needed

STORAGE
Store preferably at 15°–30° C (59°–86° F), unless otherwise directed by manufacturer. Examine parenteral preparation for particulate matter and discoloration. Do not use unless absolutely clear.

ADMINISTRATION
Note: Give 30–60 min before treatment, then repeat 90 min after treatment, and again in 3 h to prevent radiation sickness.

Intramuscular
- Give undiluted and inject deep IM into a large muscle mass appropriate for age. (see Part I)

Intravenous

PREPARE **Direct:** Dilute each 50 mg in 10 mL of NS.
ADMINISTER **Direct:** Give each 50 mg or fraction thereof over 2 min.
INCOMPATIBILITIES **Solution/Additive: Aminophylline, amobarbital, butorphanol, chlorpromazine, glycopyrrolate, hydroxyzine, midazolam, pentobarbital, prochlorperazine, promazine, promethazine, thiopental.**

ADVERSE EFFECTS CNS: *Drowsiness,* headache, incoordination, dizziness, blurred vision, nervousness, restlessness, *insomnia (especially children).* **CV:** Hypotension, palpitation. **GI:** Dry mouth, nose, throat; anorexia, constipation or diarrhea. **Urogenital:** Urinary frequency, dysuria.

DIAGNOSTIC TEST INTERFERENCE *Skin testing* procedures should not be performed within 72 h after use of an antihistamine.

INTERACTIONS Drug: Alcohol and other CNS depressants enhance CNS depression, drowsiness; TRICYCLIC ANTIDEPRESSANTS compound anticholinergic effects.

PHARMACOKINETICS Absorption: Readily absorbed from GI tract. **Onset:** 15–30 min PO; immediate IV; 20–30 min IM. **Duration:** 3–6 h. **Distribution:** Distributed into breast milk. **Elimination:** Excreted in urine.

NURSING IMPLICATIONS

Assessment & Drug Effects

- Use side rails and supervise ambulation; drug produces high incidence of drowsiness.
- Note: Tolerance to CNS depressant effects usually occurs after a few days of drug therapy; some decrease in antiemetic action may result with prolonged use.
- Monitor for dizziness, nausea, and vomiting; these may indicate drug toxicity.
- Drug is used with caution in those with seizures or taking ototoxic drugs. Monitor carefully for these adverse effects.

Patient & Family Education

- Do not drive or engage in other potentially hazardous activities until response to drug is known.
- Take 30 min before departure to prevent motion sickness; repeat before meals and upon retiring.
- Do not breast feed while taking this drug without consulting prescriber.
- Store this medication out of reach of children.

DIMERCAPROL
(dye-mer-kap′role)
BAL in Oil, British Anti-Lewisite
Classifications: CHELATING AGENT; ANTIDOTE
Pregnancy Category: D

AVAILABILITY 100 mg/mL injection

ACTIONS Dithiol compound that combines with ions of various heavy metals to form relatively stable, nontoxic, soluble complexes called chelates, which can be excreted; inhibition of enzymes by toxic metals is thus prevented. May also reactivate affected enzymes but is most effective when administered prior to enzyme damage.
THERAPEUTIC EFFECTS Neutralizes the effects of various heavy metals.

USES Acute poisoning by arsenic, gold, and mercury; as adjunct to edetate calcium disodium (EDTA) in treatment of lead encephalopathy.

UNLABELED USES Chromium dermatitis; ocular and dermatologic manifestations of arsenic poisoning, as adjunct to penicillamine to increase rate of copper excretion in Wilson's disease, and for poisoning with antimony, bismuth, chromium, copper, nickel, tungsten, zinc.

CONTRAINDICATIONS Hepatic insufficiency (with exception of postarsenical jaundice); severe renal insufficiency; poisoning due to cadmium, iron, selenium, or uranium; pregnancy (category D), lactation.
CAUTIOUS USE Hypertension, patients with G6PD deficiency.

ROUTE & DOSAGE

Arsenic or Gold Poisoning
Child/Adult: **IM** 2.5–3 mg/kg/dose q6h for first 2 days, then q12h on third day, then daily for 10 days

Mercury Poisoning
Child/Adult: **IM** 5 mg/kg initially, followed by 2.5 mg/kg 1–2 times/day for 10 days

Acute Lead Encephalopathy
Child/Adult: **IM** 4 mg/kg initially, then 3–4 mg/kg q4h with EDTA for 2–7 days depending on response

STORAGE
Store at room temperature of 15°–30° C (59°–86° F). Injection is yellow and viscous with pungent odor. Turbid solution with some visible sediment is not indicative of deterioration.

ADMINISTRATION

Intramuscular

- Initiate therapy ASAP (within 1–2 h) after ingestion of the poison because irreversible tissue damage occurs quickly, particularly in mercury poisoning.
- Give by deep IM injection only in sites appropriate for age of child (see Part I). Local pain, muscle abscess, and skin sensitization possible at injection site. Rotate injection sites and observe daily.
- Determine if a local anesthetic may be given with the injection to decrease injection site pain.
- Handle with caution; contact of drug with skin may produce erythema, edema, dermatitis.
- Note: Presence of sediment in ampule reportedly does not indicate drug deterioration.

ADVERSE EFFECTS CNS: Headache, anxiety, muscle pain or weakness, restlessness, paresthesias, tremors, *convulsions,* shock. **CV:** *Elevated BP,* tachycardia. **Special Sense:** Rhinorrhea; burning sensation, feeling of pain and constriction in throat. **GI:** Nausea, *vomiting;* burning sensation in lips and mouth, halitosis, salivation; abdominal pain, metabolic acidosis. **Urogenital:** Burning sensation in penis, renal damage. **Other:** Pains in chest or hands, pain and sterile abscess at injection site, transient leucopenia, sweating, reduction in polymorphonuclear leukocytes, dental pain.

DIAGNOSTIC TEST INTERFERENCE *I-131 thyroid uptake* values may be decreased if test is done during or immediately following dimercaprol therapy.

D

INTERACTIONS Drug: Iron, cadmium, selenium, uranium form toxic complexes with dimercaprol.

PHARMACOKINETICS Peak: 30–60 min. **Distribution:** Distributed mainly in intracellular spaces, including brain; highest concentrations in liver and kidneys. **Elimination:** Completely excreted in urine and bile within 4 h. **Half-Life:** Short.

NURSING IMPLICATIONS

Assessment & Drug Effects
- Administered with Ca-EDTA in treatment of lead poisoning.
- Monitor vital signs. Elevations of systolic and diastolic BPs accompanied by tachycardia frequently occur within a few minutes following injection and may remain elevated up to 2 h.
- Note: Fever occurs in approximately 30% of children receiving treatment and may persist throughout therapy.
- Monitor I&O. Drug is potentially nephrotoxic. Report oliguria or change in I&O ratio to physician.
- Keep urine alkaline to reduce possibility of renal damage during elimination of dimercaprol chelate.
- Check urine daily for albumin, blood, casts, and pH. Blood and urinary levels of the metal serve as guides for dosage adjustments.
- Minor adverse reactions generally reach maximum 15–20 min after drug administration and subside in 30–90 min. Ephedrine or an antihistamine is sometimes administered to prevent symptoms.

Patient & Family Education
- Drink as much fluid as prescribed.
- Instruct in safety precautions to prevent future poisonings.
- Do not breast feed while taking this drug without consulting physician.

DIPHENHYDRAMINE HYDROCHLORIDE
(dye-fen-hye′dra-meen)
Allerdryl ♣ , Banophen, Belix, Ben-Allergin, Bena-D, Benadryl, Benadryl Dye-Free, Benahist, Benoject, Benylin, Compoz, Diahist, Dihydrex, Diphen, Diphenacen-50, Fenylhist, Hyrexin, Insomnal, Nordryl, Nytol with DPH, Sleep-Eze 3, Sominex Formula 2, Tusstat, Twilite, Valdrene, Wehdryl
Classifications: ANTIHISTAMINE; H₁-RECEPTOR ANTAGONIST
Pregnancy Category: C

AVAILABILITY 25 mg, 50 mg capsules, tablets; 6.25 mg/5 mL, 12.5 mg/5 mL syrup; 50 mg/mL injection

ACTIONS H_1-receptor antagonist and antihistamine with significant anticholinergic activity. High incidence of drowsiness, but GI side effects are minor.

THERAPEUTIC EFFECTS Competes for H_1-receptor sites on effector cells, thus blocking histamine release.

USES Temporary symptomatic relief of various allergic conditions and to treat or prevent motion sickness, vertigo, and reactions to blood or plasma in susceptible patients. Also used in anaphylaxis as adjunct to epinephrine and other standard measures after acute symptoms have been controlled; in treatment of parkinsonism and drug-induced extrapyramidal reactions; as a nonnarcotic cough suppressant; as a sedative-hypnotic; and for treatment of intractable insomnia.

CONTRAINDICATIONS Hypersensitivity to antihistamines of similar structure; lower respiratory tract symptoms (including acute asthma); narrow-angle glaucoma; prostatic hypertrophy, bladder neck obstruction; GI obstruction or stenosis; pregnancy (category C), lactation, premature neonates, and neonates; use as nighttime sleep aid in children <12 y.

CAUTIOUS USE History of asthma; convulsive disorders; increased IOP; hyperthyroidism; hypertension, cardiovascular disease; diabetes mellitus; older adults, infants, and young children.

ROUTE & DOSAGE

Child: **PO/IV/IM** 0.5–1 mg/kg/dose given q6h
Adult: **PO/IM/IV** 10–50 mg t.i.d. or q.i.d. (max 400 mg/day)

STORAGE
Store in tightly covered containers at 15°–30° C (59°–86° F) unless otherwise directed by manufacturer. Keep injection and elixir formulations in light-resistant containers.

ADMINISTRATION
Oral
- Give with food or milk to reduce GI adverse effects.
- For motion sickness: Give the first dose 30 min before exposure to motion; give remaining doses before meals and at bedtime.

Intramuscular
- Give IM injection deep into large muscle mass appropriate for age (see Part I); alternate injection sites. Avoid perivascular or SC injections because of its irritating effects.
- Note: Hypersensitivity reactions (including anaphylactic shock) are more likely to occur with parenteral than PO administration.

Intravenous

PREPARE **Direct:** Give undiluted.
ADMINISTER **Direct:** Give at a rate of 25 mg or a fraction thereof over 1 min.
INCOMPATIBILITY **Y-Site: Furosemide.**

D

ADVERSE EFFECTS CNS: *Drowsiness,* dizziness, headache, fatigue, disturbed coordination, tingling, heaviness and weakness of hands, tremors, euphoria, nervousness, restlessness, insomnia; confusion; (especially in children): excitement, fever. **CV:** Palpitation, *tachycardia,* mild hypotension or hypertension, <u>cardiovascular collapse</u>. **Special Senses:** Tinnitus, vertigo, dry nose, throat, nasal stuffiness; blurred vision, diplopia, photosensitivity, dry eyes. **GI:** *Dry mouth,* nausea, epigastric distress, anorexia, vomiting, constipation, or diarrhea. **Urogenital:** Urinary frequency or retention, dysuria. **Body as a Whole:** Hypersensitivity (skin rash, urticaria, photosensitivity, <u>anaphylactic shock</u>). **Respiratory:** Thickened bronchial secretions, wheezing, sensation of chest tightness.

DIAGNOSTIC TEST INTERFERENCE In common with other antihistamines, diphenhydramine should be discontinued 4 days prior to ***skin testing*** procedures for allergy because it may obscure otherwise positive reactions.

INTERACTIONS Drug: Alcohol and other CNS DEPRESSANTS, MAO INHIBITORS compound CNS depression.

PHARMACOKINETICS Absorption: Readily absorbed from GI tract but only 40–60% reaches systemic circulation. **Onset:** 15–30 min. **Peak:** 1–4 h. **Duration:** 4–7 h. **Distribution:** Crosses placenta; distributed into breast milk. **Metabolism:** Metabolized in liver; some degradation in lung and kidney. **Elimination:** Mostly excreted in urine within 24 h.

NURSING IMPLICATIONS

Assessment & Drug Effects
- Monitor cardiovascular status especially with preexisting cardiovascular disease.
- Monitor for adverse effects especially in young children.
- Supervise ambulation and use side rails as necessary. Drowsiness is most prominent during the first few days of therapy and often disappears with continued therapy.

Patient & Family Education
- Report excess drowsiness or excitement in the child.
- Do not use alcohol and other CNS depressants because of the possible additive CNS depressant effects with concurrent use.
- Do not drive or engage in other potentially hazardous activities until the response to drug is known.
- Increase fluid intake, if not contraindicated; drug has an atropine like drying effect (thickens bronchial secretions) that may make expectoration difficult.
- Do not breast feed while taking this drug.
- Store this medication out of reach of children.

DIPHENOXYLATE HYDROCHLORIDE WITH ATROPINE SULFATE
(dye-fen-ox′i-late)
Diphenatol, Lofene, Lomanate, Lomotil, Lonox, Lo-Trol, Low-Quel, Nor-Mil
Classifications: GASTROINTESTINAL AGENT; ANTIDIARRHEAL
Pregnancy Category: C
Controlled Substance: Schedule V

AVAILABILITY 2.5 mg tablets; 2.5 mg/5 mL liquid

ACTIONS Diphenoxylate is a synthetic narcotic structurally related to meperidine. Commercially available only with atropine sulfate, added in subtherapeutic doses to discourage deliberate overdosage.
THERAPEUTIC EFFECTS Has little or no analgesic activity or risk of dependence, except in high doses. Inhibits mucosal receptors responsible for peristaltic reflex, thereby reducing GI motility.

USES Adjunct in symptomatic management of diarrhea.

CONTRAINDICATIONS Hypersensitivity to diphenoxylate or atropine; severe dehydration or electrolyte imbalance, advanced liver disease, obstructive jaundice, diarrhea caused by pseudomembranous enterocolitis associated with use of broad-spectrum antibiotics; diarrhea associated with organisms that penetrate intestinal mucosa; diarrhea induced by poisons until toxic material is eliminated from GI tract; glaucoma; children <2 y of age. Safe use during pregnancy (category C) or lactation is not established.
CAUTIOUS USE Advanced hepatic disease, abnormal liver function tests; renal function impairment, patients receiving addicting drugs, addiction-prone individuals or those whose history suggests drug abuse; ulcerative colitis; young children (particularly patients with Down syndrome).

ROUTE & DOSAGE

Diarrhea
Child: **PO** 2–12 y, 0.3–0.4 mg/kg/day of liquid in divided doses
Adult: **PO** 1–2 tablets or 1–2 teaspoons full (5 mL) 3–4 times/day (each tablet or 5 mL contains 2.5 mg diphenoxylate HCl and 0.025 mg atropine sulfate)

STORAGE
Store in tightly covered, light-resistant container, preferably 15°–30° C (59°–86° F), unless otherwise directed by manufacturer.

ADMINISTRATION
Oral
- Crush tablet if necessary and give with fluid of patient's choice.

- Reduce dosage as soon as initial control of symptoms occurs.
- Withhold drug in presence of severe dehydration or electrolyte imbalance until appropriate corrective therapy has been initiated.
- Note: Treatment is generally continued for 24–36 h before it is considered ineffective.

D

ADVERSE EFFECTS Body as a Whole: Hypersensitivity (pruritus, angioneurotic edema, giant urticaria, rash). **CNS:** Headache, sedation, drowsiness, dizziness, lethargy, numbness of extremities; restlessness, euphoria, mental depression, weakness, general malaise. **CV:** Flushing, palpitation, tachycardia. **Special Senses:** Nystagmus, mydriasis, blurred vision, miosis (toxicity). **GI:** Nausea, vomiting, anorexia, dry mouth, abdominal discomfort or distention, paralytic ileus, toxic megacolon. **Other:** Urinary retention, swelling of gums.

INTERACTIONS Drug: MAO INHIBITORS may precipitate hypertensive crisis; **alcohol** and other CNS DEPRESSANTS may enhance CNS effects; also see **atropine.**

PHARMACOKINETICS Absorption: Readily absorbed from GI tract. **Onset:** 45–60 min. **Peak:** 2 h. **Duration:** 3–4 h. **Distribution:** Distributed into breast milk. **Metabolism:** Rapidly metabolized to active and inactive metabolites in liver. **Elimination:** Excreted slowly through bile into feces; small amount excreted in urine. **Half-Life:** 4.4 h.

NURSING IMPLICATIONS

Assessment & Drug Effects

- Antidiarrheals are not recommended for patients whose diarrhea may be due to *Salmonella, Shigella, E. coli,* or pseudomembranous enterocolitis.
- Assess GI function; report abdominal distention and signs of decreased peristalsis.
- Monitor for S&S of dehydration (see Appendix D-1). It is essential to monitor young children closely; dehydration occurs more rapidly in this age group and may influence variability of response to diphenoxylate and predispose patient to delayed toxic effects.
- Monitor frequency and consistency of stools.

Patient & Family Education

- Take medication only as directed by prescriber.
- Notify prescriber if diarrhea persists or if fever, bloody stools, palpitation, or other adverse reactions occur.
- Do not drive or engage in other potentially hazardous activities until response to drug is known.
- Do not breast feed while taking this drug without consulting prescriber.
- Store this medication out of reach of children.

DIPHTHERIA AND TETANUS TOXOIDS AND ACCELULAR PERTUSSIS VACCINE (DTaP)
DIPHTHERIA AND TETANUS TOXOIDS (DT) (for pediatric use)
TETANUS AND DIPHTHERIA TOXOIDS (Td)(for adult use)
TETANUS TOXOID

Tripedia, Daptacel, Infanrix for DTaP

Classifications: ANTI-INFECTIVE, VACCINE
Pregnancy Category: X for DTaP

AVAILABILITY 0.5 mL single-dose vials; 7.5 mL multiple-dose vials
Combination Products: Pediarix (with hepatitis B and inactivated poliovirus); TriHIBit (with Haemophilus b vaccine)

ACTIONS Stimulates body production of antibodies and antitoxins against the organisms and exotoxins causing diphtheria, tetanus, and pertussis.
THERAPEUTIC EFFECTS The recommended 5-dose regimen for infants or 3-dose for older children provides protection against the diseases identified.

USES Used to provide active immunity in infants and young children under 7 years (DTaP or DT), children over 7 years and adults (Td).

CONTRAINDICATIONS Encephalopathy within 7 days of a prior dose of DTaP, DT, or Td; anaphylactic reaction to prior dose; hypersensitivity to any ingredient in formulation such as thimerosal and gelatin; severe acute illness.
CAUTIOUS USE Safety and efficacy not established under 6 mo. All of the following cautions refer to the pertussis component of the vaccine: Temperature of 40.5° C (105° F), collapse, shock, persistent and severe inconcolable crying within 48 h of a previous dose; family history of seizures; seizure within 3 days of a previous dose; presence of a condition that predisposes to seizures; progressive neurologic disorders with developmental delay or neurologic findings (defer immunization with pertussis for latter condition)

ROUTE & DOSAGE

DTaP or DT: **IM** 0.5 mL at ages 2, 4, 6, 15–18 mo and 4–6 y
Td: **IM** 0.5 mL booster dose every 10 y

STORAGE
Keep refrigerated at 2°-8° C (36°–45° F); do not freeze.

ADMINISTRATION
IM
- Shake vial well before drawing up; solution will be cloudy.
- To be given IM to infants in lateral thigh muscle.
- Use needle at least 7/8 to 1 inch for normal sized babies ages 4 mo and older in order to reach muscle mass.

- May be given in deltoid for ages 4–6 y and older.
- Schedule varies for immune compromised children and those not immunized in infancy; see Appendix H-1 and H-2.
- If a child <7 y cannot receive the pertussis component, give diphtheria and tetanus (for pediatric use) instead. For children >7 y, tetanus and diphtheria combination (for adult use) is given.
- After the initial series, a booster dose of tetanus and diphtheria is recommended every 10 y. If a wound occurs before that time and it might be contaminated with tetanus, reimmunization with Td should be given if more than 5 y have elapsed since the last dose. More frequent dosing increases incidence of side effects. Always give tetanus and diphtheria (Td) in combination (rather than tetanus toxoid alone) unless there is a prior reaction or contraindication because diphtheria can be a serious disease also.
- When both active and passive immunity are needed (such as in exposure to tetanus disease when immunization status is not up to date), DTaP or other appropriate immunization is given for active immunity at the same time as tetanus immune globulin for passive immunity at different sites.
- May be given at same time as other childhood immunizations with a different site for each IM administered.

ADVERSE EFFECTS Body as a Whole: Mild to moderate fever (fever above 40° C (105° F) is rare), irritability. **GI:** Diarrhea, vomiting, anorexia. **Skin:** Pain, tenderness, erythema. **Neurologic:** Seizures, hypotonia, hyporesponsiveness; unconsolable crying (all rare); these side effects are related to only the pertussis portion of the immunization.

INTERACTIONS Efficacy of vaccine may be reduced when child is immunosuppressed.

PHARMACOKINETICS Primary immunization with 3 doses provides protection for diseases in 70–90% of children; additional doses ensure most children are adequately immune. Immunity to diphtheria and tetanus lasts about 10 y, immunity to pertussis lasts 4–6 y.

NURSING IMPLICATIONS

Assessment & Drug Effects
- Take careful history to rule out contraindications or precautions. Instruct parents about risks and benefits of immunization. Teach side effects and to seek care immediately for those that are rare and serious (high temperature, unconsolable crying, seizures, hypotonia).
- Obtain written parental consent for immunization.
- Teach comfort measures (acetaminophen, cool compress to injection site) for mild side effects.
- Provide information about clinics and other resources to receive immunizations.
- Keep epinephrine 1:1000 and doses for children available whenever giving immunizations.

Patient and Family Education

- Return as instructed for next immunization in the series. When the child receives last dose at 4–6 y, the next dose will be tetanus and diphtheria toxoids (Td) in 10 y unless injury requiring tetanus immunization occurs earlier.
- Keep careful records of all the child's immunizations; they will be needed for entry to school.
- If no additional doses are received due to injury, tetanus and diphtheria booster should be given at ages 15 y, 25 y, 35 y, etc.

DIPYRIDAMOLE

(dye-peer-id′a-mole)

Apo-Dipyridamole ♣ , Persantine, Pyridamole, IV Persantine

Classifications: BLOOD FORMERS, COAGULATORS, AND ANTICOAGULANTS; ANTIPLATELET AGENT

Prototype: Ticlopidine

Pregnancy Category: C

AVAILABILITY 25 mg, 50 mg, 75 mg tablets; 10 mg injection

ACTIONS Nonnitrate coronary vasodilator with many properties similar to those of papaverine.

THERAPEUTIC EFFECTS Increases coronary blood flow by selectively dilating coronary arteries, thereby increasing myocardial oxygen supply. Exhibits mild inotropic action. Also has antiplatelet activity.

USES To prevent postoperative thromboembolic complications associated with prosthetic heart valves and as adjunct for thallium stress testing.

UNLABELED USES In adults, to reduce rate of reinfarction following MI; to prevent TIAs (transient ischemic attacks) and coronary bypass graft occlusion.

CONTRAINDICATIONS Pregnancy (category C), lactation.

CAUTIOUS USE Hypotension, anticoagulant therapy.

ROUTE & DOSAGE

Prevention of Thromboembolism in Cardiac Valve Replacement

Child: **PO** 1–2 mg t.i.d.
Adult: **PO** 75–100 mg q.i.d.

STORAGE

Store in tightly closed container at 15°–30° C (59°–86° F) unless otherwise directed. Protect injection from direct light.

ADMINISTRATION

Oral

- Give on an empty stomach at least 1 h before or 2 h after meals, with a full glass of water or amount appropriate for age group. Physician may prescribe with food if gastric distress persists.

Intravenous

PREPARE **Direct:** Dilute to at least a 1:2 ratio with 0.45% NaCl, NS, or D5W to yield a final volume of 20–50 mL.
ADMINISTER **Direct:** Give a single dose over 4 min (0.142 mg kg/min).

D

ADVERSE EFFECTS Usually dose related, minimal, and transient. **CNS:** Headache, dizziness, faintness, syncope, weakness. **CV:** Peripheral vasodilation, flushing. **GI:** Nausea, vomiting, diarrhea, abdominal distress. **Skin:** Skin rash, pruritus.

PHARMACOKINETICS Absorption: Readily absorbed from GI tract. **Peak:** 45–150 min. **Distribution:** Small amount crosses placenta. **Metabolism:** Metabolized in liver. **Elimination:** Mainly excreted in feces. **Half-Life:** 10–12 h.

NURSING IMPLICATIONS

Assessment & Drug Effects

- Monitor therapeutic effectiveness.
- Careful assessment of cardiovascular status and vital signs is needed.

Patient & Family Education

- Notify physician of any adverse effects.
- Make all position changes slowly and in stages, especially from recumbent to upright posture, if postural hypotension or dizziness is a problem.
- Do not breast feed while taking this drug without consulting physician.
- Store this medication out of reach of children.

DIRITHROMYCIN

(dir-ith-roe-my′sin)
Dynabac
Classifications: ANTI-INFECTIVE; MACROLIDE ANTIBIOTIC
Prototype: Erythromycin
Pregnancy Category: C

AVAILABILITY 250 mg enteric tablets

ACTIONS Dirithromycin is an analog of erythromycin. It binds reversibly to the 235 component of the 50-S ribosomal subunit of the bacteria, thus inhibiting RNA-dependent protein synthesis in bacterial cells.
THERAPEUTIC EFFECTS It is more active against gram-positive organisms than gram-negative organisms, including *Legionella, Helicobacter pylori*, and *Chlamydia trachomatis*. It is not effective against *Pseudomonas* or methicillin-resistant *Staphylococcus aureus (MRSA), S. epidermidis, Listeria monocytogenes, Legionella pneumophila, Haemophilus influenzae,* or *Neisseria gonorrhoeae*.

USES Acute bacterial exacerbations of chronic bronchitis, community-acquired pneumonia, pharyngitis/tonsillitis, uncomplicated skin/skin structure infections due to susceptible bacteria.

D

CONTRAINDICATIONS Known hypersensitivity to dirithromycin, erythromycin, or any other macrolide antibiotic; known or suspected bacteremias.

CAUTIOUS USE Concurrent administration of terfenadine, hepatic impairment, pregnancy (category C). Safety and effectiveness in lactation or children <12 y are not established.

ROUTE & DOSAGE

Bacterial Infections
Child/Adult: >12 y: **PO** 500 mg daily

STORAGE
Store at 15°–30° C (59°–86° F).

ADMINISTRATION

Oral
- Give with food or within 1 h of eating.
- Do not cut, crush, or chew tablets.

ADVERSE EFFECTS CNS: Headache, dizziness, asthenia. **CV:** Chest pain. **GI:** *Abdominal pain, nausea, diarrhea, vomiting, dyspepsia, flatulence;* elevated liver function tests (ALT, AST, GGT). **Skin:** Rash, urticaria. **Respiratory:** Dyspnea, asthma-like symptoms, rhinitis, pharyngitis, increased coughing.

INTERACTIONS Drug: May increase **theophylline** levels. May increase risk of arrhythmias with **terfenadine.**

PHARMACOKINETICS Absorption: Readily absorbed from GI tract; 60–90% hydrolyzed to active metabolite, erythromycylamine, within 35 min. **Peak:** 1.5 h. **Distribution:** High tissue concentrations of active metabolite; slowly released back into the circulation. **Metabolism:** Rapidly converted to active metabolite, erythromycylamine, in absorption and distribution phases. **Elimination:** 81–97% excreted in bile and feces. **Half-Life:** 20–50 h.

NURSING IMPLICATIONS

Assessment & Drug Effects
- Take history of previous hypersensitivity to other macrolides (e.g., erythromycin) prior to initiation of therapy.
- Withhold drug and notify physician if S&S of hypersensitivity occur (see Appendix D-1).
- Monitor liver and renal function in patients with mild liver or renal impairment.
- Monitor for S&S of superinfection (see Appendix D-1).
- Monitor theophylline levels if given concurrently with dirithromycin.
- Note: Dirithromycin may increase the blood level of theophylline, necessitating theophylline dosage adjustment.

Patient & Family Education

- Take tablets whole and within 1 h of meals.
- Monitor for and report S&S of superinfection or pseudomembranous enterocolitis (see Appendix D-1).
- Report any worsening of signs and symptoms of infection.
- Do not breast feed while taking this drug without consulting prescriber.
- Store this medication out of reach of children.

DISOPYRAMIDE PHOSPHATE

(dye-soe-peer'a-mide)
Napamide, Norpace, Norpace CR, Rythmodan ♣ , Rythmodan-LA ♣
Classifications: CARDIOVASCULAR AGENT; ANTIARRHYTHMIC, CLASS IA
Prototype: Procainamide
Pregnancy Category: C

AVAILABILITY 100 mg, 150 mg regular and sustained-release capsules

ACTIONS Class IA antiarrhythmic agent with pharmacologic actions similar to those of quinidine and procainamide, although chemically unrelated. Disopyramide shortens sinus node recovery time and increases atrial and ventricular effective refractory period but has minimal effect on refractoriness and conduction time of AV node or on conduction time of His-Purkinje system or QRS duration.
THERAPEUTIC EFFECTS Acts as myocardial depressant by reducing rate of spontaneous diastolic depolarization in pacemaker cells, thereby suppressing ectopic focal activity.

USES To suppress and prevent recurrence of premature ventricular contractions (unifocal, multifocal, paired) and ventricular tachycardia not severe enough to require cardioversion.
UNLABELED USES In combination with other antiarrhythmic drugs to treat or prevent serious refractory arrhythmias. To convert atrial fibrillation, atrial flutter, and paroxysmal atrial tachycardia to normal sinus rhythm.

CONTRAINDICATIONS Cardiogenic shock, preexisting second- or third-degree AV block (if no pacemaker is present); uncompensated or inadequately compensated CHF, hypotension (unless secondary to cardiac arrhythmia), hypokalemia. Safe use during pregnancy (category C), lactation, or in children is not established.
CAUTIOUS USE Sick sinus syndrome (bradycardia-tachycardia); Wolff-Parkinson-White (WPW) syndrome or bundle branch block, myocarditis or other cardiomyopathy, underlying cardiac conduction abnormalities; hepatic or renal impairment; urinary tract disease (especially prostatic hypertrophy); myasthenia gravis; narrow-angle glaucoma, family history of glaucoma.

Common adverse effects in *italic;* life-threatening effects underlined; generic names in **bold;** drug classifications in SMALL CAPS; ♣ Canadian drug name; ❷ Prototype drug.

469

ROUTE & DOSAGE

Arrhythmias

Child: **PO** *<1 y,* 10–30 mg/kg/day in divided doses q6h; *1–4 y,* 10–20 mg/kg/day in divided doses q6h; *4–12 y,* 10–15 mg/kg/day in divided doses q6h; *12–18 y,* 6–15 mg/kg/day in divided doses q6h
Adult: **PO** *<50 kg,* 100 mg q6h or 200 mg sustained-release q12h; *>50 kg,* 100–200 mg q6h or 300 mg sustained-release capsule q12h

STORAGE

Store at 15°–30° C (59°–86° F) unless otherwise directed.

ADMINISTRATION

Oral

- Start drug 6–12 h after last quinidine dose and 3–6 h after last procainamide dose for patients who have been receiving either quinidine or procainamide.
- Give sustained-release capsules whole.
- Do not use sustained-release capsules in loading doses when rapid control is required or in patients with creatinine clearance of ≤40 mL/min.
- Start sustained-release capsules 6 h after last dose of conventional capsule if change in drug form is made.

ADVERSE EFFECTS Body as a Whole: Hypersensitivity (pruritus, urticaria, rash, photosensitivity, <u>laryngospasm</u>). **CNS:** Dizziness, headache, fatigue, muscle weakness, convulsions, paresthesias, nervousness, acute psychosis, peripheral neuropathy. **CV:** *Hypotension,* chest pain, edema, dyspnea, syncope, bradycardia, tachycardia; worsening of CHF or cardiac arrhythmia; <u>cardiogenic shock</u>, <u>heart block</u>; edema with weight gain. **Special Senses:** *Blurred vision,* dry eyes, increased IOP, precipitation of acute angle-closure glaucoma. **GI:** *Dry mouth, constipation,* epigastric or abdominal pain, cholestatic jaundice. **Urogenital:** *Hesitancy and retention,* urinary frequency, urgency, renal insufficiency. **Other:** Dry nose and throat, drying of bronchial secretions, initiation of uterine contractions (pregnant patient); muscle aches, precipitation of myasthenia gravis, agranulocytosis (rare), thrombocytopenia.

INTERACTIONS Drug: ANTICHOLINERGIC DRUGS (e.g., TRICYCLIC ANTIDEPRESSANTS, ANTIHISTAMINES) compound anticholinergic effects; other ANTIARRHYTHMICS compound toxicities; **phenytoin, rifampin** may increase disopyramide metabolism and decrease levels; may increase **warfarin**-induced hypoprothrombinemia.

PHARMACOKINETICS Absorption: Readily absorbed from GI tract; 60–83% reaches systemic circulation. **Onset:** 30 min–3.5 h. **Peak:** 1–2 h. **Duration:** 1.5–8.5 h. **Distribution:** Distributed in extracellular fluid; crosses placenta; distributed into breast milk. **Metabolism:** Metabolized in liver. **Elimination:** 80% excreted in urine, 10% in feces. **Half-Life:** 4–10 h.

NURSING IMPLICATIONS

Assessment & Drug Effects

- Check apical pulse before administering drug. Withhold drug and notify physician if pulse rate is slower than norms established for age, or if there is any unusual change in rate, rhythm, or quality.
- Monitor ECG closely. The following signs are indications for drug withdrawal: Prolongation of QT interval and worsening of arrhythmia interval, QRS widening (>25%).
- Monitor for rapid weight gain or other signs of fluid retention.
- Lab tests: Baseline and periodic hepatic and renal function tests, blood glucose, and serum potassium. Correct hypokalemia or other imbalances before initiation of therapy.
- Monitor BP closely in all patients during periods of dosage adjustment and in those receiving high dosages.
- Monitor I&O, particularly patients with impaired renal function. Persistent urinary hesitancy or retention may necessitate lower dosage or discontinuation of drug.
- Report S&S of hyperkalemia (see Appendix D-1); it enhances drug's toxic effects.
- Measure IOP before treatment begins in patients with a family history of glaucoma.
- Monitor for S&S of CHF.
- Discontinue promptly if S&S of agranulocytosis, peripheral neuritis, or jaundice appear (see Appendix D-1).

Patient & Family Education

- Take drug precisely as prescribed to maintain regularity of heartbeat. Do not skip or stop medication or change dose without consulting physician.
- Weigh daily under standard conditions and check ankles for edema. Report to physician a weekly weight gain of ≥1–2 kg (2–4 lb).
- Make position changes slowly, particularly when getting up from lying down because of the possibility of hypotension; dangle legs for a few minutes before walking, and do not stand still for prolonged periods. If you feel light-headed, lie down or sit down.
- Do not take OTC medications unless approved by physician.
- Avoid exposure to sunlight or ultraviolet light; drug may cause photosensitivity.
- Do not drive or engage in other potentially hazardous activities until response to drug is known.
- Do not drink alcoholic beverages while taking disopyramide.
- Do not breast feed while taking this drug without consulting physician.
- Store this medication out of reach of children.

DOBUTAMINE HYDROCHLORIDE

(doe-byoo′ta-meen)

Dobutrex

Classifications: AUTONOMIC NERVOUS SYSTEM AGENT; BETA-ADRENERGIC AGONIST; CATECHOLAMINE

Prototype: Isoproterenol

Pregnancy Category: C

DOBUTAMINE HYDROCHLORIDE

AVAILABILITY 12.5 mg/mL injection

ACTIONS Produces inotropic effect by acting on beta receptors and primarily on myocardial alpha-adrenergic receptors. Increases cardiac output and decreases pulmonary wedge pressure and total systemic vascular resistance with comparatively little or no effect on BP. Also increases conduction through AV node. Has lower potential for precipitating arrhythmias than dopamine.
THERAPEUTIC EFFECTS In CHF or cardiogenic shock, increase in cardiac output enhances renal perfusion and increases renal output and renal sodium excretion.

USES Inotropic support in short term treatment of cardiac decompensation due to depressed myocardial contractility (cardiogenic shock) resulting from either organic heart disease or from cardiac surgery.
UNLABELED USES To augment cardiovascular function in children undergoing cardiac catheterization, stress thallium testing.

CONTRAINDICATIONS History of hypersensitivity to other sympathomimetic amines, ventricular tachycardia, idiopathic hypertrophic subaortic stenosis. Safe use during pregnancy (category C), lactation, children, or following acute MI is not established.
CAUTIOUS USE Preexisting hypertension, atrial fibrillation.

ROUTE & DOSAGE

Cardiac Decompensation
Child/Adult: **IV** 2.5–15 mcg/kg/min (max 40 mcg/kg/min) has been given for up to 72 h without decrease in effectiveness

STORAGE
Refrigerate reconstituted solution at 2°–15° C (36°–59° F) for 48 h or store for 6 h at room temperature.

ADMINISTRATION
Intravenous

***PREPARE* Continuous:** Reconstitute by adding 10 mL sterile water for injection or D5W to 250-mg vial; if not completely dissolved, add an additional 10 mL of diluent. ▪Further dilute to a volume of at least 50 mL with D5W, NS, LR, D5/LR, or sodium lactate injection. ▪Use IV solutions within 24 h.
***ADMINISTER* Continuous:** Rate of infusion is determined by body weight and controlled by an infusion pump (preferred) or a microdrip IV infusion set. ▪IV infusion rate and duration of therapy are determined by heart rate, blood pressure, ectopic activity, urine output, and, whenever possible, by measurements of cardiac output and central venous or pulmonary wedge pressures.

INCOMPATIBILITIES **Solution/Additive: Sodium bicarbonate, aminophylline, bretylium, bumetanide, calcium chloride, calcium gluconate, diazepam, digoxin, doxapram, epinephrine, furosemide, heparin, insulin, magnesium sulfate, phenytoin, potassium chloride, potassium phosphate. Y-Site: Acyclovir, aminophylline, sodium bicarbonate.**

D

ADVERSE EFFECTS All: Generally dose related. **CNS:** Headache, tremors, paresthesias, mild leg cramps, nervousness, fatigue (with overdosage). **CV:** *Increased heart rate and BP,* premature ventricular beats, palpitation, *anginal pain.* **GI:** Nausea, vomiting. **Other:** Nonspecific chest pain, shortness of breath.

INTERACTIONS Drug: GENERAL ANESTHETICS (especially **cyclopropane** and **halothane**) may sensitize myocardium to effects of CATECHOLAMINES such as dobutamine and lead to serious arrhythmias—used with extreme caution; BETA-ADRENERGIC BLOCKING AGENTS, e.g., **metoprolol, propranolol,** may make dobutamine ineffective in increasing cardiac output, but total peripheral resistance may increase—concomitant use generally avoided; MAO INHIBITORS, TRICYCLIC ANTIDEPRESSANTS potentiate pressor effects—use with extreme caution.

PHARMACOKINETICS Onset: 2–10 min. **Peak:** 10–20 min. **Metabolism:** Metabolized in liver and other tissues by COMT. **Elimination:** Excreted in urine. **Half-Life:** 2 min.

NURSING IMPLICATIONS

Assessment & Drug Effects
- Correct hypovolemia by administration of appropriate volume expanders prior to initiation of therapy.
- Monitor therapeutic effectiveness. At any given dosage level, drug takes 10–20 min to produce peak effects.
- Monitor ECG and BP continuously during administration.
- Note: Marked increases in blood pressure (systolic pressure is the most likely to be affected) and heart rate, or the appearance of arrhythmias or other adverse cardiac effects are usually reversed promptly by reduction in dosage.
- Observe patients with preexisting hypertension closely for exaggerated pressor response.
- Note: Tolerance has been observed with continuous or prolonged infusions; adverse reactions are no different than those seen with shorter infusions.
- Monitor I&O ratio and pattern. Urine output and sodium excretion generally increase because of improved cardiac output and renal perfusion.

Patient & Family Education
- Do not breast feed while taking this drug without consulting physician.

DOCUSATE CALCIUM (DIOCTYL CALCIUM SULFOSUCCINATE)
(dok′yoo-sate)
DCS, PMS-Docusate Calcium, Pro-Cal-Sof, Surfak

DOCUSATE POTASSIUM
Dialose, Diocto-K, Kasof

DOCUSATE SODIUM
Colace, Colace Enema, Dio-Sul, Disonate, DGSS, D-S-S, Duosol, Lax-gel, Laxinate 100, Modane Soft, Pro-Sof, Regulax ♣, Regutol, Therevac-Plus, Therevac-SB
Classifications: GASTROINTESTINAL AGENT; STOOL SOFTENER
Pregnancy Category: C

AVAILABILITY Docusate Calcium 50 mg, 240 mg capsules **Docusate Potassium** 100 mg tablets; 240 mg capsules **Docusate Sodium** 100 mg tablets; 50 mg, 100 mg, 240 mg, 250 mg, capsules; 50 mg/15 mL 60 mg/15 mL, 150 mg/15 mL syrup

ACTIONS Anionic surface-active agent with emulsifying and wetting properties.
THERAPEUTIC EFFECTS Detergent action lowers surface tension, permitting water and fats to penetrate and soften stools for easier passage.

USES Prophylactically in patients who should avoid straining during defecation and for treatment of constipation associated with hard, dry stools (e.g., following anorectal surgery, heart surgery).

CONTRAINDICATIONS Atonic constipation, nausea, vomiting, abdominal pain, fecal impaction, structural anomalies of colon and rectum, intestinal obstruction or perforation; use of docusate sodium in patients on sodium restriction; use of docusate potassium in patients with renal dysfunction; concomitant use of mineral oil; pregnancy (category C).
CAUTIOUS USE History of CHF, edema, diabetes melitus.

ROUTE & DOSAGE

Stool Softener
Child: **PO** *<3 y,* 10–40 mg/day; *3–6 y,* 20–60 mg/day; *6–12 y,* 40–150 mg/day (doses may be repeated as needed up to q.i.d.)
Adult: **PO** 50–500 mg/day **PR** 50–100 mg added to enema fluid

STORAGE
Store syrup formulations in tightly covered, light-resistant containers at 15°–30° C (59°–86° F) unless directed otherwise.

ADMINISTRATION
Oral
■ Give with a full glass of water if allowed or with fluid appropriate for age. Effective after 1–3 days.

Rectal

- Microenema: Insert full length of nozzle (half length for children) into the rectum. Squeeze entire contents of tube and remove completely before releasing grip on tube.

ADVERSE EFFECTS GI: Occasional mild abdominal cramps, *diarrhea,* nausea, bitter taste. **Other:** Throat irritation (liquid preparation), rash.

INTERACTION Drug: Docusate will increase systemic absorption of **mineral oil.**

PHARMACOKINETICS Not studied.

NURSING IMPLICATIONS

Assessment & Drug Effects

- Withhold drug if diarrhea develops and notify prescriber.
- Therapeutic effectiveness: Usually apparent 1–3 days after first dose.
- Note: A few drops of 10 mg/mL solution can be used to loosen cerumen in the ear; should only be used if tympanic membrane is intact; results observed in about 15 min.

Patient & Family Education

- Take sufficient liquid with each dose and increase fluid intake during the day, if allowed. Oral liquid (NOT syrup) may be administered in milk, fruit juice, or infant formula to mask bitter taste.
- Do not take concomitantly with mineral oil.
- Do not take for prolonged periods in lieu of proper dietary management or treatment of underlying causes of constipation.
- Store this medication out of reach of children.

DOLASETRON MESYLATE

(dol-a-se'tron)

Anzemet

Classifications: GASTROINTESTINAL AGENT; ANTIEMETIC; 5-HT₃ ANTAGONIST

Prototype: Ondansetron

Pregnancy Category: B

AVAILABILITY 50 mg, 100 mg tablets; 20 mg/mL injection

ACTIONS Dolasetron is a selective serotonin (5-HT$_3$) receptor antagonist used for control of nausea and vomiting associated with cancer chemotherapy. Serotonin receptors affected by dolasetron are located in the chemoreceptor trigger zone (CTZ) of the brain and peripherally on the vagal nerve terminal. Serotonin, released from the cells of the small intestine, activate 5-HT$_3$ receptors located on vagal efferent, neurons, thus initiating the vomiting reflex. Dolasetron causes ECG changes lasting from 6–24 h.

THERAPEUTIC EFFECTS This selective serotonin (5-HT$_3$) receptor antagonist has antiemetic properties that help patients on chemotherapy.

Common adverse effects in *italic;* life-threatening effects underlined; generic names in **bold;** drug classifications in SMALL CAPS; ♦ Canadian drug name; ◐ Prototype drug.

475

USES Prevention of nausea and vomiting from emetogenic chemotherapy, prevention and treatment of postoperative nausea and vomiting.

CONTRAINDICATIONS Hypersensitivity to dolasetron.

CAUTIOUS USE Patients who have or may develop prolongation of cardiac conduction intervals, particularly QTc (i.e., patients with hypokalemia, hypomagnesemia, diuretics, congenital QT syndrome; patients taking antiarrhythmic drugs and high-dose anthracycline therapy), pregnancy (category B), and lactation. Safety and efficacy in children <2 y are not established.

ROUTE & DOSAGE

Prevention of Chemotherapy-Induced Nausea and Vomiting

Child: **IV** >2 y, 1.8 mg/kg or 100 mg administered over 30 sec, 30 min prior to chemotherapy **PO** >2 y, 1.8 mg/kg up to 100 mg 1 h before chemotherapy
Adult: **IV** 1.8 mg/kg or 100 mg administered over 30 sec, 30 min prior to chemotherapy **PO** 100 mg 1 h prior to chemotherapy

Pre/Postoperative Nausea and Vomiting

Child: **IV** >2 y, 0.35 mg/kg up to 12.5 mg 15 min before cessation of anesthesia or when postoperative nausea and vomiting occur **PO** >2 y, 1.2 mg/kg up to 100 mg starting 2 h prior to surgery (may also mix IV formulation in apple or apple-grape juice and administer orally)
Adult: **IV** 12.5 mg 15 min before cessation of anesthesia or when postoperative nausea and vomiting occur **PO** 100 mg within 2 h prior to surgery

STORAGE

Store at 20°–25° C (66°–77° F) and protect from light. Diluted IV solution may be stored refrigerated up to 48 h.

ADMINISTRATION

Oral

- Give dissolved in apple or apple-grape juice 1 h before chemotherapy.
- Give within 2 h before surgery, when used for postoperative nausea.

Intravenous

PREPARE **Direct:** Give undiluted. **IV Infusion:** Dilute in 50 mL of any of the following: NS, D5W, D5/0.45% NaCl, LR.
ADMINISTER **Direct:** Inject undiluted drug over 30 sec. **IV Infusion:** Infuse diluted drug over 15 min.

ADVERSE EFFECTS Body as a Whole: Fever, fatigue, pain, chills or shivering. **CNS:** *Headache,* dizziness, drowsiness. **CV:** Hypertension. **GI:** *Diarrhea,* increased LFTs, abdominal pain. **Genitourinary:** Urinary retention.

PHARMACOKINETICS Absorption: Rapidly absorbed from GI tract, converted to hydrodolasetron, the active metabolite. **Peak:** 0.6 h IV, 1 h PO.

Common adverse effects in *italic;* life-threatening effects <u>underlined</u>; generic names in **bold;** drug classifications in SMALL CAPS; ◆ Canadian drug name; ◐ Prototype drug.

Distribution: Crosses placenta, distributed into breast milk. **Metabolism:** Metabolized to hydrodolasetron by carbonyl reductase. Hydrodolasetron is metabolized in the liver by CYP2D6. **Elimination:** Primarily excreted in urine as unchanged hydrodolasetron. **Half-Life:** 10 min dolasetron, 7.3 h hydrodolasetron.

D

NURSING IMPLICATIONS

Assessment & Drug Effects

- Determine serum electrolytes before initiating drug. Hypokalemia and hypomagnesemia should be correct before initiating therapy.
- Monitor closely cardiac status especially with vomiting, excess diuresis, or other conditions that may result in electrolyte imbalances.
- Monitor ECG, especially in those taking concurrent antiarrhythmic or other drugs that may cause QT prolongation.
- Monitor for and report signs of bleeding (e.g., hematuria, epistaxis, purpura, hematoma).
- Lab tests: With prolonged therapy, periodically monitor liver functions, PTT, CBC with platelet count, and alkaline phosphatase.

Patient & Family Education

- Headache requiring analgesic for relief is a common adverse effect.
- Do not breast feed while taking this drug without consulting physician.

DOPAMINE HYDROCHLORIDE

(doe'pa-meen)

Dopastat, Intropin, Revimine ♣

Classifications: AUTONOMIC NERVOUS SYSTEM AGENT; ALPHA- AND BETA-ADRENERGIC AGONIST (SYMPATHOMIMETIC)

Prototype: Epinephrine

Pregnancy Category: C

AVAILABILITY 40 mg/mL, 80 mg/mL, 160 mg/mL injection

ACTIONS Naturally occurring neurotransmitter and immediate precursor of norepinephrine. Major cardiovascular effects produced by direct action on alpha- and beta-adrenergic receptors and on specific dopaminergic receptors in mesenteric and renal vascular beds.

THERAPEUTIC EFFECTS Positive inotropic effect on myocardium increases cardiac output with increase in systolic and pulse pressure and little or no effect on diastolic pressure. Improves circulation to renal vascular bed by decreasing renal vascular resistance with resulting increase in glomerular filtration rate and urinary output. High doses stimulate alpha-adrenergic-mediated vasoconstriction

USES To correct hemodynamic imbalance in shock syndrome due to MI (cardiogenic shock), trauma, endotoxic septicemia (septic shock), open heart surgery, and CHF.

UNLABELED USES Acute renal failure; cirrhosis; hepatorenal syndrome; barbiturate intoxication.

Common adverse effects in *italic;* life-threatening effects <u>underlined;</u> generic names in **bold;** drug classifications in SMALL CAPS; ♣ Canadian drug name; ○ Prototype drug.

477

CONTRAINDICATIONS Pheochromocytoma; tachyarrhythmias, hypovolemia, or ventricular fibrillation. Safe use during pregnancy (category C), lactation, or children is not established.

CAUTIOUS USE Patients with history of occlusive vascular disease (e.g., Buerger's or Raynaud's disease); those taking phenytoin; cold injury; diabetic endarteritis, arterial embolism.

ROUTE & DOSAGE

Child/Adult: **IV** Low dose (for renal blood flow effects with minimal heart effects): 2–5 mcg/kg/min; Intermediate dose (for cardiac effect): 5–15 mcg/kg/min; High dose (for alpha-adrenergic effects; decreases renal perfusion): >20 mcg/kg/min

STORAGE

Store reconstituted solution for 24 h at 2°–15° C (36°–59° F) or 6 h at room temperature (15°–30° C; 59°–86° F).

ADMINISTRATION

Intravenous

PREPARE **Continuous:** Dilute just prior to administration. ▪ Dilute each ampule in one of the following: D5W, D5/NS, D5/LR, D5/0.45% NaCl, NS. ▪ Dilute 200-mg ampule in 250 mL, 500 mL, or 1000 mL IV solution to yield 800 mcg/mL, 400 mcg/mL, or 200 mcg/mL, respectively. Dilute 400-mg ampule in 250 mL, 500 mL, or 1000 mL IV solution to yield 1600 mcg/mL, 800 mcg/mL, or 400 mcg/mL, respectively. ▪ Dilute 800-mg ampule in 250 mL, 500 mL, or 1000 mL IV solution to yield 3200 mcg/mL, 1600 mcg/mL, or 800 mcg/mL, respectively. ▪ Consult package information for other dilutions.

ADMINISTER **Continuous:** Infusion rate is based on body weight. ▪ Infusion rate and guidelines for adjusting rate relative changes in blood pressure are prescribed by physician. ▪ Give through central line or large vein. ▪ Microdrip and other reliable metering device should be used for accuracy of flow rate.

INCOMPATIBILITIES **Solution/Additive: Sodium bicarbonate, aminophylline, amphotericin B, ampicillin, cephalothin, penicillin G. Y-Site: Acyclovir, aminophylline, amphotericin B, sodium bicarbonate.**

▪ Correct hypovolemia, if possible, with either whole blood or plasma before initiation of dopamine therapy. ▪ Monitor infusion continuously for free flow, and take care to avoid extravasation, which can result in tissue sloughing and gangrene. Use a central line if possible. ▪ Antidote for extravasation: Stop infusion promptly and remove needle. Immediately infiltrate the ischemic area with 5–10 mg phentolamine mesylate in 10–15 mL of NS, using syringe and fine needle. ▪ Protect dopamine from light. Discolored solutions should not be used.

ADVERSE EFFECTS CV: *Hypotension,* ectopic beats, *tachycardia,* anginal pain, palpitation, vasoconstriction (indicated by disproportionate rise in diastolic pressure), cold extremities; less frequent: <u>aberrant conduction,</u>

bradycardia, widening of QRS complex, elevated blood pressure. **GI:** Nausea, vomiting. **CNS:** Headache. **Skin:** Necrosis, tissue sloughing with extravasation, <u>gangrene</u>, piloerection. **Other:** Azotemia, dyspnea, dilated pupils (high doses).

DIAGNOSTIC TEST INTERFERENCE Dopamine may modify test response when histamine is used as a control for *intradermal skin tests.*

INTERACTIONS Drug: MAO INHIBITORS, ERGOT ALKALOIDS, **furazolidine** increase alpha-adrenergic effects (headache, hyperpyrexia, hypertension); **guanethidine, phenytoin** may decrease dopamine action; BETA-BLOCKERS antagonize cardiac effects; ALPHA-BLOCKERS antagonize peripheral vasoconstriction; **halothane, cyclopropane** increase risk of hypertension and ventricular arrhythmias.

PHARMACOKINETICS Onset: <5 min. **Duration:** <10 min. **Distribution:** Widely distributed; does not cross blood–brain barrier. **Metabolism:** Inactive in the liver, kidney, and plasma by monoamine oxidase and COMT. **Elimination:** Excreted in urine. **Half-Life:** 2 min.

NURSING IMPLICATIONS

Assessment & Drug Effects

- Monitor blood pressure, pulse, peripheral pulses, and urinary output continuously. Precise measurements are essential for accurate titration of dosage.
- Report the following indicators promptly to physician for use in decreasing or temporarily suspending dose: Reduced urine flow rate in absence of hypotension; ascending tachycardia; dysrhythmias; disproportionate rise in diastolic pressure (marked decrease in pulse pressure); signs of peripheral ischemia (pallor, cyanosis, mottling, coldness, complaints of tenderness, pain, numbness, or burning sensation).
- Monitor therapeutic effectiveness. In addition to improvement in vital signs and urine flow, other indices of adequate dosage and perfusion of vital organs include loss of pallor, increase in toe temperature, adequacy of nail bed capillary filling, and reversal of confusion or comatose state.

DORNASE ALFA

(dor'naze)
Pulmozyme
Classifications: ANTITUSSIVES, EXPECTORANTS, AND MUCOLYTICS AGENTS; MUCOLYTIC
Prototype: Acetylcysteine
Pregnancy Category: B

AVAILABILITY 1 mg/mL solution for inhalation

ACTIONS Dornase is a solution of recombinant human deoxyribonuclease (DNAse), an enzyme that selectively cleaves DNA. In cystic fibrosis (CF) patients, viscous, purulent secretions in the airway reduce

D

pulmonary function and lead to exacerbations of infection. Purulent pulmonary secretions contain very high concentrations of DNA released by degenerating leukocytes that are present in response to infection. **THERAPEUTIC EFFECTS** Dornase hydrolyzes the DNA in sputum of CF patients and reduces sputum viscosity. Use of dornase significantly reduces number of upper respiratory infections acquired by patients with CF.

USES In combination with standard therapies to reduce the frequency of respiratory infections in patients with CF and to improve pulmonary function.

CONTRAINDICATIONS Hypersensitivity to dornase, epoitin alpha.
CAUTIOUS USE Pregnancy (category B), lactation. Safety and efficacy in children <5 y of age are not known.

ROUTE & DOSAGE

Child/Adult: **Inhalation** >5 y, 2.5 mg (1 ampule) inhaled once daily using a recommended nebulizer, may increase to twice daily (do not mix with other agents in nebulizer)

STORAGE
Store refrigerated at 2°–8° C (36°–46° F) in protective foil pouch.

ADMINISTRATION
Inhalation
- Do not dilute or mix with any other drugs or solutions in the nebulizer.
- Use only with nebulizer systems recommended by the drug manufacturer.
- Do not shake ampules; do not use ampules that have been at room temperature longer than 24 h or have become cloudy or discolored.

ADVERSE EFFECTS Respiratory: Hoarseness, sore throat, voice alterations, pharyngitis, laryngitis, cough, rhinitis. **Other:** Conjunctivitis, chest pain, rash.

PHARMACOKINETICS Absorption: Minimal systemic absorption. **Onset:** 3–8 days. **Duration:** Benefit lasts up to 4 days after discontinuing treatment.

NURSING IMPLICATIONS

Assessment & Drug Effects
- Monitor for improvement in dyspnea and sputum clearance.
- Monitor for S&S of hypersensitivity (see Appendix D-1). Patients with a history of hypersensitivity to bovine pancreatic dornase are at high risk.
- Monitor for adverse effects; rarely, dosage adjustments may be required.

Patient & Family Education
- Report rash, hives, itching, or other signs and symptoms of hypersensitivity to prescriber immediately.
- Report adverse effects.

- Most children receive chest physiotherapy in addition; demonstrate and plan with families to accomplish this treatment.
- Take a missed dose as soon as possible; if it is almost time for the next dose, skip the missed dose.
- Do not breast feed while taking this drug without consulting physician.
- Store this medication out of reach of children.

D

DOXACURIUM CHLORIDE
(dox′a-cur-i-um)
Nuromax
Classifications: AUTONOMIC NERVOUS SYSTEM AGENT; SKELETAL MUSCLE RELAXANT, NONDEPOLARIZING AGENT
Prototype: Tubocurarine
Pregnancy Category: C

AVAILABILITY 1 mg/mL injection

ACTIONS Long-acting neuromuscular blocking agent. Binds competitively to cholinergic receptors on the motor end plate, thus resulting in a block of neuromuscular transmission. Most patients require a pharmacologic reversal prior to full spontaneous recovery from a neuromuscular block using an anticholinesterase.
THERAPEUTIC EFFECTS Produces skeletal muscle relaxation during surgery.

USES Skeletal muscle relaxation during surgery after induction with general anesthesia.
UNLABELED USES Facilitates endotracheal intubation.

CONTRAINDICATIONS Hypersensitivity to doxacurium; do not use benzyl alcohol formulation with newborns.
CAUTIOUS USE Neuromuscular diseases (e.g., myasthenia gravis); burn patients; acid–base or serum electrolyte imbalances; newborn infants, older adults, pregnancy (category C), lactation, or children <2 y of age.

ROUTE & DOSAGE

Intubation or Induction
Child: IV 2–12 y, 0.03–0.05 mg/kg with halothane general anesthesia
Adult: IV 0.05 mg/kg administered as rapid bolus injection over 5–10 sec. Use lower doses in those with renal or hepatic dysfunction

Maintenance with General Anesthesia
Child/Adult: IV 2–12 y, same dose as adult, but may have to give more frequently; 0.0005–0.01 mg/kg q60–100min administered as rapid bolus injection over 5–10 sec (dosing interval adjusted for each individual patient; use lower dosage in patients with renal or hepatic dysfunction)

Common adverse effects in *italic*; life-threatening effects underlined; generic names in **bold**; drug classifications in SMALL CAPS; ♣ Canadian drug name; ☯ Prototype drug.

481

STORAGE

Store undiluted at room temperature 15°–25° C (41°–77° F). Do not freeze. Diluted drug may be stored in polypropylene syringes for up to 24 h at 5°–25° C (41°–77° F).

ADMINISTRATION

Intravenous

PREPARE **Direct:** Dilute each 1 mL (1 mg) with 10 mL of D5W, NS, D5/NS, LR, or D5/LR to yield 0.1 mg/mL.

ADMINISTER **Direct:** Give IV push over 5–10 sec. ▪Individualize doses according to age, body size, and presence of kidney, liver, and neuromuscular diseases. ▪Note: Doxacurium contains benzyl alcohol, which has been associated with fatal complications in newborns. ▪Doxacurium should be administered under the supervision of expert clinicians. ▪See manufacturer's guidelines for dilution, compatibility, and administration.

ADVERSE EFFECTS CV: Bradycardia, hypotension, cutaneous flushing, histamine release.

INTERACTIONS Drug: VOLATILE ANESTHETICS **(isoflurane, enflurane, halothane)** potentiate the effects of doxacurium, requiring a reduced dose of doxacurium. Certain ANTIBIOTICS, including the AMINOGLYCOSIDES, **capreomycin, tetracycline, bacitracin, polymyxins, lincomycin, clindamycin,** and **colistin,** increase the neuromuscular blocking effect of doxacurium. **Carbamazepine** or **phenytoin** may increase the onset and decrease the duration of neuromuscular blockade. **Lithium, magnesium, procainamide,** or **quinidine** may enhance neuromuscular blockade.

PHARMACOKINETICS Onset: 5–10 min. **Peak:** 10 min. **Duration:** 60–160 min depending on dose. **Distribution:** 30% protein bound. **Metabolism:** Minimal to no hepatic metabolism. **Elimination:** 40–50% excreted in urine within 12 h; some excretion in bile. **Half-Life:** 1.5 h.

NURSING IMPLICATIONS

Assessment & Drug Effects

▪ Monitor for evidence of prolonged neuromuscular block, which may range from skeletal muscle weakness to prolonged paralysis with respiratory insufficiency and apnea.
▪ Monitor for full recovery of skeletal muscle function. Support ventilation until full recovery occurs.
▪ Monitor carefully, knowing that drugs used to antagonize doxacurium may wear off before the effects of doxacurium.

DOXAPRAM HYDROCHLORIDE

(dox'a-pram)

Dopram

Classifications: CENTRAL NERVOUS SYSTEM AGENT; CEREBRAL STIMULANT
Prototype: Caffeine
Pregnancy Category: B

AVAILABILITY 20 mg/mL injection

ACTIONS Short-acting analeptic capable of stimulating all levels of the cerebrospinal axis. Has minor effect on cortex. Respiratory stimulation by direct medullary action or possibly by indirect activation of peripheral chemoreceptors increases tidal volume and slightly increases respiratory rate.
THERAPEUTIC EFFECTS Decreases Pco_2 and increases Po_2 by increasing alveolar ventilation; may elevate BP and pulse rate by stimulation of brain stem vasomotor area.

USES Short-term adjunctive therapy to alleviate postanesthesia and drug-induced respiratory depression and to hasten arousal and return of pharyngeal and laryngeal reflexes. Also as a temporary measure (approximately 2 h) in hospitalized patients with COPD associated with acute respiratory insufficiency as an aid to prevent elevation of $Paco_2$ during administration of oxygen. (Not used with mechanical ventilation.)
UNLABELED USES Neonatal apnea refractory to xanthine therapy.

CONTRAINDICATIONS Epilepsy and other convulsive disorders; of ventilatory mechanism due to muscle paresis, pulmonary fibrosis, flail chest, pneumothorax, airway obstruction, extreme dyspnea, or acute bronchial asthma; severe hypertension, coronary artery disease, uncompensated heart failure, CVA. Safe use during pregnancy (category B), lactation, or in children <12 y is not established. Solution contains benzyl alcohol, which is not recommended in newborns; some clinicians have used low doses to treat neonatal apnea.
CAUTIOUS USE History of bronchial asthma, COPD; cardiac disease, severe tachycardia, arrhythmias, hypertension; hyperthyroidism; pheochromocytoma; head injury, cerebral edema, increased intracranial pressure; peptic ulcer, patients undergoing gastric surgery; acute agitation.

ROUTE & DOSAGE

Postanesthesia

Adult: **IV** 0.5–1 mg/kg single injection not to exceed 1.5 mg/kg or 2 mg/kg total dose when repeated at 5 min intervals or 1–3 mg/min infusion (max 4 mg/kg or 300 mg, not to exceed 3 g/day)

Drug-Induced CNS Depression

Adult: **IV** 1–2 mg/kg repeat in 5 min, then q1–2h until patient awakens (if relapse occurs, resume q1–2h injections (max total dose 3 g), if no response after priming dose, may give 1–3 mg/min for up to 2 h until patient awakens)

Neonatal Apnea

Neonate: **IV** 0.5–2.5 mg/kg followed by 1 mg/kg/h (titrate to max: 2.5 mg/kg/h); this use is not recommended by manufacturer

STORAGE
Store at 15°–30° C (59°–86° F) unless otherwise directed.

Common adverse effects in *italic;* life-threatening effects <u>underlined;</u> generic names in **bold;** drug classifications in SMALL CAPS; ✦ Canadian drug name; ● Prototype drug.

D

ADMINISTRATION

- IV administration to neonates: Verify correct IV concentration and rate of infusion with physician. ▪ Generally do not use in newborns because doxapram contains benzyl alcohol. ▪ Ensure adequacy of airway and oxygenation before initiation of doxapram therapy.

Intravenous

PREPARE **Direct:** Give undiluted. **IV Infusion:** Dilute 250 mg (12.5 mL) in 250 mL of D5W or NS.

ADMINISTER **Direct:** Give undiluted over 5 min. **IV Infusion:** Give at a rate of 1–3 mg/min, depending on patient response. Never exceed 3 mg/min. Give through a separate IV line from other drugs.

INCOMPATIBILITIES **Solution/Additive: Aminophylline, ascorbic acid,** CEPHALOSPORINS, **carbenicillin, dexamethasone, diazepam, digoxin, dobutamine, folic acid, furosemide, hydrocortisone, ketamine, methylprednisolone, minocycline, thiopental, ticarcillin.** Do not give through same IV line as these drugs.

ADVERSE EFFECTS CNS: Dizziness, sneezing, apprehension, confusion, *involuntary movements,* hyperactivity, paresthesias; feeling of warmth and burning, especially of genitalia and perineum; flushing, sweating, hyperpyrexia, headache, pilomotor erection, pruritus, muscle tremor, rigidity, convulsions, *increased deep-tendon reflexes,* bilateral Babinski sign, *carpopedal spasm,* pupillary dilation, mild delayed narcosis. **CV:** *Mild to moderate increase in BP, sinus tachycardia,* bradycardia, extrasystoles, lowered T waves, PVCs, chest pains, tightness in chest. **GI:** Nausea, vomiting, diarrhea, salivation, sour taste. **Urogenital:** Urinary retention, frequency, incontinence. **Respiratory:** Dyspnea, tachypnea, cough, <u>laryngospasm</u>, <u>bronchospasm</u>, hiccups, rebound hypoventilation, hypocapnia with tetany. **Other:** <u>Neonatal gasping</u> syndrome is a rare but life-threatening reaction to benzyl alcohol, which is in the doxapram drug formulation; local skin irritation, thrombophlebitis with extravasation; decreased Hgb, Hct, and RBC count; elevated BUN; albuminuria.

INTERACTIONS Drug: MAO INHIBITORS, SYMPATHOMIMETIC AGENTS add to pressor effects.

PHARMACOKINETICS Onset: 20–40 sec. **Peak:** 1–2 min. **Duration:** 5–12 min. **Metabolism:** Rapidly metabolized. **Elimination:** Excreted in urine as metabolites.

NURSING IMPLICATIONS

Assessment & Drug Effects

- Monitor IV site frequently. Extravasation or use of same IV site for prolonged periods can cause thrombophlebitis (see Appendix D-1) or tissue irritation.
- Monitor continuously and observe accurately: BP, pulse, deep tendon reflexes, airway, and arterial blood gases. All are essential guides for

determining minimum effective dosage and preventing overdosage. Make baseline determinations for comparison.

- Lab tests: Draw arterial P_{O_2} and P_{CO_2} and O_2 saturation prior to both initiation of doxapram infusion and oxygen administration, and then at least every 30 min during infusion. Infusion should not be administered for longer than 2 h.
- Discontinue doxapram if arterial blood gases show evidence of deterioration and when mechanical ventilation is initiated.
- Observe patient continuously during therapy and maintain vigilance until patient is fully alert (usually about 1 h) and protective pharyngeal and laryngeal reflexes are completely restored.
- Notify physician immediately of any adverse effects. Be alert for early signs of toxicity: Tachycardia, muscle tremor, spasticity, hyperactive reflexes.
- Note: A mild to moderate increase in BP commonly occurs.
- Discontinue if sudden hypotension or dyspnea develops.

DOXEPIN HYDROCHLORIDE
(dox'e-pin)
Adapin, Sinequan, Triadapin ♣ , Zonalon
Classifications: CENTRAL NERVOUS SYSTEM AGENT; PSYCHOTHERAPEUTIC; TRICYCLIC ANTIDEPRESSANT
Prototype: Imipramine
Pregnancy Category: C

AVAILABILITY 10 mg, 25 mg, 50 mg, 75 mg, 100 mg, 150 mg capsules; 10 mg/mL oral concentrate

ACTIONS Dibenzoxepin is a tricyclic antidepressant (TCA). Reportedly one of the most sedating of the TCAs, it inhibits serotonin reuptake from the synaptic gap; also inhibits norepinephrine reuptake to a moderate degree.

THERAPEUTIC EFFECTS Restores the level of these neurotransmitters (serotonin and norepinephrine) as the proposed mechanism of antidepressant action.

USES Psychoneurotic anxiety or depressive reactions; mixed symptoms of anxiety and depression; anxiety or depression associated with alcoholism; organic disease; psychotic depressive disorders; topical for treatment of pruritus.

UNLABELED USES Peptic ulcer disease, neuralgia.

CONTRAINDICATIONS Prior sensitivity to any TCA; during acute recovery phase following MI; glaucoma; prostatic hypertrophy; tendency for urinary retention; concurrent use of MAO inhibitors. Safe use during pregnancy (category C), lactation, or in children <12 y is not established.

CAUTIOUS USE Patients receiving electroconvulsive therapy, patients with suicidal tendency; renal, cardiovascular or hepatic dysfunction.

Common adverse effects in *italic*; life-threatening effects <u>underlined</u>; generic names in **bold**; drug classifications in SMALL CAPS; ♣ Canadian drug name; ◯ Prototype drug.

485

D

ROUTE & DOSAGE

Antidepressant

Child: **PO** 1–3 mg/kg/day in single or divided doses
Adult: **PO** 30–150 mg/day at bedtime *or* in divided doses, may gradually increase to 300 mg/day

Pruritus

Adult: **Topical** Apply a thin film q.i.d. with at least 3–4 h between applications, may use up to 8 days

STORAGE

Store all forms at 15°–30° C (59°–86° F) in tightly closed, light-resistant container.

ADMINISTRATION

Oral

- Give oral concentrate diluted with approximately 120 mL water, milk, or fruit juice.
- Empty capsule and swallow contents with fluid or mix with food as necessary if it cannot be swallowed whole or request order for oral concentrate form.
- Inform prescriber if daytime sedation is pronounced. Entire daily dose (up to 150 mg) may be prescribed for bedtime administration.

Topical

- Apply a thin file to affected areas; allow 3–4 h between applications

ADVERSE EFFECTS All: Anticholinergic. **CNS:** *Drowsiness,* dizziness, weakness, fatigue, headache, hypomania, confusion, tremors, paresthesias. **CV:** *Orthostatic hypotension,* palpitation, hypertension, tachycardia, ECG changes. **Special Senses:** Mydriasis, blurred vision, photophobia. **GI:** *Dry mouth,* sour or metallic taste, epigastric distress, constipation. **Urogenital:** Urinary retention, delayed micturition, urinary frequency. **Other:** Increased perspiration, tinnitus, weight gain, photosensitivity reaction, skin rash, agranulocytosis, *burning or stinging at application site,* edema.

INTERACTIONS Drug: May decrease antihypertensive response to ANTIHYPERTENSIVES; CNS DEPRESSANTS, **alcohol,** HYPNOTICS, BARBITURATES, SEDATIVES potentiate CNS depression; may increase hypoprothombinemic effect of ORAL ANTICOAGULANTS; **ethchlorvynol** may cause transient delirium; **levodopa,** SYMPATHOMIMETICS (e.g., **epinephrine, norepinephrine**) introduce possibility of sympathetic hyperactivity with hypertension and hyperpyrexia; MAO INHIBITORS introduce possibility of severe reactions, toxic psychosis, cardiovascular instability; **methylphenidate** increases plasma TCA levels; THYROID AGENTS may increase possibility of arrhythmias; **cimetidine** may increase plasma TCA levels. **Herbal:** Ginkgo may decrease seizure threshold; **St. John's wort** may cause **serotonin** syndrome.

PHARMACOKINETICS Absorption: Rapidly absorbed from GI sites through intact skin. **Peak:** 2 h. **Distribution:** Crosses placenta; distributed into breast milk. **Metabolism:** Metabolized in liver. **Elimination:** Primarily excreted in urine. **Half-Life:** 6–8 h.

D

NURSING IMPLICATIONS

Assessment & Drug Effects

- Monitor use of other CNS depressants, including alcohol. Danger of overdosage or suicide attempt is increased when patient uses excessive amounts of alcohol.
- Be alert to changes in voiding and evaluate patient for constipation and abdominal distention; drug has moderate to strong anticholinergic effects.
- Antidepressants increase risk of suicidal thinking and behavior in children and adolescents with major depressive disorder, obsessive compulsive disorder, and other psychiatric disorders. Observe closely for worsening of condition, suicidality, and behavior changes. Instruct family and caregivers to monitor for these symptoms and discuss with prescriber. A MedGuide describing risks and stating whether the drug is approved for the child's/adolescent's condition should be provided for all families when antidepressants are prescribed.

Patient & Family Education

- Maintain established dosage regimen and avoid change of intervals, doubling, reducing, or skipping doses.
- Report mood and behavior changes of child or adolescent to prescriber immediately.
- The actions of both alcohol and doxepin are potentiated when used together and for up to 2 wk after doxepin is discontinued.
- Do not drive or engage in other potentially hazardous activities until response to drug is known.
- Do not breast feed while taking this drug without consulting prescriber.
- Store this medication out of reach of children.

DOXORUBICIN HYDROCHLORIDE ℗ⓟ
(dox-oh-roo′bi-sin)
Adriamycin, Rubex

DOXORUBICIN LIPOSOME
Doxil
Classifications: ANTINEOPLASTIC; ANTIBIOTIC
Pregnancy Category: D

AVAILABILITY 10 mg, 20 mg, 50 mg, 100 mg, 150 mg, powder for injection; 2 mg/mL injection; 20 mg liposomal injection

ACTIONS Cytotoxic antibiotic with wide spectrum of antitumor activity and strong immunosuppressive properties. Intercalates with preformed DNA residues, blocking effective DNA and RNA transcription. A potent radiosensitizer capable of enhancing radiation reactions. No clinical cross-resistance to standard antineoplastics; therefore, it may be especially effective in patients with less advanced disease.
THERAPEUTIC EFFECTS Highly destructive to rapidly proliferating cells and slowly developing carcinomas; selectively toxic to cardiac tissue.

USES To produce regression in neoplastic conditions, including acute lymphoblastic and myeloblastic leukemias, Wilms' tumor, neuroblastoma,

---

soft-tissue and bone sarcomas, breast and ovary carcinomas, lymphomas, bronchogenic carcinoma. Generally used in combined modalities with surgery, radiation, and immunotherapy. Effective pretreatment to sensitize superficial tumors to local radiation therapy. Kaposi's sarcoma (Doxil).

D

UNLABELED USES Multiple myeloma.

CONTRAINDICATIONS Myelosuppression, impaired cardiac function, obstructive jaundice, previous treatment with complete cumulative doses of doxorubicin or daunorubicin; lactation. Safe use during pregnancy (category D) is not established.

CAUTIOUS USE Impaired hepatic or renal function; patients who have received cyclophosphamide or pelvic irradiation or radiotherapy to areas surrounding heart; history of atopic dermatitis.

ROUTE & DOSAGE

Neoplasm

Child: **IV** 35–75 mg/m^2 as single dose, repeat at 21-day interval, or 20–30 mg/m^2 once weekly
Adult: **IV** 60–75 mg/m^2 as single dose at 21-day intervals or 30 mg/m^2 on each of 3 consecutive days repeated every 4 wk (max total cumulative dose: 500–550 mg/m^2)

Kaposi's Sarcoma

Adult: **IV Doxil** 20 mg/m^2 every 3 wk. Infuse over 30 min (do not use in-line filters)

STORAGE

Store reconstituted solution for 24 h at room temperature; refrigerated at 4°–10° C (39°–50° F) for 48 h. Protect from sunlight; discard unused solution.

ADMINISTRATION

Intravenous

■ Child: Must be given under care and direction of pediatric oncology specialist. Use recommended handling techniques for hazardous medications (see Part I). ■ IV administration to infants and children: Verify correct IV concentration and rate of infusion with physician. ■ Wear gloves and use caution when preparing drug solution. If powder or solution contacts skin or mucosa, wash copiously with soap and water. ■ Exposure to doxorubicin during the first trimester of pregnancy can result in losing the fetus.

PREPARE **Direct:** Dilute the powder with NS to yield a final concentration of 2 mg/mL. Bacteriostatic diluents are not recommended.

ADMINISTER **Direct:** Administer slowly into Y-site of freely running IV infusion of NS or D5W. Tubing should be attached to a butterfly needle inserted into a large vein. Usually infused over 3–5 min. Rate will be specifically ordered. Facial flushing and local red streaking along the vein may occur if drug is administered too rapidly. ■ Avoid using antecubital vein or veins on dorsum of hand or wrist, if possible, where extravasation could damage underlying tendons and nerves. Also avoid veins in extremity with compromised venous or lymphatic drainage.

■ Note: Loposomal doxorubicin must NOT be substituted for hydrochloride preparation because severe adverse effects may occur. Loposomal dosing recommended only for Kaposi's sarcoma.

INCOMPATIBILITIES **Solution/Additive: Aminophylline, cephalothin, dexamethasone, diazepam, fluorouracil, furosemide, hydrocortisone, heparin, vinblastine. Y-Site: Furosemide, heparin,** TPN.

ADVERSE EFFECTS Body as a Whole: Hypersensitivity (red flare around injection site, erythema, skin rash, pruritus, angioedema, urticaria, eosinophilia, fever, chills, <u>anaphylactoid reaction</u>). **CV:** <u>Serious, irreversible myocardial toxicity with delayed CHF, ventricular arrhythmias, acute left ventricular failure,</u> hypertension, hypotension. **GI:** *Stomatitis,* esophagitis with ulcerations; nausea, vomiting, anorexia, inanition, diarrhea. **Hematologic:** *Severe myelosuppression* (60–85% of patients); <u>leukopenia</u> (<u>principally granulocytes</u>), thrombocytopenia, anemia. **Skin:** Hyperpigmentation of nail beds, tongue, and buccal mucosa (especially in blacks); *complete alopecia* (reversible), hyperpigmentation of dermal creases (especially in children), rash, *recall phenomenon (skin reaction due to prior radiotherapy).* **Other:** Lacrimation, drowsiness, fever, facial flush too rapid IV infusion rate, microscopic hematuria, hyperuricemia. *With extravasation: severe cellulitis, vesication, tissue necrosis,* lymphangitis, phlebosclerosis.

INTERACTIONS Drug: BARBITURATES may decrease pharmacologic effects of doxorubicin by increasing its hepatic metabolism—increase in doxorubicin dosage may be needed; **streptozocin** (Zanosar) may prolong doxorubicin half-life—dosage reduction of doxorubicin may be indicated.

PHARMACOKINETICS Distribution: Widely distributed; does not cross blood–brain barrier; crosses placenta; distribution into breast milk not known. **Metabolism:** Metabolized in liver to active metabolite. **Elimination:** Excreted primarily in bile. **Half-Life:** 16.7–31.7 h.

NURSING IMPLICATIONS

Assessment & Drug Effects

- ■ Be alert for and report signs of infection such as respiratory infections, aching, rashes, and gastrointestinal distress.
- ■ Assess immunization status prior to beginning therapy in order to be alert for diseases that pose risk.
- ■ Stop infusion, remove IV needle, and notify physician promptly if patient complains of stinging or burning sensation at the injection site.
- ■ Monitor any area of extravasation closely for 3–4 wk. If ulceration begins (usually 1–4 wk after extravasation), a plastic surgeon should be consulted.
- ■ Highly emetogenic and requires premedication with antiemetics.
- ■ Begin a flowchart to establish baseline data. Include temperature, pulse, respiration, BP, body weight, laboratory values, and I&O ratio and pattern.
- ■ Lab tests: Baseline and periodic hepatic function, renal function, CBC with differential throughout therapy.
- ■ Note: The nadir of leukopenia (an expected 1000/mm^3) typically occurs 10–14 days after single dose, with recovery occurring within 21 days.

D

- Evaluate cardiac function (ECG) prior to initiation of therapy, at regular intervals, and at end of therapy.
- Be alert to and report early signs of cardiotoxicity (see Appendix D-1). Acute life-threatening arrhythmias may occur within a few hours of drug administration. Perform frequent cardiac monitoring of children during and following treatment.
- Report promptly objective signs of hepatic dysfunction (jaundice, dark urine, pruritus) or kidney dysfunction (altered I&O ratio and pattern, local discomfort with voiding).
- Promote fastidious oral hygiene, especially before and after meals. Stomatitis, generally maximal in second week of therapy, frequently begins with a burning sensation accompanied by erythema of oral mucosa that may progress to ulceration and dysphagia in 2 or 3 days.
- Report signs of superinfection (see Appendix D-1) promptly; these may result from antibiotic therapy during leukopenic period.
- Avoid rectal medications and use of rectal thermometer; rectal trauma is associated with bloody diarrhea resulting from an antiblastic effect on rapidly growing intestinal mucosal cells.

Patient & Family Education

- Note: Complete loss of hair (reversible) is an expected adverse effect. It may also involve eyelashes and eyebrows, beard and mustache, pubic and axillary hair. Regrowth of hair usually begins 2–3 mo after drug is discontinued.
- May cause photosensitivity; avoid sunlight and uses sunscreen.
- Drug turns urine red for 1–2 days after administration.
- Report signs of infections. Avoid exposure to persons with infectious diseases.
- Keep hands away from eyes to prevent conjunctivitis. Increased tearing for 5–10 days after a single dose is possible.
- Do not breast feed while taking this drug.

DOXYCYCLINE HYCLATE

(dox-i-sye′kleen)

Adoxa, Apo-Doxy ◆ , Doryx, Doxy, Doxy-Caps, Doxychel, Doxycin ◆ , Doxy-Lemmon, Monodox, Novodoxylin ◆ , SK-Doxycycline, Vibramycin, Vibra-Tabs, Vivox

Classifications: ANTI-INFECTIVE; ANTIBIOTIC; TETRACYCLINE
Prototype: Tetracycline
Pregnancy Category: D

AVAILABILITY 50 mg, 100 mg capsules, tablets; 200 mg injection

ACTIONS Semisynthetic broad-spectrum tetracycline antibiotic derived from oxytetracycline. More completely absorbed with effective blood levels maintained for longer periods and excreted more slowly than most other tetracyclines. Thus it requires smaller and less frequent dosing.

THERAPEUTIC EFFECTS Primarily bacteriostatic in effect. Similar in use to tetracycline (e.g., effective against chlamydial and mycoplasmal infections; gonorrhea, syphilis, rickettsia).

USES Similar to those of tetracycline, e.g., chlamydial and mycoplasmal infections; gonorrhea, syphilis in penicillin-allergic patients; rickettsial diseases; acute exacerbations of chronic bronchitis.

UNLABELED USES Treatment of acute PID, leptospirosis, prophylaxis for rape victims, suppression and chemoprophylaxis of chloroquine-resistant *Plasmodium falciparum* malaria, short-term prophylaxis and treatment of travelers' diarrhea caused by enterotoxigenic strains of *Escherichia coli*. Intrapleural administration for malignant pleural effusions.

CONTRAINDICATIONS Sensitivity to any of the tetracyclines; use during period of tooth development including last half of pregnancy (category D), lactation, infants, and children <8 y (causes permanent yellow discoloration of teeth, enamel hypoplasia, and retardation of bone growth).
CAUTIOUS USE Alcoholism.

ROUTE & DOSAGE

Anti-Infective
Child: **PO/IV** >8 y, 4.4 mg/kg in 1–2 doses on day 1, then 2.2–4.4 mg/kg/day in 1–2 divided doses
Adult: **PO/IV** 100 mg q12h on day 1, then 100 mg/day as single dose (max 100 mg q12h)

Gonorrhea
Adult: **PO** 200 mg immediately, followed by 100 mg at bedtime, then 100 mg b.i.d. for 3 days

Primary and Secondary Syphilis
Adult: **PO** 300 mg/day in divided doses for at least 10 days

Travelers' Diarrhea
Adult: **PO** 100 mg/day during risk period (up to 2 wk) beginning day 1 of travel

Acne
Child: **PO** >8 y and >45 kg, 100 mg q12h on day 1, then 100 mg daily; >8 y and <45 kg, 2.2 mg/kg q12h on day 1 then 2.2 mg/kg/day
Adult: **PO** 100 mg q12h on day 1, then 100 mg daily

STORAGE
Store oral and parenteral forms (prior to reconstitution) in tightly covered, light-resistant containers at 15°–30° C (59°–86° F) unless otherwise directed. Refrigerate reconstituted solutions for up to 72 h. After this time, infusion must be completed within 12 h.

ADMINISTRATION

Oral
- Check expiration date. Degradation products of tetracycline are toxic to the kidneys.

D

- Give with food or a full glass milk to minimize nausea without significantly affecting bioavailability of drug (UNLIKE MOST TETRACYCLINES).
- Consult prescriber about ordering the oral suspension for patients who are bedridden or have difficulty swallowing.

Intravenous

PREPARE **Intermittent/Continuous:** Reconstitute by adding 10 mL sterile water for injection, or D5W, NS, LR, D5/LR or other diluent recommended by manufacturer, to each 100 mg of drug. ▪ Further dilute with 100–1000 mL (per 100 mg of drug) of compatible infusion solution to produce concentrations ranging from 0.1 to 1 mg/mL.

ADMINISTER **Intermittent/Continuous:** IV infusion rate will usually be prescribed by physician. ▪ Duration of infusion varies with dose but is usually 1–4 h. ▪ Recommended minimum infusion time for 100 mg of 0.5 mg/mL solution is 1 h. Infusion should be completed within 12 h of dilution. ▪ When diluted with LR or D5/LR, infusion must be completed within 6 h to ensure adequate stability. ▪ Protect all solutions from direct sunlight during infusion.

ADVERSE EFFECTS Special Senses: Interference with color vision. **GI:** Anorexia, *nausea,* vomiting, diarrhea, enterocolitis; esophageal irritation (oral capsule and tablet). **Skin:** Rashes, photosensitivity reaction. **Other:** Thrombophlebitis (IV use), superinfections.

DIAGNOSTIC TEST INTERFERENCE Like other *tetracyclines,* doxycycline may cause false increases in *urinary catecholamines* (fluorometric methods); false decreases in *urinary urobilinogen;* false-negative *urine glucose* with *glucose oxidase methods* (e.g., *Clinistix, TesTape*); parenteral doxycycline (containing ascorbic acid) may cause false-positive determinations using *Benedict's reagent* or *Clinitest.*

INTERACTIONS Drug: ANTACIDS, **iron** preparation, **calcium, magnesium, zinc, kaolin-pectin, sodium bicarbonate** can significantly decrease absorption; effects of both doxycycline and **desmopressin** antagonized; increases **digoxin** absorption, thus increasing risk of **digoxin** toxicity; **methoxyflurane** increases risk of renal failure.

PHARMACOKINETICS Absorption: Completely absorbed from GI tract. **Peak:** 1.5–4 h. **Distribution:** Penetrates eye, prostate, and CSF; crosses placenta; distributed into breast milk. **Metabolism:** Not metabolized. **Elimination:** 20–30% excreted in urine and 20–40% in feces in 48 h. **Half-Life:** 14–24 h.

NURSING IMPLICATIONS

Assessment & Drug Effects

- Report sudden onset of painful or difficult swallowing promptly to physician. Doxycycline (capsule and tablet forms) is associated with a comparatively high incidence of esophagitis.
- Syrup contains sodium metabisulfite, which may cause allergic reactions in susceptible individuals; ask about known allergy to sulfa products before administration.
- Report evidence of superinfections (see Appendix D-1).

Patient & Family Education

- Take capsule or tablet forms with a full glass (240 mL) of water or generous amount appropriate for age to ensure passage into stomach and prevent esophageal ulceration. Avoid taking capsule or tablet within 1 h of lying down or retiring.
- Avoid exposure to direct sunlight and ultraviolet light during and for 4 or 5 days after therapy is terminated to reduce risk of phototoxic reaction. Phototoxic reaction appears like an exaggerated sunburn. Sunscreens provide little protection.
- Do not breast feed while taking this drug.
- Store this medication out of reach of children.

DRONABINOL

(droe-nab'i-nol)
Marinol, THC
Classifications: CENTRAL NERVOUS SYSTEM AGENT; ANTIEMETIC; CANNABINOID
Pregnancy Category: B
Controlled Substance: Schedule III

AVAILABILITY 2.5 mg, 5 mg, 10 mg capsules

ACTIONS Synthetic derivative of tetrahydrocannabinol (THC), the principal psychoactive constituent of marijuana (*Cannabis sativa*). Mechanism unclear: Inhibits vomiting through control mechanism in the medulla oblongata, producing potent antiemetic effect; nontherapeutic actions are exactly like those of marijuana. Has complex CNS effect that necessitates close supervision of the patient during drug use. Decreases REM sleep; effect on BP is unpredictable; oral temperature may be decreased, and heart rate may be increased. Risk of drug abuse is high.
THERAPEUTIC EFFECTS Drug produces potent antiemetic effect and is used to treat chemotherapy induced nausea and vomiting.

USES To treat chemotherapy-induced nausea and vomiting in cancer patients who fail to respond to conventional antiemetic therapy. Appetite stimulant for AIDS patients.
UNLABELED USES Glaucoma.

CONTRAINDICATIONS Nausea and vomiting caused by other than chemotherapeutic agents; hypersensitivity to dronabinol or sesame oil; history of substance abuse; use during pregnancy (category B) only if clearly necessary; lactation.
CAUTIOUS USE First exposure, especially in hypertension, cardiovascular disorders; renal disease, epilepsy; psychiatric illness, patient receiving other psychoactive drugs; severe hepatic dysfunction.

ROUTE & DOSAGE

Chemotherapy-induced Nausea

Child/Adult: **PO** 5 mg/m^2 1–3 h before administration of chemotherapy, then q2–4h after chemotherapy for a total of 4–6 doses, dose may be increased by 2.5 mg/m^2 (max 15 mg/m^2/dose if necessary)

Appetite Stimulant
Adult: **PO** 2.5 mg b.i.d., before noon and evening meals

D

STORAGE
Store at 8°–15° C (46°–59° F).

ADMINISTRATION

Oral
- Do not repeat dose following a reaction until patient's mental state has returned to normal and the circumstances have been evaluated.

ADVERSE EFFECTS CNS: *Drowsiness,* psychologic high, dizziness, anxiety, confusion, euphoria, sensory or perceptual difficulties, impaired coordination, depression, irritability, headache, ataxia, memory lapse, paresthesias, paranoia, depersonalization, disorientation, tinnitus, nightmares, speech difficulty, facial flush, diaphoresis. **CV:** Tachycardia, orthostatic hypotension, hypertension, syncope. **GI:** Dry mouth, diarrhea, fecal incontinence. **Other:** Muscular pains.

INTERACTIONS Drug: **Alcohol** and other CNS DEPRESSANTS may exaggerate psychoactive effects of dronabinol; TRICYCLIC ANTIDEPRESSANTS, **atropine** may cause tachycardia.

PHARMACOKINETICS Absorption: Rapidly absorbed from GI tract, with bioavailability of 10–20%. **Peak:** 2–3 h. **Distribution:** Fat soluble; distributed to many organs; distributed into breast milk. **Metabolism:** Metabolized in liver; extensive first-pass metabolism. **Elimination:** Excreted principally in bile; 50% excreted in feces within 72 h; 10–15% excreted in urine. **Half-Life:** 25–36 h.

NURSING IMPLICATIONS

Assessment & Drug Effects
- Monitor patients with hypertension or heart disease for BP and cardiac status.
- Response to dronabinol is varied, and previous uneventful use does not guarantee that adverse reactions will not occur. Effects of drug may persist an unpredictably long time (days). Extended use at therapeutic dosage may cause accumulation of toxic amounts of dronabinol and its metabolites.
- Watch for disturbing psychiatric symptoms if dose is increased: Altered mental state, loss of coordination, evidence of a psychologic high (easy laughing, elation and heightened awareness), or depression.
- Note: Abrupt withdrawal are associated with symptoms (within 12 h) of irritability, insomnia, restlessness. Peak intensity occurs at about 24 h: Hot flashes, diaphoresis, rhinorrhea, watery diarrhea, hiccups, anorexia. Usually, syndrome is over in 96 h.

Patient & Family Education
- Do not drive or engage in other potentially hazardous activities that require alertness and judgment because of high incidence of dizziness and drowsiness.

Common adverse effects in *italic;* life-threatening effects <u>underlined</u>; generic names in **bold;** drug classifications in SMALL CAPS; ♣ Canadian drug name; ❷ Prototype drug.

- Understand potential (reversible) for drug-induced mood or behavior changes that may occur during dronabinol use. Report effects on mood as well as desired effect on appetite.
- Do not ingest alcohol during period of systemic dronabinol effect. Effect on blood ethanol levels are complex and unpredictable.
- Do not breast feed while taking this drug.
- Store this medication out of reach of children.

D

DROPERIDOL
(droe-per'i-dole)
Inapsine
Classifications: CENTRAL NERVOUS SYSTEM AGENT; BUTYROPHENONE; ANTIEMETIC
Prototype: Haloperidol
Pregnancy Category: C

AVAILABILITY 2.5 mg/mL injection

ACTIONS Butyrophenone derivative structurally and pharmacologically related to haloperidol. Antagonizes emetic effects of morphine-like analgesics and other drugs that act on chemoreceptor trigger zone. Mild alpha-adrenergic blocking activity and direct vasodilator effect may cause hypotension. Acts primarily at subcortical level to produce sedation.
THERAPEUTIC EFFECTS Sedative property reduces anxiety and motor activity without necessarily inducing sleep; patient remains responsive. Potentiates other CNS depressants. Also has antiemetic properties.

USES To produce tranquilizing effect and to reduce nausea and vomiting during surgical and diagnostic procedures. Also for premedication, during induction, and as adjunct in maintenance of general or regional anesthesia. Principally used in fixed combination with the potent narcotic analgesic fentanyl (Innovar) to produce neuroleptanalgesia (quiescence, reduced motor activity, and indifference to pain and environmental stimuli) to permit carrying out a variety of diagnostic and minor surgical procedures.
UNLABELED USES IV antiemetic in cancer chemotherapy.

CONTRAINDICATIONS Known intolerance to droperidol. Safe use during pregnancy (category C), lactation, or in children <2 y is not established.
CAUTIOUS USE Debilitated, patients; hypotension; liver, kidney, cardiac disease; cardiac bradyarrhythmias.

ROUTE & DOSAGE

Premedication and Antiemetic
Child: **IV/IM** 2–12 y, 0.03–0.07 mg/kg/dose over 2–5 min preoperatively or for emesis; may give up to 0.1–0.15 mg/kg/dose if needed (max 2.5 mg/dose); antiemetic dose can be repeated q3–4h prn

---

Common adverse effects in *italic;* life-threatening effects <u>underlined;</u> generic names in **bold;** drug classifications in SMALL CAPS; ♣ Canadian drug name; ✪ Prototype drug. **495**

D

Adult: **IV/IM** 2.5–5 mg 30–60 min preoperatively or for emesis; additional dose of 1.25 mg may be given if needed for premedication in 15–30 min; antiemetic dose can be repeated q3–4h prn

Maintenance of General Anesthesia

Child: **IV/IM** 2–12 y, 0.088–0.165 mg/kg
Adult: **IV/IM** *Induction,* 0.22–0.275 mg/kg; *Maintenance,* 1.25–2.5 mg

STORAGE
Store at 15°–30° C (59°–86° F), unless otherwise directed by manufacturer. Protect from light.

ADMINISTRATION

Intramuscular
■ Give deep IM into a large muscle appropriate for age (see Part I).

Intravenous
IV administration to infants and children: Verify correct rate of IV injection with physician.
PREPARE **Direct:** Give undiluted.
ADMINISTER **Direct:** Give at a rate of 10 mg or fraction thereof over 30–60 sec.
INCOMPATIBILITIES **Solution/Additive: Fluorouracil, furosemide, heparin, leucovorin, methotrexate, pentobarbital. Y-Site: Fluorouracil, furosemide, heparin, leucovorin, methotrexate, nafcillin.**

ADVERSE EFFECTS CNS: *Postoperative drowsiness, extrapyramidal symptoms:* Dystonia, akathisia, oculogyric crisis; dizziness, restlessness, anxiety, hallucinations, mental depression. **CV:** *Hypotension, tachycardia,* irregular heartbeats *(prolonged QTc interval even at low doses).* **Other:** Chills, shivering, <u>laryngospasm, bronchospasm</u>.

PHARMACOKINETICS Onset: 3–10 min. **Peak:** 30 min. **Duration:** 2–4 h; may persist up to 12 h. **Distribution:** Crosses placenta. **Metabolism:** Metabolized in liver. **Elimination:** Excreted in urine and feces.

NURSING IMPLICATIONS

Assessment & Drug Effects
■ Monitor ECG throughout therapy. Report immediately prolongation of QTc interval.
■ Monitor vital signs closely. Hypotension and tachycardia are common adverse effects.
■ Exercise care in moving medicated patients because of possibility of severe orthostatic hypotension. Avoid abrupt changes in position.
■ Observe patients for signs of impending respiratory depression carefully when receiving a concurrent narcotic analgesic carefully.
■ Note: EEG patterns are slow to return to normal during the postoperative period. Can lower seizure threshold; monitor children with history of seizures carefully.

- Observe carefully and report promptly to physician early signs of acute dystonia: Facial grimacing, restlessness, tremors, torticollis, oculogyric crisis. Extrapyramidal symptoms may occur within 24–48 h postoperatively.
- Note: Droperidol may aggravate symptoms of acute depression.

D

Patient & Family Education
- Do not breast feed while taking this drug without consulting physician.

DYPHYLLINE
(dye'fi-lin)
Dilor, Dyflex, Dyline-GG, Lufyllin, Neothylline, Protophylline ♣ , Thylline
Classifications: BRONCHODILATOR; RESPIRATORY SMOOTH MUSCLE RELAXANT; XANTHINE
Prototype: Theophylline
Pregnancy Category: C

AVAILABILITY 200 mg, 400 mg, tablets; 100 mg/15 mL, 160 mg/15 mL elixir; 250 mg/mL injection

ACTIONS Xanthine and derivative of theophylline with which it shares similar pharmacologic effects: bronchodilation, myocardial stimulation, vasodilation, diuresis, and smooth muscle relaxation. Unlike other xanthines, dyphylline is not metabolized to theophylline in body; therefore serum theophylline levels are not useful.
THERAPEUTIC EFFECTS Drug has bronchodilator effects.

USES Acute bronchial asthma and reversible bronchospasm associated with chronic bronchitis and emphysema.

CONTRAINDICATIONS Hypersensitivity to xanthine compounds; apnea in newborns. Safe use during pregnancy (category C) or lactation is not established.
CAUTIOUS USE Severe cardiac disease, hypertension, acute myocardial injury; renal or hepatic dysfunction; glaucoma; hyperthyroidism; peptic ulcer; in children; concomitant administration of other xanthine formulations or other CNS-stimulating drugs.

ROUTE & DOSAGE

Asthma
Child: **PO/IM** ≥6 y, 4.4–6.6 mg/kg/day in divided doses
Adult: **PO** 200–800 mg q6h up to 15 mg/kg q.i.d. **IM** 250–500 mg q6h (max 15 mg/kg q.i.d.)

STORAGE
Store at 15°–30° C (59°–86° F) unless otherwise directed. Protect dyphylline injection from light.

Common adverse effects in *italic;* life-threatening effects <u>underlined</u>; generic names in **bold;** drug classifications in SMALL CAPS; ♣ Canadian drug name; ❂ Prototype drug.

497

D

ADMINISTRATION

Oral

- Give oral preparation with a full glass of water or fluid amount appropriate for age on an empty stomach (e.g., 1 h before or 2 h after meals) to enhance absorption. However, administration after meals may help to relieve gastric discomfort.
- Exercise care in the amount of elixir given to children because it has a high alcohol content (18–20%).

Intramuscular

- Aspirate carefully before injecting and inject slowly. Give deep IM into a large muscle appropriate for age (see Part I).
- Do not use parenteral form if a precipitate is present.

ADVERSE EFFECTS CNS: Headache, irritability, restlessness, dizziness, insomnia, light-headedness, muscle twitching, <u>convulsions</u>. **CV:** Palpitation, *tachycardia,* extrasystoles, flushing, hypotension. **GI:** *Nausea,* vomiting, diarrhea, anorexia, epigastric distress. **Respiratory:** Tachypnea. **Other:** Albuminuria, fever, dehydration.

INTERACTIONS Drug: BETA-BLOCKERS may antagonize bronchodilating effects of dyphylline; **halothane** increases risk of cardiac arrhythmias; **probenecid** may decrease dyphylline elimination.

PHARMACOKINETICS Absorption: Readily absorbed from GI tract. **Peak:** 1 h. **Metabolism:** Metabolized in liver (but not to theophylline). **Elimination:** Excreted in urine. **Half-Life:** 2 h.

NURSING IMPLICATIONS

Assessment & Drug Effects

- Lab tests; Baseline and periodic pulmonary function tests to assess therapeutic effectiveness.
- Monitor therapeutic effectiveness; usually occurs at a ***blood level*** of at least 12 mcg/mL.
- Note: Toxic dyphylline plasma levels, although rare with normal dosage, are a risk in patients with a diminished capacity for dyphylline clearance, e.g., those with CHF or hepatic impairment or who are >55 y or <1 y of age.

Patient & Family Education

- Take medication consistently with or without food at the same time each day.
- Notify prescriber of adverse effects: Nausea, vomiting, insomnia, jitteriness, headache, rash, severe GI pain, restlessness, convulsions, or irregular heartbeat.
- Avoid alcohol and also large amounts of coffee and other xanthine-containing beverages (e.g., tea, cocoa, cola) during therapy.
- Ensure that child gets seen for regular health care visits to monitor asthma and drug effects.
- Consult prescriber before taking OTC preparations. Many OTC drugs for coughs, colds, and allergies contain ephedrine or other sympathomimetics and xanthines (e.g., caffeine, theophylline, aminophylline).
- Do not breast feed while taking this drug without consulting physician.
- Store this medication out of reach of children.

Common adverse effects in *italic;* life-threatening effects <u>underlined</u>; generic names in **bold;** drug classifications in SMALL CAPS; ✦ Canadian drug name; ☻ Prototype drug.

ECONAZOLE NITRATE

(e-kone'a-zole)
Ecostatin ♣ , Spectazole
Classifications: ANTI-INFECTIVE; ANTIBIOTIC; ANTIFUNGAL
Prototype: Fluconazole
Pregnancy Category: C

E

AVAILABILITY 1% cream

ACTIONS Synthetic imidazole derivative with broad antifungal spectrum of activity similar to that of miconazole. Exerts fungistatic action but may be fungicidal for certain microorganisms.

THERAPEUTIC EFFECTS Active against dermatophytes (including *Trichophyton mentagrophytes, T. rubrum, T. tonsurans, Epidermophyton floccosum, Microsporum audouinii, M. canis*), yeasts (e.g., *Candida albicans, Pityrosporum obiculare [tinea versicolor]*, and many other genera of fungi). Also appears to be active against some gram-positive bacteria (e.g., *Staphylococcus aureus, Streptococcus pyogenes, Corynebacterium diphtheriae*). Clinical improvement occurs within the first 1–2 wk of therapy.

USES Topically for treatment of *tinea pedis* (athlete's foot or ringworm of foot), *tinea cruris* ("jock itch" or ringworm of groin), *tinea corporis* (ringworm of body), *tinea versicolor,* and *cutaneous candidiasis* (moniliasis).

UNLABELED USES Has been used for topical treatment of erythrasma and with corticosteroids for fungal or bacterial dermatoses associated with inflammation.

CONTRAINDICATIONS Safety during pregnancy (category C) or lactation is not established.

ROUTE & DOSAGE

Tinea Cruris, Tinea Corporis, Tinea Pedis, Cutaneous Candidiasis
Child/Adult: **Topical** Apply sufficient amount and rub into affected areas twice daily, morning and evening

Tinea Versicolor
Adult: **Topical** Apply sufficient amount and rub into affected areas once daily

STORAGE
Store at less than 30° C (86° F) unless otherwise directed.

ADMINISTRATION
Topical
- Cleanse skin with soap and water and dry thoroughly before applying medication (unless otherwise directed by prescriber). Wash hands thoroughly before and after treatments.
- Do not use occlusive dressings unless prescribed by prescriber.

ADVERSE EFFECTS Skin: Burning, stinging sensation, pruritus, erythema.

INTERACTIONS Drug: No clinically significant interactions established.

PHARMACOKINETICS Absorption: Minimal percutaneous absorption through intact skin; increased absorption from denuded skin. **Peak:** 0.5–5 h. **Elimination:** <1% of applied dose is eliminated in urine and feces.

E

NURSING IMPLICATIONS

Patient & Family Education
- Use medication for the prescribed time even if symptoms improve and report to prescriber skin reactions suggestive of irritation or sensitization.
- Notify prescriber if full course of therapy does not result in improvement. Diagnosis should be reevaluated.
- Do not apply the topical cream in or near the eyes or intravaginally.
- Drug has been used safely in children ≥3 mo.
- Do not breast feed while using this drug without consulting prescriber.
- Store this medication out of reach of children.

EDETATE CALCIUM DISODIUM
(ed′e-tate)
Calcium Disodium Versenate, Calcium EDTA
Classification: CHELATING AGENT
Pregnancy Category: C

AVAILABILITY 200 mg/mL injection

ACTIONS Chelating agent that combines with divalent and trivalent metals to form stable, nonionizing soluble complexes that can be readily excreted by kidneys. Action is dependent on ability of heavy metal to displace the less strongly bound calcium in the drug molecule.
THERAPEUTIC EFFECTS Chelating agent that binds with heavy metals such as lead to form a soluble complex that can be excreted through the kidney, thereby ridding the body of the poisonous substance.

USES Principally as adjunct in treatment of acute and chronic lead poisoning (plumbism). Generally used in combination with dimercaprol (BAL) in treatment of lead encephalopathy or when blood lead level exceeds 100 mcg/dL. Also used to diagnose suspected lead poisoning.
UNLABELED USES Treatment of poisoning from other heavy metals such as chromium, manganese, nickel, zinc, and possibly vanadium; removal of radioactive and nuclear fission products such as plutonium, yttrium, uranium. Not effective in poisoning from arsenic, gold, or mercury.

CONTRAINDICATIONS Severe kidney disease, anuria; IV use in patients with lead encephalopathy not generally recommended (because of possible increase in intracranial pressure); pregnancy (category C).
CAUTIOUS USE Kidney dysfunction; active tubercular lesions; history of gout; lactation.

Common adverse effects in *italic;* life-threatening effects <u>underlined;</u> generic names in **bold;** drug classifications in SMALL CAPS; ◆ Canadian drug name; ◎ Prototype drug.

ROUTE & DOSAGE

Diagnosis of Lead Poisoning

Child: **IM** 50 mg/kg (max 1 g), then collect urine for 6–8 h (if mcg lead: mg EDTA ratio in urine is >0.5 or urine lead concentration is >1 mg/L, the test is positive)

Adult: **IV/IM** 500 mg/m² (max 1 g) over 1 h, then collect urine for 24 h (if mcg lead: mg EDTA ratio in urine is >1, the test is positive)

Treatment of Lead Poisoning

Child: For blood level >45 mcg/dL: **IM** 1000 mg/m²/day given in 2 daily doses for 5 days; if blood level remains >45 mcg, begin second 5-day course after a 3-day break. For blood level >80 mcg/dL: IV 1500 mg/m²/day by continuous infusion for 48 h (BAL is also used in combination therapy for these high lead levels). Blood levels after 48 h determine remaining therapy

Adult: **IV** 1–1.5 g/m²/day infused over 8–24 h for up to 5 days **IM** 1–1.5 g/m²/day divided into doses given q8–12h

Lead Nephropathy/Renal Impairment

Adult: **IV** Serum creatinine <2 mg/dL, give 1 g/m²/day; 2–3 mg/dL, give 500 mg/m²/day; 3.1–4 mg/dL, give 400 mg/m² 48 h; >4 mg/dL, give 500 mg/m² once/wk. Infuse over 8–24 h for 5 days, may repeat monthly until lead excretion is reduced toward normal; Child: doses reduced in renal impairment

STORAGE

Store at room temperature of 15°–30° C (59°–86° F).

ADMINISTRATION

- Note: Calcium disodium edetate can produce potentially fatal effects when higher than recommended doses are used or when it is continued after toxic effects appear.
- Use CaNa₂ EDTA, not Na₂ EDTA, which can cause tetany and life-threatening hypocalcemia.

Intramuscular

- IM route preferred for symptomatic children and recommended for patients with incipient or overt lead-induced encephalopathy. See Part I for appropriate muscle selection in children.
- Add 0.5% Procaine HCl or EMLA to minimize pain at injection site (usually 1 mL of procaine 1% to each 1 mL of concentrated drug). Consult prescriber.
- Use separate injection sites when dimercaprol (BAL) and calcium EDTA are given concurrently.

Intravenous

PREPARE **IV Infusion:** Dilute the 5-mL ampule with 250–500 mL of NS or D5W.

ADMINISTER **IV Infusion:** Warning: Rapid IV infusion may be LETHAL by suddenly increasing intracranial pressure in patients who already have cerebral edema. Manufacturer recommends total daily dose over 8–12 h. Some clinicians recommend infusing over 1–2 h. Consult prescriber for specific rate.

Common adverse effects in *italic*; life-threatening effects underlined; generic names in **bold**; drug classifications in SMALL CAPS; ✦ Canadian drug name; ○ Prototype drug.

501

INCOMPATIBILITIES **Solution/Additive: Amphotericin B, hydralazine, Ringer's lactate.**

ADVERSE EFFECTS CV: Hypotension, thrombophlebitis. **GI:** Anorexia, nausea, vomiting, diarrhea, abdominal cramps, cheilosis. **Hematologic:** Transient bone marrow depression, depletion of blood metals. **Urogenital:** Nephrotoxicity (renal tubular necrosis), proteinuria, hematuria. **Body as a Whole:** *Febrile reaction* (excessive thirst, fever, chills, severe myalgia, arthralgia, GI distress), hypocalcemia *histamine-like reactions* (flushing, throbbing headache, sweating, sneezing, nasal congestion, lacrimation, postural hypotension, tachycardia, zinc and copper deficiency).

DIAGNOSTIC TEST INTERFERENCE Edetate calcium disodium may decrease *serum cholesterol, plasma lipid* levels (if elevated), and *serum potassium* values. *Glycosuria* may occur with toxic doses.

INTERACTIONS Drug: No clinically significant interactions established.

PHARMACOKINETICS Absorption: Well absorbed IM. **Onset:** 1 h. **Peak:** Peak chelation 24–48 h. **Distribution:** Distributed to extracellular fluid; does not enter CSF. **Metabolism:** Not metabolized. **Elimination:** Chelated lead excreted in urine; 50% excreted in 1 h. **Half-Life:** 20–60 min IV, 90 min IM.

NURSING IMPLICATIONS

Assessment & Drug Effects
- If given as a continuous infusion, stop the infusion for 1 h before drawing blood for lead concentration to avoid a falsely elevated value.
- Determine adequacy of urinary output prior to therapy. This may be done by administering IV fluids before giving first dose.
- Increase fluid intake to enhance urinary excretion of chelates. Avoid excess fluid intake, however, in patients with lead encephalopathy because of the danger of further increasing intracranial pressure. Consult prescriber regarding allowable intake.
- Monitor I&O. Because drug is excreted almost exclusively via kidneys, toxicity may develop if output is inadequate. Stop therapy if urine flow is markedly diminished or absent. Report any change in output or I&O ratio to physician.
- Lab tests: Obtain serum creatinine, calcium, and phosphorus before and during each course of therapy. Monitor baseline and frequent BUN levels and ECG during therapy. With prolonged therapy determine periodic determinations of blood trace element metals (e.g., copper, zinc, magnesium).
- Be alert for occurrence of febrile reaction that may appear 4–8 h after drug infusion (see ADVERSE EFFECTS).

Patient & Family Education
- Discuss with family the sources of lead exposure for the child. Assist them to plan for a safe environment whether poisoning is due to acute or chronic ingestion. Hospital, public health, and community nurses partner to prevent cases of lead poisoning.
- Do not breast feed while taking this drug without consulting physician.

EDROPHONIUM CHLORIDE

(ed-roe-foe′nee-um)

Enlon, Reversol, Tensilon

Classifications: AUTONOMIC NERVOUS SYSTEM AGENT; CHOLINERGIC (PARASYMPATHOMIMETIC) CHOLINESTERASE INHIBITOR

Prototype: Neostigmine

Pregnancy Category: C

E

AVAILABILITY 10 mg/mL injection

ACTIONS Indirect-acting cholinesterase inhibitor similar to neostigmine that is rapidly reversible. Acts as antidote to curariform drugs by displacing them from muscle cell receptor sites, thus permitting resumption of normal transmission of neuromuscular impulses. Like neostigmine, it prolongs skeletal muscle relaxant action of succinylcholine chloride and decamethonium bromide

THERAPEUTIC EFFECTS Acts as antidote to curariform drugs by displacing them from muscle cell receptor sites, thus permitting resumption of normal transmission of neuromuscular impulses.

USES Differential diagnosis and as adjunct in evaluation of treatment requirements of myasthenia gravis, for differentiating myasthenic from cholinergic crisis, and to reverse neuromuscular blockade produced by overdosage of nondepolarizing skeletal muscle relaxants, e.g., tubocurarine, gallamine. Not recommended for maintenance therapy in myasthenia gravis because of its short duration of action.

UNLABELED USES To terminate paroxysmal atrial tachycardia, as an aid in diagnosing supraventricular tachyarrhythmias, and to evaluate function of demand pacemakers.

CONTRAINDICATIONS Hypersensitivity to anticholinesterase agents; intestinal and urinary obstruction. Safety during pregnancy (category C) or lactation is not established.

CAUTIOUS USE Bronchial asthma; cardiac arrhythmias; patients receiving digitalis.

ROUTE & DOSAGE

Edrophonium Test for Myasthenia Gravis

Newborn: 0.1 mg single dose
Infant and Child: **IV** 0.04 mg/kg/dose one time (max for child <34 kg, 1 mg; for child ≥34 kg, 2 mg); if no response in 1 min, may give 0.16 mg/kg (max total dose for child <34 kg, 5 mg; for child >34 kg, 10 mg)
Adult: **IV** Prepare 10 mg in a syringe; inject 2 mg over 15–30 sec, if no reaction after 45 sec, inject the remaining 8 mg, may repeat test after 30 min **IM** Inject 10 mg, if cholinergic reaction occurs, retest after 30 min with 2 mg to rule out false-negative reaction

Evaluation of Myasthenia Treatment

Adult: **IV** 1–2 mg administered 1 h after last PO dose of anticholinesterase medication

---

Curare Antagonist

Adult: IV 10 mg administered over 30–45 sec, may repeat q5–10min as needed up to 40 mg

STORAGE
Store at 15°–30° C (59°–86° F).

E

ADMINISTRATION
Note: Have antidote (atropine sulfate) immediately available and facilities for endotracheal intubation, tracheostomy, suction, assisted respiration, and cardiac monitoring for treatment of cholinergic reaction.

Intravenous

PREPARE **Direct:** May be given undiluted.
ADMINISTER **Direct:** USE for diagnosis of MG: Inject initial amount as described in dosage over 15–30 sec; if no reaction after 45 sec, inject additional amounts. If cholinergic reaction (increased muscle weakness) is obtained after initial 1 or 2 mg, discontinue test and give atropine IV (as ordered).

ADVERSE EFFECTS Body as a Whole: Severe adverse effects uncommon with usual doses. **CNS:** Weakness, muscle cramps, dysphoria, fasciculations, incoordination, dysarthria, dysphagia, convulsions, <u>respiratory paralysis</u>. **CV:** Bradycardia, irregular pulse, hypotension, prolonged QT interval, pulmonary edema. **Special Senses:** Miosis, blurred vision, diplopia, lacrimation. **GI:** Diarrhea, abdominal cramps, nausea, vomiting, excessive salivation. **Respiratory:** Increased bronchial secretions, <u>bronchospasm, laryngospasm</u>, pulmonary edema. **Other:** Excessive sweating, urinary frequency, incontinence, lowered seizure threshhold.

INTERACTIONS Drug: Procainamide, quinidine may antagonize the effects of edrophonium; DIGITALIS GLYCOSIDES increase the sensitivity of the heart to edrophonium; **succinylcholine, decamethonium** may prolong neuromuscular blockade.

PHARMACOKINETICS Onset: 30–60 sec IV; 2–10 min IM. **Duration:** 5–10 min IV; 5–30 min IM.

NURSING IMPLICATIONS

Assessment & Drug Effects

- Monitor vital signs. Observe for signs of respiratory distress, bradycardia, hypotension, and cardiac arrest.
- Edrophonium test for myasthenia gravis: All cholinesterase inhibitors (anticholinesterases) should be discontinued for at least 8 h before test. Positive response to edrophonium test consists of brief improvement in muscle strength unaccompanied by lingual or skeletal muscle fasciculations.
- Evaluation of myasthenic treatment: *Myasthenic response* (immediate subjective improvement with increased muscle strength, absence of fasciculations; generally indicates that patient requires larger dose of anticholinesterase agent or longer-acting drug); *cholinergic response*

Common adverse effects in *italic;* life-threatening effects <u>underlined</u>; generic names in **bold;** drug classifications in SMALL CAPS; ♣ Canadian drug name; ☻ Prototype drug.

muscarinic adverse effects (lacrimation, diaphoresis, salivation, abdominal cramps, diarrhea, nausea, vomiting; accompanied by decrease in muscle strength; usually indicates overtreatment with cholinesterase inhibitor); *adequate response* (no change in muscle strength; fasciculations may be present or absent; minimal cholinergic adverse effects (observed in patients at or near optimal dosage level).

Patient & Family Education
■ Do not breast feed while taking this drug without consulting physician.

E

EFAVIRENZ

(e-fa′vi-renz)
Sustiva
Classifications: ANTI-INFECTIVE; ANTIVIRAL; NONNUCLEOSIDE REVERSE TRANSCRIPTASE INHIBITOR (NNRTI)
Prototype: Nevirapine
Pregnancy Category: C

AVAILABILITY 50 mg, 100 mg, 200 mg capsules; 300 mg, 600 mg tablets

ACTIONS Nonnucleoside reverse transcriptase inhibitor (NNRTI) of HIV-1. Binds directly to reverse transcriptase and blocks RNA polymerase activities.
THERAPEUTIC EFFECTS Prevents replication of the HIV-1 virus. HIV-2 reverse transcriptase and DNA polymerases alpha, beta, gamma, and delta are not inhibited by efavirenz. Resistant strains appear rapidly. Effectiveness indicated by reduction in viral load (plasma HIV RNA).

USES HIV-1 infection in combination with other antiretroviral agents.

CONTRAINDICATIONS Hypersensitivity to efavirenz; pregnancy (category C), lactation.
CAUTIOUS USE Liver disease, CNS disorders. Safety and efficacy in children <3 y old or who weigh <13 kg (29 lb) are not known.

ROUTE & DOSAGE

HIV Infection
Child: **PO** ≥3 y, 10–15 kg, 200 mg daily; *15–20 kg,* 250 mg daily; *20–25 kg,* 300 mg daily; *25–32.5 kg,* 350 mg daily; *32.5–40 kg,* 400 mg daily; *>40 kg,* 600 mg daily.
Adult: **PO** 600 mg daily

STORAGE
Store at 15°–30° C (59°–86° F) in a tightly closed container and protect from light.

ADMINISTRATION
Oral
■ Use bedtime dosing to increase tolerability of CNS adverse effects.

Common adverse effects in *italic;* life-threatening effects underlined; generic names in **bold;** drug classifications in SMALL CAPS; ✦ Canadian drug name; ❷ Prototype drug.

505

▪ Give exactly as ordered. Do not skip a dose or discontinue therapy without consulting the physician. Can be given with or without food; high fat meal increases absorption.

ADVERSE EFFECTS Body as a Whole: Fatigue, fever. **CNS:** Dizziness, headache, hypoesthesia, impaired concentration, insomnia, abnormal dreams, nightmares, somnolence, depression, nervousness. **CV:** Hyper-cholesterolemia. **GI:** *Nausea,* vomiting, *diarrhea,* dyspepsia, abdominal pain, flatulence, anorexia, increased liver function tests (ALT, AST). **Respiratory:** Cough. **Skin:** *Rash* (erythematous rash, pruritus, *maculopapular rash,* <u>erythema multiforme, Stevens–Johnson syndrome, toxic epidermal necrolysis</u>), increased sweating. **Urogenital:** Renal calculus, hematuria.

DIAGNOSTIC TEST INTERFERENCE False-positive urine tests for **marijuana.**

INTERACTIONS Drug: Inhibits CYP450 enzymes so drugs metabolized by that enzyme will exhibit increased serum levels. Decreased concentrations of **clarithromycin, indinavir, nelfinavir, saquinavir;** increased concentrations of **azithromycin, ethinyl estradiol, ritonavir.** Efavirenz levels are increased by **fluconazole, ritonavir** and decreased by **saquinavir, rifampin.** Additional drugs not recommended for administration with efavirenz include **astemizole, midazolam, triazolam, cisapride,** ERGOT DERIVATIVES, **warfarin. Herbal: St. John's wort** may decrease antiretroviral activity.

PHARMACOKINETICS Peak: 5 h; steady-state 6–10 days. **Distribution:** 99% protein bound. **Metabolism:** Metabolized in liver by cytochrome P450 3A4 and 2B6; can induce (increase) its own metabolism. **Elimination:** 14–34% excreted in urine, 16–61% excreted in feces. **Half-Life:** 52–76 h after single dose, 40–55 h after multiple doses.

NURSING IMPLICATIONS

Assessment & Drug Effects

▪ Monitor GI status and evaluate ability to maintain a normal diet.
▪ Monitor for other side effects. Sever rash with blistering, desquamation, mucosal sores, and fever may necessitate discontinuation of the drug.
▪ Lab tests: Periodic liver functions and lipid profile.

Patient & Family Education

▪ The family will need assistance to plan for the complex medication regimes necessitated. Financial, emotional, and other concerns need to be addressed.
▪ Contact physician promptly if any of the following occur: Skin rash, delusions, inappropriate behavior, thoughts of suicide.
▪ Use or add barrier contraception if using hormonal contraceptive.
▪ Notify physician immediately if you become pregnant.
▪ Do not drive or engage in potentially hazardous activities until response to the drug is known. Dizziness, impaired concentration, and drowsiness usually improve with continued therapy.
▪ Do not breast feed while taking this drug.
▪ Store this medication out of reach of children.

EMLA (EUTECTIC MIXTURE OF LIDOCAINE AND PRILOCAINE)
EMLA cream
Classifications: CENTRAL NERVOUS SYSTEM AGENT; LOCAL ANESTHETIC
Prototype: Procaine
Pregnancy Category: B

E

AVAILABILITY 2.5% lidocaine/2.5% prilocaine cream

ACTIONS EMLA cream is a mixture of lidocaine and prilocaine. The mixture forms a liquid at room temperature. Concentration of anesthetic in liquid versus an emulsifier is 80% versus 20%.
THERAPEUTIC EFFECTS EMLA is a topical analgesic.

USES Topical anesthetic on normal intact skin for local anesthesia.
UNLABELED USES Topical anesthetic prior to leg ulcer debridement; treatment of post-herpetic neuralgia.

CONTRAINDICATIONS Patients with known sensitivity to local anesthetics; patients with congenital or idiopathy methemoglobinemia.
CAUTIOUS USE Acutely ill, debilitated, patients; in G6PD deficiency, severe liver or renal disease; pregnancy (category B), lactation; children <7 y of age.

ROUTE & DOSAGE

Topical Anesthetic
Child/Adult: **Topical** *> 1 mo,* apply 2.5 g of cream (½ of 5-g tube) over 20–25 cm² of skin, cover with occlusive dressing and wait at least 1 h, then remove dressing and wipe off cream, cleanse area with an antiseptic solution and prepare patient for the procedure

STORAGE
Store at 15°–30° C (59°–86° F).

ADMINISTRATION
Topical
- Apply a thick layer to skin (approximately ½ of 5-g tube per 20–25 cm² or 2 × 2 inches) at site of procedure. Apply an occlusive dressing. Do not spread out cream. Seal edges of dressing well to avoid leakage.
- Apply EMLA cream 1 h before routine procedure and 2 h before painful procedure.
- Remove EMLA cream prior to skin puncture and clean area with an aseptic solution.

ADVERSE EFFECTS Hematologic: Methemoglobinemia, especially in infants, small children, and patients with G6PD deficiency. **Skin:** *Blanching and redness,* itching, heat sensation. **Body as a Whole:** Edema, soreness, aching, numbness, heaviness. **Other:** The adverse effects of lidocaine could occur with large doses or if there is significant systemic absorption.

INTERACTIONS Drug: may cause additive toxicity with CLASS I ANTIAR-RHYTHMICS; may increase risk of developing methemoglobin when used with **acetaminophen, chloroquine, dapsone, fosphenytoin,** NITRATES and NITRITES, **nitric oxide, nitrofurantoin, nitroprusside, pamaquine, phenobarbital, phenytoin, primaquine, quinine,** or SULFONAMIDES.

PHARMACOKINETICS Absorption: Penetrates intact skin. **Onset:** 15–60 min. **Peak:** 2–3 h. **Duration:** 1–2 h after removal of cream. **Distribution:** Crosses blood–brain barrier and placenta, distributed into breast milk. **Metabolism:** Metabolized in liver. **Elimination:** 98% of absorbed dose is excreted in urine. **Half-Life:** 60–150 min.

NURSING IMPLICATIONS

Assessment & Drug Effects

- Monitor for local skin reactions including erythema, edema, itching, abnormal temperature sensations, and rash. These reactions are very common and usually disappear in 1–2 h.
- Note: Patients taking Class 1 antiarrhythmic drugs may experience toxic effects on the cardiovascular system. EMLA should be used with caution in these patients.
- Wash immediately with water or saline if contact with the eye occurs; protect the eye until sensation returns.

Patient & Family Education

- If parent applies drug at home prior to coming with child for care, instruct in correct administration.
- Skin analgesia lasts for 1 h following removal of the occlusive dressing. Analgesia may be accompanied by temporary loss of all sensation in the treated skin. Advise caution until sensation returns.
- Do not breast feed while using this drug without consulting prescriber.
- Store this medication out of reach of children.

ENALAPRIL MALEATE
(e-nal'a-pril)
Vasotec

ENALAPRILAT
Vasotec I. V.
Classifications: CARDIOVASCULAR AGENT; ANGIOTENSIN-CONVERTING ENZYME (ACE) INHIBITOR; ANTIHYPERTENSIVE
Prototype: Captopril
Pregnancy Category: D

AVAILABILITY 2.5 mg, 5 mg, 10 mg, 20 mg tablets; 1.25 mg/mL injection; 1 mg/mL suspension

ACTIONS Angiotensin-converting enzyme (ACE) inhibitor. ACE catalyzes the conversion of angiotensin I to angiotensin II, a vasoconstrictor substance. Therefore, inhibition of ACE decreases angiotensin II levels, which decreases vasopressor activity and aldosterone secretion. Both actions achieve an antihypertensive effect by suppression of the renin–angiotensin–aldosterone system. ACE inhibitors also reduce peripheral arterial resistance (afterload), pulmonary capillary wedge pressure (PCWP), a measure of preload, pulmonary vascular resistance, and improve cardiac output as well as exercise tolerance.
THERAPEUTIC EFFECTS Antihypertensive effect related to suppression of the renin–angiotensin–aldosterone system causes vasodilation and, therefore, lower blood pressure. Improvement in cardiac output results in increased exercise tolerance.

USES Management of mild to moderate hypertension as monotherapy or with a diuretic. Malignant, refractory, accelerated, and renovascular hypertension (except in bilateral renal artery stenosis or renal artery stenosis in a solitary kidney), CHF.
UNLABELED USES Hypertension or renal crisis in scleroderma.

CONTRAINDICATIONS Hypersensitivity to enalapril or captopril. There has been evidence of fetotoxicity and kidney damage in newborns exposed to ACE inhibitors during pregnancy (category D). Safety during lactation or in children is not established.
CAUTIOUS USE Renal impairment, renal artery stenosis; patients with hypovolemia, receiving diuretics, undergoing dialysis; patients in whom excessive hypotension would present a hazard (e.g., cerebrovascular insufficiency); CHF; hepatic impairment; diabetes mellitus.

ROUTE & DOSAGE

Hypertension
Neonate: **PO** 0.1 mg/kg q24h **IV** 5–10 mcg/kg q8–24h
Child: **PO** 0.08 mg/kg/day in 1–2 divided doses, may increase (max 0.5 mg/kg/day) **IV** 5–10 mcg/kg q8–24h
Adult: **PO** 5 mg/day, may increase to 10–40 mg/day in 1–2 divided doses **IV** 1.25 q6h, may give up to 5 mg q6h in hypertensive emergencies

Congestive Heart Failure
Adult: **PO** 2.5 mg 1–2 times/day, may increase up to 5–20 mg/day in 1–2 divided doses (max 40 mg/day)

STORAGE
Store tablets at 30° C (86° F); Protect from heat and light. Expiration date: 30 mo following date of manufacture if stored at <30° C.

ADMINISTRATION
Oral
- Discontinue diuretics, if possible, for 2–3 days prior to initial oral dose to reduce incidence of hypotension. If the diuretic cannot be discontinued, give initial dose of enalapril may be lowered. Keep patient under medical supervision for at least 2 h and until BP has stabilized for at least an additional hour.

- Give with food or drink of child's choice.
- Conversion from IV to oral therapy: Recommended initial dose is 5 mg once a day with a creatinine clearance of (Cl_{cr}) >30 mL/min, and 2.5 mg once daily with a Cl_{cr} <30 mL/min.

Intravenous

E Note: Verify correct IV concentration and rate of infusion/injection with physician for neonates, infants, children.
PREPARE **Direct:** Give undiluted. **Intermittent:** Dilute in 50 mL of D5W, NS, D5/NS, D5/LR.
ADMINISTER **Direct/Intermittent:** Give direct IV slowly over at least 5 min through a port of a free flowing infusion of D5W or NS or as an infusion over 5 min.
INCOMPATIBILITIES **Y-Site: Amphotericin B, amphotericin B cholesteryl, cefepime, phenytoin.**

ADVERSE EFFECTS CNS: *Headache, dizziness,* fatigue, nervousness, paresthesias, asthenia, insomnia, somnolence. **CV:** *Hypotension including postural hypotension;* syncope, palpitations, chest pain. **GI:** Diarrhea, nausea, abdominal pain, loss of taste, dyspepsia. **Hematologic:** Decreased Hgb and Hct. **Urogenital:** <u>Acute kidney failure</u>, deterioration in kidney function. **Skin:** Pruritus with and without *rash,* angioedema, erythema. **Metabolic:** Hyperkalemia. **Respiratory:** Cough.

INTERACTIONS Drug: Indomethacin and other NSAIDS may decrease antihypertensive activity; POTASSIUM SUPPLEMENTS, POTASSIUM-SPARING DIURETICS may cause hyperkalemia; may increase **lithium** levels and toxicity.

PHARMACOKINETICS Absorption: 70% absorbed from GI tract. **Onset:** 1 h PO; 15 min IV. **Peak:** 4–8 h PO; 4 h IV. **Duration:** 12–24 h PO; 6 h IV. **Distribution:** Limited amount crosses blood–brain barrier; crosses placenta. **Metabolism:** Oral dose undergoes first-pass metabolism in liver to active form, enalaprilat. **Elimination:** 60% excreted in urine, 33% in feces within 24 h. **Half-Life:** 2 h.

NURSING IMPLICATIONS

Assessment & Drug Effects

- Monitor for therapeutic effectiveness. Peak effects after the first IV dose may not occur for up to 4 h; peak effects of subsequent doses may exceed those of the first.
- Maintain bed rest and monitor BP for the first 3 h after the initial IV dose. First-dose phenomenon (i.e., a sudden exaggerated hypotensive response) may occur within 1–3 h of first IV dose, especially in the patient with very high blood pressure or one on a diuretic and controlled salt intake regimen. An IV infusion of normal saline for volume expansion may be ordered to counteract the hypotensive response. This initial response is not an indicator to stop therapy.
- Monitor BP for first several days of therapy. If antihypertensive effect is diminished before 24 h, the total dose may be given as 2 divided doses.
- Report transient hypotension with lightheadedness. Supervise ambulation until BP has stabilized.

- Lab tests: Monitor serum potassium and be alert to symptoms of hyperkalemia (K^+ >5.7 mEq/L). Patients who have diabetes, impaired kidney function, or CHF are at risk of developing hyperkalemia during enalapril treatment. Monitor kidney function closely during first few weeks of therapy.

Patient & Family Education

- Full antihypertensive effect may not be experienced until several weeks after enalapril therapy starts.
- When drug is discontinued due to severe hypotension, the hypotensive effect may persist a week or longer after termination because of long duration of drug action.
- Do not follow a low-sodium diet (e.g., low-sodium foods or low-sodium milk) without approval from physician.
- Avoid use of salt substitute (principal ingredient: potassium salt) and potassium supplements because of the potential for hyperkalemia.
- Notify physician of a persistent nonproductive cough, especially at night, accompanied by nasal congestion.
- Report to physician promptly if swelling of face, eyelids, tongue, lips, or extremities occurs. Angioedema is a rare adverse effect and, if accompanied by laryngeal edema, may be fatal.
- Do not drive or engage in other potentially hazardous activities until response to drug is known.
- Do not breast feed while taking this drug without consulting physician.
- Store this medication out of reach of children.

EPHEDRINE HYDROCHLORIDE

(e-fed′rin)
Efedron

EPHEDRINE SULFATE

Ectasule, Ephedsol, Vatronol

Classifications: AUTONOMIC NERVOUS SYSTEM AGENT; ALPHA- AND BETA-ADRENERGIC AGONIST (SYMPATHOMIMETIC); BRONCHODILATOR
Prototype: Epinephrine HCl
Pregnancy Category: C

AVAILABILITY 25 mg, capsules; 50 mg/mL injection; 0.25% nasal spray; 1% nasal gel

ACTIONS Both indirect- and direct-acting sympathomimetic amine. Thought to act indirectly by releasing tissue stores of norepinephrine and directly by stimulation of alpha-, beta$_1$-, and beta$_2$-adrenergic receptors.

THERAPEUTIC EFFECTS Like epinephrine, contracts dilated arterioles of nasal mucosa, thus reducing engorgement and edema and facilitating ventilation and drainage. Local application to eye produces mydriasis without loss of light reflexes or accommodation or change in intraocular pressure (IOP).

USES Temporary relief of congestion of hay fever, allergic rhinitis, and sinusitis; and in treatment and prophylaxis of mild cases of acute asthma

Common adverse effects in *italic;* life-threatening effects <u>underlined</u>; generic names in **bold;** drug classifications in SMALL CAPS; ✦ Canadian drug name; ⊘ Prototype drug.

511

and in patients with chronic asthma requiring continuing treatment. Also has been used for its CNS stimulant actions in treatment of narcolepsy, to improve respiration in narcotic and barbiturate poisoning, to combat hypotensive states, especially those associated with spinal anesthesia; in management of enuresis or impaired bladder control; as adjunct in treatment of myasthenia gravis; as mydriatic; to relieve dysmenorrhea; and for temporary support of ventricular rate in Adams-Stokes syndrome; for peripheral edema secondary to type 1 diabetic neuropathy.

CONTRAINDICATIONS History of hypersensitivity to ephedrine or other sympathomimetics; narrow-angle glaucoma; pregnancy (category C), lactation.

CAUTIOUS USE Exercise extreme caution if used at all in hypertension, arteriosclerosis, angina pectoris, coronary insufficiency, chronic heart disease; diabetes mellitus; hyperthyroidism; prostatic hypertrophy.

ROUTE & DOSAGE

Bronchodilator, Nasal Decongestant

Child: **PO** >2 y, 2–3 mg/kg/day in 4–6 divided doses; 6–12 y, 6.25–12.5 mg q4h (max 75 mg/24 h)
Adult: **PO** 25–50 mg q3–4h prn (max 150 mg/24 h) **IM/IV/SC** 12.5–25 mg

Hypotension

Child: **PO/IM/SC/IV** 3 mg/kg/day in 4–6 divided doses (max 75 mg/24 h)
Adult: **PO** 25 mg 1–4 times/day (max 150 mg/24 h) **IM/SC/IV** 10–50 mg IM/SC or 10–25 mg slow IV, may repeat in 5–10 min if necessary (max 150 mg/24 h)

Myasthenia Gravis

Adult: **PO** 25 mg t.i.d. or q.i.d.

Enuresis

Adult: **PO** 25 mg at bedtime

Nasal Decongestant

Adult: **Intranasal** 2–4 drops or a small amount of jelly in each nostril no more than q.i.d. for 3–4 consecutive days

STORAGE

Store at 15°–30° C (59°–86° F) in tightly closed, light-resistant containers unless otherwise directed by the manufacturer.

ADMINISTRATION

Oral

- Administer last dose a few hours before bedtime, if possible, to minimize insomnia.

Intranasal

- Have patient clear nose before instilling drops. Instruct patient to blow gently with both nostrils open. Generally, nose drops are instilled with head in lateral, head-low position to avoid entry of drug into throat. See Part I.

Common adverse effects in *italic;* life-threatening effects underlined; generic names in **bold;** drug classifications in SMALL CAPS; ✦ Canadian drug name; ◯ Prototype drug.

Intravenous

PREPARE **Direct:** Give undiluted.

ADMINISTER **Direct:** Direct IV at a rate of 10 mg or fraction thereof over 30–60 sec.

INCOMPATIBILITIES **Solution/Additive: Hydrocortisone, pentobarbital, phenobarbital, secobarbital, thiopental. Y-Site: Thiopental.**

E

ADVERSE EFFECTS CNS: Headache, insomnia, *nervousness,* anxiety, tremulousness, giddiness. **CV:** Palpitation, tachycardia, precordial pain, cardiac arrhythmias. **GU:** Difficult or painful urination, acute urinary retention (especially older men with prostatism). **GI:** Nausea, vomiting, anorexia. **Body as a Whole:** Sweating, thirst. Overdosage: Euphoria, confusion, delirium, convulsions, pyrexia, hypertension, rebound hypotension, respiratory difficulty. **Skin:** Fixed-drug eruption. Topical use: *Burning, stinging,* dryness of nasal mucosa, sneezing, rebound congestion.

DIAGNOSTIC TEST INTERFERENCE Ephedrine is generally withdrawn at least 12 h before *sensitivity tests* are made to prevent false-positive reactions.

INTERACTIONS Drug: MAO INHIBITORS, TRICYCLIC ANTIDEPRESSANTS, **furazolidone, guanethidine** may increase alpha-adrenergic effects (headache, hyperpyrexia, hypertension); **sodium bicarbonate** decreases renal elimination of ephedrine, increasing its CNS effects; **epinephrine, norepinephrine** compound sympathomimetic effects; effects of ALPHA- and BETA-BLOCKERS and ephedrine antagonized.

PHARMACOKINETICS Absorption: Readily absorbed from GI tract. **Peak:** 15 min–1 h. **Duration:** Bronchodilation 2–4 h; cardiac & pressor effects up to 4 h PO and 1 h IV. **Distribution:** Widely distributed; crosses blood–brain barrier and placenta; distributed into breast milk. **Metabolism:** Small amounts metabolized in liver. **Elimination:** Excreted in urine. **Half-Life:** 3–6 h.

NURSING IMPLICATIONS

Assessment & Drug Effects

- Supervise continuously patients receiving ephedrine IV. Take baseline BP and other vital signs. Check BP repeatedly during first 5 min, then q3–5min until stabilized.
- Monitor I&O ratio and pattern. Encourage patient to void before taking medication (SEE ADVERSE EFFECTS).
- Monitor for systemic effects of nose drops that can occur because of excessive dosage from rapid absorption of drug solution through nasal mucosa. This is most likely to occur in older adults.

Patient & Family Education

- Note: Ephedrine is a commonly abused drug. Learn adverse effects and dangers; take medication ONLY as prescribed.
- Do not take OTC medications for coughs, colds, allergies, or asthma unless approved by prescriber. Ephedrine is a common ingredient in these preparations.

- Do not breast feed while taking this drug without consulting prescriber.
- Store this medication out of reach of children.

E

EPINEPHRINE ⊖

(ep-i-ne′frin)

Bronkaid Mist, Epi-E-Zpen, Epinephrine Pediatric, EpiPen Auto-Injector, Primatene Mist Suspension

EPINEPHRINE BITARTRATE

AsthmaHaler, Bronkaid Mist Suspension, Bronitin Mist Suspension, Epitrate, Medihaler-Epi, Primatene Mist Suspension

EPINEPHRINE HYDROCHLORIDE

Adrenalin Chloride, Bronkaid Mistometer, Dysne-Inhal, Epifrin, Glaucon, SusPhrine ♣

EPINEPHRINE, RACEMIC

AsthmaNefrin, Dey-Dose Epinephrine, microNefrin, Vaponefrin ♣

EPINEPHRYL BORATE

(ep-i-ne′frill bor′ate)

Epinal, Eppy/N

Classifications: AUTONOMIC NERVOUS SYSTEM AGENT; ALPHA- AND BETA-ADRENERGIC AGONIST; BRONCHODILATOR

Pregnancy Category: C

AVAILABILITY 1:100, 1:1000, 2.25% solution for inhalation; 0.35 mg, 0.2 mg spray; 1:1000, 1:2000, 1:10,000, 1:100,000 injection; 1:200 suspension; 0.1%, 0.5%, 1%, 2% ophthalmic solution; 0.1% nasal solution

ACTIONS Naturally occurring catecholamine obtained from animal adrenal glands; also prepared synthetically. Acts directly on both alpha and beta receptors; the most potent activator of alpha receptors. Strengthens myocardial contraction; increases systolic but may decrease diastolic blood pressure; increases cardiac rate and cardiac output.

THERAPEUTIC EFFECTS Constricts bronchial arterioles and inhibits histamine release, thus reducing congestion and edema and increasing tidal volume and vital capacity. Relaxes uterine smooth musculature and inhibits uterine contractions. Imitates all actions of sympathetic nervous system except those on arteries of the face and sweat glands.

USES Temporary relief of bronchospasm, acute asthmatic attack, mucosal congestion, hypersensitivity and anaphylactic reactions, syncope due to heart block or carotid sinus hypersensitivity, and to restore cardiac rhythm in cardiac arrest. Ophthalmic preparation is used in management of simple (open-angle) glaucoma, generally as an adjunct to topical miotics and oral carbonic anhydrase inhibitors; also used as ophthalmic decongestant. Relaxes myometrium and inhibits uterine contractions; prolongs action and delays systemic absorption of local and intraspinal anesthetics. Used topically to control superficial bleeding.

Common adverse effects in *italic;* life-threatening effects <u>underlined</u>; generic names in **bold**; drug classifications in SMALL CAPS; ♣ Canadian drug name; ⊖ Prototype drug.

CONTRAINDICATIONS Hypersensitivity to sympathomimetic amines; narrow-angle glaucoma; hemorrhagic, traumatic, or cardiogenic shock; cardiac dilatation, cerebral arteriosclerosis, coronary insufficiency, arrhythmias, organic heart or brain disease; during second stage of labor; for local anesthesia of fingers, toes, ears, nose, genitalia. Safety during pregnancy (category C) or lactation is not established.

CAUTIOUS USE Debilitated patients; prostatic hypertrophy; hypertension; diabetes mellitus; hyperthyroidism; Parkinson's disease; tuberculosis; psychoneurosis; in patients with long-standing bronchial asthma and emphysema with degenerative heart disease; in children <6 y of age.

ROUTE & DOSAGE

Anaphylaxis

Neonate: **IV Intratracheal** 0.01–0.03 mg/kg (0.1–0.3 mL/kg of 1:10,000) q3–5min prn
Child: **SC** 0.01 mL/kg of 1:1000 q10–15min prn **IV** 0.01 mL/kg of 1:1000 q10–15min
Adult: **SC** 0.1–0.5 mL of 1:1000 q10–15min prn **IV** 0.1–0.25 mL of 1:1000 q10–15min

Cardiac Arrest

Child: **IV** 0.01 mg/kg (0.1 mL/kg of 1:10,000) q5min as needed; can be increased up to 0.1 mg/kg if needed **Intracardiac** 0.05–0.1 mg/kg
Adult: **IV** 0.1–1 mg (1–10 mL of 1:10,000) q5min as needed **Intracardiac** 0.1–1 mg

Asthma

Child: **SC** 0.01 mL/kg of 1:1000 q20min–4h **Inhalation** 1 inhalation q4h prn
Adult: **SC** 0.1–0.5 mL of 1:1000 q20min–4h **Inhalation** 1 inhalation q4h prn

Glaucoma

Child/Adult: **Instillation** 1–2 drops 0.25–2% solution daily or b.i.d.

Nasal Hemostasis

Child/Adult: **Instillation** 1–2 drops 0.1% ophthalmic or 0.1% nasal solution

Topical Hemostatic

Child/Adult: **Topical** 1:50,000–1:1000 applied topically or 1:500,000–1:50,000 mixed with a local anesthetic

STORAGE

Store at room temperature of 15°–30° C (59°–86° F). Protect from light. Check expiration dates frequently as many preparations have short shelf life.

ADMINISTRATION

Inhalation

- Have patient in an upright position when aerosol preparation is used. The reclining position can result in overdosage by producing large droplets instead of fine spray.

E

- Instruct patient to rinse mouth and throat with water immediately after inhalation to avoid swallowing residual drug (may cause epigastric pain and systemic effects from the propellant in the aerosol preparation) and to prevent dryness of oropharyngeal membranes.
- Do not give isoproterenol concurrently with epinephrine. Allow 4-h interval to elapse before a change is made from one drug to the other.

Instillation

- Instill nose drops with head in lateral, head-low position to prevent entry of drug into throat.
- Instruct patient to rinse nose dropper or spray tip with hot water after each use to prevent contamination of solution with nasal secretions.

Endotracheal

- Dilute with NS to produce a volume of 3–5 mL. Administer several positive-pressure ventilations after medication administration.

Ophthalmic

- Remove soft contact lenses before instilling eye drops.
- Instruct patient to apply gentle finger pressure against nasolacrimal duct immediately after drug is instilled for at least 1 or 2 min following instillation to prevent excessive systemic absorption.
- When separate solutions of epinephrine and a topical miotic are used, the miotic should be instilled 2–10 min prior to epinephrine because of the conjunctival sac's limited capacity.

Subcutaneous

- Use tuberculin syringe to ensure greater accuracy in measurement of parenteral doses.
- Protect epinephrine injection from exposure to light at all times. Do not remove ampule or vial from carton until ready to use.
- Shake vial or ampule thoroughly to disperse particles before withdrawing epinephrine suspension into syringe; then inject promptly.
- Aspirate carefully before injecting epinephrine. Inadvertent IV injection of usual SC doses can result in sudden hypertension and possibly cerebral hemorrhage.
- Rotate injection sites and observe for signs of blanching. Vascular constriction from repeated injections may cause tissue necrosis.

Intravenous

Note: Verify correct rate of IV injection to neonates, infants, children with physician.
- Note: 1:1000 solution contains 1 mg/1 mL. 1:10,000 solution contains 0.1 mg/1 mL.

PREPARE Direct: Dilute each 1 mg of 1:1000 solution with 10 mL of NS to yield 1:10,000 solution. **IV Infusion:** Further dilute in 250–500 mL of D5W.

ADMINISTER Direct: Give each 1 mg over 1 min or longer; may give more rapidly in cardiac arrest. **IV Infusion:** 1–10 mcg/min titrated according to patient's condition.

INCOMPATIBILITIES: Solution/Additive: Aminophylline, cephapirin, hyaluronidase, mephentermine, sodium bicarbonate, warfarin. Y-Site: Ampicillin, thiopental, sodium bicarbonate.

Common adverse effects in *italic;* life-threatening effects underlined; generic names in **bold;** drug classifications in SMALL CAPS; ✦ Canadian drug name; ❂ Prototype drug.

ADVERSE EFFECTS Special Senses: *Nasal burning or stinging,* dryness of nasal mucosa, sneezing, rebound congestion. *Transient stinging or burning of eyes,* lacrimation, browache, headache, rebound conjunctival hyperemia, allergy, iritis; with prolonged use: melanin-like deposits on lids, conjunctiva, and cornea; corneal edema; loss of lashes (reversible); maculopathy with central scotoma in aphakic patients (reversible). **Body as a Whole:** *Nervousness,* restlessness, sleeplessness, fear, anxiety, *tremors,* severe headache, cerebrovascular accident, weakness, dizziness, syncope, pallor, sweating, dyspnea. **Digestive:** Nausea, vomiting. **Cardiovascular:** Precordial pain, *palpitations,* hypertension, <u>MI</u>, tachyarrhythmias including <u>ventricular fibrillation</u>. **Respiratory:** Bronchial and <u>pulmonary edema</u>. **Urogenital:** Urinary retention. **Skin:** Tissue necrosis with repeated injections. **Metabolic:** Metabolic acidoses, elevated serum lactic acid, transient elevations of blood glucose. **Nervous System:** Altered state of perception and thought, psychosis.

INTERACTIONS Drug: May increase hypotension in circulatory collapse or hypotension caused by PHENOTHIAZINES, **oxytocin, entacapone.** Additive toxicities with other SYMPATHOMIMETICS **(albuterol, dobutamine, dopamine, isoproterenol, metaproterenol, norepinephrine, phenylephrine, phenylpropanolamine, pseudoephedrine, ritodrine, salmeterol, terbutaline),** MAO INHIBITORS, TRICYCLIC ANTIDEPRESSANTS. ALPHA- AND BETA-ADRENERGIC BLOCKING AGENTS (e.g., **ergotamine, propranolol**) can enhance pressor response of epinephrine; **chlorpromazine** reverses pressor response. GENERAL ANESTHETICS increase cardiac irritability.

PHARMACOKINETICS Absorption: Inactivated in GI tract. **Onset:** 3–5 min, 1 h on conjunctiva. **Peak:** 20 min, 4–8 h on conjunctiva. **Duration:** 12–24 h topically. **Distribution:** Widely distributed; does not cross blood–brain barrier; crosses placenta. **Metabolism:** Metabolized in tissue and liver by monoamine oxidase and catecholamine-methyltransferase. **Elimination:** Small amount excreted unchanged in urine; excreted in breast milk.

NURSING IMPLICATIONS

Assessment & Drug Effects

- Monitor BP, pulse, respirations, and urinary output and observe patient closely following IV administration. Epinephrine may widen pulse pressure. If disturbances in cardiac rhythm occur, withhold epinephrine and notify physician immediately.
- Keep physician informed of any changes in I&O ratio.
- Use cardiac monitor with patients receiving epinephrine IV. Have full crash cart immediately available.
- Check BP repeatedly when epinephrine is administered IV during first 5 min, then q3–5min until stabilized.
- Advise patient to report to prescriber if symptoms are not relieved in 20 min or if they become worse following inhalation.
- Advise patient to report bronchial irritation, nervousness, or sleeplessness. Dosage should be reduced.
- Monitor blood glucose & HbA_{1c} for loss of glycemic control if diabetic.

Patient & Family Education
- Be aware that intranasal application may sting slightly.
- Administer ophthalmic drug at bedtime or following prescribed miotic to minimize mydriasis, with blurred vision and sensitivity to light (possible in some patients being treated for glaucoma).
- Transitory stinging may follow initial ophthalmic administration and that headache and browache occur frequently at first but usually subside with continued use. Notify physician if symptoms persist.
- Discontinue epinephrine eye drops and consult a physician if signs of hypersensitivity develop (edema of lids, itching, discharge, crusting eyelids).
- Learn how to administer epinephrine subcutaneously. Keep medication and equipment available for home emergency. Confer with care provider for proper administration.
- Note: Inhalation epinephrine reduces bronchial secretions and thus may make mucous plugs more difficult to dislodge.
- Report tolerance to prescriber; may occur with repeated or prolonged use. Continued use of epinephrine in the presence of tolerance can be dangerous.
- Take medication only as prescribed and immediately notify prescriber of onset of systemic effects of epinephrine.
- Discard discolored or precipitated solutions. Check expiration dates regularly and replace as needed.
- Do not breast feed while taking this drug without consulting physician.
- Store this medication out of reach of children.

EPOETIN ALFA (HUMAN RECOMBINANT ERYTHROPOIETIN) ℗

(e-po′-e-tin)
Epogen, Eprex ♣, Procrit
Classifications: BLOOD FORMERS, COAGULATORS, AND ANTICOAGULANTS; HEMATOPOIETIC GROWTH FACTOR
Pregnancy Category: C

AVAILABILITY 2000 units/mL, 3000 units/mL, 4000 units/mL, 10,000 units/mL, 20,000 units/mL, 40,000 units/mL

ACTIONS Glycoprotein that stimulates RBC production. Hypoxia and anemia generally increase the production of erythropoietin.
THERAPEUTIC EFFECTS Produced in the kidney and stimulates bone marrow production of RBCs (erythropoiesis).

USES Elevates the hematocrit of patients with anemia secondary to chronic kidney failure (CRF); patients may or may not be on dialysis; other anemias related to chemotherapy treatment for malignancies and AIDS. Autologous blood donations for anticipated transfusions. Reduce need for blood in anemic surgical patients.

CONTRAINDICATIONS Uncontrolled hypertension and known hypersensitivity to mammalian cell–derived products and albumin (human).
CAUTIOUS USE Pregnancy (category C) or lactation. Safety and effectiveness in children are not established.

Common adverse effects in *italic;* life-threatening effects <u>underlined</u>; generic names in **bold;** drug classifications in SMALL CAPS; ♣ Canadian drug name; ℗ Prototype drug.

ROUTE & DOSAGE

Anemia

Child: **SC** 150 units/kg/dose 3 times/wk initially, when Hct increased to 35%, decrease dose by 25 units/kg/dose until Hct reaches 40%
Adult: **SC/IV** 3–500 units/kg/dose 3 times/wk, usually start with 50–100 units/kg/dose until target Hct range of 30–33% (max 36%) is reached, Hct should not increase by more than 4 points in any 2-wk period, rapid increase in Hct increases the risk of serious adverse reactions (hypertension, seizures), may increase dose if Hct has not increased 5–6 points after 8 wk of therapy, reduce dose after target range is reached or the Hct increases by >4 points in any 2-wk period, dose usually increased or decreased by 25 units/kg increments

STORAGE

Store at 2°–8° C (36°–46° F). Do not freeze or shake.

ADMINISTRATION

Subcutaneous

- Do not shake solution. Shaking may denature the glycoprotein, rendering it biologically inactive.
- Inspect solution for particulate matter prior to use. Do not use if solution is discolored or if it contains particulate matter.
- Use only one dose per vial, and do not reenter vial.
- Do not give with any other drug solution.

Intravenous

PREPARE Direct: Give undiluted.
ADMINISTER Direct: Give direct IV as a bolus dose over 1 min.
- Discard any unused portion of the vial. It contains no preservatives.

ADVERSE EFFECTS CNS: Seizures, *headache.* **CV:** *Hypertension.* **GI:** Nausea, diarrhea. **Hematologic:** *Iron deficiency,* thrombocytosis, *clotting of AV fistula.* **Other:** Sweating, bone pain, arthralgias.

INTERACTIONS Drug: No clinically significant interactions established.

PHARMACOKINETICS Onset: 7–14 days. **Metabolism:** Metabolized in serum. **Elimination:** Minimal recovery in urine. **Half-Life:** 4–13 h.

NURSING IMPLICATIONS

Assessment & Drug Effects

- Control BP adequately prior to initiation of therapy and closely monitor and control during therapy. Hypertension is an adverse effect that must be controlled.
- Be aware that BP may rise during early therapy as the Hct increases. Notify physician of a rapid rise in Hct (>4 points in 2 wk). Dosage will need to be reduced because of risk of serious hypertension.
- Monitor for hypertensive encephalopathy in patients with CRF during period of increasing Hct.

- Monitor for premonitory neurological symptoms (i.e., aura, and report their appearance promptly). The potential for seizures exists during periods of rapid Hct increase (>4 points in 2 wk).
- Monitor closely for thrombotic events (e.g., MI, CVA, TIA), especially for patients with CRF.
- Lab tests: Baseline transferrin and serum ferritin. Monitor aPTT & INR closely. Patients may require additional heparin during dialysis to prevent clotting of the vascular access or artificial kidney. Determine Hct twice weekly until it is stabilized in the target range (30–33%) and the maintenance dose of epoetin alfa has been determined; then monitor at regular intervals. Perform CBC with differential and platelet count regularly. Monitor BUN, creatinine, phosphorus, and potassium regularly.

Patient & Family Education

- Important to comply with antihypertensive medication and dietary restrictions.
- Do not drive or engage in other potentially hazardous activity during the first 90 days of therapy because of possible seizure activity.
- Note: As Hct increases, there is an improved sense of well-being and quality of life. It is important to continue compliance with dietary and dialysis prescriptions.
- Understand that headache is a common adverse effect. Report if severe or persistent, may indicate developing hypertension.
- Keep all follow-up appointments.
- Do not breast feed while taking this drug without consulting physician.

ERGOCALCIFEROL

(er-goe-kal-si′fe-role)
Activated Ergosterol, Calciferol, Deltalin, Drisdol, D-ViSol, Osto-forte ♣, Radiostol ♣, Radiostol Forte ♣, Vitamin D₂
Classifications: HORMONES AND SYNTHETIC SUBSTITUTES; VITAMIN D ANALOG
Prototype: Calcitriol
Pregnancy Category: C

AVAILABILITY 8000 international units/mL oral liquid; 50,000 units capsules, tablets; 500,000 international units/mL injection

ACTIONS The name vitamin D encompasses two related fat-soluble substances (sterols) that occur in nature or are synthetically prepared. Vitamin D acts like a hormone in that it is distributed through the circulation and plays a major regulatory role.
THERAPEUTIC EFFECTS Maintains normal blood calcium and phosphate ion levels by enhancing their intestinal absorption and by promoting mobilization of calcium from bone and renal tubular resorption of phosphate.

USES Familial hypophosphatemia (vitamin D–resistant rickets), osteomalacia (adult rickets), anticonvulsant-induced rickets and osteomalacia, osteoporosis, renal osteodystrophy, hypocalcemia associated with hypoparathyroidism; prophylaxis and treatment of nutritional rickets. Also hypophosphatemia in Fanconi's syndrome.

UNLABELED USES With varying clinical results in lupus vulgaris, psoriasis, and rheumatoid arthritis.

CONTRAINDICATIONS Hypersensitivity to vitamin D, hypervitaminosis D, hypercalcemia, hyperphosphatemia, renal osteodystrophy with hyperphosphatemia, malabsorption syndrome, decreased kidney function. Safe use of amounts in excess of 400 international units (10 mcg) daily during pregnancy (category C) is not established.

E

CAUTIOUS USE Coronary disease; lactation; arteriosclerosis (especially in older adults); history of kidney stones.

ROUTE & DOSAGE

Nutritional Rickets, Osteomalacia

Child: **PO/IM** 50–125 mcg/day, may need up to 250–625 mcg/day in patients with malabsorption or **PO** 2000–5000 international units/day for 6–12 wk
Adult: **PO/IM** 25–125 mcg/day for 6–12 wk, may need up to 7.5 mg/day in patients with malabsorption or **PO** 2000–5000 international units/day for 6–12 wk

Vitamin D–Dependent Rickets

Child: **PO/IM** 75–125 mcg/day, may need up to 1.5 mg/day or **PO** 3000–5000 international units/day (max 60,000 international units/day)
Adult: **PO/IM** 250 mcg–1.5 mg/day, may need up to 12.5 mg/day (prolonged therapy with >2.5 mg/day increases risk of toxicity) or **PO** 10,000–60,000 international units/day; doses up to 500,000 international units/day may be needed

Vitamin D–Resistant Rickets

Child: **PO** 400,000–800,000 international units/day; increase by 10,000–20,000 international units q3–4mo prn
Adult: **PO** 10,000–60,000 international units/day

Hypoparathyroidism, Pseudohypoparathyroidism

Child: **PO/IM** 1.25–5 mg/day (prolonged therapy with >2.5 mg/day increases risk of toxicity) or **PO** 50,000–200,000 international units/day
Adult: **PO/IM** 625 mcg–5 mg/day, may need up to 10 mg/day (prolonged therapy with >2.5 mg/day increases risk of toxicity) or **PO** 25,000–200,000 international units/day

STORAGE

Store at 15°–30° C (59°–86° F) in tightly covered light resistant containers; drug decomposes on exposure to light and air.

ADMINISTRATION

Note: 40 international units = 1 mcg. Reduce dosage, once symptoms of vitamin D deficiency are relieved, to prevent hypercalcemia.

Intramuscular

- Give injection deeply in site appropriate for age (see Part I) and inject slowly. Aspirate carefully. Rotate injection sites.

E

ADVERSE EFFECTS Body as a Whole: Fatigue, weakness, vertigo, tinnitus, ataxia, muscle and joint pain, hypotonia (infants), exanthema, rhinorrhea; pruritus; mild acidosis. **Nervous System:** Headache, drowsiness, convulsions. **Digestive:** Metallic taste, dry mouth, anorexia, nausea, vomiting, diarrhea, constipation, abdominal cramps. **Hematologic:** Anemia. **Musculoskeletal:** Calcification of soft tissues (kidneys, blood vessels, myocardium, lungs, skin). **Urogenital:** Nephrotoxicity (polyuria, hyposthenuria, polydipsia, nocturia, casts, albuminuria, hematuria), kidney failure. **Cardiovascular:** Hypertension, cardiac arrhythmias. **Special Senses:** Conjunctivitis (calcific); photophobia. **Metabolic:** Hypercalcemia, osteoporosis (adults); weight loss, chronic hypervitaminosis D in children (mental and physical retardation, suppression of linear growth).

DIAGNOSTIC TEST INTERFERENCE Vitamin D may cause false increase in *serum cholesterol* measurements *(Zlatkis-Zak reaction).*

INTERACTIONS Drug: Cholestyramine, colestipol, mineral oil may decrease absorption of vitamin D.

PHARMACOKINETICS Absorption: Readily absorbed from GI tract. **Peak activity:** After 4 wk. **Duration:** 2 mo or more. **Distribution:** Most of drug first appears in lymph, then concentrates in liver; stored chiefly in liver and to a lesser extent in skin, brain, spleen, and bones. **Metabolism:** Metabolized in liver and kidney to active metabolites. **Elimination:** About 50% of oral dose excreted in bile; may be stored in tissues for months. **Half-Life:** 12–24 h.

NURSING IMPLICATIONS

Assessment & Drug Effects

- Monitor closely patients receiving therapeutic doses of vitamin D must remain under close medical supervision.
- Lab tests: When high therapeutic doses are used, progress is followed by frequent determinations (every week or more often) of serum calcium, phosphorus, magnesium, alkaline phosphatase, BUN, and determinations of urine calcium, casts, albumin, and RBC. Blood calcium concentration is generally kept between 9 and 10 mg/dL.
- Monitor for hypercalcemia in patients with osteomalacia a decrease in serum alkaline phosphatase may signal the onset of hypercalcemia.

Patient & Family Education

- Avoid magnesium-containing antacids and laxatives with chronic kidney failure when receiving vitamin D preparations because vitamin D increases the risk of magnesium intoxication than other patients.
- Do not use OTC medications unless approved by physician.
- Do not breast feed while taking this drug without consulting physician.
- Store this medication out of reach of children.

ERYTHROMYCIN 🅟

(er-ith-roe-mye'sin)

Akne-Mycin Ery-Tab, Apo-Erythro Base ♣, A/T/S, E-Mycin, Eryc, EryDerm, Erythrocin, Erythromid ♣, Erythromycin Base, Ilotycin, Novorythro ♣, PCE, Robimycin, Ro-Mycin ♣, Staticin, T-Stat

ERYTHROMYCIN ESTOLATE

Ilosone, Nororythro ♣

ERYTHROMYCIN STEARATE

Apo-Erythro-S ♣ Eramycin, Erypar, Ethril, Erythrocin Stearate, SK-Erythromycin, Wyamycin S

Classifications: ANTI-INFECTIVE; MACROLIDE ANTIBIOTIC
Pregnancy Category: B

AVAILABILITY Erythromycin 250 mg, 333 mg, 500 mg tablets, capsules; 1.5%, 2%, topical solution; 2% gel, 2% ointment; 5% ophthalmic ointment. **Erythromycin Estolate** 250 mg capsules; 500 mg tablets; 125 mg/mL, 250 mg/mL suspension. **Erythromycin Stearate** 250 mg, 500 mg tablets

ACTIONS Macrolide antibiotic produced by a strain of *Streptomyces erythreus.* Bacteriostatic or bactericidal, depending on nature of organism and drug concentration used.

THERAPEUTIC EFFECTS More active against gram-positive than gram-negative bacteria. Effectiveness against *Chlamydia trachomatis* is basis for its topical use in prophylaxis of neonatal inclusion conjunctivitis.

USES Pneumococcal pneumonia, *Mycoplasma pneumoniae* (primary atypical pneumonia), acute pelvic inflammatory disease caused by *Neisseria gonorrhoeae* in females sensitive to penicillin, infections caused by susceptible strains of staphylococci, streptococci, and certain strains of *Haemophilus influenzae.* Also used in intestinal amebiasis, Legionnaires' disease, uncomplicated urethral, endocervical, and rectal infections caused by *C. trachomatis,* for prophylaxis of ophthalmia neonatorum caused by *N. gonorrhoeae, C. trachomatis,* and for chlamydial conjunctivitis in neonates. Considered an acceptable alternative to penicillin for treatment of streptococcal pharyngitis, for prophylaxis of rheumatic fever and bacterial endocarditis, for treatment of diphtheria as adjunct to antitoxin and for carrier state, and as alternate choice in treatment of primary syphilis in patients allergic to penicillins. **Topical applications,** Pyodermas, acne vulgaris, and external ocular infections, including neonatal chlamydial conjunctivitis and gonococcal ophthalmia.

CONTRAINDICATIONS Hypersensitivity to erythromycins; pregnancy (category B). **Estolate:** History of erythromycin-associated hepatitis; liver dysfunction; treatment of skin disorders such as acne or furunculosis; prophylaxis of rheumatic fever.

CAUTIOUS USE Impaired liver function; lactation, Cardiac disease, or with other drugs metabolized by cytochrome P-450 3A(CYP3A).

E

ROUTE & DOSAGE

Moderate to Severe Infections
Neonate: **PO** ≤*1.2 kg,* 10 mg/kg q12h; >*1.2 kg and 0–7 days,*
10 mg/kg q8–12h; >7 days, 30 mg/kg/day divided into 3 doses
Child: **PO** 30–50 mg/kg/day divided q6h
Adult: **PO** 250–500 mg q6h; 333 mg q8h

***Chlamydia trachomatis* Infections** (conjunctivitis and pneumonia)
Neonate: **PO** 50 mg/kg/day divided into doses given q6h for 14 days
Child: **IV** 20–50 mg/kg/day divided into doses given q6h **PO** 30–50
mg/kg/day divided into doses given q6–8h (max 2 g/24 h)
Adult: **IV** 15–20 mg/kg/day divided into doses given q6h **PO** 500 mg
q.i.d. *or* 666 mg q8h *or* 1–4 g/day divided into doses q6h (max 4 g/day)

Conjunctivitis
Child/Adult: **Topical** Apply ointment to infected eye 1 or more times/day

Rheumatic Fever Prophylaxis
Adult: **PO** 500 mg/day divided into doses given q12h

Properative Bowel Prep
Child/Adult: **PO** 20 mg/kg/dose erythromycin base × 3 doses, with
neomycin day before surgery

Pertussis
Child/Adult: **PO** Estolate salt 50 mg/kg/day divided into doses given
q6h for 14 days

Conjunctival Infection Prophylaxis
Neonate: **Topical** Apply 0.5–1 cm ribbon in lower conjunctival sacs
shortly after birth

STORAGE
Store all forms at 15°–30° C (59°–86° F) in tightly capped containers
unless otherwise directed by manufacturer.

ADMINISTRATION

Oral
- Give on an empty stomach 1 h before or 2 h after meals. Do not give
  with, or immediately before or after, fruit juices, and advise patient not
  to crush or chew tablets.
- Give enteric-coated tablets without regard to meals.
- Ensure that enteric-coated tablets are not chewed or crushed. They
  must be swallowed whole.
- Note: When switching from tablet to a PO liquid preparation, dosing
  may require adjustment.

Topical
- Prophylaxis for neonatal eye infection: Ribbon of ointment approximately 0.5–1 cm long is placed into lower conjunctival sac of neonate
  shortly after birth. Use a new tube of erythromycin for each neonate.
- Use only preparations labeled for ophthalmic use for treatment of eye
  infections.

Common adverse effects in *italic;* life-threatening effects <u>underlined</u>; generic names
in **bold;** drug classifications in SMALL CAPS; ♣ Canadian drug name; ❂ Prototype drug.

- IV lactobionate may contain benzyl alcohol; these formulations should be avoided in neonates. Vials are reconstituted with sterile water for injection to concentration of 50 mg/mL. Solution should be administered within 8 h of preparation.

ADVERSE EFFECTS CV: Prolonged cardiac repolarization, <u>Sudden cardiac death</u>. **GI:** *Nausea, vomiting, abdominal cramping, pseudomembranous enterocolitis,* diarrhea, heartburn, anorexia. **Body as a Whole:** Fever, eosinophilia, urticaria, skin eruptions, fixed drug eruption, anaphylaxis. Superinfections by nonsusceptible bacteria, yeasts, or fungi. **Special Senses:** Ototoxicity: reversible bilateral hearing loss, tinnitus, vertigo. **Digestive:** (Estolate) Cholestatic hepatitis syndrome. **Skin:** (topical use) Erythema, desquamation, burning, tenderness, dryness or oiliness, pruritus.

DIAGNOSTIC TEST INTERFERENCE False elevations of *urinary catecholamines, urinary steroids,* and *AST, ALT* (by *colorimetric methods*).

INTERACTIONS Drug: Many effects vary with different formulations. Serum levels and toxicities of **alfentanil, bexarotene, carbamazepine, cevimeline, cilostazol, clozapine, cyclosporine, disopyramide, estazolam, fentanyl, midazolam, methadone, modafinil, quinidine, sirolimus, digoxin, theophylline, triazolam, warfarin** are increased. Use of erythromycin with other drugs metabolized by cytochrome P-450 3A(CYP3A), such as **nitroimidazole antifungals, diltiazem, verapamil, troleandomycin** can significantly increase chance of sudden cardiac death from erythromycin. **Ergotamine** may increase peripheral vasospasm. May increase risk of arrhythmias with **astemizole, terfenadine.**

PHARMACOKINETICS Absorption: Erythromycin base is acid labile; most erythromycins are absorbed in small intestine. **Peak:** 1–4 h PO. **Distribution:** Widely distributed to most body tissues; low concentrations in CSF; concentrates in liver and bile; crosses placenta. **Metabolism:** Partially metabolized in liver. **Elimination:** Primarily excreted in bile; excreted in breast milk. **Half-Life:** 1.5–2 h.

NURSING IMPLICATIONS

Assessment & Drug Effects

- Report onset of GI symptoms after PO administration to prescriber. These are dose related; if symptoms persist after dosage reduction, prescriber may prescribe drug to be given with meals in spite of impaired absorption.
- Monitor for adverse GI effects. Pseudomembranous enterocolitis (see Appendix D-1), a potentially life-threatening condition, may occur during or after antibiotic therapy.
- Observe for S&S of superinfection by overgrowth of nonsusceptible bacteria or fungi. Emergence of resistant staphylococcal strains is highly predictable during prolonged therapy.
- Lab tests: Periodic liver function tests during prolonged therapy.
- Monitor for S&S of hepatotoxicity. Premonitory S&S include abdominal pain, nausea, vomiting, fever, leukocytosis, and eosinophilia; jaundice may or may not be present. Symptoms may appear a few days after initiation of drug but usually occur after 1–2 wk of continuous therapy. Symptoms are reversible with prompt discontinuation of erythromycin.
- Monitor cardiac status, especially if taking other drugs metabolized by cytochrome P-450 3A(CYP3A).

Common adverse effects in *italic;* life-threatening effects <u>underlined</u>; generic names in **bold;** drug classifications in SMALL CAPS; ✦ Canadian drug name; ⊘ Prototype drug.

525

- Monitor for ototoxicity that appears to develop most frequently in patients receiving 4 g/day or who have kidney or liver dysfunction. It is reversible with prompt discontinuation of drug. Perform hearing screening on children.

Patient & Family Education

- Notify physician for S&S of superinfection (see Appendix D-1).
- Notify prescriber immediately for S&S of pseudomembranous enterocolitis (see Appendix D-1), which may occur even after the drug is discontinued.
- Report any ototoxic effects including dizziness, vertigo, nausea, tinnitus, roaring noises, hearing impairment (see Appendix D-1).
- Do not breast feed while taking this drug without consulting physician.
- Store this medication out of reach of children.

ERYTHROMYCIN ETHYLSUCCINATE

(er-ith-roe-mye′sin)

Apo-Erythro-ES ♣, E. E. S., EES-200, EES-400, EryPed, Pediamycin, Wyamycin E

Classifications: ANTI-INFECTIVE; MACROLIDE ANTIBIOTIC
Prototype: Erythromycin
Pregnancy Category: B

AVAILABILITY 200 mg chewable tablet, 400 mg tablets; 100 mg/2.5 mL 200 mg/5 mL, 400 mg/5 mL suspension

ACTIONS Acid-stable ester salt of erythromycin.

THERAPEUTIC EFFECTS More active against gram-positive than gram-negative bacteria. Effectiveness against *Chlamydia trachomatis* is basis for its topical use in prophylaxis of neonatal inclusion conjunctivitis.

USES See erythromycin.

CONTRAINDICATIONS Hypersensitivity to erythromycins; history of erythromycin-associated hepatitis; preexisting liver disease.

CAUTIOUS USE Myasthenia gravis; pregnancy (category B), lactation, cardiac disease, or with other drugs metabolized by cytochrome P-450 3A (CYP3A).

ROUTE & DOSAGE

Infection

Child: **PO** 30–50 mg/kg/day in 4 divided doses (max 100 mg/kg/day) for severe infections
Adult: **PO** 400 mg q6h up to 4 g/day according to severity of infection

STORAGE
Store at 15°–30° C (59°–86° F) in tightly capped containers unless otherwise directed by manufacturer. Suspensions are stable for 14 days at room temperature unless otherwise stated by manufacturer. Note expiration date.

ADMINISTRATION
Note: 400 mg erythromycin ethylsuccinate is approximately equal to 250 mg erythromycin base.

Oral

- Chewable tablets should be chewed and not swallowed whole.

Common adverse effects in *italic;* life-threatening effects <u>underlined</u>; generic names in **bold**; drug classifications in SMALL CAPS; ♣ Canadian drug name; ❽ Prototype drug.

ADVERSE EFFECTS CV: Prolonged cardiac repolarization, <u>Sudden cardiac death</u>. **GI:** Diarrhea, *nausea,* vomiting, stomatitis, *abdominal cramps,* anorexia, hepatotoxicity. **Skin:** Skin eruptions. **Special Senses:** Ototoxicity. **Body as a Whole:** Potential for superinfections.

INTERACTIONS Drug: Serum levels and toxicities of **alfentanil, bexarotene, carbamazepine, cevimeline, cilostazol, clozapine, cyclosporine, digoxin, disopyramide, estazolam, fentanyl, midazolam, methadone, modafinil, quinidine, sirolimus, theophylline, triazolam, warfarin** are increased. Use of erythromycin with other drugs metabolized by cytochrome P-450 3A (CYP3A), such as **nitroimidazole antifungals, diltiazem, verapamil, troleandomycin** can significantly increase chance of sudden cardiac death from erythromycin. **Ergotamine** may increase peripheral vasospasm. May increase risk of arrhythmias with **astemizole, terfenadine.**

PHARMACOKINETICS Absorption: Readily absorbed from GI tract. **Peak:** 2 h. **Distribution:** Concentrates in liver; crosses placenta; distributed into breast milk. **Metabolism:** Metabolized in liver. **Elimination:** Excreted primarily in bile and feces. **Half-Life:** 2–5 h.

NURSING IMPLICATIONS

Assessment & Drug Effects

- Lab tests: Determine C&S prior to treatment. Periodic liver function tests and blood cell counts if therapy is prolonged 10 days.
- Cholestatic hepatitis syndrome is most likely to occur in those who have received erythromycin estolate for >10 days or who have had repeated courses of therapy. The condition generally clears within 3–5 days after cessation of therapy.
- Monitor cardiac status, especially if taking other drugs metabolized by cytochrome P-450 3A (CYP3A).

Patient & Family Education

- Advise patient to report immediately the onset of adverse reactions and to be on the alert for S&S associated with jaundice (see Appendix D-1).
- Ototoxicity is most likely to occur in patients receiving high dosage or who have impaired kidney function. Report immediately the onset of tinnitus, vertigo, or hearing impairment.
- Do not breast feed while taking this drug without consulting physician.
- Store this medication out of reach of children.

ERYTHROMYCIN GLUCEPTATE

(er-ith-roe-mye′sin)
Ilotycin Gluceptate

ERYTHROMYCIN LACTOBIONATE

Erythrocin Lactobionate-I. V.

Classifications: ANTI-INFECTIVE; MACROLIDE ANTIBIOTIC
Prototype: Erythromycin
Pregnancy Category: B

AVAILABILITY 500 mg, 1 g injection

ACTIONS Soluble salt of erythromycin. It binds to the 50S ribosome sub-units of susceptible bacteria, resulting in the suppression of protein synthesis of bacteria.

THERAPEUTIC EFFECTS More active against gram-positive than gram-negative bacteria. Effectiveness against *Chlamydia trachomatis* is basis for its topical use in prophylaxis of neonatal inclusion conjunctivitis.

USES When oral administration is not possible or the severity of infection requires immediate high serum levels; to enhance GI motility. See erythromycin.

CONTRAINDICATIONS Hypersensitivity to erythromycins; concurrent administration with terfenadine, astemizole, or cisapride.

CAUTIOUS USE Impaired liver function; pregnancy (category B), lactation, cardiac disease, or with other drugs metabolized by cytochrome P-450 3A (CYP3A).

ROUTE & DOSAGE

Infections
Child: **IV** 15–20 mg/kg/day in 4 divided doses up to 100 mg/kg/day for severe infections
Adult: **IV** 250 mg–1 g q6h up to 4 g/day according to severity of infection

STORAGE
Gluceptate: Reconstituted solution is stable up to 7 days if refrigerated at 2°–8° C (36°–46° F); use solution diluted for infusion within 4 h.
Lactobionate: Reconstituted solution is stable up to 14 days if refrigerated at 2°–8° C (36°–46° F); use solution diluted for infusion within 8 h.

ADMINISTRATION

Intravenous

PREPARE **Intermittent/Continuous:** Initial solution is prepared by adding 10 mL sterile water for injection without preservatives to each 500 mg or fraction thereof. Shake vial until drug is completely dissolved. **Intermittent:** Further dilute each 1 g dose in 100–250 mL of D5W or NS. **Continuous:** Further dilute each 1 g in 1000 mL D5W or NS. Give within 4 h.
ADMINISTER **Intermittent:** Give 1 g or fraction thereof over 20–60 min. Slow rate if pain develops along course of vein. **Continuous:** Continuous infusion is administered slowly, usually over 6 h.
INCOMPATIBILITIES **Solution/Additive: Dextrose**-containing solutions, **aminophylline, ampicillin,** TETRACYCLINES, **pentobarbital, secobarbital, streptomycin, heparin, cephalothin, colistimethate, floxacillin, furosemide, metaraminol, metoclopramide, vitamin B complex with C, ampicillin, amikacin. Y-Site: Aminophylline, fluconazole, heparin,** TETRACYCLINES.

ADVERSE EFFECTS CV: Prolonged cardiac repolarization, <u>Sudden cardiac death</u>. **Body as a Whole:** *Pain, venous irritation, and thrombophlebitis after IV injection;* allergic reactions, anaphylaxis (rare); superinfections. **GI:** *Nausea,* vomiting, diarrhea, *abdominal cramps,* variations in liver function tests following prolonged or repeated therapy. (See also erythromycin.)

INTERACTIONS Drug: Serum levels and toxicities of **alfentanil, bexarotene, carbamazepine, cevimeline, cilostazol, clozapine, cyclosporine, digoxin, disopyramide, estazolam, fentanyl, methadone, midazolam, modafinil, quinidine, sirolimus, theophylline, triazolam, warfarin** are increased. Use of erythromycin with other drugs metabolized by cytochrome P-450 3A (CYP3A), such as **nitroimidazole antifungals, diltiazem, verapamil, troleandomycin** can significantly increase chance of sudden cardiac death from erythromycin. **Ergotamine** may increase peripheral vasospasm. May increase risk of arrhythmias with **astemizole, terfenadine.**

E

PHARMACOKINETICS Peak: 1 h. **Distribution:** Concentrates in liver; crosses placenta; distributed into breast milk. **Metabolism:** Metabolized in liver. **Elimination:** Excreted primarily in bile and feces; 12–15% excreted in urine. **Half-Life:** 3–5 h.

NURSING IMPLICATIONS

Assessment & Drug Effects

- Lab tests: Determine C&S prior to initiation of therapy. Periodic liver function tests with daily high doses or prolonged or repeated therapy.
- Monitor hearing impairment may occur with large doses of this drug. It may occur as early as the second day and as late as the third week of therapy.
- Monitor for S&S of thrombophlebitis (see Appendix D-1). IV infusion of large doses are reported to increase risk.
- Moitor cardiac status, especially if taking other drugs metabolized by cytochrome P-450 3A (CYP3A).

Patient & Family Education

- Notify prescriber immediately of tinnitus, dizziness, or hearing impairment.
- Do not breast feed while taking this drug without consulting physician.

ETANERCEPT Pr

(e-tan′er-cept)

Enbrel

Classifications: IMMUNOMODULATOR; TUMOR NECROSIS FACTOR (TNF) RECEPTOR ANTAGONIST

Pregnancy Category: B

AVAILABILITY 25 mg injection

ACTIONS Produced by recombinant DNA technology. Binds specifically to tumor necrosis factor (TNF) and blocks it from attaching to cell surface TNF receptors.

THERAPEUTIC EFFECTS Indicated by improved RA symptomatology. This naturally occurring cytokine (e.g., IL-6) is part of the normal immune and inflammatory response. TNF mediates inflammation and modulates cellular immune responses. Elevated levels of TNF are found in the synovial fluids of rheumatoid arthritis (RA) patients.

USES Reduction of the signs and symptoms of RA in patients with inadequate response to other disease modifying antirheumatic drugs.

CONTRAINDICATIONS Patients with sepsis or other active infection; hypersensitivity to etanercept; malignancy; lactation.
CAUTIOUS USE Immunosuppression; pregnancy (category B). Safety and efficacy in children <4 y of age are not established.

ROUTE & DOSAGE

Rheumatoid Arthritis
Child: **SC** >4 y, 0.4 mg/kg (max 25 mg/dose) twice weekly
Adult: **SC** 25 mg twice weekly

STORAGE
Store reconstituted solution up to 6 h refrigerated at 2°–8° C (36°–46° F). Store unopened dose tray refrigerated at 2°–8° C (36°–46° F).

ADMINISTRATION
Subcutaneous
- Do not administer to a patient who has known or suspected sepsis.
- Reconstitute by slowly injecting the supplied diluent into the vial. Swirl gently to dissolve and do not shake. Reconstituted solution should be clear and colorless. Use within 6 h.
- Inject into thigh, abdomen, upper arm; rotate injection sites and never inject into an old injection site or where skin is tender, bruised, red, or hard.

ADVERSE EFFECTS Body as a Whole: Asthenia, serious *infections,* sepsis. **CNS:** Headache, dizziness, cerebral ischemia, depression, demyelinating disorders (multiple sclerosis, myelitis, optic neuritis). **CV:** Heart failure, <u>MI</u>, myocardial ischemia, hypertension, hypotension. **GI:** Abdominal pain, dyspepsia, cholecystitis, pancreatitis, GI hemorrhage. **Respiratory:** Rhinitis, URI, pharyngitis, cough, respiratory disorder, sinusitis, dyspnea may reactivate latent tuberculosis (TB). **Skin:** Rash; Injection site reactions (*erythema, itching, pain, swelling*). **Musculoskeletal:** Bursitis. **Hematologic:** <u>Pancytopenia</u>.

INTERACTIONS Drug: Concurrent or recent use with **azathioprine, cyclophosphamide, leflunomide, methotrexate** has been associated with pancytopenia.

PHARMACOKINETICS Onset: 1–2 wk. **Peak:** 72 h. **Half-Life:** 115 h.

NURSING IMPLICATIONS

Assessment & Drug Effects
- Monitor carefully for and immediately report S&S of infection.

Patient & Family Education
- A PPD test is recommended before starting therapy to check for TB.
- Discard all needles and syringes after use; do not reuse.
- Withhold etanercept and notify prescriber before resuming drug if you develop an infection or are exposed to varicella virus.
- Avoid vaccinations, in general, and live vaccines, in particular, while on etanercept. Plan a visit before therapy begins to get child up to date on immunizations if possible.

- Note: Injection site reactions (e.g., redness, pain, swelling) are common in the first month of therapy but generally decrease over time.
- Do not breast feed while taking this drug.

ETHACRYNIC ACID
(eth-a-krin′ik)
Edecrin

ETHACRYNATE SODIUM
Sodium Edecrin
Classifications: ELECTROLYTIC AND WATER BALANCE AGENT; LOOP DIURETIC
Prototype: Furosemide
Pregnancy Category: B

AVAILABILITY 25 mg, 50 mg tablet; 50 mg injection

ACTIONS Inhibits sodium and chloride reabsorption in proximal tubule and most segments of loop of Henle, promotes potassium and hydrogen ion excretion, and decreases urinary ammonium ion concentration and pH. Promotes calcium elimination in hypercalcemia and nephrogenic diabetes insipidus.
THERAPEUTIC EFFECTS Rapid and potent diuretic effect. Fluid and electrolyte loss may exceed that caused by thiazides. Hypotensive effect may be due to hypovolemia secondary to diuresis and in part to decreased vascular resistance.

USES Severe edema associated with CHF, hepatic cirrhosis, ascites of malignancy, kidney disease, nephrotic syndrome, lymphedema.
UNLABELED USES Treatment of nephrogenic diabetes insipidus, hypercalcemia, mild to moderate hypertension, and as adjunct in therapy of hypertensive crisis complicated by pulmonary edema.

CONTRAINDICATIONS History of hypersensitivity to ethacrynic acid; increasing azotemia, anuria; hepatic coma; severe diarrhea, dehydration, electrolyte imbalance, hypotension; pregnancy (category B), lactation, infants, parenteral use in pediatric patients.
CAUTIOUS USE Hepatic cirrhosis; cardiac patients; diabetes mellitus; history of gout; pulmonary edema associated with acute MI; hyperaldosteronism; nephrotic syndrome; history of pancreatitis.

ROUTE & DOSAGE

Edema
Child: **PO** 1 mg/kg daily, may increase to 3 mg/kg/day
Adult: **PO** 50–100 mg 1–2 times/day, may increase by 25–50 mg prn up to 400 mg/day **IV** 0.5–1 mg/kg or 50 mg up to 100 mg, may repeat if necessary

STORAGE
Store oral and parenteral form at 15°–30° C (59°–86° F) unless otherwise directed.

E

ADMINISTRATION

Oral

- Give after a meal or food to prevent gastric irritation.
- Schedule doses to avoid nocturia and thus sleep interference. Avoid administration within at least 4 h of bedtime, if possible. This recommendation may not apply to the patient who accumulates fluid and develops respiratory symptoms during sleep.

Intravenous

PREPARE **Direct/Intermittent:** Reconstitute by adding 50 mL of D5W or NS to vial. Use solution within 24 h. Vials reconstituted with D5W may turn cloudy; if so, discard the vial.
ADMINISTER **Direct:** Give at a rate of 10 mg/min. **Intermittent:** Give over 15–30 min. If a second IV dose is required, a new site should be selected to prevent thrombophlebitis.
INCOMPATIBILITIES **Solution/Additive: Hydralazine, procainamide, ranitidine, tolazoline, triflupromazine.**

ADVERSE EFFECTS CNS: Headache, fatigue, apprehension, confusion. **CV:** *Postural hypotension* (dizziness, light-headedness). **Metabolic:** Hyponatremia, *hypokalemia,* hypochloremic alkalosis, hypomagnesemia, hypocalcemia, hypercalciuria, hyperuricemia, hypovolemia, hematuria, glycosuria, hyperglycemia, gynecomastia, elevated BUN, creatinine, and urate levels. **Special Senses:** Vertigo, tinnitus, sense of fullness in ears, temporary or permanent deafness. **GI:** Anorexia, diarrhea, nausea, vomiting, dysphagia, abdominal discomfort or pain, GI bleeding (IV use), abnormal liver function tests. **Hematologic:** <u>Thrombocytopenia, agranulocytosis</u> (rare), <u>severe neutropenia</u> (rare). **Skin:** Skin rash, pruritus. **Body as a Whole:** Fever, chills, acute gout; local irritation and thrombophlebitis with IV injection.

INTERACTIONS Drug: THIAZIDE DIURETICS increase potassium loss; increased risk of **digoxin** toxicity from hypokalemia; CORTICOSTEROIDS, **amphotericin B** increase risk of hypokalemia; decreased **lithium** clearance, so increased risk of lithium toxicity; SULFONYLUREA effect may be blunted, causing hyperglycemia; ANTIHYPERTENSIVE AGENTS increase risk of orthostatic hypotension; AMINOGLYCOSIDES may increase risk of ototoxicity; **warfarin** potentiates hypoprothrombinemia.

PHARMACOKINETICS Absorption: Rapidly absorbed from GI tract. **Onset:** 30 min PO; 5 min IV. **Peak:** 2 h PO; 15–30 min IV. **Duration:** 6–8 h PO; 2 h IV. **Distribution:** Does not cross CSF. **Metabolism:** Metabolized to cysteine conjugate. **Elimination:** 30–65% excreted in urine; 35–40% excreted in bile. **Half-Life:** 30–70 min.

NURSING IMPLICATIONS

Assessment & Drug Effects

- Observe closely when receiving the drug by IV infusion. Rapid, copious diuresis following IV administration can produce hypotension.
- Monitor IV site closely. Extravasation of IV drug causes local pain and tissue irritation from dehydration and blood volume depletion.
- Monitor BP during initial therapy. Because orthostatic hypotension can occur, supervise ambulation.

- Monitor BP and pulse throughout therapy in patients with impaired cardiac function. Diuretic induced hypovolemia may reduce cardiac output, and electrolyte loss promotes cardiotoxicity in those receiving digitalis (cardiac) glycosides.
- Establish baseline weight prior to start of therapy; weigh patient under standard conditions. Keep physician informed of weight loss or gain in excess of 1 kg (2 lb)/day for child over 12 years or any weight gain for younger child.
- Monitor I&O ratio. Drug should be discontinued if excessive diuresis, oliguria, hematuria, or sudden profuse diarrhea occurs. Report signs to physician.
- Lab tests: Determine baseline and periodic blood count, serum electrolytes, CO_2, BUN, creatinine, blood glucose, uric acid, and liver function.
- Observe for and report S&S of electrolyte imbalance: Anorexia, nausea, vomiting, thirst, drymouth, polyuria, oliguria, weakness, fatigue, dizziness, faintness, headache, muscle cramps paresthesias, drowsiness, mental confusion. Instruct patient to report these symptoms promptly to physician.
- Report immediately possible signs of thromboembolic complications (see Appendix D-1).
- Impaired glucose tolerance with hyperglycemia and glycosuria has occurred in patients receiving doses in excess of 200 mg/day.

Patient & Family Education

- Learn S&S of hypokalemia and hyponatremia (see Appendix D-1), and report any of these promptly to prescriber.
- Make position changes slowly, particularly from lying to upright posture.
- Report GI adverse effects to physician; they occur most frequently after 1–3 mo of PO therapy or in patients on high dosage. The onset of loose stools or other GI symptoms at any time during therapy indicate possible need for dosage adjustment or discontinuation of drug.
- Notify physician immediately of any evidence of impaired hearing. Hearing loss may be preceded by vertigo, tinnitus, or fullness in ears; it may be transient, lasting 1–24 h, or it may be permanent.
- Do not breast feed while taking this drug.
- Store this medication out of reach of children.

ETHAMBUTOL HYDROCHLORIDE

(e-tham′byoo-tole)

Etibi ◆, Myambutol

Classifications: ANTI-INFECTIVE; ANTITUBERCULOSIS AGENT

Prototype: Isoniazid

Pregnancy Category: B

AVAILABILITY 100 mg, 400 mg tablets

ACTIONS Mode of action not completely understood, but it appears to inhibit RNA synthesis and thus arrests multiplication of tubercle bacilli. The

emergence of resistant strains is delayed by administering ethambutol in combination with other antituberculosis drugs.
THERAPEUTIC EFFECTS Synthetic antituberculosis agent with bacteriostatic effect.

USES In conjunction with at least one other antituberculosis agent in treatment of pulmonary tuberculosis.
UNLABELED USES Atypical mycobacterial infections.

CONTRAINDICATIONS Optic neuritis; hypersensitivity to ethambutol; children <13 y; lactation.
CAUTIOUS USE Patients with renal impairment; gout; ocular defects (e.g., cataract, recurrent ocular inflammatory conditions, diabetic retinopathy); pregnancy (category B).

ROUTE & DOSAGE

Tuberculosis
Child: **PO** *6–12 y,* 10–15 mg/kg/day (max 1 g/day)
Adult: **PO** 15 mg/kg q24h; for retreatment start with 25 mg/kg/day for 60 days, then decrease to 15 mg/kg/day

STORAGE
Store at 15°–30° C (59°–86° F) in tightly closed container unless otherwise directed. Protect ethambutol from light, moisture, and excessive heat.

ADMINISTRATION
Oral
▪ Give with food if GI irritation occurs.

ADVERSE EFFECTS CNS: Headache, dizziness, confusion, hallucinations, paresthesias, joint pains. **Special Senses:** Ocular toxicity: *retrobulbar optic neuritis;* possibility of anterior optic neuritis with decrease in visual acuity, temporary loss of vision, constriction of visual fields, red–green color blindness, central and peripheral scotomas, eye pain, photophobia; retinal hemorrhage and edema. **GI:** Anorexia, nausea, vomiting, abdominal pain. **Body as a Whole:** Hypersensitivity (pruritus, dermatitis, anaphylaxis).

INTERACTIONS Drug: Aluminum-containing antacids can decrease absorption.

PHARMACOKINETICS Absorption: 70–80% absorbed from GI tract. **Peak:** 2–4 h. **Distribution:** Distributes to most body tissues; highest concentrations in erythrocytes, kidney, lungs, saliva; crosses placenta; distributed into breast milk. **Metabolism:** Metabolized in liver. **Elimination:** 50% excreted in urine within 24 h; 20–22% excreted in feces. **Half-Life:** 3–4 h.

NURSING IMPLICATIONS

Assessment & Drug Effects
▪ Perform C&S prior to and periodically throughout therapy.
▪ Perform ophthalmoscopic examination prior to and at monthly intervals during therapy. Test acuity, visual fields, red–green color vision; discontinue if visual changes occur. Test eyes separately as well as together.

Common adverse effects in *italic;* life-threatening effects underlined; generic names in **bold;** drug classifications in SMALL CAPS; ✦ Canadian drug name; ◍ Prototype drug.

- Note: Ocular toxicity generally appears within 1–7 mo after start of therapy. Symptoms usually disappear within several weeks to months after drug is discontinued, depending on degree of ocular damage.
- Monitor I&O ratio in patients with renal impairment. Report oliguria or any significant changes in ratio or in laboratory reports of kidney function. Systemic accumulation with toxicity can result from delayed drug excretion.
- Lab tests: Perform liver and kidney function tests, CBC, heme, and serum uric acid levels at regular intervals throughout therapy.

E

Patient & Family Education

- Adhere to drug regimen exactly and keep follow-up appointments.
- Notify prescriber promptly of the onset of blurred vision, changes in color perception, constriction of visual fields, or any other visual symptoms. Have eyes checked regularly.
- Do not breast feed while taking this drug.
- Store this medication out of reach of children.

ETHIONAMIDE

(e-thye-on-am'ide)
Trecator-SC
Classifications: ANTI-INFECTIVE; ANTITUBERCULOSIS AGENT; ANTILEPROSY (SULFONE) AGENT
Prototype: Isoniazid
Pregnancy Category: D

AVAILABILITY 250 mg tablets

ACTIONS Bacteriostatic or bactericidal depending on concentration used and susceptibility of organism. Emergence of resistant strains may be delayed or prevented when administered concurrently with other antituberculosis drugs.

THERAPEUTIC EFFECTS Effective against human and bovine strains of *Mycobacterium tuberculosis* and *M. kansasii* and some strains of *Mycobacterium avium-intracellulare complex*. Also active against *M. leprae*.

USES Any form of active tuberculosis when treatment with primary antituberculosis drugs (e.g., isoniazid, streptomycin, ethambutol, rifampin) has failed. Must be given with at least one other effective antituberculosis agent.

UNLABELED USES Atypical mycobacterial infections and tuberculous meningitis.

CONTRAINDICATIONS Hypersensitivity to ethionamide and chemically related drugs (e.g., isoniazid, niacin [nicotinamide]); severe liver damage. Safety during pregnancy (category D), lactation, or in children and women of childbearing potential is not established.

CAUTIOUS USE Diabetes mellitus, liver dysfunction.

Common adverse effects in *italic;* life-threatening effects <u>underlined;</u> generic names in **bold;** drug classifications in SMALL CAPS; ◆ Canadian drug name; ❷ Prototype drug.

535

E

ROUTE & DOSAGE

Tuberculosis

Child: **PO** 15–20 mg/kg/day in 2–3 equally divided doses (max 1 g/day)
Adult: **PO** 0.5–1 g/day divided q8–12h.

STORAGE

Store in a cool, dry place at 8°–15° C (46°–59° F) in a tightly closed container unless otherwise directed.

ADMINISTRATION

Oral

- Give with or after meals to minimize GI adverse effects. Some patients tolerate ethionamide best when it is taken as a single dose after the evening meal or as a single dose at bedtime. GI symptoms appear to increase with divided doses, although serum concentrations may be higher.
- About 50% of patients cannot tolerate a single dose larger than 500 mg because of GI adverse effects. An antiemetic may be prescribed, but if symptoms persist, drug should be discontinued.
- Prescriber may recommend pyridoxine (vitamin B_6) concurrently to prevent or relieve peripheral neuritis and other neurotoxic effects.

ADVERSE EFFECTS CNS: Headache, restlessness, mental depression, drowsiness, dizziness, ataxia, hallucinations, paresthesias, convulsions. **GI:** Dose related and frequent; symptoms may be due to CNS stimulation rather than to GI irritation: anorexia, *epigastric distress, nausea, vomiting,* metallic taste, *diarrhea,* stomatitis, sialorrhea. **Metabolic:** Elevated ALT, AST; hepatitis (with jaundice), hypothyroidism. **Urogenital:** Menorrhagia, impotence. **Body as a Whole:** Postural hypotension.

INTERACTIONS Drug: Cycloserine, isoniazid may increase neurotoxic effects.

PHARMACOKINETICS Absorption: 80% absorbed from GI tract. **Peak:** 3 h. **Duration:** 9 h. **Distribution:** Widely distributed including CSF; crosses placenta; distribution into breast milk unknown. **Metabolism:** Metabolized in liver. **Elimination:** Excreted in urine. **Half-Life:** 3 h.

NURSING IMPLICATIONS

Assessment & Drug Effects

- Lab tests: Perform C&S prior to start of therapy. Baseline liver function tests (AST and ALT), CBC, and kidney function tests including urinalysis and every 2–4 wk during therapy.
- Report onset of skin rash. Progression to exfoliative dermatitis can occur if drug is not promptly discontinued.
- Monitor blood glucose & HbA1c closely in the diabetic until response to drug is established. These patients appear to be especially prone to hepatotoxicity (see Appendix D-1).

Patient & Family Education

- Avoid alcohol or use in moderation because ethionamide may increase potential for liver dysfunction.
- Notify physician of S&S of hepatotoxicity (see Appendix D-1); generally reversible if drug is promptly withdrawn.
- Make position changes slowly and in stages, particularly from lying to upright posture if experiencing hypotension.
- Do not breast feed while taking this drug without consulting health care provider.
- Store this medication out of reach of children.

E

ETHOSUXIMIDE ℗

(eth-oh-sux'i-mide)
Zarontin
Classifications: CENTRAL NERVOUS SYSTEM AGENT; SUCCINIMIDE ANTI-CONVULSANT
Pregnancy Category: C

AVAILABILITY 250 mg capsules; 250 mg/5 mL syrup

ACTIONS Succinimide anticonvulsant. Usually ineffective in management of psychomotor or major motor seizures.

THERAPEUTIC EFFECTS Reduces frequency of epileptiform attacks, apparently by depressing motor cortex and elevating CNS threshold to stimuli.

USES Management of absence (petit mal) seizures, myoclonic seizures, and akinetic epilepsy. May be administered with other anticonvulsants when other forms of epilepsy coexist with petit mal.

CONTRAINDICATIONS Hypersensitivity to succinimides; severe liver or kidney disease; use alone in mixed types of epilepsy (may increase frequency of grand mal seizures). Safety during pregnancy (category C), lactation, or in children <3 y is not established.

ROUTE & DOSAGE

Absence Seizures

Child: **PO** 3–6 y, 15 mg/kg/day given in two divided doses; increase prn q4–7days (max 500 mg/day). Usual maintenance dose 15–40 mg/kg/day
Child/Adult: **PO** 6–12 y and older, 250 mg b.i.d., may increase by 250 mg/day q4–7days prn (max 1.5 g/day), usual maintenance dose 20–40 mg/kg/day

STORAGE
Store all forms at 15°–30° C (59°–86° F); capsules in tight containers, and syrup in light-resistant containers; avoid freezing.

ADMINISTRATION

Oral

- Drug of choice for absence seizures; however, may increase incidence of grand mal seizures if given to child with mixed types of seizures.
- Give with food if GI distress occurs.

ADVERSE EFFECTS CNS: Drowsiness, hiccups, ataxia, dizziness, headache, euphoria, restlessness, irritability, anxiety, hyperactivity, aggressiveness, inability to concentrate, lethargy, confusion, sleep disturbances, night terrors, hypochondriacal behavior, muscle weakness, fatigue. **Special Senses:** Myopia. **GI:** Nausea, vomiting, *anorexia, epigastric distress,* abdominal pain, *weight loss,* diarrhea, constipation, gingival hyperplasia. **Urogenital:** Vaginal bleeding. **Hematologic:** Eosinophilia, leukopenia, thrombocytopenia, <u>agranulocytosis</u>, <u>pancytopenia</u>, <u>aplastic anemia</u>, positive direct Coombs' test. **Skin:** Hirsutism, pruritic erythematous skin eruptions, urticaria, alopecia, erythema multiforme, exfoliative dermatitis; lupus-like syndrome.

INTERACTIONS Drug: Carbamazepine decreases ethosuximide levels; **isoniazid** significantly increases ethosuximide levels; levels of both **phenobarbital** and ethosuximide may be altered with increased seizure frequency. **Herbal: Ginkgo** may decrease anticonvulsant effectiveness.

PHARMACOKINETICS Absorption: Readily absorbed from GI tract. **Peak:** 4 h; steady state: 4–7 days. **Metabolism:** Metabolized in liver. **Elimination:** Excreted slowly in urine; small amounts excreted in bile and feces. **Half-Life:** 30 h in children, 60 h in adults.

NURSING IMPLICATIONS

Assessment & Drug Effects

- Lab tests: Perform baseline and periodic hematologic studies, liver and kidney function.
- Monitor adverse drug effects. GI symptoms, drowsiness, ataxia, dizziness, and other neurologic adverse effects occur frequently and indicate the need for dosage adjustment.
- Observe closely during period of dosage adjustment and whenever other medications are added or eliminated from the drug regimen. Therapeutic serum levels: 40–100 mcg/mL.
- Observe patients with prior history of psychiatric disturbances for behavioral changes. Close supervision is indicated. Drug should be withdrawn slowly if these symptoms appear.

Patient & Family Education

- Discontinue drug only under prscriber supervision; abrupt withdrawal of ethosuximide (whether used alone or in combination therapy) may precipitate seizures or petit mal status. Carefully record any seizure activity and report to health care provider.
- Do not drive or engage in other potentially hazardous activities until response to drug is known.
- Monitor weight on a weekly basis. Report anorexia and weight loss to prescriber; may indicate need to reduce dosage.
- Do not breast feed while taking this drug without consulting prescriber.
- Store this medication out of reach of children.

FAMOTIDINE

(fa-moe'ti-deen)

Pepcid, Pepcid AC

Classifications: GASTROINTESTINAL AGENT; ANTISECRETORY AGENT (H$_2$-RECEPTOR ANTAGONIST)

Prototype: Cimetidine

Pregnancy Category: B

AVAILABILITY 10 mg, 20 mg, 40 mg tablets; 40 mg/5 mL suspension; 10 mg/mL, 20 mg/50 mL injection

ACTIONS Thiazole derivative, structurally similar to histamine and pharmacologically similar to cimetidine. A potent competitive inhibitor of histamine at histamine (H$_2$) receptor sites in gastric parietal cells. Inhibits basal, nocturnal, meal-stimulated, and pentagastrin-stimulated gastric secretion; also inhibits pepsin secretion. Is 20–160 times more potent than cimetidine and 3–20 times more potent than ranitidine. Does not affect gastric emptying or exocrine pancreatic function.

THERAPEUTIC EFFECTS Reduces parietal cell output of hydrochloric acid; thus, detrimental effects of acid on gastric mucosa are diminished.

USES Preferred treatment of active duodenal ulcer. Maintenance therapy for duodenal ulcer patients on reduced dosage after healing of an active ulcer. Treatment of pathologic hypersecretory conditions (e.g., Zollinger-Ellison syndrome), benign gastric ulcer, gastroesophageal reflux disease (GERD), gastritis.

UNLABELED USES Stress ulcer prophylaxis.

CONTRAINDICATIONS Safe use during pregnancy (category B), by nursing mothers.

CAUTIOUS USE Renal insufficiency.

ROUTE & DOSAGE

Duodenal Ulcer

Child: **PO** 0.5 mg/kg q8–12h (max 40 mg/day) **IV** 0.6–0.8 mg/kg/day divided into 2–3 doses (max 40 mg/day)

Adult: **PO** 40 mg at bedtime or 20 mg b.i.d. × 4–8 wk **IV** 20 mg q12h

PO Maintenance Therapy 20 mg at bedtime

Pathological Hypersecretory Conditions

Adult: **PO** 20–160 mg q6h

GERD, Gastritis

Child: **PO** 1–1.2 mg/kg/day divided into 2–3 doses (max 40 mg/day)

Adult: **PO** 10 mg b.i.d.

Renal Impairment

Cl$_{cr}$ <50 mL/min: 50% of usual dose or usual dose q36–48h for all indications

---

STORAGE

Store at 15°–30° C(59°–86° F). Protect from moisture and strong light; do not freeze. Store IV solution at 2°–8° C (36°–46° F); reconstituted IV solution is stable for 48 h at 15°–30° C (59°–86° F).

ADMINISTRATION

Oral

Doses are usually given q12h but infants and young children have faster clearance and may need q8h dosing.

- Give with liquid or food of patient's choice; an antacid may also be given if patient is also on antacid therapy.

Intravenous

Note: Verify correct IV concentration and rate of infusion/injection with prescriber before administration to infants or children.

***PREPARE* Direct:** Dilute 20 mg (2 mL) famotidine IV solution (containing 10 mg/mL) with D5W, NS, or other compatible IV diluent (see manufacturer's directions) to a total volume of 5 or 10 mL. **IV Infusion:** Dilute 2 mL famotidine IV with 100 mL compatible IV solution.

***ADMINISTER* Direct:** Give over not less than 2 min. **IV Infusion:** Infuse over 15–30 min.

***INCOMPATIBILITIES* Y-Site: Amphotericin B cholesteryl complex, cefepime.**

ADVERSE EFFECTS CNS: Dizziness, headache, confusion, depression. **GI:** Constipation, diarrhea. **Skin:** Rash, acne, pruritus, dry skin, flushing. **Hematologic:** Thrombocytopenia, **Urogenital:** Increases in BUN and serum creatinine.

INTERACTIONS Drug: No clinically significant interactions established.

PHARMACOKINETICS Absorption: Incompletely absorbed from GI tract (40–50% reaches systemic circulation). **Onset:** 1 h. **Peak:** 1–3 h PO; 0.5–3 h IV. **Duration:** 10–12 h. **Metabolism:** Metabolized in liver. **Elimination:** Excreted in urine. **Half-Life:** 2.5–4 h.

NURSING IMPLICATIONS

Assessment & Drug Effects

- Monitor for improvement in GI distress.
- Monitor for signs of GI bleeding.
- Weigh and measure children regularly and plot results on growth grids. Perform nutritional and dietary intake assessments.

Patient & Family Education

- Be aware that pain relief may not be experienced for several days after starting therapy.
- Do not breast feed while taking this drug without consulting physician.
- Store this medication out of reach of children.

FAT EMULSION, INTRAVENOUS

(fat e-mul'sion)
Intralipid, Liposyn, Nutralipid, Soyacal, Travamulsion
Classification: CALORIC AGENT
Pregnancy Category: B for Soyacal 10%; C for all others

F

AVAILABILITY 10%, 20%, 30% emulsion

ACTIONS Soybean oil in water emulsion containing egg yolk phospholipids and glycerin. Liposyn 10% is a safflower oil in water emulsion containing egg phosphatides and glycerin. Caloric value per milliliter of Intralipid 10% and Liposyn 10% is 1.1; Intralipid 20% is 2.
THERAPEUTIC EFFECTS Used as a nutritional supplement. Fat emulsions contain a mixture of neutral triglycerides, mostly unsaturated fatty acids.

USES Fatty acid deficiency. Also to supply fatty acids and calories in high-density form to patients receiving prolonged TPN therapy who cannot tolerate high dextrose concentrations or when fluid intake must be restricted as in renal failure, CHF, ascites.

CONTRAINDICATIONS Hyperlipemia; bone marrow dyscrasias; impaired fat metabolism as in pathological hyperlipemia, lipoid nephrosis, acute pancreatitis accompanied by hyperlipemia.
CAUTIOUS USE Severe hepatic or pulmonary disease; pregnancy (category C); coagulation disorders; anemia; newborns, premature neonates, infants with hyperbilirubinemia; when danger of fat embolism exists; diabetes mellitus; thrombocytopenia; history of gastric ulcer.

ROUTE & DOSAGE

Prevention of Essential Fatty Acid Deficiency

Child: **IV** 0.5–1 g/kg infused slowly over 8–12 h twice/wk (max 3–4 g/kg/day; max infusion, 0.25 g/kg/h)
Adult: **IV** 500 mL of 10% or 250 mL of 20% solution infused over 8–12 h twice/wk (max rate of 100 mL/h)

Calorie Source in Fluid-Restricted Patients

Premature neonate: **IV** 1 mg/kg/day increase by small increments as needed (max 3–4 g/kg/day; max infusion 0.15 g/kg/h)
Child: **IV** up to 4 g/kg or 60% of nonprotein calories daily infused over at least 8–12 h (max rate of 100 mL/h)
Adult: **IV** up to 2.5 g/kg or 60% of nonprotein calories daily infused over at least 8–12 h (max rate of 100 mL/h)

STORAGE

Store, unless otherwise directed by manufacturer, Intralipid 10% and Liposyn 10% at room temperature (25° C [77° F] or below); refrigerate Intralipid 20%. Do not freeze. Discard contents of partly used containers.

ADMINISTRATION

Intravenous

- Do not use if oil appears to be separating out of the emulsion.

PREPARE **IV Infusion:** Allow preparations that have been refrigerated to stand at room temperature for about 30 min before using whenever possible. Check with a pharmacist before mixing fat emulsions with electrolytes, vitamins, drugs, or other nutrient solutions.

ADMINISTER **IV Infusion:** Give fat emulsions via a separate peripheral site or by piggyback into same vein receiving amino acid injection and dextrose mixtures or give by piggyback through a Y-connector near infusion site so that the two solutions mix only in a short piece of tubing proximal to needle. ▪ Must hang fat emulsion higher than hyperalimentation solution bottle to prevent backup of fat emulsion into primary line. ▪ Do not use an in-line filter because size of fat particles is larger than pore size. Control flow rate of each solution by separate infusion pumps. Use a constant rate over 20–24 h to reduce risk of hyperlipemia in neonates and prematures because they tend to metabolize fat slowly.

INCOMPATIBILITIES **Solution/Additive: Aminophylline, amphotericin B, ampicillin, calcium chloride, calcium gluconate, gentamicin, hetastarch, magnesium chloride methicillin, penicillin G, phenytoin, ranitidine, tetracycline, vitamin B complex. Y-Site: Acyclovir, amphotericin B, cyclosporine, doxorubicin, doxycycline, droperidol, ganciclovir, haloperidol, heparin, hetastarch, hydromorphone, levorphanol, lorazepam, midazolam, minocycline, nalbuphine, ondansetron, pentobarbital, phenobarbital, phenytoin, potassium phosphate, sodium phosphate, tetracycline.**

ADVERSE EFFECTS Body as a Whole: Hypersensitivity reactions (to egg protein), irritation at infusion site. **Hematologic:** Hypercoagulability, thrombocytopenia in neonates. **GI:** *Transient increases in liver function tests, hyperlipemia.* **Long-Term Administration:** <u>Sepsis</u>, jaundice (cholestasis), hepatomegaly, <u>kernicterus</u> (infants with hyperbilirubinemia), <u>shock</u> (rare).

DIAGNOSTIC TEST INTERFERENCE Blood samples drawn during or shortly after fat emulsion infusion may produce abnormally high *hemoglobin MCH and MCHC* values. Fat emulsions may cause transient abnormalities in *liver function tests* and may interfere with estimations of *serum bilirubin* (especially in infants).

INTERACTIONS Drug: No clinically significant interactions established.

PHARMACOKINETICS: Not studied.

NURSING IMPLICATIONS

Assessment & Drug Effects

- Establish baseline weight, length, vital signs, and nutritional parameters. Perform developmental and physical assessments at baseline and

frequently during therapy. Observe patient closely. Acute reactions tend to occur within the first 2.5 h of therapy.
- Lab tests: Determine baseline values for hemoglobin, platelet count, blood coagulation, liver function, plasma lipid profile (especially serum triglycerides and cholesterol, free fatty acids in plasma). Repeat 1 or 2 times weekly during therapy in adults; more frequently in children. Report significant deviations promptly.
- Lab tests: Obtain daily platelet counts in neonates during first week of therapy, then every other day during second week, and 3 times a week thereafter because newborns are prone to develop thrombocytopenia.
- Note: Lipemia must clear after each daily infusion. Degree of lipemia is measured by serum triglycerides and cholesterol levels 4–6 h after infusion has ceased.
- See Part I for further description of nursing care for fat emulsions.

Patient & Family Education
- Report difficulty breathing, nausea, vomiting, or headache promptly.

FELBAMATE
(fel′ba-mate)
Felbatol
Classifications: CENTRAL NERVOUS SYSTEM AGENT; ANTICONVULSANT
Prototype: Phenytoin
Pregnancy Category: C

AVAILABILITY 400 mg, 600 mg tablets; 600 mg/5 mL suspension

ACTIONS Anticonvulsant mechanism has not been identified. Blocks repetitive firing of neurons and increases seizure threshold; prevents seizure spread. Less potent than phenytoin.
THERAPEUTIC EFFECTS Increases seizure threshold and prevents seizure spread.

USES Treatment of Lennox–Gastaut syndrome and partial seizures.
UNLABELED USES Monotherapy or in combination with other anticonvulsants for the treatment of generalized tonic-clonic seizures.

CONTRAINDICATIONS Hypersensitivity to felbamate or other carbamates, history of blood dyscrasia or hepatic dysfunction.
CAUTIOUS USE Pregnancy (category C), lactation. Safety and effectiveness in children other than those with Lennox–Gastaut syndrome are not established. Recommended only as second-line alternative treatment for seizures that have not responded to other medications due to reports of aplastic anemia and hepatotoxicity.

ROUTE & DOSAGE

Partial Seizures
Adult: **PO** Initiate with 1200 mg/day in 3–4 divided doses, may increase by 600 mg/day q2wk (max 3600 mg/day); when converting

to monotherapy, reduce dose of concomitant anticonvulsants by ⅓ when initiating felbamate, then continue to decrease other anticonvulsants by ⅓ with each increase in felbamate q2wk; when using as adjunctive therapy, decrease other anticonvulsants by 20% when initiating felbamate and note that further reductions in other anticonvulsants may be required to minimize side effects and drug interactions

Lennox–Gastaut Syndrome (adjunctive therapy)

Child: **PO** Start at 15 mg/kg/day divided into 3–4 doses, reduce concurrent antiepileptic drugs by 20%, further reductions may be required to minimize side effects due to drug interactions, may increase felbamate by 15 mg/kg/day at weekly intervals (max 45 mg/kg/day)

STORAGE

Store in airtight container at room temperature, 15°–30° C (59°–86° F).

ADMINISTRATION

Oral

- Do not give this drug to anyone with a history of blood dyscrasia or hepatic dysfunction.
- Titrate dose under close clinical supervision.
- Shake suspension well before giving a dose.

ADVERSE EFFECTS CNS: Mild tremors, headache, dizziness, ataxia, diplopia, blurred vision; agitation, aggression, hallucinations, fatigue, psychological disturbances. **Endocrine:** Slight elevation of serum cholesterol, hyponatremia, hypokalemia, weight gain and loss. **GI:** *Nausea and vomiting,* anorexia, constipation, hiccup, taste disturbance, indigestion, esophagitis, increased appetite, *acute liver failure*. **Hematologic:** *Aplastic anemia.*

INTERACTIONS Drug: Felbamate reduces serum **carbamazepine** levels by a mean of 25%, but increases levels of its active metabolite, increases serum **phenytoin** levels approximately 20%, and increases **valproic acid** levels. **Herbal: Gingko** may decrease anticonvulsant effectiveness.

PHARMACOKINETICS Absorption: 90% absorbed from GI tract. Absorption of tablet not affected by food. **Onset:** Therapeutic effect approximately 14 days. **Peak:** Peak plasma levels at 1–6 h. **Distribution:** 20–25% protein bound, readily crosses the blood–brain barrier. **Metabolism:** Metabolized in the liver via the cytochrome P-450 system. **Elimination:** 40–50% excreted unchanged in urine, rest excreted in urine as metabolites. **Half-Life:** 20–23 h.

NURSING IMPLICATIONS

Assessment & Drug Effects

- Drug should be prescribed only by a specialist in managing seizures.
- Lab tests: Obtain baseline values for liver function and complete hematologic studies before initiating therapy, repeat frequently during

therapy (every 12 wk), and for a lengthy period after discontinuation of felbamate. Monitor serum sodium and potassium levels periodically because hyponatremia and hypokalemia have been reported. Obtain serum levels of all anticonvulsants received.

- Report immediately any hematologic abnormalities.
- Monitor results of hepatic function tests throughout therapy.
- Note: When used concomitantly with either phenytoin or carbamazepine, carefully monitor serum levels of these drugs when felbamate is added, when adjustments in felbamate dosing are made, or when felbamate is discontinued.
- Note: A reduction in phenytoin of 10–40% is usually needed when felbamate is added to the regimen.
- Monitor weight, because both weight gain and loss have been reported. Establish baseline developmental and behavioral data and monitor frequently during therapy. Report loss of developmental progression or behavioral changes.
- Monitor for S&S of drug toxicity including GI distress and CNS toxicity.

Patient & Family Education

- Note: It is highly recommended that patients and physicians review the indication for treatment, risks associated with the drug, and the importance of undergoing regular blood monitoring.
- Report unusual changes (e.g., blurred vision, dysplopia) to physician.
- Report signs and symptoms of hypersensitivity including pruritus, urticaria, and (rarely) photosensitivity allergic reaction to physician.
- Learn adverse effects and report these to physician immediately. Record all seizure activity and report promptly.
- Do not breast feed while taking this drug.
- Store this medication out of reach of children.

FENOPROFEN CALCIUM

(fen-oh-proe′fen)

Nalfon

Classifications: CENTRAL NERVOUS SYSTEM AGENT; ANALGESIC, ANTIPYRETIC; NSAID; COX-1

Prototype: Ibuprofen

Pregnancy Category: B (D in third trimester)

AVAILABILITY 200 mg, 300 mg capsules; 600 mg tablets

ACTIONS Exhibits anti-inflammatory, analgesic, and antipyretic properties of an NSAID. Claimed to be comparable to aspirin in anti-inflammatory activity and associated with lower incidence of adverse GI symptoms.

THERAPEUTIC EFFECTS Effectiveness evidenced within a few days with peak effect in 2–3 wk. Has nonsteroidal, anti-inflammatory, antiarthritic properties which provides relief from mild to severe pain.

USES Anti-inflammatory and analgesic effects in the symptomatic treatment of acute and chronic rheumatoid arthritis and osteoarthritis; relief of mild to moderate pain.

UNLABELED USES Juvenile rheumatoid arthritis, acute gouty arthritis, ankylosing spondylitis; fever associated with pulmonary tuberculosis, type A influenza, colds; neoplasms.

CONTRAINDICATIONS History of nephrotic syndrome associated with aspirin or other NSAIDS; patient in whom urticaria, severe rhinitis, bronchospasm, angioedema, nasal polyps are precipitated by aspirin or other NSAIDS; significant renal or hepatic dysfunction; pregnancy (category B, category D in third trimester). Safety in lactation or children is not established.

CAUTIOUS USE History of upper GI tract disorders; hemophilia or other bleeding tendencies; compromised cardiac function, hypertension; impaired hearing.

ROUTE & DOSAGE

Inflammatory Disease

Child: **PO** 900 mg/m^2 in divided doses, may increase over 4 wk to 1.8 g/m^2

Adult: **PO** 300–600 mg t.i.d. or q.i.d. (max 3200 mg/day)

Mild to Moderate Pain

Adult: **PO** 200 mg q4–6h prn

STORAGE

- Store capsules and tablets in tightly closed containers at 15°–30° C (59°–86° F); avoid freezing.

ADMINISTRATION

Oral

- Give on an empty stomach 30–60 min before or 2 h after meals. Give with meals, milk, or antacid (prescribed) if patient experiences GI disturbances.
- May crush tablets or empty capsule and mix with fluid or mix with food.

ADVERSE EFFECTS CNS: *Headache, drowsiness,* dizziness, fatigue, lassitude, tremor, confusion, insomnia, nervousness, depression. **Special Senses:** Tinnitus, decreased hearing, deafness; blurred vision. **GI:** *Indigestion, nausea, vomiting,* anorexia, *constipation,* diarrhea, flatulence, abdominal pain, dry mouth; infrequent: gastritis, peptic ulcer, GI bleeding. **Urogenital:** Dysuria, cystitis, hematuria, oliguria, azotemia, anuria, allergic nephritis, papillary necrosis, nephrotoxicity (rare). **Hematologic:** (infrequent) Thrombocytopenia, hemolytic anemia, agranulocytosis, pancytopenia. **Skin** (may or may not be hypersensitivity reaction): Pruritus, rash, purpura, increased sweating, urticaria. **Body as a Whole:** Dyspnea, malaise, anaphylaxis, edema.

INTERACTIONS Drug: Fenoprofen may prolong bleeding time; should not be given with ORAL ANTICOAGULANTS, **heparin;** action and side effects of **phenytoin,** SULFONYLUREAS, SULFONAMIDES, and fenoprofen may be potentiated. **Herbal: Feverfew, garlic, ginger, gingko** may increase bleeding potential.

PHARMACOKINETICS Absorption: 80% absorbed from GI tract. **Onset:** 2 h. **Peak:** 2 h. **Duration:** 4–6 h. **Distribution:** Small amounts distributed into breast milk. **Metabolism:** Metabolized in liver. **Elimination:** Excreted primarily in urine; some biliary excretion. **Half-Life:** 3 h.

F

NURSING IMPLICATIONS

Assessment & Drug Effects

- Lab tests: Baseline evaluations of Hct and Hgb, kidney and liver function.
- Baseline and periodic auditory and ophthalmic examinations are recommended in patients receiving prolonged or high dose therapy.
- Monitor for signs and symptoms of GI bleeding.
- Note: Dosage adjustment of fenoprofen may be required when phenobarbital is added to or withdrawn from patient's drug regimen.

Patient & Family Education

- Do not drive or engage in potentially hazardous activities until response to drug is known; fenoprofen may cause dizziness and drowsiness.
- Report immediately the onset of unexplained fever, rash, arthralgia, oliguria, edema, weight gain to physician. Possible symptoms of nephrotic syndrome are rapidly reversible if drug is promptly withdrawn.
- Understand that alcohol and aspirin may increase risk of GI ulceration and bleeding tendencies; avoid both unless otherwise advised by physician.
- Inform dentist, surgeon, and other health care providers that you are taking fenoprofen because it may prolong bleeding time.
- Do not breast feed while taking this drug without consulting physician.
- Store this medication out of reach of children.

FENTANYL CITRATE

(fen'ta-nil)
Duragesic, Actiq Oralet, Sublimaze
Classifications: CENTRAL NERVOUS SYSTEM AGENT; ANALGESIC; NARCOTIC (OPIATE) AGONIST
Prototype: Morphine
Pregnancy Category: C
Controlled Substance: Schedule II

AVAILABILITY 0.05 mg/mL injection; 100 mcg, 200 mcg, 300 mcg, 400 mcg lozenges; 200 mcg, 400 mcg, 600 mcg, 800 mcg, 1200 mcg, 1600 mcg lozenges on a stick; 25 mcg/h, 50 mcg/h, 75 mcg/h, 100 mcg/h transdermal patches

ACTIONS Synthetic, potent narcotic agonist analgesic with pharmacologic actions qualitatively similar to those of morphine and meperidine, but action is more prompt and less prolonged. Principal actions: analgesia and sedation. Drug-induced alterations in respiratory rate and alveolar ventilation may persist beyond the analgesic effect. Emetic effect is less than with either morphine or meperidine.
THERAPEUTIC EFFECTS Provides analgesia and sedation.

USES Short-acting analgesic during operative and perioperative periods, as a narcotic analgesic supplement in general and regional anesthesia, and with droperidol or with diazepam to produce neuroleptoanalgesia. Also given with oxygen and a skeletal muscle relaxant (neuroleptoanesthesia) to selected high-risk patients (e.g., those undergoing open heart surgery) when attenuation of the response to surgical stress without use of additional anesthesia agents is important.

CONTRAINDICATIONS Patients who have received MAO INHIBITORS within 14 days; myasthenia gravis; labor and delivery, lactation. Safety during pregnancy (category C) or in children <12 y is not established. Safety and efficacy of transdermal patch in children is not established.
CAUTIOUS USE Head injuries, increased intracranial pressure; debilitated, poor-risk patients; COPD, other respiratory problems; liver and kidney dysfunction; bradyarrhythmias.

ROUTE & DOSAGE

Premedication

Neonate: **IV** 1–4 mcg/kg slow IV push q2–4h or 1–2 mcg/kg bolus, then infuse at 0.5–1 mcg/kg/h
Child: **IV/IM** *1–12 y,* 1–2 mcg/kg q30–60min or 1–2 mcg/kg followed by 1–3 mcg/kg/h infusion
Child: **PO** Suck on lozenge until sedated, *10–25 kg,* 200-mcg lozenge; *25–35 kg,* 300-mcg lozenge; *35–40 kg,* 400-mcg lozenge (max 400 mcg/dose)
Adult: **IM** 50–100 mcg 30–60 min before surgery **PO** Suck on 400-mcg lozenge until sedated

Adjunct for Regional Anesthesia

Adult: **IM** 50–100 mcg **IV** 2–20 mcg/kg over 1–2 min up to 50 mcg/kg

General Anesthesia

Adult: **IV** up to 150 mcg/kg as required

Postoperative Pain

Child: **IM** 1.7–3.3 mcg/kg q1–2h prn
Adult: **IM** 50–100 mcg q1–2h prn

Chronic Pain

Adult: **Transdermal** Individualize and regularly reassess doses of transdermal fentanyl; for patient not already receiving an opioid, the initial dose is 25 mcg/h patch q3days; for patients already on opioids, see package insert for conversions **Stick lozenge (Actiq)** Place in mouth between cheek and lower gum and suck on lozenge; do not chew; should be consumed over 15-min period

STORAGE
Store at 15°–30° C (59°–86° F) unless otherwise directed. Protect drug from light.

ADMINISTRATION

Intravascular

***PREPARE* Direct:** Give parenteral doses undiluted or diluted in 5 mL sterile water or NS.
***ADMINISTER* Direct:** Infuse over at least 5 min. **Oral Lozenge:** Administer to children old enough to follow directions. Instruct the child to suck, not chew the lozenge.
***INCOMPATIBILITIES* Solution/Additive: Fluorouracil, pentobarbital, thiopental.**

ADVERSE EFFECTS CNS: *Sedation,* euphoria, dizziness, diaphoresis, delirium, convulsions with high doses. **CV:** Hypotension, bradycardia, circulatory depression, cardiac arrest. **Special Senses:** Miosis, blurred vision. **GI:** *Nausea,* vomiting, constipation, ileus. **Respiratory:** Laryngospasm, bronchoconstriction, respiratory depression or arrest. **Body as a Whole:** Muscle rigidity, especially muscles of respiration after rapid IV infusion, urinary retention. **Skin:** Rash, contact dermatitis from patch.

INTERACTIONS Drug: Alcohol and other CNS DEPRESSANTS potentiate effects; MAO INHIBITORS may precipitate hypertensive crisis.

PHARMACOKINETICS Absorption: Absorbed through the skin, leveling off between 12–24 h. **Onset:** Immediate IV; 7–15 min IM; 12–24 h transdermal. **Peak:** 3–5 min IV; 24–72 h transdermal. **Duration:** 30–60 min IV; 1–2 h IM; 72 h transdermal. **Metabolism:** Metabolized in liver. **Elimination:** Excreted in urine. **Half-Life:** 17 h transdermal.

NURSING IMPLICATIONS

Assessment & Drug Effects
- Establish baseline vital signs.
- Monitor vital signs and observe patient for signs of skeletal and thoracic muscle (depressed respirations) rigidity and weakness continuously during administration and following.
- Watch carefully for respiratory depression and for movements of various groups of skeletal muscle in extremities, external eye, and neck during postoperative period. These movements may present patient management problems; report promptly.
- Note: Duration of respiratory depressant effect may be considerably longer than narcotic analgesic effect. Have immediately available oxygen, resuscitative and intubation equipment, and an opioid antagonist such as naloxone.

Common adverse effects in *italic;* life-threatening effects underlined; generic names in **bold;** drug classifications in SMALL CAPS; ✦ Canadian drug name; ❂ Prototype drug.

549

F

FERROUS SULFATE 🅟
(fer'rous sul'fate)
Feosol, Fer-In-Sol, Fer-Iron, Fero-Gradumet, Ferospace, Ferralyn, Ferra-TD, Fesofor, Hematinic, Mol-Iron, Novoferrosulfa ♣, Slow-Fe

FERROUS FUMARATE
(fer'rous foo'ma-rate)
Feco-T, Femiron, Feostat, Fersamal, Fumasorb, Fumerin, Hemocyte, Ircon-FA, Neo-Fer-50 ♣, Novofumar ♣, Palafer ♣, Palmiron

FERROUS GLUCONATE
(fer'rous gloo'koe-nate)
Fergon, Fertinic ♣, Novoferrogluc ♣, Simron
Classifications: BLOOD FORMERS, COAGULATORS, AND ANTICOAGULANTS; IRON PREPARATION
Prototype: Ferrous sulfate
Pregnancy Category: A

AVAILABILITY Ferrous Sulfate 167 mg, 200 mg, 324 mg, 325 mg tablets; 160 mg sustained-release tablets, capsules; 90 mg/5 mL syrup; 220 mg/5 mL elixir; 75 mg/0.6 mL drops **Ferrous Fumarate** 63 mg, 100 mg, 200 mg, 324 mg, 325 mg, 350 mg tablets; 100 mg/5 mL suspension; 45 mg/0.6 mL drops **Ferrous Gluconate** 240 mg, 325 mg tablets
Combination Products Available in many combination products, especially with vitamins

ACTIONS Ferrous sulfate: Standard iron preparation against which other oral iron preparations are usually measured. Corrects erythropoietic abnormalities induced by iron deficiency but does not stimulate erythropoiesis. May reverse gastric, esophageal, and other tissue changes caused by lack of iron. **Ferrous gluconate:** Claimed to cause less gastric irritation and be better tolerated than ferrous sulfate.
THERAPEUTIC EFFECTS Experienced within 48 h as a sense of well-being, increased vigor, improved appetite, and decreased irritability (in children). Improves cognitive function and learning. Reticulocyte response begins in about 4 days; it usually peaks in 7–10 days (reticulocytosis) and returns to normal after 2 or 3 wk. Hemoglobin generally increases by 2 g/dL and hematocrit by 6% in 3 wk. Iron supplements correct erythropoietic abnormalities induced by iron deficiency but do not stimulate erythropoiesis.

USES To correct simple iron deficiency and to treat iron deficiency (microcytic, hypochromic) anemias. Also may be used prophylactically during periods of increased iron needs, as in illness and pregnancy.

CONTRAINDICATIONS Peptic ulcer, regional enteritis, ulcerative colitis; hemolytic anemias (in absence of iron deficiency), hemochromatosis, hemosiderosis, patients receiving repeated transfusions, pyridoxine-responsive anemia; cirrhosis of liver.
CAUTIOUS USE Pregnancy (category A), lactation.

Common adverse effects in *italic*; life-threatening effects underlined; generic names in **bold**; drug classifications in SMALL CAPS; ♣ Canadian drug name; 🅟 Prototype drug.

ROUTE & DOSAGE

Iron Deficiency

Premature Infant: 2–4 mg elemental iron/kg/day in 1–2 PO doses (max 15 mg elemental iron/day)

Child: **PO Sulfate (30% elemental iron)** *<6 y,* 75–225 mg/day in divided doses; *6–12 y,* 600 mg/day in divided doses; **Fumarate (33% elemental iron)** 3 mg/kg t.i.d.; **Gluconate (12% elemental iron)** *<6 y,* 100–300 mg/day in divided doses; *6–12 y,* 100–300 mg t.i.d.; alternatively, calculate 3–6 mg elemental iron/kg/day in 1–3 PO doses

Adult: **PO Sulfate (30% elemental iron)** 750–1500 mg/day in 1–3 divided doses; **Fumarate (33% elemental iron)** 200 mg t.i.d. or q.i.d.; **Gluconate (12% elemental iron)** 325–600 mg q.i.d., may be gradually increased to 650 mg q.i.d. as needed and tolerated

Iron Supplement

Infants: **PO Fumarate** *Low birth weight,* 2 mg/kg/day up to 15 mg/day; *≤3 y,* 1 mg/kg/day **Sulfate** 2–6 mg/kg/day; alternatively, prematures receive 2 mg elemental iron/kg/day PO and full-term infants receive 1–2 mg elemental iron/day PO (max dose of elemental iron 15 mg/day)

Child: **PO Fumarate** 3 mg/kg daily; **Gluconate** *<6 y,* 100–300 mg/day in divided doses; *6–12 y,* 100–300 mg daily (max dose of elemental iron 15 mg/day)

Adult: **PO Sulfate** *Pregnancy,* 300–600 mg/day in divided doses; **Fumarate** 200 mg daily; **Gluconate** 325–600 mg daily (max dose of elemental iron 60 mg/day)

STORAGE

Store in tightly closed containers and protect from moisture. Store at 15°–30° C (59°–86° F). Do not use discolored tablets.

ADMINISTRATION

Oral

- Give on an empty stomach if possible because oral iron preparations are best absorbed then (i.e., between meals). Minimize gastric distress if needed by giving with or immediately after meals with adequate liquid. Vitamin C may enhance absorption.
- Do not crush tablet or empty contents of capsule when administering.
- Do not give tablets or capsules within 1 h of bedtime.
- Consult prescriber about prescribing a liquid formulation or a less corrosive form, such as ferrous gluconate, if the patient experiences difficulty in swallowing tablet or capsule.
- Dilute liquid preparations well and give through a straw or placed on the back of tongue with a dropper to prevent staining of teeth and to mask taste. Instruct the patient to rinse mouth with clear water immediately after ingestion.
- Mix ferosol elixir with water; not compatible with milk or fruit juice. Fer-In-Sol (drops) may be given in water or in fruit or vegetable juice, according to manufacturer.

ADVERSE EFFECTS GI: *Nausea, heartburn,* anorexia, *constipation,* diarrhea, epigastric pain, abdominal distress, *black stools.* **Special Senses:** Yellow-brown discoloration of eyes and teeth (liquid forms). **Large Chronic Doses in Infants** Rickets (due to interference with phosphorus absorption). **Massive Overdosage** Lethargy, drowsiness, nausea, vomiting, abdominal pain, diarrhea, local corrosion of stomach and small intestines, pallor or cyanosis, metabolic acidosis, <u>shock, cardiovascular collapse</u>, convulsions, <u>liver necrosis</u>, coma, renal failure, <u>death</u>.

DIAGNOSTIC TEST INTERFERENCE By coloring feces black, large iron doses may cause false-positive tests for ***occult blood with orthotoluidine (Hematest, Occultist, Labstix); guaiac reagent benzidine test*** is reportedly not affected.

INTERACTIONS Drug: ANTACIDS decrease iron absorption; iron decreases absorption of TETRACYCLINES, **ciprofloxacin, ofloxacin; chloramphenicol** may delay iron's effects; iron may decrease absorption of **penicillamine. Food:** Food decreases absorption of iron; **ascorbic acid (vitamin C)** may increase iron absorption.

PHARMACOKINETICS Absorption: 5–10% absorbed in healthy individuals; 10–30% absorbed in iron deficiency; food decreases amount absorbed but vitamin C may enhance absorption. **Distribution:** Transported by transferrin to bone marrow, where it is incorporated into hemoglobin; crosses placenta. **Elimination:** Most of iron released from hemoglobin is reused in body; small amounts are lost in desquamation of skin, GI mucosa, nails, and hair; 12–30 mg/mo lost through menstruation.

NURSING IMPLICATIONS

Assessment & Drug Effects

- Lab tests: Monitor Hgb and reticulocyte values before and during therapy. Investigate the absence of satisfactory response after 3 wk of drug treatment.
- Continue iron therapy for 2–3 mo after the hemoglobin level has returned to normal (roughly twice the period required to normalize hemoglobin concentration).
- Monitor bowel movements as constipation and black tarry stools are common adverse effects.
- Perform developmental and cognitive testing at beginning and periodically during therapy. Monitor sleep and alertness patterns.

Patient & Family Education

- Note: Ascorbic acid increases absorption of iron. Consuming citrus fruit or tomato juice with iron preparation (except the elixir) may increase its absorption.
- Be aware that milk, eggs, or caffeine beverages when taken with the iron preparation may inhibit absorption.
- Be aware that iron preparations cause dark green or black stools.
- Report constipation or diarrhea to prescriber; symptoms may be relieved by adjustments in dosage or diet or by change to another iron preparation.

Common adverse effects in *italic;* life-threatening effects <u>underlined</u>; generic names in **bold;** drug classifications in SMALL CAPS; ♣ Canadian drug name; ☻ Prototype drug.

- Inform families of foods that contain high amounts of iron.
- Keep this drug securely locked and out of reach of children. Poisoning can occur.
- Do not breast feed while taking this drug without consulting prescriber.

FEXOFENADINE
(fex-o-fen'a-deen)
Allegra
Classifications: ANTIHISTAMINE; H₁-RECEPTOR ANTAGONIST; NONSEDATING
Prototype: Loratidine
Pregnancy Category: C

AVAILABILITY 60 mg capsules

ACTIONS Antihistamine competitively antagonizes histamine at the H₁-receptor site; does not bind with histamine to inactivate it. Not associated with anticholinergic or sedative properties.

THERAPEUTIC EFFECTS Inhibits antigen-induced bronchospasm and histamine release from mast cells. Efficacy is indicated by reduction of the following: nasal congestion and sneezing; watery or red eyes; itching nose, palate, or eyes.

USES Relief of symptoms associated with seasonal allergic rhinitis, and chronic urticaria.

CONTRAINDICATIONS Hypersensitivity to fexofenadine; pregnancy (category C).

CAUTIOUS USE Lactation; renal and hepatic insufficiency, hypertension, diabetes mellitus, ischemic heart disease, increased ocular pressure, hyperthyroidism, renal impairment, or prostatic hypertrophy. Safety and effectiveness in children <6 y are not established.

ROUTE & DOSAGE

Allergic Rhinitis
Child: **PO** *6–11 y,* 30 mg b.i.d.
Child/Adult: >12 y, **PO** 60 mg b.i.d.

Chronic Urticaria
Child: **PO** *>6 y,* 30 mg b.i.d.
Adult: **PO** 60 mg b.i.d.

Renal Impairment
Cl_cr
Child: 30 mg daily
Adult: 60 mg daily

STORAGE
Store at 20°–25° C (68°–77° F). Protect from excess moisture.

ADMINISTRATION
Oral
- Reduce starting dose for those with decreased kidney function.

ADVERSE EFFECTS CNS: *Headache,* drowsiness, fatigue. **GI:** Nausea, dyspepsia, throat irritation.

INTERACTIONS Drug: No clinically significant interactions established.

PHARMACOKINETICS Absorption: Rapidly absorbed from GI tract, 33% reaches systemic circulation. **Onset:** 1 h. **Peak:** 2–3 h. **Duration:** At least 12 h. **Distribution:** 60–70% bound to plasma proteins. **Metabolism:** Only 5% of dose metabolized in liver. **Elimination:** 80% excreted in urine, 11% in feces. **Half-Life:** 14.4 h.

NURSING IMPLICATIONS

Assessment & Drug Effects
- Monitor therapeutic effectiveness, which is indicated by decreased nasal congestion, sneezing, watery or red eyes, and itching nose, palate, or eyes.

Patient & Family Education
- Note: Drug is well tolerated and causes minimal adverse effects.
- Do not breast feed while taking this drug without consulting prescriber.
- Store this medication out of reach of children.

FILGRASTIM
(fil-gras'tim)
Neupogen
Classifications: BLOOD FORMERS, COAGULATORS, AND ANTICOAGULANTS; HEMATOPOIETIC GROWTH FACTOR
Prototype: Epoetin alfa
Pregnancy Category: C

AVAILABILITY 300 mcg/mL injection

ACTIONS Human granulocyte colony-stimulating factor (G-CSF) produced by recombinant DNA technology. Endogenous G-CSF regulates the production of neutrophils within the bone marrow; not species specific and primarily affects neutrophil proliferation, differentiation and selected end-cell functional activity (including enhanced phagocytic activity, antibody-dependent killing, and the increased expression of some functions associated with cell-surface antigens).
THERAPEUTIC EFFECTS Increases neutrophil proliferation and differentiation within the bone marrow.

USES To decrease the incidence of infection, as manifested by febrile neutropenia, in patients with nonmyeloid malignancies receiving myelosuppressive anticancer drugs associated with a significant incidence of severe neutropenia with fever; to decrease neutropenia associated with bone marrow transplant; to treat chronic neutropenia; to mobilize peripheral blood stem cells (PBSCs) for autologous transplantation.

CONTRAINDICATIONS Hypersensitivity to *Escherichia coli*–derived proteins, simultaneous administration with chemotherapy, and myeloid cancers.

CAUTIOUS USE Pregnancy (category C), lactation.

ROUTE & DOSAGE

Neutropenia

Child/Adult: **IV** 5 mcg/kg/day by 30 min infusion, may increase by 5 mcg/kg/day if desired effect is not present in 7 days (max 30 mcg/kg/day) **SC** 5 mcg/kg/day as single dose, may increase by 5 mcg/kg/day (max 20 mcg/kg/day) Note: discontinue when ANC >10,000/mm^3

F

STORAGE

Store refrigerated at 2°–8° C (36°–46° F). Do not freeze. Avoid shaking.

ADMINISTRATION

Subcutaneous & Intravenous

- Do not administer filgrastim 24 h before or after cytotoxic chemotherapy.
- Use only one dose per vial; do not reenter the vial.
- Prior to injection, filgrastim may be allowed to reach room temperature for a maximum of 6 h. Discard any vial left at room temperature for >6 h.

PREPARE **Intermittent/Continuous:** May dilute with 10–50 mL D5W to yield 15 mcg/mL or greater. If more diluent is used to yield concentrations of 5–15 mcg/mL, 2 mL of 5% human albumin must be added for each 50 mL D5W (prior to adding filgrastim) to prevent adsorption to plastic IV infusion materials.

ADMINISTER **Intermittent:** Give a single dose over 15–30 min. **Continuous:** Give a single dose over 4–24 h.

INCOMPATIBILITIES **Y-Site: Amphotericin B, cefepime, cefoperazone, cefotaxime, cefoxitin, ceftizoxime, ceftriaxone, cefuroxime, clindamycin, dactinomycin, etoposide, fluorouracil, furosemide, gentamicin, heparin, imipenem, mannitol, methylprednisolone, metronidazole, mitomycin, piperacillin, prochlorperazine, thiotepa.**

ADVERSE EFFECTS CV: Abnormal ST segment depression. **Hematologic:** Anemia. **GI:** Nausea, anorexia. **Body as a Whole:** *Bone pain,* hyperuricemia, *fever.*

DIAGNOSTIC TEST INTERFERENCE Elevations in **leukocyte alkaline phosphatase, serum alkaline phosphatase, lactate dehydrogenase,** and **uric acid** have been reported. These elevations appear to be related to increased bone marrow activity.

INTERACTIONS Drug: Can interfere with activity of CYTOTOXIC AGENTS, do not use 24 h before or after CYTOTOXIC AGENTS

PHARMACOKINETICS Absorption: Readily absorbed from SC site. **Onset:** 4 h. **Peak:** 1 h. **Elimination:** Probably excreted in urine. **Half-Life:** 1.4–7.2 h.

Common adverse effects in *italic;* life-threatening effects <u>underlined</u>; generic names in **bold**; drug classifications in SMALL CAPS; ♣ Canadian drug name; ❷ Prototype drug.

555

NURSING IMPLICATIONS

Assessment & Drug Effects

- Lab tests: Obtain a baseline CBC with differential and platelet count prior to administering drug. Obtain CBC twice weekly during therapy to monitor neutrophil count and leukocytosis. Monitor Hct and platelet count regularly.
- Discontinue filgrastim when absolute neutrophil count exceeds 10,000/mm^3 after the chemotherapy-induced nadir. Neutrophil counts should then return to normal.
- Obtain baseline uric acid and liver function studies and monitor during therapy.
- Monitor patients with preexisting cardiac conditions closely. MI and arrhythmias have been associated with a small percent of patients receiving filgrastim.
- Monitor temperature q4h. Incidence of infection should be reduced after administration of filgrastim.
- Assess degree of bone pain if present. Consult physician if nonnarcotic analgesics do not provide relief.

Patient & Family Education

- Report bone pain and, if necessary, to request analgesics to control pain.
- Note: Proper drug administration and disposal is important. A puncture-resistant container for the disposal of used syringes and needles should be available to the patient if administered at home. All equipment must be stored out of reach of children.
- Do not breast feed while taking this drug without consulting physician.

FLECAINIDE 🅿️

(fle-kay'nide)
Tambocor
Classifications: CARDIOVASCULAR AGENT; ANTIARRHYTHMIC; CLASS IC
Pregnancy Category: C

AVAILABILITY 50 mg, 100 mg, 150 mg tablets

ACTIONS Local (membrane) anesthetic and antiarrhythmic with electrophysiologic properties similar to other class IC antiarrhythmic drugs. Slows conduction velocity throughout myocardial conduction system, increases ventricular refractoriness; little effect on repolarization. Prolongs His-ventricular (HQ) and QRS intervals at therapeutic doses.

THERAPEUTIC EFFECTS Clinically, causes both hypotension and negative entropy (in higher dose ranges) and is an effective suppressant of PVCs and a variety of atrial and ventricular arrhythmias.

USES Life-threatening ventricular arrhythmias.
UNLABELED USES Atrial tachycardia and other arrhythmias unresponsive to standard agents (e.g., quinidine), Wolff-Parkinson-White syndrome, and recurrent ventricular tachycardias.

CONTRAINDICATIONS Hypersensitivity to flecainide; preexisting second- or third-degree AV block, right bundle branch block when associated with a left hemiblock unless a pacemaker is present; cardiogenic shock, significant hepatic impairment. Safety during pregnancy (category C), lactation, or in children <18 y is not established.
CAUTIOUS USE CHF, sick sinus syndrome, renal impairment.

ROUTE & DOSAGE

Life-Threatening Ventricular Arrhythmias
Child: **PO** 1–3 mg/kg/day in 3 divided doses (max 8 mg/kg/day); increase as needed) usual dose 3–6 mg/kg/day; dosage adjusted downward in renal failure
Adult: **PO** 100 mg q12h, may increase by 50 mg b.i.d. q4 days (max 600 mg/day)

STORAGE
Store in tightly covered, light-resistant containers at 15°–30° C (59°–86° F) unless otherwise directed.

ADMINISTRATION

Oral
- Do not increase dosage more frequently than every 4 days.

ADVERSE EFFECTS CNS: *Dizziness,* headache, light-headedness, unsteadiness, paresthesias, fatigue. **CV:** Arrhythmias, chest pain, worsening of CHF. **Special Senses:** *Blurred vision, difficulty in focusing,* spots before eyes. **GI:** *Nausea,* constipation, change in taste perception. **Body as a Whole:** Dyspnea, fever, edema.

INTERACTIONS Drug: Cimetidine may increase flecainide levels; may increase **digoxin** levels 15–25%; BETA-BLOCKERS may have additive negative inotropic effects.

PHARMACOKINETICS Absorption: Readily absorbed from GI tract. **Peak:** 2–3 h. **Distribution:** Crosses placenta; distributed into breast milk. **Metabolism:** Metabolized in liver. **Elimination:** Excreted mainly in urine. **Half-Life:** 7–22 h.

NURSING IMPLICATIONS

Assessment & Drug Effects
- Correct preexisting hypokalemia or hyperkalemia before treatment is initiated.
- Note: ECG monitoring, including Holter monitor for ambulating patients, is essential because of the possibility of drug-induced arrhythmias.
- Determine pacing threshold for patients with pacemakers before initiation of therapy, after 1 wk of therapy, and at regular intervals thereafter.
- Monitor plasma level recommended, especially in patients with severe CHF or renal failure because drug elimination may be delayed in these patients.

- Note: Effective trough plasma levels are between 0.7–1 mcg/mL. The probability of adverse reactions increases when trough levels exceed 1 mcg/mL.
- Attempt dosage reduction with caution after arrhythmia is controlled.

Patient & Family Education
- Note: it is VERY important to take this drug at the prescribed times.
- Report visual disturbances to physician.
- Do not breast feed while taking this drug without consulting physician.
- Store this medication out of reach of children.

FLUCONAZOLE ⊘
(flu-con'a-zole)
Diflucan
Classifications: ANTI-INFECTIVE; ANTIBIOTIC; ANTIFUNGAL
Pregnancy Category: C

AVAILABILITY 50 mg, 100 mg, 150 mg, 200 mg tablets; 10 mg/mL, 40 mg/mL suspension; 2 mg/mL injection

ACTIONS Fungistatic; may also be fungicidal depending on concentration. Interferes with formation of ergosterol, the principal sterol in the fungal cell membrane that when depleted interrupts membrane function. **THERAPEUTIC EFFECTS** Antifungal properties are related to the drug effect on the fungal cell membrane functioning.

USES Cryptococcal meningitis and oropharyngeal and systemic candidiasis, both commonly found in AIDS and other immunocompromised patients; vaginal candidiasis.

CONTRAINDICATIONS Hypersensitivity to fluconazole or other azole antifungals.
CAUTIOUS USE Pregnancy (category C).

ROUTE & DOSAGE

Oropharyngeal Candidiasis
Child: **PO/IV** 3–6 mg/kg/day
Adult: **PO/IV** 200 mg on day 1, then 100 mg daily × 2 wk

Esophageal Candidiasis
Child: **PO/IV** 3–6 mg/kg/day
Adult: **PO/IV** 200 mg on day 1, then 100 mg daily × 3 wk

Systemic Candidiasis
Child: **PO/IV** 3–6 mg/kg/day
Adult: **PO/IV** 400 mg on day 1, then 200 mg daily × 4 wk

Vaginal Candidiasis
Adult: **PO** 150 mg for 1 dose

Common adverse effects in *italic;* life-threatening effects underlined; generic names in **bold;** drug classifications in SMALL CAPS; ♣ Canadian drug name; ⊘ Prototype drug.

Cryptococcal Meningitis

Newborn: <29 wk postconception, 5–6 mg/kg/dose q48h (for >14 days age) or q72h (for 0–14 days age); 30–36 wk postconception, 3–6 mg/kg/dose q24h (for >14 days age) or q48h (for 0–14 days age); 37–44 wk postconception, 3–6 mg/kg/dose q24h (for >7 days age) or q48h (for 0–7 days age); >45 wk postconception, 3–6 mg/kg/dose q24h

Child: **PO/IV** 6–12 mg/kg/day as loading dose and then maintenance of 200–400 mg QD starting 24 h later

Adult: **PO/IV** 400 mg on day 1, then 200 mg daily × 10–12 wk

F

STORAGE

Store in light-resistant containers at less than 30° C (86° F). Protect injection solution from freezing.

ADMINISTRATION

Oral

- Take this medication for the full course of therapy, which may take weeks or months.
- Take next dose as soon as possible if you miss a dose, however, do not take a dose if it is almost time for next dose. Do not double dose.

Intravenous

PREPARE Continuous: Packaged ready for use as a 2 mg/mL solution. Remove wrapper just prior to use.

ADMINISTER Continuous: Give at a maximum rate of approximately 200 mg/h. Give after hemodialysis is completed. ▪ Do not use IV admixtures of fluconazole and other medications.

INCOMPATIBILITIES Solution/Additive: Trimethoprim-sulfamethoxazole. Y-Site: Amphotericin B, amphotericin B cholesteryl, ampicillin, calcium gluconate, ceftazidime, ceftriaxone, cefuroxime, chloramphenicol, clindamycin, diazepam, digoxin, erythromycin, furosemide, haloperidol, hydroxyzine, imipenem-cilastatin, pentamidine, piperacillin, ticarcillin, trimethoprim-sulfamethoxazole.

ADVERSE EFFECTS CNS: Headache. **GI:** Nausea, vomiting, abdominal pain, diarrhea, increase in AST in patients with cryptococcal meningitis and AIDS. **Skin:** Rash.

INTERACTIONS Drug: Increased PT in patients on **warfarin;** may increase **alosetron, bexarotene, cevimeline, cilostazol, cyclosporine, dofetilide, haloperidol, levobupivicaine, modafinil, phenytoin, zonisamide** levels and toxicity; hypoglycemic reactions with ORAL SULFONYLUREAS; decreased fluconazole levels with **rifampin, cimetidine;** may prolong the effects of **alfentanil, fentanyl, methadone.**

PHARMACOKINETICS Absorption: 90% absorbed from GI tract. **Peak:** 1–2 h. **Distribution:** Widely distributed, including CSF. **Metabolism:** 11% of dose metabolized in liver. **Elimination:** Excreted in urine. **Half-Life:** 20–50 h.

Common adverse effects in *italic;* life-threatening effects underlined; generic names in **bold;** drug classifications in SMALL CAPS; ♣ Canadian drug name; ⦿ Prototype drug.

NURSING IMPLICATIONS

Assessment & Drug Effects

- Monitor for allergic response. Patients allergic to other azole antifungals may be allergic to fluconazole.
- Lab tests: Monitor BUN, serum creatinine, and liver function.
- Note: Drug may cause elevations of the following laboratory serum values: ALT, AST, alkaline phosphatase, bilirubin.
- Monitor for S&S of hepatotoxicity (see Appendix D-1).

Patient & Family Education

- Monitor carefully for loss of glycemic control if diabetic.
- Inform prescriber of all medications being taken.
- Store this medication out of reach of children.

FLUCYTOSINE
(floo-sye'toe-seen)
Ancobon, Ancotil ♣, 5-FC, 5-Fluorocytosine
Classifications: ANTI-INFECTIVE; ANTIBIOTIC; ANTIFUNGAL
Prototype: Fluconazole
Pregnancy Category: C

AVAILABILITY 250 mg, 500 mg capsules

ACTIONS Ineffective for cancerous tumors possibly because it does not enter mammalian cells. Selectively penetrates fungal cell and is converted to fluorouracil, an antimetabolite believed to be responsible for antifungal activity.
THERAPEUTIC EFFECTS Has antifungal activity against *Cryptococcus* and *Candida* as well as *Chromomycosis*.

USES Alone or in combination with amphotericin B for serious systemic infections caused by susceptible strains of *Cryptococcus* and *Candida* species.
UNLABELED USES *Chromomycosis*.

CONTRAINDICATIONS Safety during pregnancy (category C) or lactation is not established.
CAUTIOUS USE Extreme caution in impaired kidney function; bone marrow depression, hematologic disorders, patients being treated with or having received radiation or bone marrow depressant drugs.

ROUTE & DOSAGE

Fungal Infection
Neonate: **PO** 80–160 mg/kg/day divided into 4 doses
Child: **PO** <50 kg, 1.5–4.5 g/m²/day divided into doses given q6h; >50 kg, 50–150 mg/kg/day in doses q6h divided into doses given q6h
Adult: **PO** 50–150 mg/kg/day divided every hour

Common adverse effects in *italic*; life-threatening effects underlined; generic names in **bold**; drug classifications in SMALL CAPS; ♣ Canadian drug name; ◑ Prototype drug.

STORAGE
Store in light-resistant containers at 15°–30° C (59°–86° F).

ADMINISTRATION

Oral

- Give lower dosages with longer dosage intervals in patients with serum creatinine of 1.7 mg/dL or higher. Check with physician.
- Give capsules a few at a time over 15 min to decrease incidence and severity of nausea and vomiting.

ADVERSE EFFECTS CNS: Confusion, hallucinations, headache, sedation, vertigo. **GI:** Nausea, vomiting, diarrhea, abdominal bloating, enterocolitis. **Hematologic:** Hypoplasia of bone marrow: anemia, leukopenia, thrombocytopenia, <u>agranulocytosis</u>, eosinophilia. **Skin:** Rash. **Metabolic:** Elevated levels of serum alkaline phosphatase, AST, ALT, BUN, serum creatinine. **GI:** Hepatomegaly, hepatitis.

DIAGNOSTIC TEST INTERFERENCE False elevations of *serum creatinine* can occur with *Ektachem analyzer.*

INTERACTIONS Drug: Amphotericin B produces additive or synergistic effects and can increase flucytosine toxicity by inhibiting its renal clearance.

PHARMACOKINETICS Absorption: Readily absorbed from GI tract. **Peak:** 2 h. **Distribution:** Widely distributed in body tissues including aqueous humor and CSF; crosses placenta. **Metabolism:** Minimally metabolized. **Elimination:** 75–90% excreted in urine unchanged. **Half- Life:** 3–6 h.

NURSING IMPLICATIONS

Assessment & Drug Effects

- C&S tests should be performed before initiation of therapy and at weekly intervals during therapy. Organism resistance has been reported.
- Lab tests: Obtain baseline hematology, kidney and liver function on all patients before and at frequent intervals during therapy. Twice weekly leukocyte and differential counts with WBC with differential and platelet counts are recommended.
- Do frequent assays of blood drug level, especially in patients with impaired kidney function to determine adequacy of drug excretion (*therapeutic range:* 25–100 mg/mL).
- Monitor I&O. Report change in I&O ratio or pattern. Because most of drug is eliminated unchanged by kidneys, compromised function can lead to drug accumulation.

Patient & Family Education

- Report fever, sore mouth or throat, and unusual bleeding or bruising tendency to physician.
- Be aware that the general duration of therapy is 4–6 wk, but it may continue for several months.
- Do not breast feed while taking this drug without consulting prescriber.
- Store this medication out of reach of children.

F

FLUDROCORTISONE ACETATE

(floo-droe-kor'ti-sone)

Florinef Acetate

Classifications: HORMONE AND SYNTHETIC SUBSTITUTE; ADRENAL CORTICOSTEROID; MINERALOCORTICOID; ANTI-INFLAMMATORY AGENT

Prototype: Hydrocortisone

Pregnancy Category: C

AVAILABILITY 0.1 mg tablets

ACTIONS Long-acting synthetic steroid with potent mineralocorticoid and moderate glucocorticoid activity. Small doses produce marked sodium retention, increased urinary potassium excretion, and elevated BP.

THERAPEUTIC EFFECTS Synthetic corticosteroid replacement product for adrenocortical insufficiency.

USES Partial replacement therapy for adrenocortical insufficiency and for treatment of salt-losing forms of congenital adrenogenital syndrome.

UNLABELED USES To increase systolic and diastolic blood pressure in patients with severe hypotension secondary to diabetes mellitus or to levodopa therapy.

CONTRAINDICATIONS Hypersensitivity to glucocorticoids, idiopathic thrombocytopenic purpura, psychoses, acute glomerulonephritis, viral or bacterial diseases of skin, infections not controlled by antibiotics, active or latent amebiasis, hypercorticism (Cushing's syndrome), smallpox vaccination or other immunologic procedures. Topical steroids are contraindicated in presence of varicella, vaccinia, on surfaces with compromised circulation, and in children <2 y.

CAUTIOUS USE Children; diabetes mellitus; chronic, active hepatitis positive for hepatitis B surface antigen; hyperlipidemia; cirrhosis; stromal herpes simplex; glaucoma, tuberculosis of eye; osteoporosis; convulsive disorders; hypothyroidism; diverticulitis; nonspecific ulcerative colitis; fresh intestinal anastomoses; active or latent peptic ulcer; gastritis; esophagitis; thromboembolic disorders; CHF; metastatic carcinoma; hypertension; renal insufficiency; history of allergies; active or arrested tuberculosis; systemic fungal infection; myasthenia gravis. Safety in pregnancy (category C) or lactation is not established.

ROUTE & DOSAGE

Adrenocortical Insufficiency

Infant: 0.05–0.1 mg/day
Child: **PO** 0.05–0.25 mg/day
Adult: **PO** 0.1 mg/day, may range from 0.1 mg 3 times/wk to 0.25 mg/day

Salt-Losing Adrenogenital Syndrome

Child: **PO** 0.05–0.1 mg/day
Adult: **PO** 0.1–0.2 mg/day

Common adverse effects in *italic;* life-threatening effects <u>underlined</u>; generic names in **bold;** drug classifications in SMALL CAPS; ♣ Canadian drug name; ◑ Prototype drug.

STORAGE
Store in airtight containers at 15°–30° C (59°–86° F). Protect from light.

ADMINISTRATION

Oral

- Note: Concomitant oral cortisone or hydrocortisone therapy may be advisable to provide substitute therapy approximating normal adrenal activity.

ADVERSE EFFECTS CNS: Vertigo, headache, nystagmus, increased intracranial pressure with papilledema (usually after discontinuation of medication), mental disturbances, aggravation of preexisting psychiatric conditions, insomnia, ataxia (rare). **CV:** CHF, hypertension, thromboembolism (rare), tachycardia. **Endocrine:** Suppressed linear growth in children, decreased glucose tolerance; hyperglycemia, manifestations of latent diabetes mellitus; hypocorticism; amenorrhea and other menstrual difficulties. **Special Senses:** Posterior subcapsular cataracts (especially in children), glaucoma, exophthalmos, increased intraocular pressure with optic nerve damage, perforation of the globe. **Metabolic:** Hypocalcemia; *sodium and fluid retention;* hypokalemia and hypokalemic alkalosis, negative nitrogen balance, decreased serum concentration of vitamins A and C. **GI:** *Nausea,* increased appetite, ulcerative esophagitis, pancreatitis, abdominal distension, peptic ulcer with perforation and hemorrhage, melena. **Hematologic:** Thrombocytopenia. **Musculoskeletal:** Long-term use: Osteoporosis, compression fractures, muscle wasting and weakness, tendon rupture, aseptic necrosis of femoral and humeral heads. **Skin:** Skin thinning and atrophy, *acne, impaired wound healing;* petechiae, ecchymosis, easy bruising; suppression of skin test reaction; hypopigmentation or hyperpigmentation, hirsutism, acneiform eruptions, subcutaneous fat atrophy; allergic dermatitis, urticaria, angioneurotic edema, increased sweating. **Body as a Whole:** <u>Anaphylactoid reactions</u> (rare), aggravation or masking of infections; malaise, weight gain, obesity. **Urogenital:** Increased or decreased motility and number of sperm.

INTERACTIONS Drug: The antidiabetic effects of **insulin** and SULFONYLUREAS may be diminished; **amphotericin B,** DIURETICS may increase **potassium** loss; **warfarin** may decrease prothrombin time; **indomethacin, ibuprofen** can potentiate the pressor effect of fludrocortisone; ANABOLIC STEROIDS increase risk of edema and acne; **rifampin** may increase the hepatic metabolism of fludrocortisone.

PHARMACOKINETICS Absorption: Readily absorbed from GI tract. **Peak:** 1.7 h. **Metabolism:** Metabolized in liver. **Half-Life:** 3.5 h.

NURSING IMPLICATIONS

Assessment & Drug Effects

- Monitor weight and I&O ratio to observe onset of fluid accumulation, especially if patient is on unrestricted salt intake and without potassium supplement. Report weight gain of 2 kg (5 lb)/wk for older children (>12 years) or any weight gain for children <12 years.

- Monitor and record BP daily. If hypertension develops as a consequence of therapy, report to physician. Usually, the dose will be reduced to 0.05 mg/day.
- Check BP q4–6h and weight at least every other day during periods of dosage adjustment.
- Lab tests: Periodic serum electrolytes and ABGs during prolonged therapy.
- Monitor for S&S of hypokalemia and hyperkalemic metabolic alkalosis (see Appendix D-1).
- Monitor for signs of overdosage (hypercorticism): psychosis, excess weight gain, edema, congestive heart failure, ravenous appetite, severe insomnia, and increase in BP.
- Note: Signs of insufficient dosage (hypocorticism) are loss of weight and appetite, nausea, vomiting, diarrhea, muscular weakness, increased fatigue, and hypotension.

Patient & Family Education

- Report signs of hypokalemia (see Appendix D-1).
- Be aware of signs of potassium depletion associated with high sodium intake: Muscle weakness, paresthesias, circumoral numbness; fatigue, anorexia, nausea, mental depression, polyuria, delirium, diminished reflexes, arrhythmias, cardiac failure, ileus, ECG changes.
- Advise patient to eat foods with high potassium content.
- Signs of edema should be reported immediately. Sodium intake may or may not require regulation, depending on individual needs and clinical situation.
- Weigh child daily each day under standard conditions and report steady weight gain.
- Report intercurrent infection, trauma, or unexpected stress of any kind promptly when taking maintenance therapy.
- Medication must not be suddenly stopped. Notify prescriber if child is ill or vomiting and cannot take drug.
- Carry medical identification at all times. It needs to indicate medical diagnosis, medication(s), physician's name, address, and telephone number.
- Do not breast feed while taking this drug without consulting physician.
- Store this medication out of reach of children.

FLUMAZENIL ●

(flu-ma′ze-nil)

Mazicon ♣ , Romazicon

Classifications: CENTRAL NERVOUS SYSTEM AGENT; BENZODIAZEPINE ANTAGONIST

Pregnancy Category: C

AVAILABILITY 0.1 mg/mL injection

ACTIONS Antagonizes the effects of benzodiazepine on the CNS, including sedation, impairment of recall, and psychomotor impairment. Does not reverse the effects of opioids.

THERAPEUTIC EFFECTS Reverses the action of a benzodiazepine.

USES Complete or partial reversal of sedation induced by benzodiazepine for anesthesia or diagnostic or therapeutic procedures and through overdose.

UNLABELED USES Seizure disorders, alcohol intoxication, hepatic encephalopathy, facilitation of weaning from mechanical ventilation.

CONTRAINDICATIONS Hypersensitivity to flumazenil or to benzodiazepines; patients given a benzodiazepine for control of a life-threatening condition; patients showing signs of cyclic antidepressant overdose; seizure-prone individuals during labor and delivery. Effects on children are not established.

CAUTIOUS USE Hepatic function impairment, older adults, pregnancy (category C), lactation, intensive care patients, head injury, drug- and alcohol-dependent patients, and physical dependence upon benzodiazepines.

ROUTE & DOSAGE

Reversal of Sedation

Child: **IV** 0.01 mg/kg initially, then 0.005–0.01 mg/kg (max dose 0.2 mg) given q1min (max total cumulative dose 1 mg). Doses may be repeated in 20 min (max 3 mg in 1 h)
Adult: **IV** 0.2 mg over 15 sec, may repeat 0.2 mg q60sec for 4 additional doses or a cumulative dose of 1 mg

Benzodiazepine Overdose

Adult: **IV** 0.2 mg over 30 sec, if no response after 30 sec, then 0.3 mg over 30 sec, may repeat with 0.5 mg q60sec (max cumulative dose of 3 mg)

STORAGE
Store at 15°–30° C (59°–86° F).

ADMINISTRATION
Intravenous

***PREPARE* Direct:** May give undiluted or diluted. If diluted use D5W, lactated Ringer's, NS.

***ADMINISTER* Direct:** ■ Ensure patency of IV before administration of flumazenil, since extravasation will cause local irritation. ■ Give through an IV that is freely flowing into a large vein. Give each 0.2 mg dose in small quantities over 15 sec each 0.2 mg dose should be given in small quantities over 15 sec. Repeat at 60-sec intervals (see ROUTE & DOSAGE). Do not give as a bolus dose. In high-risk patients, slow the rate to intervals of 6–10 min to provide the smallest effective dose. ■ Give repeat doses at 20 min intervals if resedation occurs (max 1 mg given at a rate of 0.2 mg/min, not to exceed 3 mg in any 1-h period). ■ Use all diluted solutions within 24 h of dilution.

ADVERSE EFFECTS CNS: Emotional lability, headache, *dizziness,* agitation, *resedation,* seizures esp if taking benzodiazepines for seizure control, blurred vision. **GI:** *Nausea, vomiting,* hiccups. **Other:** Shivering, pain at injection site, hypoventilation.

INTERACTIONS Drug: May antagonize effects of **zaleplon, zolpidem;** may cause convulsions or arrhythmias with TRICYCLIC ANTIDEPRESSANTS.

PHARMACOKINETICS Onset: 1–5 min. **Peak:** 6–10 min. **Duration:** 2–4 h. **Metabolism:** Metabolized in the liver to inactive metabolites. **Elimination:** 90–95% excreted in urine, 5–10% in feces within 72 h. **Half-Life:** 54 min.

NURSING IMPLICATIONS

Assessment & Drug Effects

- Note: Effect is seen in 1–3 min. If no effect consider if another drug was taken; flumazenil does not reverse narcotics. Because excretion is rapid, effects of flumazenil may wear off before benzodiazepine reversal is complete.
- Monitor respiratory status carefully until risk of resedation is unlikely (up to 120 min). Drug may not fully reverse benzodiazepine-induced ventilatory insufficiency.
- Monitor carefully for seizures and take appropriate precautions.

Patient & Family Education

- Do not drive or engage in potentially hazardous activities until at least 18–24 h after discharge following a procedure.
- Do not ingest alcohol or nonprescription drugs for 18–24 h after flumazenil is administered or if the effects of the benzodiazepine persist.
- Do not breast feed while taking this drug without consulting physician.

FLUOCINOLONE ACETONIDE

(floo-oh-sin'oh-lone)
Fluoderm ✦, Fluolar, Fluonid, Flurosyn, Synalar, Synalar-HP, Synemol
Classifications: SKIN AND MUCOUS MEMBRANE AGENT; ANTI-INFLAMMATORY; ADRENAL CORTICOSTEROID
Prototype: Hydrocortisone
Pregnancy Category: C

AVAILABILITY 0.025% ointment, cream; 0.2% cream; 0.01% cream, solution, shampoo, oil. **See Appendix** I-1.

FLUORESCEIN SODIUM

(flure'e-seen)
Fluorescite, Fluor-I-Strip, Fluor-I-Ful-Glo, Funduscein
Classification: OPHTHALMIC DIAGNOSTIC AGENT
Pregnancy Category: C

Common adverse effects in *italic;* life-threatening effects <u>underlined;</u> generic names in **bold;** drug classifications in SMALL CAPS; ✦ Canadian drug name; ⊘ Prototype drug.

AVAILABILITY 10%, 25% injection; 2% ocular solution; 0.6 mg, 1 mg, 9 mg strips

ACTIONS Mildly antiseptic fluorescent dye related chemically to phenolphthalein that demonstrates defects of the corneal epithelium.
THERAPEUTIC EFFECTS Any break in the epithelial tissue allows the dye to enter the tissue. Epithelial damage will appear as a bright green area.

USES An aid in fitting hard contact lenses, applanation tonometry, detecting corneal epithelial defects, and testing potency of lacrimal system. Used IV as a diagnostic aid in retinal angiography. Also used as an antidote for aniline dye.

CONTRAINDICATIONS Topical use with soft contact lenses not recommended.
CAUTIOUS USE History of hypersensitivity, allergies, bronchial asthma; pregnancy (category C), lactation.

ROUTE & DOSAGE

Diagnostic Aid
Adult: **Instillation** Instill 1–2 drops then have patient keep eyelid closed for 60 sec or moisten strip with sterile water, touch conjunctiva or fornix with moistened tip, and have patient blink to distribute

Retinal Angiography
Child: **IV** 7.5 mg/kg injected rapidly in antecubital vein
Adult: **IV** 5 mL of 10% solution or 3 mL of 25% solution injected rapidly in antecubital vein.

STORAGE
Store below 27° C (80° F); keep tightly closed when not in use and protect from light and freezing.

ADMINISTRATION

Instillation
- Avoid touching eyelids or surrounding area with eyedropper when instilling medication.
- Fit hard contact lenses: Instill drug with contact lenses in place. Have patient blink several times to distribute dye. Under blue light, areas that lack fluorescein will appear black, indicating that contact lens is touching cornea at these points.
- Test for potency of lacrimal system: One drop of 2% solution is instilled into conjunctival sac. Have patient blink at least 4 times. After 6 min, nasal secretions are examined under blue light. Traces of dye in secretions indicate that nasolacrimal drainage system is open.

ADVERSE EFFECTS Special Senses: *Temporary stinging, burning sensation,* conjunctival redness. **CNS:** (IV administration) Headache, paresthesias, pyrexia, convulsions. **CV:** (IV administration) Hypotension, transient dyspnea, acute pulmonary edema, basilar artery ischemia, syncope, <u>severe shock, cardiac arrest</u>. **GI:** (IV administration) Nausea, vomiting, strong metallic taste following high dosage. **Body as a Whole:**

Common adverse effects in *italic;* life-threatening effects <u>underlined</u>; generic names in **bold;** drug classifications in SMALL CAPS; ♣ Canadian drug name; ● Prototype drug.

567

(IV administration) Hypersensitivity (urticaria, pruritus, angioneurotic edema, <u>anaphylactic reaction</u>). **Skin:** (IV administration) Thrombophlebitis at injection site, temporary discoloration of skin and urine.

INTERACTIONS Drug: No clinically significant interactions established.

NURSING IMPLICATIONS

Assessment & Drug Effects

- Have facilities for treatment of anaphylactic reaction immediately available (e.g., epinephrine 1:1000 for IV or IM use, an antihistamine, and oxygen).
- Discontinue fluorescein immediately if signs and symptoms of sensitivity develop.

Patient & Family Education

- Note: IV administration may impart a yellowish orange discoloration to skin and to urine. Skin discoloration usually fades in 6–12 h; urine clears in 24–36 h.
- Do not breast feed while taking this drug without consulting physician.

FLUORIDE, SODIUM

(flo′rid)

Fluorinse, Fluoritab, Flura-Drops, Karidium, Pediaflor, Point-Two, Thera-Flur-N

Classifications: ELECTROLYTE AND WATER BALANCE AGENT: DENTAL PROPHYLACTIC

Pregnancy Category: C

AVAILABILITY 0.25 mg, 0.5 mg, 1 mg tablets; 0.125 mg, 0.25 mg, 0.5 mg drops; 0.2 mg/mL solution; 0.02%, 0.04%, 0.09%, 2% rinse; 0.5%, 1.2% gel

ACTIONS Source of the fluorine ion, a trace element. Incorporates into developing tooth enamel hardens surfaces and increases resistance to cariogenic microbial processes. Topical application reduces acid production by bacteria in dental plaque and promotes remineralization of acid-damaged enamel. Application to exposed root surfaces supports formation of insoluble materials within dentinal tubules, thereby blocking transport of offending stimuli. Arrests rapid dental decay associated with drug-, radiation-, or age-related xerostomia. One of the few agents known that stimulates osteoblastic activity, leading to increased bone mass.

THERAPEUTIC EFFECTS Topical application reduces acid production by bacteria in dental plaque and promotes remineralization of enamel.

USES When fluoride ion concentration in drinking water is 0.6 ppm or less, to prevent periodontal disease and dental caries, to treat dental cervical hypersensitivity, and to control dental caries associated with xerostomia.

UNLABELED USES Adjunctive treatment of osteoporosis; management of bone lesions in multiple myeloma; to reduce bone pain in patient with metastatic prostatic carcinoma; to stabilize progression of hearing loss in a limited number of patients with otosclerosis.

CONTRAINDICATIONS When daily intake of fluoride from drinking water exceeds 0.7 ppm; low-sodium or sodium-free diets; hypersensitivity to fluoride; gels or dental rinses by children <6 y, 1 mg tablet or rinse in children <3 y, or 1 mg rinse in children <6 y, pregnancy (category C).

ROUTE & DOSAGE

Prevent Periodontal Disease (Drinking Water Concentration <0.3 ppm)
Child: **PO** *6 mo–3 y,* 0.25 mg/day; *3–6 y,* 0.5 mg/day; *6–16 y,* 1 mg/day

Prevent Periodontal Disease (Drinking Water Concentration 0.3–0.6 ppm)
Child: **PO** *Birth–3 y,* no supplementation; *3–6 y,* 0.25 mg/day; *6–16 y,* 0.5 mg/day
NOTE: fluoride supplementation is not recommended before 6 months of age or if local water supply contains >0.6 ppm

Prevent Dental Caries
Child: **Topical** *6–12 y,* 5 mL of 0.2% solution daily; *>12 y,* 10 mL of 0.2% solution daily

Desensitization of Exposed Root Surfaces
Child: **Topical** 0.2% rinsing solution once nightly after brushing and flossing

STORAGE
Store all forms in tight plastic or paraffin-lined glass containers (sodium fluoride reacts with ordinary glass at a slow but appreciable rate) at 15°–30° C (59°–86° F). Avoid freezing.

ADMINISTRATION
Oral
- Avoid giving sodium fluoride with milk or dairy products. Calcium from these products combines with fluorine, decreasing its absorption.
- Give drops preferably after meals. Give undiluted or mixed with fluids or foods.
- Dissolve tablets in the mouth or chew before swallowing. Administer at bedtime (after brushing the teeth).

Topical
- Apply all fluorine preparations after thoroughly brushing and flossing; preferably at bedtime.
- Do not swallow topical or rinse preparations.
- If patient's mouth is sore, the neutral preparation (Thera-Flur N) is better tolerated.
- Use as treatment for dental cervical hypersensitivity: Thoroughly brush teeth; then swish PO solution around and between teeth for 1 min; expectorate. If gel is used, apply a few drops to toothbrush and brush gently onto affected surfaces.
- Apply gel-drops with applicators supplied by the dentist. Spread gel on inner surfaces of applicators, which are placed over lower and upper teeth at the same time. User bites down lightly for 6 min, then removes applicators and rinses mouth thoroughly. Applicators are cleaned with cold water.

ADVERSE EFFECTS Skin: Rash, atopic dermatitis, urticaria, stomatitis. **Body as a Whole:** GI and respiratory allergic reactions, salty or soapy taste, dehydration, thirst, excessive salivation, muscle weakness, tremors, <u>shock, death from cardiac and respiratory failure.</u> **Musculoskeletal:** Dental fluorosis (brown or white mottling of tooth enamel), osseous fluorosis (patchy mineralization and possible decrease in bone strength).

INTERACTIONS Drug: Aluminum, calcium, magnesium-containing products may decrease **fluoride** absorption.

PHARMACOKINETICS Absorption: Readily absorbed from GI tract. **Distribution:** Fluoride is stored in bones and teeth; crosses placenta; distributed into breast milk. **Elimination:** Rapidly excreted, primarily in urine with small amounts in feces.

NURSING IMPLICATIONS

Assessment & Drug Effect
- Monitor therapeutic effectiveness.

Patient & Family Education
- Do not eat, drink, or rinse mouth for at least 30 min after using the rinsing solution.
- Do not exceed recommended dosage. If mottling of teeth occurs, notify dentist.
- Apply sodium fluoride gel or solution used in orthodontic treatment regimen immediately before attachment or reattachment of the tooth-encircling bands.
- To be effective, fluorine supplementation must be consistent and continuous from infancy until 12–14 y.
- Consult dentist about continuing fluoride therapy if you move or there is a change in water supply (mottling may occur if drinking water has fluorine content >1.5 ppm).
- Do not breast feed while taking or using this drug without consulting physician.
- Store this medication out of reach of children.

FLUOXETINE HYDROCHLORIDE ⊕

(flu'ox-e-tine)

Prozac, Prozac Weekly, Sarafem

Classifications: CENTRAL NERVOUS SYSTEM AGENT; PSYCHOTHERAPEUTIC; SEROTONIN-REUPTAKE INHIBITOR (SSRI)

Pregnancy Category: B

AVAILABILITY 10 mg tablets; 10 mg, 20 mg capsules; 20 mg/5 mL solution; **Prozac Weekly:** 90 mg sustained-release capsules

ACTIONS Oral antidepressant chemically unrelated to tricyclic, tetracyclic, MAOI, or other available antidepressants. Antidepressant effect is presumed to be linked to its inhibition of CNS neuronal uptake of serotonin, a neurotransmitter. Known as a selective serotonin reuptake inhibitor (SSRI).

THERAPEUTIC EFFECTS Effectiveness may take from several days to 5 wk to develop fully. Drug has antidepressant, antiobsessive-compulsive, and antibulimic actions.

USES Depression, obsessive-compulsive disorder (OCD), bulimia nervosa, premenstrual dysphoric disorder.
UNLABELED USES Obesity.

CONTRAINDICATIONS Hypersensitivity to fluoxetine, or other SSRI drugs.
CAUTIOUS USE Hepatic and renal impairment, anorexia, hyponatremia, diabetes, patients with history of suicidal ideations. Older adults may require dose adjustments. Safety in pregnancy (category B), lactation, and in children is not established.

ROUTE & DOSAGE

Depression, Obsessive-Compulsive Disorder
Child: **PO** >8 y, 10–20 mg/day in a.m. (max 60 mg/day)
Adult: **PO** 20 mg/day in a.m., may increase by 20 mg/day at weekly intervals (max 80 mg/day); 20 mg/day in a.m., when stable may switch to 90 mg sustained-release capsule weekly (max 90 mg/wk)

Premenstrual Dysphoric Disorder
Adult: **PO** 10–20 mg daily (max 60 mg/day)

Bulimia Nervosa
Adult: **PO** 60 mg daily

STORAGE
Store at 15°–25° C (59°–77° F).

ADMINISTRATION
Oral
- Give as a single dose in morning. Give in two divided doses; one in a.m. and one at noon to prevent insomnia, when more than 20 mg/day prescribed.
- Provide suicidal or potentially suicidal patient with small quantities of prescription medication.

ADVERSE EFFECTS CNS: *Headache, nervousness, anxiety, insomnia,* drowsiness, fatigue, tremor, dizziness. **CV:** Palpitations, hot flushes, chest pain. **GI:** *Nausea, diarrhea,* anorexia, dyspepsia, increased appetite, dry mouth. **Skin:** Rash, pruritus, sweating, hypersensitivity reactions. **Special Senses:** Blurred vision. **Body as a Whole:** Myalgias, arthralgias, flu-like syndrome, hyponatremia, **Urogenital:** Sexual dysfunction, menstrual irregularities.

INTERACTIONS Drug: Concurrent use of **tryptophan** may cause agitation, restlessness, and GI distress; MAO INHIBITORS, **selegiline** may increase risk of severe hypertensive reaction and death; increases half-life of **diazepam;** may increase toxicity of TRICYCLIC ANTIDEPRESSANTS; AMPHETAMINES, **cilostazol, nefazodone, pentazocine, propafenone,**

sibutramine, tramadol, venlafaxine may increase risk of serotonin syndrome; may inhibit metabolism of **carbamazepine, phenytoin, ritonavir;** increased ergotamine toxicity with **dihydroergotamine, ergotamine. Herbal: St. John's wort** may cause serotonin syndrome.

PHARMACOKINETICS Absorption: 60–80% absorbed from GI tract. **Onset:** 1–3 wk. **Peak:** 4–8 h. **Distribution:** Widely distributed, including CNS. **Metabolism:** Metabolized in liver to active metabolite, norfluoxetine. **Elimination:** >80% excreted in urine; 12% in feces. **Half-life:** Fluoxetine 2–3 days, norfluoxetine 7–9 days.

NURSING IMPLICATIONS

Assessment & Drug Effects

- Use with caution in children especially those with impaired renal or hepatic function (may need lower dose).
- Use with caution in anorexic patient, because weight loss is a possible side effect.
- Monitor for S&S of anaphylactoid reaction (see Appendix D-1).
- Lab tests: Periodic serum electrolytes; monitor closely plasma glucose in diabetes.
- Monitor serum sodium level for development of hyponatremia, especially in patients who are taking diuretics or are otherwise hypovolemic.
- Monitor diabetics for loss of glycemic control; hypoglycemia has occurred during initiation of therapy, and hyperglycemia during drug withdrawal.
- Monitor for S&S of improved affect. Requires approximately 2–3 wk for therapeutic effects to be felt.
- Weigh weekly to monitor weight loss, particularly in the nutritionally compromised patient. Report significant weight loss to prescriber.
- Observe for and promptly report rash or urticaria and signs and symptoms of fever, leukocytosis, arthralgias, carpal tunnel syndrome, edema, respiratory distress, and proteinuria. Drug may have to be discontinued or adjunctive therapy instituted with steroids or antihistamines.
- Observe for dizziness and drowsiness and employ safety measures (up with assistance, side rails, etc.) as indicated.
- Monitor for and report increased anxiety, nervousness, or insomnia; may need modification of drug dose.
- Monitor for seizures in patients with a history of seizures. Use appropriate safety precautions.
- Antidepressants increase risk of suicidal thinking and behavior in children and adolescents with major depressive disorder, obsessive compulsive disorder, and other psychiatric disorders. Observe closely for worsening of condition, suicidality, and behavior changes. Instruct family and caregivers to monitor for these symptoms and discuss with prescriber. A MedGuide describing risks and stating whether the drug is approved for the child's/adolescent's condition should be provided for all families when antidepressants are prescribed.
- Monitor patients with hepatic or renal impairment carefully for signs and symptoms of toxicity (e.g., agitation, restlessness, nausea, vomiting, seizures).

Common adverse effects in *italic;* life-threatening effects <u>underlined</u>; generic names in **bold**; drug classifications in SMALL CAPS; ✦ Canadian drug name; ⊘ Prototype drug.

Patient & Family Education

- Notify prescriber of intent to become pregnant.
- Notify prescriber of any rash; possible sign of a serious group of adverse effects.
- Do not drive or engage in potentially hazardous activities until response to drug is known; especially if dizziness noted.
- Monitor blood glucose for loss of glycemic control if diabetic.
- Keep scheduled appointments with health care provider. Report immediately increasing depression and any thoughts of suicide.
- Note: Drug may increase seizure activity in those with history of seizure.
- Do not breast feed while taking this drug without consulting physician.
- Store this medication out of reach of children.

FLUTICASONE

(flu-ti-ca′sone)
Flonase, Flovent, Cutivate
Classifications: SKIN AND MUCOUS MEMBRANE AGENT; ANTI-INFLAMMATORY; HORMONES AND SYNTHETIC SUBSTITUTES; ADRENAL CORTICOSTEROID
Prototype: Hydrocortisone
Pregnancy Category: C

AVAILABILITY 44 mcg, 110 mcg, 220 mcg aerosol; 50 mcg, 100 mcg, 250 mcg powder; 0.05%, 0.005% cream; 0.005% ointment. **See Appendix I-1.**

FLUVOXAMINE

(flu-vox′a-meen)
Luvox
Classifications: CENTRAL NERVOUS SYSTEM AGENT; PSYCHOTHERAPEUTIC; SELECTIVE SEROTONIN-REUPTAKE INHIBITOR (SSRI)
Prototype: Fluoxetine
Pregnancy Category: B

AVAILABILITY 25 mg, 50 mg, 100 mg tablets

ACTIONS Antidepressant with potent, selective, inhibitory activity on neuronal (5-HT) serotonin-reuptake inhibitor (SSRI); structurally unrelated to TCAs. Compared with TCAs, shows fewer anticholinergenic effects and no severe cardiovascular effects.

THERAPEUTIC EFFECTS Effective as an antidepressant and for control of obsessive-compulsive disorders.

USES Treatment of depression and obsessive-compulsive disorders.
UNLABELED USES Chronic tension type headaches, panic attacks.

CONTRAINDICATIONS Hypersensitivity to fluvoxamine or fluoxetine.
CAUTIOUS USE Pregnancy (category B), lactation, liver disease, renal impairment, history of seizures.

F

ROUTE & DOSAGE

Depression, Obsessive-Compulsive Disorder

Child: **PO** *8–11 y,* start with 25 mg q at bedtime, may increase by 25 mg q4–7days (max 200 mg/day in divided doses; divide doses >50 mg/day into b.i.d. dosing)
Adult: **PO** Start with 50 mg daily, may increase slowly up to 300 mg/day given q at bedtime, or divided b.i.d. (max 200 mg/day; divide doses >50 mg/day into b.i.d. dosing)

STORAGE

Store at room temperature, 15°–30° C (59°–86° F), away from moisture and light.

ADMINISTRATION

Oral

- Give starting doses at bedtime to improve tolerance to nausea and vomiting; both are common early in therapy. Titrate dose to lowest possible to achieve effect.

ADVERSE EFFECTS CNS: *Somnolence, headache, agitation, insomnia, dizziness,* seizures. **CV:** Orthostatic hypotension, slight bradycardia. **GI:** *Nausea, vomiting, dry mouth, constipation, anorexia.* **Urogenital:** Sexual dysfunction. **Skin:** Stevens-Johnson syndrome, toxic epidermal necrolysis (rare).

DIAGNOSTIC TEST INTERFERENCE *Gamma-glutamyl transferase* increased by more than 3-fold following 3 wk of therapy.

INTERACTIONS Drug: Fluvoxamine has been shown to significantly increase plasma levels of **amitriptyline, clomipramine,** and other TRICYCLIC ANTIDEPRESSANTS to mildly increase levels of their metabolites. May antagonize the blood pressure–lowering effects of **atenolol** and other BETA-BLOCKERS. May increase levels and toxicity of **carbamazepine, mexiletine.** May increase **lithium** levels causing neurotoxicity, **serotonin** syndrome, somnolence, and mania. One report of increased **theophylline** levels with toxicity. Increases prothrombin time in patients on **warfarin. Herbal: Melatonin** may increase and prolong drowsiness; **St. John's wort** may cause **serotonin** syndrome.

PHARMACOKINETICS Absorption: Almost completely absorbed from GI tract. **Onset:** 4–7 days. **Distribution:** Approximately 77% bound to plasma proteins; excreted in human breast milk but in an amount that poses little risk to the nursing infant. **Metabolism:** Metabolized in liver. **Elimination:** Completely excreted in urine. **Half-Life:** 16–24 h.

NURSING IMPLICATIONS

Assessment & Drug Effects

- Monitor for significant nausea and vomiting, especially during initial therapy.

Common adverse effects in *italic;* life-threatening effects underlined; generic names in **bold;** drug classifications in SMALL CAPS; ♣ Canadian drug name; ⦾ Prototype drug.

- Assess safety; drowsiness and dizziness are common adverse effects.
- Monitor PT and INR carefully with concurrent warfarin therapy; adjust warfarin as needed.
- Antidepressants increase risk of suicidal thinking and behavior in children and adolescents with major depressive disorder, obsessive compulsive disorder, and other psychiatric disorders. Observe closely for worsening of condition, suicidality, and behavior changes. Instruct family and caregivers to monitor for these symptoms and discuss with prescriber. A MedGuide describing risks and stating whether the drug is approved for the child's/adolescent's condition should be provided for all families when antidepressants are prescribed.

Patient & Family Education
- Note: Nausea and vomiting are common in early therapy. Notify physician if these adverse effects last more than a few days.
- Exercise caution with hazardous activity until response to the drug is known.
- Keep scheduled appointments with health care provider. Report immediately increasing depression and any thoughts of suicide.
- Do not breast feed while taking this drug without consulting prescriber.
- Store this medication out of reach of children.

FOLIC ACID (VITAMIN B₉, PTEROYLGLUTAMIC ACID)
(fol'ic)
Apo-Folic ♣ , Folacin, Folvite, Novofolacid ♣

FOLATE SODIUM
Folvite Sodium
Classification: VITAMIN B₉
Pregnancy Category: A

AVAILABILITY 0.4 mg, 0.8 mg, 1 mg tablets; 5 mg/mL injection

ACTIONS Vitamin B complex essential for nucleoprotein synthesis and maintenance of normal erythropoiesis. Acts against folic acid deficiency that impairs thymidylate synthesis and results in production of defective DNA that leads to megaloblast formation and arrest of bone marrow maturation.
THERAPEUTIC EFFECTS Stimulates production of RBCs, WBCs, and platelets in patients with megaloblastic anemias. Include improved symptoms of glossitis, diarrhea, constipation, weight loss, irritability, fatigue, restless legs, diffuse muscular pain, insomnia, forgetfulness, mental depression, pallor. Adequate intake by pregnant women is associated with lowered rates of birth defects such as spina bifida and cleft palate.

USES Folate deficiency, macrocytic anemia, and megaloblastic anemias associated with malabsorption syndromes, alcoholism, primary liver disease, inadequate dietary intake, pregnancy, infancy, and childhood.

CONTRAINDICATIONS Folic acid alone for pernicious anemia or other vitamin B₁₂ deficiency states; normocytic, refractory, aplastic, or undiagnosed anemia.
CAUTIOUS USE Pregnancy (category A), lactation.

FOLIC ACID (VITAMIN B₉, PTEROYLGLUTAMIC ACID)

ROUTE & DOSAGE

Treatment of Deficiency

Infant: **PO/IM/SC/IV** 15 mcg/kg/dose (max 50 mcg/day)
Child: **PO/IM/SC/IV** 1 mg/day
Adult: **PO/IM/SC/IV** 1–3 mg/day

Maintenance

Pregnant/Lactating: **PO/IM/SC/IV** 0.8 mg/day
Infants: **PO/IM/SC/IV** 30–45 mcg/day
Child: **PO/IM/SC/IV** 0.1–0.4 mg/day
Adult: **PO/IM/SC/IV** 0.5 mg/day

STORAGE

Store at 15°–30° C (59°–86° F) in tightly closed containers protected from light, unless otherwise directed.

ADMINISTRATION

Intravenous

PREPARE **Direct or Continuous:** Given undiluted.
ADMINISTER **Direct or Continuous:** Give over 30–60 sec. May also add to a continuous infusion.
INCOMPATIBILITIES **Solution/Additive: Doxapram.**

ADVERSE EFFECTS Reportedly nontoxic. Slight flushing and feeling of warmth following IV administration.

DIAGNOSTIC TEST INTERFERENCE Falsely low serum *folate levels* may occur with *Lactobacillus casei assay* in patients receiving antibiotics such as TETRACYCLINES.

INTERACTIONS Drug: Chloramphenicol may antagonize effects of **folate** therapy; **phenytoin** metabolism may be increased, thus decreasing its levels in **folate**-deficient patients.

PHARMACOKINETICS Absorption: Readily absorbed from proximal small intestine. **Peak:** 30–60 min PO. **Distribution:** Distributed to all body tissues; high concentrations in CSF; crosses placenta; distributed into breast milk. **Metabolism:** Metabolized in liver to active metabolites. **Elimination:** Small amounts eliminated in urine in folate-deficient patients; large amounts excreted in urine with high doses.

NURSING IMPLICATIONS

Assessment & Drug Effects

- *Normal serum level* is >3 ng/mL and RBC Folate level is 153–605 ng/mL.
- Obtain a careful history of dietary intake and drug and alcohol usage prior to start of therapy. Drugs reported to cause folate deficiency include oral contraceptives, alcohol, barbiturates, methotrexate, phenytoin, primidone, and trimethoprim. Folate deficiency may also result from renal dialysis. Many young women may not ingest adequate amounts to meet recommended intake during pregnancy. Large doses

may mask the hematalogic effects of vitamin B$_{12}$ deficiency, while allowing the neurologic complications of vitamin B$_{12}$ deficiency to progress.
- Keep physician informed of patient's response to therapy.
- Monitor patients on phenytoin for subtherapeutic plasma levels.

Patient & Family Education
- Instruct all families of young children about adequate intake of folate. Females of childbearing age and who are pregnant or lactating should receive careful instruction and supplements if indicated. Fortified grains, liver, yeast, and leafy vegetables are common sources.
- Remain under close medical supervision while taking folic acid therapy. Adjustment of maintenance dose should be made if there is threat of relapse.
- Do not breast feed while taking this drug without consulting physician.
- Store this medication out of reach of children.

FORMOTEROL FUMARATE
(for-mo-ter'ol)
Foradil Aerolizer
Classifications: AUTONOMIC NERVOUS SYSTEM AGENT; BETA-ADRENERGIC AGONIST (SYMPATHOMIMETIC); BRONCHODILATOR
Prototype: Albuterol
Pregnancy Category: C

AVAILABILITY 12 mcg inhalation capsules

ACTIONS Long-acting selective beta$_2$-adrenergic receptor agonist. Stimulates production of intracellular cyclic AMP, which causes relaxation of bronchial smooth muscle. Also inhibits release of mediators of immediate hypersensitivity (e.g., histamine and leukotrienes) from mast cells in the lung.
THERAPEUTIC EFFECTS Acts locally in lung as a bronchodilator; prevents bronchoconstriction that occurs during an asthma attack.

USES Treatment of asthma, prevention of exercise-induced asthma, prevention of bronchospasm in COPD.
UNLABELED USES Bronchitis.

CONTRAINDICATIONS Hypersensitivity to formoterol; significantly worsening or acutely deteriorating asthma; severe asthmatic attacks; paradoxical bronchospasm; pregnancy (category C); lactation. Safety and efficiency in children <5 y are not established.
CAUTIOUS USE Cardiovascular disorders (especially coronary insufficiency, cardiac arrhythmias, and hypertension); convulsive disorders; thyrotoxicosis; heightened responsiveness to sympathomimetic amines; diabetes mellitus.

ROUTE & DOSAGE

Treatment of Asthma, COPD
Child/Adult: **Inhaled** ≥5 y, inhale contents of 1 capsule q12h

---

Prevention of Exercise-Induced Asthma
Child/Adult: **Inhaled** ≥*12 y*, inhale contents of 1 capsule at least 15 min before exercise, do not repeat for at least 12 h

STORAGE
Store capsules in the blister at 20°–25° C (62°–77° F).

ADMINISTRATION

Oral Inhalation
- Remove capsule from blister IMMEDIATELY before use.
- Avoid exposing capsules to moisture.
- Give capsules only by the oral inhalation route and only by using the Aerolizer Inhaler™. Review use of the Aerolizer Inhaler in *Patient Instructions for Use* provided by manufacturer. Do not use a spacer with the Aerolizer.
- Instruct patient not to swallow capsule and not to exhale into the Aerolizer.
- Patients who have been taking the inhaled form, short-acting beta$_2$-agonists regularly (e.g., 3–4 times a day) are usually instructed to use these drugs ONLY for symptomatic relief of acute asthma symptoms. Check with physician.

ADVERSE EFFECTS Body as a Whole: *Viral infections,* chest infection, chest pain, fatigue, hyperglycemia. **CNS:** Headache, tremor, dizziness, insomnia. **GI:** Abdominal pain, dyspepsia, nausea. **Respiratory:** Pharyngitis, bronchitis, dyspnea, tonsillitis, dysphonia, <u>fatal exacerbation of asthma</u>. **Skin:** Rash.

INTERACTIONS Drug: Effects may be antagonized by NON-SELECTIVE BETA-BLOCKERS; XANTHINES, STEROIDS; DIURETICS may potentiate hypokalemia.

PHARMACOKINETICS Absorption: Rapidly absorbed into plasma after oral inhalation. **Onset:** 1–3 min. **Peak:** 1–3 h. **Metabolism:** Metabolized by glucuronidation in the liver. **Elimination:** 60% excreted in urine, 33% in feces. **Half-Life:** 10 h.

NURSING IMPLICATIONS

Assessment & Drug Effects
- Monitor cardiovascular status with periodic ECG, BP, and HR determinations.
- Withhold drug and notify physician immediately of signs and symptoms of bronchospasm.
- Lab tests: Monitor serum potassium and blood glucose periodically.
- Monitor diabetics closely for loss of glycemic control.

Patient & Family Education
- Do not take this drug more frequently than every 12 h.
- Use a short-acting inhaler if symptoms develop between doses of formoterol.
- Seek medical care immediately if a previously effective dosage regimen fails to provide the usual response, or if swelling about the face and neck and difficulty breathing develop.

Common adverse effects in *italic;* life-threatening effects <u>underlined</u>; generic names in **bold**; drug classifications in SMALL CAPS; ♣ Canadian drug name; ☉ Prototype drug.

- Report any of the following immediately to the physician: Rash, hives, palpitations, chest pain, rapid heart rate, tremor or nervousness.
- Note to diabetics: Monitor blood glucose levels carefully because hyperglycemia is a possible adverse reaction.
- Do not breast feed while taking this drug.
- Store this medication out of reach of children.

FOSPHENYTOIN SODIUM

(fos-phen'i-toin)
Cerebyx
Classifications: CENTRAL NERVOUS SYSTEM AGENT; HYDANTOIN ANTI-CONVULSANT AGENT
Prototype: Phenytoin
Pregnancy Category: D

AVAILABILITY 150 mg, 750 mg vials

ACTIONS Prodrug of phenytoin that converts to the anticonvulsant, phenytoin, after parenteral administration. Thought to modulate the sodium channels of neurons, calcium flux across neuronal membranes, and enhance the sodium–potassium ATPase activity of neurons and glial cells.
THERAPEUTIC EFFECTS The cellular mechanism of phenytoin is thought to be responsible for the anticonvulsant activity of fosphenytoin.

USES Control of generalized convulsive status epilepticus and the prevention and treatment of seizures during neurosurgery, or as a parenteral short-term substitute for oral phenytoin.
UNLABELED USES Antiarrhythmic agent especially in treatment of digitalis-induced arrhythmia; treatment of trigeminal neuralgia (tic douloureux).

CONTRAINDICATIONS Hypersensitivity to hydantoin products, rash, seizures due to hypoglycemia, sinus bradycardia, complete or incomplete heart block; Adams–Stokes syndrome; pregnancy (category D), lactation.
CAUTIOUS USE Impaired liver or kidney function, alcoholism, hypotension, heart block, bradycardia, severe CAD, diabetes mellitus, hyperglycemia, respiratory depression, acute intermittent porphyria. Safety in children not fully established.

ROUTE & DOSAGE

Status Epilepticus
Child: Use phenytoin doses with conversion of 1 mg phenytoin = 1 mg PE (PE = phenytoin sodium equivalents)
Adult: **IV Loading Dose** 15–20 mg PE/kg administered at 100–150 mg PE/min (nonemergent loading dose, 10–20 PE/kg) **IV Maintenance Dose** 4–6 mg PE/kg/day

Substitution for Oral Phenytoin Therapy
Child/Adult: **IV/IM** Substitute fosphenytoin at the same total daily dose in mg PE as the oral dose at a rate of infusion not greater than 150 mg PE/min

F

STORAGE
Store at 2°–8° C (36°–46° F); may store at room temperature not to exceed 48 h.

ADMINISTRATION
Note: All dosing is expressed in phenytoin sodium equivalents (PE) to avoid the need to calculate molecular weight adjustments between fosphenytoin and phenytoin sodium doses. **ALWAYS** prescribe and fill fosphenytoin in PE units.

Intramuscular

- Follow institutional policy regarding maximum volume to inject into one IM site. Not the recommended route in status epilepticus.

Intravenous

PREPARE **Direct:** Dilute in DSW or NS to a concentration of 1.5–25 mg PE/mL.
ADMINISTER **Direct:** Do not administer at a rate >150 mg PE/min.

ADVERSE EFFECTS CNS: Usually dose related. Paresthesia, tinnitus, *nystagmus, dizziness, somnolence, drowsiness,* ataxia, mental confusion, tremors, insomnia, headache, seizures, increased reflexes, dysarthria, intracranial hypertension. Abrupt withdrawal can cause status epilepticus. **CV:** Bradycardia, tachycardia, asystole, hypotension, hypertension, <u>cardiovascular collapse, cardiac arrest</u>, heart block, ventricular fibrillation, phlebitis. **Special Senses:** Photophobia, conjunctivitis, diplopia, blurred vision. **GI:** *Gingival hyperplasia,* nausea, vomiting, constipation, epigastric pain, dysphagia, loss of taste, weight loss, hepatitis, liver necrosis. **Hematologic:** Thrombocytopenia, leukopenia, leukocytosis, <u>agranulocytosis</u>, pancytopenia, eosinophilia; megaloblastic, hemolytic, or <u>aplastic anemias</u>. **Metabolic:** Fever, hyperglycemia, glycosuria, weight gain, edema, transient increase in serum thyrotropic (TSH) level, hyperkalemia, osteomalacia or rickets associated with hypocalcemia and elevated alkaline phosphatase activity. **Skin:** Alopecia, hirsutism (especially in young female); <u>rash: scarlatiniform, maculopapular, urticarial, morbilliform (may be fatal)</u>; bullous, exfoliative, or purpuric dermatitis; <u>Stevens–Johnson syndrome, toxic epidermal necrolysis</u>, keratosis, neonatal hemorrhage, *pruritus*. **Urogenital:** Acute renal failure, Peyronie's disease. **Respiratory:** Acute pneumonitis, pulmonary fibrosis. **Musculoskeletal:** Periarteritis nodosum, acute systemic lupus erythematosus, craniofacial abnormalities (with enlargement of lips). **Other:** Lymphadenopathy, injection site pain, chills.

DIAGNOSTIC TEST INTERFERENCE Fosphenytoin may produce lower than normal values for ***dexamethasone*** or ***metyrapone*** tests; may increase serum levels of ***glucose, BSP,*** and ***alkaline phosphatase*** and may decrease ***PBI*** and ***urinary steroid*** levels.

INTERACTIONS Drug: Alcohol decreases fosphenytoin effects; other ANTICONVULSANTS may increase or decrease fosphenytoin levels; fosphenytoin may decrease absorption and increase metabolism of ORAL ANTICOAGULANTS; fosphenytoin increases metabolism of CORTICOSTEROIDS and ORAL CONTRACEPTIVES, thus decreasing their effectiveness; **amiodarone, chloramphenicol, omeprazole** increase fosphenytoin levels; ANTITUBERCULOSIS AGENTS decrease fosphenytoin levels. **Food: Folic acid, calcium, vitamin D** absorption may be decreased by fosphenytoin; fosphenytoin absorption may be decreased by enteral nutrition supplements. **Herbal: Ginkgo** may decrease anticonvulsant effectiveness.

PHARMACOKINETICS Absorption: Completely absorbed after IM administration. **Peak:** 30 min IM. **Distribution:** 95–99% bound to plasma proteins, displaces phenytoin from protein binding sites; crosses placenta, small amount in breast milk. **Metabolism:** Converted to phenytoin by phosphatases; phenytoin is oxidized in liver to inactive metabolites. **Elimination:** Half-life 15 min to convert fosphenytoin to phenytoin, 22 h phenytoin; phenytoin metabolites excreted in urine.

NURSING IMPLICATIONS

Note: See **phenytoin** for additional nursing implications.

Assessment & Drug Effects

- Monitor ECG, BP, and respiratory function continuously during and for 10–20 min after infusion.
- Discontinue infusion and notify physician if rash appears. Be prepared to substitution alternative therapy rapidly to prevent withdrawal-precipitated seizures.
- Lab tests: Monitor CBC with differential, platelet count, serum electrolytes, and blood glucose.
- Allow at least 2 h after IV infusion and 4 h after IM injection before monitoring total plasma phenytoin concentration.
- ***Therapeutic serum level*** is 10–20 mg/L of free and bound phenytoin or 1–2 mg/L of free phenytoin only.
- Monitor diabetics for loss of glycemic control.
- Consider total amount of phosphate administered in drug for those on phosphate restrictions.
- Monitor carefully for adverse effects, especially in patients with renal or hepatic disease or hypoalbuminemia.

Patient & Family Education

- Be aware of potential adverse effects. Itching, burning, tingling, or paresthesia are common during and for some time following IV infusion.
- Do not breast feed while taking this drug.

FURAZOLIDONE

(fur-a-zoe'li-done)
Furoxone
Classifications: ANTI-INFECTIVE; NITROFURAN ANTIBIOTIC; MAO INHIBITOR
Pregnancy Category: C

AVAILABILITY 100 mg tablets; 50 mg/15 mL liquid

ACTIONS Synthetic nitrofuran with antibacterial and antiprotozoal properties. Acts by interfering with several bacterial enzyme systems including cell wall synthesis of the bacteria.

THERAPEUTIC EFFECTS A MAO INHIBITOR that is cumulative and dose related (occurring after 4 or 5 days of therapy). Bactericidal against majority of GI pathogens, including species of *Enterobacter aerogenes, Escherichia coli, Giardia lamblia, Proteus, Salmonella, Shigella, Staphylococcus,* and *Vibrio cholerae.*

F

USES Bacterial or protozoal diarrhea and enteritis caused by susceptible organisms.

CONTRAINDICATIONS Hypersensitivity to furazolidone, concurrent use with alcohol, other MAO INHIBITORS, tyramine-containing foods, indirect-acting sympathomimetic amines; infants <1 mo. Safety during pregnancy (category C) or lactation is not established.

CAUTIOUS USE If at all, patients with G6PD deficiency.

ROUTE & DOSAGE

Diarrhea and Enteritis

Child: **PO** *1 mo–1 y*, 8–17 mg q.i.d.; *1–4 y*, 17–25 mg q.i.d.; *≥5 y*, 25–50 mg q.i.d. (max 8.8 mg/kg/day)
Adult: **PO** 100 mg q.i.d.

STORAGE

Store in tight, light-resistant containers (drug darkens on exposure to light) at 15°–30° C (59°–86° F). Protect from excessive heat.

ADMINISTRATION

Oral

- Diarrhea should respond in 2–5 days.
- Some patients taking the drug who also ingested alcohol had flushing, temperature elevation, hypotension, dyspnea, chest constriction (disulfiram-type reaction). Symptoms improve 24 h after alcohol ingestion.

ADVERSE EFFECTS GI: *Nausea, vomiting,* abdominal pain, diarrhea. **Hypersensitivity:** Fever, arthralgia, hypotension, urticaria, angioedema, vesicular or morbilliform rash. **Body as a Whole:** Headache, malaise, dizziness, hypoglycemia. **Hematologic:** Intravascular hemolysis in patients with G6PD deficiency, <u>agranulocytosis</u> (rare). **Special Senses:** Partial deafness.

DIAGNOSTIC TEST INTERFERENCE Furazolidone metabolite reportedly may cause false-positive reactions for **_urine glucose_** with **_copper sulfate reduction methods,_** e.g., **_Benedict's reagent, Clinitest,_** and **_Fehling's solution._**

INTERACTIONS Drug: Alcohol may elicit disulfiram-type reaction up to 4 days after the drug is stopped; MAO INHIBITORS, NARCOTICS, SYMPATHOMIMETIC AMINES, **ephedrine, phenylpropanolamine** may cause a hypertensive reaction; TRICYCLIC ANTIDEPRESSANTS may cause toxic psychosis. **Food:** May interact with tyramine-containing foods, resulting in flushing, tachycardia, and hypertensive crisis. See **phenelzine** (MAO INHIBITOR prototype). **Herbal: Ginseng** may cause hypertension, manic symptoms, headaches, nervousness; **ma-huang, ephedra, St. John's wort** may lead to hypertensive crisis.

PHARMACOKINETICS Absorption: Poorly absorbed from GI tract. **Metabolism:** Metabolized in intestines. **Elimination:** Excreted in urine.

NURSING IMPLICATIONS

Assessment & Drug Effects

- Monitor for nausea and vomiting. Dosage reduction may be needed.
- Note: Bed rest, fluid and electrolyte replacement (as indicated) are important adjuncts to therapy. Consult physician regarding dietary allowances.
- Keep prescriber informed of S&S of dehydration (see Appendix D-1) and electrolyte imbalance.
- Monitor patients for lost glycemic control because drug may cause hypoglycemia (see Appendix D-1). Use glucose oxidase methods for urine testing (e.g., Clinistix, Diastix, TesTape).

Patient & Family Education

- Report the following to prescriber: Faintness, weakness, and lightheadedness. These may be symptoms of hypersensitivity reaction or hypoglycemia.
- Be aware of and avoid foods high in tyramine (e.g., aged and fermented food and drinks) that may produce hypertensive reaction. Hypertensive crisis is most likely to occur when drug is continued beyond 5 days or when large doses are given.
- Do not drink alcohol during furazolidone therapy and for at least 4 days after drug is stopped. Ingestion of alcohol may cause disulfiram-type reaction (see Appendix D-1); symptoms may last up to 24 h.
- Note: Drug may impart a harmless brown color to urine.
- Monitor blood glucose for loss of glycemic control if diabetic.
- Do not breast feed while taking this drug without consulting physician.
- Store this medication out of reach of children.

FUROSEMIDE ℗

(fur-oh′se-mide)

Fumide ♣, Furomide ♣, Lasix, Luramide ♣

Classifications: ELECTROLYTIC AND WATER BALANCE AGENT; LOOP DIURETIC
Pregnancy Category: C

AVAILABILITY 20 mg, 40 mg, 80 mg tablets; 10 mg/mL, 40 mg/5 mL oral solution; 10 mg/mL injection

ACTIONS Rapid-acting potent sulfonamide "loop" diuretic and antihypertensive with pharmacologic effects and uses almost identical to those of ethacrynic acid. Exact mode of action not clearly defined; decreases renal vascular resistance and may increase renal blood flow.

THERAPEUTIC EFFECTS Inhibits reabsorption of sodium and chloride primarily in loop of Henle and also in proximal and distal renal tubules; an antihypertensive that decreases edema and intravascular volume. Reportedly less ototoxic than ethacrynic acid.

USES Treatment of edema associated with CHF, cirrhosis of liver, and kidney disease, including nephrotic syndrome. May be used for management of hypertension, alone or in combination with other antihypertensive agents, and for treatment of hypercalcemia. Has been used concomitantly with mannitol for treatment of severe cerebral edema, particularly in meningitis.

CONTRAINDICATIONS History of hypersensitivity to furosemide or sulfonamides; increasing oliguria, anuria, fluid and electrolyte depletion states; hepatic coma; pregnancy (category C), lactation.
CAUTIOUS USE Infants, older adults; hepatic cirrhosis, nephrotic syndrome; cardiogenic shock associated with acute MI; history of SLE, history of gout; patients receiving digitalis glycosides or potassium-depleting steroids.

ROUTE & DOSAGE

Edema

Neonate: **PO** 0.5–1 mg/kg/dose given q8–24h and titrated upward if needed (max 6 mg/kg/dose) **IV/IM** 1–2 mg/kg q12–24h (max IV dose, 2 mg/kg/dose)
Child: **PO** 0.5–2 mg/kg, may be increased by 1–2 mg/kg q6–8h (max 6 mg/kg/dose) **IV/IM** 1 mg/kg, may be increased by 1 mg/kg q2h if needed (max 6 mg/kg/dose)
Adult: **PO** 20–80 mg in 1 or more divided doses up to 600 mg/day if needed **IV/IM** 20–40 mg in 1 or more divided doses up to 600 mg/day

Hypertension

Adult: **PO** 10–40 mg b.i.d. (max 480 mg/day)

STORAGE

■ Store tablets at controlled room temperature, preferably at 15°–30° C (59°–86° F) unless otherwise directed. Protect from light. ■ Store oral solution in refrigerator, preferably at 2°–8° C (36°–46° F). Protect from light and freezing. ■ Store parenteral solution at controlled room temperature, preferably at 15°–30° C (59°–86° F) unless otherwise directed. Protect from light. Use infusion solutions within 24 h.

ADMINISTRATION

Oral

■ Give with food or milk to reduce possibility of gastric irritation.
■ Schedule doses to avoid sleep disturbance (e.g., a single dose is generally given in the morning; twice-a-day doses at 8 a.m. and 2 p.m.).
■ Note: Slight discoloration of tablets reportedly does not alter potency.

Intramuscular

■ Protect syringes from light once they are removed from package.
■ Discard yellow or otherwise discolored injection solutions.

Common adverse effects in *italic;* life-threatening effects <u>underlined</u>; generic names in **bold;** drug classifications in SMALL CAPS; ✤ Canadian drug name; ❂ Prototype drug.

Intravenous

Note: Verify correct IV concentration and rate of infusion/injection with physician before administration to infants or children. Intermittent infusion rate should not exceed 0.5 mg/kg/min.

PREPARE Direct: Give undiluted.

ADMINISTER Direct: Give undiluted at a rate of 20 mg or a fraction thereof over 1 min. With high doses and in infants/young children a rate of 4 mg/min is recommended to decrease risk of ototoxicity.

INCOMPATIBILITIES Solution/Additive: Buprenorphine, chlorpromazine, ciprofloxacin, diazepam, diphenhydramine, dobutamine, doxapram, doxorubicin, droperidol, erythromycin, gentamicin, isoproterenol, labetalol, meperidine, metoclopramide, milrinone, netilmicin, pancuronium, prochlorperazine, promethazine, quinidine, thiamine vinblastine, vincristine. Y-Site: Amrinone, amsacrine, ciprofloxacin, diazepam, diltiazem, dobutamine, diphenhydramine, dopamine, doxorubicin, droperidol, esmolol, filgrastim, fluconazole, gemcitabine, gentamicin, hydralazine, idarubicin, methocarbamol, metoclopramide, midazolam, milrinone, morphine, netilmicin, nicardipine, ondansetron, quinidine, thiopental, tobramycin, vecuronium, vinblastine, vincristine, vinorelbine, TPN.

ADVERSE EFFECTS CV: Postural hypotension, dizziness with excessive diuresis, acute hypotensive episodes, circulatory collapse. **Metabolic:** Hypovolemia, dehydration, hyponatremia, *hypokalemia*, hypochloremia metabolic alkalosis, hypomagnesemia, hypocalcemia (tetany) from increased calcium excretion, hyperglycemia, glycosuria, elevated BUN, hyperuricemia;. **GI:** Nausea, vomiting, oral and gastric burning, anorexia, diarrhea, constipation, abdominal cramping, acute pancreatitis, jaundice. **Urogenital:** Allergic interstitial nephritis, irreversible renal failure, urinary frequency; nephrocalcinosis with prolonged use in premature infants. **Hematologic:** Anemia, leukopenia, thrombocytopenic purpura; aplastic anemia, agranulocytosis (rare). **Special Senses:** Tinnitus, vertigo, feeling of fullness in ears, hearing loss (rarely permanent but more common in presence of renal disease), blurred vision. **Skin:** Pruritus, urticaria, exfoliative dermatitis, purpura, photosensitivity, porphyria cutanea tarde, necrotizing angiitis (vasculitis). **Body as a Whole:** Increased perspiration; paresthesias; activation of SLE, muscle spasms, weakness; thrombophlebitis, pain at IM injection site.

DIAGNOSTIC TEST INTERFERENCE Furosemide may cause elevations in *BUN, serum amylase, cholesterol, triglycerides, uric acid* and *blood glucose* levels, and may decrease *serum calcium, magnesium, potassium,* and *sodium* levels.

INTERACTIONS Drug: OTHER DIURETICS enhance diuretic effects; with **digoxin**, increased risk of toxicity because of hypokalemia; NONDEPOLARIZING NEUROMUSCULAR BLOCKING AGENTS (e.g., **tubocurarine**) prolong neuromuscular blockage; CORTICOSTEROIDS, **amphotericin B** potentiate hypokalemia; decreased **lithium** elimination and increased toxicity; SULFONYLUREAS, **insulin** blunt hypoglycemic effects; NSAIDS may attenuate diuretic effects.

PHARMACOKINETICS Absorption: 60% of oral dose absorbed from GI tract. **Peak:** 60–70 min PO; 20–60 min IV. **Onset:** 30–60 min PO; 5 min IV. **Duration:** 2 h. **Distribution:** Crosses placenta. **Metabolism:** Small amount metabolized in liver. **Elimination:** Rapidly excreted in urine; 50% of oral dose and 80% of IV dose excreted within 24 h; excreted in breast milk. **Half-Life:** 30 min.

F

NURSING IMPLICATIONS

Assessment & Drug Effects

- Observe patients receiving parenteral drug carefully; closely monitor BP and vital signs. Sudden death from cardiac arrest has been reported.
- Monitor BP during periods of diuresis and through period of dosage adjustment.
- Observe patients closely during period of rapid diuresis. Sudden alteration in fluid and electrolyte balance may precipitate significant adverse reactions. Report symptoms to physician.
- Lab tests: Obtain frequent blood count, serum and urine electrolytes, CO_2, BUN, blood sugar, and uric acid values during first few months of therapy and periodically thereafter.
- Monitor for S&S of hypokalemia (see Appendix D-1).
- Monitor I&O ratio and pattern. Report decrease or unusual increase in output. Excessive diuresis can result in dehydration and hypovolemia, circulatory collapse, and hypotension. Weigh patient daily under standard conditions.
- Monitor urine and blood glucose & HbA_{1c} closely in diabetics and patients with decompensated hepatic cirrhosis. Drug may cause hyperglycemia.
- Note: Excessive dehydration is most likely to occur in infants, those with chronic cardiac disease on prolonged salt restriction, or those receiving sympatholytic agents.

Patient & Family Education

- Review correct administration for infants and young children. Because children with heart defects may also be taking digoxin, correct administration and scheduling of drugs and awareness of side effects is very important.
- Consult physician regarding allowable salt and fluid intake.
- Ingestion potassium-rich foods daily (e.g., bananas, oranges, peaches, dried dates) to reduce or prevent potassium depletion.
- Learn S&S of hypokalemia (see Appendix D-1). Report muscle cramps or weakness to physician.
- Make position changes slowly because high doses of antihypertensive drugs taken concurrently may produce episodes of dizziness or imbalance.
- Avoid replacing fluid losses with appropriate amounts of water.
- Avoid prolonged exposure to direct sun.
- Keep securely locked away and out of reach of young children. Be aware that this drug has potential for abuse by persons with anorexia or bulimia who are attempting weight loss.
- Do not breast feed while taking this drug.

GABAPENTIN

(gab-a-pen'tin)
Neurontin
Classifications: CENTRAL NERVOUS SYSTEM AGENT; ANTICONVULSANT
Prototype: Phenytoin
Pregnancy Category: C

AVAILABILITY 100 mg, 300 mg, 400 mg capsules; 600 mg, 800 mg tablets; 250 mg/5 mL solution.

ACTIONS Gabapentin is a GABA neurotransmitter analog; however, it does not interact with GABA receptors, and it does not inhibit GABA uptake or degradation. Mechanism of action is unknown. An effect of gabapentin on central serotonin metabolism has been postulated.
THERAPEUTIC EFFECTS Gabapentin is used in conjunction with other anticonvulsants to control certain types of seizures in patients with epilepsy.

USES Adjunctive therapy for partial seizures with or without secondary generalization in adults, post-herpetic neuralgia.
UNLABELED USES Add-on therapy for generalized seizures.

CONTRAINDICATIONS Hypersensitivity to gabapentin; pregnancy (category C), lactation.
CAUTIOUS USE Status epilepticus, renal impairment, older adults. Safety and efficacy in children <3 y are not established.

ROUTE & DOSAGE

Adjunctive Therapy for Seizure Disorder

Child: **PO** *3–12 y,* initiate with 10–15 mg/kg/day in 3 divided doses, titrate q3 days to target dose of 40 mg/kg/day in child 3–4 y and 25–35 mg/kg/day in child ≥5 y in 3 divided doses
Child/Adult: **PO** *>12 y,* initiate with 300 mg on day 1, 300 mg b.i.d. on day 2, 300 mg t.i.d. on day 3, and continue to increase over a week to an initial total dose of 400 mg t.i.d. (1200 mg/day); may increase to 1800–2400 mg/day depending on response (most patients receive 600–1800 mg/day in 3 divided doses) 400 mg t.i.d. (1200 mg/day); may increase to 1800–2400 mg/day depending on response (most patients receive 600–1800 mg/day in 3 divided doses) new content

Post-Herpetic Neuralgia

Adult: **PO** Initiate with 300 mg day 1, 300 mg b.i.d. day 2, and 300 mg t.i.d. day 3; may increase up to 600 mg t.i.d. if needed

Renal Impairment

Cl_{cr} >60 mL/min: 400 mg t.i.d.; 30–60 mL/min: 300 mg b.i.d.; 15–30 mL/min: 300 mg daily; <15 mL/min: 300 mg every other day; hemodialysis: 200–300 mg following dialysis

STORAGE

Store at 15°–30° C (59°–86° F); protect from heat, moisture, and direct light.

ADMINISTRATION

Oral

- Adjust dosage for patients with creatinine clearance of 60 mL/min or less. See manufacturer's recommendations.
- Separate doses of gabapentin and antacids by 2 h.
- Withdraw drug gradually over 1 wk; abrupt discontinuation may cause status epilepticus. For t.i.d. dosing, interval between doses should not exceed 12 h.

ADVERSE EFFECTS CNS: *Drowsiness, fatigue,* dizziness, tremor, slurred speech, impaired concentration, headache, increased frequency of partial seizures. **Endocrine:** Weight gain. **GI:** Nausea, gastric upset, vomiting. **Special Senses:** Blurred vision, nystagmus. **Skin:** Rash, eczema.

INTERACTIONS Drug: Increase in **phenytoin** levels at higher doses (300–600 mg/day gabapentin). Does not appear to affect serum levels of other ANTICONVULSANTS. ANTACIDS reduce absorption of gabapentin about 20%. **Herbal: Ginkgo** may decrease anticonvulsant effectiveness.

PHARMACOKINETICS Absorption: 50–60% absorbed from GI tract. **Peak:** Peak level 1–3 h; peak effect 2–4 wk. **Distribution:** Crosses the blood–brain barrier comparable to other anticonvulsants; readily passes into cerebrospinal fluid; is not bound to plasma proteins; highest concentrations (in animal studies) found in pancreas and kidneys. **Metabolism:** Does not appear to be metabolized. **Elimination:** 76–81% excreted unchanged in 96 h; 10–23% recovered in feces. **Half-Life:** 5–6 h.

NURSING IMPLICATIONS

Assessment & Drug Effects

- Monitor for therapeutic effectiveness; May not occur until several weeks following initiation of therapy.
- Assess frequency of seizures: In rare cases, the drug has increased the frequency of partial seizures. Drug must be withdrawn slowly if discontinued.
- Assess safety: Vision, concentration, and coordination may be impaired by gabapentin.

Patient & Family Education

- Learn potential adverse effects of drug.
- Notify physician immediately if any of the following occur: Increased seizure frequency, visual changes, unusual bruising or bleeding.
- Do not drive or engage in other potentially hazardous activities until response to drug is known.
- Do not abruptly discontinue use of drug; do not take drug within 2 h of an antacid.
- Do not breast feed while taking this drug.
- Store this medication out of reach of children.

Common adverse effects in *italic;* life-threatening effects <u>underlined;</u> generic names in **bold;** drug classifications in SMALL CAPS; ♣ Canadian drug name; ⊘ Prototype drug.

GANCICLOVIR

(gan-ci'clo-vir)
Cytovene
Classifications: ANTI-INFECTIVE; ANTIVIRAL AGENT
Prototype: Acyclovir
Pregnancy Category: C

AVAILABILITY 250 mg, 500 mg capsules; 500 mg powder for injection

ACTIONS Ganciclovir is an antiviral drug active against cytomegalovirus (CMV). It prevents the replication CMV DNA.
THERAPEUTIC EFFECTS Sensitive human viruses include CMV, herpes simplex virus-1 and -2 (HSV-1, HSV-2), Epstein–Barr virus, and varicella-zoster virus.

USES CMV retinitis, prophylaxis and treatment of systemic CMV infections in immunocompromised patients including HIV-positive and transplant patients.

CONTRAINDICATIONS Hypersensitivity to ganciclovir or acyclovir, lactation.
CAUTIOUS USE Renal impairment, older adults, pregnancy (category C). Safety and efficacy in children are not established; use with extreme caution in children <12 y.

ROUTE & DOSAGE

Induction Therapy

Child/Adult: **IV** *>3 mo,* 5 mg/kg over 1 h q12h for 14–21 days (doses may range from 2.5–5.0 mg/kg over 1 h q8–12h for 10–35 days)

Maintenance Therapy

Adult: **IV** 5 mg/kg over 1 h daily or 6 mg/kg over 1 h daily 5 days/wk
PO 1000 mg t.i.d. or 500 mg 6 times/day q3h while awake

Prevention of CMV Disease in Transplant Recipients

Child/Adult: **IV** 5 mg/kg q12h 7–14 days, then 5 mg/kg daily or 6 mg/kg/day 5 days/wk

CMV Infection after Bone Marrow Transplant

Child: **IV** 7.5–19.5 mg/kg/day divided into doses given q8h

Renal Impairment

See prescribing information for dosing in patients with renal impairment

STORAGE
- Store reconstituted solutions refrigerated at 4° C (40° F); use within 12 h.
- Store infusion solution refrigerated up to 24 h of preparation.

ADMINISTRATION
Note: Do not administer if neutrophil count falls below 500/mm^3 or platelet count falls below 25,000/mm^3.

- Avoid direct contact of powder in capsules or solution with skin and mucous membranes. Wash thoroughly with soap and water if contact occurs. See Part I for handling of hazardous substances.

Oral

- Give with food.

Intravenous

IV administration to infants and children: Verify correct IV concentration and rate of infusion with physician.

PREPARE **Intermittent:** Reconstitute the 500-mg vial using only 10 mL of sterile water (supplied) for injection immediately before use to yield 50 mg/mL. Shake well to dissolve. Withdraw the ordered amount and add to 100 mL of NS, D5W, or RL (volume less than 100 mL may be used, but the final concentration should be <10 mg/mL).

ADMINISTER **Intermittent:** Give at a constant rate over 1 h. Avoid rapid infusion or bolus injection.

INCOMPATIBILITIES **Solution/Additive:** Amino acid solutions (TPN), bacteriostatic water for injection, **fludarabine, foscarnet, ondansetron. Y-Site: Total parenteral nutrition.**

ADVERSE EFFECTS CNS: *Fever,* headache, disorientation, mental status changes, ataxia, <u>coma</u>, confusion, dizziness, paresthesia, nervousness, somnolence, tremor. **CV:** Edema, phlebitis. **GI:** *Nausea, diarrhea,* anorexia, elevated liver enzymes. **Hematologic:** <u>*Bone marrow suppression*</u>, *thrombocytopenia, granulocytopenia, eosinophilia, leukopenia*, hyperbilirubinemia. **Metabolic:** Hyperthermia, hypoglycemia. **Urogenital:** Infertility. **Skin:** Rash. **Special Senses:** retinal detachment.

INTERACTIONS Drug: ANTINEOPLASTIC AGENTS, **amphotericin B, didanosine, trimethoprim-sulfamethoxazole (TMP-SMZ), dapsone, pentamidine, probenecid, zidovudine** may increase bone marrow suppression and other toxic effects of ganciclovir; may increase risk of nephrotoxicity from **cyclosporine;** may increase risk of seizures due to **imipenemcilastatin.**

PHARMACOKINETICS Onset: 3–8 days. **Duration:** Clinical relapse can occur 14 days to 3.5 mo after stopping therapy; positive blood and urine cultures recur 12–60 days after therapy. **Distribution:** Distributes throughout body including CSF, eyes, lungs, liver, and kidneys; crosses placenta in animals; not known if distributed into breast milk. **Metabolism:** Not metabolized. **Elimination:** 94–99% of dose is excreted unchanged in urine. **Half-Life:** 2.5–4.2 h.

NURSING IMPLICATIONS

Assessment & Drug Effects

- Lab tests: Neutrophil and platelet counts at least every other day during twice-daily dosing and weekly thereafter; more frequent monitoring may be indicated in certain patients. Monitor serum creatinine or creatinine clearance at least q2wk. Closely monitor renal function in the older adult.
- Inspect IV insertion site throughout infusion for signs and symptoms of phlebitis.

Patient & Family Education

- Note: Drug is not a cure for CMV retinitis; follow regular ophthalmologic examination schedule.
- Drink lots of fluids during therapy.
- Use barrier contraception throughout therapy and for at least 90 days afterwards.
- Maintain frequent hematologic monitoring.
- Do not breast feed while taking this drug.
- Store this medication out of reach of children.

G

GENTAMICIN SULFATE ℞

(jen-ta-mye'sin)

Garamycin, Garamycin Ophthalmic, Genoptic

Classifications: ANTI-INFECTIVE; AMINOGLYCOSIDE ANTIBIOTIC

Pregnancy Category: C

AVAILABILITY 10 mg/mL, 40 mg/mL injection; 0.1% ointment, cream; 3 mg/mL ophthalmic solution; 3 mg/g ophthalmic ointment

ACTIONS Broad-spectrum aminoglycoside antibiotic derived from *Micromonospora purpurea*. Action is usually bacteriocidal.

THERAPEUTIC EFFECTS Active against a wide variety of gram-negative bacteria, including *Citrobacter, Escherichia coli, Enterobacter, Klebsiella, Proteus* (including indole-positive and indole-negative strains), *Pseudomonas aeruginosa,* and *Serratia* sp. Also effective against certain gram-positive organisms, particularly penicillin-sensitive and some methicillin-resistant strains of *Staphylococcus aureus* (MRSA).

USES Parenteral use restricted to treatment of serious infections of GI, respiratory, and urinary tracts, CNS, bone, skin, and soft tissue (including burns) when other less toxic antimicrobial agents are ineffective or are contraindicated. Has been used in combination with other antibiotics. Also used topically for primary and secondary skin infections and for superficial infections of external eye and its adnexa.

UNLABELED USES Prophylaxis of bacterial endocarditis in patients undergoing operative procedures or instrumentation.

CONTRAINDICATIONS History of hypersensitivity to or toxic reaction with any aminoglycoside antibiotic. Safe use during pregnancy (category C) or lactation is not established.

CAUTIOUS USE Impaired renal function; history of eighth cranial (acoustic) nerve impairment; preexisting vertigo or dizziness or tinnitus; dehydration, fever; use in older adults, premature infants, neonates, and infants; obesity, neuromuscular disorders: myasthenia gravis, parkinsonian syndrome; hypocalcemia, heart failure, topical applications to widespread areas.

ROUTE & DOSAGE

Moderate to Severe Infection

Neonate: **IV/IM** 2.5 mg/kg q12–24h; dosed once daily if postconceptual age is <30 wk and the infant is under 2 wk of age; dosed q12h if

Common adverse effects in *italic;* life-threatening effects <u>underlined</u>; generic names in **bold;** drug classifications in SMALL CAPS; ✦ Canadian drug name; ℗ Prototype drug.

591

G

postconceptual age is 30 wks and infant is older than 2 wk of age, or if postconceptual age is >37 wk and infant is under 1 wk of age; dosed q8h if postconceptual age is >37 wk and infant is over 1 wk of age
Child: **IV/IM** 6–7.5 mg/kg/day in 3–4 divided doses. **Intrathecal** *>3 mo,* 1–2 mg preservative free daily
Adult: **IV/IM** 1.5–2 mg/kg; Loading dose 5–7 mg/kg one time, and then frequency is determined by setting. Commonly, 3–6 mg/kg/day in 2–3 divided doses depending on clearance rate. Alternatively, extended dosing of 5–7 mg/kg one time, with future dosing determined by clearance rate; usually dosed q24–48h. **Intrathecal** 4–8 mg preservative free daily **Topical** 1–2 drops of solution in eye q4h up to 2 drops q1h or small amount of ointment b.i.d. or t.i.d.

Acute Pelvic Inflammatory Disease
Adult: **IV/IM** 2 mg/kg followed by 1.5 mg/kg q8h

Infection with Cystic Fibrosis
Child/Adult: 7.5–10.5 mg/kg/day divided into doses given q8h

Prophylaxis of Bacterial Endocarditis
Child: **IV/IM** *<27 kg,* 2 mg/kg 30 min before procedure, may repeat in 8 h
Adult: **IV/IM** 1.5 mg/kg 30 min before procedure, may repeat in 8 h

STORAGE
Store all gentamicin solutions at 2°–30° C (36°–86° F) unless otherwise directed by manufacturer.

ADMINISTRATION

Ophthalmic
- Apply pressure to inner canthus for 1 min immediately after instillation of drops.
- Have patient keep eyes closed for 1–2 min after administration of ophthalmic ointment to assure medication contact. Caution patient that vision will be blurred for a few minutes.

Topical
- Wash affected area with mild soap and water, rinse, and dry thoroughly. Gently apply small amount of medication to lesions; cover with sterile gauze.
- Do not apply topical preparations, particularly cream, to large denuded body surfaces because systemic absorption and toxicity are possible.

Intramuscular
- Give deep into a large muscle appropriate for age of child (see Part I).
- Do not use solutions that are discolored or that contain particulate matter; drug for IV or IM is clear and colorless or slightly yellow.

Intrathecal
- Note: Intrathecal formulation is a clear and colorless solution.
- Use promptly after opening; contains no preservatives and any unused portion should be discarded.

Common adverse effects in *italic;* life-threatening effects <u>underlined;</u> generic names in **bold;** drug classifications in SMALL CAPS; ♣ Canadian drug name; ● Prototype drug.

Intravenous

***PREPARE* Intermittent:** Dilute a single dose with 50–200 mL of D5W or NS. For pediatric patients, amount of infusion fluid may be proportionately smaller depending on patient's needs but should be sufficient to be infused over the same time period as for adults.
***ADMINISTER* Intermittent:** Give over 30 min–2 h.
***INCOMPATIBILITIES* Solution/Additive:** Fat emulsion, TPN, **amphotericin B, ampicillin, carbenicillin,** CEPHALOSPORINS, **cytarabine, heparin. Y-Site:** Furosemide, iodipamide.

ADVERSE EFFECTS Special Senses: Ototoxicity (vestibular disturbances, impaired hearing), optic neuritis. **CNS:** Neuromuscular blockade: skeletal muscle weakness, apnea, respiratory paralysis (high doses); arachnoiditis (intrathecal use). **CV:** Hypotension or hypertension. **GI:** Nausea, vomiting, transient increase in AST, ALT, and serum LDH and bilirubin; hepatomegaly, splenomegaly. **Hematologic:** Increased or decreased reticulocyte counts; granulocytopenia, thrombocytopenia, thrombocytopenic purpura, anemia. **Body as a Whole:** Hypersensitivity (rash, pruritus, urticaria, exfoliative dermatitis, eosinophilia, burning sensation of skin, drug fever, joint pains, laryngeal edema, anaphylaxis). **Urogenital:** Nephrotoxicity: proteinuria, tubular necrosis, cells or casts in urine, hematuria, rising BUN, nonprotein nitrogen, serum creatinine; *decreased creatinine clearance.* **Other:** Local irritation and pain following IM use; thrombophlebitis, abscess, superinfections, syndrome of hypocalcemia (tetany, weakness, hypokalemia, hypomagnesemia). **Topical and Ophthalmic:** Photosensitivity, sensitization, erythema, pruritus; burning, stinging, and lacrimation (ophthalmic formulation).

INTERACTIONS Drug: Amphotericin B, capreomycin, cisplatin, methoxyflurane, polymyxin B, vancomycin increase risk of nephrotoxicity. **Ethacrynic acid** and **furosemide** may increase risk of ototoxicity. GENERAL ANESTHETICS and NEUROMUSCULAR BLOCKING AGENTS (e.g., **succinylcholine**) potentiate neuromuscular blockade. **Indomethacin** may increase gentamicin levels in neonates.

PHARMACOKINETICS Absorption: Well absorbed from IM site. **Peak:** 30–90 min IM. **Distribution:** Widely distributed in body fluids, including ascitic, peritoneal, pleural, synovial, and abscess fluids; poor CNS penetration; concentrates in kidney and inner ear; crosses placenta. **Metabolism:** Not metabolized. **Elimination:** Excreted unchanged in urine; small amounts accumulate in kidney and are eliminated over 10–20 days; small amount excreted in breast milk. **Half-Life:** 2–4 h.

NURSING IMPLICATIONS

Assessment & Drug Effects

- Lab tests: Perform C&S and renal function prior to first dose and periodically during therapy; therapy may begin pending test results. Determine creatinine clearance and serum drug concentrations at frequent intervals, particularly for patients with impaired renal function, infants (renal immaturity), patients receiving high doses or therapy beyond 10 days, patients with fever or extensive burns, edema, obesity.

- Repeat C&S if improvement does not occur in 3–5 days; reevaluate therapy.
- Monitor peak and trough levels. **Peak level** for most infections should be 6–10 mg/L; for pulmonary infection, neutropenia, and severe sepsis it should be 8–10 mg/L. **Peak level** above 12 mg/L or **trough above** 2 mg/L indicates toxicity.
- Draw blood specimens for peak serum gentamicin concentration 30 min–1 h after IM administration, and 30 min after completion of a 30–60 min IV infusion, preferably after third consecutive dose. Draw blood specimens for trough levels just before the next IM or IV dose, preferably prior to third consecutive dose. Use nonheparinized tubes to collect blood.
- Check baseline weight and vital signs; determine vestibular and auditory function before therapy and at regular intervals. Check vestibular and auditory function again 3–4 wk after drug is discontinued (the time that deafness is most likely to occur).
- Monitor I&O. Keep patient well hydrated to prevent chemical irritation of renal tubules. Report oliguria, unusual appearance of urine, change in I&O ratio or pattern, and presence of edema (prolongs elimination time).
- Note: Ototoxic effect (see Appendix D-1) is greatest on the vestibular branch of eighth cranial (acoustic) nerve (symptoms: headache, dizziness or vertigo, nausea and vomiting with motion, ataxia, nystagmus). However, damage to the auditory branch (tinnitus, roaring noises, sensation of fullness in ears, hearing impairment) may also occur. Report promptly to prevent permanent damage.
- Watch for signs and symptoms of bacterial overgrowth (opportunistic infections) with resistant or nonsusceptible organisms (diarrhea, anogenital itching, vaginal discharge, stomatitis, glossitis).

Patient & Family Education

- Note: When using topical applications: Avoid excessive exposure to sunlight because of danger of photosensitivity; withhold medication and notify physician if condition fails to improve within 1 wk, worsens, or signs of irritation or sensitivity occur; and apply medication as directed and only for length of time prescribed (overuse can result in superinfections).
- Do not breast feed while taking this drug without consulting physician.
- Store this medication out of reach of children.

GLUCAGON
(gloo′ka-gon)
GlucaGen
Classifications: HORMONES AND SYNTHETIC SUBSTITUTES
Pregnancy Category: B

AVAILABILITY 1 mg powder for injection

ACTIONS Polypeptide hormone produced by alpha cells of islets of Langerhans. Stimulates uptake of amino acids and their conversion to glucose precursors.

THERAPEUTIC EFFECTS Promotes lipolysis in liver and adipose tissue with release of free fatty acid and glycerol, which further stimulates ketogenesis and hepatic gluconeogenesis. Action in hypoglycemia relies on presence of adequate liver glycogen stores.

USES Emergency treatment of severe hypoglycemic reactions in diabetic patients who are unconscious or unable to swallow food or liquids and in psychiatric patients receiving insulin shock therapy. Also radiologic studies of GI tract to relax smooth muscle and thereby allow finer detail of mucosa; to diagnose insulinoma.
UNLABELED USES GI disturbances associated with spasm, cardiovascular emergencies, and to overcome cardiotoxic effects of beta blockers, quinidine, tricyclic antidepressants; as an aid in abdominal imaging.

CONTRAINDICATIONS Hypersensitivity to glucagon or protein compounds. Safe use during pregnancy (category B) or lactation is not established.
CAUTIOUS USE Insulinemia, pheochromocytoma.

ROUTE & DOSAGE

Hypoglycemia
Neonate/Infant: **IM/IV/SC** 0.025–0.3 mg/kg/dose q30min prn (max 1 mg)
Child: **IM/IV/SC** 0.03–0.1 mg/kg/dose q20min prn (max 1 mg/dose)
Adult: **IM/IV/SC** 0.5–1 mg, may repeat q5–20 min if no response for 1–2 more doses

Insulin Shock Therapy
Adult: **IM/IV/SC** 0.5–1 mg usually 1 h after coma develops, may repeat in 25 min if no response

Diagnostic Aid to Relax Stomach or Upper GI Tract
Adult: **IM/IV/SC** 0.25–2 mg 10 min before the procedure

Diagnostic Aid for Examination of Colon
Adult: **IM/IV/SC** 2 mg 10 min before the procedure

STORAGE
Store unreconstituted vials and diluent at 20°–25° C (68°–77° F).

ADMINISTRATION
Note: 1 mg = 1 unit

Subcutaneous/Intramuscular
- Dilute 1 unit (1 mg) of glucagon with 1 mL of diluent supplied by manufacturer.
- Use immediately after reconstitution of dry powder. Discard any unused portion.
- Note: Glucagon is incompatible in syringe with any other drug.

Common adverse effects in *italic;* life-threatening effects underlined; generic names in **bold;** drug classifications in SMALL CAPS; ♣ Canadian drug name; ⊕ Prototype drug.

595

Intravenous

PREPARE Direct: Prepare as noted. Do not use a concentration >1 unit/mL.
ADMINISTER Direct: Give 1 unit or fraction thereof over 1 min. May be given through a Y-site D5W (not NS) infusing.
INCOMPATIBILITY Solution/Additive: Sodium chloride.

ADVERSE EFFECTS GI: Nausea and vomiting. **CV:** Cardiac stimulatory effect. **Body as a Whole:** Hypersensitivity reactions. **Skin:** <u>Stevens–Johnson syndrome</u> (erythema multiforme), urticaria. **Metabolic:** Hyperglycemia, hypokalemia.

PHARMACOKINETICS Onset: 5–20 min. **Peak:** 30 min. **Duration:** 1–1.5 h. **Metabolism:** Metabolized in liver, plasma, and kidneys. **Half-Life:** 3–10 min.

NURSING IMPLICATIONS

Assessment & Drug Effects
- Be prepared to give IV glucose if patient fails to respond to glucagon. Notify physician immediately.
- Hypoglycemia treatment may require dextrose 25% solution.
- Note: Patient usually awakens from (diabetic) hypoglycemic coma 5–20 min after glucagon injection. Give PO carbohydrate as soon as possible after patient regains consciousness. Complex carbohydrate and protein will follow with careful monitoring of condition and blood glucose levels.
- Note: After recovery from hypoglycemic reaction, symptoms such as headache, nausea, and weakness may persist.

Patient & Family Education
- Note: Physician may request that a responsible family member be taught how to administer glucagon SC or IM for patients with frequent or severe hypoglycemic reactions. Store this medication out of reach of children. Notify physician promptly whenever a hypoglycemic reaction occurs so the reason for the reaction can be determined.
- Review package insert and directions (see ADMINISTRATION).
- Do not breast feed while taking this drug without consulting physician.

GLYCERIN
(gli′ser-in)
Fleet Babylax, Glycerol, Osmoglyn
GLYCERIN ANHYDROUS
Ophthalgan
Classifications: FLUID AND ELECTROLYTE AGENT; HYPEROSMOTIC LAXATIVE; ANTIGLAUCOMA
Pregnancy Category: C

AVAILABILITY 50% oral solution; suppositories; 4 mL/applicator, ophthalmic solution

ACTIONS When administered orally, glycerin raises plasma osmotic pressure by withdrawing fluid from extravascular spaces; lowers ocular tension by decreasing volume of intraocular fluid. Also may decrease CSF pressure and produce slight diuresis. Topical application to eye reduces edema by hydroscopic effect. Glycerin suppositories apparently work by causing dehydration of exposed tissue, which produces an irritant effect, and by absorbing water from tissues, thus creating more mass. Both actions stimulate peristalsis in the large bowel and thus increases peristalsis. **THERAPEUTIC EFFECTS** Also reduces intraocular pressure by lowering intraocular fluid. Relieves constipation by absorption of water and stimulation of peristalsis.

G

USES Orally to reduce elevated intraocular pressure (IOP) before or after surgery in patients with acute narrow-angle glaucoma, retinal detachment, or cataract and to reduce elevated CSF pressure. Sterile glycerin (anhydrous) is used topically to reduce superficial corneal edema resulting from trauma, surgery, or disease and to facilitate ophthalmoscopic examination. Used rectally (suppository or enema) to relieve constipation.

CONTRAINDICATIONS Safe use during pregnancy (category C) or lactation is not established.
CAUTIOUS USE Cardiac, renal, or hepatic disease; diabetes mellitus; dehydrated patients.

ROUTE & DOSAGE

Decrease IOP
Child/Adult: **PO** 1–1.8 g/kg 1–1.5 h before ocular surgery, may repeat q5h

Constipation
Neonate: **PR** 0.5 mL of rectal solution (enema) or one suppository "chip"
Child: **PR** <6 y, insert 1 infant suppository or 2–5 mL of enema high into rectum and retain for 15 min
Child/Adult: **PR** ≥6 y, insert 1 suppository or 5–15 mL of enema high into rectum and retain for 15 min

Reduction of Corneal Edema
Adult: **Topical** 1–2 drops instilled into eye q3–4h

STORAGE
Store oral solutions, enema, suppository in tightly covered containers at 15°–30° C (59°–86° F); avoid freezing. Ophthalmic solution is stored in tightly covered containers and protected from light. Do not use if crystals or precipitate are present; discard 6 mo after dropper is placed in container.

ADMINISTRATION

Oral
- Pour commercially available flavored solution over crushed ice, then sip through a straw. Lemon or lime juice and NS (if allowed) may be added to unflavored solution for palatability.

■ Prevent or relieve headache (from cerebral dehydration) by having patient lie down during and after administration of drug.

Rectal

■ Ensure that suppository is inserted beyond rectal sphincter.

ADVERSE EFFECTS CNS: Headache, dizziness, disorientation. **CV:** Irregular heartbeat. **GI:** Nausea, vomiting, thirst, diarrhea, abdominal cramps, rectal discomfort, hyperemia of rectal mucosa. **Metabolic:** Hyperglycemia, glycosuria, dehydration, <u>hyperosmolar nonketotic coma</u>.

PHARMACOKINETICS Absorption: Readily absorbed from GI tract after oral administration; rectal preparations are poorly absorbed. **Onset:** 10 min PO. **Peak:** 30 min–2 h. **Duration:** 4–8 h. **Metabolism:** 80% metabolized in liver; 10–20% metabolized in kidneys to CO_2 and water or utilized in glucose or glycogen synthesis. **Elimination:** 7–14% excreted unchanged in urine. **Half-Life:** 30–40 min.

NURSING IMPLICATIONS

Assessment & Drug Effects

■ Consult physician regarding fluid intake in patients receiving drug for elevated IOP. Although hypotonic fluids will relieve thirst and headache caused by the dehydrating action of glycerin, these fluids may nullify its osmotic effect.

■ Monitor glycemic control in diabetics. Drug may cause hyperglycemia (see Appendix D-1).

Patient & Family Education

■ Evacuation usually comes 15–30 min after administration of glycerin rectal suppository or enema.

■ Note: Slight hyperglycemia and glycosuria may occur with PO use; adjustment in antidiabetic medication dosage may be required.

■ Do not breast feed while taking this drug without consulting prescriber.

■ Store this medication out of reach of children.

GLYCOPYRROLATE

(glye-koe-pye'roe-late)

Robinul, Robinul Forte

Classifications: AUTONOMIC NERVOUS SYSTEM AGENT; ANTICHOLINERGIC (PARASYMPATHOLYTIC); ANTIMUSCARINIC, ANTISPASMODIC

Prototype: Atropine

Pregnancy Category: B

AVAILABILITY 1 mg, 2 mg tablets; 0.2 mg/mL injection

ACTIONS Synthetic anticholinergic (antimuscarinic) compound with pharmacologic effects similar to those of atropine. Inhibits muscarinic action of acetylcholine or autonomic neuroeffector sites innervated by postganglionic cholinergic nerves.

THERAPEUTIC EFFECTS Inhibits motility of GI tract and genitourinary tract and decreases volume of gastric and pancreatic secretions, saliva, and perspiration.

USES Adjunctive management of peptic ulcer and other GI disorders associated with hyperacidity, hypermotility, and spasm. Also used parenterally as preanesthetic and intraoperative medication and to reverse neuromuscular blockade.

CONTRAINDICATIONS Glaucoma; asthma; prostatic hypertrophy, obstructive uropathy; obstructive lesions or atony of GI tract; severe ulcerative colitis; myasthenia gravis; tachycardia; during cyclopropane anesthesia; children <12 y (except parenteral use in conjunction with anesthesia). Safe use during pregnancy (category B) or lactation is not established.
CAUTIOUS USE Autonomic neuropathy, hepatic or renal disease.

ROUTE & DOSAGE

Peptic Ulcer
Adult: **PO** 1 mg t.i.d. or 2 mg b.i.d. or t.i.d. in equally divided intervals (max 8 mg/day), then decrease to 1 mg b.i.d. **IM/IV** 0.1–0.2 mg as single dose t.i.d. or q.i.d.

Reversal of Neuromuscular Blockade
Child/Adult: **IV** 0.2 mg glycopyrrolate administered with 1 mg of neostigmine or 5 mg pyridostigmine

Control of Secretions
Child: **PO** 0.04–0.1 mg/kg/dose given q4–8h (max 0.2 mg/dose or 0.8 mg/24 h) **IM/IV** 0.004–0.01 mg/kg/dose given q4–8h
Adult: **PO** 1–2 mg/dose; administer b.i.d. or t.i.d. **IM/IV** 0.1–0.2 mg/dose given q4–8h

STORAGE
Store at 20°–25° C (68°–77° F).

ADMINISTRATION

Oral
- Give without regard to meals.

Intramuscular
- Give undiluted, deep into a large muscle mass appropriate for age. (see Part I)

Intravenous
PREPARE **Direct:** Give undiluted. Inspect for cloudiness and discoloration. Discard if present.
ADMINISTER **Direct:** Give 0.2 mg or fraction thereof over 1–2 min.
INCOMPATIBILITIES **Solution/Additive: Chloramphenicol, dexamethasone, diazepam, dimenhydrinate, methohexital, methylprednisolone, pentazocine, phenobarbital, secobarbital, sodium bicarbonate, thiopental. Y-Site: Diazepam, dimenhydrinate, methohexital, pentazocine, phenobarbital, secobarbital, thiopental.**

ADVERSE EFFECTS Body as a Whole: *Decreased sweating,* weakness, atropine-like effects. **CNS:** Dizziness, drowsiness, overdosage (<u>neuromuscular blockade</u> with curare-like action leading to muscle weakness and <u>paralysis</u> is possible). **CV:** Palpitation, tachycardia. **GI:** *Xerostomia,* nausea, constipation. **GU:** *Urinary hesitancy or retention.* **Special Senses:** Blurred vision, mydriasis.

INTERACTIONS Drug: Amantadine, ANTIHISTAMINES, TRICYCLIC ANTIDEPRESSANTS, **quinidine, disopyramide, procainamide** compound anticholinergic effects; decreases **levodopa** effects; **methotrimeptrazine** may precipitate extrapyramidal effects; decreases antipsychotic effects (decreased absorption) of PHENOTHIAZINES.

PHARMACOKINETICS Absorption: Poorly and incompletely absorbed from GI tract. **Onset:** 1 min IV; 15–30 min IM/SC; 1 h PO. **Peak:** 30–45 min IM/SC; 1 h PO. **Duration:** 2–7 h IM/SC; 8–12 h PO. **Distribution:** Crosses placenta. **Metabolism:** Minimally metabolized in liver. **Elimination:** 85% excreted in urine.

NURSING IMPLICATIONS

Assessment & Drug Effects
- Incidence and severity of adverse effects are generally dose related.
- Monitor I&O ratio and pattern particularly in young children. Watch for urinary hesitancy and retention.
- Monitor vital signs, especially when drug is given parenterally. Report any changes in heart rate or rhythm.

Patient & Family Education
- Avoid high environmental temperatures (heat prostration can occur because of decreased sweating).
- Do not drive or engage in other potentially hazardous activities requiring mental alertness until response to drug is known.
- Use good oral hygiene, rinse mouth with water frequently and use a saliva substitute to lessen effects of dry mouth.
- Do not breast feed while taking this drug without consulting physician.
- Store this medication out of reach of children.

GOLD SODIUM THIOMALATE

(thye-oh-mah'late)
Myochrysine
Classification: GOLD COMPOUND
Prototype: Aurothioglucose
Pregnancy Category: C

AVAILABILITY 50 mg/mL injection

ACTIONS Water-soluble gold compound similar to aurothioglucose in actions and uses. Has immunomodulatory and anti-inflammatory effects. Action mechanism unclear. Drug appears to act by suppression of

phagocytosis, altered immune responses, and possibly by inhibition of prostaglandin synthesis.
THERAPEUTIC EFFECTS Has immunomodulatory and anti-inflammatory effects.

USES Selected patients (adults and juveniles) with acute rheumatoid arthritis.
UNLABELED USES Psoriatic arthritis, Felty's syndrome.

CONTRAINDICATIONS History of severe toxicity from previous exposure to gold or other heavy metals; severe debilitation; SLE, Sjögren's syndrome in rheumatoid arthritis; renal disease; hepatic dysfunction, history of infectious hepatitis or hematologic disorders; uncontrolled diabetes or CHF. Safe use during pregnancy (category C) and lactation is not established.
CAUTIOUS USE History of drug allergies or hypersensitivity, hypertension.

ROUTE & DOSAGE

Rheumatoid Arthritis

Child: **IM** 10 mg test dose, then 1 mg/kg/wk or 2.5–5 mg for wk 1 and 2, followed by 1 mg/kg q1–4wk (max single dose, 50 mg)
Adult: **IM** 10 mg wk 1, 25 mg wk 2, then 25–50 mg/wk to a cumulative dose of 1 g (if improvement occurs, continue at 25–50 mg q2wk for 2–20 wk, then q3–4wk indefinitely or until adverse effects occur)

STORAGE
Store in tight, light-resistant containers at 15°–30° C (59°–86° F).

ADMINISTRATION

Intramuscular

- Agitate vial before withdrawing dose to ensure uniform suspension.
- Give deep into muscle mass appropriate for age (Part I). Patient should remain recumbent for at least 30 min after injection because of the danger of "nitritoid reaction" (transient giddiness, vertigo, facial flushing, fainting).
- Observe for allergic reactions. Do not use if any darker than pale yellow.

ADVERSE EFFECTS CNS: Dizziness, syncope, sweating, flushing. **CV:** Bradycardia. **GI:** Hepatitis, metallic taste, *stomatitis,* nausea, vomiting. **Hematologic:** <u>Agranulocytosis, aplastic anemia,</u> eosinophilia (all rare). **Urogenital:** Nephrotic syndrome, glomerulitis with hematuria, *proteinuria.* **Skin:** Transient pruritus, *erythema, dermatitis,* fixed drug eruption, alopecia, shedding of nails, gray to blue pigmentation of skin (chrysiasis). **Special Senses:** Gold deposits in ocular tissues, *photosensitivity.* **Body as a Whole:** Peripheral neuritis, angioneurotic edema, interstitial pneumonitis, <u>anaphylaxis</u> (rare). **Respiratory:** Pulmonary fibrosis.

INTERACTIONS Drug: ANTIMALARIALS, IMMUNOSUPPRESSANTS, **penicillamine, phenylbutazone** increase risk of blood dyscrasias.

Common adverse effects in *italic;* life-threatening effects <u>underlined;</u> generic names in **bold;** drug classifications in SMALL CAPS; ✦ Canadian drug name; ❶ Prototype drug.

601

PHARMACOKINETICS Absorption: Slowly and irregularly absorbed from IM site. **Peak:** 3–6 h. **Distribution:** Widely distributed, especially to synovial fluid, kidney, liver, and spleen; does not cross blood–brain barrier; crosses placenta. **Metabolism:** Not studied. **Elimination:** 60–90% of dose ultimately excreted in urine; also eliminated in feces; traces may be found in urine for 6 mo. **Half-Life:** 3–168 days.

NURSING IMPLICATIONS

Assessment & Drug Effects

- Lab tests: Prior to each injection, urinalysis for protein, blood, and sediment. Withhold drug and notify physician promptly if proteinuria or hematuria develops. Also do baseline Hgb and RBC, WBC count, differential count, platelet count before initiation of therapy and at regular intervals.
- Note: Rapid reduction in hemoglobin level, WBC count below 4000/mm^3, eosinophil count above 5%, and platelet count below 100,000/mm^3 signify possible toxicity.
- Interview and examine patient and family before each injection to detect occurrence of transient pruritus or dermatitis (both are common early indications of toxicity), stomatitis (sore tongue, palate, or throat), metallic taste, indigestion, or other signs and symptoms of possible toxicity. Interrupt treatment immediately and notify physician if any of these reactions occurs.
- Observe for allergic reaction, which may occur almost immediately after injection, 10 min after injection, or at any time during therapy. Withhold drug and notify physician if observed. Keep antidote dimercaprol (BAL) on hand during time of injection.

Patient & Family Education

- Therapeutic effects may not appear until after 2 mo of therapy.
- Notify physician of rapid improvement in joint swelling; this is indicative that you are closely approaching drug tolerance level.
- Use protective measures in sunlight. Exposure to sunlight may aggravate gold dermatitis.
- Notify physician at the appearance of purpura or ecchymoses; this is always an indication for doing a platelet count.
- Know possible adverse reactions and report any symptom suggestive of toxicity immediately to physician.
- Do not breast feed while taking this drug without consulting physician.

GRANISETRON

(gran′i-se-tron)
Kytril
Classifications: GASTROINTESTINAL AGENT; ANTIEMETIC; 5-HT$_3$ ANTAGONIST
Prototype: Ondansetron
Pregnancy Category: B

AVAILABILITY 1 mg tablets; 1 mg/mL injection

ACTIONS Granisetron is a selective serotonin (5-HT$_3$) receptor antagonist. Serotonin receptors of the 5-HT$_3$ type are located centrally in the chemoreceptor trigger zone, and peripherally on the vagal nerve terminals. Serotonin is released from the wall of the small intestine, stimulates the vagal afferent neurons through the serotonin (5-HT$_3$) receptors, and initiates the vomiting reflex.

THERAPEUTIC EFFECTS This selective serotonin (5-HT$_3$) receptor antagonist is used for the prevention of nausea and vomiting associated with cancer chemotherapy.

USES Prevention of nausea and vomiting associated with initial and repeat courses of emetogenic cancer therapy, including high-dose cisplatin.

CONTRAINDICATIONS Hypersensitivity to granisetron.
CAUTIOUS USE Liver disease, pregnancy (category B), lactation, children <2 y.

ROUTE & DOSAGE

Nausea and Vomiting

Child/Adult: **IV** >2 y, 10 mcg/kg infused over 30 sec–5 min, beginning at least 30 min before initiation of chemotherapy (up to 40 mcg/kg per dose has been used) **PO** 1 mg b.i.d., start 1 mg up to 1 h prior to chemotherapy, then second tab 12 h later or 2 mg daily

STORAGE
Store at 15°–30° C (59°–86° F) for 24 h after dilution under normal lighting conditions.

ADMINISTRATION

Oral
- Give only on the day of chemotherapy.

Intravenous

PREPARE **Direct:** Give undiluted. **IV Infusion:** Dilute in NS or D5W to a total volume of 20–50 mL. Prepare infusion at time of administration; do not mix in solution with other drugs.
ADMINISTER **Direct:** Give a single dose over 30 sec. **IV Infusion:** Infuse diluted drug over 5 min or longer; complete infusion 20–30 min prior to initiation of chemotherapy.

ADVERSE EFFECTS CNS: *Headache,* dizziness, somnolence, insomnia, labile mood, anxiety, fatigue. **GI:** Constipation, diarrhea, elevated liver function tests.

PHARMACOKINETICS Onset: Several minutes. **Duration:** Approximately 24 h. **Distribution:** Widely distributed in body tissues. **Metabolism:** Appears to be metabolized in liver. **Elimination:** Excreted in urine as metabolites. **Half-Life:** 10–11 h in cancer patients, 4–5 h in healthy volunteers.

Common adverse effects in *italic;* life-threatening effects underlined; generic names in **bold;** drug classifications in SMALL CAPS; ♣ Canadian drug name; ⊘ Prototype drug.

603

NURSING IMPLICATIONS

Assessment & Drug Effects

- Monitor the frequency and severity of nausea and vomiting.
- Perform baseline weight and nutrition assessments of children and monitor closely during chemotherapy.
- Lab tests: Monitor liver function; elevated AST and ALT values usually normalize within 2 wk of last dose.
- Assess for headache, which usually responds to nonnarcotic analgesics.

Patient & Family Education

- Note: Headache requiring an analgesic for relief is a common adverse effect.
- Learn ways to manage constipation.
- Meet with health care providers as needed to enhance nutritional state of child.
- Do not breast feed while taking this drug without consulting physician.
- Store this medication out of reach of children.

GRISEOFULVIN MICRO-SIZE

(gri-see-oh-ful′vin)

Fulvicin-U/F, Grifulvin V, Grisactin, Grisovin-FP ♣

GRISEOFULVIN ULTRAMICROSIZE

Fulvicin P/G, Grisactin Ultra, Gris-PEG

Classifications: ANTI-INFECTIVE; ANTIBIOTIC; ANTIFUNGAL
Prototype: Fluconazole
Pregnancy Category: C

AVAILABILITY Griseofulvin Micro-Size 250 mg, 500 mg tablets; 250 mg capsules; 125 mg/5 mL suspension **Griseofulvin Ultramicrosize** 125 mg, 165 mg, 250 mg, 330 mg tablets

ACTIONS Fungistatic antibiotic derived from species of *Penicillium.* Arrests metaphase of cell division by disrupting mitotic spindle structure in fungal cells. Deposits in keratin precursor cells and has special affinity for diseased tissue. It is tightly bound to new keratin of skin, hair, and nails, which becomes highly resistant to fungal invasion. Theoretically cross-sensitivity with penicillin is a possibility.

THERAPEUTIC EFFECTS Effective against various species of *Epidermophyton, Microsporum,* and *Trichophyton* (has no effect on other fungi, including *Candida,* bacteria, and yeasts).

USES Mycotic disease of skin, hair, and nails not amenable to conventional topical measures. Concomitant use of appropriate topical agent may be required, particularly for tinea pedis.

UNLABELED USES Raynaud's disease, angina pectoris, and gout.

CONTRAINDICATIONS Porphyria; hepatic disease; SLE. Safe use during pregnancy (category C), lactation, children ≤2 y, or for prophylaxis against fungal infections is not established.

CAUTIOUS USE Penicillin-sensitive patients (possibility of cross-sensitivity with penicillin exists; however, reportedly penicillin-sensitive patients have been treated without difficulty).

ROUTE & DOSAGE

Tinea Corporis, Tinea Cruris, Tinea Capitis
Child: **PO** 10–20 mg/kg/day microsize or 5–10 mg/kg/day ultramicrosize in single or divided doses
Adult: **PO** 500 mg microsize or 330–375 mg ultramicrosize daily in single or divided doses

Tinea Pedis, Tinea Unguium
Child: **PO** 10–20 mg/kg/day microsize or 5–10 mg/kg/day ultramicrosize in single or divided doses
Adult: **PO** 0.75–1 g microsize or 660–750 mg ultramicrosize daily in single or divided doses (decrease microsize dose to 500 mg/day after response is noted)

G

STORAGE
Store at 15°–30° C (59°–86° F) in tightly covered containers unless otherwise directed.

ADMINISTRATION

Oral
- Give with or after meals to allay GI disturbances.
- Give the microsize formulations with a high fat content meal (increases drug absorption rate) to enhance serum levels. Consult prescriber for recommendations.
- Note: Duration of treatment depends on time required to replace infected skin, hair, or nails, and thus varies with infection site. Average duration of treatment for tinea capitis (scalp ringworm), 4–6 wk; tinea corporis (body ringworm), 2–4 wk; tinea pedis (athlete's foot), 4–8 wk; tinea unguium (nail fungus), 4–6 mo for fingernails, depending on rate of growth, and 6 mo or more for toenails.

ADVERSE EFFECTS Body as a Whole: Hypersensitivity (urticaria, photosensitivity, skin rashes, pruritus, fixed drug eruption, serum sickness syndromes, severe angioedema). **CNS:** *Severe headache,* insomnia, fatigue, mental confusion, impaired performance of routine functions, psychotic symptoms, vertigo. **GI:** Heartburn, nausea, vomiting, diarrhea, flatulence, dry mouth, thirst, decreased taste acuity, anorexia, unpleasant taste, furred tongue, oral thrush hepatotoxicity. **Hematologic:** Leukopenia, neutropenia, granulocytopenia, punctate basophilia, monocytosis. **Urogenital:** Nephrotoxicity (proteinuria) estrogen-like effects (in children); aggravation of SLE. **Other:** Overgrowth of nonsusceptible organisms; candidal intertrigo.

INTERACTIONS Drug: Alcohol may cause flushing and tachycardia; BARBITURATES may decrease activity of griseofulvin; may decrease hypoprothrombinemic effects of ORAL ANTICOAGULANTS; may increase **estrogen** metabolism, resulting in break through bleeding, and decrease contraceptive efficacy of ORAL CONTRACEPTIVES; may decrease level of **cyclosporine, warfarin.**

PHARMACOKINETICS Absorption: Absorbed primarily from duodenum; microsize is variably and unpredictably absorbed; ultramicrosize is almost completely absorbed. **Peak:** 4–8 h. **Distribution:** Concentrates in skin, hair, nails, fat, and skeletal muscle; crosses placenta. **Metabolism:** Metabolized in liver. **Elimination:** Excreted mainly in urine; some excretion in perspiration. **Half-Life:** 9–24 h.

NURSING IMPLICATIONS

Assessment & Drug Effects

- Inquire about history of sensitivity to griseofulvin, penicillins, or other allergies prior to initiating treatment.
- Monitor food intake. Drug may alter taste sensations, and this may cause appetite suppression and inadequate nutrient intake.
- Lab tests: WBC with differential at least once weekly during first month of therapy or longer; periodic renal and hepatic function tests are also advised.
- Continue treatment until there is clinical improvement or until 2 or 3 consecutive weekly cultures are negative.

Patient & Family Education

- Continue treatment as prescribed to prevent relapse, even if you experience symptomatic relief after 48–96 h of therapy.
- Avoid exposure to intense natural or artificial sunlight, because photosensitivity-type reactions may occur.
- Note: Headaches often occur during early therapy but frequently disappear with continued drug administration.
- Disulfiram-type reactions (see Appendix D-1) are possible with ingestion of alcohol during therapy.
- Pharmacologic effects of oral contraceptives may be reduced. Breakthrough bleeding and pregnancy may occur. Alternative forms of birth control should be used during therapy.
- Do not breast feed while taking this drug without consulting prescriber.
- Store this medication out of reach of children.

GUAIFENESIN 🅿️

(gwye-fen'e-sin)

Amonidrin, Anti-Tuss, Breonesin, Gee-Gee, GG-Cen, Glyceryl Guaiacolate, Glycotuss, Glytuss, Guaituss, Hytuss, Malotuss, Mytussin, Mucinex, Nortussin, Resyl ♣, Robitussin

Classifications: ANTITUSSIVE; EXPECTORANT
Pregnancy Category: C

AVAILABILITY 100 mg/5 mL syrup; 100 mg/5 mL, 200 mg/5 mL liquid; 200 mg capsules; 300 mg sustained-release capsules; 100 mg, 200 mg, 1200 mg tablets; 600 mg sustained-release tablets

Combination Products: Available in many combination products

ACTIONS Enhances reflex outflow of respiratory tract fluids by irritation of gastric mucosa.
THERAPEUTIC EFFECTS Aids in expectoration by reducing adhesiveness and surface tension of secretions.

USES To combat dry, nonproductive cough associated with colds and bronchitis. A common ingredient in cough mixtures.

CONTRAINDICATIONS Hypersensitivity to guaifenesin; pregnancy (category C), lactation.

ROUTE & DOSAGE

Cough
Child: **PO** *<2 y,* 12 mg/kg/day in 6 divided doses; *2–5 y,* 50–100 mg q4h up to 600 mg/day; *6–11 y,* 100–200 mg q4h up to 1.2 g/day
Adult: **PO** 200–400 mg q4h up to 2.4 g/day or 1200 mg b.i.d. of the sustained-release dosage form

STORAGE
Store at 15°–30° C (59°–86° F) in light resistant container.

ADMINISTRATION
Oral
- Ensure that sustained-release form of drug is not chewed or crushed. It must be swallowed whole.
- Follow dose with a full glass of water if not contraindicated or with amount appropriate for age.
- Carefully observe maximum daily doses for adults and children.

ADVERSE EFFECTS GI: Low incidence of nausea. **CNS:** Drowsiness.

DIAGNOSTIC TEST INTERFERENCE Guaifenesin may produce color interference with certain laboratory determinations of *urinary 5-hydroxyindoleacetic acid (5-HIAA)* and *vanillylmandelic acid (VMA).*

INTERACTIONS Drug: By inhibiting platelet function, guaifenesin may increase risk of hemorrhage in patients receiving **heparin** therapy.

PHARMACOKINETICS Not studied.

NURSING IMPLICATIONS

Assessment & Drug Effects
- Monitor for therapeutic effectiveness. Persistent cough may indicate a serious condition requiring further diagnostic work.
- Notify prescriber if high fever, rash, or headaches develop.

Patient & Family Education
- Increase fluid intake to help loosen mucus.
- Contact prescriber if cough persists beyond 1 wk.
- Contact prescriber if high fever, rash, or headache develops.
- Because this product is present in several combination remedies, be

---

Common adverse effects in *italic;* life-threatening effects <u>underlined</u>; generic names in **bold;** drug classifications in SMALL CAPS; ♣ Canadian drug name; ✪ Prototype drug.

607

sure to inform health care provider of all medications, both prescribed and OTC.
- Do not breast feed while taking this drug.
- Store this medication out of reach of children.

GUANETHIDINE SULFATE

(gwahn-eth'i-deen)
Ismelin, Apo-Guanethidine ♣
Classifications: CARDIOVASCULAR AGENT; CENTRALLY ACTING ANTIHYPERTENSIVE
Prototype: Methyldopa
Pregnancy Category: C

AVAILABILITY 10 mg, 25 mg tablets

ACTIONS Potent, long-acting, adrenergic blocking agent. Competes with norepinephrine for reuptake into adrenergic neurons; displaces stored norepinephrine, thus exposing it to degradation by MAO. Produces a gradual prolonged fall in BP, usually associated with bradycardia and decreased pulse pressure. Drug-induced sodium retention and expansion of plasma volume, with resulting tolerance to antihypertensive effect, may occur unless concomitant diuretic therapy is administered.

THERAPEUTIC EFFECTS It is more effective in lowering orthostatic than supine BP. Antihypertensive effect results from venous dilatation with peripheral pooling, decreased venous return, and decreased cardiac output.

USES Stepped-care approach to treatment of moderate to severe hypertension either alone or in conjunction with a thiazide diuretic or hydralazine.

UNLABELED USES Chronic open-angle glaucoma, endocrine ophthalmopathy. **Orphan Drug:** Reflex sympathetic dystrophy syndrome; causalgia.

CONTRAINDICATIONS Pheochromocytoma, frank CHF (not due to hypertension). Safe use during pregnancy (category C) is not established.

CAUTIOUS USE Diabetes mellitus, impaired renal or hepatic function, sinus bradycardia, limited cardiac reserve, coronary disease with insufficiency, recent MI, cerebrovascular insufficiency, febrile illnesses, older adults; lactation; history of peptic ulcer, colitis, or bronchial asthma.

ROUTE & DOSAGE

Hypertension

Child: **PO** 0.2 mg/kg/day, may increase by 0.2 mg/kg q1–3wk if needed (max 1–1.6 mg/kg/day)
Adult: **PO** 10 mg daily, may be increased by 10 mg q5–7days up to 300 mg/day (start with 25–50 mg/day in hospitalized patients, increase by 25–50 mg q1–3days)

STORAGE

Store in tightly covered containers at room temperature.

Common adverse effects in *italic;* life-threatening effects underlined; generic names in **bold;** drug classifications in SMALL CAPS; ♣ Canadian drug name; �𝗣 Prototype drug.

ADMINISTRATION

Oral

- Crush tablet before administration if needed to enable swallowing and give with small amount of fluid of child's choice.
- Increase dosage slowly (at intervals of no less than 5–7 days for adults and 1–3 wk in children) and only if there has been no reduction in standing BP from previous levels. BP should be monitored during dosage adjustment period.

ADVERSE EFFECTS CV: *Marked orthostatic and exertional hypotension* with dizziness, light-headedness; bradycardia, symptomatic sick sinus syndrome (weakness, dizziness, blurred vision); angina, *edema with weight gain,* CHF, complete heart block. **Special Senses:** Blurred vision, ptosis of eyelids, parotid tenderness, nasal congestion. **GI:** *Severe diarrhea,* nausea, vomiting, constipation, dry mouth. **Urogenital:** Nocturia, urinary retention, incontinence, inhibition of ejaculation, impotence. **Skin:** Skin eruptions, loss of scalp hair. **Other:** Dyspnea, psychic depression, weakness, fatigue, myalgia, tremor, chest paresthesias, asthma, rise in BUN, polyarteritis nodosa.

INTERACTIONS Drug: Alcohol, levodopa, DIURETICS and other HYPOTENSIVE AGENTS increase hypotensive effects; MAO INHIBITORS may antagonize hypotensive effects; **norepinephrine, pseudoephedrine,** other DECONGESTANTS, TRICYCLIC ANTIDEPRESSANTS, PHENOTHIAZINES block hypotensive effects. **Herbal: Mahuang, ephedra** may cause enhanced sympathomimetic effects.

PHARMACOKINETICS Absorption: Completely absorbed, but undergoes significant first-pass metabolism by liver; 3–50% of dose reaches systemic circulation. **Peak effect:** 1–3 wk. **Distribution:** Rapidly distributed to adrenergic neuron storage sites; does not cross blood–brain barrier. **Metabolism:** Metabolized in liver to inactive metabolites. **Elimination:** Excreted in urine. **Half-Life:** 5 days.

NURSING IMPLICATIONS

Assessment & Drug Effects

- Take BP first in supine position and then again after patient has been standing for 10 min. Ideal dosage reduces standing BP to within normal range without faintness, dizziness, weakness, or fatigue.
- Monitor I&O, especially in patients with limited cardiac reserve or impaired renal function. Report changes in I&O ratio.
- Observe for evidence of edema and weight gain. Sudden weight gain of 1 kg (2 lb) in 24 h or more for child over 12 years or any weight gain in younger child should be reported to prescriber. Patients with limited cardiac reserve are particularly susceptible to guanethidine-induced sodium and water retention, with resulting edema, CHF, and drug resistance.
- Observe patients on antidiabetic therapy closely for signs of hypoglycemia.

Patient & Family Education

- Do not stop drug without consulting prescriber.
- Ask for assistance with walking.

Common adverse effects in *italic;* life-threatening effects underlined; generic names in **bold;** drug classifications in SMALL CAPS; ♣ Canadian drug name; ⊘ Prototype drug.

609

■ Understand that orthostatic hypotension is most prominent shortly after arising from sleep and when too rapid changes are made to sitting or upright positions. Move gradually to sitting position and make all position changes slowly and in stages. Flex arms and legs slowly before standing to augment venous return. Orthostatic hypotension is intensified by prolonged standing, hot baths or showers, hot tubs or saunas, hot weather, alcohol ingestion, and strenuous physical exercise (particularly if followed by immobility).

■ Lie down or sit down (in head-low position) immediately at the onset of dizziness, weakness, or faintness.

■ Consult prescriber regarding allowable salt intake.

■ Reduced dosage in presence of febrile illnesses. Report fever to prescriber.

■ Consult health care professional before taking any OTC drug; guanethidine may sensitize the patient to some sympathomimetic agents found in OTC cold remedies and cause hypertensive crisis.

■ Do not breast feed while taking this drug.

■ Store this medication out of reach of children.

HAEMOPHILUS b CONJUGATE VACCINE (Hib)
(hee-mof'il-us)
HibTITER, PedvaxHIB, ProHIBiT
Classifications: ANTI-INFECTIVE; VACCINE
Prototype: Hepatitis B vaccine
Pregnancy Category: C

AVAILABILITY 7.5 mcg, 10 mcg, 15 mcg, 25 mcg injection

ACTIONS A highly purified capsular polysaccharide extracted from *Haemophilus influenzae* type b (Hib). Hib capsular polysaccharide, principal antigen in the vaccine, promotes production of Hib anticapsular antibodies. It mediates complement-dependent bacteriolyses of *H. influenzae* type b organism. Serum antibody response is age dependent; i.e., response is poor in infants, increasing significantly between 12–24 mo.

THERAPEUTIC EFFECTS The vaccine produces antibodies effective against <u>Haemophilus influenzae</u> type b.

USES To provide active immunity to *H. influenzae* type b (Hib) infection in children 2 mo–5 y.
UNLABELED USES Adults at risk of Hib infection who have Hodgkin's disease, before immunosuppressive chemotherapy.

CONTRAINDICATIONS Hypersensitivity to any component of vaccine (e.g., thiomersal); febrile illness (other than upper respiratory tract infection); active infection. Safe use during pregnancy (category C) or lactation is not established.

ROUTE & DOSAGE

Immunoprophylaxis for *H. influenzae* type b Infection

Child: **IM** *2–6 mo,* HibTITER 0.5 mL, 3 doses 2 mo apart with booster at 15 mo; PedvaxHIB 0.5 mL, 2 doses 2 mo apart with booster at 12 mo; *7–11 mo* at time of first dose, HibTITER 0.5 mL, 2 doses 2 mo apart with booster at 15 mo; PedvaxHIB 0.5 mL, 2 doses 2 mo apart with booster at 15 mo; *12–14 mo* at time of first dose, HibTITER 0.5 mL, 1 dose with booster at 15 mo; PedvaxHIB 0.5 mL, 1 dose with booster at 15 mo; *15 mo–5 y* at time of first dose, all vaccines 0.5 mL as 1 dose See Appendix H-1 for immunization schedule.

STORAGE

Store vaccine at 2°–8° C (36°–46° F); may be frozen without loss of potency. Diluent can be stored at room temperature. Do not freeze the diluent.

ADMINISTRATION

Intramuscular

- Reconstitute lyophilized powder with supplied diluent to yield 25 mcg/0.5 mL.
- Note: Use different sites when giving Hib polysaccharide vaccine and DPT (diphtheria, pertussis, tetanus) at the same time. See Part I for site selection.
- Note: The initial series for HibTITER is 4 doses and that for PedvaxHIB is 3 doses. Read package inserts carefully for product uses and follow directions precisely.

ADVERSE EFFECTS Skin: Irritation at injection site (4–9%). **Other:** Acute febrile reactions (13%), irritability, anorexia, <u>anaphylactoid reaction</u> (rare).

DIAGNOSTIC TEST INTERFERENCE Hib polysaccharide vaccine may interfere with interpretation of ***antigen detection tests*** (e.g., latex agglutination) used in diagnosis of systemic Hib disease.

INTERACTIONS Drug: IMMUNOSUPPRESSANT DRUGS, STEROIDS may decrease antibody response.

PHARMACOKINETICS Onset: Antibody levels detected within 2 wk. **Peak:** 3 wk. **Duration:** 1.5–3.5 y. **Distribution:** Crosses placenta; distributed into breast milk.

NURSING IMPLICATIONS

Assessment & Drug Effects

- Be prepared for anaphylactoid reaction (see Appendix D-1) by having epinephrine 1:1000 available.
- U.S. law requires that parents be given teaching on risks and benefits of immunization. Medication amount, site, route, date, company, lot number, and parent consent must be recorded. Inform parents of next scheduled immunizations and make an appointment for this visit.

Patient & Family Education

- Note: Local reactions to the vaccine at the injection site (erythema, tenderness, induration, swelling, pain) may appear within 6 h after administration; usually symptoms are mild and disappear in 24 h.
- Monitor temperature after injection. An acute febrile reaction with temperature above 38.3° C (101° F) may follow vaccination (less than 1% of recipients). Notify health care professional.
- Do not breast feed when administered this immunization without consulting health care professional.

HALCINONIDE
(hal-sin'oh-nide)
Halog
Classifications: SKIN AND MUCOUS MEMBRANE AGENT; ANTI-INFLAMMATORY STEROID
Prototype: Hydrocortisone
Pregnancy Category: C

AVAILABILITY 0.1% ointment, cream, solution; 0.025% cream

ACTIONS Fluorinated steroid with substituted 17-hydroxyl group, chemically similar to flurandrenolide (Cordran).
THERAPEUTIC EFFECTS Crosses cell membranes, complexes with nuclear DNA, and stimulates synthesis of enzymes thought to be responsible for anti-inflammatory effects.

USES Relief of pruritic and inflammatory manifestations of corticosteroid-responsive dermatoses.

CONTRAINDICATIONS Use on large body surface area; long-term use.
CAUTIOUS USE Children, lactation, pregnancy (category C).

ROUTE & DOSAGE

Inflammation

Child: **Topical** Apply thin layer daily
Adult: **Topical** Apply thin layer b.i.d. or t.i.d.

STORAGE
Store at 15°–30° C (59°–86° F).

ADMINISTRATION

Topical
- Wash skin gently and dry thoroughly before each application.
- Note: Ointment is preferred for dry scaly lesions. Moist lesions are best treated with solution.
- Do not apply in or around the eyes.
- Do not apply occlusive dressings over areas covered with halcinonide unless specifically prescribed.

Common adverse effects in *italic;* life-threatening effects underlined; generic names in **bold;** drug classifications in SMALL CAPS; ◆ Canadian drug name; ❷ Prototype drug.

ADVERSE EFFECTS Endocrine: Reversible HPA axis suppression, hyperglycemia, glycosuria. **Skin:** Burning, itching, irritation, erythema, dryness, folliculitis, hypertrichosis, pruritus, acneiform eruptions, hypopigmentation, perioral dermatitis, allergic contact dermatitis, stinging cracking/tightness of skin, secondary infection, skin atrophy, striae, miliaria, telangiectasia.

PHARMACOKINETICS Absorption: Minimum absorption through intact skin; increased absorption from axilla, eyelid, face, scalp, scrotum, or with occlusive dressing.

NURSING IMPLICATIONS

Assessment & Drug Effects
- Discontinue if signs of infection or irritation occur.
- Monitor for systemic corticosteroid effects that may occur with occlusive dressings or topical applications over large areas of skin.

Patient & Family Education
- Do not medicate infants and young children without prescription.
- Do not breast feed while using this drug without consulting physician.
- Store this medication out of reach of children.

HALOPERIDOL 🅟
(ha-loe-per′i-dole)
Haldol, Peridol ♣

HALOPERIDOL DECANOATE
Haldol LA
Classifications: CENTRAL NERVOUS SYSTEM AGENT; PSYCHOTHERAPEUTIC; ANTIPSYCHOTIC; BUTYROPHENONE
Pregnancy Category: C

AVAILABILITY 0.5 mg, 1 mg, 2 mg, 5 mg, 10 mg, 20 mg tablets; 2 mg/mL oral solution; 5 mg/mL (lactate), 50 mg/mL (decanoate), 100 mg/mL (decanoate) injection

ACTIONS Potent, long-acting butyrophenone derivative with pharmacologic actions similar to those of piperazine phenothiazines but with higher incidence of extrapyramidal effects and less hypotensive and relatively low sedative activity.

THERAPEUTIC EFFECTS Decreases psychotic manifestations and exerts strong antiemetic effect.

USES Management of manifestations of psychotic disorders and for control of tics and vocal utterances of Gilles de la Tourette's syndrome; for treatment of agitated states in acute and chronic psychoses. Used for short-term treatment of hyperactive children and for severe behavior problems in children of combative, explosive hyperexcitability.

UNLABELED USES Cancer chemotherapy as an antiemetic in doses smaller than those required for antipsychotic effects; treatment of autism; alcohol dependence; chorea.

CONTRAINDICATIONS Parkinson's disease, parkinsonism, seizure disorders, coma; alcoholism; severe mental depression, CNS depression; thyrotoxicosis. Safe use during pregnancy (category C), lactation, or in children <3 y is not established.

CAUTIOUS USE Older adult or debilitated patients, urinary retention, glaucoma, severe cardiovascular disorders; patients receiving anticonvulsant, anticoagulant, or lithium therapy.

ROUTE & DOSAGE

Psychosis

Child: 3–12 y, **PO** 0.025–0.05 mg/day divided into 2–3 doses may be increased by 0.25–0.5 mg q5–7days (max 0.15 mg/kg/day); usual dose 0.01–0.03 mg/kg/day **IM** (lactate formulation) 6–12 y, 1–3 mg/kg/dose q4–8h (max 0.15 mg/kg/day)
Adult: **PO** 0.2–5 mg b.i.d. or t.i.d. **IM** 2–5 mg repeated q4h prn; Decanoate: 50–100 mg q4wk

Severe Psychosis

Child: **PO** 0.05–0.15 mg/kg/day in 2–3 divided doses. Usual dose 0.05–0.15 mg/kg/day divided into 2–3 doses
Adult: **PO** 3–5 mg b.i.d. or t.i.d., may need up to 100 mg/day **IM** 2–5 mg, may repeat q.h. prn; Decanoate: 50–100 mg q4wk

Tourette's Disorder

Child: **PO** 0.05–0.075 mg/kg/day in 2–3 divided doses
Adult: **PO** 0.5–2 mg/dose given 2–3 times/day

STORAGE

Store in light-resistant container at 15°–30° C (59°–86° F), unless otherwise specified by manufacturer. Discard darkened solutions.

ADMINISTRATION

Oral

- Give with a full glass (240 mL) of water or with amount appropriate for age, or with food or milk.
- Taper dosing regimen when discontinuing therapy. Abrupt termination can initiate extrapyramidal symptoms.

Intramuscular

- Note that lactate is available as 5 mg/mL and deconoate or long acting is 50 and 100 mg/mL. Read labels carefully and clarify orders for proper formulation and amount.
- Give by deep injection into a large muscle. Consult Part I for site selection in children. Do not exceed 3 mL per injection site or maximum allowed for size of child.
- Have patient recumbent at time of parenteral administration and for about 1 h after injection. Assess for orthostatic hypotension.

ADVERSE EFFECTS CNS: *Extrapyramidal reactions:* Parkinsonian symptoms, dystonia, akathisia, <u>tardive dyskinesia</u> (after long-term use); insomnia, restlessness, anxiety, euphoria, agitation, drowsiness, mental depression, lethargy, fatigue, weakness, tremor, ataxia, headache, confusion, vertigo; neuroleptic malignant syndrome, hyperthermia, grand mal seizures, exacerbation of psychotic symptoms. **CV:** Tachycardia, ECG changes, hypotension, hypertension (with overdosage). **Endocrine:** Menstrual irregularities, galactorrhea, lactation, gynecomastia, impotence, increased libido, hyponatremia, hyperglycemia, hypoglycemia. **Special Senses:** Blurred vision. **Hematologic:** Mild transient leukopenia, agranulocytosis (rare). **GI:** Dry mouth, anorexia, nausea, vomiting, constipation, diarrhea, hypersalivation. **Urogenital:** Urinary retention, priapism. **Respiratory:** Laryngospasm, bronchospasm, increased depth of respiration, bronchopneumonia, respiratory depression. **Skin:** Diaphoresis, maculopapular and acneiform rash, photosensitivity. **Other:** Cholestatic jaundice, variations in liver function tests, decreased serum cholesterol.

INTERACTIONS Drug: CNS DEPRESSANTS, OPIATES, **alcohol** increase CNS depression; may antagonize activity of ORAL ANTICOAGULANTS; ANTICHOLINERGICS may increase intraocular pressure; **methyldopa** may precipitate dementia.

PHARMACOKINETICS Absorption: Well absorbed from GI tract; 60% reaches systemic circulation. **Onset:** 30–45 min IM. **Peak:** 2–6 h PO; 10–20 min IM; 6–7 days decanoate. **Distribution:** Distributes mainly to liver with lower concentration in brain, lung, kidney, spleen, heart. **Metabolism:** Metabolized in liver. **Elimination:** 40% excreted in urine within 5 days; 15% eliminated in feces; excreted in breast milk. **Half-Life:** 13–35 h.

NURSING IMPLICATIONS

Assessment & Drug Effects

- Monitor for therapeutic effectiveness. Because of long half-life, therapeutic effects are slow to develop in early therapy or when established dosing regimen is changed. "Therapeutic window" effect (point at which increased dose or concentration actually decreases therapeutic response) may occur after long period of high doses. Close observation is imperative when doses are changed.
- Target symptoms expected to decrease with successful haloperidol treatment include hallucinations, insomnia, hostility, agitation, and delusions.
- Monitor patient's mental status daily.
- Monitor for neuroleptic malignant syndrome (NMS) (see Appendix D-1), especially in those with hypertension or taking lithium. Symptoms of NMS can appear suddenly after initiation of therapy or after months or years of taking neuroleptic (antipsychotic) medication. Immediately discontinue drug if NMS suspected.
- Monitor for parkinsonism and tardive dyskinesia (see Appendix D-1). Risk of tardive dyskinesia appears to be greater in women receiving high doses. It can occur after long-term therapy and even after therapy is discontinued.
- Monitor for extrapyramidal (neuromuscular) reactions that occur frequently during first few days of treatment. Symptoms are usually dose related and are controlled by dosage reduction or concomitant administration of antiparkinson drugs.

- Be alert for behavioral changes in patients who are concurrently receiving antiparkinson drugs.
- Monitor for exacerbation of seizure activity.
- Observe patients closely for rapid mood shift to depression when haloperidol is used to control mania or cyclic disorders. Depression may represent a drug adverse effect or reversion from a manic state.
- Lab tests: Monitor WBC count with differential and liver function in patients on prolonged therapy.

Patient & Family Education

- Avoid use of alcohol during therapy.
- Do not drive or engage in other potentially hazardous activities until response to drug is known.
- Discuss oral hygiene with health care provider; dry mouth may promote dental problems. Drink adequate fluids.
- Avoid overexposure to sun or sunlamp and use a sunscreen; drug can cause a photosensitivity reaction.
- Do not breast feed while taking this drug without consulting physician.
- Store this medication out of reach of children.

HEPARIN SODIUM ●

Hepalean ♣, Heparin Sodium Lock Flush Solution, Hep-Lock, Lipo-Hepin, Liquaemin Sodium

Classifications: BLOOD FORMERS, COAGULATORS, AND ANTICOAGULANTS
Pregnancy Category: C

AVAILABILITY 10 units/mL, 100 units/mL, 1000 units/mL, 2000 units/mL, 5000 units/mL, 10,000 units/mL, 20,000 units/mL, 40,000 units/mL injection

ACTIONS Strongly acidic, high-molecular-weight mucopolysaccharide with rapid anticoagulant effect. Prepared from bovine lung tissue or porcine intestinal mucosa.

THERAPEUTIC EFFECTS Exerts direct effect on blood coagulation (clotting) by enhancing the inhibitory actions of antithrombin III (heparin cofactor) on several factors essential to normal blood clotting, thereby blocking the conversion of prothrombin to thrombin and fibrinogen to fibrin. Does not lyse already existing thrombi but may prevent their extension and propagation. Inhibits formation on new clots.

USES Prophylaxis and treatment of venous thrombosis and pulmonary embolism and to prevent thromboembolic complications arising from cardiac and vascular surgery, frostbite, and during acute stage of MI. Also used in treatment of disseminated intravascular coagulation (DIC), atrial fibrillation with embolization, and as anticoagulant in blood transfusions, extracorporeal circulation, and dialysis procedures.

UNLABELED USES Prophylaxis in hip and knee surgery. Heparin Sodium Lock Flush Solution is used to maintain potency of indwelling IV catheters in intermittent IV therapy or blood sampling. It is not intended for anticoagulant therapy.

CONTRAINDICATIONS History of hypersensitivity to heparin (white clot syndrome); active bleeding, bleeding tendencies (hemophilia, purpura, thrombocytopenia); jaundice; ascorbic acid deficiency; inaccessible ulcerative lesions; visceral carcinoma; open wounds, extensive denudation of skin, suppurative thrombophlebitis; advanced kidney, liver, or biliary disease; active tuberculosis; bacterial endocarditis; continuous tube drainage of stomach or small intestines; threatened abortion; suspected intracranial hemorrhage, severe hypertension; recent surgery of eye, brain, or spinal cord; spinal tap; shock.

CAUTIOUS USE Alcoholism; history of allergy (asthma, hives, hay fever, eczema); during menstruation; pregnancy (category C), especially the last trimester, and immediate postpartum period; patients with indwelling catheters; older adults; use of acid-citrate-dextrose (ACD)-converted blood (may contain heparin); patients in hazardous occupations; cerebral embolism.

ROUTE & DOSAGE

Treatment of Thromboembolism

Child: **IV** 50 units/kg bolus, then 20,000 units/m^2/24 h or 50–100 units/kg q4h or 15–25 units/kg/h
Adult: **IV** 5000 units/bolus dose, then 18 units/kg/h; adjust to maintain desired PTT (1.5–2.5 times control) **SC** 10,000–20,000 units followed by 8000–20,000 units q8–12h

Open Heart Surgery

Adult: **IV** 150–300 units/kg

Prophylaxis of Embolism

Adult: **SC** 5000 units q8–12h until ambulatory

STORAGE
Store at 15°–30° C (59°–86° F). Protect from freezing.

ADMINISTRATION
Note: Before administration, check coagulation test values; if results are not within therapeutic range, notify physician for dosage adjustment. Do not use solutions of heparin or heparin lock-flush that contain benzyl alcohol preservative in neonates.

Subcutaneous

- Use more concentrated heparin solutions for SC injection.
- Make injections into the fatty layer of the abdomen or just above the iliac crest. Avoid injecting within 5 cm (2 in) of umbilicus or in a bruised area. Insert needle into tissue roll perpendicular to skin surface. Do not withdraw plunger to check entry into blood vessel. Systematically rotate injection sites and keep record.
- Exercise caution to avoid IM injection.

Intravenous

PREPARE **Direct:** Give undiluted. **Intermittent/Continuous:** May add to any amount of NS, D5W, or Ringer's for injection. Invert IV solution container at least 6 times to ensure adequate mixing.

ADMINISTER **Direct:** Give a single dose over 60 sec. **Intermittent/Continuous:** Use infusion pump and give over 4–24 h.

INCOMPATIBILITIES **Solution/Additive:** Amikacin, chlorpromazine, codeine, cytarabine, diazepam, dobutamine, doxorubicin, droperidol, erythromycin, gentamicin, haloperidol, hyaluronidase, hydrocortisone, kanamycin, levorphanol, meperidine, methadone, methicillin, methotrimeprazine, morphine, netilmicin, nitroglycerin, pentazocine, polymyxin B, promethazine, streptomycin, tetracycline, tobramycin, triflupromazine, vancomycin. **Y-Site:** Amikacin, dacarbazine, diazepam, diphenhydramine, doxycycline, doxorubicin, droperidol, ergotamine, erythromycin, gentamicin, haloperidol, kanamycin, methotrimeprazine, netilmicin, nitroglycerin, phenytoin, polymyxin B, streptomycin, tobramycin, triflupromazine, vancomycin.

ADVERSE EFFECTS Hematologic: <u>Spontaneous bleeding</u>, *transient thrombocytopenia,* hypofibrinogenemia, "white clot syndrome." **Body as a Whole:** Fever, chills, urticaria, pruritus, skin rashes, itching and burning sensations of feet, numbness and tingling of hands and feet, elevated BP, headache, nasal congestion, lacrimation, conjunctivitis, chest pains, arthralgia, <u>bronchospasm, anaphylactoid reactions</u>. **Endocrine:** Osteoporosis, hypoaldosteronism, suppressed renal function, hyperkalemia; rebound hyperlipidemia (following termination of heparin therapy). **GI:** Increased AST, ALT. **Urogenital:** Priapism (rare). **Skin:** Injection site reactions: pain, itching, ecchymoses, tissue irritation and sloughing; cyanosis and pains in arms or legs (vasospasm), reversible transient alopecia (usually around temporal area).

DIAGNOSTIC TEST INTERFERENCE Notify laboratory that patient is receiving heparin, when a test is to be performed. Possibility of false-positive rise in *BSP* test and in *serum thyroxine;* and increases in *resin T_3 uptake;* false-negative ^{125}I *fibrinogen uptake.* Heparin prolongs *PT.* Valid readings may be obtained by drawing blood samples at least 4–6 h after an IV dose (but at any time during heparin infusion) and 12–24 h after an SC heparin dose.

INTERACTIONS Drug: May prolong PT, which is used to monitor therapy with ORAL ANTICOAGULANTS; **aspirin,** NSAIDS increase risk of bleeding; **nitroglycerin** IV may decrease anticoagulant activity; **protamine** antagonizes effects of heparin. **Herbal: Feverfew, ginkgo, ginger, valerian** may potentiate bleeding.

PHARMACOKINETICS Onset: 20–60 min SC. **Peak:** Within minutes. **Duration:** 2–6 h IV; 8–12 h SC. **Distribution:** Does not cross placenta; not distributed into breast milk. **Metabolism:** Metabolized in liver and by reticuloendothelial system. **Elimination:** Excreted slowly in urine. **Half-Life:** 90 min.

NURSING IMPLICATIONS

Assessment & Drug Effects

- Lab tests: Baseline blood coagulation tests, Hct, Hgb, RBC, and platelet counts prior to initiation of therapy and at regular intervals throughout therapy.
- Monitor APTT levels closely.

Common adverse effects in *italic;* life-threatening effects <u>underlined</u>; generic names in **bold;** drug classifications in SMALL CAPS; ✦ Canadian drug name; ● Prototype drug.

- Note: In general, dosage is adjusted to keep APTT between 1.5–2.5 times normal control level.
- Draw blood for coagulation test 30 min before each scheduled SC or intermittent IV dose and approximately q4h for patients receiving continuous IV heparin during dosage adjustment period. After dosage is established, tests may be done once daily.
- Patients vary widely in their reaction to heparin; risk of hemorrhage appears greatest in women, and patients with liver disease or renal insufficiency.
- Monitor vital signs. Report fever, drop in BP, rapid pulse, and other S&S of hemorrhage.
- Observe all needle sites daily for hematoma and signs of inflammation (swelling, heat, redness, pain).
- Antidote: Have on hand protamine sulfate (1% solution), specific heparin antagonist.

Patient & Family Education

- Protect from injury and notify physician of pink, red, dark brown, or cloudy urine; red or dark brown vomitus; red or black stools; bleeding gums or oral mucosa; ecchymoses, hematoma, epistaxis, bloody sputum; chest pain; abdominal or lumbar pain or swelling; unusual increase in menstrual flow; pelvic pain; severe or continuous headache, faintness, or dizziness.
- Note: Menstruation may be somewhat increased and prolonged; usually, this is not a contraindication to continued therapy if bleeding is not excessive.
- Correct technique for SC administration is a needed skill for those discharged from hospital on heparin.
- Engage in normal activities such as shaving with a safety razor in the absence of a low platelet (thrombocyte) count. Usually, heparin does not affect bleeding time.
- Caution: Smoking and alcohol consumption may alter response to heparin and are not advised.
- Do not take aspirin or any other OTC or herbal medication without physician's approval.

HEPATITIS A VACCINE

(hep′a-ti-tis)

Havrix, Vaqta, Twinrix (with hepatitis B)

Classifications: ANTI-INFECTIVE; VACCINE

Prototype: Hepatitis B vaccine

Pregnancy Category: C

AVAILABILITY 720 EL·units/0.5 mL, 1440 EL·units/1 mL (Havrix); 25 units/0.5 mL, 50 units/1 mL (Vaqta).

Combination Products: Available in combination with hepatitis B (Twinrix).

ACTIONS Anti-hepatitis A virus antibody titers following administration of hepatitis A vaccine (inactivated) are comparable to those observed after natural hepatitis A virus infection.

THERAPEUTIC EFFECTS Antibody levels are 50- to 300-fold higher with inactivated hepatitis A vaccine than with passive immunity with human immune globulin.

USES Active immunization against hepatitis A. Recommended as part of immunization schedule for young children in states with high incidence of the disease.

CONTRAINDICATIONS Hypersensitivity to any component in vaccine, pregnancy (category C), children <2 y.
CAUTIOUS USE Lactation.

ROUTE & DOSAGE

Hepatitis A Immunization

Child receiving Twinrix (combination with hepatitis B): **IM** *2–18 y,*
2 doses of 0.5 mL in deltoid muscle given 1 mo apart; booster dose
(0.5 mL) at 6–12 mo after primary doses
Child/Adult >2 y: **IM** *1 mL in deltoid muscle; booster dose (1 mL) at*
6–12 mo after primary dose
See Appendix H-1 for immunization schedule.

STORAGE
Store at 2°–8° C (36°–47° F). Discard vaccine if it has been frozen.

ADMINISTRATION
Intramuscular
- Give only in deltoid for adults and children older than 2 y. Do NOT give IV, SC, or intradermally.
- Use vaccine as packaged without dilution.
- Shake vial and syringe well before withdrawal and injection, respectively. Vaccine should be an opaque white suspension; discard if it looks otherwise.
- U.S. law requires that parents be given teaching on risks and benefits of immunization. Medication amount, site, route, date, company, lot number, and parent consent must be recorded. Inform parents of next scheduled immunizations and make an appointment for this visit.

ADVERSE EFFECTS CNS: *Headache,* fatigue, fever, malaise, somnolence vertigo, insomnia, photophobia, convulsions, neuropathy, paresthesia.
GI: Anorexia, nausea, abdominal pain, diarrhea, dysgeusia, vomiting.
Skin: Pruritus, rash, urticaria, erythema multiforme, hyperhidrosis, <u>angioedema</u> (rare). **Other:** *Soreness at injection site, pain, swelling, redness at injection site,* pharyngitis, lymphadenopathy.

INTERACTIONS Drug: No clinically significant interactions established

PHARMACOKINETICS Onset: 3 wk. **Duration:** 1–3 y with single dose, 5–10 y with booster.

Common adverse effects in *italic;* life-threatening effects <u>underlined</u>; generic names in **bold;** drug classifications in SMALL CAPS; ✥ Canadian drug name; ● Prototype drug.

NURSING IMPLICATIONS

Assessment & Drug Effects

- Do not administer during a severe infection.
- Assess for S&S of anaphylaxis and have epinephrine 1:1000 available.

Patient & Family Education

- Note: Injection site soreness is common; most adverse reactions are mild and usually last less than 24 h.
- Get booster injection within 6–12 mo.
- Instruct parents about next recommended immunizations and make appointment with health care provider if possible.
- Do not breast feed while taking this drug without consulting health care provider.

H

HEPATITIS B IMMUNE GLOBULIN

(hep′a-ti-tis)
H-BIG, Hep-B-Gammagee, HyperHep
Classifications: ANTI-INFECTIVE; VACCINE
Prototype: Hepatitis B vaccine
Pregnancy Category: C

AVAILABILITY 1 mL, 4 mL, 5 mL vials

ACTIONS Sterile solution of immunoglobulins (immunoglobulin G [IgG]) prepared by a special process using pooled human plasma. Serum has also been tested for and found free of antibody to HIV. The possibility of transmission of hepatitis infection or AIDS from H-BIG is remote.

THERAPEUTIC EFFECTS Preparation contains a high antibody titer specific to hepatitis B surface antigen (anti-HBs); plasma does not show serologic evidence of hepatitis B surface antigen (HBsAg).

USES Prophylactically to provide passive immunity to hepatitis B infection in individuals exposed to HBV or HBsAg-positive materials (blood plasma, serum). Also as postexposure prophylaxis after bite or percutaneous exposure, ingestion, direct mucous membrane contact, sexual or intimate contact, and in neonates born to HBsAg-positive women.

CONTRAINDICATIONS Pregnancy (category C).
CAUTIOUS USE History of systemic allergic reactions to immune globulin, concurrent administration of immunosuppression drugs; thrombocytopenia or bleeding disorders, HBsAg-positive individuals, patients with specific immunoglobulin A (IgA) deficiency; lactation.

ROUTE & DOSAGE

Hepatitis B Prophylaxis

Child/Adult: **IM** 0.06 mL/kg as soon as possible after exposure, preferably within 24 h, but no later than 7 days, repeat 28–30 days after exposure

---

Newborn Exposure

Child: IM 0.5 mL within 12 hours of birth when baby's mother is HBsAg positive, repeat dose 3 and 6 mo later
See Appendix H-1 for immunization schedule.

STORAGE

Store at 2°–8° C (36°–46° F) unless otherwise directed. Avoid freezing.

ADMINISTRATION

Intramuscular

- Give Hepatitis B immune globulin at the same time or up to 1 mo preceding hepatitis B vaccination (hepatitis B vaccine). Does not impair the active immune response from the vaccination. Give within 12 h of birth to all infants born to mothers with HBsAg positive status; hepatitis B vaccine is given at same time at a second site (see hepatitis B vaccine below).
- Give preferably into deltoid muscle or anterolateral aspect of thigh.
- Note: For neonates and small children the injection site should be the anterolateral aspect of the thigh.
- Do NOT administer by IV; inadvertent IV or intravascular administration can cause a precipitous fall in BP and an anaphylactic reaction.

ADVERSE EFFECTS Body as a Whole: Muscle stiffness; pain, tenderness, swelling, erythema of injection site, nausea, faintness, fever, dizziness, malaise, lassitude, body and joint pain, leg cramps. **Skin:** Urticaria, rash, angioedema, pruritus, erythema, sensitization (following large or repeated doses), anaphylaxis (rare).

INTERACTIONS Drug: May interfere with immune response to LIVE-VIRUS VACCINES (measles/mumps/rubella/poliovirus).

PHARMACOKINETICS Absorption: Slowly absorbed from IM site. **Onset:** 1–6 days. **Peak:** 3–11 days. **Duration:** 2–6 mo. **Elimination:** Half-life 21 days.

NURSING IMPLICATIONS

Assessment & Drug Effects

- Have epinephrine 1:1000 readily available; hypersensitivity reactions are most likely to occur in patients receiving large doses or repeated injections.

Patient & Family Education

- Learn potential adverse reactions.
- Do not breast feed after taking this drug without consulting care provider.

HEPATITIS B VACCINE (RECOMBINANT) 🅟

(hep'a-ti-tis)
Engerix-B, Recombivax HB
Classifications: ANTI-INFECTIVE; VACCINE
Pregnancy Category: C

AVAILABILITY 10 mcg/mL, 5 mcg/0.5 mL, 40 mcg/mL (Recombivax); 20 mcg/mL, 10 mcg/0.5 mL (Engerix-B)

ACTIONS Suspension of inactivated and purified hepatitis B surface antigen (HBsAg) derived from human plasma of screened asymptomatic HBsAg-positive carriers of hepatitis B virus. Hepatitis B vaccine recombinant is the first vaccine produced by gene splicing. No human plasma is used in its production.

THERAPEUTIC EFFECTS The recommended 3-dose regimen produces active immunity against hepatitis B infection by inducing protective antibody (anti-HBs) formation.

USES To promote active immunity in individuals at high risk of potential exposure to hepatitis B virus or HBsAg-positive materials. Has been used simultaneously (into different sites) with hepatitis B immune globulin (H-BIG) for postexposure prophylaxis in selected patients. Must be given within 12 h of birth to all infants born to mothers with positive or unknown HbsAg status. For infants of mothers with negative HbsAg status, infant should be immunized before discharge from the hospital.

CONTRAINDICATIONS History of allergic reaction to hepatitis B vaccine or to any ingredient in the formulation; HBsAg carriers. Safe use during pregnancy (category C) and lactation is not established.

CAUTIOUS USE Compromised cardiopulmonary status, serious active infection or fever; thrombocytopenia or other bleeding disorders.

ROUTE & DOSAGE

Hepatitis B Prevention

Child: **IM** Recombivax 0.5 mL (5 mcg) at 0, 1, and 6 mo; Engerix-B 0.5 mL (10 mcg) at 0, 1, and 6 mo or 0, 1, 2, and 12 mo
NOTE: Give first dose within 12 hours of birth if baby's mother is HBsAg positive, with second dose given at 1–2 months of age.
Adult: **IM** Recombivax 1 mL (10 mcg) at 0, 1, and 6 mo; Engerix-B 1 mL (20 mcg) at 0, 1, and 6 mo or 0, 1, 2, and 12 mo

Dialysis and Immunodeficient Patients

Adult: **IM** Recombivax 2mL (20 mcg) at 0, 1, and 6 mo; Engerix-B 2 mL (40 mcg) at 0, 1, and 6 mo or 0, 1, 2, and 12 mo

STORAGE
Store unopened and opened vials at 2°–8° C (36°–46° F) unless otherwise directed. Avoid freezing (freezing destroys potency).

ADMINISTRATION

Intramuscular

- Give preferably into the deltoid and in neonates and infants into the anterolateral thigh, avoiding blood vessels and nerves. Carefully aspirate to prevent inadvertent intravascular injection.
- Have epinephrine 1:1000 immediately available to treat anaphylaxis.
- Shake vial well before withdrawing dose to assure uniform suspension.

ADVERSE EFFECTS Body as a Whole: *Mild local tenderness at injection site, local inflammatory reaction* (swelling, heat, redness, induration, pain);

---

fever, malaise, fatigue, headache, dizziness, faintness, leg cramps, myalgia, arthralgia. **GI:** Nausea, vomiting, diarrhea. **Skin:** Rash, urticaria, pruritus.

INTERACTIONS Drug: No clinically significant interactions established.

PHARMACOKINETICS Absorption: Slowly absorbed from IM site. **Onset:** 2 wk. **Peak:** 6 mo. **Duration:** At least 3 y.

NURSING IMPLICATIONS

Assessment & Drug Effects

- Note: The ACIP recommends serologic confirmation of post vaccination immunity in patients undergoing dialysis and in immunodeficient patients.
- Monitor temperature. Some patients develop a temperature elevation of 38.3° C (101° F) following vaccination that may last 1 or 2 days.
- Babies born to mothers who are HbsAg positive must receive this vaccine and receive a dose of hepatitis B immune globulin at a separate site within 12 h of birth. If the mother is HbsAg negative, baby should receive the vaccine before discharge from the hospital. If the mother's hepatitis B status is unknown, the baby should receive the vaccine within 12 h of birth. Inquire about hepatitis B vaccine during health care encounters with adolescents; the vaccine may not have been required when they were young and they are at high risk from sexual activity and blood transfer. Begin immunization series immediately if needed.
- U.S. law requires that parents be given teaching on risks and benefits of immunization. Medication amount, site, route, date, company, lot number, and parent consent must be recorded. Inform parents of next scheduled immunizations and make an appointment for this visit.

Patient & Family Education

- Learn potential adverse reaction and benefits of vaccine.
- Teach about next recommended immunizations and make appointment with health care provider if possible.
- Do not breast feed while taking this drug without consulting physician.

HETASTARCH
(het′a-starch)
HES, Hespan, Hydroxyethyl Starch, Hextend
Classifications: PLASMA VOLUME EXPANDER
Prototype: Albumin
Pregnancy Category: C

AVAILABILITY 6 g/100 mL injection

ACTIONS Synthetic starch closely resembling human glycogen. Acts much like albumin and dextran but is claimed to be less likely to produce anaphylaxis or to interfere with cross-matching or blood-typing procedures. Causes no significant alterations in fibrinogen or clotting time but may prolong the PTT and PT. Not a substitute for blood or plasma.

THERAPEUTIC EFFECTS Colloidal osmotic properties are approximately equal to those of human serum albumin. In hypovolemic patients, it increases arterial and venous pressures, heart rate, cardiac output, urine output, and colloidal osmotic pressure.

USES Early fluid replacement and plasma volume expansion when whole blood is not available or when there is no time for necessary cross-matching. Used to expand plasma volume during cardiopulmonary bypass and in adjunctive treatment of shock caused by hemorrhage, burns, surgery, sepsis, or other trauma. Also used as sedimenting agent in preparation of granulocytes by leukopheresis.
UNLABELED USES As a priming fluid in pump oxygenators for perfusion during extracorporeal circulation and as a cryoprotective agent for long-term storage of whole blood.

H

CONTRAINDICATIONS Severe bleeding disorders, CHF, renal failure with oliguria and anuria, treatment of shock not accompanied by hypovolemia, pregnancy (category C). Safe use in children is not established.
CAUTIOUS USE Hepatic or renal insufficiency, pulmonary edema in the very young or older adults, patients on sodium restriction.

ROUTE & DOSAGE

Plasma Volume Expansion
Child: **IV** 10 mL/kg/dose (max 20 mL/kg/24 h)
Adult: **IV** 500–1000 mL at a maximum rate of 20 mL/kg/h (max 1500 mL/day)

Leukapheresis
Adult: **IV** 250–750 mL infused at a constant fixed ratio of 8:1 to venous whole blood

STORAGE
Store at room temperature; avoid extremes of heat or cold. Discard partially used bags.

ADMINISTRATION

Intravenous

PREPARE **IV Infusion:** Use undiluted as prepared by manufacturer.
ADMINISTER **IV Infusion:** Specific flow rate is prescribed by physician. Rate may be as high as 20 mL/kg/h in acute hemorrhagic shock. Rate is usually reduced in patients with burns or septic shock.

ADVERSE EFFECTS CV: Peripheral edema, circulatory overload, heart failure. **Hematologic:** With large volumes, prolongation of PT, PTT, clotting time, and bleeding time; decreased Hct, Hgb, platelets, calcium, and fibrinogen; dilution of plasma proteins, hyperbilirubinemia, increased sedimentation rate. **Body as a Whole:** Pruritus, anaphylactoid reactions (periorbital edema, urticaria, wheezing), vomiting, mild fever, chills, influenza-like symptoms, headache, muscle pains, submaxillary and parotid glandular swelling.

INTERACTIONS Drug: No clinically significant interactions established.

PHARMACOKINETICS Duration: 24–36 h. **Distribution:** Remains in intravascular space. **Metabolism:** Metabolized in reticuloendothelial system. **Elimination:** Excreted in urine with some biliary excretion.

NURSING IMPLICATIONS

Assessment & Drug Effects

- Monitor for S&S of hypersensitivity reaction (see Appendix D-1).
- Measure and record I&O. Report oliguria or significant changes in I&O ratio.
- Monitor BP and vital signs and observe patient for unusual bruising or bleeding.
- Lab tests: Monitor WBC count with differential, platelet count, and PT & PTT during leukapheresis.
- Observe for signs of circulatory overload (see Appendix D-1).
- Check laboratory reports of Hct values. Notify physician if there is an appreciable drop in Hct or if value approaches 30% by volume. Hct should not be allowed to drop below 30%.

Patient & Family Education

- Notify physician for any of the following:
  Difficulty breathing, nausea, chills, headache, itching.

HUMAN GROWTH HORMONE

Nutropin AQ, Genotropin, Humatrope, Norditropin, Saizen, Serostim
See Somatotropin.

HYDRALAZINE HYDROCHLORIDE ⓟⓡ
(hye-dral′a-zeen)
Alazine, Apresoline
Classifications: CARDIOVASCULAR AGENT; NONNITRATE VASODILATOR; ANTIHYPERTENSIVE
Pregnancy Category: C

AVAILABILITY 10 mg, 25 mg, 50 mg, 100 mg tablets; 20 mg/mL vial

ACTIONS Reduces BP mainly by direct effect on vascular smooth muscles of arterial resistance vessels, resulting in vasodilation. Has little effect on venous capacitance vessels. Hypotensive effect may be limited by sympathetic reflexes, which increase heart rate, stroke volume, and cardiac output.
THERAPEUTIC EFFECTS Diastolic response is often greater than systolic response. Vasodilation reduces peripheral resistance and substantially improves cardiac output, and renal and cerebral blood flow. Postural hypotensive effect is reportedly less than that produced by ganglionic blocking agents.

USES Most commonly in stepped-care approach to treat moderate to severe hypertension. Also in early malignant hypertension and resistant hypertension that persists after sympathectomy.

UNLABELED USES Conjunctively with cardiac glycosides and other vasodilators in short-term treatment of acute CHF; unexplained pulmonary hypertension.

CONTRAINDICATIONS Coronary artery disease, mitral valvular rheumatic heart disease, MI, tachycardia, SLE. Safe use during pregnancy (category C) or lactation is established.

CAUTIOUS USE Cerebrovascular accident, advanced renal impairment, use with MAO INHIBITORS.

ROUTE & DOSAGE

Hypertension

Child: **PO** 0.75–1 mg/kg/day given in 4 divided doses (max 25 mg/dose or 5 mg/kg/day for infants and 7.5 mg/kg/day for children) **IV/IM** (in hypertensive crisis) 0.1–0.2 mg/kg/dose given q4–6h (max 20 mg/dose)
Adjust doses in renal disease.
Adult: **PO** 10–50 mg q.i.d. **IM** 10–50 mg q4–6h **IV** 10–20 mg q4–6h

STORAGE

Store at 15°–30° C (59°–86° F) in tight, light-resistant containers unless otherwise directed. Avoid freezing.

ADMINISTRATION

Oral

- Give with food; bioavailability is increased by taking it with food.
- Discontinue gradually to avoid sudden rise in BP and acute heart failure.
- Inform patients of the dangers of abrupt withdrawal.

Intramuscular

- Give deep into a large muscle appropriate for age. See Part I for site selection.

Intravenous

***PREPARE* Direct:** Give undiluted. Use immediately after being drawn into syringe. Do not add to IV solutions.
***ADMINISTER* Direct:** Give each 10 mg or fraction thereof over 1 min.
***INCOMPATIBILITIES* Solution/Additive: Aminophylline, ampicillin, chlorothiazide, edetate calcium disodium, hydrocortisone, mephentermine, methohexital, nitroglycerin, phenobarbital, verapamil.**

ADVERSE EFFECTS Body as a Whole: Hypersensitivity (rash, urticaria, pruritus, fever, chills, arthralgia, eosinophilia, cholangitis, hepatitis, obstructive jaundice). **CNS:** *Headache,* dizziness, tremors. **CV:** *Palpitation,* angina, *tachycardia,* flushing, paradoxical pressor response. Overdose: arrhythmia, <u>shock</u>. **Special Senses:** Lacrimation, conjunctivitis. **GI:** Anorexia, nausea, vomiting, diarrhea, constipation, abdominal pain, paralytic ileus. **Urogenital:** Difficulty in urination, glomerulonephritis. **Hematologic:** Decreased hematocrit and hemaglobin, anemia, agranulocytosis (rare). **Other:** Nasal congestion, muscle cramps, SLE-like syndrome, fixed drug eruption, edema.

DIAGNOSTIC TEST INTERFERENCE Positive *direct Coombs' tests* in patients with hydralazine-induced SLE. Hydralazine interferes with urinary *17-OHCS* determinations *(modified Glenn-Nelson technique).*

INTERACTIONS Drug: BETA-BLOCKERS and other ANTIHYPERTENSIVE AGENTS compound hypotensive effects.

PHARMACOKINETICS Absorption: Readily absorbed from GI tract. **Onset:** 20–30 min. **Peak:** 2 h. **Duration:** 2–6 h. **Distribution:** Crosses placenta; distributed into breast milk. **Metabolism:** Metabolized in intestinal wall and liver. **Elimination:** 90% rapidly excreted in urine; 10% excreted in feces. **Half-Life:** 2–8 h.

NURSING IMPLICATIONS

Assessment & Drug Effects
- Lab tests: Determine antinuclear antibody titer before initiation of therapy and periodically during prolonged therapy. Make baseline and periodic determinations of BUN, creatinine clearance, uric acid, serum potassium, blood glucose, and ECG.
- Monitor for S&S of SLE, especially with prolonged therapy.
- Monitor BP and HR closely. Check every 5 min until it is stabilized at desired level, then every 15 min thereafter throughout hypertensive crisis.
- Monitor I&O when drug is given parenterally and in those with renal dysfunction.

Patient & Family Education
- Monitor weight, check for edema, and report weight gain to physician.
- Note: Some patients experience headache and palpitations within 2–4 h after first PO dose; symptoms usually subside spontaneously.
- Make position changes slowly and to avoid standing still, hot baths/showers, strenuous exercise, and excessive alcohol intake.
- Do not drive or engage in other potentially hazardous activities until response to drug is known.
- Do not breast feed while taking this drug without consulting prescriber.
- Store this medication out of reach of children.

HYDROCHLOROTHIAZIDE ⊕

(hye-droe-klor-oh-thye′a-zide)

Apo-Hydro ♣, Diaqua, Esidrix, Hydro-Chlor, HydroDIURIL, Hydromal, Hydro-T, Oretic, SKHydrochlorothiazide, HCTZ, Urozide ♣

Classifications: ELECTROLYTIC AND WATER BALANCE AGENT; DIURETIC, THIAZIDE
Pregnancy Category: B

AVAILABILITY 12.5 mg capsules; 25 mg, 50 mg, 100 mg tablets; 50 mg/ 5 mL oral solution

ACTIONS Similar to chlorothiazide. Diuretic action is associated with drug interference with absorption of sodium ions across the distal renal tubular segment of the nephron. This enhances excretion of sodium, chloride, potassium, bicarbonates, and water.

THERAPEUTIC EFFECTS It has hypotensive action and elevates plasma renin activity.

USES Adjunct in treatment of edema associated with CHF, hepatic cirrhosis, renal failure, and in the stepped-care management of hypertension (step 1 and 2 agent).

UNLABELED USES Nephrogenic diabetes insipidus, hypercalciuria, and treatment of electrolyte disturbances associated with renal tubular acidosis.

CONTRAINDICATIONS Hypersensitivity to thiazides or other sulfonamides; anuria, pregnancy (category B), lactation.

CAUTIOUS USE Bronchial asthma, allergy; hepatic cirrhosis; renal dysfunction; history of gout, SLE; diabetes mellitus; older adults.

ROUTE & DOSAGE

Edema
Adult: **PO** 25–100 mg/day in 1–3 divided doses (max 200 mg/day)

Hypertension
Neonate/Infant <6 mo: **PO** 2–4 mg/kg/day divided into 2 doses
Infant/Child >6 mo: **PO** 2 mg/kg/day divided into 2 doses
Adult: **PO** 12.5–100 mg/day in 1–2 divided doses

STORAGE
Store tablets in tightly closed container at 15°–30° C (59°–86° F) unless otherwise directed.

ADMINISTRATION
Oral
- Give with food or milk to reduce GI upset.
- Schedule doses to avoid nocturia and interrupted sleep. If given in 2 doses, schedule second dose no later than 3 p.m.

ADVERSE EFFECTS CNS: Mood changes, unusual tiredness or weakness, dizziness, light-headedness, paresthesias. **CV:** Irregular heartbeat, weak pulse, orthostatic hypotension. **GI:** Dry mouth, increased thirst, nausea, vomiting, anorexia, diarrhea, pancreatitis, jaundice. **Hematologic:** <u>Agranulocytosis</u>, thrombocytopenia, <u>aplastic anemia</u>, leukopenia. **Metabolic:** *Hyperglycemia,* glycosuria, *hyperuricemia, hypokalemia.* **Other:** Hypersensitivity reactions, photosensitivity, blurred vision, yellow vision (xanthopsia), muscle spasm.

DIAGNOSTIC TEST INTERFERENCE Falsely decreased value in ***total urinary estrogen*** by ***spectrophotometric assay.*** See chlorothiazide.

INTERACTIONS Drug: Amphotericin B, CORTICOSTEROIDS increase hypokalemic effects; SULFONYLUREAS, **insulin** may antagonize hypoglycemic effects; **cholestyramine, colestipol** decrease THIAZIDE absorption;

diazoxide intensifies hypoglycemic and hypotensive effects; increased **potassium** and **magnesium** loss may cause **digoxin** toxicity; decreases **lithium** excretion and increases toxicity; increases risk of NSAID-induced renal failure and may attenuate diuresis.

PHARMACOKINETICS Absorption: Incompletely absorbed. **Onset:** 2 h. **Peak:** 4 h. **Duration:** 6–12 h. **Distribution:** Distributed throughout extracellular tissue; concentrates in kidney; crosses placenta; distributed in breast milk. **Metabolism:** Does not appear to be metabolized. **Elimination:** Excreted in urine. **Half-Life:** 45–120 min.

NURSING IMPLICATIONS

Assessment & Drug Effects

- Monitor for therapeutic effectiveness. Antihypertensive effects may be noted in 3–4 days; maximal effects may require 3–4 wk. Take baseline weight and weigh frequently during therapy.
- Lab tests: Baseline and periodic determinations of serum electrolytes, blood counts, BUN, blood glucose, uric acid, CO_2, are recommended.
- Check BP before initiation of therapy and at regular intervals.
- Monitor closely for hypokalemia; it increases the risk of digoxin toxicity.
- Monitor I&O and check for edema.
- Note: Drug may cause hyperglycemia and loss of glycemic control in diabetics.
- Note: Drug may cause orthostatic hypotension, dizziness.

Patient & Family Education

- Consult prescriber before using OTC drugs. Many contain large amounts of sodium as well as potassium.
- Monitor weight daily.
- Note: Diabetic patients need to monitor blood glucose closely. This drug causes impaired glucose tolerance.
- Report signs of hypokalemia (see Appendix D-1) to prescriber.
- Change positions slowly; avoid hot baths or showers, extended exposure to sunlight, and sitting or standing still for long periods.
- Note: Photosensitivity reaction may occur 10–14 days after initial sun exposure.
- Do not breast feed while taking this drug.
- Store this medication out of reach of children.

HYDROCODONE BITARTRATE

(hye-droe-koe'done)
Dihydrocodeinone Bitartrate, Hycodan, Robidone A, Vicodin (with acetaminophen)
Classifications: CENTRAL NERVOUS SYSTEM AGENT; NARCOTIC (OPIATE) AGONIST ANALGESIC; ANTITUSSIVE
Prototype: Morphine
Pregnancy Category: C
Controlled Substance: Schedule III

Common adverse effects in *italic;* life-threatening effects <u>underlined;</u> generic names in **bold;** drug classifications in SMALL CAPS; ✦ Canadian drug name; ⦿ Prototype drug.

AVAILABILITY Hydrocodone tablets of various strengths (5, 7.5, 10 mg) with various strengths of acetaminophen.
Combination Products: Also available in combination with other drugs such as chlorpheniramine, phenylephrine, and brompheniramine. Available in several combinations as syrups also.

ACTIONS Morphine derivative similar to codeine but more addicting and with slightly greater antitussive activity, and analgesic effect. CNS depressant with moderate to severe relief of pain. Available in the United States only in combination with other drugs.
THERAPEUTIC EFFECTS Suppresses cough reflex by direct action on cough center in medulla. CNS depressant with moderate to severe relief of pain.

USES Symptomatic relief of hyperactive or nonproductive cough and for relief of moderate to moderately severe pain. A common ingredient in a variety of proprietary mixtures.

CONTRAINDICATIONS Hypersensitivity to hydrocodone or any opioid derivative; lactation.
CAUTIOUS USE Respiratory depression, asthma, emphysema; history of drug abuse or dependence; postoperative patients; debilitated patients; children <1 y; pregnancy (category C); patients with preexisting increased intracranial pressure.

ROUTE & DOSAGE

Mild to Moderate Pain, Cough
Child: **PO** *2–12 y,* 1.25–5 mg q4–6h (max 10 mg/dose)
Adult: **PO** 5–10 mg q4–6h prn (max 15 mg/dose)

STORAGE
Preserve at room temperature in tight, light-resistant containers.

ADMINISTRATION
Oral
▪ Give with food or milk to prevent GI irritation.

ADVERSE EFFECTS GI: Dry mouth, *constipation, nausea,* vomiting. **CNS:** Light-headedness, sedation, dizziness, *drowsiness,* euphoria, dysphoria, **Respiratory:** <u>Respiratory depression</u>. **Skin:** Urticaria, rash, pruritus.

INTERACTIONS Drug: Alcohol and other CNS DEPRESSANTS compound sedation and CNS depression. **Herbal: St. John's wort** increases sedation.

PHARMACOKINETICS Onset: 10–20 min. **Duration:** 3–6 h. **Distribution:** Crosses placenta; distributed into breast milk. **Metabolism:** Metabolized in liver. **Elimination:** Excreted in urine. **Half-Life:** 3.8 h.

NURSING IMPLICATIONS

Assessment & Drug Effects
- Monitor for effectiveness of drug for pain relief.
- Monitor for nausea and vomiting, especially in ambulatory patients.
- Monitor respiratory status and bowel elimination.

Patient & Family Education
- Avoid hazardous activities until response to drug is determined.
- Do not use alcohol or other CNS depressants; may cause additive CNS depression.
- Drink plenty of liquids for adequate hydration. Adjust to amount appropriate for age.
- Do not to take larger doses than prescribed because abuse potential is high. Take only amount prescribed to avoid overdosage with acetaminophen or other products in combination.
- Do not breast feed while taking this drug.
- Store this medication out of reach of children.

HYDROCORTISONE ⓟ
(hye-droe-kor′ti-sone)

Aeroseb-HC, Alphaderm, Cetacort, Cortaid, Cort-Dome, Cortenema, Cortril, Dermacort, Dermolate, Hydrocortone, Hytone, Proctocort, Rectocort ◆, Synacort

HYDROCORTISONE ACETATE

Anusol HC, CaldeCort, Carmol HC, Colifoam, Cortaid, Cortamed, Cort-Dome, Cortef Acetate, Corticaine, Cortifoam, Cortiment ◆, Epifoam, Hydrocortone Acetate

HYDROCORTISONE CYPIONATE

Cortef Fluid

HYDROCORTISONE SODIUM PHOSPHATE

Hydrocortone Phosphate

HYDROCORTISONE SODIUM SUCCINATE

A-Hydrocort, Solu-Cortef

HYDROCORTISONE VALERATE

Westcort

Classifications: SKIN AND MUCOUS MEMBRANE AGENT; ANTI-INFLAMMATORY; SYNTHETIC HORMONE; ADRENAL CORTICOSTEROIDS; GLUCOCORTICOID; MINERALOCORTICOID
Pregnancy Category: C

AVAILABILITY Hydrocortisone 5 mg, 10 mg, 20 mg tablets; 0.5%, 1%, 2.5% cream, lotion, ointment, spray **Hydrocortisone Acetate** 25 mg/mL, 50 mg/mL suspension; 0.5%, 1% cream, ointment **Hydrocortisone Cypionate** 10 mg/5 mL oral suspension **Hydrocortisone Sodium**

Phosphate 50 mg/mL injection **Hydrocortisone Sodium Succinate** 100 mg/2 mL, 250 mg/2 mL, 500 mg/4 mL, 1000 mg/8 mL vials **Hydrocortisone Valerate** 0.2% cream, ointment

ACTIONS Short-acting synthetic steroid with both glucocorticoid and mineralocorticoid properties that affect nearly all systems of the body. **Anti-inflammatory (Glucocorticoid) Action:** Stabilizes leukocyte lysosomal membranes; inhibits phagocytosis and release of allergic substances; suppresses fibroblast formation and collagen deposition; reduces capillary dilation and permeability; and increases responsiveness of cardiovascular system to circulating catecholamines. **Immunosuppressive Action:** Modifies immune response to various stimuli; reduces antibody titers; and suppresses cell-mediated hypersensitivity reactions. **Mineralocorticoid Action:** Promotes sodium retention, but under certain circumstances (e.g., sodium loading), enhances sodium excretion; promotes potassium excretion; and increases glomerular filtration rate (GFR). **Metabolic Action:** Promotes hepatic gluconeogenesis, protein catabolism, redistribution of body fat, and lipolysis.
THERAPEUTIC EFFECTS Hydrocortisone has anti-inflammatory, immunosuppressive, and metabolic functions in the body.

USES Replacement therapy in adrenocortical insufficiency; to reduce serum calcium in hypercalcemia, to suppress undesirable inflammatory or immune responses, to produce temporary remission in nonadrenal disease, and to block ACTH production in diagnostic tests. Use as antiinflammatory or immunosuppressive agent largely replaced by synthetic glucocorticoids that have minimal mineralocorticoid activity.

CONTRAINDICATIONS Hypersensitivity to glucocorticoids, idiopathic thrombocytopenic purpura, psychoses, acute glomerulonephritis, viral or bacterial diseases of skin, infections not controlled by antibiotics, active or latent amebiasis, hypercorticism (Cushing's syndrome), smallpox vaccination or other immunologic procedures. Topical steroids contraindicated in presence of varicella, vaccinia, on surfaces with compromised circulation, and in children <2 y. Safe use during pregnancy (category C) or lactation is not established.
CAUTIOUS USE Children; diabetes mellitus; chronic, active hepatitis positive for hepatitis B surface antigen; hyperlipidemia; cirrhosis; stromal herpes simplex; glaucoma, tuberculosis of eye; osteoporosis; convulsive disorders; hypothyroidism; diverticulitis; nonspecific ulcerative colitis; fresh intestinal anastomoses; active or latent peptic ulcer; gastritis; esophagitis; thromboembolic disorders; CHF; metastatic carcinoma; hypertension; renal insufficiency; history of allergies; active or arrested tuberculosis; systemic fungal infection; myasthenia gravis.

ROUTE & DOSAGE

Adrenal Insufficiency, Anti-Inflammatory
Child: **PO** 2.5–10 mg/kg/day in 3–4 divided doses **IV/IM** 1–5 mg/kg/day divided q12–24h
Adult: **PO** 15–240 mg/dose given q12h **IV/IM** 15–800 mg/day in 3–4 divided doses (max 2 g/day) **SC** Sodium phosphate only, 15–240 mg/day

Status Asthmaticus
Child: **IV** 4–8 mg/kg/dose (max dose 250 mg) for loading dose, then 8 mg/kg/day divided into doses given q6h.
Adult: **IV** 100–500 mg/dose given q6h

Intra-Articular, Intralesional (Acetate Salt)
Adult: **IM** 5–50 mg q3– 5days for bursae; 5–50 mg once q1–4wk for joints

Anti-Inflammatory Agent
Adult: **Topical** apply a small amount to the affected area 1–4 times/day **PR** insert 1% cream, 10% foam, 10–25 mg suppository, or 100 mg enema nightly

H

STORAGE
Store medication at 15°–30° C (59°–86° F) unless otherwise directed by manufacturer; protect from light and freezing.

ADMINISTRATION
Note: Hydrocortisone phosphate may be given SC, IM, or IV. Hydrocortisone succinate may be given IM or IV.

Oral
Give oral drug with food.

Rectal
■ Administer retention enema preferably after a bowel movement; retain at least 1 h or all night if possible.

Topical
■ Apply medication sparingly, rub until it disappears, and then reapply, leaving a thin coat over lesion. Completely cover area with transparent plastic or other occlusive device or vehicle when so ordered. Use gloves to apply cream and wash hands thoroughly after removing gloves.
■ Avoid covering a weeping or exudative lesion. Do not get the medication in or near the eye.
■ Note: Occlusive dressings usually are not applied to face, scalp, scrotum, axilla, and groin.
■ Inspect skin carefully between applications for ecchymotic, petechial, and purpuric signs, maceration, secondary infection, skin atrophy, striae or miliaria; if present, stop medication and notify physician.

Intramuscular
■ Inject deep into muscle mass appropriate for age. See Part I.

Intravenous
IV administration to infants, children: Verify correct IV concentration and rate of infusion/injection with physician.
PREPARE **Direct:** Give undiluted (preferred). **Intermittent:** Dilute in 50–100 mL of D5W, NS, or D5/NS.
ADMINISTER **Direct:** Give each dose at a rate of 25 mg or fraction thereof (phosphate) or 500 mg or fraction thereof (succinate) over 1 min. **Intermittent:** Give over 10 min. Administer solutions that have been diluted for IV infusion within 24 h.

INCOMPATIBILITIES Solution/Additive: **Amobarbital, ampicillin, bleomycin, colistimethate, dimenhydrinate, doxapram, doxorubicin, ephedrine, heparin, hydralazine, metaraminol, methicillin, nafcillin, pentobarbital, phenobarbital, prochlorperazine, promethazine, secobarbital,** TETRACYCLINES. Y-Site: **Ergotamine, phenytoin.**

ADVERSE EFFECTS Body as a Whole: Hypersensitivity or <u>anaphylactoid reactions; aggravation or masking of infections;</u> malaise, weight gain, obesity; urogenital urinary frequency and urgency, enuresis increased or decreased motility and number of sperm. **CNS:** Vertigo, headache, nystagmus, ataxia (rare), increased intracranial pressure with papilledema (usually after discontinuation of medication), mental disturbances, aggravation of preexisting psychiatric conditions, insomnia, anxiety, mental confusion, depression. **CV:** Syncopal episodes, thrombophlebitis, thromboembolism or fat embolism, palpitation, tachycardia, necrotizing angiitis, CHF, hypertension edema. **Endocrine:** Suppressed linear growth in children, decreased glucose tolerance; hyperglycemia, manifestations of latent diabetes mellitus; hypocorticism; amenorrhea and other menstrual difficulties moonfacies. **GI:** Cramping, bleeding. **Special Senses:** Posterior subcapsular cataracts (especially in children), glaucoma, exophthalmos, increased intraocular pressure with optic nerve damage, perforation of the globe, fungal infection of the cornea, decreased or blurred vision. **Metabolic:** Hypocalcemia; *sodium and fluid retention;* hypokalemia and hypokalemic alkalosis decreased serum concentration of vitamins A and C; hyperglycemia, hypernatremia. **GI:** *Nausea,* increased appetite, ulcerative esophagitis, -pancreatitis, abdominal distention, peptic ulcer with perforation and hemorrhage, melena. **Hematologic:** Thrombocytopenia, polycythemia, ecchymoses. **Musculoskeletal:** Osteoporosis, compression fractures, muscle wasting and weakness, tendon rupture, aseptic necrosis of femoral and humeral heads. **Skin:** Skin thinning and atrophy, *acne, impaired wound healing;* petechiae, ecchymosis, easy bruising; suppression of skin test reaction; hypopigmentation or hyperpigmentation, hirsutism, acneiform eruptions, subcutaneous fat atrophy; allergic dermatitis, urticaria, angioneurotic edema, increased sweating. With parenteral therapy at IV site, pain, irritation, necrosis, atrophy, sterile abscess; Charcot-like arthropathy following intraarticular use; burning and tingling in perineal area (after IV injection).

DIAGNOSTIC TEST INTERFERENCE Hydrocortisone (corticosteroids) may increase serum ***cholesterol, blood glucose,*** serum ***sodium, uric acid*** (in acute leukemia) and ***calcium*** (in bone metastasis). It may decrease serum ***calcium, potassium, PBI, thyroxin (T_4), triiodothyronine (T_3) and reduce thyroid*** ^{131}I uptake. It increases ***urine glucose*** level and ***calcium*** excretion; decreases ***urine 17-OHCS*** and **17-KS** levels. May produce false-negative results with **nitroblue tetrazolium test** for systemic bacterial infection and may suppress reactions to skin tests.

INTERACTIONS Drug: BARBITURATES, **phenytoin, rifampin** may increase hepatic metabolism, thus decreasing cortisone levels; ESTROGENS potentiate the effects of hydrocortisone; NSAIDS compound ulcerogenic effects; **cholestyramine, colestipol** decrease hydrocortisone absorption;

Common adverse effects in *italic;* life-threatening effects <u>underlined;</u> generic names in **bold;** drug classifications in SMALL CAPS; ♣ Canadian drug name; ◐ Prototype drug.

635

DIURETICS, **amphotericin b** exacerbate hypokalemia; ANTICHOLINESTERASE AGENTS (e.g., **neostigmine**) may produce severe weakness; immune response to VACCINES and TOXOIDS may be decreased.

PHARMACOKINETICS Absorption: Readily absorbed from GI tract and IM injection site. **Onset:** 1–2 h PO; immediately IV; 3–5 days PR. **Peak:** 1 h PO; 4–8 h IM. **Duration:** 1–1.5 day PO/IM; 0.5–4 wk intra-articular. **Distribution:** Distributed primarily to muscles, liver, skin, intestines, kidneys; crosses placenta. **Metabolism:** Hepatically metabolized. **Elimination:** HPA suppression 8–12 h; metabolites excreted in urine; excreted in breast milk. **Half-Life:** 1.5–2 h.

H

NURSING IMPLICATIONS

Assessment & Drug Effects

- Establish baseline and continuing data on BP, weight, fluid and electrolyte balance, and blood glucose.
- Lab tests: Periodic serum electrolytes, blood glucose, Hct and Hgb, platelet count, and WBC with differential.
- Monitor for adverse effects. Those with low serum albumin are especially susceptible to adverse effects.
- Be alert to signs of hypocalcemia (see Appendix D-1).
- Ophthalmoscopic examinations are recommended every 2–3 mo, especially if patient is receiving ophthalmic steroid therapy.
- Monitor for persistent backache or chest pain; compression and spontaneous fractures of long bones and vertebrae present hazards.
- Monitor for and report changes in mood and behavior, emotional instability, or psychomotor activity, especially with long-term therapy.
- Be alert to possibility of masked infection and delayed healing (antiinflammatory and immunosuppressive actions).
- Note: Dose adjustment may be required if patient is subjected to severe stress (serious infection, surgery, or injury).
- Note: Single doses of corticosteroids or use for a short period (<1 wk) do not produce withdrawal symptoms when discontinued, even with moderately large doses.

Patient & Family Education

- Expect a slight weight gain with improved appetite. After dosage is stabilized, notify prescriber of a sudden slow but steady weight increase such as (2 kg [5 lb]/wk) for older children and adults, or any steady increase by younger children.
- Avoid alcohol and caffeine; may contribute to steroid-ulcer development in long-term therapy.
- Do not ignore dyspepsia with hyperacidity. Report symptoms to physician and do NOT self medicate to find relief.
- Do NOT use aspirin or other OTC drugs unless prescribed specifically by the physician.
- Note: A high protein, calcium, and vitamin D diet is advisable to reduce risk of corticosteroid induced osteoporosis.
- Notify prescriber of slow healing, any vague feeling of being sick, or return to pretreatment symptoms.
- Do not abruptly discontinue drug; doses are gradually reduced to prevent withdrawal symptoms.

- Report exacerbation of disease during drug withdrawal.
- Carry medical identification at all times. It needs to indicate medical diagnosis, drug therapy, and name of prescriber.
- Apply topical preparations sparingly in small children. The hazard of systemic toxicity is higher because of the greater ratio of skin surface area to body weight.
- Check shelf-life date on topical corticosterone during long-term use.
- Do not breast feed while taking this drug without consulting physician.
- Store this medication out of reach of children.

HYDROFLUMETHIAZIDE

(hye-droe-floo-meth-eye′a-zide)

Diucardin, Saluron

Classifications: ELECTROLYTIC AND WATER BALANCE AGENT; DIURETIC, THIAZIDE

Prototype: Hydrochlorothiazide

Pregnancy Category: B

AVAILABILITY 50 mg tablets

ACTIONS Thiazide diuretic chemically related to sulfonamides. Diuretic action results in excretion of sodium, chloride, potassium bicarbonate, and water.

THERAPEUTIC EFFECTS Results in antihypertensive activity and decreased edema.

USES Mild hypertension, management of edema associated with CHF.

CONTRAINDICATIONS Hypersensitivity to other thiazides or sulfonamide derivatives; anuria; lactation; hypokalemia.

CAUTIOUS USE Pregnancy (category B).

ROUTE & DOSAGE

Edema

Adult: **PO** 25 mg–200 mg/day in 1–2 divided doses

Hypertension

Child: **PO** 1 mg/kg/day given daily
Adult: **PO** 50–100 mg/day in 1–2 divided doses

STORAGE

Store tablets in tightly closed container at 15°–30° C (59°–86° F) unless otherwise directed

ADMINISTRATION

Oral

- Give diuretic dose early in the morning to prevent interrupted sleep. If two doses are taken each day, schedule second dose no later than 3 p.m.

ADVERSE EFFECTS CV: Postural hypotension, **Skin:** Photosensitivity, **Metabolic:** *Hypokalemia, hyperglycemia,* hyponatremia, *asymptomatic hyperuricemia.* (See also hydrochlorothiazide.)

INTERACTIONS Drug: Amphotericin B, CORTICOSTEROIDS increase hypokalemic effects; may antagonize hypoglycemic effects of ORAL HYPO-GLYCEMIC AGENTS, **insulin; cholestyramine, colestipol** decrease thiazide absorption; **diazoxide** intensifies hypoglycemic and hypotensive effects; increased potassium and magnesium loss may cause **digoxin** toxicity; decreases **lithium** excretion, thus increasing **lithium** toxicity; increases risk of NSAID-induced renal failure (NSAIDS may attenuate diuresis).

PHARMACOKINETICS Absorption: Incompletely absorbed. **Onset:** 1–2 h. **Peak:** 3–4 h. **Duration:** 18–24 h. **Distribution:** Distributed throughout extracellular tissue; concentrates in kidney; crosses placenta; distributed in breast milk. **Metabolism:** Does not appear to be metabolized. **Elimination:** Excreted in urine. **Half-Life:** 17 h.

NURSING IMPLICATIONS

Assessment & Drug Effects

- Monitor for therapeutic effectiveness. Antihypertensive effects may be noted in 3–4 days, maximal effects may require 3–4 wk.
- Lab tests: Make baseline and periodic determinations for serum electrolytes, blood counts, BUN, blood glucose, uric acid, and CO_2.
- Monitor patient for hypokalemia and hyponatremia (see Appendix D-1).
- Report onset of joint pain and limitation of motion to physician; asymptomatic hyperuricemia can result from interference with uric acid excretion.
- Monitor for S&S of diabetes. Watch diabetic patients for loss of glycemic control.

Patient & Family Education

- Note: Thiazide-related photosensitivity is considered a photoallergy. It occurs 1½–2 wk after initial sun exposure. Inform physician.
- Do not breast feed while taking this drug.
- Store this medication out of reach of children.

HYDROMORPHONE HYDROCHLORIDE

(hye-droe-mor′fone)
Dilaudid, Dilaudid-HP
Classifications: CENTRAL NERVOUS SYSTEM AGENT; ANALGESIC; NARCOTIC (OPIATE) AGONIST
Prototype: Morphine
Pregnancy Category: C
Controlled Substance: Schedule II

AVAILABILITY 1 mg, 2 mg, 3 mg, 4 mg, 8 mg tablets; 5 mg/5 mL oral liquid; 1 mg/mL, 2 mg/mL, 4 mg/mL, 10 mg/mL injection; 3 mg suppositories

ACTIONS Semisynthetic derivative structurally similar to morphine but with 8–10 times more potent analgesic effect. Has more rapid onset and shorter duration of action than morphine and is reported to have less hypnotic action and less tendency to produce nausea and vomiting.
THERAPEUTIC EFFECTS Is a narcotic analgesic that controls mild to moderate pain. Has antitussive properties.

USES Relief of moderate to severe pain and control of persistent nonproductive cough.

CONTRAINDICATIONS Hypersensitivity to hydromorphone is a contraindication, intolerance to other opiate agonists; lactation.
CAUTIOUS USE Safe use in pregnancy (category C) or in children is not established.

ROUTE & DOSAGE

Moderate to Severe Pain

Child: **PO** 0.03–0.08 mg/kg q4–6h (max 5 mg/dose) **IV** 0.015 mg/kg q4–6h
Adult: **PO** 1–4 mg q4–6h prn **SC/IM/IV** 1–2 mg q4–6h prn
Rectal 3 mg q4–6h

Antitussive

Child: **PO** 6–12 y, 0.5 mg q3–4h prn
Adult: **PO** 1 mg q3–4h prn

STORAGE

Store in tight, light-resistant containers at 15°–30° C (59°–86° F).

ADMINISTRATION

Note: A fixed schedule when narcotic therapy is initiated provides more effective management than a prn schedule.

Intravenous

IV administration to infants, children: Verify correct IV concentration and rate of infusion with physician.
PREPARE **Direct:** Dilute each dose in at least 5 mL of sterile water or NS.
IV Infusion: Using Dilaudid-HP, reconstitute 250-mg dry powder vial immediately prior to use with 25 mL sterile water for injection to yield 10 mg/mL. Final dilution of Dilaudid-HP 250 and HP 500 (supplied 500 mg/50 mL) must be ordered by physician.
ADMINISTER **Direct:** Give 2 mg or fraction thereof over 3–5 min. **IV Infusion:** Both final volume and rate of infusion must be ordered by physician.
INCOMPATIBILITIES **Solution/Additive: Prochlorperazine, sodium bicarbonate, thiopental. Y-Site: Minocycline, prochlorperazine, tetracycline.**

- A slight discoloration in ampules or multidose vials causes no loss of potency.

ADVERSE EFFECTS GI: Nausea, vomiting, constipation. **CNS:** Euphoria, dizziness, sedation, *drowsiness.* **CV:** Hypotension, bradycardia or tachycardia. **Respiratory:** <u>Respiratory depression.</u> **Special Senses:** Blurred vision.

INTERACTIONS Drug: Alcohol and other CNS DEPRESSANTS compound sedation and CNS depression. **Herbal: St. John's wort** may increase sedation.

PHARMACOKINETICS Onset: 15–30 min. **Peak:** 30–90 min. **Duration:** 4–5 h. **Distribution:** Crosses placenta; distributed into breast milk. **Metabolism:** Metabolized in liver. **Elimination:** Excreted in urine.

NURSING IMPLICATIONS

Assessment & Drug Effects

- Note baseline respiratory rate, rhythm, and depth and size of pupils before administration. Respirations of 12/min or less (or lower level appropriate for age of child) and mitosis are signs of toxicity. Withhold drug and promptly notify physician.
- Monitor vital signs at regular intervals. Drug-induced respiratory depression may occur even with small doses and increases progressively with higher doses.
- Assess effectiveness of pain relief 30 min after medication administration.
- Monitor drug effects carefully in very young children and those with impaired renal and hepatic function.
- Assess effectiveness of cough. Drug depresses cough and sigh reflexes and may induce atelectasis, especially in postoperative patients and those with pulmonary disease.
- Note: Nausea and orthostatic hypotension most often occur in ambulatory patients or when a supine patient assumes the head-up position.
- Monitor I&O ratio and pattern. Assess lower abdomen for bladder distension. Report oliguria or urinary retention.
- Monitor bowel pattern; drug-induced constipation may require treatment.

Patient & Family Education

- Request medication at the onset of pain and do not wait until pain is severe.
- Use caution with activities requiring alertness; drug may cause drowsiness, dizziness, and blurred vision.
- Avoid alcohol and other CNS depressants while taking this drug.
- Do not breast feed while taking this drug.
- Store this medication in locked area out of reach of children; this is a Schedule II drug.

HYDROXOCOBALAMIN (VITAMIN B$_{12alpha}$)
(hye-drox-oh-koe-bal'a-min)
Hydrobexan, Hydroxo-12, LA-12
Classifications: HORMONES AND SYNTHETIC SUBSTITUTES; VITAMIN B$_{12}$
Prototype: Cyanocobalamin
Pregnancy Category: A (C if >RDA)

AVAILABILITY 1000 mcg/mL injection

ACTIONS Cobalamin derivative similar to cyanocobalamin (vitamin B$_{12}$). More slowly absorbed from injection site than cyanocobalamin and may be taken up by liver in larger quantities. Essential for normal cell growth, cell reproduction maturation of RBCs, myelin synthesis, and believed to be involved in protein synthesis.

THERAPEUTIC EFFECTS Vitamin B$_{12}$ deficiency results in megaloblastic anemia.

USES Treatment of Vitamin B$_{12}$ deficiency.
UNLABELED USES Cyanide poisoning and tobacco amblyopia.

CONTRAINDICATIONS History of sensitivity to vitamin B$_{12}$, other cobalamins, or cobalt; indiscriminate use in folic acid deficiency.
CAUTIOUS USE Safe use during pregnancy [category A, category C (parenteral)], lactation, or in children is not established.

ROUTE & DOSAGE

Vitamin B$_{12}$ Deficiency
Child: **IM** 100 mcg doses to a total of 1–5 mg over 2 wk and then 30–50 mcg/mo
Adult: **IM** 30 mcg/day for 5–10 days, then 100–200 mcg/mo or 1000 mcg every other day until remission and then 1000 mcg/mo

STORAGE
Store at 15°–30° C (59°–86° F).

ADMINISTRATION
Intramuscular
- Give deep into a large muscle mass appropriate for age (see Part I).

ADVERSE EFFECTS Generally safe; all side effects are very rare. **Body as a Whole:** Itching, urticaria, feeling of swelling, <u>anaphylaxis</u>. **GI:** Transient diarrhea. **Resp:** Pulmonary edema. **CV:** Congestive heart failure, vascular thrombosis.

INTERACTION Drug: Chloramphenicol may interfere with therapeutic response to hydroxocobalamin.

PHARMACOKINETICS Distribution: Widely distributed; principally stored in liver, kidneys, and adrenals; crosses placenta. **Metabolism:** Converted in tissues to active coenzymes; enterohepatically cycled. **Elimination:** 50–95% of doses ≥100 mcg are excreted in urine in 48 h; excreted in breast milk.

NURSING IMPLICATIONS
Assessment & Drug Effects
- Monitor for therapeutic effectiveness: Response to drug therapy is usually dramatic, occurring within 48 h. Effectiveness is measured by laboratory values and improvement in manifestations of vitamin B$_{12}$ deficiency. Characteristically, reticulocyte concentration rises in 3–4 days, peaks in 5–8 days, and then gradually declines as erythrocyte count and hemoglobin rise to normal levels (in 4–6 wk).

- Lab tests: Prior to therapy determine reticulocyte and erythrocyte counts, Hgb, Hct, vitamin B$_{12}$, and serum folate levels; repeated 5–7 days after start of therapy and at regular intervals during therapy.
- Obtain a careful history of sensitivities. Sensitization can take as long as 8 y to develop.
- Monitor potassium levels during the first 48 h, particularly in patients with Addisonian pernicious anemia or megaloblastic anemia. Conversion to normal erythropoiesis increases erythrocyte potassium requirement and can result in severe hypokalemia and sudden death.
- Monitor vital signs in patients with cardiac disease and in those receiving parenteral cyanocobalamin, and be alert to symptoms of pulmonary edema; generally occur early in therapy.
- Note: Some patients experience mild pain at injection site after administration.
- Monitor bowel function. Bowel regularity is essential for consistent absorption of oral preparations.
- Note: Smokers appear to have increased requirements for vitamin B$_{12}$.

Patient & Family Education

- Notify physician of any intercurrent disease or infection. Increased dosage may be required.
- Note: It is imperative to understand that drug therapy must be continued throughout life for pernicious anemia to prevent irreversible neurologic damage.
- Neurologic damage is considered irreversible if there is no improvement after 1–1½ y of adequate therapy.
- Dietary deficiency of vitamin B$_{12}$ has been observed in strict vegetarians (vegans) and their breast-fed infants.
- Do not breast feed while taking this drug without consulting prescriber.

HYDROXYCHLOROQUINE SULFATE

(hye-drox-ee-klor'oh-kwin)
Plaquenil Sulfate
Classifications: ANTI-INFECTIVE; ANTIMALARIAL
Prototype: Chloroquine
Pregnancy Category: C

AVAILABILITY 200 mg tablets

ACTIONS Derivative closely related to chloroquine. Antimalarial activity is believed to be based on ability to form complexes with DNA of parasite, thereby inhibiting replication and transcription to RNA and DNA synthesis of the parasite.
THERAPEUTIC EFFECTS of the parasite. Effective against *Plasmodium vivax* and *Plasmodium malariae.*

USES Suppressive prophylaxis and treatment of acute malarial attacks due to all forms of susceptible malaria. Used adjunctively with primaquine for eradication of *Plasmodium vivax* and *Plasmodium malariae.* More commonly prescribed than chloroquine for treatment of rheumatoid arthritis and lupus erythematosus (usually in conjunction with salicylate or corticosteroid therapy).

UNLABELED USES Porphyria cutanea tarda.

CONTRAINDICATIONS Known hypersensitivity to, or retinal or visual field changes associated with quinoline compounds; psoriasis, porphyria, long-term therapy in children; pregnancy (category C). Safe use in juvenile arthritis or lactation is not established.

CAUTIOUS USE Hepatic disease; alcoholism, use with hepatotoxic drugs; impaired renal function; metabolic acidosis; patients with tendency to dermatitis.

ROUTE & DOSAGE

Note: Doses are expressed in terms of hydroxychloroquine base: 400 mg tablet = 310 mg base; 800 mg tablet = 620 mg base

Acute Malaria

Child: **PO** 10 mg base/kg, then 5 mg base/kg at 6, 18, and 24 h
Adult: **PO** 620 mg base followed by 310 mg base at 6, 18, and 24 h

Malaria Suppression

Child: **PO** 5 mg base/kg the same day each week starting 2 wk before exposure and continuing for 4–6 wk after leaving the area of exposure
Adult: **PO** 310 mg base the same day each week starting 2 wk before exposure and continuing for 4–6 wk after leaving the area of exposure

Lupus Erythematosus

Child: **PO** 3–5 mg/kg/day in 1–2 divided doses (max 400 mg/day or 7 mg/kg/day)
Adult: **PO** 310 mg base 1–2 times/day

Rheumatoid Arthritis

Child: **PO** 3–5 mg/kg/day in 1–2 divided doses (max 400 mg/day or 7 mg/kg/day)
Adult: **PO** 400–600 mg/day until response, then decrease to lowest maintenance levels possible

STORAGE
Store at 15°–30° C (59°–86° F) unless otherwise directed.

ADMINISTRATION

Oral
- Give drug with meals or milk to reduce incidence of GI distress.
- Give antacids and laxatives at least 4 h before or after hydroxychloroquine.

ADVERSE EFFECTS CNS: Fatigue, vertigo, headache, mood or mental changes, anxiety, *retinopathy,* blurred vision, difficulty focusing. **GI:** Anorexia, nausea, vomiting, diarrhea, abdominal cramps, weight loss. **Hematologic:** Hemolysis in patients with G6PD deficiency, <u>agranulocytosis</u> (rare), <u>aplastic anemia</u> (rare), thrombocytopenia. **Skin:** Bleaching or loss of hair, unusual pigmentation (blueblack) of skin or inside mouth, skin rash, itching.

INTERACTIONS Drug: **Aluminum-** and **magnesium**-containing ANTACIDS and LAXATIVES decrease hydroxychloroquine absorption; separate administrations by at least 4 h; hydroxychloroquine may interfere with response to **rabies vaccine.**

PHARMACOKINETICS Absorption: Rapidly and almost completely absorbed. **Peak:** 1–2 h. **Distribution:** Widely distributed; concentrates in lungs, liver, erythrocytes, eyes, skin, and kidneys; crosses placenta. **Metabolism:** Partially metabolized in liver to active metabolite. **Elimination:** Eliminated in urine; excreted in breast milk. **Half-Life:** 70–120 h.

NURSING IMPLICATIONS

Assessment & Drug Effects

- Monitor for therapeutic effectiveness; may not appear for several weeks, and maximal benefit may not occur for 6 mo.
- Do baseline and periodic ophthalmoscopic examinations and blood cell counts on all patients on long-term therapy.
- Discontinue drug if weakness, visual symptoms, hearing loss, unusual bleeding, bruising, or skin eruptions occur.

Patient & Family Education

- Learn about adverse effects and their symptoms when taking prolonged therapy.
- Follow drug regimen exactly as prescribed by the prescriber.
- Do not breast feed while taking this drug without consulting prescriber.
- Store this medication out of reach of children.

HYDROXYZINE HYDROCHLORIDE ⓟⓡ
(hye-drox′i-zeen)
Atarax, Hyzine-50, Quiess, Vistaril Intramuscular, Vistacon, Vistaject-25 & -50

HYDROXYZINE PAMOATE
Hy-Pam, Vamate, Vistaril Oral
Classifications: ANTIHISTAMINE; ANTIPRURITIC
Pregnancy Category: C

AVAILABILITY Hydroxyzine HCl 10 mg, 25 mg, 50 mg, 100 mg tablets; 10 mg/5 mL syrup; 25 mg/5 mL oral suspension; 25 mg/mL, 50 mg/mL injection **Hydroxyzine Pamoate** 25 mg, 50 mg, 100 mg capsules

ACTIONS Piperazine derivative structurally and pharmacologically related to other cyclizines (e.g., buclizine, chlorcyclizine). In common with such agents, it causes CNS depression.
THERAPEUTIC EFFECTS Its tranquilizing (ataractic) effect is produced primarily by depression of hypothalamus and brain-stem reticular formation, rather than cortical areas. In addition it is an effective agent for pruritus.

USES Emotional or psychoneurotic states characterized by anxiety, tension, or psychomotor agitation; to relieve anxiety, control nausea and emesis, and reduce narcotic requirements before or after surgery or delivery. Also used in management of pruritus due to allergic conditions, e.g., chronic urticaria, atopic and contact dermatoses, and in treatment of acute and chronic alcoholism with withdrawal symptoms or delirium tremens.

CONTRAINDICATIONS Known hypersensitivity to hydroxyzine; use as sole treatment in psychoses or depression. Safe use during early pregnancy (category C) or lactation is not established.

CAUTIOUS USE History of allergies.

ROUTE & DOSAGE

Anxiety
Child: **PO** 0.5 mg/kg/dose q6–8h **IM** 0.5–1 mg/kg/dose q4–6h
Adult: **PO** 25–100 mg t.i.d. or q.i.d. **IM** 25–100 mg q4–6h (max 600 mg/day)

Pruritus
Child: **PO** >6 y, 50–100 mg/day in divided doses; <6 y, 50 mg/day in divided doses **IM** 1.1 mg/kg q4–6h
Adult: **PO** 25 mg t.i.d. or q.i.d. **IM** 25 mg q4–6h

Nausea
Child: **IM** 1.1 mg/kg q4–6h
Adult: **IM** 25–100 mg q4–6h

STORAGE
Protect all forms from light. Store at 15°–30° C (59°–86° F) unless otherwise specified.

ADMINISTRATION

Oral
- Tablets may be crushed and taken with fluid of choice. Capsule may be emptied and contents swallowed with water or mixed with food. Liquid formulations are available.

Intramuscular
- Give deep into body of a large muscle. The Z-track technique of injection is recommended to prevent SC infiltration.
- Recommended site: In adult, the gluteus maximus or vastus lateralis; in children, the vastus lateralis.

INCOMPATIBILITIES **Solution/Additive: Aminophylline, amobarbital, chloramphenicol, dimenhydrinate, penicillin G, pentobarbital, phenobarbital.**

ADVERSE EFFECTS CNS: *Drowsiness* (usually transitory), sedation, dizziness, headache, **CV:** Hypotension. **GI:** *Dry mouth.* **Body as a Whole:** Urticaria, dyspnea, chest tightness, wheezing, involuntary

Common adverse effects in *italic;* life-threatening effects <u>underlined</u>; generic names in **bold;** drug classifications in SMALL CAPS; ♦ Canadian drug name; ◐ Prototype drug.

645

motor activity (rare). **Hematologic:** Phlebitis, hemolysis, thrombosis. **Skin:** Erythematous macular eruptions, erythema multiforme, digital gangrene from inadvertent IV or intra-arterial injection, injection site reactions.

DIAGNOSTIC TEST INTERFERENCE Possibility of false-positive *urinary 17-hydroxycorticosteroid* determinations **(modified Glenn-Nelson technique).**

INTERACTIONS Drug: Alcohol and CNS DEPRESSANTS add to CNS depression; TRICYCLIC ANTIDEPRESSANTS and other ANTICHOLINERGICS have additive anticholinergic effects; may inhibit pressor effects of **epinephrine.**

PHARMACOKINETICS Absorption: Readily absorbed from GI tract. **Onset:** 15–30 min PO. **Duration:** 4–6 h. **Distribution:** Not known if it crosses placenta or is distributed into breast milk. **Metabolism:** Metabolized in liver. **Elimination:** Probably excreted in bile.

NURSING IMPLICATIONS

Assessment & Drug Effects

- Evaluate alertness. Drowsiness may occur and usually disappears with continued therapy or following reduction of dosage.
- Monitor condition of oral membranes daily when patient is on high dosage of hydroxyzine.
- Reevaluate usefulness of drug periodically.
- Reduce dosage of the depressant up to 50% when CNS depressants are prescribed concomitantly.

Patient & Family Education

- Do not drive or engage in other potentially hazardous activities until response to drug is known.
- Do NOT take alcohol and hydroxyzine at the same time.
- Notify physician immediately if you become pregnant.
- Relieve dry mouth by frequent warm water rinses, increasing fluid intake, and use of a salivary substitute (e.g., Moi-Stir, Xero-Lube).
- Give teeth scrupulous care. Avoid irritation or abrasion of gums and other oral tissues.
- Consult prescriber before self dosing with OTC medications.
- Do not breast feed while taking this drug without consulting prescriber.
- Store this medication out of reach of children.

HYOSCYAMINE SULFATE

(hye-oh-sye'a-meen)

Anaspaz, Cystospaz, Levsin, Levsinex, Neoquess, NuLev

Classifications: ANTICHOLINERGIC (PARASYMPATHOLYTIC); ANTIMUSCARINIC, ANTISPASMODIC

Prototype: Atropine

Pregnancy Category: C

AVAILABILITY 0.125 mg, 0.150 mg tablets; 0.125 mg sublingual tablets; 0.375 sustained-release capsules; 0.125 mg orally disintegrating tablet; 0.125 mg/mL oral solution; 0.125 mg/5 mL elixir; 0.5 mg/mL injection

ACTIONS Extremely potent belladonna alkaloid with anticholinergic and antispasmodic activity. Anticholinergic effect chiefly related to the levo isomer.
THERAPEUTIC EFFECTS Anticholinergic and antispasmodic action is produced by competitive inhibition of acetylcholine at the parasympathetic neuroeffector junctions.

USES GI tract disorders caused by spasm and hypermotility, as conjunct therapy with diet and antacids for peptic ulcer management, and as an aid in the control of gastric hypersecretion and intestinal hypermotility. Also symptomatic relief of biliary and renal colic, as a "drying agent" to relieve symptoms of acute rhinitis, to control preanesthesia salivation and respiratory tract secretions, to treat symptoms of parkinsonism, and to reduce pain and hypersecretion in pancreatitis.

CONTRAINDICATIONS Hypersensitivity to belladonna alkaloids, narrow-angle glaucoma, prostatic hypertrophy, obstructive diseases of GI or GU tract, paralytic ileus or intestinal atony, myasthenia gravis.
CAUTIOUS USE Diabetes mellitus, cardiac disease; pregnancy (category C).

ROUTE & DOSAGE

GI Spasms
Child: **PO** *2–12 y,* 0.0625–0.125 mg q4h prn (max 0.75 mg/day)
Adult: **IV/IM/SC** 0.25–0.5 mg q6h **PO/SL** 0.125–0.25 mg t.i.d. or q.i.d. prn

STORAGE
Store at 15°–30° C (59°–86° F).

ADMINISTRATION
Oral
- Give preparations about 1 h before meals and at bedtime (at least 2 h after last meal).
- Ensure that sustained-release form of drug is not chewed or crushed. It must be swallowed whole.

Intravenous

PREPARE **Direct:** Give undiluted.
ADMINISTER **Direct:** Give a single dose over 60 sec.

ADVERSE/SIDE EFFECTS CNS: Headache, unusual tiredness or weakness, confusion, *drowsiness,* excitement. **CV:** Palpitations, tachycardia. **Special Senses:** *Blurred vision,* increased intraocular tension, cycloplegia, mydriasis. **GI:** *Dry mouth, constipation,* paralytic ileus. **Other:** *Urinary retention,* anhidrosis, suppression of lactation.

INTERACTIONS Drug: Amantadine, ANTIHISTAMINES, TRICYCLIC ANTIDEPRESSANTS, **quinidine, disopyramide, procainamide** add anticholinergic effects; decreases **levodopa** effects; **methotrimeprazine** may precipitate extrapyramidal effects; decreases antipsychotic effects of PHENOTHIAZINES (decreased absorption).

PHARMACOKINETICS Absorption: Well absorbed from all administration sites. **Onset:** 2–3 min IV; 20–30 min PO. **Peak effect:** 15–30 min IV; 30–60 min PO. **Duration:** 4–6 h (up to 12 h with sustained-release form). **Distribution:** Distributed in most body tissues; crosses blood–brain barrier and placenta; distributed in breast milk. **Metabolism:** Metabolized in liver. **Elimination:** Excreted in urine. **Half-Life:** 3.5–13 h.

NURSING IMPLICATIONS

Assessment & Drug Effects
- Monitor bowel elimination; may cause constipation.
- Monitor urinary output.
- Lessen risk of urinary retention by having patient void prior to each dose.
- Assess for dry mouth and recommend good practices of oral hygiene.

Patient & Family Education
- Avoid excessive exposure to high temperatures; drug-induced heatstroke can develop.
- Do not drive or engage in other potentially hazardous activities until response to drug is known.
- Use dark glasses if experiencing blurred vision, but if this adverse effect persists, notify prescriber for dose adjustment or possible drug change.
- Do not breast feed while taking this drug without consulting prescriber.
- Store this medication out of reach of children.

IBUPROFEN ⊘

(eye-byoo′proe-fen)
Advil, Amersol ♣, Children's Motrin, Haltran, Ibuprin, Junior Strength Motrin Caplets, Medipren, Motrin, Nuprin, Pediaprofen, Pamprin-IB, Rufen, Trendar
Classifications: CENTRAL NERVOUS SYSTEM AGENT; NSAID (COX-1); ANALGESIC; ANTIPYRETIC
Pregnancy Category: B

AVAILABILITY 100 mg, 200 mg, 400 mg, 600 mg, 800 mg tablets; 50 mg, 100 mg chewable tablets; 100 mg/5 mL, 100 mg/2.5 mL suspension; 40 mg/mL drops

ACTIONS Prototype of the propionic acid NSAIDS (COX-1) inhibitor with nonsteroidal antiinflammatory activity and significant antipyretic and analgesic properties. Blocks prostaglandin synthesis. Ibuprofen activity also includes modulation of T-cell function, inhibition of inflammatory cell chemotaxis, decreased release of superoxide radicals, or increased scavenging of these compounds at inflammatory sites.

THERAPEUTIC EFFECTS Has nonsteroidal anti-inflammatory, analgesic, and antipyretic effects. Inhibits platelet aggregation and prolongs bleeding time but does not affect prothrombin or whole blood clotting times. Cross-sensitivity with aspirin and other nonsteroidal anti-inflammatory drugs has been reported.

USES Chronic, symptomatic rheumatoid arthritis and osteoarthritis; relief of mild to moderate pain; primary dysmenorrhea; reduction of fever.
UNLABELED USES Gout, juvenile rheumatoid arthritis, psoriatic arthritis, ankylosing spondylitis, vascular headache.

CONTRAINDICATIONS Patient in whom urticaria, severe rhinitis, bronchospasm, angioedema, nasal polyps are precipitated by aspirin or other NSAIDs; active peptic ulcer, bleeding abnormalities. Safe use during pregnancy (category B, category D in third trimester), lactation, or children <6 mo is not established.
CAUTIOUS USE Hypertension, dehydration, history of GI ulceration, impaired hepatic or renal function, chronic renal failure, cardiac decompensation, those taking anticoagulants, patients with SLE.

ROUTE & DOSAGE

Inflammatory Disease
Child: **PO** *<20 kg,* up to 400 mg/day in divided doses; *20–30 kg,* up to 600 mg/day in divided doses; *30–40 kg,* up to 800 mg/day in divided doses; alternatively, 5–10 mg/kg/dose given q6–8h
Adult: **PO** 400–800 mg t.i.d. or q.i.d. (max 3200 mg/day)

Juvenile Rheumatoid Arthritis
Child: 30–50 mg/kg/day divided into doses given q6h

Mild to Moderate Pain, Dysmenorrhea, Antipyresis
Adult: **PO** 200–400 mg q4–6h (max 3.2 g/day)

Fever
Child: **PO** *6 mo–12 y,* 5–10 mg/kg q4–6h up to 40 mg/kg/day
Adult: **PO** 200–400 mg t.i.d. or q.i.d. (max 1200 mg/day)

STORAGE
Store in tightly closed, light-resistant containers at 15°–30° C (59°–86° F).

ADMINISTRATION
Oral
- Take with meals or milk to decrease incidence of GI upset.
- Ensure that chewable tablets are chewed or crushed before being swallowed.
- Note: Tablet may be crushed if child is unable to swallow it whole and mixed with small amount of food or liquid before swallowing. Alternately, suspension or drops may be used.

ADVERSE EFFECTS CNS: Headache, dizziness, light-headedness, anxiety, emotional lability, fatigue, malaise, drowsiness, anxiety, confusion, depression, aseptic meningitis. **CV:** Hypertension, palpitation, congestive heart failure (patient with marginal cardiac function); peripheral edema.

Special Senses: Amblyopia (blurred vision, decreased visual acuity, scotomas, changes in color vision); nystagmus, visual-field defects; tinnitus, impaired hearing. **GI:** Dry mouth, gingival ulcerations, dyspepsia, *heartburn, nausea,* vomiting, anorexia, diarrhea, constipation, bloating, flatulence, epigastric or abdominal discomfort or pain, GI ulceration, *occult blood loss.* **Hematologic:** Thrombocytopenia, neutropenia, hemolytic or <u>aplastic anemia</u>, leukopenia; decreased Hgb, Hct; transitory rise in AST, ALT, serum alkaline phosphatase; rise in (Ivy) bleeding time. **GU:** Acute renal failure, polyuria, azotemia, cystitis, hematuria, nephrotoxicity, decreased creatinine clearance. **Skin:** Maculopapular and vesicobullous skin eruptions, erythema multiforme, pruritus, rectal itching, acne. **Body as a Whole:** Fluid retention with edema, Stevens-Johnson syndrome, <u>toxic hepatitis</u>, hypersensitivity reactions, <u>anaphylaxis</u>, bronchospasm, serum sickness, SLE, angioedema.

INTERACTIONS Drug: ORAL ANTICOAGULANTS, **heparin** may prolong bleeding time; may increase **lithium, digoxin,** and **methotrexate** levels and toxicity. **Herbal: Fever few, garlic, ginger, ginkgo** may increase bleeding potential.

PHARMACOKINETICS Absorption: 80% absorbed from GI tract. **Onset:** 1 h antipyretic effect. **Peak:** 1–2 h. **Duration:** 6–8 h. **Metabolism:** Metabolized in liver. **Elimination:** Excreted primarily in urine; some biliary excretion. **Half-Life:** 2–4 h.

NURSING IMPLICATIONS

Assessment & Drug Effects

- Monitor for therapeutic effectiveness. Optimum response generally occurs within 2 wk (e.g., relief of pain, stiffness, or swelling; or improved joint flexion and strength).
- Observe patients with history of cardiac decompensation closely for evidence of fluid retention and edema.
- Lab tests: Baseline and periodic evaluations of Hgb, renal and hepatic function, and auditory and ophthalmologic examinations are recommended in patients receiving prolonged or high-dose therapy.
- Monitor for GI distress and S&S of GI bleeding.
- Note: Symptoms of acute toxicity in children include apnea, cyanosis, response only to painful stimuli, dizziness, and nystagmus.

Patient & Family Education

- Notify prescriber immediately of passage of dark tarry stools, "coffee-grounds" emesis, frankly bloody emesis, or other GI distress, as well as blood or protein in urine, and onset of skin rash, pruritus, jaundice.
- Do not drive or engage in other potentially hazardous activities until response to the drug is known.
- Do not self-medicate with ibuprofen if taking prescribed drugs or being treated for a serious condition without consulting prescriber.
- Do not take aspirin concurrently with ibuprofen. Many OTC drugs contain aspirin and other compounds; check all OTC drugs with prescriber.
- Avoid alcohol and NSAIDS unless otherwise advised by prescriber. Concurrent use may increase risk of GI ulceration and bleeding tendencies.

Common adverse effects in *italic;* life-threatening effects <u>underlined;</u> generic names in **bold;** drug classifications in SMALL CAPS; ✦ Canadian drug name; ⦿ Prototype drug.

- Do not breast feed while taking this drug without consulting prescriber.
- Store this medication out of reach of children.

IDARUBICIN
(i-da-a-roo'bi-cin)
Idamycin, Idamycin PFS
Classifications: ANTINEOPLASTIC, ANTIBIOTIC
Prototype: Doxorubicin
Pregnancy Category: D

AVAILABILITY 5 mg, 10 mg, 20 mg vials; 1 mg/mL injection

ACTIONS Cytotoxic anthracycline antibiotic and derivative of daunorubicin. Potency of idarubicin is greater than that of daunorubicin or doxorubicin. It may be less cardiotoxic than other anthracyclines. Idarubicin exhibits inhibitory effects on DNA and RNA polymerase and, therefore, on nucleic acid synthesis. Intensive maintenance with idarubicin is not recommended due to its considerable toxicity, including deaths while patient was in remission of acute myelogenous leukemia (AML).
THERAPEUTIC EFFECTS Idarubicin exhibits inhibitory effects on DNA and RNA polymerase and, therefore, on nucleic acid synthesis.

USES In combination with other antineoplastic drugs for treatment of AML.
UNLABELED USES Breast cancer, other solid tumors.

CONTRAINDICATIONS Myelosuppression, hypersensitivity to idarubicin or doxorubicin, pregnancy (category D), lactation.
CAUTIOUS USE Impaired renal or hepatic function; patients who have received irradiation or radiotherapy to areas surrounding heart. Safety and efficacy in children not established.

ROUTE & DOSAGE

Acute Myelogenous Leukemia (AML)
Adult: **IV** 8–12 mg/m^2 daily for 3 days injected slowly over 10–15 min
Acute Nonlymphocytic Leukemia, Acute Lymphocytic Leukemia
Child: **IV** 10–12 mg/m^2/day for 3 days

STORAGE
Store reconstituted solutions up to 7 days refrigerated at 2°–8° C (36°–46° F) and 72 h at room temperature (15°–30° C [59°–86° F]).

ADMINISTRATION
- Child: Must be given under care and direction of pediatric oncology specialist. Use recommended handling techniques for hazardous medications (see Part I)

Common adverse effects in *italic;* life-threatening effects <u>underlined</u>; generic names in **bold**; drug classifications in SMALL CAPS; ◆ Canadian drug name; ❂ Prototype drug.

651

Intravenous

IV administration to infants, children: Verify correct IV concentration and rate of infusion with physician.

PREPARE **IV Infusion:** Reconstitute 5- and 10-mg vials with 5 and 10 mL, respectively, of nonbacteriostatic NS to yield 1 mg/mL. Vials are under negative pressure, therefore, carefully insert needle into vial to reconstitute. Wash skin accidentally exposed with soap and water.

ADMINISTER **IV Infusion:** Give slowly over 10–15 min into tubing of free flowing IV of NS or D5W. If extravasation is suspected, immediately stop infusion, elevate the arm, and apply ice pack for ½ h then q.i.d. for ½ h × 3 day.

INCOMPATIBILITIES **Solution/Additive: Acyclovir,** ALKALINE SOLUTIONS (i.e., **sodium bicarbonate), ampicillin/sulbactam, cefazolin, ceftazidime, clindamycin, dexamethasone, etoposide, furosemide, gentamicin, heparin, hydrocortisone, imipenem/cilastatin, meperidine, methotrexate, mezlocillin, sargramostim, sodium bicarbonate, vancomycin, vincristine.** Y-Site: Same as above.

ADVERSE EFFECTS CV: CHF, atrial fibrillation, chest pain, MI. **GI:** *Nausea, vomiting, diarrhea, abdominal pain,* mucositis. **Hematologic:** <u>*Anemia, leukopenia*</u>, thrombocytopenia. **Other:** Nephrotoxicity, hepatotoxicity, *alopecia,* rash.

INTERACTIONS Drug: IMMUNOSUPPRESSANTS cause additive bone marrow suppression; ANTICOAGULANTS, NSAIDS, SALICYLATES, **aspirin,** THROMBOLYTIC AGENTS increase risk of bleeding; idarubicin may blunt the effects of **filgrastim, sargraostim.**

PHARMACOKINETICS Onset: Median time to remission 28 days. **Peak:** Serum level 4 h. **Duration:** Serum levels 120 h. **Distribution:** Concentrates in nucleated blood and bone marrow cells. **Metabolism:** Metabolized in liver to idarubicinol, which may be as active as idarubicin. **Elimination:** 16% excreted in urine; 17% excreted in bile. **Half-Life:** Idarubicin 15–45 h, idarubicinol 45 h.

NURSING IMPLICATIONS

Assessment & Drug Effects

- Monitor infusion site closely, because extravasation can cause severe local tissue necrosis. Notify physician if pain, erythema, or edema develops at insertion site.
- Lab tests: Monitor hepatic and renal function, CBC with differential and coagulation studies periodically.
- Monitor cardiac status closely, especially in those with preexisting cardiac disease.
- Monitor hematologic status carefully; during the period of myelosuppression, patients are at high risk for bleeding and infection.
- Monitor for development of hyperuricemia secondary to lysis of leukemic cells.
- Be alert for and report signs of infection such as respiratory infections, aching, rashes, and gastrointestinal distress.

- Assess immunization status prior to beginning therapy in order to be alert for diseases that pose risk.

Patient & Family Education
- Learn all potential adverse reactions to idarubicin.
- Anticipate possible hair loss.
- Report signs of infections. Avoid exposure to persons with infectious diseases.
- May discolor urine (pink or red).
- Discuss interventions to minimize nausea, vomiting, diarrhea, and stomatitis with health care providers.
- Do not breast feed while taking this drug.

IDOXURIDINE (IDU)
(eye-dox-yoor′i-deen)
Herplex Liquifilm, IDU, Stoxil
Classifications: ANTI-INFECTIVE; ANTIVIRAL
Prototype: Acyclovir
Pregnancy Category: C

AVAILABILITY 0.1% ophthalmic solution

ACTIONS Topical antiviral agent. Pyrimidine nucleoside structurally related to thymidine, a nucleic acid essential for synthesis of viral DNA. Antiviral activity is primarily due to inhibition of viral replication.
THERAPEUTIC EFFECTS Inhibits growth of *Herpes simplex types I* and *II, varicella-zoster, vaccinia, cytomegalovirus,* and small animal viruses containing DNA. Not effective against RNA viruses. Epithelial viral infections characterized by a dendritic figure respond well to the antiviral activity especially during initial attacks. Chronic or recurrent viral infections that involve deep stromal structures (e.g., herpetic iritis) respond less well and do not heal. Some resistant strains of *Herpes simplex* have been reported.

USES *Herpes simplex* keratitis as single agent or conjunctively with a corticosteroid.
UNLABELED USES Cutaneous *Herpes simplex.*

CONTRAINDICATIONS Hypersensitivity to idoxuridine, iodine or iodine-containing preparations, or any components in the formulation, lactation.
CAUTIOUS USE Pregnancy (category C), corticosteroid therapy.

ROUTE & DOSAGE

Herpes Simplex Keratitis
Child/Adult: **Topical** 1 drop instilled in conjunctival sac q1h during the day and q2h at night until improvement occurs, then decrease to q2h during the day and q4h at night; use ointment q4h during the day with the last dose at bedtime (5 applications/day)

Common adverse effects in *italic;* life-threatening effects <u>underlined</u>; generic names in **bold;** drug classifications in SMALL CAPS; ◆ Canadian drug name; ❷ Prototype drug.

653

STORAGE

Store ophthalmic solution refrigerated at 2°–8° C (36°–46° F) in a tightly covered, light-resistant container unless otherwise directed. The ointment should be stored at 2°–15° C (36°–59° F).

ADMINISTRATION

Topical

- Prevent the possibility of systemic absorption by applying light finger pressure to head of lacrimal duct for 1 min when eye drop is instilled.
- Follow manufacturer's directions regarding storage. Decomposed idoxuridine not only has reduced antiviral activity but also may be toxic.

ADVERSE EFFECTS Body as a Whole: (Sensitization, systemic absorption [stomatitis, anorexia, nausea, vomiting, alopecia, leukopenia, thrombocytopenia, iodism, hepatotoxicity].) **Special Senses:** (Local irritation, pain, burning, lacrimation, pruritus, inflammation, or edema of eyes, lids, and surrounding face; follicular), conjunctivitis, photophobia; corneal ulceration and swelling; delayed healing, small defects in corneal epithelium (local overdosage).

INTERACTIONS Drug: Boric acid-containing solutions may cause precipitation.

PHARMACOKINETICS Absorption: Poorly absorbed from eye tissues. **Distribution:** Crosses placenta. **Metabolism:** Metabolized in liver.

NURSING IMPLICATIONS

Assessment & Drug Effects

- Monitor for therapeutic effectiveness. Epithelial infections usually improve within 7–8 days. If patient continues to improve, therapy is generally continued ≤21 days.
- Supervise patients closely by ophthalmologist.

Patient & Family Education

- Learn proper technique for eye drop instillation (see Part I).
- Do not exceed the recommended frequency and duration of therapy.
- Wear sunglasses if photosensitivity is troublesome.
- Do not breast feed while taking this drug.
- Store this medication out of reach of children.

IMIPENEM-CILASTATIN SODIUM 🅟

(i-mi-pen'em sye-la-stat'in)

Primaxin

Classifications: ANTI-INFECTIVE; BETA-LACTAM ANTIBIOTIC

Pregnancy Category: C

AVAILABILITY 250 mg, 500 mg, 750 mg vials

ACTIONS Fixed combination of imipenem, a beta-lactam antibiotic, and cilastatin. Action of imipenem: Inhibition of mucopeptide synthesis in bacterial cell walls leading to cell death. Cilastatin increases the serum half-life of imipenem.

THERAPEUTIC EFFECTS Has the greatest microbiologic spectrum of any beta-lactam antibiotic, surpassing that of all the third-generation cephalosporins. Acts synergistically with aminoglycoside antibiotics against some isolates of *Pseudomonas aeruginosa*. Infections resistant to cephalosporins, penicillins, and aminoglycosides have responded to treatment with this combination.

USES Treatment of serious infections caused by susceptible organisms in the urinary tract, lower respiratory tract, bones and joints, skin and skin structures; also intra-abdominal, gynecologic, and mixed infections; bacterial septicemia and endocarditis; infections in children with cystic fibrosis.

CONTRAINDICATIONS Hypersensitivity to any component of product, multiple allergens. Safe use in pregnancy (category C) is not established.
CAUTIOUS USE Lactation; patients with CNS disorders (e.g., seizures, brain lesions, history of recent head injury); renal impairment; patients with history of penicillin allergies.

ROUTE & DOSAGE

Serious Infections

Neonate: <1 wk, **IV** 40–50 mg/kg/day divided into doses given q12h; *1–4 wk,* **IV** 60–75 mg/kg/day divided into doses given q8h
Child: 4 wk–3 mo, **IV** 100 mg/kg/day divided into doses given q6h; *>3 mo,* **IV** 60–100 mg/kg/day divided into doses given q6h **IM** 15–25 mg/kg q12h
Adult: **IV** 250–1000 mg infused over 20–30 min q6–8h, up to 1 g infused over 40–60 min q6h (max 4 g/day or 50 mg/kg/day, whichever is less) **IM** 500 or 750 mg q12h

Renal Impairment

Cl_{cr} 20–30 mL/min, dose q8–12h; <20 mL/min, dose q12h

STORAGE
Store according to manufacturer's recommendations; stability of IV solutions depends on diluent used for reconstitution. Most IV solutions retain potency for 4 h at 15°–30° C (59°–86° F) or for 24 h if refrigerated at 4° C (39° F). Avoid freezing.

ADMINISTRATION
Caution: IM and IV solutions are NOT interchangeable; do NOT give IM solution by IV, and do NOT give IV solution as IM.

Intramuscular
- Reconstitute powder for IM injection as follows: Add 2 mL or 3 mL of 1% lidocaine HCl solution without epinephrine, respectively, to the 500-mg vial or the 750-mg vial. Agitate to form a suspension, then withdraw and inject entire contents of the vial IM.

- Give IM suspension by deep injection into the gluteal muscle (older child) or lateral thigh (young child). See Part I for site selection in children.
- Use reconstituted IM injection within 1 h after preparation.

Intravenous

PREPARE **Intermittent:** Dilute each dose with 10 mL of D5W, NS, or other compatible infusion solution. Agitate the solution until clear. Color should range from colorless to yellow. Further dilute with 100 mL of same solution used for initial dilution.

ADMINISTER **Intermittent:** Give each 500 mg or fraction thereof over 30–60 min. Do NOT give as a bolus dose. Nausea appears to be related to infusion rate, and if it presents during infusion, slow the rate (occurs most frequently with 1-g doses).

INCOMPATIBILITIES **Solution/Additive: Ringer's lactate,** stable in **dextrose**-containing solutions for only 4 h.

ADVERSE EFFECTS Body as a Whole: Hypersensitivity (rash, fever, chills, dyspnea, pruritus), weakness, oliguria/anuria, polyuria, polyarthralgia; *phlebitis and pain at injection site,* superinfections. **CNS:** Seizures, dizziness, confusion, somnolence, encephalopathy, myoclonus, tremors, paresthesia, headache. **GI:** *Nausea, vomiting,* diarrhea, <u>pseudomembranous colitis,</u> hemorrhagic colitis, gastroenteritis, abdominal pain, glossitis, heartburn. **Respiratory:** Chest discomfort, hyperventilation, dyspnea. **Skin:** Rash, pruritus, urticaria, candidiasis, flushing, increased sweating, skin texture change, facial edema. **Metabolic:** Hyponatremia, hyperkalemia. **Special Senses:** Transient hearing loss increased WBC, AST, ALT, alkaline phosphatase, BUN, LDH, creatinine; decreased Hgb, Hct, eosinophilia.

INTERACTIONS Drug: Aztreonam, cephalosporins, penicillins may antagonize the antibacterial effects.

PHARMACOKINETICS Distribution: Widely distributed; limited concentrations in CSF; crosses placenta; in breast milk. **Elimination:** 70% of dose excreted in urine within 10 h. **Half-Life:** 1 h.

NURSING IMPLICATIONS

Assessment & Drug Effects

- Determine previous hypersensitivity reaction to beta-lactam antibiotics (penicillins and cephalosporins) or to other allergens.
- Monitor for S&S of hypersensitivity (see Appendix D-1). Discontinue drug and notify physician if signs and symptoms occur.
- Monitor closely patients vulnerable to CNS adverse effects.
- Notify physician if focal tremors, myoclonus, or seizures occur; dosage adjustment may be needed.
- Monitor for S&S of superinfection (see Appendix D-1).
- Notify physician promptly to rule out pseudomembranous enterocolitis if severe diarrhea accompanied by abdominal pain and fever occurs (see Appendix D-1).
- Note: Sodium content derived from drug is high; consider in patient on restricted sodium intake.
- Monitor renal, hematologic, and liver function periodically.

Common adverse effects in *italic;* life-threatening effects <u>underlined</u>; generic names in **bold;** drug classifications in SMALL CAPS; ♣ Canadian drug name; ⊘ Prototype drug.

Patient & Family Education

- Notify physician immediately to report pruritus or symptoms of respiratory distress.
- Report pain or discomfort at IV infusion site.
- Report loose stools or diarrhea promptly.
- Do not breast feed while taking this drug without consulting physician.

IMIPRAMINE HYDROCHLORIDE
(im-ip′ra-meen)
Impril ♣, Janimine, Novopramine ♣, Tofranil

IMIPRAMINE PAMOATE
Tofranil-PM
Classifications: CENTRAL NERVOUS SYSTEM AGENT; PSYCHOTHERAPEUTIC; TRICYCLIC ANTIDEPRESSANT
Pregnancy Category: C

AVAILABILITY 10 mg, 25 mg, 50 mg tablets; 75 mg, 100 mg, 125 mg, 150 mg capsules

ACTIONS Tricyclic antidepressant (TCA) and tertiary amine, structurally related to the phenothiazines. In contrast with phenothiazines, which act on dopamine receptors, TCAs potentiate both norepinephrine and serotonin in the CNS by blocking their reuptake by presynaptic neurons. Decreases number of awakenings from sleep, markedly reduces time in REM sleep, and increases stage 4 sleep.

THERAPEUTIC EFFECTS As a TCA antidepressant, imipramine potentiates the effects of both norepinephrine and serotonin in the CNS by blocking their reuptake by the neurons. Relief of nocturnal enuresis is perhaps due to anticholinergic activity and to nervous system stimulation, resulting in earlier arousal to sensation of full bladder.

USES Endogenous depression and occasionally for reactive depression. Imipramine is the only TCA used as temporary adjuvant treatment of enuresis in children >6 y.

UNLABELED USES Certain syndromes that mimic or overlap diagnostically with depression: Alcoholism, cocaine withdrawal; attention deficit disorder with or without hyperactivity (children >6 y and adolescents); with amphetamines or methylphenidate for narcolepsy; phobic anxiety syndromes such as panic disorders and agoraphobia; obsessive-compulsive neurosis; chronic intractable pain.

CONTRAINDICATIONS Hypersensitivity to tricyclic drugs; acute recovery period after MI, defects in bundle-branch conduction; severe renal or hepatic impairment; use of imipramine HCl in children <12 y except to treat enuresis; use of pamoate in children of any age. Safe use during pregnancy (category D) or lactation is not established.

CAUTIOUS USE Children, adolescents, older adults; respiratory difficulties; cardiovascular, hepatic, or GI diseases; blood disorders; increased intraocular pressure, narrow-angle glaucoma; schizophrenia, hypomania or manic episodes, patient with suicidal tendency, seizure disorders; urinary retention; alcoholism, hyperthyroidism; electroshock therapy.

ROUTE & DOSAGE

Depression

Child <12 y: **PO** 1.5 mg/kg/day, may increase by 1 mg/kg/day q3–4days (max 5 mg/kg/day)
Child ≥12 y: 25–50 mg/day given in 1–3 doses (should not usually exceed 100 mg/day)
Adult: **PO** 75–100 mg/day (max 300 mg/day) in 1 or more divided doses **IM** 50–100 mg/day in divided doses

Enuresis in Childhood

Child: **PO** 10–25 mg 1 h before bedtime; *6–12 y,* may increase to 50 mg at bedtime (max 2.5 mg/kg); *>12 y,* may increase to 75 mg at bedtime (max 2.5 mg/kg)

STORAGE

ADMINISTRATION

Oral

- Do NOT make dosage adjustments more frequently than q4days.
- Give with or immediately after food.
- Note: Single doses can be given at bedtime or q.a.m., respectively, if drowsiness or insomnia results.

Intramuscular

- Use IM form only for those unable/unwilling to take oral form.
- Dissolve crystals by immersing intact ampule in warm water for about 1 min.

ADVERSE EFFECTS Body as a Whole: Hypersensitivity (skin rash, erythema, petechiae, urticaria, pruritus, photosensitivity, <u>angioedema</u> of face, tongue, or generalized; drug fever). **CNS:** *Sedation, drowsiness,* dizziness, headache, fatigue, numbness, tingling (paresthesias) of extremities; incoordination, ataxia, tremors, peripheral neuropathy, extrapyramidal symptoms (including parkinsonism effects and tardive dyskinesia); lowered seizure threshold, altered EEG patterns, delirium, disturbed concentration, confusion, hallucinations, anxiety, nervousness, insomnia, vivid dreams, restlessness, agitation, shift to hypomania, mania; exacerbation of psychoses; hyperpyrexia. **CV:** *Orthostatic hypotension,* mild sinus tachycardia; *arrhythmias,* hypertension or hypotension, palpitation, <u>MI</u>, CHF, *heart block,* ECG changes, stroke, flushing, cold cyanotic hands and feet (peripheral vasospasm). **Endocrine:** Testicular swelling, gynecomastia (men), galactorrhea and breast enlargement (women), increased or decreased libido, ejaculatory and erectile disturbances, delayed or absent orgasm (male and female); elevation or depression of blood glucose levels. **Special Senses:** Nasal congestion, tinnitus; *Blurred vision,* disturbances of accommodation, *slight mydriasis,* nystagmus. **GI:** *Dry mouth,* constipation, heartburn, excessive appetite, weight gain, nausea, vomiting, diarrhea, slowed gastric emptying time, flatulence, abdominal cramps, esophageal reflux, anorexia, stomatitis, increased salivation, black tongue, peculiar taste, paralytic ileus. **Urogenital:** *Urinary retention,* delayed micturition, nocturia, paradoxic urinary frequency. **Hematologic:** Bone marrow depression; <u>agranulocytosis</u>, eosinophilia, thrombocytopenia. **Other:** Excessive perspiration, cholestatic jaundice, precipitation of acute intermittent porphyria; dyspnea, changes in heat and cold tolerance, hair loss, syndrome of inappropriate antidiuretic hormone secretion (SIADH).

DIAGNOSTIC TEST INTERFERENCE Imipramine elevates ***serum bilirubin, alkaline phosphatase*** and may increase or decrease ***blood glucose.*** It decreases ***urinary 5-HIAA*** and ***VMA*** excretion and may falsely increase excretion of ***urinary catecholamines.***

INTERACTIONS Drug: MAO INHIBITORS may precipitate hyperpyrexic crisis, tachycardia, or seizures; ANTIHYPERTENSIVE AGENTS potentiate orthostatic hypotension; CNS DEPRESSANTS, **alcohol** add to CNS depression; **norepinephrine** and other SYMPATHOMIMETICS may increase cardiac toxicity; **cimetidine** decreases hepatic metabolism, thus increasing imipramine levels; **methylphenidate** inhibits metabolism of imipramine and thus may increase its toxicity. **Herbal: Ginkgo** may decrease seizure threshold; **St. John's wort** may cause **serotonin** syndrome.

PHARMACOKINETICS Absorption: Completely absorbed from GI tract. **Peak:** 1–2 h PO; 30 min IM. **Metabolism:** Metabolized to the active metabolite desipramine in liver. **Elimination:** Primarily excreted in urine, small amount in feces; crosses placenta; may be secreted in breast milk. **Half-Life:** 8–16 h.

NURSING IMPLICATIONS

Assessment & Drug Effects

- Monitor for therapeutic effectiveness; may not occur for 2 wk or more.
- Prevent serious adverse effects by accurate early reporting to prescriber about patient's response to drug.
- Antidepressants increase risk of suicidal thinking and behavior in children and adolescents with major depressive disorder, obsessive compulsive disorder, and other psychiatric disorders. Observe closely for worsening of condition, suicidality, and behavior changes. Instruct family and caregivers to monitor for these symptoms and discuss with prescriber. A MedGuide describing risks and stating whether the drug is approved for the child's/adolescent's condition should be provided for all families when antidepressants are prescribed.
- Note: Dose sensitivity and adverse effects are most likely to occur in adolescents, use a lower initial dose in these cases.
- ***Therapeutic serum level*** is 150–250 ng/mL. ***Toxic level*** is 1000 ng/mL but toxic effects may be seen with levels as low as 300 ng/mL. Obtain trough sample within 30 min of next scheduled dose after 5–7 days of medication.
- Lab tests: Monitor hepatic and renal function, CBC with differential, and fluid and electrolyte balance periodically.
- Monitor HR and BP frequently. Orthostatic hypotension may be marked in pretreatment hypertensive or cardiac patients.

Common adverse effects in *italic;* life-threatening effects <u>underlined</u>; generic names in **bold**; drug classifications in SMALL CAPS; ♣ Canadian drug name; ⊘ Prototype drug.

659

- Monitor for potential signs of toxicity: QRS prolongation (to 100 ms or greater), arrhythmias, hypotension, respiratory depression, altered level of consciousness, seizures. Overdose onset may be sudden.
- Weigh patient under standard conditions biweekly; report a gain of 0.5–1.0 kg (1½–2 lb) within 2–3 days and frank edema for older children or any weight gain for younger children.
- Monitor urinary and bowel elimination, at least until maintenance dosage is stabilized, to detect urinary retention or frequency, constipation, or paralytic ileus.
- Report promptly early signs of agranulocytosis (see Appendix D-1).
- Report signs of cholestatic jaundice: Flu-like symptoms, yellow skin or sclerae, dark urine, light colored stools, pruritus.
- Notify prescriber of extrapyramidal symptoms (tremors, twitching, ataxia, incoordination, hyperreflexia, drooling) in patients receiving large doses.
- Monitor diabetic patients for loss of glycemic control. Hyperglycemia or hypoglycemia (see Appendix D-1) occur in some patients.
- Inspect oral mucosa frequently, especially gingival surfaces.
- For high-dose therapy, drug should be withdrawn slowly when discontinued.

Patient & Family Education
- Change position slowly and in stages, especially from lying down to upright posture and dangle legs over bed for a few minutes before walking.
- Note: Effectiveness can decrease with continued drug administration in some patients. Inform physician if this occurs.
- Keep scheduled appointments with health care provider. Report immediately increasing depression and any thoughts of suicide.
- Do NOT use OTC drugs or herbal products while on a TCA without prescriber approval.
- Do not drive or engage in other potentially hazardous activities until response to drug is known.
- Avoid exposure to strong sunlight because of potential photosensitivity. Use sunscreen with at least SPF of 12–15 if allowed.
- Do not breast feed while taking this drug without consulting prescriber.
- Store this medication out of reach of children.

IMMUNE GLOBULIN INTRAMUSCULAR (IGIM, GAMMA GLOBULIN, IMMUNE SERUM GLOBULIN [ISG])

(im'mune glob'u-lin)
BayGam

IMMUNE GLOBULIN INTRAVENOUS (IGIV)

Gamimune N, Gammagard, Gammar-P IV, IGIV, Iveegam, Sandoglobulin, Venoglobulin-S
Classifications: SERUM; IMMUNIZING AGENT; IMMUNE GLOBULINS
Pregnancy Category: C

Common adverse effects in *italic;* life-threatening effects <u>underlined</u>; generic names in **bold;** drug classifications in SMALL CAPS; ♣ Canadian drug name; ● Prototype drug.

AVAILABILITY IGIM 2 mL, 10 mL vials **IGIV** 5%, 10% solution; 50 mg/mL powder for injection

ACTIONS Sterile concentrated solution containing globulin (primarily IgG) prepared from large pools of normal human plasma of either venous or placental origin and processed by a special fractionating technique.
THERAPEUTIC EFFECTS Like hepatitis B immune globulin (H-BIG), contains antibodies specific to hepatitis B surface antigen but in lower concentrations. Therefore, not considered treatment of first choice for postexposure prophylaxis against hepatitis B but usually an acceptable alternative when H-BIG is not available. Also much less expensive than H-BIG. Nonreactive when tested for hepatitis B.

USES IGIM: In susceptible persons to provide passive immunity or to modify severity of certain infectious diseases, e.g., rubeola (measles), rubella (German measles), varicella-zoster (chickenpox), type A (infectious) hepatitis, and as replacement therapy in congenital agammaglobulinemia or IgG deficiency diseases. May be used as an alternative to HBIG to provide passive immunity in hepatitis B infection. Also for postexposure prophylaxis of hepatitis non-A, non-B, and nonspecific hepatitis.
IGIV: Principally as maintenance therapy in patients unable to manufacture sufficient quantities of IgG antibodies, in patients requiring an immediate increase in immunoglobulin levels, and when IM injections are contraindicated as in patients with bleeding disorders or who have small muscle mass. Also in chronic autoimmune thrombocytopenia and idiopathic thrombocytopenic purpura (ITP).
UNLABELED USES Kawasaki syndrome, chronic lymphocytic leukemia, AIDS, premature and low birth-weight neonates, autoimmune neutropenia or hemolytic anemia.

CONTRAINDICATIONS History of anaphylaxis or severe reaction to human immune serum globulin (IG) or to any ingredient in the formulation such as thimerosal (mercury derivative) preservative in IM formulations and maltose (stabilizing agent) in IV formulations; persons with clinical hepatitis A; IGIV for patients with class-specific anti-IgA deficiencies; IGIM in severe thrombocytopenia or other bleeding disorders.
CAUTIOUS USE Safe use during pregnancy (category C) or lactation is not established.

ROUTE & DOSAGE

Hepatitis A Exposure
Child/Adult: **IM** 0.02 mL/kg as soon as possible after exposure; if period of exposure will be ≥3 mo, give 0.05–0.06 mL/kg once q4–6mo

Hepatitis B Exposure
Child/Adult: **IM** 0.02–0.06 mL/kg as soon as possible after exposure if H-BIG is unavailable

Rubella Exposure
Adult: **IM** 20 mL as single dose in susceptible pregnant women

Rubeola Exposure
Child/Adult: **IM** 0.25 mL/kg within 6 days of exposure

Varicella-Zoster Exposure
Child/Adult: **IM** 0.6–1.2 mL/kg promptly

Immunoglobulin Deficiency
Child/Adult: **IV** Gammagard, Gamimune, 100 mg/kg/mo;
Sandoglobulin, Venoglobulin-S 200 mg/kg/mo

Idiopathic Thrombocytopenia Purpura
Child/Adult: **IV** 400 mg/kg/day for 5 consecutive days or 1 g/kg
every other day for up to 3 doses

Kawasaki Disease
Child/Adult: **IV** 2 g/kg given over 10–12 h or 400 mg/kg/day on
4 consecutive days

STORAGE
Store Gamimune N at 2°–8° C (36°–46° F); store Sandoglobulin below
20° C (68° F) unless otherwise directed. Avoid freezing. Do not use if turbidity has occurred or if product has been frozen. Do not mix with other
drugs. Discard partially used vial.

ADMINISTRATION
Note: In hepatitis A (infectious hepatitis), immune globulin is most effective when given before or as soon as possible after exposure but not
more than 2 wk after (incubation period for hepatitis A is 15–50 days). Do
not give immune globulin to those presenting clinical manifestations of
hepatitis A. For hepatitis B (serum hepatitis), give immune globulin
within 24 h and not more than 7 days after exposure. IGIM and IGIV formulations are NOT interchangeable.

Intramuscular
- Give adults and older children injections into deltoid or anterolateral aspect of thigh; neonates and small children, into anterolateral aspect of
  thigh. See Part I for site selection.
- Avoid gluteal injections; however, when large volumes of immune globulin are prescribed or when large doses must be divided into several injections, the upper outer quadrant of the gluteus has been used in adults.

Intravenous

PREPARE **IV Infusion:** Refer to manufacturer's directions for information
on reconstitution, dilution, and flow IV rates. Venoglobulin-S and
Gammagard are packaged with the diluent and transfer device.
Gamimune N may be given undiluted or diluted to a 5% solution. Sandoglobulin is provided with enough diluent to make a 3% solution.
ADMINISTER **IV Infusion:** Flow rates vary with product being infused.
Gamimune N is generally started at 0.01–0.02 mL/kg/min for 30 min; if
tolerated, rate is increased to 0.02–0.04 mL/kg/min. The initial flow
rate for Sandoglobulin is 0.5–1 mL/min; if tolerated after 15–30 min,
rate is increased to 1.5–2.5 mL/min.

ADVERSE EFFECTS Body as a Whole: *Pain, tenderness, muscle stiffness
at IM site;* local inflammatory reaction, erythema, urticaria, angioedema,
headache, malaise, fever, arthralgia, nephrotic syndrome, <u>hypersensiti-</u>

vity (fever, chills, anaphylactic shock), infusion reactions (*nausea, flushing, chills,* headache, chest tightness, wheezing, skeletal pain, back pain, abdominal cramps, anaphylaxis).

INTERACTIONS Drug: May interfere with antibody response to LIVE-VIRUS VACCINES (measles/mumps/rubella); give VACCINES 14 days before or 3 mo after IMMUNE GLOBULINS.

PHARMACOKINETICS Peak: 2 days. **Distribution:** Rapidly and evenly distributed to intravascular and extravascular fluid compartments. **Half-Life:** 21–23 days.

NURSING IMPLICATIONS

Assessment & Drug Effects

- Make sure emergency drugs and appropriate emergency facilities are immediately available for treatment of anaphylaxis or sensitization.
- Note: Hypersensitivity reactions (see Appendix D-1) are most likely in patients receiving large IM doses, repeated injections, or rapid IV infusion.
- Monitor vital signs and infusion rate closely when patient is receiving IGIV.
- Note: IGIV has a mild diuretic effect in some patients due to presence of maltose.

Patient & Family Education

- Stop infusion and report immediately S&S of hypersensitivity (see Appendix D-1).
- Report immediately infusion symptoms of nausea, chills, headache, and chest tightness.
- Note: Passive immunity to measles (rubeola) lasts about 3–4 wk after immune globulin. In general, children ≤15 mo need active immunization with measles virus vaccine 3 mo after IGIM.
- Report signs of infections of any type.
- Do not breast feed while taking this drug without consulting physician.

INDINAVIR SULFATE

(in-din′a-vir)
Crixivan
Classifications: ANTI-INFECTIVE; ANTIVIRAL; PROTEASE INHIBITOR
Prototype: Saquinavir
Pregnancy Category: C

AVAILABILITY 100 mg, 200 mg, 333 mg, 400 mg capsules

ACTIONS Indinavir is an HIV protease inhibitor. HIV protease is an enzyme required to produce the polyprotein precursors of the functional proteins in infectious HIV.
THERAPEUTIC EFFECTS Protease inhibitors prevent cleavage of the HIV viral polyproteins, resulting in formation of immature noninfectious virus particles. Indinavir binds to the protease active site and thus inhibits activity of the enzyme.

USES Treatment of HIV infection, usually in combination with other antiretroviral agents or protease inhibitors.

Common adverse effects in *italic;* life-threatening effects underlined; generic names in **bold;** drug classifications in SMALL CAPS; ♣ Canadian drug name; ◑ Prototype drug.

663

CONTRAINDICATIONS Hypersensitivity to indinavir, lactation.
CAUTIOUS USE Hepatic dysfunction, renal impairment, history of nephrolithiasis, history of adverse responses to other protease inhibitors, pregnancy (category C). Safety and efficacy in children are not established.

ROUTE & DOSAGE

HIV

Child: PO 500 mg/m^2/dose given q8h
Adult: PO 800 mg (2 × 400 mg) q8h, 1 h before or 2 h after meal

STORAGE
Store tightly closed with desiccant in original bottle.

ADMINISTRATION

Oral

- Give with water on an empty stomach 1 h before or 2 h after meal; if needed, may be given with a very light meal or beverage.
- Note: When didanosine and indinavir are ordered concurrently, give each on empty stomach at least 1 h apart.
- Do not administer concurrently with astemizole, cisapride, midazolam, terfenadine, or triazolam.

ADVERSE EFFECTS CNS: Fatigue, headache, insomnia, dizziness, somnolence, nervousness, agitation, anxiety, paresthesia, peripheral neuropathy, tremor, vertigo. **CV:** Palpitations. **Hematologic:** Anemia, splenomegaly, lymphadenopathy. **GI:** *Nausea,* diarrhea, abdominal discomfort, dyspepsia, stomatitis, anorexia, dry mouth, cholecystitis, cholestasis, constipation, flatulence. **Skin:** Body odor, rash, pruritus, seborrhea, skin ulceration, dry skin, sweating, urticaria. **Other:** Myalgia, allergic reaction, bronchitis, cough, rhinitis, taste alterations, visual disturbances, hyperglycemia, diabetes, kidney stones.

INTERACTIONS Drug: Rifabutin, rifampin significantly decrease indinavir levels. **Ketoconazole** significantly increases indinavir levels. Indinavir could inhibit the metabolism and increase the toxicity of **astemizole, cisapride, midazolam, terfenadine, triazolam.** Indinavir and **didanosine** should be administered at least 1 h apart on empty stomach to permit full absorption of each; increased ergotamine toxicity with **dihydroergotamine, ergotamine. Herbal: St. John's wort** decreases antiretroviral activity of indinavir.

PHARMACOKINETICS Absorption: Rapidly absorbed from GI tract; a meal high in calories, fat, and protein significantly reduces absorption. **Distribution:** 60% protein bound. **Metabolism:** Metabolized in liver by cytochrome P4503A4 (CYP3A4). **Elimination:** Excreted primarily in feces (>80%), 20% excreted in urine.

NURSING IMPLICATIONS

Assessment & Drug Effects

- Lab tests: Monitor CBC with differential and platelet count, liver function tests, CPK, urinalysis, and serum amylase periodically.

- Assess for S&S of renal dysfunction, respiratory dysfunction, GI distress, and other common adverse effects.

Patient & Family Education
- Learn drug interactions and potential adverse reactions. Drink plenty of liquid to minimize risk of renal stones.
- Notify physician of flank pain, hematuria, S&S of jaundice, or other distressing adverse effects. Be alert for signs of infection. Encourage adequate nutrition.
- Do not breast feed while taking this drug.
- Store this medication out of reach of children.

INDOMETHACIN

(in-doe-meth′a-sin)
Indameth, Indocid ♦, Indocin, Indocin SR
Classifications: CENTRAL NERVOUS SYSTEM AGENT; ANALGESIC, ANTIPYRETIC; NSAID
Prototype: Ibuprofen
Pregnancy Category: B (D in third trimester or if used for more than 48 h)

AVAILABILITY 25 mg, 50 mg capsules; 75 mg sustained-release capsules; 25 mg/5 mL oral suspension; 50 mg suppositories; 1 mg injection

ACTIONS Potent nonsteroidal compound with anti-inflammatory, analgesic, and antipyretic effects similar to those of aspirin. Appears to reduce motility of polymorphonuclear leukocytes, development of cellular exudates, and vascular permeability in injured tissue resulting in its anti-inflammatory effects.
THERAPEUTIC EFFECTS Antipyretic and anti-inflammatory actions may be related to its ability to inhibit prostaglandin biosynthesis. It is a potent analgesic.

USES Palliative treatment in active stages of moderate to severe rheumatoid arthritis, ankylosing rheumatoid spondylitis, and other types of arthritis in those intolerant to or unresponsive to adequate trials with salicylates and other therapy. Also used IV to close patent ductus arteriosus in the premature infant.
UNLABELED USES To relieve biliary pain and dysmenorrhea, Paget's disease, athletic injuries, juvenile arthritis, idiopathic pericarditis.

CONTRAINDICATIONS Allergy to indomethacin, aspirin, or other NSAID; nasal polyps associated with angioedema, history of GI lesions; pregnancy (category B; D in third trimester or if used >48 h), lactation, children ≤14 y.
CAUTIOUS USE History of psychiatric illness, epilepsy, parkinsonism; impaired renal or hepatic function; uncontrolled infections; coagulation defects, CHF; older adults, persons in hazardous occupations.

Common adverse effects in *italic;* life-threatening effects <u>underlined</u>; generic names in **bold;** drug classifications in SMALL CAPS; ♦ Canadian drug name; ❷ Prototype drug.

665

ROUTE & DOSAGE

Rheumatoid Arthritis

Adult: **PO** 25–50 mg b.i.d. or t.i.d. (max 200 mg/day) or 75 mg sustained release 1–2 times/day

Pediatric Arthritis

Child: **PO** 1–2 mg/kg/day in 2–4 divided doses (max 4 mg/kg/day) or 150–200 mg/day

Close Patent Ductus Arteriosus

Premature neonate: **IV** *<48 h,* 0.2 mg/kg followed by 2 doses of 0.1 mg/kg q12–24h; *2–7 days,* 0.2 mg/kg followed by 2 doses of 0.2 mg/kg q12–24h; *>7 days,* 0.2 mg/kg followed by 2 doses of 0.25 mg/kg q12–24h

STORAGE

Store oral and rectal forms in tight, light-resistant containers unless otherwise directed. Do not freeze.

ADMINISTRATION

Oral

- Give immediately after meals, or with food, milk, or antacid (if prescribed) to minimize GI side effects.

Rectal

- Indomethacin rectal suppository use is contraindicated with history of proctitis or recent bleeding.

Intravenous

PREPARE **Direct:** Dilute 1 mg with 1 mL of NS or sterile water for injection without preservatives. Resulting concentration (1 mg/mL) may be further diluted with an additional 1 mL for each 1 mg to yield 0.5 mg/mL.

ADMINISTER **Direct:** Give by direct IV with a single dose given over 5–10 sec. Avoid extravasation or leakage; drug can be irritating to tissue. Discard any unused drug, because it contains no preservative. Rapid infusions have been associated with an increased risk of necrotizing enterocolitis. Infusion should be given over 30 min–24 h to decrease risk of this potentially fatal side effect.

ADVERSE EFFECTS Body as a Whole: Hypersensitivity (rash, purpura, pruritus, urticaria, angioedema, angiitis, rapid fall in blood pressure, dyspnea, asthma syndrome in aspirin-sensitive patients), edema, weight gain, flushing, sweating. **CNS:** Headache, *dizziness,* vertigo, lightheadedness, syncope, fatigue, muscle weakness, ataxia, insomnia, nightmares, drowsiness, confusion, coma, convulsions, peripheral neuropathy, psychic disturbances (hallucinations, depersonalization, depression), aggravation of epilepsy, parkinsonism. **CV:** Elevated BP, palpitation, chest pains, tachycardia, bradycardia, CHF. **Special Senses:** Blurred vision, lacrimation, eye pain, visual field changes, corneal deposits, retinal disturbances including macula, *tinnitus,* hearing disturbances, epistaxis. **GI:** *Nausea, vomiting,* diarrhea, anorexia, bloating,

Common adverse effects in *italic;* life-threatening effects <u>underlined;</u> generic names in **bold;** drug classifications in SMALL CAPS; ♣ Canadian drug name; ⊘ Prototype drug.

abdominal distention, ulcerative stomatitis, proctitis, rectal bleeding, <u>GI ulceration, hemorrhage, perforation,</u> *toxic hepatitis,* necrotizing entero-colitis. **Hematologic:** Hemolytic anemia, <u>aplastic anemia</u> (sometimes fatal), <u>agranulocytosis,</u> leukopenia, thrombocytopenic purpura, inhibited platelet aggregation. **Urogenital:** Renal function impairment, hematuria, urinary frequency; vaginal bleeding, breast changes. **Skin:** Hair loss, exfoliative dermatitis, erythema nodosum, tissue irritation with extravasation. **Metabolic:** Hyponatremia, hypokalemia, hyperkalemia, hypoglycemia or hyperglycemia, glycosuria (rare).

DIAGNOSTIC TEST INTERFERENCE Increased *AST, ALT, bilirubin, BUN;* positive **direct *Coombs' test.***

INTERACTIONS Drug: ORAL ANTICOAGULANTS, **heparin, alcohol** may prolong bleeding time; may increase **lithium** toxicity; effects of ORAL ANTICO-AGULANTS, **phenytoin,** SALICYLATES, SULFONAMIDES, SULFONYLUREAS increased because of protein binding displacement; increased toxicity including GI bleeding with SALICYLATES, NSAIDS; may blunt effects of ANTIHYPERTENSIVES and DIURETICS. **Herbal: Feverfew, garlic, ginger, ginkgo** may increase bleeding potential.

PHARMACOKINETICS Absorption: Completely absorbed from GI tract. **Onset:** 1–2 h. **Peak:** 3 h. **Duration:** 4–6 h. **Metabolism:** Metabolized in liver. **Elimination:** Excreted primarily in urine. **Half-Life:** 2.5–124 h.

NURSING IMPLICATIONS

Assessment & Drug Effects

- Monitor for therapeutic effectiveness: In acute gouty attack, relief of joint tenderness and pain is usually apparent in 24–36 h; swelling generally disappears in 3–5 days. In rheumatoid arthritis: Reduced fever, increased strength, reduced stiffness, and relief of pain, swelling, and tenderness.
- Question patient carefully regarding aspirin sensitivity before initiation of therapy.
- Observe patients carefully; instruct to report adverse reactions promptly to prevent serious and sometimes irreversible or fatal effects.
- Lab tests: Monitor renal function, hepatic function, CBC with differential, BP and HR, visual and hearing acuity periodically.
- Monitor weight and observe dependent areas for signs of edema in patients with underlying cardiovascular disease.
- Monitor I&O closely and keep physician informed during IV administration for patent ductus arteriosus. Significant impairment of renal function is possible; urine output may decrease by 50% or more. Also monitor BUN, serum creatinine, glomerular filtration rate, creatinine clearance, and serum electrolytes.

Patient & Family Education

- Notify physician of S&S of GI bleeding, visual disturbance, tinnitus, weight gain, or edema.
- Do not take aspirin or other NSAIDS; they increase possibility of ulcers.
- Note: Frontal headache is the most frequent CNS adverse effect; if it persists, dosage reduction or drug withdrawal may be indicated. Take

drug at bedtime with milk to reduce the incidence of morning headache.
- Do not drive or engage in other potentially hazardous activities until response to drug is known.
- Do not breast feed while taking this drug.
- Store this medication out of reach of children.

INFLIXIMAB
(in-flix'i-mab)
Remicade
Classifications: IMMUNOSUPPRESSANT; TUMOR NECROSIS FACTOR-ALPHA RECEPTOR ANTAGONIST
Prototype: Etanercept
Pregnancy Category: C

AVAILABILITY 100 mg powder for injection

ACTIONS IgG_1-K monoclonal antibody that binds specifically to tumor necrosis factor-alpha (TNF-alpha), a cytokine. Thus it prevents TNF-alpha from binding to its receptors. TNF-alpha induces proinflammatory cytokines such as interleukin-1 (IL-1) and IL-6.

THERAPEUTIC EFFECTS Treatment with infliximab reduces infiltration of inflammatory cells and TNF-alpha production in inflamed areas of the intestine. Elevated concentrations of TNF-alpha have been found in the stools of Crohn's disease patients and correlated with disease activity.

USES Moderately to severely active Crohn's disease, including fistulizing Crohn's disease, rheumatoid arthritis.

CONTRAINDICATIONS Hypersensitivity to infliximab; CHF; pregnancy (category C); lactation.

CAUTIOUS USE History of allergic phenomena or untoward responses to monoclonal antibody preparation; renal or hepatic impairment; multiple sclerosis (potential exacerbation); immunosuppressed patients; older adults. Safety and effectiveness in pediatric patients is not established although it has been successfully used in children 6–18 y with Crohn's disease.

ROUTE & DOSAGE

Crohn's Disease
Child ≥6 y: **IV** 5 mg/kg infused over at least 2 h, may be repeated 2 times at 4-wk intervals
Adult: **IV** 5 mg/kg infused over at least 2 h, may repeat at 2 and 6 wk for fistulizing disease

Rheumatoid Arthritis
Adult: **IV** 3 mg/kg infused over at least 2 h, followed by 2 mg/kg on weeks 2 and 6, then 2 mg/kg q8wk

STORAGE
Store unopened vials at 2°–8° C (36°–46° F).

Common adverse effects in *italic*; life-threatening effects <u>underlined</u>; generic names in **bold**; drug classifications in SMALL CAPS; ✦ Canadian drug name; ❷ Prototype drug.

ADMINISTRATION

Note: Do not administer to a patient who has known or suspected sepsis.

Intravenous

PREPARE **IV Infusion:** Reconstitute each vial with 10 mL of sterile water for injection using a 21-gauge or smaller syringe. Inject sterile water against wall of vial, then gently swirl to dissolve but do not shake. Let stand for 5 min. Solution should be colorless to light yellow with a few translucent particles. Discard if particles are opaque. Further dilute by first removing from a 250-mL IV bag of NS a volume of NS equal to the volume of reconstituted infliximab to be added to the IV bag. Slowly add the total volume of reconstituted infliximab solution to the 250-mL infusion bag and gently mix. Infusion concentration should be 0.4 to 4 mg/mL. Begin infusion within 3 h of preparation.

ADMINISTER **IV Infusion:** Give over at least 2 h using a polyethylene-lined infusion set with an in-line, low-protein-binding filter (pore size 1.2 micron or less). Infliximab is INCOMPATIBLE with PVC equipment or devices. Discard unused infusion solution.

INCOMPATIBILITIES **Solution/Additive:** Incompatible with **PVC** bags and tubing. **Y-Site:** Do not infuse with any other drugs.

ADVERSE EFFECTS Body as a Whole: Fatigue, fever, pain, myalgia, back pain, chills, hot flashes, arthralgia; infusion-related reactions (fever, chills, pruritus, urticaria, chest pain, hypotension, hypertension, dyspnea). Increased risk of opportunistic infections, including tuberculosis. **CNS:** Headache, dizziness, involuntary muscle contractions, paresthesias, vertigo, anxiety, depression, insomnia. **CV:** Chest pain, peripheral edema, hypotension, hypertension, tachycardia, anemia, CHF. **GI:** Nausea, diarrhea, abdominal pain, vomiting, constipation, dyspepsia, flatulence, intestinal obstruction, ulcerative stomatitis, increased hepatic enzymes. **Respiratory:** URI, pharyngitis, bronchitis, rhinitis, coughing, sinusitis, dyspnea. **Skin:** Rash, pruritus, acne, alopecia, fungal dermatitis, eczema, dry skin, increased sweating, urticaria. **Other:** Infections, development of autoantibodies, lupus-like syndrome, conjunctivitis, dysuria, urinary frequency.

INTERACTIONS Drug: May decrease effectiveness of VACCINES given concurrently.

PHARMACOKINETICS Distribution: Distributed primarily to the vascular compartment. **Half-Life:** 9.5 days.

NURSING IMPLICATIONS

Assessment & Drug Effects

- Discontinue IV infusion and notify physician for fever, chills, pruritus, urticaria, chest pain, dyspnea, hypo/hypertension.
- Monitor for and immediately report signs and symptoms of local IV site or more generalized infection.

Patient & Family Education

- Report any infection to your physician promptly.
- Report symptoms of Crohn's and any improvement.
- Do not breast feed while taking this drug.

INSULIN GLARGINE
(in′-su-lin glar′-geen)
Lantus

INSULIN (REGULAR)
Humulin R, Novolin R, Regular Insulin, Pork Regular Iletin II, Regular Purified Pork Insulin, Velosulin, Velosulin BR, Velosulin Human

INSULIN INJECTION CONCENTRATED
Iletin II Regular (Concentrated), U-500

INSULIN, ISOPHANE (NPH)
Humulin N, Iletin II (pork), Insulatard NPH, Mixtard, Novolin 70/30, Novolin

INSULIN LISPRO
Humalog

INSULIN, PROTAMINE ZINC (PZI)
Iletin II

INSULIN ZINC SUSPENSION (LENTE)
Humulin L, Lente Iletin II (pork), Lente Purified Pork Insulin, Novolin

INSULIN ZINC SUSPENSION, EXTENDED (ULTRALENTE)
Humulin U, Ultralente, Ultralente Insulin

INSULIN ZINC SUSPENSION, PROMPT (SEMILENTE)
Semilente Insulin, Semilente Purified Pork Insulin

Classifications: HORMONE AND SYNTHETIC SUBSTITUTE; ANTIDIABETIC AGENT; INSULIN
Pregnancy Category: B

AVAILABILITY 100 units/mL injection; 500 units/mL injection (concentrated injection only)

ACTIONS Solution of insulin extracted from beta cells in pork pancreas or synthesized by recombinant DNA technology (human). Pork insulin can be modified with protamine and/or zinc to delay absorption and promote long action. Enhances transmembrane passage of glucose across cell membranes of most body cells and by unknown mechanism may enter the cell to activate selected intermediary metabolic process. Promotes conversion of glucose to glycogen. Types and their sources include:
Glargine—recombinant human insulin, long acting
Regular—pork or synthetic recombinant DNA technology, short acting
Concentrated—pork, higher dose than any other forms, intermediate acting
Isophane (NPH)—pork or human, purified to cause less allergic reactions, zinc and protamine added, intermediate acting

Lispro—human recombinant DNA technology, rapid acting
Protamine Zinc (PZI)—pork, zinc and protamine added, long acting
Zinc Suspension (Lente)—pork, zinc added, intermediate acting
Zinc Suspension, Extended (Lente)—pork, zinc added, long acting
Zin Suspension, Prompt (Semilente)—pork, zinc added, rapid acting
THERAPEUTIC EFFECTS Lowers blood glucose levels by stimulating peripheral glucose passage across cell membranes and uptake into cells, especially in muscle and fat cells. Inhibits hepatic glucose production from glycogen.

USES For routine daily management of type 1 and type 2 diabetes, and for emergency care of ketoacidosis.

CONTRAINDICATIONS Prior hypersensitivity to the particular type of insulin or its additives; hypoglycemia
CAUTIOUS USE Renal and hepatic impairment; pregnancy (category B for all types except glargine which is C), hyper- or hypothyroidism, lactation, not at all types have safety and efficacy established for children (glargine not established <6 y, regular and PZI <2 y, concentrated, Lente and Semilente <12 y, NPH <3 y, Lispro and Ultralente <3 y.

ROUTE & DOSAGE

Diabetes

Note: Doses vary depending on a variety of factors such as age of child, activity level, and combination of types of insulins used. Doses are based on blood glucose levels. Some starting doses are:
Child: **SC** 2–4 units regular insulin 15–30 minutes before meals and at bed time
Adult: **SC** 5–10 units regular insulin 15–30 minutes before meals and at bed time
Regular doses are adjusted as needed when other intermediate and long acting insulins are added to regimen.

Diabetic Ketoacidosis

Child/Adult: **IV** 0.1 unit/kg/h as continuous drip; an initial bolus of 0.1 unit/kg may be infused more rapidly to begin therapy

STORAGE
Store in refrigerator at 2°–8° C (36°–46° F). May be stored at room temperature 15°–30° C (59°–86° F). Discard opened refrigerated vials after 28 days and unrefrigerated vials after 14 days. Do not expose to excessive heat or sunlight, and do not freeze.

ADMINISTRATION
Subcutaneous

■ Do not give this SC products IV. Use an insulin syringe for accurate measurement. Insulin types should be mixed only when prescribed. If missed, regular is drawn up first into the syringe. Any change in the strength, brand, purity, type, or species (pork, human), or mixing sequence should be prescribed by the physician as availability in the body may be altered. Do not give cold insulin as lipodystrophy, reduced absorption, and local discomfort can result. Rotate injection sites;

common sites are upper arms, thighs, abdomen, buttocks and upper back. Insulin pump injections are given into abdomen.

Pump

To calculate total daily insulin pump dose, take 90% of the usual daily insulin dose given by injection, and use that number to calculate pump dose. First take 50% of the total daily pump dose and then divide by 24 to obtain hourly basal pump dose. Then use the other 50% and divide it into 4 daily doses that are given by bolus at meal times. For example, 20% may be given at breakfast, 10% at midday meal, 15% at evening meal, and 5% at evening snack.

Intravenous

Use only preparations intended for IV use.
PREPARE Direct: Give undiluted. **Continuous:** Diluted in NS or 0.45% NaCl. When 100 unit insulin is added to 1000 mL, solution yields 0.1 unit/mL.
ADMINISTER Direct: Give 50 units or a fraction thereof over 1 min. **Continuous:** Rate ordered by physician. When starting IV infusion, fill tubing with insulin infusion and wait 30 minutes. Flush the line, and connect line to the patient to start infusion. Insulin is absorbed into the container and tubing in amounts that vary according to concentration of insulin, infusion setup, and flow rate. The initial wait allows the potential biding sites to be saturated. Monitor patient response closely during IV insulin infusions because of the variable availability of medication.
INCOMPATIBILITIES Solution/Additive: Aminophylline, amobarbital, chlorothiazide, cytarabine, dobutamine, pentobarbital, phenobarbital, phenytoin, secobarbital, sodium bicarbonate, thiopental. **Y-Site:** Dobutamine.

ADVERSE EFFECTS Body as a Whole: Most adverse effects are related to hypoglycemia, <u>anaphylaxis</u> (rare), hyperinsulinemia; *Profuse sweating,* hunger, headache, *nausea, tremulousness,* tremors, *palpitation,* tachycardia, weakness, fatigue, nystagmus, circumoral pallor, numb mouth, tongue, and other paresthesias, visual disturbances (diplopia, blurred vision, mydriasis), staring expression, confusion, personality changes, ataxia, incoherent speech apprehension, irritability, inability to concentrate, personality changes, uncontrolled yawning, loss of consciousness, delirium, hypothermia, convulsions, abnormal Babinski reflex, coma. **CNS:** With overdose, psychic disturbances (i.e., aphasia, personality changes, maniacal behavior). **Metabolic:** Posthypoglycemia or rebound hyperglycemia (Somogyi effect), hypokalemia, lipoatrophy and lipohypertrophy of injection sites, insulin resistance. **Skin:** Localized allergic reactions at injection site, generalized urticaria or bullae, lymphadenopathy.

DIAGNOSTIC TEST INTERFERENCE Large doses of insulin may increase urinary excretion of VMA. Insulin can cause alterations in thyroid function tests and liver function test and may decrease serum potassium and serum calcium.

INTERACTIONS Drug: Alcohol, anabolic steroids, MAO inhibitors, guanethidine, salicylates may potentiate corticosteroids, epinephrine may antagonize hypoglycemic effects, furosemide, thiazine diuretics increase serum glucose levels, propranolol and other beta blockers may mask symptoms of hypoglycemic reaction. **Herbal:** Garlic, ginseng may potentiate hypoglycemic effects.

PHARMACOKINETICS Absorption: Rapid. **Distribution:** Throughout extracellular fluids. **Metabolism:** Metabolized primarily in liver with some metabolism in kidneys. **Elimination:** <2% excreted in urine. **Half-Life:** Biological, up to 13 h.

	Onset (h)	Peak (h)	Effective duration (h)	Maximum duration (h)
PORK				
Regular	0.5–2	3–4	4–6	6–8
Semi-Lente	1–1.5	5–10	12–16	
NPH	4–6	8–14	16–20	20–24
Lente	4–6	8–14	16–20	20–24
Untralente	8–14	Minimal	24–36	24–36
HUMAN				
Lispro	0.15–0.25	0.5–1.5	3	4
Regular	0.5–1	2–3	3–6	4–6
NPH	2–4	4–10	10–16	14–18
Lente	3–4	4–12	12–18	16–20
Ultralente	6–10	None	18–20	20–30

(Data from American Diabetes Association http://www.diabetes.org)

NURSING IMPLICATIONS

Assessment & Drug Effects

- A comprehensive teaching program for the child and family is needed. Diet, physical activity, insulin injections and other lifestyle adjustments are needed by children with newly diagnosed diabetes.
- Frequency of blood glucose monitoring is determined by the type of insulin and the health status. Several times daily is the norm in usual management.
- Lab Tests: Periodic postprandial blood glucose, HbA1C. Test urine for ketones in new, unstable, and type 1 diabetes; if there is weight loss, vigorous exercise, in illness, or if blood glucose is elevated. Notify prescriber promptly for presence of acetone with glucose in the urine; may indicate onset of ketoacidosis. Acetone without glucose in the urine may signify insufficient carbohydrate intake. Monitor for S&S of hypoglycemia (see Appendix D-1) at time of peak actions of insulin. Onset of hypoglycemia may be rapid and sudden.
- Ketoacidosis: Check BP, I&O, and blood glucose and ketones every hour during treatment for ketoacidosis with IV infusion. Glucose should not fall faster than 80–100 mg/dL/h. Dehydration of 5–10% is common with diabetic ketoacidosis so 10–20 mL/kg bolus of NS or LR over 1 h may be used, followed by IV insulin injection and 0.45 NS over next 48 hours to restore imbalance and provide for maintenance fluid needs. Once blood glucose is 250–300 mg/dL, add dextrose 5% to IV infusion fluids. Patients with severe hypoglycemia may be given glucagons, epinephrine, or IV glucose. When fully conscious oral carbohydrate is given. Laboratory studies include sodium, potassium, phosphate, bicarbonate.

Patient & Family Education

- Learn correct injection technique for SC or insertion of needles for pump. Inject into the abdomen during sports activities to ensure more steady absorption. Notify prescriber of local reactions at injection site. Recognize a variety of factors as possible causes of hypoglycemia: Insufficient food intake, vomiting, diarrhea, unaccustomed exercise, infection, illness, nervous or emotional tension, overindulgence in alcohol. Seek regulation by care provider. Respond promptly to signs of hypoglycemia. Take 4 oz (120 mL) or other ordered amount of fruit juice or carbonated beverage; child commonly requires 1.5–3 oz (45–90 L), followed by complex carbohydrate and protein food. Obtain emergency care if there is failure to show immediate improvement. Carry simple sugar source at all times, such as a lump of sugar or a candy. Be sure the child has access to these sources at school. Inform teachers of the S&S of hypoglycemia and hyperglycemia and how to treat each. Check blood glucose frequently on prescribed timetable. Notify care provider of blood glucose <80 and >120 mg/dL. Bring log of blood glucose to each health care visit.
- Avoid OTC medications unless prescribed by health care provider.
- Do not breast feed while taking this drug without consulting physician.
- Store this medication and syringes out of reach of children.

INTERFERON ALFA-2b

(in-ter-feer′on)

Intron A

Classifications: IMMUNOMODULATOR; INTERFERON
Prototype: Interferon alfa-2a
Pregnancy Category: C

AVAILABILITY 5 million international units, 10 million international units, 18 million international units, 25 million international units, 50 million international units vials

ACTIONS Alpha (leukocyte) interferon is a natural product induced virally in peripheral WBC or lymphoblastoid cells. The drug interferon alfa-2b is obtained by recombinant DNA technology from a strain of *Escherichia coli* bearing an interferon alfa-2b gene from human leukocytes.
THERAPEUTIC EFFECTS Has the same actions (antiviral, immunomodulating, antiproliferative) as interferon alfa-2a.

USES Hairy cell leukemia in splenectomized and nonsplenectomized patients ≥18 y, chronic myelogenous leukemia, renal cell carcinoma, melanoma, chronic hepatitis B or C.
UNLABELED USES Multiple sclerosis, condylomata acuminata, AIDS-related Kaposi's sarcoma.

CONTRAINDICATIONS Hypersensitivity to interferon alfa-2b or to any components of the product. Safe use during pregnancy (category C), lactation, or children <18 y is not established.
CAUTIOUS USE Severe, preexisting cardiac, renal, or hepatic disease; pulmonary disease (e.g., COPD); diabetes mellitus patients prone to

---

Common adverse effects in *italic*; life-threatening effects <u>underlined</u>; generic names in **bold**; drug classifications in SMALL CAPS; ♣ Canadian drug name; ❷ Prototype drug.

ketoacidosis; coagulation disorders; severe myelosuppression; recent MI; previous dysrhythmias, children.

ROUTE & DOSAGE

Hairy Cell Leukemia
Adult: **IM/SC** 2 million units/m^2 3 times/wk

Kaposi's Sarcoma
Adult: **IM/SC** 30 million units/m^2 3 times/wk

Condylomata Acuminata
Adult: **IM/SC** 1 million units/m^2 3 times/wk

Chronic Hepatitis B or C
Adult: **SC** 3 million units 3 times/wk × 18–24 mo

Chronic Myelogenous Leukemia
Child/Adult: **IM/SC** 2.5–5 million units/m^2/day

STORAGE
Store vials and reconstituted solutions at 2°–8° C (36°–46° F); remains stable for 1 mo.

ADMINISTRATION
- Child: Interferon alfa-2b must be given under care and direction of pediatric oncology specialist. Use recommended handling techniques for hazardous medications (see Part I).
- Although not approved for or tested widely in children, some children with adult-type chronic myelogenous leukemia have been successfully treated with this drug.

Subcutaneous/Intramuscular
- Reconstitution: The final concentration with the amount of required diluent is determined by the condition being treated (see manufacturer's directions). Inject diluent (bacteriostatic water for injection) into interferon alfa-2b vial; gently agitate solution before withdrawing dose with a sterile syringe.
- Make sure reconstituted solution is clear and colorless to light yellow and free of particulate material; discard if there are particles or solution is discolored.

ADVERSE EFFECTS Body as a Whole: *Flu-like syndrome (fever, chills) associated with myalgia and arthralgia,* leg cramps. **CNS:** Depression, nervousness, anxiety, confusion, *dizziness, fatigue,* somnolence, insomnia, altered mental states, ataxia, tremor, paresthesias, *headache.* **CV:** Hypertension, dyspnea, *hot flushes.* **Special Senses:** Epistaxis, pharyngitis, sneezing; abnormal vision. **GI:** Taste alteration, *anorexia,* weight loss, *nausea,* vomiting, stomatitis, *diarrhea,* flatulence. **Hematologic:** Mild thrombocytopenia, transient granulocytopenia, <u>leukemia</u>. **Skin:** Mild pruritus, mild alopecia, rash, dry skin, herpetic eruptions, nonherpetic cold sores, urticaria.

INTERACTIONS May increase **theophylline** levels; additive myelosuppression with ANTINEOPLASTICS, **zidovudine** may increase hematologic toxicity, increase **doxorubicin** toxicity, increase neurotoxicity with **vinblastine.**

Common adverse effects in *italic;* life-threatening effects <u>underlined</u>; generic names in **bold**; drug classifications in SMALL CAPS; ✦ Canadian drug name; ❷ Prototype drug.

675

PHARMACOKINETICS Peak: 6–8 h. **Metabolism:** Metabolized in kidneys. **Half-Life:** 6–7 h.

NURSING IMPLICATIONS

Assessment & Drug Effects

- Be alert for and report additional signs of infection such as respiratory infections, aching, rashes, and gastrointestinal distress.
- Assess immunization status prior to beginning therapy in order to be alert for diseases that pose risk.
- Lab tests: Monitor CBC with differential and platelet counts closely.
- Monitor for ecchymoses, petechiae, and bruising.
- Assess hydration status; patient should be well hydrated especially during initial stage of treatment and if vomiting or diarrhea occurs.
- Assess for flu-like symptoms, which may be relieved by acetaminophen (if prescribed).
- Monitor level of GI distress and ability to consume fluids and food.
- Monitor mental status and alertness; implement safety precautions if needed.

Patient & Family Education

- Report signs of infections. Avoid exposure to persons with infectious diseases.
- Learn techniques for reconstitution and administration of drug.
- Do NOT change brands of interferon without first consulting the physician.
- Note: If flu-like symptoms develop, take acetaminophen as advised by physician and take interferon at bedtime.
- Note: Fertile, nonpregnant woman need to use effective contraception.
- Use caution with hazardous activities until response to drug is known.
- Learn about adverse effects and notify physician about those that cause significant discomfort.
- Do not breast feed while taking this drug without consulting physician.

IODOQUINOL
(eye-oh-do-kwin′ole)
Diiodohydroxyquin, Dioquinol, Sebaquin, Yodoxin
Classifications: ANTI-INFECTIVE; AMEBICIDE; ANTIPROTOZOAL
Prototype: Emetine
Pregnancy Category: C

AVAILABILITY 210 mg, 650 mg tablets

ACTIONS Direct-acting (contact) amebicide.
THERAPEUTIC EFFECTS Effective against both trophozoites and cyst forms of *Entamoeba histolytica* in intestinal lumen. Not useful for extraintestinal amebiasis. Range of antiprotozoal action includes *Trichomonas vaginalis* and *Balantidium coli;* also has some antibacterial and antifungal properties.

USES Intestinal amebiasis and for asymptomatic passers of cysts. Commonly used either concurrently or in alternating courses with another intestinal amebicide.

UNLABELED USES *Balantidiasis* and *Acrodermatitis enteropathica;* traveler's diarrhea; shampoo preparation (Sebaquin) used for control of seborrheic dermatitis of scalp.

CONTRAINDICATIONS Hypersensitivity to any 8-hydroxyquinoline or to iodine-containing preparations or foods; hepatic or renal damage; preexisting optic neuropathy. Safe use during pregnancy (category C) or lactation is not established.

CAUTIOUS USE Severe thyroid disease; minor self-limiting problems; prolonged high-dosage therapy.

ROUTE & DOSAGE

Intestinal Amebiasis

Child: **PO** 30–40 mg/kg/day in 2–3 divided doses for 20 days (max 1.95 g/day), may repeat after a 2–3 wk drug-free interval
Adult: **PO** 630–650 mg t.i.d. for 20 days (max 2 g/day), may repeat after a 2–3 wk drug-free interval

STORAGE

Store at room temperature unless otherwise directed.

ADMINISTRATION

Oral

- Give drug after meals. If patient has difficulty swallowing tablet, crush and mix with applesauce.

ADVERSE EFFECTS Body as a Whole: Hypersensitivity (urticaria, pruritus). **CNS:** Headache, agitation, retrograde amnesia, vertigo, ataxia, peripheral neuropathy (especially in children); muscle pain, weakness usually below T_{12} vertebrae, dysesthesias especially of lower limbs, paresthesias, increased sense of warmth. **Special Senses:** Blurred vision, optic atrophy, optic neuritis, permanent loss of vision. **GI:** Nausea, vomiting, anorexia, abdominal cramps, diarrhea, constipation, rectal irritation and itching. **Skin:** Discoloration of hair and nails, acne, hair loss, urticaria, various forms of skin eruptions. **Hematologic:** Agranulocytosis (rare). **Endocrine:** Thyroid hypertrophy, iodism (generalized furunculosis [iodine toxiderma], skin eruptions, fever, chills, weakness).

DIAGNOSTIC TEST INTERFERENCE Iodoquinol can cause elevations of *PBI* and decrease of *I-131 uptake* (effects may last for several weeks to 6 mo even after discontinuation of therapy). *Ferric chloride test for PKU* (phenylketonuria) may yield false-positive results if iodoquinol is present in urine.

INTERACTIONS No clinically significant interactions established.

PHARMACOKINETICS Absorption: Small amount absorbed from GI tract. **Elimination:** Excreted in feces.

NURSING IMPLICATIONS

Assessment & Drug Effects

- Monitor I&O ratio. Record characteristics of stools: Color, consistency, frequency, presence of blood, mucus, or other material.

Common adverse effects in *italic*; life-threatening effects underlined; generic names in **bold**; drug classifications in SMALL CAPS; ♣ Canadian drug name; ☻ Prototype drug.

677

- Note: Ophthalmologic examinations are recommended at regular intervals during prolonged therapy.
- Monitor and report immediately the onset of blurred or decreased vision or eye pain. Also report symptoms of peripheral neuropathy: Pain, numbness, tingling, or weakness of extremities.

Patient & Family Education

- Report skin S&S of agranulocytosis (see Appendix D-1).
- Complete full course of treatment. Stool needs to be examined again 1, 3, and 6 mo after termination of treatment.
- Note: Intestinal amebiasis is spread mainly by contaminated water, raw fruits or vegetables, flies, roaches, and hand-to-mouth transfer of infected feces. It is very important to wash hands after defecation and before eating.
- Do not breast feed while taking this drug without consulting prescriber.
- Store this medication out of reach of children.

IPRATROPIUM BROMIDE

(i-pra-troe′pee-um)

Atrovent

Classifications: AUTONOMIC NERVOUS SYSTEM AGENT; ANTICHOLINERGIC (PARASYMPATHOLYTIC); BRONCHODILATOR

Prototype: Atropine

Pregnancy Category: B

AVAILABILITY 0.02% solution for inhalation; 18 mcg inhaler; 0.03%, 0.06% nasal spray

ACTIONS Quaternary compound, chemically related to atropine, with low solubility; does not cross blood–brain barrier. Produces local, site-specific effects on the larger central airways including bronchodilation and prevention of bronchospasms.

THERAPEUTIC EFFECTS Bronchodilation inhibits acetylcholine at its receptor sites, thereby blocking cholinergic bronchomotor tone (bronchoconstriction); also abolishes vagally mediated reflex bronchospasm triggered by such nonspecific agents as cigarette smoke, inert dusts, cold air, and a range of inflammatory mediators (e.g., histamine).

USES Maintenance therapy in COPD including chronic bronchitis and emphysema; nasal spray for perennial rhinitis and symptomatic relief of rhinorrhea associated with the common cold.

UNLABELED USES Perennial nonallergic rhinitis.

CONTRAINDICATIONS Use as primary treatment for acute episodes; hypersensitivity to atropine or derivatives. Safe use in children <12 y is not established.

CAUTIOUS USE Pregnancy (category B), lactation; narrow-angle glaucoma; prostatic hypertrophy, bladder neck obstruction.

ROUTE & DOSAGE

COPD

Child: **Inhalation** *3–12 y,* 1–2 inhalations t.i.d. (max 6/day) **Nebulizer** 125–250 mcg t.i.d.
Adult: **Inhalation** 2 inhalations of MDI q.i.d. at no less than 4 h intervals (max 12 inhalations in 24 h) **Nebulizer** 500 mcg (1 unit dose vial) q6–8h

Rhinitis

Adult: **Intranasal** ≥5 y, 2 sprays of 0.03% each nostril b.i.d. or t.i.d.

Common Cold

Adult: **Intranasal** 2 sprays of 0.06% each nostril t.i.d. or q.i.d. up to 4 days

STORAGE

Store from 15°–30° C (59°–86° F) and avoid humidity.

ADMINISTRATION

Intranasal/Inhalation/Nebulizer

- Shake inhaler well before use.
- Effect of medication decreases if canister is cold.
- Demonstrate aerosol use and check return demonstration (see Part I).
- Wait 3 min between inhalations if more than one inhalation per dose is ordered.
- Avoid contact with eyes.

ADVERSE EFFECTS Special Senses: Blurred vision (especially if sprayed into eye), difficulty in accommodation, acute eye pain, worsening of narrow-angle glaucoma. **GI:** Bitter taste, dry oropharyngeal membranes. With higher doses; nausea, constipation. **Respiratory:** *Cough,* hoarseness, exacerbation of symptoms, drying of bronchial secretions, mucosal ulcers, epistaxis, nasal dryness. **Skin:** Rash, hives. **Urogenital:** Urinary retention. **CNS:** Headache.

PHARMACOKINETICS Absorption: 10% of inhaled dose reaches lower airway; approximately 0.5% of dose is systemically absorbed. **Peak effect:** 1.5–2 h. **Duration:** 4–6 h. **Elimination:** 48% of dose excreted in feces; <5% excreted in urine. **Half-Life:** 1.5–2 h.

NURSING IMPLICATIONS

Assessment & Drug Effects

- Monitor respiratory status; auscultate lungs before and after inhalation.
- Report treatment failure (exacerbation of respiratory symptoms) to physician.

Patient & Family Education

- Note: This medication is not an emergency agent because of its delayed onset and the time required to reach peak bronchodilation.
- Review patient information sheet on proper use of nasal spray.

- Allow 30–60 sec between puffs for optimum results. Do not let medication contact your eyes.
- Wait 5 min between this and other inhaled medications. Check with prescriber about sequence of administration.
- Take medication only as directed, noting some leniency in number of puffs within 24 h. Supervise child's administration until certain all of dose is being administered.
- Rinse mouth after medication puffs to reduce bitter taste.
- Discuss changes in normal urinary pattern with the prescriber.
- Call prescriber if you note changes in sputum color or amount, ankle edema, or significant weight gain.
- Do not breast feed while taking this drug without consulting physician.
- Store this medication out of reach of children.

IRON DEXTRAN
(i'ern dek'stran)
Dexferrum, Imfed, Imferon
Classifications: BLOOD FORMERS, COAGULATORS, AND ANTICOAGULANTS; IRON PREPARATION
Prototype: Ferrous sulfate
Pregnancy Category: C

AVAILABILITY 50 mg/mL

ACTIONS A dark brown, slightly viscous liquid complex of ferric hydroxide with dextran in 0.9% NaCl solution for injection.
THERAPEUTIC EFFECTS Reticuloendothelial cells of liver, spleen, and bone marrow dissociate iron from iron dextran complex. The released ferric ion combines with transferrin and is transported to bone marrow, where it is incorporated into hemoglobin.

USES Only in patients with clearly established iron deficiency anemia when oral administration of iron is unsatisfactory or impossible. Each milliliter of iron dextran contains 50 mg elemental iron.

CONTRAINDICATIONS Hypersensitivity to the product; all anemias except iron-deficiency anemia. Not recommended for children <4 mo of age. Safe use during pregnancy (category C) is not established.
CAUTIOUS USE Lactation; rheumatoid arthritis, ankylosing spondylitis; impaired hepatic function; history of allergies or asthma.

ROUTE & DOSAGE

Iron Deficiency
Total replacement dose of iron dextran (mL) = 0.0476 × weight (kg) × (desired Hgb [g/dL] − measured Hgb [g/dL]) + 1 mL/5 kg body weight (max 14 mL)
Child: **IM/IV** <5 kg, no more than 0.5 mL (25 mg)/day; 5–10 kg, no more than 1 mL (50 mg)/day; >10 kg, no more than 2 mL (100 mg)/day
Adult: **IM/IV** dose is individualized and determined as above (see package insert for more detail); do not administer more than 100 mg (2 mL) of iron dextran within 24 h

Acute Blood Loss

Total replacement dose of iron dextran (mL) $= 0.02 \times$ blood loss (mL) $\times$ hematocrit expressed as fraction. Assumes 1 mL RBC $= 1$ mg elemental iron.

STORAGE
Store below 30° C (86° F) unless otherwise directed.

ADMINISTRATION
Note: The multiple-dose vial is used ONLY for IM injections. It is not suitable for IV use because it contains a preservative (phenol).

Test Dose

- Give a test dose of 0.5 mL (0.25 mL for infants) over a 5-min period before the first IM or IV therapeutic dose to observe patient's response to the drug. Have epinephrine (0.5 mL of a 1:1000 solution) immediately available for hypersensitivity emergency.
- Note: Although anaphylactic reactions (see Appendix D-1) usually occur within a few minutes after injection, it is recommended that 1 h or more elapse before remainder of initial dose is given following test dose.

Intramuscular

- Give injection only into the muscle mass in upper outer quadrant of buttock (never in the upper arm). In small child, use the lateral thigh. See Part I for site selection. Use a 2- or 3-inch, 19- or 20-gauge needle. The Z-track technique is recommended. Use one needle to withdraw drug from container and change to a new needle for injection. Techniques important to prevent brown tissue staining.
- Note: If patient is receiving IM in standing position, patient should be bearing weight on the leg opposite the injection site; if in bed, patient should be in the lateral position with injection site uppermost.

Intravenous

Ensure that ONLY the vial for IV use is selected.
***PREPARE* Direct:** If the IV injection does not exceed 100 mg, it is administered undiluted. **IV Infusion:** Dilute in 250–1000 mL of NS.
***ADMINISTER* Direct:** Give 50 mg (1 mL) or fraction thereof over 60 sec or longer. Do not give IV push. **IV Infusion:** Give test dose of 25 mg (0.5 mL) over 5 min. If no adverse reactions occur after 1 h, infuse remainder of calculated dose over 1–8 h. After infusion is completed, flush vein with 10 mL of NS. Have patient remain in bed for at least 30 min after IV administration to prevent orthostatic hypotension. Monitor BP and pulse.

ADVERSE EFFECTS Body as a Whole: Hypersensitivity (urticaria, skin rash, allergic purpura, pruritus, fever, chills, dyspnea, arthralgia, myalgia; anaphylaxis). **CNS:** Headache, shivering, transient paresthesias, syncope, dizziness, coma, seizures. **CV:** *Peripheral vascular flushing (rapid IV), hypotension,* precordial pain or pressure sensation, tachycardia, fatal cardiac arrhythmias, circulatory collapse. **GI:** Nausea, vomiting, transient loss of taste perception, metallic taste, diarrhea, melena, abdominal pain, hemorrhagic gastritis, intestinal necrosis, hepatic damage. **Skin:** Sterile abscess and brown skin discoloration (IM site), local phlebitis (IV site), lymphadenopathy, *pain at IM injection site.* **Metabolic:** Hemosiderosis, metabolic acidosis, hyperglycemia, reactivation of quiescent rheumatoid

---

arthritis, exogenous hemosiderosis. **Hematologic:** Bleeding disorder with severe toxicity.

DIAGNOSTIC TEST INTERFERENCE Falsely elevated *serum bilirubin* and falsely decreased *serum calcium* values may occur. Large doses of iron dextran may impart a brown color to serum drawn 4 h after iron administration. *Bone scans* involving Tc-99m diphosphonate have shown dense areas of activity along contour of iliac crest 1–6 days after IM injections of iron dextran.

INTERACTIONS May decrease absorption of oral **iron, chloramphenicol** may decrease effectiveness of iron, a toxic complex may form with **dimercaprol.**

PHARMACOKINETICS Absorption: 60% absorbed from IM site by 3 days; 90% absorbed by 1–3 wk. **Distribution:** Crosses placenta; distributed into breast milk. **Metabolism:** Metabolized in reticuloendothelial system. **Half-Life:** 6 h.

NURSING IMPLICATIONS

Assessment & Drug Effects
- Oral iron is preferred whenever possible due to side effects of injectable forms.
- Monitor for therapeutic effectiveness: Anticipated response to parenteral iron therapy is an average weekly hemoglobin rise of about 1 g/day. Peak levels are generally reached in about 4–8 wk.
- Note: Systemic reactions may occur over 24 h after parenteral iron has been administered. Large IV dose are associated with increased frequency of adverse effects.
- Lab tests: Periodic determinations of Hgb and Hct, and reticulocyte count should be made.

Patient & Family Education
- Do not take oral iron preparations when receiving iron injections.
- Eat foods high in iron and vitamin C.
- Notify physician of any of the following: Backache or muscle ache, chills, dizziness, fever, headache, nausea or vomiting, paresthesias, pain or redness at injection site, skin rash or hives, or difficulty breathing.
- Do not breast feed while taking this drug without consulting physician.

ISOETHARINE HYDROCHLORIDE
(eye-soe-eth′a-reen)
Arm-a-Med Isoetharine, Beta-2, Bronkosol, Dey-Lute, Dispos-a-Med Isoetharine
Classifications: AUTONOMIC NERVOUS SYSTEM AGENT; BETA-ADRENERGIC AGONIST (SYMPATHOMIMETIC); BRONCHODILATOR
Prototype: Albuterol
Pregnancy Category: C

AVAILABILITY 1% solution

ACTIONS Synthetic sympathomimetic stimulant with relatively rapid onset and long duration of action. Has selective affinity for beta$_2$ adrenoreceptors on bronchial and selected arteriolar musculature.
THERAPEUTIC EFFECTS Relieves reversible bronchospasm and by bronchodilation facilitates expectoration of pulmonary secretions. Increases vital capacity and decreases airway resistance.

USES Bronchial asthma and reversible bronchospasm occurring with bronchitis and emphysema.

CONTRAINDICATIONS Known hypersensitivity to sympathomimetic amines and to bisulfites; concomitant use with epinephrine or other sympathomimetic amines; patients with preexisting cardiac arrhythmias associated with tachycardia. Use during pregnancy (category C) or lactation requires judgment of risk/benefit ratio.
CAUTIOUS USE Older adults; hypertension; acute coronary artery disease; CHF; cardiac asthma; hyperthyroidism, diabetes mellitus; tuberculosis; history of seizures.

ROUTE & DOSAGE

Bronchospasm

Child: **Inhalation** 0.01 mL/kg of 1% solution (max 0.5 mL) diluted in 2–3 mL normal saline
Adult: **Inhalation** 0.5–1 mL 0.5% or 0.5 mL 1% solution diluted 1:3 with normal saline *or* 2–4 mL 0.125% solution undiluted *or* 2–5 mL 0.2% solution undiluted *or* 2 mL 0.25% solution undiluted per nebulizer q4h (max 5 times/day); 1–2 inhalations from an MDI q4h up to 5 times/day

STORAGE
Store at 15°–30° C (59°–86° F).

ADMINISTRATION
Inhalation
- Give on arising in morning and before meals to reduce fatigue from activity by improving lung ventilation.
- Wait 1 full min after initial 1 or 2 inhalations (Bronkometer) to be sure of necessity for another dose. Action should begin immediately and peak within 5–15 min.
- Alternate therapy with concurrent epinephrine administration, but do not administer simultaneously because of danger of excessively rapid heartbeat.
- Do not use discolored or precipitated solutions.
- Protect solutions from light, freezing, and heat.

ADVERSE EFFECTS CV: *Tachycardia, palpitations,* changes in BP, cardiac arrest. **GI:** Nausea, vomiting. **CNS:** Headache, *anxiety,* tension, restlessness, insomnia, *tremor,* weakness, dizziness, excitement. **Respiratory:** Cough, bronchial irritation and edema; tachyphylaxis.

INTERACTIONS Drug: Epinephrine, other SYMPATHOMIMETIC BRONCHODILATORS possibly have additive effects; MAO INHIBITORS, TRICYCLIC ANTIDEPRESSANTS potentiate action on vascular system; effects of both BETA-ADRENERGIC BLOCK-ERS and isoetharine antagonized when given together.

PHARMACOKINETICS Onset: Immediate. **Peak effect:** 5–15 min. **Duration:** 1–4 h. **Metabolism:** Metabolized in lungs, liver, GI tract, and other tissues. **Elimination:** Excreted by kidneys.

NURSING IMPLICATIONS

Assessment & Drug Effects
- Do not use this product if patient has a history of allergy to sulfite agents. The preservative sodium bisulfite is in the hydrochloride formulation.
- Monitor cardiac status and report tachycardia and palpitations.

Patient & Family Education
- Close eyes when actuating the nebulizer.
- Use inhalation therapy according to prescribed regimen. Overuse may decrease desired effect and cause symptoms including tachycardia, palpitations, headache, nausea, dizziness.
- Read information and instructions furnished with the aerosol form of isoetharine.
- Increase daily fluid intake to aid in liquefaction of bronchial secretions.
- Discontinue drug and notify prescriber if a sudden increase in dyspnea occurs.
- Do not discard drug applicator.
- Refill units are available.
- Work with school personnel to arrange child access to drug during school hours.
- Do not breast feed while taking this drug without consulting prescriber.
- Store this medication out of reach of children.

ISONIAZID (ISONICOTINIC ACID HYDRAZIDE) ⊙
(eye-soe-nye′a-zid)
INH, Isotamine ♦, Laniazid, Nydrazid, PMS Isoniazid ♦, Teebaconin
Classifications: ANTI-INFECTIVE; ANTITUBERCULOSIS AGENT
Pregnancy Category: C

AVAILABILITY 50 mg, 100 mg, 300 mg tablets; 50 mg/5 mL syrup; 100 mg/mL injection

ACTIONS Hydrazide of isonicotinic acid with highly specific action against *Mycobacterium tuberculosis*. Postulated to act by interfering with biosynthesis of bacterial proteins, nucleic acid, and lipids.

THERAPEUTIC EFFECTS Exerts bacteriostatic action against actively growing tubercle bacilli; may be bactericidal in higher concentrations.

USES Treatment of all forms of active tuberculosis caused by susceptible organisms and as preventive in high-risk persons (e.g., household members, persons with positive tuberculin skin test reactions). May be used alone or with other tuberculostatic agents.

UNLABELED USES Treatment of atypical mycobacterial infections; tuberculous meningitis; action tremor in multiple sclerosis.

CONTRAINDICATIONS History of isoniazid-associated hypersensitivity reactions, including hepatic injury; acute liver damage of any etiology; pregnancy (category C) unless risk is warranted.

CAUTIOUS USE Chronic liver disease; renal dysfunction; history of convulsive disorders; chronic alcoholism; persons over 35 y; lactation.

ROUTE & DOSAGE

Treatment of Active Tuberculosis
Child: **PO** 10–15 mg/kg/day or 20–30 mg/kg given 2 times/wk (max 900 mg dose; max 300–500 mg/day)
Adult: **PO** 5–10 mg/kg/day or 15 mg/kg given 2 times/wk (max 900 mg dose; max 300 mg/day)

Preventive Therapy
Child: **PO** 10 mg/kg up to 300 mg/day or 15 mg/kg 3 times/wk or 20–40 mg/kg 2 times/wk (max 900 mg dose)
Adult: **PO** 300 mg/day. Same doses may be given only, if oral therapy is not possible.

STORAGE
Store in tightly closed, light-resistant containers.

ADMINISTRATION

Oral
- Give on an empty stomach at least 1 h before or 2 h after meals. If GI irritation occurs, drug may be taken with meals.
- Administered with rifampin in most cases. Supplemental pyridoxine is recommended at 1–2 mg/kg/day.

Intramuscular
- Note: Isoniazid solution for IM injection tends to crystallize at low temperatures; if this occurs, solution should be allowed to warm to room temperature to redissolve crystals before use. This route is not preferred.
- Give deep into a large muscle mass appropriate for age. (see Part I) and rotate injection sites; local transient pain may follow IM injections.

ADVERSE EFFECTS Body as a Whole: Drug-related fever, rheumatic and lupus erythematosus-like syndromes, irritation at injection site; hypersensitivity (fever, chills, skin eruption, vasculitis). **CNS:** *Paresthesias, peripheral neuropathy,* headache, unusual tiredness or weakness, tinnitus, dizziness, hallucinations. **Special Senses:** Blurred vision, visual disturbances, optic neuritis, atrophy. **GI:** Nausea, vomiting, epigastric distress, dry mouth, constipation; hepatotoxicity (*elevated AST, ALT;* bilirubinemia, jaundice, <u>hepatitis</u>). **Hematologic:** Agranulocytosis, hemolytic or <u>aplastic anemia</u>, thrombocytopenia, eosinophilia, methemoglobinemia. **Metabolic:** Decreased vitamin B_{12} absorption, pyridoxine (vitamin B_6) deficiency, pellagra, gynecomastia, hyperglycemia, glycosuria, hyperkalemia, hypophosphatemia, hypocalcemia, acetonuria, metabolic acidosis, proteinuria. **Other:** Dyspnea, urinary retention (males).

DIAGNOSTIC TEST INTERFERENCE Isoniazid may produce false-positive results using **copper sulfate tests** (e.g., **Benedict's solution, Clinitest**) but not with **glucose oxidase methods** (e.g., **Clinistix, Dextrostix, TesTape**).

INTERACTIONS Drug: Cycloserine, ethionamide enhance CNS toxicity; may increase **phenytoin** levels, resulting in toxicity; ALUMINUM-CONTAINING ANTACIDS decrease GI absorption; **disulfiram** may cause coordination difficulties or psychotic reactions; **alcohol** increases risk of hepatotoxicity. **Food:** Food decreases rate and extent of isoniazid absorption; should be taken 1 h before meals.

PHARMACOKINETICS Absorption: Readily absorbed from GI tract; food may reduce rate and extent of absorption. **Peak:** 1–2 h. **Distribution:** Distributed to all body tissues and fluids including the CNS; crosses placenta. **Metabolism:** Inactivated by acetylation in liver. **Elimination:** 75–96% excreted in urine in 24 h; excreted in breast milk. **Half-Life:** 1–4 h.

NURSING IMPLICATIONS

Assessment & Drug Effects

- Arrange home visit if possible to gather data on family and obtain skin test results.
- Monitor for therapeutic effectiveness: Evident within the first 2–3 wk of therapy. More than 90% of patients receiving optimal therapy have negative sputum by the sixth month.
- Perform appropriate susceptibility tests before initiation of therapy and periodically thereafter to detect possible bacterial resistance.
- Lab tests: Monitor hepatic function periodically. Isoniazid hepatitis (sometimes fatal) usually develops during the first 3–6 mo of treatment, but may occur at any time during therapy; especially in those who ingest alcohol daily.
- Monitor for visual disturbance. An eye examination may be warranted.
- Note: Inactivation of the drug is genetically determined. Slow inactivation leads to high plasma drug levels and increased risk of toxicity.
- Isoniazid-induced pyridoxine (vitamin B_6) depletion causes neurotoxic effects. B_6 supplementation (10–50 mg day for adults) usually accompanies isoniazid use.
- Peripheral neuritis, the most common toxic effect, is usually preceded by paresthesias of feet and hands (numbness, tingling, burning). Patients particularly susceptible include alcoholics and patients with liver disease, malnourished patients, diabetics, slow inactivators, pregnant women.
- Monitor BP during period of dosage adjustment. Some experience orthostatic hypotension; therefore, caution against rapid positional changes.
- Monitor diabetics for loss of glycemic control.
- Check weight at least twice weekly under standard conditions.

Patient & Family Education

- Note: Eating tyramine-containing foods (e.g., aged cheeses, smoked fish) may cause palpitation, flushing, and blood pressure elevation. Histamine-containing foods (e.g., skipjack, tuna, sauerkraut juice, yeast extracts) may cause exaggerated drug response (headache, hypotension, palpitation, sweating, itching, flushing, diarrhea).

- Withhold medication and notify physician if S&S of hepatotoxicity develop (e.g., dark urine, jaundice, clay-colored stools).
- Avoid or at least reduce alcohol intake while on isoniazid therapy because of increased risk of hepatotoxicity.
- Withhold all drugs and notify physician of hypersensitivity reaction immediately; generally occurs within 3–7 wk after initiation of therapy.
- Do not breast feed while taking this drug without consulting physician.
- Store this medication out of reach of children.

ISOPROTERENOL HYDROCHLORIDE

(eye-soe-proe-ter′e-nole)

Dispos-a-Med, Isoproterenol, Isuprel

ISOPROTERENOL SULFATE

Medihaler-Iso

Classifications: AUTONOMIC NERVOUS SYSTEM AGENT; BETA-ADRENERGIC AGONIST (SYMPATHOMIMETIC); BRONCHODILATOR

Prototype: Albuterol

Pregnancy Category: C

AVAILABILITY Isoproterenol HCl 0.5%, 1% solution for inhalation; 103 mcg aerosol; 0.2 mg/mL, 0.02 mg/mL injection **Isoproterenol Sulfate** 80 mcg aerosol

ACTIONS Synthetic sympathomimetic amine. Acts directly on beta$_1$-adrenergic receptors with little or no effect on alpha-adrenoceptors. Drug-induced stimulation of beta$_1$-adrenergic receptors results in increased cardiac output and cardiac work by increasing strength of contraction and, to a slight degree, rate of contraction of the heart. Produces slight increase in systolic BP and decrease in diastolic pressure.

THERAPEUTIC EFFECTS Reduces total peripheral resistance and increases venous return to the heart by mobilizing blood from vascular reservoirs and increases cardiac contractions. Stimulation of beta$_2$-adrenoceptors relaxes bronchospasm and, by increasing ciliary motion, facilitates expectoration of pulmonary secretions. May dilate trachea and main bronchi past the resting diameter.

USES Bronchodilator in treatment of bronchial asthma and reversible bronchospasm induced by anesthesia. Also used as cardiac stimulant in cardiac arrest, carotid sinus hypersensitivity, cardiogenic and bacteremic shock, Adams-Stokes syndrome, or ventricular arrhythmias. Used in treatment of shock that persists after replacement of blood volume.

UNLABELED USES Treatment of status asthmaticus in children.

CONTRAINDICATIONS Preexisting cardiac arrhythmias associated with tachycardia; tachycardia caused by digitalis intoxication, central hyperexcitability, cardiogenic shock secondary to coronary artery occlusion and MI; simultaneous administration with epinephrine. Safe use during pregnancy (category C) or lactation is not established.

ISOPROTERENOL HYDROCHLORIDE

CAUTIOUS USE Sensitivity to sympathomimetic amines; debilitated patients, hypertension, coronary insufficiency and other cardiovascular disorders, renal dysfunction, hyperthyroidism, diabetes, glaucoma, tuberculosis, during anesthesia by cyclopropane.

ROUTE & DOSAGE

Bronchospasms

Child/Adult: **MDI** 1–2 inhalations 4–6 times/day (max 6 inhalations in any hour during a 24 h period). **Compressed Air or IPPB** 0.5 mL of 0.5% solution diluted to 2–2.5 mL with water or saline over 10–20 min up to 5 times/day
Adult: **IV** 0.01–0.02 mg prn

Cardiac Arrhythmias/Cardiac Resuscitation

Child: **IV** 2.5 mcg/min *or* 0.1–2 mcg/kg/min by continuous infusion
Adult: **IV** 0.02–0.06 mg bolus, followed by 5 mcg/min infusion
SC 0.15–0.2 mg prn

STORAGE
Store all formulations in tightly covered, light-resistant containers.

ADMINISTRATION

MDI
- Shake MDI thoroughly to activate.
- Breathe out through nose expelling as much air from lungs as possible.
- Close lips and teeth around open end of mouthpiece placed well into mouth aimed at back of throat.
- Inhale deeply while pressing down on canister to activate spray mechanism.
- Try to hold breath for 10 sec; then slowly exhale through nose or pursed lips. Spacers may be used in children.
- Wait 2 full min before starting a second inhalation, if it is necessary (see Part I).

IPPB
- Follow IPPB manufacturer's instructions.
- Have patient sit erect in chair or, if not able, lie in semi-Fowler's position.
- Instruct patient to ALLOW MACHINE TO DO THE WORK (deliver medication into air passages and breathe for the patient).
- Rinse mouth immediately after inhalation therapy to prevent dryness and throat irritation.

Intravenous

PREPARE Direct: Dilute 1 mL of 1:5000 solution with 9 mL NS or D5W to produce a 1:50,000 (0.02 mg/mL) solution. **IV Infusion:** Dilute 10 mL of 1:5000 solution in 500 mL D5W to produce a 1:250,000 (4 mcg/mL) solution.
ADMINISTER Direct: Give each 1 mL of 1:50,000 solution over 1 min. Flush with 15–20 mL NS. **IV Infusion:** Infusion rate is generally decreased or infusion may be temporarily discontinued if heart rate exceeds 110 bpm (verify excess rate for child), because of the danger of precipitating

arrhythmias. Microdrip or constant-infusion pump is recommended to prevent sudden influx of large amounts of drug. IV administration is regulated by continuous ECG monitoring. Patient must be observed and response to therapy must be monitored continuously.

INCOMPATIBILITIES **Solution/Additive:** Sodium bicarbonate, **aminophylline.** Isoproterenol solutions lose potency with standing. Discard if precipitate or discoloration is present.

ADVERSE EFFECTS CNS: Headache, mild tremors, nervousness, anxiety, insomnia, excitement, fatigue. **CV:** Flushing, palpitations, tachycardia, unstable BP, anginal pain, <u>ventricular arrhythmias</u>. **GI:** Swelling of parotids (prolonged use), bad taste, buccal ulcerations (sublingual administration), nausea. **Other:** Severe prolonged asthma attack, sweating, bronchial irritation and edema. **Acute Poisoning:** Overdosage, especially after excessive use of aerosols (*tachycardia,* palpitations, nervousness, nausea, vomiting).

INTERACTIONS Drug: Epinephrine and other SYMPATHOMIMETIC AMINES increase effects and cause cardiac toxicity. HALOGENATED GENERAL ANESTHETICS exacerbate arrhythmias, whereas BETA-BLOCKERS antagonize effects.

PHARMACOKINETICS Absorption: Rapidly absorbed from oral inhalation or parenteral administration. **Onset:** Immediate. **Duration:** 1 h oral inhalation; 2 h SC. **Metabolism:** Action terminated by tissue uptake and metabolized by COMT in liver, lungs, and other tissues. **Elimination:** 40–50% excreted in urine unchanged.

NURSING IMPLICATIONS

Assessment & Drug Effects

- Check pulse before and during IV administration. Rate >110 for adults usually indicates need to slow infusion rate or discontinue infusion (verify upper limit of allowed child pulse rate). Consult prescriber for guidelines. Incidence of arrhythmias is high, particularly when drug is administered IV to patients with cardiogenic shock or ischemic heart disease, digitalized patients, or to those with electrolyte imbalance.
- Note: Tolerance to bronchodilating effect and cardiac stimulant effect may develop with prolonged use.
- Discontinue drug if parotid swelling occurs; has been reported after prolonged use.
- Note: Once tolerance has developed, continued use can result in serious adverse effects including rebound bronchospasm.

Patient & Family Education

- Take medication as prescribed; (i.e., do not increase, decrease, or omit doses or change intervals between doses). Notify prescriber if treatment fails to give satisfactory relief.
- Child and parents should be informed about adverse effects and report onset of such reactions to prescriber.
- Be aware that saliva and sputum may appear pink after inhalation treatment.
- Work with school to arrange child's access to medication during school hours.

- Do not breast feed while taking this drug without consulting prescriber.
- Store this medication out of reach of children.

ISOTRETINOIN (13-*cis*-RETINOIC ACID) ⓟ
(eye-soe-tret'i-noyn)
Accutane, Claravis
Classifications: SKIN AND MUCOUS MEMBRANE AGENT; ANTIACNE; RETINOID
Pregnancy Category: X

AVAILABILITY 10 mg, 20 mg, 40 mg capsules

ACTIONS Highly toxic metabolite of retinol (vitamin A). Principal actions: Regulation of cell (e.g., epithelial) differentiation and proliferation and of altered lipid composition on skin surface.
THERAPEUTIC EFFECTS Decreases sebum secretion by reducing sebaceous gland size; inhibits gland cell differentiation; blocks follicular keratinization. Has antiacne properties and may be used as a chemotherapeutic agent for epithelial carcinomas

USES Treatment of severe recalcitrant cystic or conglobate acne in patient unresponsive to conventional treatment, including systemic antibiotics.
UNLABELED USES Lamellar ichthyosis, oral leukoplakia, hyperkeratosis, acne rosacea, scarring gram negative folliculitis; adjuvant therapy of basal cell carcinoma of lung and cutaneous T-cell lymphoma (mycosis fungoides); psoriasis; chemoprevention for prostate cancer.

CONTRAINDICATIONS Pregnancy (category X); sensitivity to parabens (preservatives in the formulation), lactation.
CAUTIOUS USE Coronary artery disease; diabetes mellitus; obesity; alcoholism; rheumatologic disorders; history of pancreatitis, hepatitis; retinal disease; elevated triglycerides.

ROUTE & DOSAGE

Cystic Acne
Adult: **PO** 0.5–1 mg/kg/day in 2 divided doses (max recommended dose, 2 mg/kg/day)
Disorders of Keratinization
Adult: **PO** up to 4 mg/kg/day in divided doses

STORAGE
Store in tight, light-resistant container. Capsules remain stable for 2 y.

ADMINISTRATION
Oral
- Give with or shortly after meals.
- Reassess regimen after 2 wk of treatment and dose adjusted as warranted.

■ Note: A single course of therapy provides adequate control in many patients. If a second course is necessary, it is delayed at least 8 wk because improvement may continue without the drug.

ADVERSE EFFECTS Body as a Whole: Most are dose-related (i.e., occurring at doses >1 mg/kg/day), reversible with termination of therapy. **CNS:** Lethargy, headache, fatigue, visual disturbances, pseudotumor cerebri, paresthesias, dizziness, depression, psychosis, <u>suicide</u> (rare). **Special Senses:** Reduced night vision, dry eyes, papilledema, eye irritation, *conjunctivitis,* corneal opacities. **GI:** *Dry mouth,* anorexia, nausea, vomiting, abdominal pain, nonspecific GI symptoms, <u>acute hepatotoxic reactions</u> (rare), inflammation and bleeding of gums, increased AST, ALT, acute pancreatitis. **Hematologic:** Decreased Hct, Hgb, elevated sedimentation rate. **Musculoskeletal:** Arthralgia; bone, joint, and muscle pain and stiffness; chest pain, skeletal hyperostosis (especially in athletic people and with prolonged therapy), mild bruising. **Skin:** *Cheilitis,* skin fragility, dry skin, pruritus, peeling of face, palms, and soles; photosensitivity (photoallergic and phototoxic), erythema, skin infections, petechiae, rash, urticaria, exaggerated healing response (painful exuberant granulation tissue with crusting), brittle nails, thinning hair. **Respiratory:** Epistaxis, *dry nose.* **Metabolic:** Hyperuricemia, *increased serum concentrations of triglycerides by 50–70%,* serum cholesterol by 15–20%, VLDL cholesterol by 50–60%, LDL cholesterol by 15–20%.

INTERACTION Drug: VITAMIN A SUPPLEMENTS increase toxicity.

PHARMACOKINETICS Absorption: Rapid absorption after slow dissolution in GI tract; 25% of administered drug reaches systemic circulation. **Peak:** 3.2 h. **Distribution:** Not fully understood; appears in liver, ureters, adrenals, ovaries and lacrimal glands. **Metabolism:** Metabolized in liver; enterohepatically cycled. **Elimination:** Excreted in urine and feces in equal amounts. **Half-Life:** 10–20 h.

NURSING IMPLICATIONS

Assessment & Drug Effects

■ Lab tests: Determine baseline blood lipids at outset of treatment, then at 2 wk, 1 mo, and every month thereafter throughout course of therapy; liver function tests at 2- or 3-wk intervals for 6 mo and once a month thereafter during treatment. Rule out pregnancy.
■ Report signs of liver dysfunction (jaundice, pruritus, dark urine) promptly.
■ Monitor closely for loss of glycemic control in diabetic and diabetic prone patients.
■ Be certain that adolescent females understand that they must not get pregnant while on this drug. Offer access to birth control if desired.
■ Note: Persistence of hypertriglyceridemia (levels above 500–800 mg/dL) despite a reduced dose indicates necessity to stop drug to prevent onset of acute pancreatitis.

Patient & Family Education

■ Maintain drug regimen even if during the first few weeks transient exacerbations of acne occur. Recurring symptoms may signify response of deep unseen lesions.

- Discontinue medication at once and notify prescriber to rule out benign intracranial hypertension if visual disturbances occur along with nausea, vomiting, and headache.
- Note: Visual disturbances may also signify development of corneal opacities, which should be ruled out by ophthalmic examination. Discontinue drug if corneal opacities are present. Return for a follow-up examination.
- Rule out pregnancy within 2 wk of starting treatment. Use a reliable contraceptive 1 mo before, throughout, and 1 mo after therapy is discontinued.
- Reduce weight and restrict alcohol and dietary fat intake as prophylactic measures against development of hypertriglyceridemia.
- Do not self-medicate with multivitamins, which usually contain vitamin A. Toxicity of isotretinoin is enhanced by vitamin A supplements.
- Avoid or minimize exposure of the treated skin to sun or sunlamps. Photosensitivity (photoallergic and phototoxic) potential is high; risk of skin cancer may be increased by this drug.
- Notify prescriber of abdominal pain, rectal bleeding, or severe diarrhea, which are possible symptoms of drug-induced inflammatory bowel disease. Drug treatment will be discontinued.
- Keep lips moist and softened (use thin layer of lubricant such as petroleum jelly); dry mouth and cheilitis (inflamed, chapped lips), frequent adverse effects of isotretinoin, are distressing and are potential preconditions to infections.
- Notify prescriber of joint pain, such as pain in the great toe (symptom of gout and hyperuricemia).
- Do not share drug with friend(s) because it is associated with adverse effects that necessitate medical supervision.
- Do not breast feed while taking this drug.
- Store this medication out of reach of children.

ITRACONAZOLE

(i-tra-con′a-zole)
Sporanox
Classifications: ANTI-INFECTIVE; ANTIBIOTIC; ANTIFUNGAL
Prototype: Fluconazole
Pregnancy Category: C

AVAILABILITY 100 mg capsules; 10 mg/mL oral solution; 10 mg/mL injection

ACTIONS Synthetic antifungal agent active against many fungi, including yeast and dermatophytes.
THERAPEUTIC EFFECTS Antifungal spectrum of activity is similar to fluconazole.

USES Treatment of systemic fungal infections caused by blastomycosis, histoplasmosis, aspergillosis, onychomycosis due to dermatophytes of the toenail with or without fingernail involvement; oropharyngeal and esophageal candidiasis; orally to treat superficial mycoses (*Candida*, pityriasis versicolor). IV for treatment of blastomycosis, histoplasmosis, and aspergillosis.
UNLABELED USES Systemic and vaginal candidiasis.

CONTRAINDICATIONS Coadministration of terfenadine, astemizole, cisapride; hypersensitivity to itraconazole; lactation.

CAUTIOUS USE Hypersensitivity to other azole antifungal agents, hepatitis, HIV infection, pregnancy (category C). Safety and efficacy in children are not established.

ROUTE & DOSAGE

Pulmonary and Extrapulmonary Blastomycosis, Nonmeningeal Histoplasmosis
Child: **PO** 3–5 mg/kg/day for 3–6 mo
Adult: **PO** 200 mg once daily (increase to max: 200 mg b.i.d. if no apparent improvement) Continue for at least 3 mo; for life-threatening infections, start with 200 mg t.i.d. for 3 days, then 200–400 mg/day **IV** 200 mg b.i.d. infused over 1 h for 4 doses, then 200 mg daily

Oropharyngeal Candidiasis
Adult: **PO** 200 mg daily for 1–2 wk

Esophageal Candidiasis
Adult: **PO** 100 mg daily for at least 3 wk (max 200 mg/day)

Vaginal Candidiasis
Adult: **PO** 200 mg daily for 3 days

Onychomycosis
Adult: **PO** 200 mg daily for 3 mo

STORAGE
Store liquid at or below 25° C (77° F).

ADMINISTRATION

Oral
- Give capsules with a full meal.
- Give oral solution without food. Liquid should be vigorously swished for several seconds and swallowed.
- Do not interchange oral solution and capsules.
- Divide dosages greater than 200 mg/day into 2–3 doses.

Intravenous

***PREPARE* Intermittent:** Withdraw 25 mL from the ampule and add to infusion bag provided (contains 50 mL of NS). Mix gently to disperse evenly. IV solution contains 3.33 mg/mL.

***ADMINISTER* Intermittent:** Use a flow control device and the infusion set provided to infuse 60 mL (200 mg) of the diluted solution over 60 min. Stop the infusion and flush set with 15–20 mL NS over 1–15 min via the 2-way stopcock. Then discard the entire infusion set.

***INCOMPATIBILITIES* Solution/Additive or Y-Site:** Do not mix with any other drugs or infuse other drugs concomitantly through the same line.

ADVERSE EFFECTS CV: Hypertension with higher doses. **CNS:** Headache, dizziness, fatigue, somnolence (euphoria, drowsiness <1%). **Endocrine:** Gynecomastia, hypokalemia (especially with higher doses), hypertriglyceridemia. **GI:** *Nausea, vomiting, dyspepsia, abdominal pain, diarrhea, anorexia, flatulence, gastritis;* elevations of serum transaminases, alkaline

---

Common adverse effects in *italic;* life-threatening effects <u>underlined</u>; generic names in **bold;** drug classifications in SMALL CAPS; ♣ Canadian drug name; ✪ Prototype drug.

phosphatase, and bilirubin. **Urogenital:** Decreased libido, impotence. **Skin:** Rash, pruritus. **Acute Poisoning:** Severe toxicity (doses exceeding 400 mg daily have been associated with higher risk of hypokalemia, hypertension, adrenal insufficiency).

INTERACTIONS Drug: Itraconazole may increase levels and toxicity of ORAL HYPOGLYCEMIC AGENTS **warfarin, terfenadine, ritonavir, indinavir, vinca alkaloids, busulfan, midazolam, triazolam, diazepam, nifedipine, nicardipine, amlodipine, felodipine, lovastatin, simvastatin, cyclosporine, tacrolimus, methylprednisolone, digoxin.** Combination with **astemizole, cisapride, pimozide, quinidine** may cause severe cardiac events including cardiac arrest or sudden death. Itraconazole levels are decreased by **carbamazepine, phenytoin, phenobarbital, isoniazid, rifabutin, rifampin.**

PHARMACOKINETICS Absorption: Well absorbed from GI tract when taken with food. **Onset:** 2 wk–3 mo. **Peak:** Peak levels at 1.5–5 h. Steady-state concentrations reached in 10–14 days. **Distribution:** Highly protein bound, minimal concentrations in CSF. Higher concentrations in tissues than in plasma. **Metabolism:** Extensively metabolized in liver by CYP3A4, may undergo enterohepatic recirculation. **Elimination:** 35% in urine, 55% excreted in feces. **Half-Life:** 34–42 h.

NURSING IMPLICATIONS

Assessment & Drug Effects

- Lab tests: C&S tests should be done before initiation of therapy. Drug may be started pending results. Monitor hepatic functions especially in those with preexisting hepatic abnormalities.
- Monitor for digoxin toxicity when given concurrently with digoxin.
- Monitor PT and INR carefully when given concurrently with warfarin.
- Monitor for S&S of hypersensitivity (see Appendix D-1); discontinue drug and notify prescriber if noted.

Patient & Family Education

- Take capsules, but NOT oral solution, with food.
- Notify prescriber promptly for S&S of liver dysfunction, including anorexia, nausea, and vomiting; weakness and fatigue; dark urine and clay-colored stool.
- Note: Risk of hypoglycemia may increase in diabetics on oral hypoglycemic agents.
- Do not breast feed while taking this drug.
- Store this medication out of reach of children.

IVERMECTIN

(i-ver-mec′tin)
Stromectol
Classifications: ANTI-INFECTIVE; ANTHELMINTIC
Prototype: Mebendazole
Pregnancy Category: C

AVAILABILITY 6 mg tablets

ACTIONS A semisynthetic anthelmintic agent that is a broad-spectrum antiparasitic agent with a unique mode of action. It leads to an increase in the permeability to chloride ions of the cell membrane of the parasites, resulting in hyperpolarization of the nerve or muscle cell.

THERAPEUTIC EFFECTS Hyperpolarization of nerve and muscle cells of the parasites results in its paralysis and death.

USES Treatment of strongyloidiasis of the intestinal tract, onchocerciasis.

CONTRAINDICATIONS Hypersensitivity to ivermectin.
CAUTIOUS USE Pregnancy (category C), lactation. Safety and efficacy in children ≤15 kg are not established.

ROUTE & DOSAGE

Strongyloides
Child/Adult: **PO** ≥*15 kg,* 200 mcg/kg times 1 dose (supplied as 6 mg tablets)

Onchocerciasis
Child/Adult: **PO** ≥*15 kg,* 150 mcg/kg times 1 dose, may repeat q3–12mo prn

STORAGE
Store below 30° C (86° F).

ADMINISTRATION

Oral
- Give tablets with water rather than any other type of liquid.

ADVERSE EFFECTS Body as a Whole: *Fever,* peripheral edema. **CNS:** Dizziness. **CV:** Tachycardia. **GI:** Diarrhea, nausea. **Skin:** *Pruritus, rash.* **Other:** Arthralgia/synovitis, lymphadenopathy.

INTERACTIONS No clinically significant interactions established.

PHARMACOKINETICS Peak: 4 h. **Distribution:** Distributed into breast milk. **Metabolism:** Metabolized in the liver. **Elimination:** Excreted in feces over 12 days. **Half-Life:** 16 h.

NURSING IMPLICATIONS

Assessment & Drug Effects
- Monitor for therapeutic effectiveness: Indicated by negative stool samples.
- Monitor for cardiovascular effects such as orthostatic hypotension and tachycardia.
- Monitor for and report inflammatory conditions of the eyes.

Patient & Family Education
- Get a follow-up stool examination to determine effectiveness of treatment. Treatment for worms does not kill adult parasites; repeated follow-up and retreatment are usually needed.
- Notify prescriber if eye discomfort develops.
- Do not breast feed while taking this drug without consulting physician.
- Store this medication out of reach of children.

KANAMYCIN
(kan-a-mye′sin)
Kantrex
Classifications: ANTI-INFECTIVE; ANTIBIOTIC; AMINOGLYCOSIDE
Prototype: Gentamicin
Pregnancy Category: D

AVAILABILITY 75 mg, 500 mg tablets, 1 g vials

ACTIONS Broad-spectrum, aminoglycoside antibiotic derived from *Streptomyces kanamyceticus.* Usually bactericidal in action.
THERAPEUTIC EFFECTS Active against many gram-negative microorganisms, especially *Acinetobacter, Escherichia coli, Enterobacter aerogenes, Klebsiella pneumoniae, Proteus* sp., and *Serratia marcescens.* Also effective against many strains of *Staphylococcus aureus,* but it is not the drug of choice. Inhibits growth of *Mycobacterium tuberculosis in vitro.*

USES Orally to reduce ammonia producing bacteria in intestinal tract, as adjunctive treatment of hepatic coma, and for preoperative bowel antisepsis; parenterally for short-term treatment of serious infections; intraperitoneally after fecal spill during surgery; as irrigation solution; and as aerosol treatment. In conjunction with other drugs to treat tuberculosis in patients resistant to conventional therapy.

CONTRAINDICATIONS History of hypersensitivity to kanamycin or other aminoglycosides; history of drug-induced ototoxicity, preexisting hearing loss, vertigo, or tinnitus; long-term therapy; PO use in intestinal obstruction or ulcerative bowel lesions; intraperitoneally to patients under effects of inhalation anesthetics or skeletal muscle relaxants. Safety during pregnancy (category D) or lactation is not established.
CAUTIOUS USE Impaired renal function; older adults, neonates, and infants (immature renal systems); myasthenia gravis.

ROUTE & DOSAGE

Preoperative Intestinal Antisepsis
Child: 150–250 mg/kg/day divided into doses given q6h (max 4 g/day)
Adult: **PO** 1 g q1h for 4 doses then q6h for 36–72 h

Hepatic Coma
Adult: **PO** 8–12 g/day in divided doses

Serious Infection
Newborn: birthweight <2 kg and <7 days of age, 15 mg/kg/day divided into 2 doses; birthweight ≤2 kg and ≥7 days of age, 22.5 mg/kg/day divided into 3 doses; birthweight >2 kg and <7 days of age, 20 mg /kg/day divided into 2 doses; birthweight >2 kg and >7 days of age, 30 mg/kg/day divided into 3 doses
Child/Adult: **IV/IM** 15–30 mg/kg/day in equally divided doses q8–12h

Common adverse effects in *italic;* life-threatening effects underlined; generic names in **bold;** drug classifications in SMALL CAPS; ✦ Canadian drug name; ● Prototype drug.

Adult: **Intraperitoneal** 500 mg diluted in 20 mL sterile water instilled through wound catheter **Inhalation** 250 mg diluted in 3 mL NS administered per nebulizer q6–12h **Irrigation** 0.25% solution prn

STORAGE

Store capsules at 15°–30° C (59°–86° F) unless otherwise directed. Store vials at 15°–30° C (59°–86° F) unless otherwise directed. Some vials may darken with time, but this does not affect potency. Discard partially used vials within 48 h.

ADMINISTRATION

Oral

■ Give on a full or empty stomach.

Intramuscular

■ Administer IM injection deep into muscle mass appropriate for child (see Part I) and for adults into upper outer quadrant of gluteal muscle (often painful).
■ Observe sites daily for signs of irritation; rotate injection sites.

Intravenous

PREPARE **Intermittent:** Dilute each 500 mg with at least 100 mL NS, D5W, D5/NS.
ADMINISTER **Intermittent:** Over 30–60 min.
INCOMPATIBILITIES **Solution/Additive: Cephalothin, cephapirin, chlorpheniramine, colistimethate, heparin, hydrocortisone, methohexital, ampicillin, carbenicillin, methicillin, penicillin, mezlocillin, piperacillin. Y-site: Heparin, methohexital.**

ADVERSE EFFECTS All: Dose related. **Body as a Whole:** Eosinophilia, maculopapular rash, pruritus, urticaria, drug fever, <u>anaphylaxis</u>. **CNS:** Dizziness, circumoral and other paresthesias, optic neuritis, peripheral neuritis, headache, restlessness, tremors, lethargy, convulsions; <u>neuromuscular paralysis, respiratory depression</u> (rarely). **Special Senses:** Deafness (can be irreversible), *tinnitus, vertigo* or *dizziness,* ataxia, nystagmus. **GI:** Nausea, vomiting, diarrhea, appetite changes, abdominal discomfort, stomatitis, proctitis, malabsorption syndrome (with prolonged oral administration). **Hematologic:** Anemia, increased or decreased reticulocytes, granulocytopenia, <u>agranulocytosis</u>, thrombocytopenia, purpura. **Urogenital:** <u>Nephrotoxicity</u>; hematuria, urine casts and cells, proteinuria; elevated serum creatinine and BUN. **Other:** Superinfections; local pain; nodular formation at injection site.

INTERACTIONS Drug: Amphotericin B, cisplatin, methoxyflurane, vancomycin add to nephrotoxicity; general anesthetics, skeletal muscle relaxants add to neuromuscular blocking effects; **capreomycin** compounds ototoxicity and nephrotoxicity; loop and thiazide diuretics may increase risk of ototoxicity.

PHARMACOKINETICS Absorption: Poorly absorbed from GI tract; readily absorbed from peritoneal cavity, bronchial tree, and wounds. **Peak:** 1–2 h. **Distribution:** Crosses placenta; distributed into breast milk. **Elimination:** 80–90% excreted in urine within 24 h. **Half-Life:** 2–4 h.

NURSING IMPLICATIONS

Assessment & Drug Effects

- Lab tests: Monitor baseline C&S, urinalysis, and kidney function prior to initiation of therapy and periodically thereafter. Monitor serum sodium, potassium, calcium, and magnesium.
- Monitor peak and trough serum kanamycin concentrations: ***Therapeutic serum levels*** are peak 15–30 mg/L and trough <5–10 mg/L. Draw peak 30–60 min after the 3rd IM dose or 30 min after IV infusion. Draw trough in 30 min before IM or IV dose.
- Notify physician immediately of signs of renal irritation: Albuminuria, casts, red and white cells in urine, increasing BUN, and serum creatinine, decreasing creatinine clearance, oliguria, and edema.
- Keep patient well hydrated to prevent chemical irritation of renal tubules.
- Monitor I&O. Report decrease in urine output or change in I&O ratio.
- Determine baseline weight and vital signs and monitor at regular intervals during therapy.
- Report signs of superinfection (see Appendix D-1).
- Monitor for hearing and balance problems; stop drug if ototoxicity occurs. Tinnitus is not a reliable index of ototoxicity. Risk of ototoxicity is high in patients with impaired renal function, children, poorly hydrated patients, and with therapy ≥5 days.
- Note: Deafness has occurred 2–7 days or more after termination of therapy in patients with impaired renal function.

Patient & Family Education

- Report ototoxic symptoms such as dizziness, hearing loss, weakness, or loss of balance; drug may need to be discontinued.
- Do not breast feed while taking this drug without consulting physician.
- Store this medication out of reach of children.

KAOLIN AND PECTIN

(kay'oh-lin and pek'tin)
Kao-Span, Kolain w/Pectin, K-C
Classifications: GASTROINTESTINAL AGENT; ANTIDIARRHEAL
Prototype: Diphenoxylate with atropine
Pregnancy Category: C

AVAILABILITY 5.2 g kaolin/260 mg pectin/30 mL, 90 g kaolin/2 g pectin/30 mL

ACTIONS Kaolin is hydrated aluminum silicate. Efficacy of kaolin or pectin in diarrhea is not clearly established.
THERAPEUTIC EFFECTS Kaolin is reported to have adsorbent, protectant, and demulcent properties. Mechanism of action of pectin may help consolidate stool.

USES Adjunct in symptomatic treatment of mild to moderately severe acute diarrhea. Commonly used in antidiarrheal combination products.

CONTRAINDICATIONS Suspected obstructive bowel lesion, pseudomembranous colitis, diarrhea associated with bacterial toxins; presence of fever;

K

use for more than 48 h without medical direction. Safety during pregnancy (category C), lactation, or in children <3 y is not established.

ROUTE & DOSAGE

Diarrhea

Child: **PO** *3–5 y,* 15–30 mL regular suspension or 15 mL concentrated suspension after each loose bowel movement; *6–11 y,* 30–60 mL regular suspension or 30 mL concentrated suspension after each loose bowel movement; *≥12 y,* 60 mL regular suspension or 45 mL concentrated suspension after each loose bowel movement
Adult: **PO** 60–120 mL of regular suspension or 45–90 mL of concentrated suspension after each loose bowel movement

STORAGE
Store in tightly closed container at 15°–30° C (59°–86° F) unless otherwise directed. Protect from freezing.

ADMINISTRATION
- Administer at least 2–4 h before other oral medications.
- Shake suspension well before pouring.

ADVERSE EFFECTS GI: Constipation usually mild and transient.

INTERACTIONS Drug: Chloroquine, digoxin, penicillamine, tetracycline, ciprofloxacin, and most other drugs.

PHARMACOKINETICS Absorption: Not absorbed from GI tract.

NURSING IMPLICATIONS

Assessment & Drug Effects
- Assess for abdominal distention and number of stools per day.
- Note: Fecal impaction may result from taking kaolin and pectin.
- Note: Drug may decrease absorption of any orally administered medication.

Patient & Family Education
- Do not exceed prescribed dosage.
- Notify prescriber if diarrhea is not controlled within 48 h or if fever develops.
- Not for use in children <3 y of age unless under supervision of health care professional.
- Do not breast feed while taking this drug without consulting physician.
- Store this medication out of reach of children.

KETOCONAZOLE
(ke-to-con′a-zol)
Nizoral, Nizoral A–D
Classifications: ANTI-INFECTIVE; ANTIBIOTIC; ANTIFUNGAL
Prototype: Fluconazole
Pregnancy Category: C

Common adverse effects in *italic;* life-threatening effects <u>underlined;</u> generic names in **bold;** drug classifications in SMALL CAPS; ♦ Canadian drug name; ● Prototype drug.

699

K

AVAILABILITY 200 mg tablets; 2% cream; 2% shampoo

ACTIONS Synthetic imidazole derivative and broad-spectrum antifungal agent closely related to miconazole. Studies suggest mode of action interferes with synthesis of ergosterol, which results in an increase in cell membrane permeability and ultimately inhibition of fungal growth.
THERAPEUTIC EFFECTS Usually fungistatic, but may be fungicidal in high concentrations.

USES Oral: Severe systemic fungal infections including candidiasis (e.g., oral thrush, candiduria), chronic mucocutaneous candidiasis, pulmonary and disseminated coccidioidomycosis, histoplasmosis, paracoccidioidomycosis, blastomycosis, and chromomycosis. **Topical:** Tinea corporis and tinea cruris (caused by *Epidermophyton floccosum, Trichophyton mentagrophytes,* and *Trichophyton rubrum*) and in treatment of tinea versicolor (pityriasis) caused by *Malassezia furfur (Pityrosporum obiculare),* seborrheic dermatitis.
UNLABELED USES Oral: Onychomycosis, vaginal candidiasis, Cushing's syndrome associated with adrenal or pituitary adenoma; precocious puberty, dysfunctional hirsutism, and as swish and swallow preparation for prophylaxis against fungal infections in patients with neutropenia induced by cancer chemotherapy and in patients with AIDS.

CONTRAINDICATIONS Hypersensitivity to ketoconazole or any component in the formulation; chronic alcoholism, fungal meningitis. Safety during pregnancy (category C), lactation, or in children <2 y is not established.
CAUTIOUS USE Achlorhydria, history of hepatic disease.

ROUTE & DOSAGE

Fungal Infections
Child: **PO** >2 y, 3.3–6.6 mg/kg/day as single dose
Adult: **PO** 200–400 mg once daily **Topical** Apply 1–2 times/day to affected area and surrounding skin

Dandruff
Child/Adult: **Topical** Shampoo twice a week for 4 wk with at least 3 days between shampoos

STORAGE
Store in tightly covered container at 15°–30° C (59°–86° F) unless otherwise directed.

ADMINISTRATION
Oral
- Give with water, fruit juice, coffee, or tea; drug requires an acid medium for dissolution and absorption.
- Relieve nausea and vomiting during early therapy by taking drug with food and dividing into 2 daily doses.
- Do not give with antacids.

Topical

- Apply sufficient shampoo to produce lather to wash scalp and hair and gently massage over entire scalp area for 1 min, rinse hair thoroughly, and repeat, leaving shampoo on scalp for 3 min. Rinse thoroughly.

ADVERSE EFFECTS Oral—Body as a Whole: Skin rash, erythema, urticaria, pruritus, angioedema, <u>anaphylaxis</u>. **GI:** *Nausea, vomiting,* anorexia, epigastric or abdominal pain, constipation, diarrhea, transient elevation in serum liver enzymes, <u>fatal hepatic necrosis</u> (rare). **Hematologic:** With high doses, lowers serum testosterone and ACTH-induced corticosteroid serum levels, transient decreases in serum cholesterol and triglycerides; hyponatremia (rare). **Urogenital:** Gynecomastia (males), breast pain; uterine bleeding, loss of libido, impotence, oligospermia, hair loss. **Other:** <u>Acute hypoadrenalism</u> (<u>reduction of adrenal stress syndrome</u>), renal hypofunction. **Topical—Skin:** Mild transient erythema, severe irritation, pruritus, stinging.

INTERACTIONS Drug: Alcohol may cause sunburnlike reaction; antacids, anticholinergics, h2-receptor antagonists decrease ketoconazole absorption; **isoniazid, rifampin** increase ketoconazole metabolism, thus decreasing its activity; levels of **phenytoin** and ketoconazole decreased; may increase **cyclosporine** levels and toxicity; **warfarin** may potentiate hypoprothrombinemia; may increase levels of **carbamazepine, cisapride,** resulting in arrhythmias. **Herbal: Echinacea** may increase risk of hepatotoxicity.

PHARMACOKINETICS Absorption: Erratically absorbed from GI tract (needs an acid pH); minimal absorption topically. **Peak:** 1–2 h. **Distribution:** Distributed to saliva, urine, sebum, and cerumen; CSF levels unpredictable; distributed into breast milk. **Metabolism:** Metabolized in liver. **Elimination:** Primarily excreted in feces, 13% in urine. **Half-Life:** 8 h.

NURSING IMPLICATIONS

Assessment & Drug Effects

- Lab tests: Monitor baseline liver function tests (AST, ALT, alkaline phosphatase, and bilirubin) and repeat at least monthly throughout therapy.
- Monitor for S&S of hepatotoxicity (see Appendix D-1). Discontinue drug immediately to prevent irreversible liver damage and report to prescriber.

Patient & Family Education

- Report signs and symptoms of hepatotoxicity promptly to health care provider (see Appendix D-1).
- Note: Drowsiness and dizziness are early and time-limited adverse effects.
- Do not drive or engage in potentially hazardous activities until response to drug is known.
- Avoid OTC drugs for gastric distress, such as Rolaids, Tums, Alka-Seltzer and check with physician before taking any other nonprescribed medicines.
- Do not alter dose or dose interval and do not stop taking ketoconazole before consulting the prescriber.
- Notify prescriber if skin condition fails to respond to topical therapy or worsens or if signs of irritation or sensitivity occur.

- Do not breast feed infants while taking this drug without consulting prescriber.
- Store this medication out of reach of children.

KETOROLAC TROMETHAMINE
(ke-tor'o-lac)
Toradol, Acular, Acular LS
Classifications: CENTRAL NERVOUS SYSTEM AGENT; NSAID, ANALGESIC; ANTIPYRETIC
Prototype: Ibuprofen
Pregnancy Category: B

AVAILABILITY 10 mg tablets; 15 mg/mL, 30 mg/mL injection; 0.4%, 0.5% ophthalmic solution

ACTIONS Inhibits synthesis of prostaglandins and is a peripherally acting analgesic. Ketorolac does not have any known effects on opiate receptors.
THERAPEUTIC EFFECTS Ketorolac exhibits analgesic, anti-inflammatory, and antipyretic activity.

USES *Short-term* management of pain; ocular itching due to seasonal allergic conjunctivitis, reduction of postoperative pain and photophobia after refractive surgery.

CONTRAINDICATIONS Hypersensitivity to ketorolac; individuals with complete or partial syndrome of nasal polyps, angioedema, and bronchospastic reaction to aspirin or other NSAIDS; during labor and delivery; patients with severe renal impairment or at risk for renal failure due to volume depletion; patients with risk of bleeding; active peptic ulcer disease; hepatitc disease, pre- or intraoperatively; intrathecal or epidural administration; in combination with other NSAIDS; lactation.
CAUTIOUS USE History of peptic ulcers; impaired renal or hepatic function; debilitated patients; pregnancy (category B). Safety and effectiveness in children is not established.

ROUTE & DOSAGE

Pain
Child: **IM/IV** 0.5 mg/kg/dose given q6h (max 30 mg q6h or 120 mg/day) **PO** >50 kg 10 mg q6h prn (max 40 mg/day)
Adult: **IV Loading Dose** 30 mg (15 mg <50 kg) **IM** 30–60 mg loading dose, then 15–30 mg q6h (max 150 mg/day on first day, then 120 mg subsequent day [30 mg load, then 15 mg q6h if <50 kg]) **PO** 10 mg q6hs prn (max 40 mg/day), max duration all routes 5 days

Allergic Conjunctivitis
Adult: **Ophthalmic** 1 drop 0.5% solution q.i.d.

Pain after Refractive Surgery
Adult: **Ophthalmic** *Acular LS only* 1 drop in operative eye q.i.d. up to 4 days

STORAGE
Store all forms at 15°–30° C (59°–86° F).

ADMINISTRATION
WARNING: Do not administer IV, IM, or PO ketorolac longer than 5 days

Oral
- Give with food to reduce GI effects.

Instillation
- Do not touch container to the eye when applying ophthalmic drops.

Intramuscular
- Inject IM drug slowly and deeply into a large muscle appropriate for age (see Part I).
- Rotate injection sites to avoid injection site pain in patients receiving multiple doses.

Intravenous
PREPARE **Direct:** Give undiluted.
ADMINISTER **Direct:** Give IV bolus dose over at least 15 sec. Give through a Y-tube in a free-flowing IV is preferred.

K

ADVERSE EFFECTS CNS: *Drowsiness,* dizziness, headache. **GI:** *Nausea,* dyspepsia, GI pain, <u>hemorrhage</u>. **Other:** Edema, sweating, pain at injection site.

INTERACTIONS Drug: May increase **methotrexate** levels and toxicity; may increase **lithium** levels and toxicity. **Herbal: Feverfew, garlic, ginger, ginkgo** increased bleeding potential.

PHARMACOKINETICS Peak: 45–60 min. **Distribution:** Distributed into breast milk. **Metabolism:** Metabolized in liver. **Elimination:** Excreted in urine. **Half-Life:** 4–6 h.

NURSING IMPLICATIONS

Assessment & Drug Effects
- Correct hypovolemia prior to administration of ketorolac.
- Lab tests: Periodic serum electrolytes and liver functions; urinalysis (hematuria and proteinuria) with long-term use.
- Monitor urine output esp in those with a history of cardiac decompensation, renal impairment, heart failure, or liver dysfunction as well as those taking diuretics. Discontinuation of drug will return urine output to pretreatment level.
- Monitor for S&S of GI distress or bleeding including nausea, GI pain, diarrhea, melena, or hematemesis. GI ulceration with perforation can occur anytime during treatment. Drug decreases platelet aggregation and thus may prolong bleeding time.
- Monitor for fluid retention and edema in patients with a history of CHF.

Patient & Family Education
- Watch for S&S of GI ulceration and bleeding (e.g., bloody emesis, black tarry stools) during long-term therapy.

- Note: Possible CNS adverse effects (e.g., light-headedness, dizziness, drowsiness).
- Do not drive or engage in potentially hazardous activities until response to drug is known.
- Do not use other NSAIDs while taking this drug.
- Do not breast feed while taking this drug.
- Store this medication out of reach of children.

LABETALOL HYDROCHLORIDE
(la-bet′a-lole)
Normodyne, Trandate
Classifications: AUTONOMIC NERVOUS SYSTEM AGENT; ALPHA- AND BETA-ADRENERGIC ANTAGONIST (SYMPATHOLYTIC); ANTIHYPERTENSIVE AGENT
Prototype: Propranolol
Pregnancy Category: C, D if used in 2nd or 3rd trimesters

AVAILABILITY 100 mg, 200 mg, 300 mg tablet; 5 mg/mL injection

ACTIONS The alpha blockade results in vasodilation, decreased peripheral resistance, and orthostatic hypotension and only slightly affects cardiac output and coronary artery blood flow. It has beta-blocking effects on the sinus node, AV node, and ventricular muscle, which lead to bradycardia, delay in AV conduction, and depression of cardiac contractility.

THERAPEUTIC EFFECTS Acts as an adrenergic receptor blocking agent that combines selective alpha activity and nonselective beta-adrenergic blocking actions. Both actions contribute to blood pressure reduction.

USES Mild, moderate, and severe hypertension. May be used alone or in combination with other antihypertensive agents, especially thiazide diuretics.

CONTRAINDICATIONS Bronchial asthma; uncontrolled cardiac failure, heart block (greater than first degree), cardiogenic shock, severe bradycardia. Safe use during pregnancy (category C, D in 2nd and 3rd trimesters), lactation, or in children is not established.

CAUTIOUS USE Nonallergic bronchospastic disease (COPD), well-compensated patients with history of heart failure; pheochromocytoma; impaired liver function, jaundice; diabetes mellitus; peripheral vascular disease.

ROUTE & DOSAGE

Hypertension

Child: **PO** 4 mg/kg/day divided into doses b.i.d.; increase up to 40 mg/kg/day **IV** in hypertensive emergency 0.2–1 mg/kg/dose q10min (max 20 mg/dose) *or* infusion rate of 0.4–1 mg/kg/h (max 3 mg/kg/h)
Adult: **PO** 100 mg b.i.d., may gradually increase to 200–400 mg b.i.d. (max 1200–2400 mg/day). **IV** 20 mg slowly over 2 min, with 40–80 mg q10min if needed up to 300 mg total or 2 mg/min continuous infusion (max 300 mg total dose)

STORAGE

Store at 2°–30° C (36°–86° F) unless otherwise advised. Do not freeze. Protect tablets from moisture.

ADMINISTRATION

Oral

- Give with or immediately after food consistently. Food increases drug bioavailability.

Intravenous

Note: Amount of IV solution may be changed depending on patient status.

PREPARE Direct: Give undiluted. **Continuous:** Dilute 300 mg in 240 of D5W, NS, D5/NS, RL, or other compatible IV solution to yield 1 mg/mL. **ADMINISTER Direct:** Give a 20-mg dose slowly over 2 min. Maximum hypotensive effect occurs 5–15 min after each administration. **Continuous:** Normal rate is 2 mg/min. Keep patient supine when receiving labetalol IV. Take BP immediately before administration. Rate is adjusted according to BP response. Discontinue drug once the desired BP is attained.

INCOMPATIBILITIES Solution/Additive: Sodium bicarbonate. **Y-Site:** Furosemide, heparin, nafcillin, thiopental, warfarin.

- Controlled infusion pump device is recommended for maintaining accurate flow rate during IV infusion. Usually administered at rate of 2 mg/min.

ADVERSE EFFECTS CNS: Dizziness, fatigue/malaise, headache, tremors, transient paresthesias (especially scalp tingling), hypoesthesia (numbness) following IV, mental depression, drowsiness, sleep disturbances, nightmares. **CV:** *Postural hypotension,* angina pectoris, palpitation, bradycardia, syncope, pedal or peripheral edema, pulmonary edema, CHF, flushing, cold extremities, arrhythmias (following IV), paradoxical hypertension (patients with pheochromocytoma). **Special Senses:** Dry eyes, vision disturbances, nasal stuffiness, rhinorrhea. **GI:** Nausea, vomiting, dyspepsia, constipation, diarrhea, taste disturbances, cholestasis with or without jaundice, increases in serum transaminases, dry mouth. **Urogenital:** Acute urinary retention, difficult micturition, impotence, ejaculation failure, loss of libido, Peyronie's disease. **Respiratory:** Dyspnea, <u>bronchospasm</u>. **Skin:** Rashes of various types, increased sweating, pruritus. **Body as a Whole:** Myalgia, muscle cramps, toxic myopathy, antimitochondrial antibodies, positive antinuclear antibodies (ANA), SLE syndrome, pain at IV injection site.

DIAGNOSTIC TEST INTERFERENCE False increases in ***urinary catecholamines*** when measured by ***nonspecific trihydroxyindole (THI) reaction*** (due to labetalol metabolites) but not with specific ***radioenzymatic*** or ***high-performance liquid chromatography assay techniques.***

INTERACTIONS Drug: Cimetidine may increase effects of labetalol; **glutethimide** decreases effects of labetalol; **halothane** adds to hypotensive effects; may mask symptoms of hypoglycemia caused by ORAL SULFONYLUREAS, **insulin;** BETA AGONISTS antagonize effects of labetalol.

PHARMACOKINETICS Absorption: Readily absorbed from GI tract, but only 25% reaches systemic circulation because of first pass metabolism. **Onset:** 20 min–2 h PO; 2–5 min IV. **Peak:** 1–4 h PO; 5–15 min IV. **Duration:** 8–24 h PO; 2–4 h IV. **Distribution:** Crosses placenta; distributed into breast milk. **Metabolism:** Metabolized in liver. **Elimination:** 60% excreted in urine, 40% in bile. **Half-Life:** 3–8 h.

NURSING IMPLICATIONS

Assessment & Drug Effects

- Monitor BP and pulse during dosage adjustment period. Use standing BP as indicator for making dosage adjustments for oral drugs and assessing patient's tolerance of dosage increases. Take after patient stands for 10 min. Clarify with prescriber.
- Monitor BP at 5-min intervals for 30 min after IV administration; then at 30-min intervals for 2 h; then hourly for about 6 h; and as indicated thereafter.
- Monitor diabetic patients closely; drug may mask usual cardiovascular response to acute hypoglycemia (e.g., tachycardia).
- Convert from IV to PO therapy only when supine diastolic pressure rises about 10 mmHg.
- Maintain patient in supine position for at least 3 h after IV administration. Then determine patient's ability to tolerate elevated and upright positions before allowing ambulation. Manage this slowly.

Patient & Family Education

- Note: Postural hypotension is most likely to occur during peak plasma levels (i.e., 2–4 h after drug administration).
- Make all position changes slowly and in stages, particularly from lying to upright position.
- Do not drive or engage in other potentially hazardous activities until response to drug is known.
- Note: Most adverse effects (e.g., scalp tingling) are mild, transient, and dose related and occur early in therapy.
- Be sure to keep follow-up appointments. Get liver and kidney function tests periodically during therapy.
- Discontinue drug gradually over 1–2 wk period after chronic administration. Close monitoring during this time is very important.
- Do not breast feed while taking this drug without consulting physician.
- Store this medication out of reach of children.

LACTULOSE

(lak'tyoo-lose)
Cephulac, Chronulac
Classifications: GASTROINTESTINAL AGENT; HYPEROSMOTIC LAXATIVE
Pregnancy Category: C

AVAILABILITY 10 g/15 mL solution, syrup

ACTIONS Reduces blood ammonia; appears to involve metabolism of lactose to organic acids by resident intestinal bacteria.

THERAPEUTIC EFFECTS Acidifies colon contents, which retards diffusion of nonionic ammonia (NH_3) from colon to blood while promoting its migration from blood to colon. In the acidic colon, NH_3 is converted to nonabsorbable ammonium ions (NH_4) and is then expelled in feces by laxative action. Decreased blood ammonia in a patient with hepatic encephalopathy is marked by improved EEG patterns and mental state (clearing of confusion, apathy, and irritation). Osmotic effect of organic acids causes laxative action, which moves water from plasma to intestines, softens stools, and stimulates peristalsis by pressure from water content of stool.

USES Prevention and treatment of portal-systemic encephalopathy (PSE), including stages of hepatic precoma and coma, and by prescription for relief of chronic constipation.
UNLABELED USES to restore regular bowel habit posthemorrhoidectomy; to evacuate bowel after barium studies; and for treatment of chronic constipation in children.

CONTRAINDICATIONS Galactosemia; low galactose diet; pregnancy (category C). Safe use in lactation or children is not established.
CAUTIOUS USE Diabetes mellitus; concomitant use with electrocautery procedures (proctoscopy, colonoscopy); debilitated patients; pediatric use.

L

ROUTE & DOSAGE

Prevention and Treatment of Portal-Systemic Encephalopathy

Infant: **PO** 2.5–10 mL/day in 3–4 divided doses adjusted to produce 2–3 soft stools/day
Child/Adolescent: **PO** 40–90 mL/day in divided doses adjusted to produce 2–3 soft stools/day
Adult: **PO** 30–45 mL t.i.d. or q.i.d. adjusted to produce 2–3 soft stools/day

Management of Acute Portal-Systemic Encephalopathy

Adult: **PO** 30–45 mL q1–2h until laxation is achieved, then adjusted to produce 2–3 soft stools/day. **Rectal** 300 mL diluted with 700 mL water given via rectal balloon catheter, and retained for 30–60 min, may repeat in 4–6 h if necessary or until patient can take PO

Chronic Constipation

Child: **PO** 7.5 mL/day after breakfast
Adult: **PO** 30–60 mL/day prn

STORAGE

Do not freeze. Avoid prolonged exposure to temperatures above 30° C (86° F) or to direct light. Normal darkening does not affect action, but discard solution that is very dark or cloudy.

ADMINISTRATION

Oral

- Give with fruit juice, water, or milk (if not contraindicated) to increase palatability. Laxative effect is enhanced by taking with ample liquids. Avoid meal times.

Rectal

▪ Administer as a retention enema via a rectal balloon catheter. If solution is evacuated too soon, instillation may be promptly repeated.

ADVERSE EFFECTS GI: Flatulence, borborygmi, belching, abdominal cramps, pain, and distention (initial dose); *diarrhea* (excessive dose); nausea, vomiting, colon accumulation of hydrogen gas; hypernatremia.

INTERACTIONS Drug: LAXATIVES may incorrectly suggest therapeutic action of lactulose.

PHARMACOKINETICS Absorption: Poorly absorbed from GI tract. **Metabolism:** Metabolized in gut by intestinal bacteria.

NURSING IMPLICATIONS

Assessment & Drug Effects

▪ In portal systemic encephalopathy, serum potassium is measured. Weigh daily and monitor I&O.
▪ In children if the initial dose causes diarrhea (>2–3 soft stools/day), dosage is reduced immediately. Discontinue if diarrhea persists.
▪ Promote fluid intake (≥1500–2000 mL/day for adults; appropriate fluid level for child) during drug therapy for constipation. Lactulose-induced osmotic changes in the bowel support intestinal water loss and potential hypernatremia. Discuss strategy with prescriber.

Patient & Family Education

▪ Laxative action is not instituted until drug reaches the colon; therefore, about 24–48 h is needed.
▪ Do not self-medicate with another laxative due to slow onset of drug action.
▪ Notify prescriber if diarrhea (i.e., more than 2 or 3 soft stools/day) occurs. Diarrhea is a sign of overdosage. Dose adjustment may be indicated.
▪ Do not breast feed while taking this drug without consulting physician.
▪ Store this medication out of reach of children.

LAMIVUDINE

(lam-i-vu′deen)
Epivir, Epivir-HBV, Heptovir ✦
Classifications: ANTI-INFECTIVE; ANTIRETROVIRAL AGENT
Prototype: Zidovudine (AZT)
Pregnancy Category: C

AVAILABILITY 100 mg, 150 tablets; 5 mg/mL, 10 mg/mL oral solution
Combination Products: Available in combination with zidovudine (Combivir)

ACTIONS Lamivudine (formerly 3TC) is a synthetic nucleoside analogue.
THERAPEUTIC EFFECTS Its phosphorylated metabolite (L-TP) inhibits the transcription of the HIV viral DNA chain.

USES HIV infection in combination with zidovudine; treatment of chronic hepatitis B.

CONTRAINDICATIONS Hypersensitivity to lamivudine, lactation.
CAUTIOUS USE Renal impairment, pregnancy (category C), children. Safety of using product for more than 1 y has not been tested.

ROUTE & DOSAGE

HIV Infection

Neonate: Epivir **PO** 2 mg/kg/dose given q.i.d.
Child: Epivir **PO** *3 mo–16 y,* 4 mg/kg b.i.d. (max 150 mg b.i.d.)
Adult: Epivir **PO** ≥*50 kg,* 150 mg b.i.d.; <*50 kg,* 2 mg/kg/dose b.i.d.

Chronic Hepatitis B

Child: Epivir-HBV 3 mg/kg/day
Adult: Epivir-HBV: **PO** 100 mg daily

Needle-Stick Prophylaxis

Adolescent/Adult: 150 mg/dose given b.i.d. × 28 days; used in combination with zidovudine (AZT) and indinavir

Renal Impairment

Cl_{cr} 30–49=100% normal dose;
    15–29=66% normal dose;
    5–14=33% normal dose;
    <5=17% normal dose

STORAGE

Store solution at 2°–25° C (36°–77° F) tightly closed.

ADMINISTRATION

Oral

- Give Epivir b.i.d. in combination with AZT. Note that the recommended dose for adults who weigh <50 kg (110 lb) is 2 mg/kg. Give Epivir-HBV daily; do NOT give in combination with AZT.
- Strawberry-banana flavor oral solution used for children.

ADVERSE EFFECTS CNS: *Neuropathy, insomnia,* sleep disorders, *dizziness,* depression, *headache,* fatigue, *fever, chills.* **GI:** *Pancreatitis (more common in children), nausea, diarrhea,* vomiting, anorexia, abdominal pain, cramps, dyspepsia, increased LFTs (ALT, amylase), <u>hepatomegaly with steatosis.</u> **Hematologic:** Neutropenia, anemia, thrombocytopenia. **Musculoskeletal:** Myalgia, arthralgia, malaise, pain. **Skin:** Rash. **Respiratory:** Nasal symptoms, cough. **Metabolic:** <u>Lactic acidosis.</u>

INTERACTIONS Drug: Increases the C_{max} of **zidovudine. Trimethoprim-sulfamethoxazole** increases serum levels of lamivudine. Increased risk of lactic acidosis in combination with other REVERSE TRANSCRIPTASE INHIBITORS and ANTIRETROVIRAL AGENTS.

PHARMACOKINETICS Absorption: Rapidly absorbed from GI tract (86% reaches systemic circulation). **Distribution:** Low binding to plasma proteins. **Metabolism:** Minimal metabolism. **Elimination:** Excreted primarily unchanged in urine. **Half-Life:** 2–4 h.

NURSING IMPLICATIONS

Assessment & Drug Effects

- Monitor children closely for S&S of pancreatitis; if they occur, immediately stop drug and notify physician.
- Lab tests: Monitor CBC with differential, kidney & liver function, and serum amylase throughout therapy.
- Monitor for and report all significant adverse reactions.

Patient & Family Education

- Report any of the following immediately: Nausea, vomiting, anorexia, abdominal pain, jaundice.
- Note: The long-term effects of lamivudine are unknown.
- Management of the child's disease and medication regimen can be difficult. Families need much support and many resources.
- Do not breast feed while taking this drug.
- Store this medication out of reach of children.

LAMOTRIGINE

(la-mo′tri-geen)
Lamictal
Classifications: CENTRAL NERVOUS SYSTEM AGENT; ANTICONVULSANT
Prototype: Phenytoin
Pregnancy Category: C

AVAILABILITY 25 mg, 100 mg, 150 mg, 200 mg tablets; 5 mg, 25 mg chewable tablets

ACTIONS Anticonvulsant. The exact mechanism of action is not known; thought to act by inhibiting the release of glutamate, an excitatory neurotransmitter, at voltage-sensitive sodium channels.
THERAPEUTIC EFFECTS Stabilizes neuronal membranes and inhibits neurotransmitter release (i.e., glutamate) in brain tissue.

USES Adjunctive therapy for partial seizures in adults (>16 y). Generalized tonic–clonic, absence, or myoclonic seizures in adults.

CONTRAINDICATIONS Hypersensitivity to lamotrigine, lactation.
CAUTIOUS USE Renal insufficiency, concomitant administration of other anticonvulsants, pregnancy (category C), cardiac or liver function impairment. Safety and efficacy in children <16 y for conditions other than Lennox-Gastaut syndrome are not established. Fatal rash has been reported in children <16 y.

ROUTE & DOSAGE

Partial Seizures, Patients Receiving Enzyme Inducing Antiepileptic Drugs (AEDs) But Not Valproic Acid

Child: **PO** 2–16 y, 1 mg/kg b.i.d. times 2 wk, then 2.5 mg/kg b.i.d. times 2 wk, then 5 mg/kg b.i.d.; usual range 5–15 mg/kg/day (max 15 mg/kg/day or 400 mg/day)
Adult: **PO** Start with 50 mg daily for 2 wk, then 50 mg b.i.d. for 2 wk, may titrate up to 300–500 mg/day in 2 divided doses (max 700 mg/day)

Partial Seizures, Patients Receiving Valproic Acid and an Enzyme Inducing AED

Child: **PO** 2–16 y, 0.2 mg/kg/day times 2 wk, then 0.5 mg/kg/day × 2 wk, then 1 mg/kg/day (max 5 mg/kg/day or 250 mg/day)
Adult: **PO** Start with 25 mg every other day for 2 wk, then 25 mg daily for 2 wk, may titrate up to 150 mg/day in 2 divided doses (max 200 mg/day)

Patients Receiving Valproic Acid But No Enzyme Inducing AED

Child: **PO** 0.1–0.2 mg/kg/day given 2 wk, then 0.2–0.5 mg/kg/day given daily × 2 wk, then 0.5–1.0 mg/kg/day given daily (max 2 mg/kg/day or 150 mg/day)

STORAGE
Store at 15°–30° C (59°–86° F) in a dry environment; protect from light.

ADMINISTRATION
Oral

- Note: Doses are carefully calibrated depending on other antiepileptic drugs. Lamotrigine may be given (1) with enzyme inducing antiepileptic drugs (AEDs) but not with valproic acid, (2) with enzyme inducing AEDs AND valproic acid, or (3) without enzyme inducing AEDs but with valproic acid. Enzyme inducing AEDs include carbamazepine, phenytoin, and phenobarbital.
- Note: Reduced dose may be warranted with renal and hepatic impairment.
- Ensure that chewable tablets are chewed or crushed before being swallowed with a liquid.
- When discontinued, drug should be tapered off gradually over a 2-wk period, unless patient safety is at risk.

ADVERSE EFFECTS CNS: *Dizziness, ataxia, somnolence, headache,* aphasia, vertigo, confusion, slurred speech, irritability, depression, incoordination, hostility. **GI:** *Nausea,* vomiting, anorexia, abdominal pain, diarrhea, dyspepsia, constipation. **Urogenital:** Hematuria, dysmenorrhea, vaginitis. **Special Senses:** *Diplopia, blurred vision.* **Musculoskeletal:** Peripheral neuropathy, chills, tremor, arthralgia. **Skin:** Rash (including Stevens-Johnson syndrome, toxic epidermal Necrolysis; these side effects more common in children), urticaria, pruritus, alopecia, acne. **Respiratory:** *Rhinitis,* pharyngitis, cough.

INTERACTIONS Drug: Carbamazepine, phenobarbital, primidone, phenytoin, fosphenytoin may decrease lamotrigine levels. **Valproic**

Common adverse effects in *italic;* life-threatening effects <u>underlined</u>; generic names in **bold**; drug classifications in SMALL CAPS; ♣ Canadian drug name; ✿ Prototype drug.

711

acid, acetaminophen, carbamazepine, phenytoin may increase lamotrigine levels. Lamotrigine may decrease serum levels of **valproic acid. Herbal: Ginkgo** may decrease anticonvulsant effectiveness.

PHARMACOKINETICS Absorption: Readily absorbed from GI tract; 98% reaches systemic circulation. **Onset:** 12 wk. **Peak:** 1–4 h. **Distribution:** 55% protein bound; crosses placenta; distributed into breast milk. **Metabolism:** Metabolized in liver to inactive metabolite. **Elimination:** Can induce own metabolism; excreted in urine. **Half-Life:** 25–30 h.

NURSING IMPLICATIONS

Assessment & Drug Effects

- Withhold drug if rash develops and immediately report to physician.
- Monitor the plasma levels of lamotrigine and other anticonvulsants when given concomitantly. Monitor and carefully record/report seizure activity.
- Monitor for adverse reactions when lamotrigine is used with other anticonvulsants, especially valproic acid (fatigue, skin rash, ataxia are more common with this combination of drugs).
- Be aware of drug interactions and closely monitor when interacting drugs are added or discontinued.

Patient & Family Education

- Notify physician for any of the following: Worsening seizure control, skin rash, ataxia, blurred vision or diplopia, fever or flu-like symptoms.
- Do not drive or engage in other potentially hazardous activities until response to the drug is known.
- Use protection from sunlight or ultraviolet light until tolerance is known; drug increases photosensitivity.
- Schedule periodic ophthalmologic exams with long-term use.
- Do not discontinue lamotrigine abruptly.
- Do not breast feed while taking this drug.
- Store this medication out of reach of children.

LANSOPRAZOLE

(lan'so-pra-zole)
Prevacid
Classifications: GASTROINTESTINAL AGENT; ANTISECRETORY (H$_2$-RECEPTOR ANTAGONIST); PROTON PUMP INHIBITOR
Prototype: Omeprazole
Pregnancy Category: C

AVAILABILITY 15 mg, 30 mg sustained-release capsules; 15 mg, 30 mg packets for suspension

ACTIONS Belongs to a class of antisecretory compounds that are gastric acid pump inhibitors. Specifically, it suppresses gastric acid secretion by inhibiting the H$^+$, K$^+$-ATPase enzyme (the acid [proton H$^+$] pump) in the parietal cells. Lansoprazole does not exhibit anticholinergic or H$_2$-histamine antagonist properties.

THERAPEUTIC EFFECTS Suppresses gastric acid formation in the stomach.

USES Short-term treatment of duodenal ulcer (up to 4 wk) and erosive esophagitis (up to 8 wk), pathologic hypersecretory disorders, gastric ulcers; in combination with clarithromycin and amoxicillin for *Helicobacter pylori*. Gastroesophageal reflux disease.

CONTRAINDICATIONS Hypersensitivity to lansoprazole, lactation. Severe hepatic impairment, pregnancy (category C).

ROUTE & DOSAGE

Duodenal Ulcer
Adult: **PO** 15 mg daily times 4 wk
Erosive Esophagitis
Child: **PO** 1–11 y, 1.5 mg/kg/day (max 30 mg/day)
Adult: **PO** 30 mg daily times 8 wk, then decrease to 15 mg daily
GERD
Child 1–11y: 1.5 mg/kg/day (max 30 mg/day)
Adult: 15 mg daily for up to 8 wk
Hypersecretory Disorder
Adult: **PO** 60 mg daily (max 120 mg/day in divided doses), may need to be adjusted for hepatic impairment
H. pylori
Adult: **PO** 30 mg b.i.d. times 2 wk, in combination with 2 antibiotics

STORAGE
Store at 15°–30° C (59°–86° F) in tightly closed container in dry environment.

ADMINISTRATION
Oral
- Give before a meal.
- Give at least 30 min prior to any concurrent sucralfate therapy.
- Do not crush or chew capsules. Capsules can be opened and granules sprinkled on food or mixed with 40 mL of apple juice and administered through a NG tube. Do not crush or chew granules.

ADVERSE EFFECTS CNS: Fatigue, dizziness, headache. **GI:** Nausea, *diarrhea,* constipation, anorexia, increased appetite, thirst elevated serum transaminases (AST, ALT). **Skin:** Rash.

INTERACTIONS Drug: May decrease **theophylline** levels. **Sucralfate** decreases lansoprazole bioavailability. May interfere with absorption of **ketoconazole, digoxin, ampicillin,** or IRON SALTS. **Food:** Food reduces peak lansoprazole levels by 50%.

PHARMACOKINETICS Absorption: Rapidly absorbed from GI tract after leaving stomach; unstable in acidic media. **Onset:** Acid reduction within 2 h; ulcer relief within 1 wk. **Peak:** 1.5–3 h. **Duration:** 24 h. **Distribution:** 97% bound to plasma proteins. **Metabolism:** Metabolized in liver by cytochrome P-450 system. **Elimination:** 14–25% excreted in urine as metabolites; part of dose eliminated in bile and feces. **Half-Life:** 1.5 h.

NURSING IMPLICATIONS

Assessment & Drug Effects
- Lab tests: Monitor CBC, kidney and liver function tests, and serum gastric levels periodically.
- Monitor for therapeutic effectiveness of concurrently used drugs that require an acid medium for absorption (e.g., digoxin, ampicillin, ketoconazole).

Patient & Family Education
- Inform prescriber of diarrhea.
- Do not breast feed while taking this drug.
- Store this medication out of reach of children.

LEUCOVORIN CALCIUM
(loo-koe-vor'in)
Calcium Folinate, Citrovorum Factor, Folinic Acid, Wellcovorin
Classifications: BLOOD FORMERS, COAGULATORS, AND ANTICOAGULANTS; ANTIANEMIC AGENT; ANTIDOTE
Pregnancy Category: C

AVAILABILITY 5 mg, 15 mg, 25 mg tablets; 3 mg/mL ampule; 50 mg, 100 mg, 350 mg vials

ACTIONS A reduced form of folic acid; unlike folic acid, it does not require enzymatic reduction and therefore is readily available to participate in reactions.
THERAPEUTIC EFFECTS Functions as an essential cell growth factor. When given during antineoplastic therapy, it prevents serious toxicity by protecting cells from the action of folic acid antagonists such as methotrexate.

USES Folate-deficient megaloblastic anemias due to sprue, pregnancy, and nutritional deficiency when oral therapy is not feasible. Also to prevent or diminish toxicity of antineoplastic folic acid antagonists, particularly methotrexate; and as adjunct with antifols (e.g., pyrimethamine) in pneumocystosis or toxoplasmosis to prevent significant bone marrow toxicity.

CONTRAINDICATIONS Undiagnosed anemia, pernicious anemia, or other megaloblastic anemias secondary to vitamin B_{12} deficiency. Safe use during pregnancy (category C) or lactation is not established.
CAUTIOUS USE Renal dysfunction.

ROUTE & DOSAGE

Megaloblastic Anemia
Child/Adult: **IV/IM** No more than 1 mg/day
Leucovorin Rescue for Methotrexate Toxicity
Child/Adult: **PO/IM/IV** 10–100 mg/m² based on serum methotrexate concentrations and creatinine levels

Common adverse effects in *italic;* life-threatening effects <u>underlined</u>; generic names in **bold**; drug classifications in SMALL CAPS; ♣ Canadian drug name; ⊘ Prototype drug.

Leucovorin Rescue for Other Folate Antagonist Toxicity
Child/Adult: **PO/IM/IV** 5–15 mg/day
Adjunct for Treatment of Pneumocystosis or Toxoplasmosis
Child/Adult: **PO/IM/IV** 3–6 mg t.i.d.

STORAGE
Store powder for injection and tablets at 15°–30° C (59°–86° F) and protect from light.

ADMINISTRATION
- Child: When given for methotrexate rescue, must be given under care and direction of pediatric oncology specialist. Use recommended handling techniques for hazardous medications (see Part I)
- When used for methotrexate rescue, leucovorin should start within 24 h of methotrexate. It is continued until methotrexate level has declined to $<10^{-8}$ M. Leucovorin doses are adjusted based on methotrexate levels and creatinine clearance.
- Oral route is NOT recommended for doses higher than 25 mg or if patient is likely to vomit. Doses usually begin with IV and then later doses may be oral.

Intramuscular
- Use 3-mg ampules for IM injection.
- Give deep into a large muscle appropriate for age of child (see Part I).

Intravenous

PREPARE **Direct:** Give 1 mL (3 mg) ampules, which contain benzyl alcohol, undiluted. **IV Infusion:** For doses <10 mg/m², reconstitute each 50 mg in 5 mL (10 mg per 1 mL in 10 mL) of bacteriostatic water for injection with benzyl alcohol. For doses >10 mg/m² reconstitute, as above, but with sterile water for injection without a preservative. Final concentration is 10 mg/mL. Further dilute in 100–500 mL of IV solutions (e.g., D5W, NS, RL) to yield a concentration of 10–20 mg/mL of IV solution.
ADMINISTER **Direct:** Give 160 mg or fraction thereof over 1 min. **IV Infusion:** Do not exceed direct IV rate. Give more slowly if the volume of IV solution to be infused is large; over 15–60 min, depending on the volume of solution.
INCOMPATIBILITIES **Solution/Additive: Droperidol, fluorouracil. Y-Site: Amphotericin B cholesteryl complex, droperidol, foscarnet, sodium bicarbonate.** ■ Use solution reconstituted with bacteriostatic water within 7 days. Use solution reconstituted with sterile water for injection immediately. ■ Protect from light.

ADVERSE EFFECTS Body as a Whole: Allergic sensitization (urticaria, pruritus, rash, wheezing). **Hematologic:** Thrombocytosis.

INTERACTIONS Drug: May enhance adverse effects of **fluorouracil;** may reverse therapeutic effects of **methotrexate, trimethoprim-sulfamethoxazole.**

PHARMACOKINETICS Onset: Within 30 min. **Duration:** 3–6 h. **Distribution:** Crosses placenta; distributed into breast milk. **Metabolism:** Metabolized in liver and intestinal mucosa to tetrahydrofolic acid derivatives. **Elimination:** 80–90% excreted in urine, 5–8% in feces.

NURSING IMPLICATIONS

Assessment & Drug Effects

- Monitor neurologic status. Use of leucovorin alone in treatment of pernicious anemia or other megaloblastic anemias associated with vitamin B_{12} deficiency can result in an apparent hematological remission while allowing already present neurologic damage to progress.
- Lab tests: Do Cl_{cr} determinations prior to initiation of leucovorin, urine pH prior to and about every 6 h throughout therapy; daily serum creatinine levels are recommended to detect onset of kidney function impairment.

Patient & Family Education

- Notify physician of S&S of a hypersensitivity reaction immediately (see Appendix D-1).
- Do not breast feed while taking this drug without consulting physician.

LEUPROLIDE ACETATE ⊕

(loo-proe'lide)

Eligard, Lupron, Lupron Depot, Lupron Depot-Ped, Viadur

Classifications: HORMONE AND SYNTHETIC SUBSTITUTE; GONADOTROPIN-RELEASING HORMONE ANALOG

Pregnancy Category: X

AVAILABILITY 5 mg/mL injection; 3.75 mg, 7.5 mg, 11.25 mg, 15 mg, 22.5 mg, 30 mg microspheres for injection (depot formulations); 65 mg implant

ACTIONS Occupies and desensitizes pituitary GnRH receptors, resulting initially in release of gonadotropins LH and FSH and stimulation of ovarian and testicular steroidogenesis.

THERAPEUTIC EFFECTS Long-term administration suppresses both gonadotropin secretion and steroidogenesis and leads to prostatic and testicular atrophy. **Antitumor Effect:** May inhibit growth of hormone-dependent tumors as indicated by reduction in concentrations of PSA and serum testosterone to levels equal to or less than pretreatment levels. **Contraceptive Effect:** By inhibiting gonadotropin release, ovulation or spermatogenesis is suppressed.

USES Palliative treatment of advanced prostatic carcinoma as alternative to orchiectomy or estrogen administration; endometriosis; anemia caused by leiomyomata.

UNLABELED USES Breast cancer; male contraceptive; delayed puberty.

CONTRAINDICATIONS Following orchiectomy or estrogen therapy; metastatic cerebral lesions; pregnancy (category X), lactation.

CAUTIOUS USE Life-threatening carcinoma in which rapid symptomatic relief is necessary; known hypersensitivity to benzyl alcohol.

ROUTE & DOSAGE

Endometriosis, Anemia
Adult: **IM** 3.75 mg every mo or 11.25 mg q3mo

Precocious Puberty
Child: **IM** Depot-Ped, 0.15–0.3 mg/kg q28days (minimum 7.5 mg), titrate by 3.75 mg increments q4wk

STORAGE
Refrigerate unopened vials. Store vial in use at room temperature for several months without loss of potency. Protect from light and freezing.

ADMINISTRATION

Subcutaneous
- Do not use Depot-Ped form for SC injection.
- Rotate injection sites.

Intramuscular
- Prepare solution for Depot-Ped injection using a 22-gauge needle (or syringe provided by manufacturer), withdraw 1.5 mL of diluent from the supplied ampule and inject it into the vial. Shake well to form a uniform suspension. Withdraw entire contents and administer immediately.
- Do not administer parenteral drug formulation if particulate matter or discoloration is present.

ADVERSE EFFECTS Body as a Whole: *Disease flare,* injection site irritation, asthenia, fatigue, fever, facial swelling. **CNS:** Dizziness, pain, headache, paresthesia. **CV:** *Peripheral edema,* cardiac arrhythmias, <u>MI</u>. **Endocrine:** *Hot flushes, impotence, decreased libido,* gynecomastia, breast tenderness, amenorrhea, vaginal bleeding, thyroid enlargement, hypoglycemia. **GI:** Nausea, vomiting, constipation, anorexia, sour taste, GI bleeding, diarrhea. **Musculoskeletal:** Increased bone pain, myalgia. **Renal:** Increased hematuria, dysuria, flank pain. **Respiratory:** Pleural rub, pulmonary fibrosis flare. **Hematologic:** Decreased Hct, Hgb. **Skin:** Pruritus, rash, hair loss.

INTERACTIONS Drug: ANDROGENS, ESTROGENS would counteract therapeutic effects.

PHARMACOKINETICS Absorption: Readily absorbed from SC or IM sites. **Metabolism:** Metabolized by enzymes in hypothalamus and anterior pituitary. **Half-Life:** 3 h.

NURSING IMPLICATIONS

Assessment & Drug Effects
- Monitor hemoglobin and hematocrit. Evaluate symptoms of endometriosis.
- Do baseline and periodic weight, height, and Tanner puberty stage evaluations (see Part I for Tanner stages).

- Inspect injection site. If local hypersensitivity reactions occur (erythema, induration), suspect sensitivity to benzyl alcohol. Report to prescriber.
- Monitor I&O ratio and pattern. Report hematuria and decreased output. Carefully monitor voiding problems.

Patient & Family Education
- Hot flushes may be experienced.
- Notify prescriber of neurologic signs and symptoms (paresthesia and weakness in lower limbs). Exercise caution when walking without assistance.
- When used for endometriosis, continuous treatment may cause amenorrhea and other menstrual irregularities.
- Do not breast feed while taking this drug.

LEVALBUTEROL HYDROCHLORIDE
(lev-al-bu'ter-ole)
Xopenex
Classifications: AUTONOMIC NERVOUS SYSTEM AGENT (SYMPATHOMIMETIC); BETA-ADRENERGIC AGONIST; BRONCHODILATOR (RESPIRATORY SMOOTH MUSCLE RELAXANT)
Prototype: Albuterol
Pregnancy Category: C

AVAILABILITY 0.63 mg/3 mL, 1.25 mg/3 mL inhalation solution

ACTIONS An isomer of albuterol with beta$_2$-adrenergic agonist properties, drug acts on the beta$_2$-receptors of the smooth muscles of the bronchial tree, thus resulting in bronchodilation.
THERAPEUTIC EFFECTS Decreases airway resistance, facilitates mucous drainage, and increases vital capacity.

USES Treatment or prevention of bronchospasm in patients with reversible obstructive airway disease.

CONTRAINDICATIONS Hypersensitivity to levalbuterol or albuterol; pregnancy (category C); lactation.
CAUTIOUS USE Cardiovascular disorders especially coronary insufficiency, cardiac arrhythmias, and hypertension; convulsive disorders; diabetes mellitus, diabetic ketoacidosis; hypersensitivity to sympathetic amines; hyperthyroidism.

ROUTE & DOSAGE

Bronchospasm
Child: **Inhalation** 6–11 y, 0.31 mg by nebulization t.i.d. q6–8h (max 0.63 mg t.i.d.)
Adult: **Inhalation** 0.63 mg by nebulization t.i.d. q6–8h, may increase to 1.25 mg t.i.d. if needed

Common adverse effects in *italic;* life-threatening effects <u>underlined</u>; generic names in **bold;** drug classifications in SMALL CAPS; ◆ Canadian drug name; ☻ Prototype drug.

STORAGE
Store at 15°–25° C (59°–77° F) in protective foil pouch.

ADMINISTRATION

Inhalation
- Use vials within 2 wk of opening pouch. Protect vial from light and use within 1 wk after removal from pouch. Use only if solution in vial is colorless.
- Give thorough instruction on proper use of inhaler and have child demonstrate (see Part I).

INCOMPATIBILITIES Solution/Additive: Compatibility when mixed with other drugs in a nebulizer has not been established.

ADVERSE EFFECTS Body as a Whole: Allergic reactions, flu syndrome, pain. **CNS:** Migraine, dizziness, nervousness, tremor, anxiety. **CV:** Tachycardia. **GI:** Dyspepsia. **Respiratory:** Increased cough, viral infection, rhinitis, sinusitis, turbinate edema, paradoxical bronchospasm. **Endocrine:** Increase in serum glucose, hypokalemia.

INTERACTIONS Drug: BETA-ADRENERGIC BLOCKERS may antagonize **levalbuterol** effects; MAOI, TRICYCLIC ANTIDEPRESSANTS may potentiate **levalbuterol** effects on vascular system; ECG changes or hypokalemia may be exacerbated by LOOP or THIAZIDE DIURETICS.

PHARMACOKINETICS Onset: 5–15 min. **Duration:** 3–6 h. **Half-life:** 3.3 h.

NURSING IMPLICATIONS

Assessment & Drug Effects
- Monitor for S&S of CNS or cardiovascular stimulation (e.g., BP, HR, respiratory status).
- Perform careful respiratory assessment.
- Lab tests: Periodic serum potassium levels especially with coadministered loop or thiazide diuretics.
- Monitor diabetics for loss of glycemic control.

Patient & Family Education
- Seek medical advice immediately if a previously effective dose becomes ineffective.
- Record respiratory symptoms and report to health care provider.
- Report immediately to prescriber: Chest pains or palpitations, swelling of the eyelids, tongue, lips or face; increased wheezing or difficulty breathing.
- Do not use drug more frequently than prescribed.
- Exercise caution with hazardous activities; dizziness and vertigo are possible side effects.
- Check with prescriber before taking OTC cold medication.
- Work with school to arrange for child to have access to drug during school hours.
- Do not breast feed while taking this drug.
- Store this medication out of reach of children.

LEVOFLOXACIN
(lev-o-flox′a-sin)
Levaquin, Quixin
Classifications: ANTI-INFECTIVE; ANTIBIOTIC; QUINOLONE
Prototype: Ciprofloxacin
Pregnancy Category: C

AVAILABILITY 250 mg, 500 mg tablets; 250 mg, 500 mg injection; 0.5% ophthalmic solution

ACTIONS A broad-spectrum fluoroquinolone antibiotic that inhibits DNA bacterial topoisomerase II, an enzyme required for DNA replication, transcription, repair, and recombination.

THERAPEUTIC EFFECTS Prevents replication of certain bacteria resistant to beta-lactam antibiotics.

USES Treatment of maxillary sinusitis, acute exacerbations of bacterial bronchitis, community-acquired pneumonia, uncomplicated skin/skin structure infections, UTI, acute pyelonephritis caused by susceptible bacteria; chronic bacterial prostatitis; bacterial conjunctivitis.

CONTRAINDICATIONS Hypersensitivity to levofloxacin and quinolone antibiotics; lactation.

CAUTIOUS USE Known or suspected CNS disorders predisposed to seizure activity (e.g., severe cerebral atherosclerosis), risk factors associated with potential seizures (e.g., some drug therapy, renal insufficiency), diabetes; pregnancy (category C); patients receiving theophylline or caffeine. Safety and efficacy in children <18 y are not established (see note in ADMINISTRATION section).

ROUTE & DOSAGE

Infections
Adult: **PO** 500 mg q24h times 10 days **IV** 500 mg infused over 60 min q24h times 7–14 days

Uncomplicated UTI
Adult: **PO** 250 mg q24h times 14 days

Complicated UTI, Pyelonephritis
Adult: **PO** 250 mg q24h times 10 days **IV** 250 mg infused over 60 min q24h times 10 days

Chronic Bacterial Prostatitis
Adult: **PO** 500 mg q24h times 28 days

Renal Impairment
Give an initial dose of 500 mg with adjusted maintenance doses as follows: Cl$_{cr}$ 20–50 mg/min: 250 mg q24h; <20 mL/min: 250 mg q48h

Skin & Skin Structure Infections
Adult: **PO** 750 mg q24h times 14 days

Renal Impairment

Give an initial dose of 250 mg with adjusted maintenance doses as follows: Cl_{cr} <20 mL/min: 250 mg q48h

Bacterial Conjunctivitis

Adult: **Ophthalmic** Days 1–2, 1–2 drops in affected eye(s) q2h while awake (max 8 times/day); days 3–7, 1–2 drops in affected eye(s) q4h while awake (max 4 times/day)

STORAGE

Store tablets in a tightly closed container. IV solution is stable for 72 h at 25° C (77° F).

ADMINISTRATION

Note: The manufacturer states that drug is contraindicated in children <18 y because it and other fluoroquinolones cause arthropathy in young animals of various types. The American Academy of Pediatrics states quinolones may be justified in children in special circumstances but only after careful assessment of risk and benefit. A physician trained in such use should be the prescriber and should monitor the child. The drugs should only be used in children when no other agent can effectively treat their infection.

Oral

- Do not give oral drug within 2 h of drugs containing aluminum or magnesium (antacids), iron, zinc, or sucralfate.

Intravenous

PREPARE **Intermittent:** Withdraw the desired dose from 500-mg (25 mg/mL) single-use vial. Add to enough D5W, NS, D5/NS, D5/RL, or other compatible solutions to produce a concentration of 5 mg/mL (e.g., 500 mg [or 20 mL] added to 80 mL). Discard any unused drug remaining in the vial.

ADMINISTER **Intermittent:** Give over ≥60 min. Do NOT give a bolus dose nor infuse too rapidly.

INCOMPATIBILITIES **Y-Site:** Do not add any drugs to levofloxacin solution or infuse simultaneously through the same line (manufacturer recommendation).

ADVERSE EFFECTS CNS: Headache, insomnia, dizziness. **GI:** Nausea, diarrhea, constipation, vomiting, abdominal pain, dyspepsia. **Skin:** Rash, pruritus. **Special Senses:** Decreased vision, foreign body sensation, transient ocular burning, ocular pain, photophobia. **Urogenital:** Vaginitis. **Body as a Whole:** Injection site pain or inflammation, chest or back pain, fever, pharyngitis.

DIAGNOSTIC TEST INTERFERENCE May cause false positive on *opiate screening tests.*

INTERACTIONS Drug: Magnesium or **aluminum-containing antacids, sucralfate, iron, zinc** may decrease **levofloxacin** absorption; NSAIDS may increase risk of CNS reactions, including seizures; may cause hyper- or hypoglycemia in patients on ORAL HYPOGLYCEMIC AGENTS.

PHARMACOKINETICS Absorption: Rapidly absorbed from GI tract. **Peak:** 1–2 h PO. **Distribution:** Penetrates lung tissue, 24–38% protein bound. **Metabolism:** Minimally metabolized in the liver. **Elimination:** Primarily excreted unchanged in urine. **Half-Life:** 6–8 h.

NURSING IMPLICATIONS

Assessment & Drug Effects

- Lab tests: Do C&S test prior to beginning therapy and periodically.
- Withhold therapy and report to physician immediately any of the following: Skin rash or other signs of a hypersensitivity reaction (see Appendix D-1); CNS symptoms such as seizures, restlessness, confusion, hallucinations, depression; skin eruption following sun exposure; symptoms of colitis such as persistent diarrhea; joint pain, inflammation, or rupture of a tendon; hypoglycemic reaction in diabetic on an oral hypoglycemic agent.

Patient & Family Education

- Learn important indications for discontinuing drug and immediately notifying physician.
- Consume fluids liberally while taking levofloxacin.
- Allow a minimum of 2 h between drug dosage and taking any of the following: Aluminum or magnesium antacids, iron supplements, multivitamins with zinc, or sucralfate.
- Avoid exposure to excess sunlight or artificial UV light.
- Avoid NSAIDs while taking levofloxacin, if possible.
- Do not breast feed while taking this drug.
- Store this medication out of reach of children.

LEVOTHYROXINE SODIUM (T₄) ℗

(lee-voe-thye-rox′een)

Eltroxin ♣ , Levothroid, Levoxyl, Levo-T, Synthroid

Classifications: HORMONES AND SYNTHETIC SUBSTITUTES; THYROID AGENT
Pregnancy Category: A

AVAILABILITY 25 mcg, 50 mcg, 75 mcg, 88 mcg, 100 mcg, 112 mcg, 125 mcg, 137 mcg, 150 mcg, 175 mcg, 200 mcg, 300 mcg tablets; 200 mcg, 500 mcg vials

ACTIONS Synthetically prepared monosodium salt and levo-isomer of thyroxine, with similar actions and uses (thyroxine, principal component of thyroid gland secretions, determines normal thyroid function).

THERAPEUTIC EFFECTS Principal effects include diuresis, loss of weight and puffiness, increased sense of well-being and activity tolerance, and rise of T_3 and T_4 serum levels toward normal.

USES Specific replacement therapy for diminished or absent thyroid function resulting from primary or secondary atrophy of gland, surgery, excessive radiation or antithyroid drugs, congenital defect. Administered orally for hypothyroid state; administered IV for myxedematous coma or

Common adverse effects in *italic*; life-threatening effects <u>underlined</u>; generic names in **bold**; drug classifications in SMALL CAPS; ♣ Canadian drug name; ℗ Prototype drug.

other thyroid dysfunctions demanding rapid replacement, as well as in failure to respond to oral therapy.

CONTRAINDICATIONS Hypersensitivity to levothyroxine; thyrotoxicosis, severe cardiovascular conditions, adrenal insufficiency.
CAUTIOUS USE Angina pectoris, hypertension, impaired kidney function, pregnancy (category A), lactation.

ROUTE & DOSAGE

Thyroid Replacement

Child: **PO** 0–6 mo, 8–10 mcg/kg/day or 25–50 mcg/day; 6–12 mo, 6–8 mcg/kg/day or 50–75 mcg/day; 1–5 y, 5–6 mcg/kg/day or 75–100 mcg/day; 6–12 y, 4–5 mcg/kg/day or 100–150 mcg/day; >12 y, 2–3 mcg/kg/day or >150 mcg/day **IV** 50–75% of usual PO dose
Adult: **PO** 25–50 mcg/day, gradually increased by 25–50 mcg/day q2–4wk to usual dose of 100–200 mcg/day **IV** 50% of usual PO dose

Myxedema Coma

Adult: **IV** 200–500 mcg IV stat, then 100–300 mcg after 24 h if needed, then 50–200 mcg/day until patient is stable and can take drug PO

STORAGE
Store in tightly covered, light-resistant container.

ADMINISTRATION

Oral
■ Give as a single dose, preferably 1 h before or 2 h after breakfast, to prevent insomnia. Give consistently with respect to meals.

Intravenous

***PREPARE* Direct:** Reconstitute by adding 5 mL NS for injection immediately before administration. Shake vial until solution is clear. Do NOT mix with IV solutions. Discard unused portion.
***ADMINISTER* Direct:** Give at a rate of 0.1 mg or a fraction thereof over 1 min into a Y-site closest to needle insertion. Give IMMEDIATELY after reconstitution.

ADVERSE EFFECTS CNS: Irritability, nervousness, *insomnia,* headache (pseudotumor cerebri in children), tremors, craniosynostosis (excessive doses in children). **CV:** Palpitations, tachycardia, arrhythmias, angina pectoris, hypertension. **GI:** Nausea, diarrhea, change in appetite. **Urogenital:** Menstrual irregularities. **Body as a Whole:** Weight loss, heat intolerance, sweating, fever, leg cramps, temporary hair loss (children), anaphylaxis to tartrazine in 0.1 and 0.3 mg tablets.

INTERACTIONS Drug: Cholestyramine, colestipol decrease absorption of levothyroxine; **epinephrine, norepinephrine** increase risk of cardiac insufficiency; ORAL ANTICOAGULANTS may potentiate hypoprothrombinemia.

PHARMACOKINETICS Absorption: Variable and incompletely absorbed from GI tract (50–80%). **Peak:** 3–4 wk. **Duration:** 1–3 wk. **Distribution:** Gradually released into tissue cells. **Half-Life:** 6–7 days.

NURSING IMPLICATIONS

Assessment & Drug Effects

- Monitor pulse before each dose during dose adjustment. If rate is >100 or level determined for child, consult prescriber.
- Monitor for adverse effects during early adjustment. If metabolism increases too rapidly, especially in heart disease patients, symptoms of angina or cardiac failure may appear.
- Note: Levothyroxine may aggravate severity of previously obscured symptoms of diabetes mellitus, Addison's disease, or diabetes insipidus. Therapy for these disorders may require adjustment.
- Lab tests: Baseline and periodic tests of thyroid function. Closely monitor PT/INR and assess for evidence of bleeding if patient is receiving concurrent anticoagulant therapy. A decrease in anticoagulant dosage may be needed 1–4 wk after concurrent levothyroxine is started.
- Monitor bone age, growth, and psychomotor function in children.
- Some children have partial hair loss after a few months; it returns even with continued therapy.
- Synthroid 0.1- and 0.3-mg tablets contain tartrazine, which may cause an allergic-type reaction in certain patients, particularly those who are hypersensitive to aspirin.

Patient & Family Education

- Thyroid replacement therapy is usually lifelong.
- Learn how to self-monitor pulse rate. Notify prescriber if rate begins to increase above 100 (or level determined for child) or if rhythm changes are noted.
- Notify prescriber immediately of signs of toxicity (e.g., chest pain, palpitations, nervousness).
- Avoid OTC medications unless approved by prescriber.
- Be sure child visits health care provider regularly for growth and other measurements.
- Do not breast feed while taking this drug without consulting physician.
- Store this medication out of reach of children.

LIDOCAINE HYDROCHLORIDE ⊘

(lye'doe-kane)

Anestacon, Dilocaine, L-Caine, Lidoderm, Lida-Mantle, Lidoject-1, LidoPen Auto Injector, Nervocaine, Octocaine, Xylocaine, Xylocard ♣

Classifications: CARDIOVASCULAR AGENT; ANTIARRHYTHMIC, CLASS IB; CENTRAL NERVOUS SYSTEM AGENT; LOCAL ANESTHETIC (AMIDE TYPE)
Pregnancy Category: B

AVAILABILITY Antidysrhythmic 300 mg/3 mL auto-injector; 0.2%, 0.4%, 0.8%, 1%, 2%, 4%, 10%, 20% injections **Local Anesthetic** 0.5%, 1%,

1.5%, 2%, 4% **Topical** 2%, 2.5%, 4%, 5% solution; 2.5%, 5% ointment; 0.5%, 4% cream; 0.5%, 2.5% gel; 0.5%, 10% spray; 2% jelly; 0.5% patch

ACTIONS Similar to those of procainamide and quinidine, but has little effect on myocardial contractility, AV and intraventricular conduction, cardiac output, and systolic arterial pressure in equivalent doses. Exerts antiarrhythmic action (Class IB) by suppressing automaticity in His-Purkinje system and by elevating electrical stimulation threshold of ventricle during diastole. Action as local anesthetic is more prompt, more intense, and longer lasting than that of procaine.

THERAPEUTIC EFFECTS Suppresses automaticity in His-Purkinje system and elevates electrical stimulation threshold of ventricle during diastole. Prompt, intense and long-lasting local anesthetic.

USES Rapid control of ventricular arrhythmias occurring during acute MI, cardiac surgery, and cardiac catheterization and those caused by digitalis intoxication. Also as surface and infiltration anesthesia and for nerve block, including caudal and spinal block anesthesia and to relieve local discomfort of skin and mucous membranes. Patch for relief of pain associated with post-herpetic neuralgia.

UNLABELED USES Refractory status epilepticus.

CONTRAINDICATIONS History of hypersensitivity to amide-type local anesthetics; application or injection of lidocaine anesthetic in presence of severe trauma or sepsis, blood dyscrasias, supraventricular arrhythmias, Stokes-Adams syndrome, untreated sinus bradycardia, severe degrees of sinoatrial, atrioventricular, and intraventricular heart block. Safe use during pregnancy (category B), lactation, or in children is not established.

CAUTIOUS USE Liver or kidney disease, CHF, marked hypoxia, respiratory depression, hypovolemia, shock; myasthenia gravis; debilitated patients, older adults; family history of malignant hyperthermia (fulminant hypermetabolism). Topical use in eyes, over large body areas, over prolonged periods, in severe or extensive trauma or skin disorders.

ROUTE & DOSAGE

Ventricular Arrhythmias

Child: **IV** 0.5–1 mg/kg bolus dose, then 10–50 mcg/kg/min infusion (max dose in 1st hr, 3–5 mg/kg)
Adult: **IV** 50–100 mg bolus at a rate of 20–50 mg/min, may repeat in 5 min, then start infusion of 20–50 mcg/kg/min (1–4 mg/min) immediately after first bolus **IM/SC** 200–300 mg IM, may repeat once after 60–90 min

Anesthetic Uses

Child: **Infiltration** max dose (solutions without epinephrine) 4.5 mg/kg/dose (or up to 300 mg) **Infiltration** max dose (solution with epinephrine) 7 mg/kg/dose (or up to 500 mg), not to be repeated within 2 h **Topical** 3 mg/kg/dose, not to be repeated within 2 h
Adult: **Infiltration** 0.5–1% solution **Nerve Block** 1–2% solution **Epidural** 1–2% solution **Caudal** 1–1.5% solution **Spinal** 5% with glucose **Saddle Block** 1.5% with dextrose **Topical** 2.5–5% jelly, ointment, cream, or solution

---

Post-Herpetic Neuralgia

Adult: **Topical** Apply up to 3 patches over intact skin in most painful areas once for up to 12 h per 24-h period

STORAGE

Store all products at room temperature 15°–30° C (59°–86° F).

ADMINISTRATION

Intramuscular

- Give in deltoid muscle or anterolateral thigh as preferred sites. See Part I for site selection.

Topical

- Do not apply topical lidocaine to large areas of skin or to broken or abraded surfaces. Consult prescriber about covering area with a dressing.
- Avoid topical preparation contact with eyes.

Intravenous

Note: Do not use lidocaine solutions containing preservatives for spinal or epidural (including caudal) block. Use ONLY lidocaine HCl injection without preservatives or epinephrine that is specifically labeled for IV injection or infusion. Do not use preparation with epinephrine for arrhythmia. Prolonged administration to infants may cause toxicity.

PREPARE **Direct:** Give undiluted. **IV Infusion:** Use D5W for infusion. For adults, add 1 g to 250 or 500 mL to yield 2 or 4 mg/mL, respectively; for children, add 120 mg to 100 mL to yield 1.2 mg/mL. ■ Do not use solutions with particulate matter or discoloration.

ADMINISTER **Direct:** Give at a rate of 50 mg or fraction thereof over 1 min. **IV Infusion:** Use microdrip and infusion pump. Rate of flow is usually ≤4 mg/min.

INCOMPATIBILITIES: **Solution/Additive: Phenytoin, ampicillin, cefazolin. Y-Site: Amphotericin B cholesteryl complex, phenytoin, thiopental.** ■ Discard partially used solutions of lidocaine without preservatives.

ADVERSE EFFECTS CNS: Drowsiness, dizziness, light-headedness, restlessness, confusion, disorientation, irritability, apprehension, euphoria, wild excitement, numbness of lips or tongue and other paresthesias including sensations of heat and cold, chest heaviness, difficulty in speaking, difficulty in breathing or swallowing, muscular twitching, tremors, psychosis. With high doses: convulsions, respiratory depression and arrest. **CV:** With high doses, hypotension, bradycardia, conduction disorders including heart block, cardiovascular collapse, cardiac arrest. **Special Senses:** Tinnitus, decreased hearing; blurred or double vision, impaired color perception. **Skin:** Site of topical application may develop erythema, edema. **GI:** Anorexia, nausea, vomiting. **Body as a Whole:** Excessive perspiration, soreness at IM site, local thrombophlebitis (with prolonged IV infusion), hypersensitivity reactions (urticaria, rash, edema, anaphylactoid reactions).

DIAGNOSTIC TEST INTERFERENCE Increases in ***creatine phosphokinase (CPK)*** level may occur for 48 h after IM dose and may interfere with test for presence of MI.

INTERACTIONS Drug: Lidocaine patch may increase toxic effects of **tocainide, mexiletine;** BARBITURATES decrease lidocaine activity; **cimetidine,** BETA-BLOCKERS, **quinidine** increase pharmacologic effects of lidocaine; **phenytoin** increases cardiac depressant effects; **procainamide** compounds neurologic and cardiac effects.

PHARMACOKINETICS Absorption: Topical application is 3% absorbed through intact skin. **Onset:** 45–90 sec IV; 5–15 min IM; 2–5 min topical. **Duration:** 10–20 min IV; 60–90 min IM; 30–60 min topical; >100 min injected for anesthesia. **Distribution:** Crosses blood–brain barrier and placenta; distributed into breast milk. **Metabolism:** Metabolized in liver. **Elimination:** Excreted in urine. **Half-Life:** 1.5–2 h; 3.2 h in premature infants.

NURSING IMPLICATIONS

Assessment & Drug Effects

- Stop infusion immediately if ECG indicates excessive cardiac depression (e.g., prolongation of PR interval or QRS complex and the appearance or aggravation of arrhythmias).
- Monitor BP and ECG constantly; assess respiratory and neurologic status frequently to avoid potential overdosage and toxicity.
- Auscultate lungs for basilar rales, especially in patients who tend to metabolize the drug slowly (e.g., CHF, cardiogenic shock, hepatic dysfunction).
- Watch for neurotoxic effects (e.g., drowsiness, dizziness, confusion, paresthesias, visual disturbances, excitement, behavioral changes) in patients receiving IV infusions or with high lidocaine blood levels.
- Note: Lidocaine *therapeutic serum levels* are 1.5–5 mg/L to treat arrhythmia. Levels greater than 7 mg/L are potentially toxic; toxicity level in premature infants is 5 mg/L.

Patient & Family Education

- Swish and spit out when using lidocaine solution for relief of mouth discomfort; gargle for use in pharynx, may be swallowed (follow prescriber instructions). Evaluate ability of child to follow directions and use drug correctly.
- Oral topical anesthetics (e.g., Xylocaine Viscous) may interfere with swallowing reflex. Should NOT be used for teething discomfort in infants. Do NOT ingest food within 60 min after drug application, especially pediatric, or debilitated patients. Do not chew gum while buccal and throat membranes are anesthetized to prevent biting trauma.
- Do not breast feed while taking this drug without consulting physician.
- Store this medication out of reach of children.

LINCOMYCIN HYDROCHLORIDE

(lin-koe-mye′sin)
Lincocin
Classifications: ANTI-INFECTIVE; CLINDAMYCIN ANTIBIOTIC
Prototype: Clindamycin
Pregnancy Category: B

LINCOMYCIN HYDROCHLORIDE

AVAILABILITY 500 mg capsules; 300 mg injection

ACTIONS Derived from *Streptomyces lincolnensis*. Similar to clindamycin in antibacterial activity and demonstrates some cross-resistance with it. Bacteriostatic or bactericidal depending on concentration used and sensitivity of organism.

THERAPEUTIC EFFECTS Effective against most of the common gram-positive pathogens, particularly streptococci, pneumococci, and staphylococci. Also effective against Bacteroides and other anaerobes; however, it has little activity against most gram-negative organisms and ineffective against viruses, yeasts, or fungi. Resistance by *Staphylococcus* is acquired in stepwise manner.

USES Reserved for treatment of serious infections caused by susceptible bacteria in penicillin-allergic patients or patients for whom penicillin is inappropriate.

CONTRAINDICATIONS Previous hypersensitivity to lincomycin and clindamycin; impaired liver function, known monilial infections (unless treated concurrently); use in newborns. Safe use in pregnancy (category B) or lactation is not established.

CAUTIOUS USE Impaired kidney function; history of GI disease, particularly colitis; history of liver, endocrine, or metabolic diseases; history of asthma, hay fever, eczema, drug or other allergies; older adult patients.

ROUTE & DOSAGE

Infections

Child: PO >1 mo, 30–60 mg/kg in 3–4 divided doses **IM** 10 mg/kg q12–24h **IV** 10–20 mg/kg/day in 2–3 divided doses
Adult: PO 500 mg q6–8h (max 8 g/day) **IM** 600 mg q12–24h **IV** 600 mg–1 g q8–12h
Patients with renal disease (Cl_{cr} <10 mL/min) should receive 25–30% usual dose.

STORAGE

Store capsules and injection solution at 20°–25° C (68°–77° F). Store capsules in tightly covered containers and avoid freezing solution.

ADMINISTRATION

Oral/Intramuscular

- Give with a full glass (240 mL [8 oz]) of water or generous amount for age at least 1 h before or 2 h after meals; absorption is reduced and delayed by presence of food in stomach.
- Give injection deep into large muscle mass appropriate for age (see Part I); inject slowly to minimize pain. Rotate injection sites.

Intravenous

PREPARE Intermittent: Dilute 1 g of lincomycin in at least 100 mL of D5W, NS, or other compatible solution.
ADMINISTER Intermittent: Give at a rate ≤1 g/h.

Common adverse effects in *italic;* life-threatening effects <u>underlined</u>; generic names in **bold;** drug classifications in SMALL CAPS; ✦ Canadian drug name; ❂ Prototype drug.

INCOMPATIBILITIES **Solution/Additive: Penicillin G, phenytoin, ampicillin, carbenicillin, methicillin.** ▪ Follow manufacturer's directions for further information on reconstitution, storage time, compatible IV fluids, and IV administration rates.

ADVERSE EFFECTS Body as a Whole: Hypersensitivity (pruritus, urticaria, skin rashes, exfoliative and vesiculobullous dermatitis, erythema multiforme [rare], angioedema, photosensitivity, <u>anaphylactoid reaction</u>, serum sickness); superinfections (proctitis, pruritus ani, vaginitis); vertigo, dizziness, headache, generalized myalgia, thrombophlebitis following IV use; pain at IM injection site. **CV:** Hypotension, syncope, <u>cardiopulmonary arrest</u> (particularly after rapid IV). **GI:** Glossitis, stomatitis, *nausea, vomiting,* anorexia, decreased taste acuity, unpleasant or altered taste, abdominal cramps, *diarrhea,* acute enterocolitis, <u>pseudomembranous colitis</u> (potentially fatal). **Hematologic:** Neutropenia, leukopenia, <u>agranulocytosis</u>, thrombocytopenic purpura, <u>aplastic anemia</u>. **Special Senses:** Tinnitus.

INTERACTIONS Drug: Kaolin/pectin decreases lincomycin absorption; **tubocurarine, pancuronium** may enhance neuromuscular blockade.

PHARMACOKINETICS Absorption: Partially absorbed from GI tract (20–30%). **Peak:** 2–4 h PO; 30 min IM. **Duration:** 6–8 h PO; 12–14 h IM; 14 h IV. **Distribution:** High concentrations in bone, aqueous humor, bile, and peritoneal, pleural, and synovial fluids; crosses placenta; distributed into breast milk. **Metabolism:** Partially metabolized in liver. **Elimination:** Excreted in urine and feces. **Half-Life:** 5 h.

NURSING IMPLICATIONS

Assessment & Drug Effects
▪ Lab tests: Perform C&S initially and during therapy to determine continued microbial susceptibility. Periodic liver & kidney function tests and CBC are indicated during prolonged drug therapy.
▪ Take a careful history of previous sensitivities to drugs or other allergens.
▪ Monitor BP and pulse. Have patient remain recumbent following drug administration until BP stabilizes.
▪ Monitor closely and report changes in bowel frequency. Discontinue drug if significant diarrhea occurs.
▪ Diarrhea, acute colitis, or pseudomembranous colitis (see Appendix D-1) may occur up to several weeks after cessation of therapy.
▪ Examine IM/IV injection sites daily for signs of inflammation.
▪ Monitor serum drug levels closely in patients with severe impairment of kidney function (levels tend to be higher).
▪ Superinfections by nonsusceptible organisms are most likely to occur when duration of therapy exceeds 10 days (see Appendix D-1).

Patient & Family Education
▪ Notify prescriber immediately of symptoms of hypersensitivity (see Appendix D-1). Drug should be discontinued.
▪ Notify prescriber promptly of the onset of perianal irritation, diarrhea, or blood and mucus in stools. Do not self-medicate for diarrhea; antidiarrheal agents may prolong and worsen diarrhea by delaying removal of toxins from colon.

Common adverse effects in *italic*; life-threatening effects <u>underlined</u>; generic names in **bold;** drug classifications in SMALL CAPS; ♣ Canadian drug name; ✪ Prototype drug.

- Take drug as prescribed for full course of therapy.
- Do not breast feed while taking this drug without consulting prescriber.
- Store this medication out of reach of children.

LINDANE ●

(lin'dane)

Gamma Benzene, Kwell, Scabene

Classifications: SKIN AND MUCOUS MEMBRANE AGENT; SCABICIDE; PEDI-CULICIDE

Pregnancy Category: C

AVAILABILITY 1% lotion, shampoo

ACTIONS Related to its direct absorption by parasites and ova (nits). Drug absorption through the exoskeleton stimulates the nervous system of the parasites, resulting in seizures and death.

THERAPEUTIC EFFECTS Has ectoparasitic and ovicidal activity against the two variants of *Pediculus humanus, P. capitis* (head louse), and *P. pubis* (crab louse), and the arthropod *Sarcoptes scabiei* (scabies). Lindane is not prophylactic for pediculosis.

USES To treat head and crab lice and scabies infestations and to eradicate their ova.

CONTRAINDICATIONS Premature neonates, patient with known seizure disorders; application to eyes, face, mucous membranes, urethral meatus, open cuts or raw, weeping surfaces; prolonged or excessive applications or simultaneous application of creams, ointments, oils. Use during pregnancy (category B), in children <2 y, or lactation is not recommended by CDC.

CAUTIOUS USE Children <10 y.

ROUTE & DOSAGE

Pediculosis and Scabies Infestation

Child/Adult <2 y: **Topical** Apply to all body areas except the face, urethra, mucous membranes, or nonintact skin; leave lotion on 8–12 h for adults, 6–8 h for children, then rinse off; leave shampoo on 5 min, then rinse thoroughly; may repeat once in 7 days if needed

Pediculosis Capitis

Topical Apply 15–30 mL shampoo, lather 4–5 min, rinse, and comb with fine-toothed comb; repeat once in 7 days if needed

STORAGE

Store in tight container away from direct light and heat. Protect from freezing.

ADMINISTRATION

Note: Caregiver needs to wear plastic disposable or rubber gloves when applying lindane, especially if pregnant or applying medication to more than one patient, to avoid prolonged skin contact. Permethrin, not lindane, is to be used in infants and young children and during pregnancy.

Topical

- Remove all skin lotions, creams, and oil-based hair dressings completely and allow skin to dry and cool before applying lindane; this will reduce percutaneous absorption.
- Shake cream or lotion container well. *Scabies:* Apply thin film from neck down over entire body surface including soles of feet. Avoid face and urethral meatus. Pay particular attention to intertriginous areas (finger webs and other body creases and folds), wrists, elbows, axilla, groin, and belt line. Rub drug in; allow skin to dry and cool after application. After 8–12 h (6–8 h for children), remove medication by bath or shower. Change all clothing and bedding; treat family members. *Pediculosis pubis:* Apply thin film of drug to hair and skin of pubic area and, if infected, to thighs, trunk, axillary areas. Leave in place 8–12 h and follow with bath or shower. Observation of living lice after 7 days indicates the need for reapplication. Sexual contacts should be treated.
- Shampoo *Pediculosis capitis:* Apply sufficient quantity to wet hair and skin. Work drug thoroughly onto hair shafts and scalp and allow to remain in place 4 min. Add small amounts of water sufficient to make a thick lather; then rinse well with water. Pay particular attention to areas above and behind ears and occipital region. Use fine-tooth comb or tweezers to remove remaining nit shells. If necessary, treatment may be repeated after 7 days. *Pediculosis pubis:* See above. Repeat treatment after 7 days only if live lice are present.

ADVERSE EFFECTS CNS: CNS stimulation (usually after accidental ingestion or misuse of product): Restlessness, dizziness, tremors, seizures. **Hematologic:** Aplastic anemia. **Body as a Whole:** Inhalation (headache, nausea, vomiting, irritation of ENT). **Skin:** Eczematous eruptions, rash.

INTERACTIONS Drug: No clinically significant interactions established.

PHARMACOKINETICS Absorption: Slowly and incompletely absorbed through intact skin; maximum absorption from face, scalp, axillae. **Distribution:** Stored in body fat. **Metabolism:** Metabolized in liver. **Elimination:** Excreted in urine and feces.

NURSING IMPLICATIONS

Assessment & Drug Effects

- Suspect scabies if a person complains of nocturnal itching (classic symptom). Infestation sources: Sex partner, other family members, people and animals in close contact.
- Identify and treat the sex partner simultaneously because both scabies and *P. pubis* infestation are sexually transmitted diseases.
- Burrows made by scabies mites (may or may not be visible) appear as grayish black straight or S-shaped lines with a papule containing the mite at one end and surrounded by a mild erythematous area.

Patient & Family Education

- Lindane is a highly toxic drug if topical applications are excessive or if swallowed or inhaled, and when administered to infants and young children. Keep out of reach of children.
- Cover hands of young children to prevent accidental ingestion from thumb sucking.
- Note: Lindane shampoo is an effective disinfectant for personal items such as combs, brushes.
- Skin penetration with scabies mites causes an intolerable itching that may persist 2–3 wk after they have been killed.
- Discontinue medication and notify prescriber if skin eruptions appear.
- Do not apply medication to face, mouth, open skin lesions, or to eyelashes; avoid contact with eyes. If accidental eye contact occurs, flush with water.
- Recurring limited infestations of scabies may indicate a domestic animal source (e.g., cat, dog, cattle, poultry).
- Perform related teaching to manage infections (e.g., washing bedding, care of toys, avoiding sharing of hair care supplies).
- Do not breast feed while taking this drug.
- Store this medication out of reach of children.

LINEZOLID ⊕

(lin-e-zo_lid)
Zyvox, Zyvoxam ♦
Classifications: ANTI-INFECTIVE; ANTIBIOTIC; OXAZOLIDINONE
Pregnancy Category: C

AVAILABILITY 400 mg, 600 mg tablets; 100 mg/5 mL suspension; 200 mg, 400 mg, 600 mg injection

ACTIONS Synthetic antibiotic of a new class, the oxazolidinone group, that is bacteriocidal against gram-positive, gram-negative, and anaerobic bacteria. It binds to a site on the bacterial 23S ribosomal RNA of the bacteria, which prevents the bacterial RNA translation process.

THERAPEUTIC EFFECTS Bacteriostatic against *enterococci* and *staphylococci,* and bacteriocidal against *streptococci.* These include *Enterococcus faecium* (vancomycin-resistant strains only), *Staphylococcus aureus* (including methicillin-resistant) strains.

USES Treatment of vancomycin-resistant *Enterococcus faecium,* nosocomial pneumonia, complicated and uncomplicated skin and skin structure infections, community-acquired pneumonia due to susceptible gram-positive organisms.

CONTRAINDICATIONS Hypersensitivity to linezolid, pregnancy (category C). Safety and effectiveness in children <18 y not established, but has been used in cases where other therapy is not available.

CAUTIOUS USE Lactation, previous thrombocytopenia; patients on MAOI, or serotonin-reuptake inhibitors, or adrenergic agents, hypertension; phenylketonuria; carcinoid syndrome.

ROUTE & DOSAGE

Vancomycin-Resistant *Enterococcus faecium*

Child: **PO/IV** *2–11 y,* 10 mg/kg q8h times 14–28 days
Adolescents/Adult: **PO/IV** *≥12 y,* 600 mg q12h times 14–28 days

Nosocomial or Community-Acquired Pneumonia, Complicated Skin Infections

Child: **PO/IV** *2–11 y,* 10 mg/kg q8h times 10–14 days
Adolescents/Adult: **PO/IV** *≥12 y,* 600 mg q12h times 10–14 days

Uncomplicated Skin Infections

Child: **PO** *5–11 y,* 10 mg/kg q12h times 10–14 days
Adolescents/Adult: **PO** *≥12 y,* 400–600 mg q12h times 10–14 days

STORAGE
Store at 25° C (77° F) preferred; 15°–30° C (59°–86° F) permitted. Protect from light and keep bottles tightly closed.

ADMINISTRATION
Note: No dosage adjustment is necessary when switching from IV to oral administration.

Oral
- Reconstitute suspension by adding 123 mL distilled water in two portions; after adding first half, shake to wet all of the powder, then add second half of water and shake vigorously to produce a uniform suspension with a concentration of 100 mg/5 mL.
- Before each use, mix suspension by inverting bottle 3–5 times, but DO NOT SHAKE. Discard unused suspension after 21 days.

Intravenous
***PREPARE* Intermittent:** IV solution is supplied in a single-use, ready-to-use infusion bag. Remove from protective wrap immediately prior to use. Check for minute leaks by firmly squeezing bag. Discard if leaks are detected.
***ADMINISTER* Intermittent:** Do not use infusion bag in a series connection. Give over 30–120 min. If IV line is used to infuse other drugs, flush before and after with D5W, or NS, or LR.
***INCOMPATIBILITIES* Solution/Additive:** Ceftriaxone, erythromycin, trimethoprim-sulfamethoxazole. **Y-Site:** Amphotericin B, ceftriaxone, chlorpromazine, diazepam, pentamidine, erythromycin, phenytoin, trimethoprim-sulfamethoxazole.

ADVERSE EFFECTS Body as a Whole: Fever. **GI:** *Diarrhea, nausea, vomiting, constipation, taste alteration,* abnormal LFTs, tongue discoloration. **Hematologic:** Thrombocytopenia, leukopenia. **CNS:** *Headache, insomnia, dizziness.* **Skin:** Rash. **Urogenital:** Vaginal moniliasis.

INTERACTIONS Drug: MAO INHIBITORS may cause hypertensive crisis; **pseudoephedrine** may cause elevated BP. **Food:** TYRAMINE-CONTAINING FOOD may cause elevated BP. **Herbal: Ginseng, ephedra, ma huang** may lead to elevated BP, headache, nervousness.

PHARMACOKINETICS Absorption: Rapidly or extensively absorbed, 100% bioavailable. **Peak:** 1–2 h PO. **Distribution:** 31% protein bound. **Metabolism:** Metabolized by oxidation. **Elimination:** Primarily excreted in urine. **Half-Life:** 6–7 h.

NURSING IMPLICATIONS

Assessment & Drug Effects

- Monitor for S&S of bleeding, hypertension, or pseudomembranous colitis that begins with diarrhea.
- Lab tests: C&S before initiating therapy and during therapy as indicated; drug may be started pending results. Monitor complete blood count, including platelet count and Hgb & Hct, in those at risk for bleeding or with >2 wk of linezolid therapy.

Patient & Family Education

- Report any of the following to physician promptly: Onset of diarrhea; easy bruising or bleeding of any type; or S&S of superinfection (see Appendix D-1).
- Avoid foods and beverages high in tyramine (e.g., aged, fermented, pickled or smoked foods and beverages). Limit tyramine intake to >100 mg per meal (see *Information for Patients* provided by the manufacturer).
- Do not take OTC cold remedies or decongestants without consulting physician.
- Note for phenylketonurics: Each 5-mL oral suspension contains 20 mg phenylalanine.
- Do not breast feed while taking this drug without consulting physician.
- Store this medication out of reach of children.

LIOTHYRONINE SODIUM (T₃)

(lye-oh-thye'roe-neen)
Cytomel, Triostat
Classifications: HORMONE AND SYNTHETIC SUBSTITUTE; THYROID AGENT
Prototype: Levothyroxine sodium
Pregnancy Category: A

AVAILABILITY 5 mcg, 25 mcg, 50 mcg tablets; 10 mcg/mL injection

ACTIONS Synthetic form of natural thyroid hormone. Shares actions and uses of thyroid but has more rapid action and more rapid disappearance of effect, permitting quick dosage adjustment if necessary.
THERAPEUTIC EFFECTS Used in T₃ suppression test to differentiate suspected hyperthyroidism from euthyroidism. Principal effect: Increase in the metabolic rate of all body tissues.

USES Replacement or supplemental therapy for cretinism, myxedema, goiter, secondary (pituitary) or tertiary (hypothalamic) hypothyroidism, and T₃ suppression test.

CONTRAINDICATIONS Hypersensitivity to liothyronine; thyrotoxicosis, severe cardiovascular conditions, adrenal insufficiency.

Common adverse effects in *italic;* life-threatening effects <u>underlined</u>; generic names in **bold**; drug classifications in SMALL CAPS; ♦ Canadian drug name; ☻ Prototype drug.

CAUTIOUS USE Angina pectoris, hypertension, impaired kidney function; pregnancy (category A), lactation.

ROUTE & DOSAGE

Thyroid Replacement
Child: **PO** 5 mcg/day gradually increased by 5 mcg/day q3–4days until desired response
Adult: **PO** 25–75 mcg/day

Myxedema
Adult: **PO** 5–100 mcg/day **IV** 25–50 mcg, may repeat >4 h and <12 h after previous dose. Target dose >65 mcg/day (max 100 mcg/day)

Goiter
Child: **PO** 5 mcg/day, increase by 5 mcg q1–2wk (usual maintenance dose 15–20 mcg/day)
Adult: **PO** 5–75 mcg/day

T₃ Suppression Test
Adult: **PO** 75–100 mcg/day times 7 days

L

STORAGE
Store tablets in heat-, light-, and moisture-proof container.

ADMINISTRATION

Oral
- Give daily before breakfast.
- Discontinue other thyroid drug when changing to liothyronine; initiate liothyronine at low dosage with gradual increases according to patient's response.

Intravenous

PREPARE Direct: Give undiluted.
ADMINISTER Direct: Give each 10 mcg or fraction thereof over 1 min.

ADVERSE EFFECTS Endocrine: Result from overdosage evidenced as S&S of hyperthyroidism (see Appendix D-1). **Musculoskeletal:** Accelerated rate of bone maturation in children.

INTERACTIONS Drug: Cholestyramine, colestipol decrease absorption; **epinephrine, norepinephrine** increase risk of cardiac insufficiency; ORAL ANTICOAGULANTS may potentiate hypoprothrombinemia.

PHARMACOKINETICS Absorption: Completely absorbed from GI tract. **Peak:** 24–72 h. **Duration:** Up to 72 h. **Distribution:** Gradually released into tissue cells. **Half-Life:** 6–7 days.

NURSING IMPLICATIONS

Assessment & Drug Effects
- Watch for possible additive effects during the early period of liothyronine substitution for another preparation, particularly in children and

Common adverse effects in *italic;* life-threatening effects underlined; generic names in **bold;** drug classifications in SMALL CAPS; ♣ Canadian drug name; ❷ Prototype drug.

735

patients with cardiovascular disease. Residual actions of other thyroid preparations may persist for weeks.

- Monitor and evaluate child's growth and developmental patterns.
- Metabolic effects of liothyronine persist a few days after drug withdrawal.
- Withhold drug for 1–2 days at onset of overdosage symptoms (hyperthyroidism, see Appendix D-1); usually therapy can be resumed with lower dosage.

Patient & Family Education

- Take medication exactly as ordered.
- Learn S&S of hyperthyroidism (see Appendix D-1); notify prescriber promptly if they appear.
- Ensure that child is seen in health supervision visits for monitoring of growth and development.
- Do not breast feed while taking this drug without consulting physician.
- Store this medication out of reach of children.

LIOTRIX (T₃-T₄)

(lye'oh-trix)

Euthroid, Thyrolar

Classifications: HORMONE AND SYNTHETIC SUBSTITUTE; THYROID AGENT

Prototype: Levothyroxine sodium

Pregnancy Category: A

AVAILABILITY ¼ grain, ½ grain, 1 grain, 2 grain, 3 grain tablets

ACTIONS Synthetic levothyroxine (T_4) and liothyronine (T_3) combined in a constant 4:1 ratio by weight. Products by different manufacturers differ in total amounts of each drug included in the formulation.

THERAPEUTIC EFFECTS Increases metabolic rate of all body tissues.

USES Replacement or supplemental therapy for cretinism, myxedema, goiter, and secondary (pituitary) or tertiary (hypothalamic) hypothyroidism. Also with antithyroid agents in thyrotoxicosis and to prevent goitrogenesis and hypothyroidism.

CONTRAINDICATIONS Thyrotoxicosis, acute MI, morphologic hypogonadism, nephrosis, adrenal deficiency due to hypopituitarism.

CAUTIOUS USE Concomitant anticoagulant therapy; myxedema; angina pectoris, hypertension, arteriosclerosis; kidney dysfunction, pregnancy (category A), lactation.

ROUTE & DOSAGE

Thyroid Replacement

Child/Adult: **PO** 12.5–30 mcg/day, gradually increase to desired response

STORAGE

Store in heat-, light-, and moisture-proof container. Shelf-life: 2 y.

ADMINISTRATION

Oral

- Give as a single daily dose, preferably before breakfast.
- Make dose increases at 1- to 2-wk intervals.

ADVERSE EFFECTS CNS: Nervousness, headache, tremors, insomnia. **CV:** Palpitation, tachycardia, angina pectoris, cardiac arrhythmias, hypertension, CHF. **GI:** Nausea, abdominal cramps, diarrhea. **Body as a Whole:** Weight loss, heat intolerance, fever, sweating, menstrual irregularities. **Musculoskeletal:** Accelerated rate of bone maturation in infants and children.

INTERACTIONS Drug: Cholestyramine, colestipol decrease absorption; **epinephrine, norepinephrine** increase risk of cardiac insufficiency; ORAL ANTICOAGULANTS may potentiate hypoprothrombinemia.

PHARMACOKINETICS Not studied.

NURSING IMPLICATIONS

Assessment & Drug Effects

- Watch for possible additive effects during the early period of liothyronine substitution for another preparation, particularly in children, and patients with cardiovascular disease. Residual actions of other thyroid preparations may persist for weeks.
- Monitor and evaluate child's growth and developmental patterns.
- Note: Metabolic effects of liotrix persist a few days after drug withdrawal.
- Withhold drug for 1–2 days at onset of overdosage symptoms (hyperthyroidism; see Appendix D-1); usually therapy can be resumed with lower dosage.
- Monitor diabetics for glycemic control; an increase in insulin or oral hypoglycemic may be required.

Patient & Family Education

- Follow directions for taking this drug (see ADMINISTRATION).
- Notify prescriber of headache (euthyroid patients); may indicate need for dosage adjustment or change to another thyroid preparation.
- Take medication exactly as ordered.
- Learn S&S of hyperthyroidism (see Appendix D-1); notify prescriber if they appear.
- Ensure that child is seen in health supervision visits for monitoring of growth and development.
- Do not breast feed while taking this drug without consulting physician.
- Store this medication out of reach of children.

LISINOPRIL

(ly-sin′o-pril)

Prinivil, Zestril

Classifications: CARDIOVASCULAR AGENT; ANGIOTENSIN-CONVERTING ENZYME INHIBITOR; ANTIHYPERTENSIVE AGENT

Prototype: Captopril

Pregnancy Category: D

AVAILABILITY 2.5 mg, 5 mg, 10 mg, 20 mg, 40 mg tablets

ACTIONS Lowers BP by specific inhibition of the angiotensin-converting enzyme (ACE). This interrupts conversion sequences initiated by renin that form angiotensin II, a potent vasoconstrictor. ACE inhibition alters hemodynamics without compensatory reflex tachycardia or changes in cardiac output (except in patients with CHF).
THERAPEUTIC EFFECTS Improved cardiac output and exercise tolerance due to inhibition of ACE also decreases circulating aldosterone, which is normally released in response to angiotensin II stimulation. Reduced aldosterone is associated with a potassium-sparing effect. Also decreases peripheral resistance (afterload) and pulmonary vascular resistance.

USES Hypertension, alone or concomitantly with other classes of antihypertensive agents; CHF; to improve MI survival.

CONTRAINDICATIONS Patients with a history of angioedema related to treatment with an angiotensin converting enzyme inhibitor, pregnancy (category D), children <6 y; lactation.
CAUTIOUS USE Impaired kidney function, hyperkalemia, patients on diuretic therapy; autoimmune diseases, especially systemic lupus erythematosus (SLE).

ROUTE & DOSAGE

Hypertension

Child: **PO** 6–16 y, start at 0.07 mg/kg (max 5 mg) daily (max dose 40 mg/day)
Adult: **PO** 10 mg daily, may increase up to 20–40 mg 1–2 times/day (max 80 mg/day)

STORAGE
Store away from both moisture and heat.

ADMINISTRATION
Oral

- Give an initial dose of 5 mg for diuretic-treated patients. Monitor drug effect for 2 h or until the BP is stabilized for at least 1 additional hour. Concurrent administration with a diuretic may compound hypotensive effect.
- Give before dialysis; lisinopril is removed from blood by hemodialysis.

ADVERSE EFFECTS CNS: Headache, dizziness, fatigue. **CV:** Hypotension, chest pain. **GI:** Nausea, vomiting, diarrhea, anorexia, constipation. **Hematologic:** <u>Neutropenia</u>. **Respiratory:** Dyspnea, cough. **Skin:** Rash. **Metabolic:** Azotemia, hyperkalemia, increased BUN and creatinine levels. **Body as a Whole:** Hypersensitivity (hoarseness, swelling of mouth, hands, feet or face, trouble breathing).

INTERACTIONS Drug: Indomethacin and other NSAIDS may decrease antihypertensive activity; POTASSIUM SUPPLEMENTS, POTASSIUM-SPARING

DIURETICS may cause hyperkalemia; may increase **lithium** levels and toxicity.

PHARMACOKINETICS Absorption: 25% absorbed from GI tract. **Onset:** 1 h. **Peak:** 6–8 h. **Duration:** 24 h. **Distribution:** Limited amount crosses blood–brain barrier; crosses placenta; small amount distributed in breast milk. **Metabolism:** Is not metabolized. **Elimination:** Excreted primarily in urine. **Half-Life:** 12 h.

NURSING IMPLICATIONS

Assessment & Drug Effects

- Place patient in supine position and notify physician if sudden and severe hypotension occurs within the first 1–5 h after initial drug dose; possible particularly in patients who are sodium or volume depleted because of diuretic therapy.
- Measure BP just prior to dosing to determine whether satisfactory control is being maintained for 24 h. If the antihypertensive effect is diminished in less than 24 h, an increase in dosage may be necessary.
- Monitor closely for angioedema of extremities, face, lips, tongue, glottis, and larynx. Discontinue drug promptly and notify physician if such symptoms appear; carefully monitor for airway obstruction until swelling is relieved.
- Monitor serum sodium and serum potassium levels for hyponatremia and hyperkalemia.
- Lab tests: Determine WBC count prior to initiation of treatment, every month for the first 3–6 mo of therapy, and at periodic intervals for 1 y. Withhold therapy and notify physician if neutropenia (neutrophil count <1000/mm^3) develops; kidney function tests at periodic intervals, especially in patients with severe volume or sodium replacement or those with severe CHF.

Patient & Family Education

- Discontinue drug and contact physician immediately for severe hypersensitivity reaction (e.g., hoarseness, swelling of the face, mouth, hands, or feet, or sudden trouble breathing).
- Be aware of importance of proper diet, including sodium and potassium restrictions. Do NOT use salt substitute containing potassium.
- Continued compliance with high BP medication is very important. If a dose is missed, take it as soon as possible but not too close to next dose.
- Do not drive or engage in other potentially hazardous activities until response to the drug is known.
- With concomitant therapy lisinopril increases the risk of lithium toxicity.
- Notify physician promptly of any indication of infection (e.g., sore throat, fever).
- Do not store drug in a moist area. Heat and moisture may cause the medicine to break down.
- Do not breast feed while taking this drug.
- Store this medication out of reach of children.

Common adverse effects in *italic;* life-threatening effects underlined; generic names in **bold;** drug classifications in SMALL CAPS; ♣ Canadian drug name; ☮ Prototype drug.

739

LITHIUM CARBONATE 🅟

(li'thee-um)

Eskalith, Eskalith CR, Lithane, Lithobid, Lithonate, Lithotabs

LITHIUM CITRATE

Cibalith-S

Classifications: CENTRAL NERVOUS SYSTEM AGENT; PSYCHOTHERAPEUTIC AGENT; ANTIMANIC

Pregnancy Category: D

AVAILABILITY Lithium Carbonate 150 mg, 300 mg, 600 mg capsules; 300 mg tablets; 300 mg, 450 mg sustained-release tablets **Lithium Citrate** 300 mg/5 mL syrup

ACTIONS The lithium ion behaves in the body much like the sodium ion, but its exact mechanism of action is unclear. Competes with various physiologically important cations: Na^+, K^+, Ca^{2+}, Mg^{2+}; therefore, it affects cell membranes, body water, and neurotransmitters. At the synapse, it accelerates catecholamine destruction, inhibits the release of neurotransmitters and decreases sensitivity of postsynaptic receptors.

THERAPEUTIC EFFECTS Inhibits neurotransmitters; decreases overactivity of receptors involved in stimulating manic states. Response evidenced by changed facial affect, improved posture, assumption of self-care, improved ability to concentrate, improved sleep pattern.

USES Control and prophylaxis of acute mania and the acute manic phase of mixed bipolar disorder.

UNLABELED USES Acute and recurrent depression (unipolar affective disorder), schizophrenic disorders, disorders of impulse control, alcohol dependence, antineoplastic drug-induced neutropenia, aplastic anemia, SIADH, cyclic neutropenia.

CONTRAINDICATIONS Significant cardiovascular or kidney disease, brain damage, severe debilitation, dehydration or sodium depletion; patients on low-salt diet or receiving diuretics; pregnancy, especially first trimester (category D), lactation, children <12 y.

CAUTIOUS USE Older adults; thyroid disease; epilepsy; concomitant use with haloperidol and other antipsychotics; parkinsonism; diabetes mellitus; severe infections; urinary retention.

ROUTE & DOSAGE

Mania

Child: **PO** 15–60 mg/kg/day divided into 3–4 doses; adjust as needed weekly to reach therapeutic effects
Adult: 300 mg t.i.d. or q.i.d. or 15–20 mL (24–32 mEq) solution in 2–4 divided doses; adjust as needed to reach therapeutic effects (max 2.4 g/day)

STORAGE

Store tablets and capsules at 15°–30° C (59°–86° F). Protect from light and moisture.

Common adverse effects in *italic;* life-threatening effects <u>underlined</u>; generic names in **bold;** drug classifications in SMALL CAPS; ♣ Canadian drug name; 🅟 Prototype drug.

ADMINISTRATION

Oral

- Give with meals.
- Ensure that sustained-release tablets are not chewed or crushed; must be swallowed whole.

ADVERSE EFFECTS CNS: Dizziness, *headache, lethargy,* drowsiness, *fatigue,* slurred speech, psychomotor retardation, giddiness, incontinence, restlessness, seizures, confusion, blackout spells, disorientation, *recent memory loss,* stupor, coma, EEG changes. **CV:** Arrhythmias, hypotension, vasculitis, <u>peripheral circulatory collapse</u>, ECG changes. **Special Senses:** Impaired vision, transient scotomas, tinnitus. **Endocrine:** Diffuse thyroid enlargement, hypothyroidism, *nephrogenic diabetes insipidus,* transient hyperglycemia, glycosuria, hyponatremia. **GI:** *Nausea, vomiting, anorexia, abdominal pain, diarrhea, dry mouth,* metallic taste. **Musculoskeletal:** *Fine hand tremors,* coarse tremors, choreoathetotic movements; fasciculations, clonic movements, incoordination including ataxia, *muscle weakness,* hyperreflexia, encephalopathic syndrome (weakness, lethargy, fever, tremors, confusion, extrapyramidal symptoms). **Skin:** Thought to be toxicity rather than allergy: Pruritus, maculopapular rash, hyperkeratosis, chronic folliculitis, transient acneiform papules (face, neck, intertriginous areas), anesthesia of skin, cutaneous ulcers, drying and thinning of hair, allergic vasculitis. **Hematologic:** *Reversible leukocytosis* (14,000 to 18,000/mm^3). **Urogenital:** Albuminuria, oliguria, urinary incontinence, polyuria, polydipsia, increased uric acid excretion. **Body as a Whole:** Edema, weight gain (common) or loss, exacerbation of psoriasis; flu-like symptoms.

INTERACTIONS Drug: Carbamazepine, haloperidol, PHENOTHIAZINES increase risk of neurotoxicity, extrapyramidal effects, and tardive dyskinesias; DIURETICS, NSAIDS, **methyldopa, probenecid,** TETRACYCLINES decrease renal clearance of lithium, increasing pharmacologic and toxic effects; THEOPHYLLINES, **urea, sodium bicarbonate, sodium or potassium citrate** increase renal clearance of lithium, decreasing its pharmacologic effects.

PHARMACOKINETICS Absorption: Readily absorbed from GI tract. **Peak:** 0.5–3 h carbonate; 15–60 min citrate. **Distribution:** Crosses blood–brain barrier and placenta; distributed into breast milk. **Metabolism:** Not metabolized. **Elimination:** 95% excreted in urine, 1% in feces, 4–5% in sweat. **Half-Life:** 20–27 h; longer with renal impairment.

NURSING IMPLICATIONS

Assessment & Drug Effects

- Monitor response to drug. Usual lag of 1–2 wk precedes response to lithium therapy. Keep prescriber informed of progress.
- Monitor lithium level: *Therapeutic level* is 0.6–1.6 mEq/L. *Toxic level* is 2–2.5 mEq/L; seizures or death may occur by 2.5 mEq/L. Blood sample to determine serum lithium level is drawn within 30 min prior to next dose (8–12 h after last dose) when lithium level is fairly stable (after 4–6 days on the drug). When lithium levels are above 2.0 mEq/L, symptoms may include ataxia, blurred vision, giddiness, tinnitus, muscle twitching or coarse tremors, and a large output of dilute urine.

- Monitor for S&S of impending lithium toxicity, such as vomiting, diarrhea, lack of coordination, drowsiness, muscular weakness, slurred speech. Withhold next dose and call prescriber. Drug should not be stopped abruptly.
- Weigh patient daily; check ankles, tibiae, and wrists for edema. Report changes in I&O ratio, sudden weight gain, or edema.
- Polydipsia and polyuria, apparently not dose related, are common early adverse effects. Symptoms may lessen but reappear after several months or even years of maintenance.
- Report early signs of extrapyramidal reactions promptly to prescriber. The encephalopathic syndrome may be induced when lithium is given concomitantly with haloperidol or with other antipsychotic medication, particularly in older adults.
- Keep prescriber informed of all presenting S&S. The fine tremor of hand or jaw, polyuria, mild thirst, transient mild nausea, and general discomfort that may occur in early treatment of mania sometimes persist throughout therapy. Usually, however, symptoms subside with temporary reduction of dose. If symptoms persist, drug is withdrawn.
- Monitor thyroid function periodically. Be alert to and report symptoms of hypothyroidism (see Appendix D-1).
- Neonates born of mothers who took lithium during pregnancy may have high serum lithium level manifested by flaccidity, poor reflexes, cardiac dysrhythmia, and chronic twitching. Care by a neonatoligist is needed.
- Lithane contains tartrazine, which may cause an allergic-type reaction in susceptible patients.

Patient & Family Education

- Be alert to increased output of dilute urine and persistent thirst. Dose reduction may be indicated.
- Contact prescriber if diarrhea or fever develops. Avoid practices that may encourage dehydration: Hot environment, excessive caffeine beverages, excessive exercise.
- Drink generous amounts of liquids during stabilization period and during ongoing therapy.
- Avoid self-prescribed low-salt regimen, self-dosing with Rolaids, Sodamints, or other sodium antacids, high-sodium foods (e.g., prepared meats and diet soda). Avoid also crash diets or diet pills that reduce appetite and food, salt, and fluid intake.
- Reduced intake of fluid and sodium can accelerate lithium retention with subsequent toxicity. Conversely, marked increase in sodium intake can increase lithium excretion and reduce drug effect.
- Do not drive or engage in other potentially hazardous activities until response to drug is known. Lithium may impair both physical and mental ability.
- Use effective contraceptive measures during lithium therapy. If therapy is continued during pregnancy, serum lithium levels must be closely monitored to prevent toxicity. Kidney clearance of lithium increases during pregnancy but reverts to lower rate immediately after delivery; dosage is reduced to prevent toxicity.
- Follow a regular clinical evaluation schedule on serum lithium levels to ensure safe and effective treatment. It is important to you and your family to keep all clinic appointments.

Common adverse effects in *italic*; life-threatening effects underlined; generic names in **bold**; drug classifications in SMALL CAPS; ♣ Canadian drug name; ๑ Prototype drug.

- Do not breast feed while taking this drug.
- Store this medication out of reach of children.

LOMUSTINE
(loe-mus'teen)
CeeNU, CCNU
Classifications: ANTINEOPLASTIC; ALKYLATING AGENT
Prototype: Cyclophosphamide
Pregnancy Category: D

AVAILABILITY 10 mg, 40 mg, 100 mg capsules

ACTIONS Lipid-soluble alkylating nitrosourea with actions like those of carmustine (e.g., cell-cycle nonspecific activity against rapidly proliferating cell populations).
THERAPEUTIC EFFECTS Inhibits synthesis of both DNA and RNA; has antineoplastic and myelosuppressive effect.

USES Palliative therapy in addition to other modalities or with other chemotherapeutic agents in primary and metastatic brain tumors and as secondary therapy in Hodgkin's disease.
UNLABELED USES GI, lung, and renal carcinomas, non-Hodgkin's lymphomas, malignant melanoma, and multiple myelomas.

CONTRAINDICATIONS Immunization with live-virus vaccines, viral infections. Safe use during pregnancy (category D) or lactation is not established. Reported to be carcinogenic in laboratory animals.
CAUTIOUS USE Patients with decreased circulating platelets, leukocytes, or erythrocytes; kidney or liver function impairment; infection; previous cytotoxic or radiation therapy.

ROUTE & DOSAGE

Palliative Therapy
Child: **PO** 75–150 mg/m^2 q6wk
Adult: **PO** 130 mg/m^2 as single dose, repeated in 6 wk; subsequent doses based on hematologic response (WBC > 4000/mm^3, platelets > 100,000/mm^3)

STORAGE
Store capsules away from excessive heat (over 40° C or 115° F).

ADMINISTRATION
Child: Must be given under care and direction of pediatric oncology specialist. Use recommended handling techniques for hazardous medications (see Part I).
Oral
- Give on an empty stomach to reduce possibility of nausea; may also give an antiemetic before drug to prevent nausea.

ADVERSE EFFECTS CNS: Lethargy, ataxia, disorientation. **GI:** Anorexia, *nausea, vomiting,* stomatitis, transient elevations of LFTs. **Hematologic:**

Delayed (cumulative) myelosuppression: <u>thrombocytopenia, leukopenia</u>; anemia. **Skin:** Alopecia, skin rash, itching. **Urogenital:** Nephrotoxicity. **Respiratory:** Pulmonary toxicity (rare).

INTERACTIONS Drug: Cimetidine can increase bone marrow toxicity; ANTICOAGULANTS, NSAIDS, SALICYLATES increase risk of bleeding. **Phenobarbital** may decrease response to lomustine.

PHARMACOKINETICS Absorption: Readily absorbed from GI tract. **Peak:** 1–6 h. **Distribution:** Readily crosses blood–brain barrier; crosses placenta; distributed into breast milk. **Metabolism:** Metabolized in liver to several active metabolites. **Elimination:** Excreted in urine. **Half-Life:** 16–48 h.

NURSING IMPLICATIONS

Assessment & Drug Effects
- Lab tests: Monitor blood counts weekly for at least 6 wk after last dose. Liver and kidney function tests should be performed periodically.
- A repeat course is not given until platelets have returned to above 100,000/mm^3 and leukocytes to above 4000/mm^3.
- Avoid invasive procedures during nadir of platelets.
- Thrombocytopenia occurs about 4 wk and leukopenia about 6 wk after a dose, persisting 1–2 wk.
- Be alert for and report signs of infection such as respiratory infections, aching, rashes, and gastrointestinal distress.
- Assess immunization status prior to beginning therapy in order to be alert for diseases that pose risk.
- Inspect oral cavity daily for S&S of superinfections (see Appendix D-1) and stomatitis or xerostomia.

Patient & Family Education
- Nausea and vomiting may occur 3–5 h after drug administration, usually lasting less than 24 h.
- Anorexia may persist for 2 or 3 days after a dose.
- Notify physician of signs of sore throat, cough, fever. Also report unexplained bleeding or easy bruising.
- Report signs of infections. Avoid exposure to persons with infectious diseases.
- Use reliable contraceptive measures during therapy.
- Be aware of the possibility of hair loss while taking this drug.
- A given dose may include capsules of different colors; the pharmacist prepares prescribed dose by combining various capsule strengths.
- Do not breast feed while taking this drug without consulting physician.
- Store this medication out of reach of children.

LOPERAMIDE

(loe-per′a-mide)
Imodium, Imodium AD, Kaopectate III, Maalox Anti-diarrheal, Pepto Diarrhea Control
Classifications: GASTROINTESTINAL AGENT; ANTIDIARRHEAL
Prototype: Diphenoxylate HCl with atropine sulfate
Pregnancy Category: B

AVAILABILITY 2 mg tablets, capsules; 1 mg/mL, 1 mg/5 mL liquid

ACTIONS Effective antidiarrheal; synthetic piperidine derivative chemically related to diphenoxylate and to meperidine. Reportedly has longer duration of action.

THERAPEUTIC EFFECTS Inhibits GI peristaltic activity by direct action on circular and longitudinal intestinal muscles. Prolongs transit time of intestinal contents, increases consistency of stools, and reduces fluid and electrolyte loss.

USES Acute nonspecific diarrhea, chronic diarrhea associated with inflammatory bowel disease, and to reduce fecal volume from ileostomies.

CONTRAINDICATIONS Conditions in which constipation should be avoided, severe colitis, acute diarrhea caused by broad-spectrum antibiotics (pseudomembranous colitis) or associated with microorganisms that penetrate intestinal mucosa (e.g., toxigenic *Escherichia coli, Salmonella,* or *Shigella*). Safe use during pregnancy (category B), lactation, or in children <2 y is not established.

CAUTIOUS USE Dehydration; diarrhea caused by invasive bacteria; impaired liver function; prostatic hypertrophy; history of narcotic dependence.

ROUTE & DOSAGE

Acute Diarrhea

Child: **PO** 2–6 y, 1 mg t.i.d.; 6–8 y, 2 mg b.i.d.; 8–12 y, 2 mg t.i.d. (max single dose 2 mg); follow with 0.1 mg/kg/dose after each loose stool
Adult: **PO** 4 mg followed by 2 mg after each unformed stool (max 16 mg/day)

Chronic Diarrhea

Child: **PO** 0.08–0.24 mg/kg divided into 2–3 daily doses (max 2 mg/dose)
Adult: **PO** 4 mg followed by 2 mg after each unformed stool until diarrhea is controlled (max 16 mg/day)

STORAGE
Store at room temperature in tightly closed containers. Oral solution should not be added to other solutions.

ADMINISTRATION

Oral
- Do not give prn doses to a child with acute diarrhea.

ADVERSE EFFECTS Body as a Whole: Hypersensitivity (skin rash); fever. **CNS:** Drowsiness, fatigue, dizziness, CNS depression (overdosage). **GI:** Abdominal discomfort or pain, abdominal distention, bloating, constipation, nausea, vomiting, anorexia, dry mouth; toxic megacolon (patients with ulcerative colitis).

INTERACTIONS Drug: No clinically significant interactions established.

Common adverse effects in *italic;* life-threatening effects underlined; generic names in **bold;** drug classifications in SMALL CAPS; ♣ Canadian drug name; ● Prototype drug.

745

PHARMACOKINETICS Absorption: Poorly absorbed from GI tract. **Onset:** 30–60 min. **Peak:** 2.5 h solution; 4–5 h capsules. **Duration:** 4–5 h. **Metabolism:** Metabolized in liver. **Elimination:** Primarily excreted in feces, <2% excreted in urine. **Half-Life:** 11 h.

NURSING IMPLICATIONS

Assessment & Drug Effects

- Monitor therapeutic effectiveness. Chronic diarrhea usually responds within 10 days. If improvement does not occur within this time, it is unlikely that symptoms will be controlled by further administration.
- Discontinue if there is no improvement after 48 h of therapy for acute diarrhea.
- Monitor fluid and electrolyte balance.
- Notify prescriber promptly if the patient with ulcerative colitis develops abdominal distention or other GI symptoms (possible signs of potentially fatal toxic megacolon).

Patient & Family Education

- Notify prescriber if diarrhea does not stop in a few days or if abdominal pain, distention, or fever develops.
- Record number and consistency of stools.
- Do not drive or engage in other potentially hazardous activities until response to drug is known.
- Do not take alcohol and other CNS depressants concomitantly unless otherwise advised by physician; may enhance drowsiness.
- Learn measures to relieve dry mouth; rinse mouth frequently with water, suck hard candy.
- Do not breast feed while taking this drug without consulting prescriber.
- Store this medication out of reach of children.

LOPINAVIR/RITONAVIR

(lop-i-na′ver/rit-o-na′ver)
Kaletra

Classifications: ANTI-INFECTIVE; ANTIRETROVIRAL AGENT; PROTEASE INHIBITOR
Prototype: Saquinavir Mesylate
Pregnancy Category: C

AVAILABILITY Combination Products: 133.3 mg lopinavir/33.3 mg ritonavir capsules; 400 mg lopinavir/100 mg ritonavir/5 mL suspension

ACTIONS Lopinavir is an HIV protease inhibitor that inhibits the activity of HIV protease and prevents the cleavage of viral polyproteins essential for the maturation of HIV. Ritonavir in the formulation inhibits the CYP3A metabolism of lopinavir, thereby, increasing the blood level of lopinavir. **THERAPEUTIC EFFECTS** Decreases plasma HIV RNA level; elevates CD_4 cell counts as a result of the combined therapy of the two drugs in HIV-infected patients.

USES Treatment of HIV infection in combination with other antiretroviral agents.

CONTRAINDICATIONS Hypersensitivity to lopinavir or ritonavir; concurrent administration with drugs that utilize CYP3A or CYP2D6 for metabolism (e.g., ergotamine, pimozide); lactation.
CAUTIOUS USE Hepatic impairment, patients with hepatitis B or C, older adults; pregnancy (category C). Safety and efficacy in children <6 mo are not established.

ROUTE & DOSAGE

HIV Infection

Note: All doses are in lopinavir/ritonavir ratio. For example 400/100 mg = 400 mcg lopinavir and 100 mg ritonavir combination product.
Child: **PO** 6 mo–12 y, 7–15 kg, 12/3 mg/kg; 15–40 kg, 10/2.5 mg/kg; >40 kg, 400/100 mg b.i.d., increase dose 7–15 kg, 13/3.25 mg/kg; 15–40 kg, 11/2.75 mg/kg; >40 kg, 533/133 mg b.i.d., with concurrent efavirenz or nevirapine
Adult: **PO** 400/100 mg (3 capsules or 5 mL suspension) b.i.d., increase dose to 533/133 mg (4 capsules or 6.5 mL) b.i.d., with concurrent efavirenz or nevirapine

L

STORAGE
Store refrigerated at 2°–8° C (36°–46° F). If stored at room temperature ≤25° C (77° F), discard after 2 mo.

ADMINISTRATION
Note: Take with food.

Oral
- Give with a meal or light snack.
- Note: If didanosine is concurrently ordered, give didanosine 1 h before or 2 h after lopinavir/ritonavir.

ADVERSE EFFECTS Body as a Whole: Asthenia, pain. **GI:** Abdominal pain, abnormal stools, *diarrhea, nausea, <u>pancreatitis</u>,* vomiting. **CNS:** Headache, insomnia. **Skin:** Rash.

INTERACTIONS Drug: Flecainide, propafenone, pimozide may lead to life-threatening arrhythmias; **rifampin** may decrease antiretroviral response; **dihydroergotamine, ergonovine, ergotamine, methylergonovine** may lead to acute ergot toxicity; HMG-COA REDUCTASE INHIBITORS may increase risk of myopathy and rhabdomyolysis; BENZODIAZEPINES may have prolonged sedation or respiratory depression; **efavirenz, nevirapine,** ANTICONVULSANTS, STEROIDS may decrease lopinavir levels; **delavirdine, ritonavir** may increase lopinavir levels; may increase levels of **amprenavir, indinavir, saquinavir, ketoconazole, itraconazole, midazolam, triazolam, rifabutin, sildenafil, atorvastatin, cerivastatin,** IMMUNOSUPPRESSANTS; may decrease levels of **atovaquone, methadone, ethinyl estradiol.** Also see INTERACTIONS in **ritonavir** monograph. **Herbal: St. John's wort** may decrease antiretroviral activity.

PHARMACOKINETICS Absorption: Increased absorption when taken with food. **Peak:** 4 h. **Distribution:** 98–99% protein bound. **Metabolism:**

Extensively metabolized by CYP3A. **Elimination:** Excreted primarily in feces. **Half-Life:** 5–6 h lopinavir.

NURSING IMPLICATIONS

Assessment & Drug Effects

- Monitor for S&S of pancreatitis, especially with marked triglyceride elevations; new onset diabetes or loss of glycemic control; hypothyroidism or Cushing's syndrome.
- Monitor for signs of alcohol toxicity especially in high doses because the drug formulation contains alcohol.
- Lab test: Periodically monitor fasting blood glucose, AST & ALT, total cholesterol & triglycerides, serum amylase, inorganic phosphorus, CBC with differential, and thyroid functions.

Patient & Family Education

- Report all prescription and nonprescription drugs being taken. Do not use herbal products, especially St. John's wort, without first consulting the physician.
- Become familiar with the potential adverse effects of this drug; report those that are bothersome to physician.
- Concurrent use of sildenafil (Viagra) increases risk for adverse effects such as hypotension, changes in vision, and sustained erection; promptly report any of these to the physician.
- Use additional or alternative contraceptive measures if estrogen based hormonal contraceptives are being used.
- Do not breast feed while taking this drug.
- Store this medication out of reach of children.

LORACARBEF
(lor-a-car′bef)
Lorabid
Classifications: ANTI-INFECTIVE; ANTIBIOTIC; BETA-LACTAM
Prototype: Imipenem
Pregnancy Category: B

AVAILABILITY 200 mg, 400 mg capsules; 100 mg/5 mL, 200 mg/5 mL suspension

ACTIONS Second-generation cephalosporin antibiotic with drug structure characterized by a beta-lactam ring (like the penicillin structure). Generally resistant to hydrolysis by beta-lactamases.

THERAPEUTIC EFFECTS Effective against gram-positive and gram-negative bacteria including *staphylococci, beta-hemolytic streptococci, Streptococcus pneumoniae, Haemophilus influenzae, Moraxella catarrhalis.*

USES Upper and lower respiratory tract infections, skin and skin structure infections, urinary tract infections.

CONTRAINDICATIONS Hypersensitivity to cephalosporins and related antibiotics.

Common adverse effects in *italic;* life-threatening effects <u>underlined</u>; generic names in **bold;** drug classifications in SMALL CAPS; ♣ Canadian drug name; ⊘ Prototype drug.

CAUTIOUS USE Renal impairment, seizures, patients with penicillin allergy, pregnancy (category B), lactation.

ROUTE & DOSAGE

Upper & Lower Respiratory Tract Infections
Child: **PO** 15–30 mg/kg/day divided q12h taken 1 h after meals or 2 h before meals
Adult: **PO** 200–400 mg q12h taken 1 h after meals or 2 h before meals

Skin & Skin Structure Infections
Child: **PO** 15 mg/kg/day divided q12h taken 1 h after meals or 2 h before meals
Adult: **PO** 200 mg q12h taken 1 h after meals or 2 h before meals

Urinary Tract Infections
Adult: **PO** 200 mg q24h or 400 mg q12h taken 1 h after meals or 2 h before meals

Otitis Media
Child: **PO** 30 mg/kg/day divided into doses given q12h taken 1 h after meals or 2 h before meals

Renal Impairment
Cl_{cr} 10–49 mL/min: Reduce recommended dose by 50% or give standard dose q24h; <10 mL/min: extend dosing interval to every 3–5 days

L

STORAGE
Store suspension in a tightly closed container. Discard after 14 days.

ADMINISTRATION
Oral
- Reconstitute suspension by adding 30 or 60 mL of water to the 50- or 100-mL bottles, respectively, of dry mixture. Add the water in 2 portions and shake bottle after each portion.
- Give at least 1 h before or 2 h after meals.
- Give half of the normal dose if Cl_{cr} lies between 10 and 49 mL/min.

ADVERSE EFFECTS CNS: Headache. **GI:** Nausea, vomiting, diarrhea, diaper rash, abdominal pain. **Other:** Rash, candidiasis.

INTERACTIONS Drug: May have prolonged bleeding time with **warfarin.**

PHARMACOKINETICS Absorption: Readily absorbed from GI tract. **Peak:** 45–60 min. **Distribution:** Distributes into middle ear fluid. **Elimination:** Excreted in urine. **Half-Life:** 0.78–0.85 h.

NURSING IMPLICATIONS

Assessment & Drug Effects
- Take a careful history to determine previous hypersensitivity reaction to beta-lactam antibiotics (penicillins and cephalosporins) or to other allergens.

- Discontinue drug and notify the prescriber immediately if allergic reaction occurs (e.g., hives, wheezing, rash, pruritus).
- Inspect patient's mouth on a regular basis to detect superinfection (see Appendix D-1).
- Rule out pseudomembranous enterocolitis (see Appendix D-1) if severe diarrhea accompanied by abdominal pain and fever occurs. Notify prescriber immediately.
- Monitor kidney function throughout therapy with concurrent diuretic use.

Patient & Family Education
- Notify prescriber immediately of rash or any other allergic reaction.
- Report loose stools or diarrhea promptly.
- Do not breast feed while taking this drug without consulting physician.
- Store this medication out of reach of children.

LORATADINE 🅟

(lor'a-ti-deen)
Claritin, Claritin Reditabs
Classifications: ANTIHISTAMINE; H_1-RECEPTOR ANTAGONIST; NONSEDATING
Pregnancy Category: B

AVAILABILITY 10 mg tablets; 1 mg/mL syrup
Combination Products: Available with pseudoephedrine.

ACTIONS Long-acting antihistamine with selective peripheral H_1-receptor sites, thus blocking histamine release.
THERAPEUTIC EFFECTS Long-acting H_1-receptor antagonist of histamine that disrupts capillary permeability and edema formation and constriction of respiratory, GI, and vascular smooth muscle.

USES Relief of symptoms of seasonal allergic rhinitis; idiopathic chronic urticaria.

CONTRAINDICATIONS Hypersensitivity to loratadine.
CAUTIOUS USE Hepatic and renal impairment, pregnancy (category B), lactation. Safety and effectiveness in children <2 y are not established.

ROUTE & DOSAGE

Allergic Rhinitis
Child: **PO** <30 kg, 5 mg daily; >30 kg, 10 mg daily
Adult: **PO** 10 mg once daily on an empty stomach; start patients with liver disease with 10 mg every other day

Timed Release Tablets with Loratidine and Pseudoephedrine
Child/Adults >12 y: **PO** 1 tab b.i.d. (Claritin-D 12 h) or **PO** 1 tab daily (Claritin-D 24 h)

STORAGE
Store in a tightly closed container.

Common adverse effects in *italic;* life-threatening effects <u>underlined</u>; generic names in **bold**; drug classifications in SMALL CAPS; ♣ Canadian drug name; 🅞 Prototype drug.

ADMINISTRATION

Oral

■ Give on an empty stomach 1 h before or 2 h after a meal.

ADVERSE EFFECTS CNS: Dizziness, dry mouth, fatigue, headache, *sedation,* somnolence, altered salivation and lacrimation, thirst, flushing, anxiety, depression, impaired concentration. **CV:** Hypotension, hypertension, palpitations, syncope, tachycardia. **GI:** Nausea, vomiting, flatulence, abdominal distress, constipation, diarrhea, weight gain, dyspepsia. **Body as a Whole:** Arthralgia, myalgia. **Special Senses:** Blurred vision, earache, eye pain, tinnitus. **Skin:** Rash, pruritus, photosensitivity.

INTERACTIONS Drug: No clinically significant interactions established.

PHARMACOKINETICS Absorption: Readily absorbed from GI tract. **Onset:** 1–3 h. **Peak:** 8–12 h; reaches steady state levels in 3–5 days. **Duration:** 24 h. **Distribution:** Distributed into breast milk. **Metabolism:** Metabolized to active metabolite, descarboethoxyloratidine, in the liver. **Elimination:** Excreted in urine and feces. **Half-Life:** 12–15 h.

NURSING IMPLICATIONS

Assessment & Drug Effects

■ Assess carefully for and report distressing or dangerous S&S that occur with sedation after initiation of the drug. A variety of adverse effects, although not common, are possible. Some are an indication to discontinue the drug.
■ May be given at night to reduce problems with side effect of sedation.
■ Monitor cardiovascular status and report significant changes in BP and palpitations or tachycardia.

Patient & Family Education

■ Drug may cause significant drowsiness in those with liver or kidney impairment.
■ Note: Concurrent use of alcohol and other CNS depressants may have an additive effect.
■ Do not breast feed while taking this drug without consulting prescriber.
■ Store this medication out of reach of children.

LORAZEPAM 🅟

(lor-a′ze-pam)
Ativan
Classifications: CENTRAL NERVOUS SYSTEM AGENT; ANXIOLYTIC; SEDATIVE-HYPNOTIC; BENZODIAZEPINE
Pregnancy Category: D
Controlled Substance: Schedule IV

AVAILABILITY 0.5 mg, 1 mg, 2 mg tablets; 2 mg/mL oral solution; 2 mg/mL, 4 mg/mL injection

ACTIONS Most potent of the available benzodiazepines. Effects (anxiolytic, sedative, hypnotic, and skeletal muscle relaxant) are mediated by the inhibitory neurotransmitter GABA. Action sites: Thalamic, hypothalamic, and limbic levels of CNS.

THERAPEUTIC EFFECTS Antianxiety agent that also causes mild suppression of REM sleep, while increasing total sleep time.

USES Management of anxiety disorders and for short-term relief of symptoms of anxiety. Also used for preanesthetic medication to produce sedation and to reduce anxiety and recall of events related to day of surgery; for management of status epilepticus.

UNLABELED USES Chemotherapy-induced nausea and vomiting; anticipatory nausea and vomiting.

CONTRAINDICATIONS Known sensitivity to benzodiazepines; acute narrow-angle glaucoma; primary depressive disorders or psychosis; coma, shock, acute alcohol intoxication; pregnancy (category D), and lactation; children <12 y (PO preparation).

CAUTIOUS USE Renal or hepatic impairment; organic brain syndrome; myasthenia gravis; narrow angle glaucoma; suicidal tendency; GI disorders; debilitated patients; limited pulmonary reserve; monitor for propylene glycol toxicity with long-term infusion.

ROUTE & DOSAGE

Antianxiety

Child: **PO/IV** 0.05 mg/kg q4–8h (max 2 mg/dose)
Adult: **PO** 2–6 mg/day in divided doses (max 10 mg/day)

Insomnia

Adult: **PO** 2–4 mg at bedtime

Premedication

Child: **PO/IV/IM** 0.05 mg/kg (range: 0.02–0.08 mg/kg)
Adult: **IM** 2–4 mg (0.05 mg/kg) at least 2 h before surgery **IV** 0.044 mg/kg up to 2 mg 15–20 min before surgery

Status Epilepticus

Neonate: **IV** 0.05 mg/kg over 2–5 min, may repeat in 10–15 min
Child: **IV** 0.05–0.1 mg/kg slow IV over 2–5 min (max 4 mg/dose), may repeat with 0.05 mg/kg × 1 in 10–15 min if needed (max 4 mg/dose)
Adult: **IV** 4 mg injected slowly at 2 mg/min, may repeat dose once if inadequate response after 10 min (max in 12 h is 8 mg)

STORAGE

Refrigerate at 2°–8° C (36°–46° F) and protect from light.

ADMINISTRATION

Oral

■ Increase the evening dose when higher oral dosage is required, before increasing daytime doses.

Intramuscular

■ Injected undiluted, deep into a large muscle mass appropriate for age (see Part I).

Intravenous

- IV administration to neonates, infants, children: Verify correct IV concentration and rate of infusion with physician.

PREPARE **Direct:** Prepare lorazepam immediately before use. Dilute with an equal volume of sterile water, D5W, or NS.

ADMINISTER **Direct:** Inject directly into vein or into IV infusion tubing at rate not to exceed 2 mg/min and with repeated aspiration to confirm IV entry. Take extreme precautions to PREVENT intra-arterial injection and perivascular extravasation.

INCOMPATIBILITY **Y-Site: Idarubicin, omeprazole, ondansetron, sargramostim, sufentanil, TPN with albumin.**

- Keep parenteral preparation in refrigerator; do not freeze.
- Do not use a discolored solution or one with a precipitate.

ADVERSE EFFECTS Body as a Whole: Usually disappear with continued medication or with reduced dosage. **CNS:** Anterograde amnesia, *drowsiness, sedation,* dizziness, weakness, unsteadiness, disorientation, depression, sleep disturbance, restlessness, confusion, hallucinations. **CV:** Hypertension or hypotension. **Special Senses:** Blurred vision, diplopia; depressed hearing. **GI:** Nausea, vomiting, abdominal discomfort, anorexia.

INTERACTIONS Drug: Alcohol, CNS DEPRESSANTS, ANTICONVULSANTS potentiate CNS depression; **cimetidine** increases lorazepam plasma levels, increases toxicity; lorazepam may decrease antiparkinsonism effects of **levodopa;** may increase **phenytoin** levels; smoking decreases sedative and antianxiety effects. **Herbal: Kava-kava, valerian** may potentiate sedation.

PHARMACOKINETICS Absorption: Readily absorbed from GI tract. **Onset:** 1–5 min IV; 15–30 min IM. **Peak:** 60–90 min IM; 2 h PO. **Duration:** 12–24 h. **Distribution:** Crosses placenta; distributed into breast milk. **Metabolism:** Not metabolized in liver. **Elimination:** Excreted in urine. **Half-Life:** 10–20 h.

NURSING IMPLICATIONS

Assessment & Drug Effects

- Have equipment for maintaining patent airway immediately available before starting IV administration.
- IM or IV lorazepam injection of 2–4 mg is usually followed by a depth of drowsiness or sleepiness that permits patient to respond to simple instructions whether patient appears to be asleep or awake.
- Supervise for at least 8 h after lorazepam injection to prevent falling and injury.
- Monitor for propylene glycol toxicity with long-term infusion.
- Lab tests: Assess CBC and liver function tests periodically for patients on long-term therapy.
- Supervise patient who exhibits depression with anxiety closely; the possibility of suicide exists, particularly when there is apparent improvement in mood.

Patient & Family Education

- Do not drive or engage in other hazardous activities for a least 24–48 h after receiving IM injection of lorazepam.

- Do not drink large volumes of coffee. Anxiolytic effects of lorazepam can significantly be altered by caffeine.
- Do not consume alcoholic beverages for at least 24–48 h after an injection and avoid when taking an oral regimen.
- Notify prescriber if daytime psychomotor function is impaired; a change in regimen or drug may be needed.
- Terminate regimen gradually over a period of several days. Do not stop long-term therapy abruptly; withdrawal may be induced with feelings of panic, tonic-clonic seizures, tremors, abdominal and muscle cramps, sweating, vomiting.
- Do not self-medicate with OTC drugs; seek prescriber guidance.
- Discuss discontinuation of drug with prescriber if you wish to become pregnant.
- Do not breast feed while taking this drug.
- Store this medication out of reach of children.

LYMPHOCYTE IMMUNE GLOBULIN

(lymph'o-site)

Antithymocyte Globulin, ATG, Atgam

Classifications: IMMUNOSUPPRESSANT; SERUM IMMUNE GLOBULIN

Prototype: Cyclosporine

Pregnancy Category: C

AVAILABILITY 50 mg/mL injection

ACTIONS An immunoglobulin (IgG) and lymphocyte-selective immunosuppressant derived from serum of healthy horses that have been immunized with human thymus lymphocytes. Action mechanism is not clear. Produces little effect on B-lymphocyte cells and is not associated with severe lymphopenia. Increases susceptibility of patient to viral infections; it may reactivate or support infection with cytomegalovirus, herpes simplex virus (especially labial infections), or with Epstein-Barr virus (EBV). As with other immunosuppressant agents, carcinogenicity of this drug may be expressed.

THERAPEUTIC EFFECTS Alters the formation of T lymphocytes (killer cells) and reduces their number.

USES Primarily to prevent or delay onset or to reverse acute renal allograft rejection.

UNLABELED USES Moderate and severe aplastic anemia in patients unsuitable for bone marrow transplantation, T-cell malignancy, acute and chronic graft-vs-host disease, and to prevent rejection of skin allografts.

CONTRAINDICATIONS Hypersensitivity to thimerosal (preservative) or to other equine gamma globulin preparations; history of previous systemic reaction to ATG, hemorrhagic diatheses; use in kidney transplant patient not receiving a concomitant immunosuppressant. Safe use during pregnancy (category C) or lactation is not established.

CAUTIOUS USE Children (experience limited).

ROUTE & DOSAGE

Renal Allotransplantation
Child: **IV** 5–25 mg/kg/day by slow IV infusion
Adult: **IV** 10–30 mg/kg/day by slow IV infusion

Prevention of Allograft Rejection
Adult: **IV** 15 mg/kg/day for 14 days followed by 15 mg/kg every other day for 14 days

Treatment of Allograft Rejection
Adult: **IV** 10–15 mg/kg/day for 14 days followed by 15 mg/kg every other day for 14 days if needed

Aplastic Anemia
Child: **IV** 10–20 mg/kg/day for 8–14 days, then 10–30 mg/kg every other day for 7 more doses
Adult: **IV** 15 mg/kg/day for 14 days followed by 15 mg/kg every other day for 14 days or 15 mg/kg/day for 10 days

STORAGE
Refrigerate ampules and diluted solutions (if prepared before time of infusion) at 2°–8° C (35°–46° F). Do not freeze.

ADMINISTRATION

Intravenous

- Administer lymphocyte immune globulin (ATG) ONLY if experienced with immunosuppressant therapy and management of transplant patients.
- Do an intradermal skin test to rule out allergy to the drug before first dose. Inject 0.1 mL of a 1:1000 dilution (5 mcg equine IgG in normal saline) and a saline control. If local reaction occurs (wheal or erythema more than 10 mm) or if there is pseudopod formation, itching, or local swelling, use caution during infusion. Discontinue infusion if systemic reaction develops (generalized rash, tachycardia, dyspnea, hypotension, anaphylaxis).

PREPARE IV Infusion: Withdraw required dose of ATG concentrate and inject into IV solution container of 0.45% NaCl or NS. Invert IV container during injection of ATG to prevent its contact with air inside container. Use enough IV solution to create a concentration ≤4 mg/mL.
- Inspect concentrate and diluted solution for particulate matter (may develop during storage) and discoloration; discard if present.

ADMINISTER IV Infusion: Give through an in-line 0.2–1.0 mcm filter into a high-flow vein to decrease potential for phlebitis and thrombosis. Give over ≥4 h (usually 4–8 h). Must finish infusion within 12 h of preparation.
- Total storage time for diluted solutions: No MORE than 12 h (including storage time and actual infusion time).

ADVERSE EFFECTS CNS: Headache, paresthesia, seizures. **CV:** Peripheral thrombophlebitis, hypotension, <u>hypertension</u>. **GI:** Nausea, vomiting,

Common adverse effects in *italic;* life-threatening effects <u>underlined;</u> generic names in **bold;** drug classifications in SMALL CAPS; ✦ Canadian drug name; ● Prototype drug.

755

diarrhea, stomatitis, hiccups, epigastric pain, abdominal distension. **Hematologic:** *Leukopenia, thrombocytopenia.* **Musculoskeletal:** Arthralgia, myalgias, chest or back pain. **Respiratory:** Dyspnea, <u>laryngospasm, pulmonary edema</u>. **Skin:** *Rash, pruritus,* urticaria, wheal and flare. **Body as a Whole:** <u>Anaphylaxis</u> (may occur at any time during the infusion); *chills, fever,* night sweats, pain at infusion site, hyperglycemia, systemic infection, wound dehiscence; *serum sickness,* herpes simplex virus reactivation.

INTERACTIONS Drug: Azathioprine, CORTICOSTEROIDS, other IMMUNO-SUPPRESSANTS increase degree of immunosuppression.

PHARMACOKINETICS Distribution: Poorly distributed into lymphoid tissues (spleen, lymph nodes); probably crosses placenta and into breast milk. **Elimination:** About 1% of dose is excreted in urine. **Half-Life:** Approximately 6 days.

NURSING IMPLICATIONS

Assessment & Drug Effects

- Discontinue infusion and initiate appropriate therapy promptly with onset of anaphylactic response (respiratory distress; pain in chest, flank, back; hypotension, anxiety).
- Monitor BP, vital signs, and patient's complaints during entire administration period carefully. Prompt treatment is indicated for observed and reported symptoms of anaphylaxis (incidence: 1%), serum sickness, or allergic response. Always have equipment for assisted respiration, epinephrine, antihistamines, corticosteroid, and vasopressor available at bedside.
- Predictive value of skin test is not proven. Observe patient carefully; allergic reaction can occur even when test is negative.
- Watch closely for S&S of serum sickness: Fever, malaise, arthralgia, nausea, vomiting, lymphadenopathy and morbilliform eruptions on trunk and extremities. Rash begins as asymptomatic pale pink macules in periumbilical region, axilla, and groin, then rapidly becomes generalized, erythematous, and confluent. Bands of progressive erythema along the sides of hands, fingers, feet, toes, and at margins of palm or plantar skin are characteristic. In ATG-induced serum sickness, when platelet count is low, petechiae and purpura rapidly replace rash distribution over the body. Petechial areas are especially noticeable on legs but also on palms and soles. Serum sickness usually occurs 6–18 days after initiation of therapy; may occur during drug administration or when treatment is stopped.
- Monitor carefully for S&S of thrombocytopenia, concurrent infection, and leukopenia; patient usually receives concomitant corticosteroids and antimetabolites.
- Monitor patient's temperature and attend to complaints of sore throat or rhinorrhea. Report to physician; ATG treatment may be stopped.

Patient & Family Education

- Notify physician immediately of pain in chest, flank, or back; chills; pruritus; night sweats; sore throat.
- Do not breast feed while taking this drug without consulting physician.

MAGNESIUM CITRATE

(mag-nes'i-um)

Citrate of Magnesia, Citroma, Citro-Nesia

Classifications: GASTROINTESTINAL AGENT; SALINE CATHARTIC

Prototype: Magnesium hydroxide

Pregnancy Category: B

AVAILABILITY 1.75 g/30 mL solution

ACTIONS Promotes bowel evacuation by causing osmotic retention of fluid, which distends colon and stimulates peristaltic activity.

THERAPEUTIC EFFECTS Evacuates bowels.

USES To evacuate bowel prior to certain surgical and diagnostic procedures and to help eliminate parasites and toxic materials after treatment with a vermifuge.

CONTRAINDICATIONS Kidney disease; nausea, vomiting, diarrhea, abdominal pain, acute surgical abdomen; intestinal impaction, obstruction or perforation; rectal bleeding; use of solutions containing sodium bicarbonate in patients on sodium-restricted diets; lactation.

CAUTIOUS USE Pregnancy (category B); renal insufficiency; those receiving digoxin.

ROUTE & DOSAGE

Bowel Evacuation

Child: **PO** 2–6 y, 2–4 mL/kg given in 1–2 doses; 6–12 y, 100–150 mL/day given in 1–2 doses

Adult: **PO** 150–300 mL/day given in 1–2 doses

STORAGE

Store at 2°–30° C (36°–86° F) in tightly covered containers.

ADMINISTRATION

Oral

- Give on an empty stomach with a full (240 mL or 8 oz) glass of water or amount appropriate for age of child. Time dosing so that it does not interfere with sleep. Drug produces a watery or semifluid evacuation in 2–6 h.
- Chill solution by pouring it over ice or refrigerate it until ready to use to increase palatability.
- Be aware that once container is opened, effervescence will decrease. This does not affect the quality of preparation.

ADVERSE EFFECTS GI: Abdominal cramps, nausea, fluid and electrolyte imbalance. **CV:** Hypotension. **Respiratory:** Respiratory depression. **Body as a Whole:** Hypermagnesemia (prolonged use); muscle weakness.

INTERACTIONS Drug: May decrease effectiveness of **digoxin**, ORAL ANTI-COAGULANTS, PHENOTHIAZINES; will decrease absorption of H_2 antagonists, phenytoin, iron salts, steroids, benzodiazepines, **ciprofloxacin,** TETRACYCLINES; **sodium polystyrene sulfonate** will bind magnesium, decreasing its effectiveness.

PHARMACOKINETICS Onset: 0.5–2 h; about 30% of dose is absorbed so magnesium content may be important to consider.

NURSING IMPLICATIONS

Assessment & Drug Effects

- Monitor for dehydration, hypokalemia, and hyponatremia (see Appendix D-1) because drug may cause intense bowel evacuation. Monitor for hypermagnesemia. Carefully monitor vital signs.

Patient & Family Education

- Do not use for routine treatment of constipation.
- Expect some degree of abdominal cramping.
- Do not breast feed while using this drug.
- Store this medication out of reach of children.

M

MAGNESIUM HYDROXIDE 🅟

(mag-nes'i-um)

Magnesia, Magnesia Magma, Milk of Magnesia, M.O.M.

Classifications: GASTROINTESTINAL AGENT; SALINE CATHARTIC; ANTACID

Pregnancy Category: B

AVAILABILITY 311 mg tablets; 400 mg/5 mL, 800 mg/5 mL suspension

ACTIONS Aqueous suspension of magnesium hydroxide with rapid and long-acting neutralizing action. May cause slight acid rebound.

THERAPEUTIC EFFECTS Acts as antacid in low doses and as mild saline laxative at higher doses. Causes osmotic retention of fluid, which distends colon, resulting in mechanical stimulation of peristaltic activity.

USES Short-term treatment of occasional constipation, for relief of GI symptoms associated with hyperacidity, and as adjunct in treatment of peptic ulcer. Also has been used in treatment of poisoning by mineral acids and arsenic, and as mouthwash to neutralize acidity.

CONTRAINDICATIONS Abdominal pain, nausea, vomiting, diarrhea, severe kidney dysfunction, fecal impaction, intestinal obstruction or perforation, rectal bleeding, colostomy, ileostomy, lactation. Safety during pregnancy (category B) and in children <2 y is not established.

ROUTE & DOSAGE

Laxative

Child: **PO** <2 y, 0.5 mL/kg; 2–5 y, 0.4–1.2 g (5–15 mL)/day in 1–4 divided doses; 6–11 y, 1.2–2.4 g (15–30 mL)/day in 1–4 divided doses

Common adverse effects in *italic;* life-threatening effects <u>underlined</u>; generic names in **bold;** drug classifications in SMALL CAPS; ♣ Canadian drug name; 🅞 Prototype drug.

Adult: **PO** 2.4–4.8 g (30–60 mL)/day in 1–4 divided doses

Antacid

Child: **PO** 2.5–5 mL/dose given 1–4 times daily (suspension form)
Adult: **PO** 5–15 mL/dose given 1–4 times daily (suspension form);
622–1244 mg/dose given 1–4 times daily (tablets)

STORAGE

Store at 15°–30° C (59°–86° F) in tightly covered container. Slowly absorbs carbon dioxide on exposure to air. Avoid freezing.

ADMINISTRATION

Oral

- Shake bottle well before pouring to ensure mixing of suspension.
- Follow drug with at least a full glass of water to enhance drug action for laxative effect. Administer in the morning or at bedtime. Most effective when taken on an empty stomach.

ADVERSE EFFECTS GI: Nausea, vomiting, abdominal cramps, *diarrhea*. **Urogenital:** Alkalinization of urine. **Body as a Whole:** Weakness, lethargy, mental depression, hyporeflexia, dehydration, <u>coma</u>. **Metabolic:** Electrolyte imbalance with prolonged use; hypermagnesemia. **CV:** Hypotension, bradycardia, <u>complete heart block</u> and <u>other ECG abnormalities</u>. **Respiratory:** <u>Respiratory depression</u>.

INTERACTIONS Drug: Milk of Magnesia decreases absorption of **chlordiazepoxide, dicumarol, digoxin, isoniazid,** QUINOLONES, TETRACYCLINES.

PHARMACOKINETICS Absorption: 15–30% of magnesium is absorbed. **Onset:** 3–6 h. **Distribution:** Small amounts of magnesium distributed in saliva and breast milk. **Elimination:** Excreted in feces; some renal excretion.

NURSING IMPLICATIONS

Assessment & Drug Effects

- Evaluate the patient's continued need for drug. Prolonged and frequent use of laxative doses may lead to dependence. Additionally, even therapeutic doses can raise urinary pH and thereby predispose susceptible patients to urinary infection and urolithiasis.
- Lab tests: Monitor serum magnesium with signs of hypermagnesemia such as bradycardia (see Appendix D-1), especially with frequent use or any degree of renal impairment.

Patient & Family Education

- Investigate the cause of persistent or recurrent constipation or gastric distress with prescriber.
- Do not breast feed while using this drug.
- Store this medication out of reach of children.

Common adverse effects in *italic;* life-threatening effects <u>underlined</u>; generic names in **bold;** drug classifications in SMALL CAPS; ♣ Canadian drug name; ✪ Prototype drug.

759

MAGNESIUM SULFATE

(mag-nes'i-um)

Epsom Salt

Classifications: GASTROINTESTINAL AGENT; SALINE CATHARTIC; REPLACEMENT AGENT; ANTICONVULSANT

Prototype: Magnesium hydroxide

Pregnancy Category: A

AVAILABILITY 0.8 mEq/mL, 1 mEq/mL, 4 mEq/mL injection

ACTIONS *Orally:* Acts as a laxative by osmotic retention of fluid, which distends colon, increases water content of feces, and causes mechanical stimulation of bowel activity. *Parenterally:* Acts as a CNS depressant and also as a depressant of smooth, skeletal, and cardiac muscle function. Anticonvulsant properties thought to be produced by CNS depression, principally by decreasing the amount of acetylcholine liberated from motor nerve terminals, thus producing peripheral neuromuscular blockade.

THERAPEUTIC EFFECTS Effective parenterally as a CNS depressant, smooth muscle relaxant and anticonvulsant in labor and delivery, and cardiac disorders. It is a laxative when taken orally.

USES Orally to relieve acute constipation and to evacuate bowel in preparation for x-ray of intestines. Parenterally to control seizures in toxemia of pregnancy, epilepsy, and acute childhood nephritis and for prophylaxis and treatment of hypomagnesemia such as in total parenteral nutrition (added to infusion solution). Topically to reduce edema, inflammation, and itching.

UNLABELED USES To inhibit premature labor (tocolytic action) and as adjunct in hyperalimentation, treatment of barium poisoning, status asthmaticus refractory to other agents.

CONTRAINDICATIONS Myocardial damage; heart block; cardiac arrest except for certain arrhythmias; IV administration during the 2 h preceding delivery; PO use in patients with abdominal pain, nausea, vomiting, fecal impaction, or intestinal irritation, obstruction, or perforation.

CAUTIOUS USE Impaired kidney function; digitalized patients; concomitant use of other CNS depressants; neuromuscular blocking agents, or cardiac glycosides; pregnancy (category A), lactation, children.

ROUTE & DOSAGE

Laxative

Child: **PO** 0.25 g/kg/dose given 1–4 times daily
Adult: **PO** 10–30 g once daily

Preterm Labor

Adult: **IM/IV** 4–6 g in 250 mL D5W infused slowly over at least 20 min, followed by 2–4 g/h for 12–24 h

Hypomagnesemia Seizures

Child: **IV** 20–100 mg/kg q4–6h prn

Common adverse effects in *italic*; life-threatening effects <u>underlined</u>; generic names in **bold**; drug classifications in SMALL CAPS; ♣ Canadian drug name; ✿ Prototype drug.

Adult: **IM/IV** *Mild,* 1 g q6h for 4 doses; *Severe,* 250 mg/kg infused over 4 h

Total Parenteral Nutrition

Infants: **IV in TPN solution** 0.25–0.6 mEq/kg MgSO₄/day
Adult: **IV in TPN solution** 5–6 mEq MgSO₄/day

ADMINISTRATION

Oral

- Give in the morning or midafternoon in a glass of water for laxative action. Disguise bitter, salty taste by chilling or flavoring with lemon or orange juice.

Intramuscular

- Give deep using the 50% concentration for adults and the 20% concentration for children.

Intravenous

Note: Verify correct IV concentration and rate of infusion for administration to infants, children with physician.

PREPARE **Direct/IV Infusion:** Give solutions with concentrations of ≤20% undiluted.

ADMINISTER **Direct:** Give at a rate of 150 mg over at least 1 min. Note: 20% solution contains 200 mg/mL, 10% solution contains 100 mg/mL.
IV Infusion: Give required dose over 4 h. Do not exceed the direct rate. Maximum infusion rate 1 mEq/kg/h or 125 mg MgSO₄ salt/kg/h.

INCOMPATIBILITIES **Solution/Additive: 10% fat emulsion; amphotericin B, calcium gluceptate, clindamycin, cyclosporine, dobutamine, polymyxin B sulfate, procaine, sodium bicarbonate. Y-Site: Amphotericin B cholesteryl, cefepime.**

ADVERSE EFFECTS Body as a Whole: Flushing, sweating, extreme thirst, sedation, confusion, depressed reflexes or no reflexes, muscle weakness, flaccid paralysis, hypothermia. **CV:** Hypotension, depressed cardiac function, complete heart block, circulatory collapse. **Respiratory:** Respiratory paralysis. **Metabolic:** Hypermagnesemia, hypocalcemia, dehydration, electrolyte imbalance including hypocalcemia with repeated laxative use.

INTERACTIONS Drug: NEUROMUSCULAR BLOCKING AGENTS add to respiratory depression and apnea.

PHARMACOKINETICS Onset: 1–2 h PO; 1 h IM. **Duration:** 30 min IV; 3–4 h PO. **Distribution:** Crosses placenta; distributed into breast milk. **Elimination:** Eliminated in kidneys.

NURSING IMPLICATIONS

Assessment & Drug Effects

- Observe constantly when given IV. Check BP and pulse q10–15min or more often if indicated. Have calcium gluconate IV available as antidote.
- Lab tests: Monitor *plasma magnesium levels* in patients receiving drug parenterally (normal: 1.8–3.0 mEq/L). *Plasma levels* in excess of

3 mEq/L are reflected in CNS depression, those >5 mEq/L in depressed deep-tendon reflexes and >12 in respiratory arrest and heart block. Be familiar with all symptoms of magnesium intoxication (see ADVERSE EFFECTS). Monitor calcium and phosphorus levels also.

- Early indicators of magnesium toxicity (hypermagnesemia) include cathartic effect, profound thirst, feeling of warmth, sedation, confusion, depressed deep-tendon reflexes, and muscle weakness.
- Monitor respiratory rate closely. Report immediately if rate falls below 12 for adults or below normal level for age of child.
- Test patellar reflex before each repeated parenteral dose. Depression or absence of reflexes is a useful index of early magnesium intoxication.
- Check urinary output, especially in patients with impaired kidney function. Therapy is generally not continued if urinary output is less than 100 mL during the 4 h preceding each dose.
- Observe newborns of mothers who received parenteral magnesium sulfate within a few hours of delivery for signs of toxicity, including respiratory and neuromuscular depression. IV calcium may be administered to reverse magnesium toxicity in newborns.
- Observe patients receiving drug for hypomagnesemia for improvement in these signs of deficiency: Irritability, choreiform movements, tremors, tetany, twitching, muscle cramps, tachycardia, hypertension, psychotic behavior.

Patient & Family Education

- Drink sufficient water during the day when drug is administered orally to prevent net loss of body water.
- Recommended daily allowances of magnesium are obtained in a normal diet. Rich sources are whole-grain cereals, legumes, nuts, meats, seafood, milk, most green leafy vegetables, and bananas.
- Do not breast feed while taking this drug without consulting physician.
- Store this medication out of reach of children.

MANNITOL ⊕

(man′i-tole)
Osmitrol
Classifications: ELECTROLYTIC AND WATER BALANCE AGENT; OSMOTIC DIURETIC
Pregnancy Category: C

AVAILABILITY 5%, 10%, 15%, 20%, 25% injection

ACTIONS In large doses, increases rate of electrolyte excretion by the kidney, particularly sodium, chloride, and potassium.
THERAPEUTIC EFFECTS Induces diuresis by raising osmotic pressure of glomerular filtrate, thereby inhibiting tubular reabsorption of water and solutes. Reduces elevated intraocular and cerebrospinal pressures by increasing plasma osmolality, thus inducing diffusion of water from these fluids back into plasma and extravascular space.

USES To promote diuresis in prevention and treatment of oliguric phase of acute kidney failure following cardiovascular surgery, severe traumatic injury, surgery in presence of severe jaundice, hemolytic transfusion reaction. Also used to reduce elevated intraocular (IOP) and intracranial pressure (ICP), to measure glomerular filtration rate (GFR), to promote excretion of toxic substances, to relieve symptoms of pulmonary edema, and as irrigating solution in transurethral prostatic reaction to minimize hemolytic effects of water. Commercially available in combination with sorbitol for urogenital irrigation.

CONTRAINDICATIONS Anuria; marked pulmonary congestion or edema; severe CHF; severe renal disease; metabolic edema; organic CNS disease, intracranial bleeding; shock, severe dehydration, history of allergy; pregnancy (category C), lactation; concomitantly with blood.

ROUTE & DOSAGE

Acute Kidney Failure

Child: **IV Test Dose** 200 mg/kg (max 12.5 g) over 3–5 min **Positive Response** Urine flow of 1 mL/kg/h for 1–2 h **Maintenance** 0.25–0.5 g/kg q4–6h
Adult: **IV Test Dose** 0.2 g/kg or 12.5 g as a 15–20% solution over 3–5 min **Positive Response** 30–50 mL of urine over next 2–3 h, may repeat test dose 1 time. If still negative, do not use. **Treatment** 50–100 g as 15–20% solution over 90 min to several hours

Cerebral Edema

Child: 0.25 g/kg/dose over 20–30 min; increase gradually to 1 g/kg/dose as needed
Adult: 1–2 g/kg/dose given over 30–60 min

STORAGE

Store at 15°–30° C (59°–86° F) unless otherwise directed. Avoid freezing.

ADMINISTRATION

Intravenous

Note: Verify correct IV concentration and rate of infusion for administration to infants, children with physician.
PREPARE **IV Infusion:** Give undiluted.
ADMINISTER **IV Infusion:** Give a single dose over 30–90 min. Oliguria: A test dose is given to patients with marked oliguria to check adequacy of kidney function. Response is considered satisfactory if urine flow of at least 30–50 mL/h is produced over 2–3 h after drug administration; then rate is adjusted to maintain urine flow at 30–50 mL/h with a single dose usually being infused over ≥90 min. Concentrations higher than 15% have a greater tendency to crystallize. Use an administration set with an in-line IV filter when infusing concentrations of 15% or above.
INCOMPATIBILITIES **Solution/Additive: Imipenem-cilastatin. Y-Site: Cefepime, doxorubicin liposome, filgrastim.**

ADVERSE EFFECTS CNS: Headache, tremor, convulsions, dizziness, transient muscle rigidity. **CV:** Edema, CHF, angina-like pain, hypotension, hypertension, thrombophlebitis. **Eye:** Blurred vision. **GI:** Dry mouth, nausea, vomiting. **Urogenital:** Marked diuresis, urinary retention, nephrosis,

Common adverse effects in *italic;* life-threatening effects underlined; generic names in **bold;** drug classifications in SMALL CAPS; ♣ Canadian drug name; ❷ Prototype drug.

763

uricosuria. **Metabolic:** *Fluid and electrolyte imbalance,* especially <u>hyponatremia</u>; dehydration, acidosis. **Other:** With extravasation (local edema, skin necrosis; chills, fever, allergic reactions).

INTERACTIONS Drug: Increases urinary excretion of **lithium,** SALICYLATES, BARBITURATES, **imipramine, potassium.**

PHARMACOKINETICS Onset: 1–3 h diuresis; 30–60 min IOP; 15 min ICP. **Duration:** 4–6 h IOP; 3–8 h ICP. **Distribution:** Confined to extracellular space; does not cross blood–brain barrier except with very high plasma levels in the presence of acidosis. **Metabolism:** Small quantity metabolized to glycogen in liver. **Elimination:** Rapidly excreted by kidneys. **Half-Life:** 100 min.

NURSING IMPLICATIONS

Assessment & Drug Effects

- Take care to avoid extravasation. Observe injection site for signs of inflammation or edema.
- Lab tests: Monitor closely serum and urine electrolytes/osmolality and kidney function during therapy.
- Measure I&O accurately and record to achieve proper fluid balance.
- Monitor vital signs closely. Report significant changes in BP and signs of CHF.
- Perform thorough and frequent neurological assessments, especially for increased ICP.
- Monitor for possible indications of fluid and electrolyte imbalance (e.g., thirst, muscle cramps or weakness, paresthesias, and signs of CHF).
- Be alert to the possibility that a rebound increase in ICP sometimes occurs about 12 h after drug administration. Patient may complain of headache or confusion.
- Take accurate daily weight.

Patient & Family Education

- Report any of the following: Thirst, muscle cramps or weakness, paresthesia, dyspnea, or headache.
- Family members should immediately report any evidence of confusion.
- Do not breast feed while using this drug.

MEASLES, MUMPS, AND RUBELLA VACCINES (MMR)

(mē′sels-mamps-roo-bel′a)

MMR-II

Classifications: ANTI-INFECTIVE, VACCINE
Pregnancy Category: C

AVAILABILITY Single-dose vials with powder; single-dose 0.5 mL vials of diluent for mixing

ACTIONS Stimulates body production of antibodies against the viruses causing measles, mumps, and rubella.
THERAPEUTIC EFFECTS The recommended two-dose regimen provides protection against the diseases identified.

Common adverse effects in *italic;* life-threatening effects <u>underlined</u>; generic names in **bold**; drug classifications in SMALL CAPS; ✦ Canadian drug name; ⦾ Prototype drug.

USES Used to provide active immunity in children or adults who are not immune.

CONTRAINDICATIONS Hypersensitivity to any of the vaccines or components such as gelatin and neomycin; pregnant females; previous anaphylaxis to this vaccine; serious acute illness; most immunodeficiency states; recent administration of blood products.

CAUTIOUS USE History of cerebral injury, hypersensitivity to eggs, thrombocytopenia; safety and efficacy in children <6 mo not established.

ROUTE & DOSAGE

SC 0.5 mL (entire contents of reconstituted vial) at 12–15 mo and 4–6 y

STORAGE

Keep vaccine refrigerated at 2°–8° C (36°–45° F); do not freeze. Diluent may be kept at room temperature. Once reconstituted, vaccine must be kept refrigerated and in the dark and must be used within 8 h.

ADMINISTRATION

Subcutaneous

- First dose given into SC tissue in thigh of infant, can be given into arm for 4–6 y dose.
- Variable length of time is needed after administration of blood products; see Appendix H-1.
- Each of the vaccine components is produced singly also. Women who are found to be not immune to rubella during pregnancy tests are given rubella vaccine singly after delivery to aid in preventing the risk of rubella syndrome in subsequent pregnancies. During an outbreak of measles, the single measles vaccine may be given as early as 6 mo of age, with reimmunization with MMR at recommended ages. Cases of measles imported in international adopted infants necessitates extreme caution with adoptees and careful, prompt administration of immunizations on arrival in new home country.
- These are live-virus vaccines and must be maintained in manner described in package insert to preserve potency. This includes administration within 8 h of reconstitution, refrigeration for powder or reconstituted solutions, and maintaining darkness for powder or reconstituted solutions.

ADVERSE EFFECTS Body as a Whole: Atypical measles with rash, fever, headache, malaise, <u>anaphylaxis</u>. **GI:** Nausea, vomiting, diarrhea. **Skin:** Tenderness, swelling, erythema (all mild). **Hematologic:** Thrombocytopenia. **Musculoskeletal:** Arthritis (acute or chronic), arthralgia, myalgia (these effects most common in adult females). **Neurologic:** <u>Encephalitis</u>, encephalopathy (rare).

INTERACTIONS Efficacy of vaccine may be reduced when child is immunosuppressed or has received blood products in past months.

PHARMACOKINETICS Highly effective in producing immunity in most individuals; no booster needed after initial series.

NURSING IMPLICATIONS

Assessment & Drug Effects

- Take careful history to rule out contraindications, lowered immunity, or recent blood product administration.
- Instruct parents about risks and benefits of immunization. Teach side effects and to seek care immediately for those that are unexpected or serious. Obtain written parental consent for immunization.
- Teach comfort measures (acetaminophen, cool compress to injection site) for mild side effects.
- Provide information about clinics and other resources to receive immunizations.
- Keep epinephrine 1:1000 and recommended doses for children available whenever giving immunizations.

Patient and Family Education

- Return as directed for second dose in the series. No further booster doses are currently recommended after initial 2-dose series.

MEBENDAZOLE ⊘

(me-ben′da-zole)

Vermox

Classifications: ANTI-INFECTIVE; ANTHELMINTIC

Pregnancy Category: C

AVAILABILITY 100 mg tablets

ACTIONS Carbamate with unusually broad spectrum of anthelmintic activity. Mechanism of action not known.

THERAPEUTIC EFFECTS Inhibits formation of worm's microtubules and inhibits glucose and other nutrient uptake by susceptible helminths.

USES Treatment of *Trichuris trichiura* (whipworm), *Enterobius vermicularis* (pinworm), *Ascaris lumbricoides* (roundworm), *Ancylostoma duodenale* (common hookworm), *Necator americanus* (American hookworm) in single or mixed infections.

UNLABELED USES Beef, dwarf, and pork tapeworm and threadworm infections.

CONTRAINDICATIONS Safety during pregnancy (category C), lactation, or in children <2 y is not established.

ROUTE & DOSAGE

Pinworms

Child/Adult: **PO** 100 mg as single dose; repeat in 2 wk prn

Hookworms, Roundworms (<u>Ascaris</u>), Whipworm (<u>Trichuris</u>)

Child/Adult: **PO** 100 mg b.i.d. × 3 days; repeat in 3–4 wk prn

Capillariasis

Child/Adult: **PO** 200 mg b.i.d. × 20 days

Common adverse effects in *italic*; life-threatening effects <u>underlined</u>; generic names in **bold**; drug classifications in SMALL CAPS; ◆ Canadian drug name; ⊘ Prototype drug.

STORAGE
Store at 15°–25° C (59°–77° F) in tightly closed container.

ADMINISTRATION

Oral
- Allow tablets to be chewed and swallowed, or crushed and mixed with food if needed.

ADVERSE EFFECTS GI: Transient abdominal pain, diarrhea, nausea, vomiting. **Body as a Whole:** Dizziness, fever (possibly due to tissue necrosis in cysts); rash, pruritis, alopecia; flushing.

INTERACTIONS Drug: Carbamazepine, phenytoin can increase metabolism of mebendazole; **cimetidine** may inhibit metabolism, thereby increasing level of mebendezole.

PHARMACOKINETICS Absorption: Minimal absorption from GI tract (2–10% of oral dose). **Metabolism:** Metabolized to inactive metabolite. **Elimination:** Primarily eliminated in feces. **Half-Life:** 3–9 h.

NURSING IMPLICATIONS

Assessment & Drug Effects
- Initiate second course of treatment if cure does not occur within time frame indicated for specific infection.
- Examine and treat all family members who may be infected simultaneously because pinworms are readily transmitted from person to person.

Patient & Family Education
- Practice thorough hand washing after touching any potentially contaminated item.
- Change underclothing, bedclothes, towels, and facecloths daily; bathe frequently, preferably by showering. Infected person should sleep alone.
- Do not breast feed while taking this drug without consulting prescriber.
- Store this medication out of reach of children.

MEDROXYPROGESTERONE ACETATE/ESTRADIOL CYPIONATE

(med-rox′y-pro-ges′te-rone/es-tra-di′ol)
Lunelle
Classifications: HORMONE AND SYNTHETIC SUBSTITUTE; ESTROGEN; PROGESTIN
Prototype: Estradiol/progesterone
Pregnancy Category: X

AVAILABILITY 25 mg medroxyprogesterone/5 mg estradiol cypionate per 0.5 mL

ACTIONS Progesterone prevents follicular maturation and ovulation. In addition, it induces morphological changes in the endometrium including thinning of its lining, which may result in decreased likelihood of implantation. Mechanism of action is not fully understood.

THERAPEUTIC EFFECTS Contraceptive that may act by preventing follicular maturation and ovulation, thickening of the cervical mucus, which prevents passage of sperm into the uterus, and decreases ability of sperm to survive in an environment of altered endometrium.

USES Hormonal contraception.

CONTRAINDICATIONS Hypersensitivity of any component of the product; pregnancy (category X), suspicion of pregnancy; genital bleeding of unknown etiology; thrombophlebitis or history of thrombophlebitic disorders: CVA or coronary artery disease (CAD); women smokers >35 y; liver dysfunction, jaundice associated with pregnancy or contraceptive use; carcinoma of the endometrium, breast or other known estrogen-dependent neoplasia; severe hypertension; diabetes with vascular involvement; headaches with focal neurologic symptoms; valvular heart disease with complications; history of hypertension or hypertensive-related diseases (i.e., renal disease or renal failure); liver dysfunction; lactation.
CAUTIOUS USE Diabetes mellitus; history of depression; disorders involving fluid retention; history of hyperlipidemia; history of smoking (tobacco use).

ROUTE & DOSAGE

Contraception

Adolescent/Adult: **IM** 0.5 mL every mo or 28 days

STORAGE
Store at 20°–25° C (68°–77° F).

ADMINISTRATION

Intramuscular
- Shake vial or prefilled syringe vigorously before use to ensure a uniform suspension.
- Give into the deltoid, gluteus maximus, or anterior thigh.

ADVERSE EFFECTS Body as a Whole: Asthenia, dizziness. **CV:** Hypertension, MI, thrombophlebitis. **GI:** Abdominal pain, nausea, gallbladder disease, hepatic adenomas or benign liver tumors, enlarged abdomen. **Endocrine:** Breast tenderness/pain. **Hematologic:** Arterial thromboembolism. **Metabolic:** Weight gain. **CNS:** <u>Cerebral hemorrhage, cerebral thrombosis</u>, depression, emotional lability, headache, nervousness. **Respiratory:** Pulmonary embolism. **Skin:** Acne, alopecia. **Urogenital:** Amenorrhea, dysmenorrhea, menorrhagia, metrorrhagia, decreased libido, vaginal moniliasis, vulvovaginal disorders. [Also see ORAL CONTRACEPTIVES.]

DIAGNOSTIC TEST INTERFERENCE Increase ***BSP*** retention, ***prothrombin, platelet aggregability, thyroid-binding globulin, PBI, T$_4$, transcortin, corticosteroid, triglyceride, phospholipid*** levels; may increase ***ceruloplasmin, aldosterone, amylase transferrin, renin*** activity; May decrease ***antithrombin III, T$_3$ resin uptake, serum folate, glucose tolerance, albumin, vitamin B$_{12}$;*** may reduce ***metapyrone*** test response.

Common adverse effects in *italic;* life-threatening effects <u>underlined</u>; generic names in **bold;** drug classifications in SMALL CAPS; ♣ Canadian drug name; ❂ Prototype drug.

INTERACTIONS Drug: Aminoglutethimide, ANTIBIOTICS, BARBITURATES, **carbamazepine, fosphenytoin, griseofulvin, modafinil, oxcarbazepine, phenytoin, pioglitazone, primidone,** PROTEASE INHIBITORS, **rifabutin, rifampin, rifapentine, topiramate, troglitazone** may decrease contraceptive effectiveness; may decrease effectiveness of ORAL HYPOGLYCEMIC AGENTS, **clofibrate;** may increase toxicity of **cyclosporine;** may increase hypercoagulability with **aminocaproic acid;** may interfere with activity of AROMATASE INHIBITORS. **Herbal: St. John's wort** may decrease contraceptive effectiveness.

PHARMACOKINETICS Absorption: Slowly absorbed from IM site. **Peak:** 1–10 days. **Duration:** 1 mo. **Distribution:** 86% protein bound. **Metabolism:** Extensively metabolized by hydrolysis in liver. **Elimination:** Primarily excreted in urine. **Half-Life:** 14–15 days.

NURSING IMPLICATIONS

Assessment & Drug Effects

- Monitor for and report immediately signs and symptoms of thrombophlebitis or thromboembolism (e.g., pulmonary embolism, CVA, TIA, retinal embolism).
- Monitor BP especially with preexisting hypertension.
- Monitor weight and degree of fluid retention.
- Monitor for signs and symptoms of bronchospasm in asthma patients; notify physician immediately.
- Lab tests: HgA$_{1C}$ q3mo, and frequent fasting blood glucose and postprandial blood glucose in diabetics; periodic lipid profile and liver function tests.

Patient & Family Education

- Follow the schedule for receiving this drug. Drug must be administered every 28–30 days to remain effective.
- Use alternative forms of barrier contraception while taking antibiotics.
- Avoid smoking while using this form of contraception. Smoking greatly increases the risk of serious cardiovascular adverse effects.
- Diabetics should closely monitor blood glucose for loss of glycemic control.
- Do not use OTC drugs, including St. John's wort, vitamin C, or acetaminophen without consulting the prescriber.
- Report episodes of calf pain or tenderness, shortness of breath, chest pain, visual disturbances, drooping eyelid, double vision, or any other unusual symptom to the prescriber.
- Do not breast feed while taking this drug.
- Store this medication out of reach of children.

MEFLOQUINE HYDROCHLORIDE

(me-flo'quine)

Lariam

Classifications: ANTI-INFECTIVE; ANTIMALARIAL
Prototype: Chloroquine
Pregnancy Category: C

AVAILABILITY 250 mg tablets

ACTIONS Antimalarial agent, structurally related to quinine.
THERAPEUTIC EFFECTS Effective against all types of malaria, including chloroquine-resistant malaria.

USES Treatment of mild to moderate acute malarial infections, prevention of chloroquine-resistant malaria caused by *Plasmodium falciparum* and *P. vivax.*

CONTRAINDICATIONS Hypersensitivity to mefloquine or a related compound; with a calcium channel blocking agent, severe heart arrhythmias, history of QTc prolongation; psychiatric depression; seizure disorders; pregnancy (category C); infancy.
CAUTIOUS USE Lactation, persons piloting aircraft or operating heavy machinery. Safety and efficacy in children are not established.

ROUTE & DOSAGE

Note: FDA has NOT approved use of mefloquine in children, and the U.S. Public Health Service does NOT recommend its use in children <15 kg or in pregnant women.

Treatment of Malaria

Child >15 kg: PO 15–25 mg/kg as single dose (max 1250 mg/dose)
Adult: PO 1250 mg (5 tablets) as single oral dose taken with at least 8 oz (120 mL) of water

Prophylaxis for Malaria

Child: PO 15–19 kg, ¼ tablet; 20–30 kg, ½ tablet; 31–45 kg, ¾ tablet; >45 kg, 250 mg (1 tablet).
All doses given once weekly starting 1 wk before exposure and continuing for 4 wk after leaving endemic area.
Adult: PO 250 mg once a week times 4 wk (beginning 1 wk before travel), then 250 mg every other week for duration of exposure and for 2 doses after leaving endemic area

STORAGE
Store at 15°–30° C (59°–86° F).

ADMINISTRATION
Oral
- Give with food and at least 8 oz (120 mL) water.
- Do not give concurrently with quinine or quinidine; wait at least 12 h beyond last dose of either drug before administering mefloquine.

ADVERSE EFFECTS Body as a Whole: Arthralgia, chills, fatigue, fever. **CNS:** Dizziness, nightmares, visual disturbances, headache, syncope, confusion, psychosis. **CV:** Bradycardia, ECG changes (including QTc prolongation), first-degree AV block. **GI:** Nausea, vomiting, abdominal pain, anorexia, diarrhea. **Skin:** Rash, itching.

DIAGNOSTIC TEST INTERFERENCE Transient increase in liver transaminases.

INTERACTIONS Drug: Mefloquine can prolong cardiac conduction in patients taking BETA-BLOCKERS, CALCIUM CHANNEL BLOCKERS, and possibly **digoxin. Quinine and metoclopramide** may decrease plasma mefloquine concentrations. Mefloquine may decrease **valproic acid** serum concentrations by increasing its hepatic metabolism. Administration with **chloroquine** may increase risk of seizures. Increase risk of cardiac arrest and seizures with **quinidine.**

PHARMACOKINETICS Absorption: 85% absorbed, concentrates in red blood cells. **Onset:** 59 and 28 h for parasite and fever clearance times in patients with *P. vivax* infections, respectively; 166 and 93 h in patients with *P. malariae* infections. **Distribution:** Concentrated in red blood cells due to high affinity binding to red blood cell membranes; 98% protein bound; distributed minimally into breast milk. **Metabolism:** Metabolized in liver. **Elimination:** Eliminated primarily in bile and feces. **Half-Life:** 10–21 days (shorter in patients with acute malaria).

NURSING IMPLICATIONS

Assessment & Drug Effects

- Monitor carefully during prophylactic use for development of unexplained anxiety, depression, restlessness, or confusion; such manifestations may indicate a need to discontinue the drug.
- Evaluate cardiac and liver functions periodically with prolonged use.
- Lab tests: Monitor periodically CBC with differential during prolonged use.
- Monitor closely blood levels of anticonvulsants with concomitant therapy.
- Consult the latest edition of the American Academy of Pediatrics Redbook for current recommendations on malaria and other infectious disease treatment.

Patient & Family Education

- Take drug on the same day each week when used for malaria prophylaxis.
- Do not perform potentially hazardous activities until response to drug is known.
- Report any of the following immediately: Fever, sore throat, muscle aches, visual problems, anxiety, confusion, mental depression, hallucinations.
- Do not breast feed while taking this drug without consulting prescriber.
- Store this medication out of reach of children.

MENINGOCOCCAL VACCINE

men-in-goe-coc'al
Menomune-A/C/Y/W-135
Classifications: ANTI-INFECTIVE, VACCINE
Pregnancy Category: Used only when clearly needed

AVAILABILITY Single dose vial with 0.78 mL and 10-dose vial with 6 mL.

ACTIONS Stimulates body production of antibodies against *Neisseria meningitides* serogroups A, C, Y, and W-135.

THERAPEUTIC EFFECTS The recommended single-dose regimen provides protection against the specified serotypes of mengococcal infection.

USES Used to provide active immunity in susceptible individuals.

CONTRAINDICATIONS Allergy to the vaccine or any of its components, such as thimerosal; severe acute illness; immunosuppression
CAUTIOUS USE Safety and efficacy in children <2 y not established.

ROUTE & DOSAGE

SC 0.5 mL in single dose at 2 y of age or older

STORAGE
Keep vaccine and diluent refrigerated at 2°–8° C (36°–45° F); do not freeze. After reconstitution, keep single-dose vials refrigerated and use within 30 min; reconstituted 10-dose vials can be refrigerated for up to 35 days.

ADMINISTRATION
Subcutaneous
- Given into SC tissue in thigh of 2-y-old; can be given into arm for older children and adolescents.
- Recommended for those with complement deficiency, properdin deficiency, asplenia, travelers to areas of *N. meningitides* disease, military personnel, college students or others living in dormitory-type arrangements, contacts of those with the disease if it is type C, some health care and laboratory personnel.

ADVERSE EFFECTS Body as a Whole: Fever, fatigue, headache, chills, rash, anaphylaxis (rare). **Skin:** Tenderness, erythema, induration.

INTERACTIONS Efficacy of vaccine may be lessened when child is immunosuppressed.

PHARMACOKINETICS Immunity to each of the vaccine serotypes is 87–100% by 4 wk after immunization; immunity to W-135 type may be less in children. Duration of immunity is unknown but appears variable; no routine booster doses are recommended.

NURSING IMPLICATIONS

Assessment & Drug Effects
- Take careful history to rule out contraindications or lowered immunity.
- Instruct parents about risks and benefits of immunization. Teach side effects and to seek care immediately for those that are unexpected or serious. Obtain written parental consent for immunization.
- Teach comfort measures (acetaminophen, cool compress to injection site) for mild side effects.
- Provide information about clinics and other resources to receive immunizations.
- Keep epinephrine 1:1000 and doses recommended for children available whenever giving immunizations.

Common adverse effects in *italic;* life-threatening effects <u>underlined</u>; generic names in **bold;** drug classifications in SMALL CAPS; ♣ Canadian drug name; ✪ Prototype drug.

Patient & Family Education

- No booster doses are currently recommended after initial immunization. Realize that only four types of meningococcal disease are available in vaccine; there are several other types.
- Recommended for adolescents who have not received vaccine and are headed to college.

MEPERIDINE HYDROCHLORIDE

(me-per'i-deen)
Demerol, Pethadol ✦, Pethidine Hydrochloride ✦
Classifications: CENTRAL NERVOUS SYSTEM AGENT; NARCOTIC (OPIATE) AGONIST ANALGESIC
Prototype: Morphine
Pregnancy Category: B (D at term)
Controlled Substance: Schedule II

AVAILABILITY 50 mg, 100 mg tablets; 50 mg/5 mL syrup; 10 mg/mL, 25 mg/mL, 50 mg/mL, 75 mg/mL, 100 mg/mL injection

ACTIONS Synthetic morphine-like compound. Chemically dissimilar to morphine, but in equianalgesic doses it is qualitatively comparable. Usual doses produce either no pupillary change or slight miosis, but overdosage results in marked miosis or mydriasis. Also, unlike morphine, has little or no antidiarrheic or antitussive action. Produces CNS stimulation in toxic doses.
THERAPEUTIC EFFECTS Control of moderate to severe pain.

USES Relief of moderate to severe pain, for preoperative medication, for support of anesthesia, and for obstetric analgesia.

CONTRAINDICATIONS Hypersensitivity to meperidine; convulsive disorders; acute abdominal conditions prior to diagnosis; pregnancy prior to labor (category B), at term (category D), lactation.
CAUTIOUS USE Head injuries, increased intracranial pressure; asthma and other respiratory conditions; sicle cell disease; supraventricular tachycardias; prostatic hypertrophy; urethral stricture; glaucoma; debilitated patients; impaired kidney or liver function, hypothyroidism, Addison's disease.

ROUTE & DOSAGE

Moderate to Severe Pain
Child: **PO/SC/IM/IV** 1–1.5 mg/kg q3–4h (max ≤100 mg q4h) prn
Adult: **PO/SC/IM/IV** 50–150 mg q3–4h prn

Preoperative
Child: **IM/SC** 1–2.2 mg/kg 30–90 min before surgery
Adult: **IM/SC** 50–150 mg 30–90 min before surgery

Obstetric Analgesia
Adult: **IM/SC** 50–100 mg when pains become regular, may be repeated q1–3h
Note: Adjust doses in renal failure.

STORAGE

Store at 15°–30° C (59°–86° F) in tightly closed, light-resistant containers unless otherwise directed by manufacturer.

ADMINISTRATION

Oral

▪ Give syrup formulation in half a glass of water. Undiluted syrup may cause topical anesthesia of mucous membranes.

Subcutaneous and Intramuscular Injections

▪ Be aware that SC route is painful and can cause local irritation. IM route is preferred.
▪ Consult Part I for IM site selection in children.
▪ Aspirate carefully before giving IM injection to avoid inadvertent IV administration. IV injection of undiluted drug can cause a marked increase in heart rate and syncope.

Intravenous

Note: Verify correct IV concentration and rate of infusion/injection for administration to infants or children with physician.

PREPARE **Direct:** Dilute 50 mg in at least 5 mL of NS or sterile water to yield 10 mg/mL. **IV Infusion:** Dilute to a concentration of 1–10 mg/mL in NS, D5W, or other compatible solution.

ADMINISTER **Direct:** Give at a rate not to exceed 25 mg/min. Slower injection preferred. **IV Infusion:** Usually given through a controlled infusion device at a rate not to exceed 25 mg/min.

INCOMPATIBILITIES **Solution/Additive: Aminophylline,** BARBITURATES, **floxacillin, furosemide, heparin, methicillin, morphine, phenytoin, sodium bicarbonate. Y-Site: Allopurinol, amphotericin B cholesteryl complex, cefepime, cefoperazone, doxorubicin liposome, furosemide, heparin, idarubicin, imipenem-cilastatin, mezlocillin, minocycline, tetracycline.**

ADVERSE EFFECTS Body as a Whole: Allergic (*pruritus,* urticaria, skin rashes, wheal and flare over IV site), profuse perspiration. **CNS:** *Dizziness,* weakness, euphoria, dysphoria, *sedation,* headache, uncoordinated muscle movements, disorientation, decreased cough reflex, miosis, corneal anesthesia, respiratory depression. Toxic doses: Muscle twitching, tremors, hyperactive reflexes, excitement, hypersensitivity to external stimuli, agitation, confusion, hallucinations, dilated pupils, convulsions. Seizures result from the metabolite (normeperidine) and are more common in renal disease, sickle cell disease, and in those with history of seizures. **CV:** Facial flushing, light-headedness, hypotension, syncope, palpitation, bradycardia, tachycardia, cardiovascular collapse, cardiac arrest (toxic doses). **GI:** Dry mouth, *nausea,* vomiting, *constipation,* biliary tract spasm. **Urogenital:** Oliguria, urinary retention. **Respiratory:** Respiratory depression in newborn, bronchoconstriction (large doses). **Skin:** Phlebitis (following IV use), pain, tissue irritation and induration, particularly following subcutaneous injection. **Metabolic:** Increased levels of serum amylase, BSP retention, bilirubin, AST, ALT.

DIAGNOSTIC TEST INTERFERENCE High doses of meperidine may interfere with *gastric emptying studies* by causing delay in gastric emptying.

INTERACTIONS Drug: Alcohol and other CNS DEPRESSANTS, **cimetidine** cause additive sedation and CNS depression; AMPHETAMINES may potentiate CNS STIMULATION; MAO INHIBITORS, **selegiline, furazolidone** may cause excessive and prolonged CNS depression, convulsions, cardiovascular collapse; **phenytoin** may increase toxic meperidine metabolites. **Herbal: St. John's wort** may increase sedation.

PHARMACOKINETICS Absorption: 50–60% absorbed from GI tract. **Onset:** 15 min PO; 10 min IM, SC; 5 min IV. **Peak:** 1 h PO, IM, SC. **Duration:** 2–4 h PO, IM, SC; 2 h IV. **Distribution:** Crosses placenta; distributed into breast milk. **Metabolism:** Metabolized in liver. **Elimination:** excreted in urine. **Half-Life:** 3–5 h.

NURSING IMPLICATIONS

Assessment & Drug Effects

- Give narcotic analgesics in the smallest effective dose and for the least period of time compatible with patient's needs.
- Assess patient's need for prn medication. Record time of onset, duration, and quality of pain.
- Note respiratory rate, depth, and rhythm and size of pupils in patients receiving repeated doses. If respirations are 12/min or below for adults or below a preestablished rate for children, and pupils are constricted or dilated (see ACTIONS AND USES) or breathing is shallow, or if signs of CNS hyperactivity are present, consult physician before administering drug.
- Monitor vital signs closely. Heart rate may increase markedly, and hypotension may occur. Meperidine may cause severe hypotension in postoperative patients and those with depleted blood volume.
- Schedule deep breathing, coughing (unless contraindicated), and changes in position at intervals to help to overcome respiratory depressant effects.
- Chart patient's response to drug and evaluate continued need.
- Repeated use can lead to tolerance as well as psychic and physical dependence of the morphine type.
- Be aware that abrupt discontinuation following repeated use results in morphine-like withdrawal symptoms. Symptoms develop more rapidly (within 3 h, peaking in 8–12 h) and are of shorter duration than with morphine. Nausea, vomiting, diarrhea, and pupillary dilatation are less prominent, but muscle twitching, restlessness, and nervousness are greater than produced by morphine.

Patient & Family Education

- Do not smoke and walk without assistance after receiving the drug. Bed side rails and cribs for children are advised.
- Be aware that nausea, vomiting, dizziness, and faintness associated with fall in BP are more pronounced when walking than when lying down. Symptoms are aggravated when the head is positioned upward.
- Do not drive or engage in potentially hazardous activities until any drowsiness and dizziness have passed.
- Do not take other CNS depressants or drink alcohol because of their additive effects.
- Do not breast feed while using this drug unless directed by physician.
- Store this medication in locked area out of reach of children; this is a Schedule II drug.

MEPHENTERMINE SULFATE
(me-fen'ter-meen)
Wyamine
Classifications: AUTONOMIC NERVOUS SYSTEM AGENT; BETA-ADRENERGIC AGONIST (SYMPATHOMIMETIC)
Prototype: Isoproterenol
Pregnancy Category: D

AVAILABILITY 15 mg/mL, 30 mg/mL injection

ACTIONS Synthetic sympathomimetic with alpha- and predominant beta-adrenergic activity. Acts by releasing norepinephrine from tissue storage sites. Produces a positive inotropic action and increases cardiac output. Elevation of BP results primarily from increased cardiac output, and to a lesser extent from increased peripheral vasoconstriction. Antiarrhythmic action results from decrease in AV conduction time, atrial refractory period, and conduction time in ventricular muscle.
THERAPEUTIC EFFECTS Heart rate may be reflectively slowed; BP elevated. Antiarrhythmic.

USES Mainly as pressor agent in treatment of hypotension secondary to ganglionic blockade or spinal anesthesia. Also has been used as an emergency measure in therapy of shock secondary to hemorrhage until whole blood replacement is available; as adjunct in treatment of cardiogenic shock, and to abolish certain cardiac arrhythmias.

CONTRAINDICATIONS Shock secondary to hemorrhage (except in emergency). Safety during pregnancy (category D) or lactation is not established.
CAUTIOUS USE Arteriosclerosis; cardiovascular disease; hypovolemia; hypertension; hyperthyroidism; patients with known hypersensitivities; chronically ill patients.

ROUTE & DOSAGE

Hypotension
Child: **IM/IV** 0.4 mg/kg
Adult: **IM/IV** 10–80 mg

Hypotensive Emergency
Adult: **IV** 20–60 mg as an IV infusion (1.2 mg/mL in D5W)

STORAGE
Store at 15°–30° C (59°–86° F) in tightly closed, light-resistant containers unless otherwise directed by manufacturer.

ADMINISTRATION

Intravenous

PREPARE Direct: May give undiluted. **IV Infusion:** Further dilute by adding 600 mg to 50 mL of D5W.

***ADMINISTER* Direct:** Give at a rate of 30 mg/min. **IV Infusion:** Give at a rate of 1–5 mg/min (rate is usually prescribed by physician).
***INCOMPATIBILITIES* Solution/Additive:** Epinephrine, hydralazine.

ADVERSE EFFECTS CNS: Euphoria, anorexia, weeping, nervousness, anxiety, tremor, seizures, incoherence, drowsiness. **CV:** Tachycardia. With large doses: Cardiac arrhythmias, marked elevation of BP.

INTERACTIONS Drug: Mephentermine may be ineffective in patients receiving **reserpine, guanethidine,** PHENOTHIAZINES; MAO INHIBITORS, SYMPATHOMIMETIC AMINES, **furazolidone, isoniazid** may potentiate pressor response; **methyldopa,** TRICYCLIC ANTIDEPRESSANTS may potentiate or inhibit pressor response; **cyclopropane, halothane** may cause serious arrhythmia; may increase risk of **digoxin**-induced arrhythmias.

PHARMACOKINETICS Onset: 5–15 min IM; immediate IV. **Duration:** 1–4 h IM; 15–30 min IV. **Metabolism:** Rapidly metabolized in liver. **Elimination:** Excreted in urine.

NURSING IMPLICATIONS

Assessment & Drug Effects
- Observe and monitor BP, HR, ECG, and CVP carefully.
- IV administration: Check BP and pulse q2min until stabilized at prescribed level, then q5min during therapy. Continue monitoring vital signs for at least 45–60 min and longer if indicated after therapy.

MEPHOBARBITAL

(me-foe-bar'bi-tal)
Mebaral, Methylphenobarbital
Classifications: CENTRAL NERVOUS SYSTEM AGENT; ANTICONVULSANT; BARBITURATE; SEDATIVE-HYPNOTIC
Prototype: Phenobarbital
Pregnancy Category: D
Controlled Substance: Schedule IV

AVAILABILITY 32 mg, 50 mg, 100 mg tablets

ACTIONS Long-acting barbiturate with pharmacologic properties similar to those of phenobarbital; however, larger doses are required to produce comparable anticonvulsant effects.
THERAPEUTIC EFFECTS Limits the spread of seizure activity by increasing the threshold for motor cortex stimuli. Exerts strong sedative effect, but relatively mild hypnotic effect.

USES To control grand mal and petit mal epilepsy, alone or in combination with other anticonvulsant agents, and for sedative effect in management of delirium tremens and other acute agitation and anxiety states.

CONTRAINDICATIONS Hypersensitivity to barbiturates; lactation. Safety during pregnancy (category D) is not established.
CAUTIOUS USE Fever, hyperthyroidism, alcoholism; liver, kidney, or cardiac dysfunction.

ROUTE & DOSAGE

Anticonvulsant

Child: **PO** ≤5 y, 16–32 mg t.i.d. or q.i.d.; ≥5 y, 32–64 mg t.i.d. or q.i.d. *or* 4–10 mg/kg/day
Adult: **PO** 400–600 mg/day in divided doses

Sedative

Child: **PO** ≤5 y, 16–32 mg t.i.d. or q.i.d.; ≥5 y, 32–64 mg t.i.d. or q.i.d.
Adult: **PO** 32–100 mg t.i.d. or q.i.d.

Delirium Tremens

Adult: **PO** 200 mg t.i.d. or q.i.d.

STORAGE

Store tightly covered at 15°–30° C (59°–86° F) unless directed otherwise by manufacturer.

ADMINISTRATION

Oral

- Change from other anticonvulsant by gradually tapering off the former as mephobarbital doses are increased to maintain seizure control.
- When prescribed concurrently with phenobarbital, dose should be about one-half the amount of each used alone. When prescribed concurrently with phenytoin, the dose of phenytoin is usually reduced.
- Reduce discontinued drug dosage gradually over 4 or 5 days to avoid precipitating seizures of status epilepticus.

ADVERSE EFFECTS CNS: *Drowsiness,* dizziness, unsteadiness, hangover, paradoxical excitement. **GI:** Nausea, vomiting, constipation. **Body as a Whole:** Hypersensitivity reactions, respiratory depression.

INTERACTIONS Drug: Alcohol, CNS DEPRESSANTS compound CNS depression; may decrease absorption and increase metabolism of ORAL ANTICOAGULANTS; increases metabolism of CORTICOSTEROIDS, ORAL CONTRACEPTIVES, ANTICONVULSANTS, **digitoxin,** possibly decreasing their effects; ANTIDEPRESSANTS potentiate adverse effects; **griseofulvin** decreases absorption of mephobarbitol. **Herbal: Kava-kava, valerian** may potentiate sedation.

PHARMACOKINETICS Absorption: 50% absorbed from GI tract. **Onset:** 60 min. **Duration:** 10–12 h. **Metabolism:** Metabolized in liver to phenobarbital. **Elimination:** Excreted in urine. Alkalinization of urine or increase of urinary flow significantly increases the rate of phenobarbital excretion. **Half-Life:** 34 h.

NURSING IMPLICATIONS

Assessment & Drug Effects

- Monitor respiratory status, especially with concurrent CNS therapy with other drugs.
- Be prepared for paradoxical response to barbiturate therapy (i.e., irritability, marked excitement [aggression in children], depression, confusion) in older adults, debilitated patients, or children.

Common adverse effects in *italic;* life-threatening effects <u>underlined</u>; generic names in **bold;** drug classifications in SMALL CAPS; ♣ Canadian drug name; ☻ Prototype drug.

Patient & Family Education

- Be aware that abrupt cessation after prolonged therapy may result in withdrawal symptoms (tremulousness, weakness, insomnia, delirium, convulsions).
- Avoid driving and potentially hazardous activities until response to drug has stabilized.
- Do not take alcohol in any amount with a barbiturate.
- Do not breast feed while using this drug.
- Store this medication out of reach of children.

MEPROBAMATE ℗

(me-proe-ba′mate)

Equanil, Meprospan, Miltown

Classifications: CENTRAL NERVOUS SYSTEM AGENT; PSYCHOTHERAPEUTIC; CARBAMATE; ANXIOLYTIC; SEDATIVE-HYPNOTIC

Pregnancy Category: D

Controlled Substance: Schedule IV

AVAILABILITY 200 mg, 400 mg, 600 mg tablets

ACTIONS Propanediol carbamate derivative structurally and pharmacologically related to carisoprodol. CNS depressant actions similar to those of barbiturates. Acts on multiple sites in CNS and appears to block corticothalamic impulses. No effect on medulla, reticular activating system, or autonomic nervous system.

THERAPEUTIC EFFECTS Antianxiety agent. Hypnotic doses suppress REM sleep.

USES To relieve anxiety and tension of psychoneurotic states and as adjunct in disease states associated with anxiety and tension. Also used to promote sleep in anxious, tense patients.

CONTRAINDICATIONS History of hypersensitivity to meprobamate or related carbamates such as carisoprodol and tybamate; history of acute intermittent porphyria; pregnancy (category D), lactation, children <6 y.

CAUTIOUS USE Impaired kidney or liver function; convulsive disorders; history of alcoholism or drug abuse; patients with suicidal tendencies.

ROUTE & DOSAGE

Sedative

Child: **PO** 100–200 mg b.i.d. or t.i.d. *or* 25 mg/kg/day in 2–3 divided doses *or* 700 mg/m²/day in 2–3 divided doses
Adult: **PO** 1.2–1.6 g/day in 3–4 divided doses (max 2.4 g/day)

Preoperative

Child: **PO** 200 mg
Adult: **PO** 400 mg

STORAGE

Store at 15°–30° C (59°–86° F) unless otherwise specified by manufacturer.

ADMINISTRATION

Oral

- Give with food to minimize gastric distress.
- Treat physical dependence by gradual drug withdrawal over 1–2 wk to prevent onset of withdrawal symptoms.

ADVERSE EFFECTS Body as a Whole: Allergy or idiosyncratic reactions (itchy, urticarial, or erythematous maculopapular rash; <u>exfoliative dermatitis</u>, petechiae, purpura, ecchymoses, eosinophilia, peripheral edema, angioneurotic edema, adenopathy, fever, chills, proctitis, bronchospasm, oliguria, anuria, <u>Stevens-Johnson syndrome</u>); <u>anaphylaxis</u>. **CNS:** *Drowsiness and ataxia,* dizziness, vertigo, slurred speech, headache, weakness, paresthesias, impaired visual accommodation, paradoxic euphoria and rage reactions, seizures in epileptics, panic reaction, rapid EEG activity. **CV:** Hypotensive crisis, syncope, palpitation, tachycardia, arrhythmias, transient ECG changes, <u>circulatory collapse</u> (toxic doses). **GI:** Anorexia, nausea, vomiting, diarrhea. **Hematologic:** <u>Aplastic anemia</u> (rare): Leukopenia, <u>agranulocytosis, thrombocytopenia</u>, exacerbation of acute intermittent porphyria. **Respiratory:** <u>Respiratory depression</u>.

DIAGNOSTIC TEST INTERFERENCE Meprobamate may cause falsely high *urinary steroid* determinations. *Phentolamine* tests may be falsely positive; meprobamate should be withdrawn at least 24 h and preferably 48–72 h before the test.

INTERACTIONS Drug: Alcohol entacapone, TRICYCLIC ANTIDEPRESSANTS, ANTIPSYCHOTICS, OPIATES, SEDATING ANTIHISTAMINES, **pentazocine, tramadol,** MAOIS, SEDATIVE-HYPNOTICS, ANXIOLYTICS may potentiate CNS depression. **Herbal: Kava-kava, valerian** may potentiate sedation.

PHARMACOKINETICS Absorption: Well absorbed from GI tract. **Peak:** 1–3 h. **Onset:** 1 h. **Distribution:** Uniformly distributed throughout body; crosses placenta. **Metabolism:** Rapidly metabolized in liver. **Elimination:** Renally excreted; excreted in breast milk. **Half-Life:** 10–11 h.

NURSING IMPLICATIONS

Assessment & Drug Effects

- Supervise ambulation, if necessary.
- Utilize safety precautions for hospitalized patients. Hypnotic doses may cause increased motor activity during sleep.
- Consult prescriber if daytime psychomotor function is impaired. A change in regimen or drug may be indicated.
- Withdraw gradually in physically dependent patients to prevent preexisting symptoms or withdrawal reactions within 12–48 h: Vomiting, ataxia, muscle twitching, mental confusion, hallucinations, convulsions, trembling, sleep disturbances, increased dreaming, nightmares, insomnia. Symptoms usually subside within 12–48 h.

Patient & Family Education

- Take drug as prescribed. Psychic or physical dependence may occur with long-term use of high doses.
- Be aware that tolerance to alcohol will be lowered.

Common adverse effects in *italic;* life-threatening effects <u>underlined</u>; generic names in **bold;** drug classifications in SMALL CAPS; ♣ Canadian drug name; ⊘ Prototype drug.

- Make position changes slowly, especially from lying down to upright; dangle legs for a few minutes before standing.
- Avoid driving or engaging hazardous activities until response to drug is known.
- Report immediately onset of skin rash, sore throat, fever, bruising, unexplained bleeding.
- Do not breast feed while using this drug.
- Store this medication out of reach of children.

MERCAPTOPURINE (6-MP, 6-MERCAPTOPURINE)

(mer-kap-toe-pyoor′een)
Purinethol
Classifications: ANTINEOPLASTIC; ANTIMETABOLITE; IMMUNOSUPPRESSANT
Prototype: Fluorouracil
Pregnancy Category: D

AVAILABILITY 50 mg tablets

ACTIONS Antimetabolite and purine antagonist. Inhibits purine metabolism by unclear mechanism. Blocks conversion of inosinic acid to adenine and xanthine ribotides within sensitive tumor cells. Also inhibits adenine-containing coenzymes, suggesting an influence over multiple cellular reactions.
THERAPEUTIC EFFECTS Delayed immunosuppressive properties and carcinogenic potential.

USES Primarily for acute lymphocytic and myelogenous leukemia. Response in adults is less than in children, but mercaptopurine is initial drug of choice. In chronic granulocytic leukemia, produces temporary remission.
UNLABELED USES Prevention of transplant graft rejection; SLE; rheumatoid arthritis; Crohn's disease.

CONTRAINDICATIONS Prior resistance to mercaptopurine; first trimester of pregnancy (category D); lactation; infections.
CAUTIOUS USE Impaired kidney or liver function; concomitant use with allopurinol.

ROUTE & DOSAGE

Leukemias
Child/Adult: **PO Loading Dose** 2.5 mg/kg/day, may increase up to 5 mg/kg/day after 4 wk if needed **PO Maintenance Dose** 1.25–2.5 mg/kg/day

STORAGE
Store tablets in light- and air-resistant container.

ADMINISTRATION
Child: Must be given under care and direction of pediatric oncology specialist. Use recommended handling techniques for hazardous medications (see Part I).

Oral

- Give total daily dose at one time.
- Reduce dose of mercaptopurine usually by ⅓ – ¼ when given concurrently with allopurinol.

ADVERSE EFFECTS GI: Stomatitis, esophagitis, anorexia, nausea, vomiting, diarrhea, intestinal ulcerations, impaired liver function, <u>hepatic necrosis</u>. **Hematologic:** Leukopenia, anemia, eosinophilia, pancytopenia, <u>thrombocytopenia</u>, abnormal bleeding, bone marrow hypoplasia. **Urogenital:** Hyperuricemia, oliguria, renal impairment. **Skin:** Rash. **Body as a Whole:** Drug fever.

INTERACTIONS Drug: Allopurinol may inhibit metabolism and thus increase toxicity of mercaptopurine; may potentiate or antagonize anticoagulant effects of **warfarin.**

PHARMACOKINETICS Absorption: Approximately 50% absorbed from GI tract. **Peak:** 2 h. **Distribution:** Distributes into total body water. **Metabolism:** Rapidly metabolized by xanthine oxidase in liver. **Elimination:** 11% excreted in urine within 6 h. **Half-Life:** 20–50 min.

NURSING IMPLICATIONS

Assessment & Drug Effects

- Lab tests: Monitor CBC with differential, platelet count, Hgb, Hct, and liver functions daily.
- Monitor for S&S of liver damage. Hepatic toxicity occurs most often when dose exceeds 2.5 mg/kg/day. Jaundice signals onset of hepatic toxicity and may necessitate terminating use.
- Be alert for and report signs of infection such as respiratory infections, aching, rashes, and gastrointestinal distress.
- Assess immunization status prior to beginning therapy in order to be alert for diseases that pose risk.
- Withhold drug and notify physician at the first sign of an abnormally large or rapid fall in platelet and leukocyte counts.
- Record baseline data related to I&O ratio and pattern and body weight.
- Check vital signs daily. Report febrile states promptly.
- Protect patient from exposure to trauma, infections, or other stresses (restrict visitors and personnel who have colds) during periods of leukopenia.
- Report nausea, vomiting, or diarrhea. These may signal excessive dosage, especially in adults.
- Watch for signs of abnormal bleeding (ecchymoses, petechiae, melena, bleeding gums) if thrombocytopenia develops; report immediately.

Patient & Family Education

- Report any signs of bleeding (e.g., hematuria, bruising, bleeding gums).
- Report signs of hepatic toxicity (see Appendix D-1).
- Increase hydration (10–12 glasses of fluid daily or amount ordered by physician) to reduce risk of hyperuricemia.
- Notify physician of onset of chills, nausea, vomiting, flank or joint pain, swelling of legs or feet, or symptoms of anemia. Report signs of infections. Avoid exposure to persons with infectious diseases.

- Do not breast feed while using this drug.
- Store this medication out of reach of children.

MEROPENEM
(mer-o'pe-nem)
Merrem
Classifications: ANTI-INFECTIVE; CARBAPENEM ANTIBIOTIC
Prototype: Imipenem
Pregnancy Category: B

AVAILABILITY 500 mg, 1 g injection

ACTIONS Broad-spectrum carbapenem antibiotic that inhibits the cell wall synthesis of gram-positive and gram-negative bacteria by its strong affinity for penicillin-binding proteins of bacterial cell wall.
THERAPEUTIC EFFECTS Effective against both gram-positive and gram-negative bacteria. High resistance to most bacterial beta-lactamases. Do not use to treat methicillin-resistant *Staphylococci* (MRSA), corynebacterium, certain strains of enterococcus.

USES Complicated appendicitis and peritonitis, bacterial meningitis caused by susceptible bacteria.
UNLABELED USES Other intra-abdominal infections, skin/soft tissue infections, febrile neutropenia.

CONTRAINDICATIONS Hypersensitivity to meropenem, other carbapenem antibiotics including imipenem, penicillins, cephalosporins, or other beta-lactams; lactation.
CAUTIOUS USE History of asthma or allergies, renal impairment, epileptics, history of neurologic disorders, older adult, pregnancy (category B). Safety and effectiveness in infants <3 mo not established.

ROUTE & DOSAGE

Intra-Abdominal Infections
Child: **IV** ≥3 mo, 20 mg/kg q8h (max 1 g q8h)
Adult: **IV** 1 g q8h

Bacterial Meningitis
Child: **IV** ≥3 mo, 40 mg/kg q8h (max 2 g q8h)
Adult: **IV** 2 g q8h

Renal Impairment
Cl_{cr} 26–50 mL/min: 1 g q12h; 10–25 mL/min: 500 mg q12h; <10 mL/min: 500 mg q24h

STORAGE
Store undiluted at 15°–30° C (59°–86° F), diluted IV solutions should generally be used within 1 h of preparation.

ADMINISTRATION

Intravenous

PREPARE Direct: Reconstitute the 500-mg or 1-g vial, respectively, by adding 10 or 20 mL sterile water for injection to yield approximately 50 mg/mL. Shake to dissolve and let stand until clear. **IV Infusion:** Further dilute in 50–100 mL of D5W, NS, or D5/NS.
ADMINISTER Direct: Give over 3–5 min. **IV Infusion:** Give over 15–30 min.
INCOMPATIBILITIES Solution/Additive: Ringer's lactate, mannitol, amphotericin B, metronidazole, multivitamins. Y-Site: Amphotericin B, diazepam, metronidazole.

ADVERSE EFFECTS GI: Diarrhea, nausea, vomiting, constipation. **Other:** Inflammation at injection site, phlebitis, thrombophlebitis. **CNS:** Headache. **Skin:** Rash, pruritus, diaper rash. **Body as a Whole:** Apnea, oral moniliasis, sepsis, shock. **Hematologic:** Anemia.

INTERACTION Drug: Probenecid will delay meropenem excretion; may decrease **valproic acid** serum levels.

PHARMACOKINETICS Distribution: Attains high concentrations in bile, bronchial secretions, cerebrospinal fluid. **Metabolism:** Undergoes renal and extrarenal metabolism via dipeptidases or nonspecific degradation. **Elimination:** Excreted primarily in urine. **Half-Life:** 0.8–1 h.

NURSING IMPLICATIONS

Assessment & Drug Effects

- Lab tests: Perform C&S tests prior to therapy. Monitor periodically liver and kidney function.
- Determine history of hypersensitivity reactions to other beta-lactams, cephalosporins, penicillins, or other drugs.
- Discontinue drug and immediately report S&S of hypersensitivity (see Appendix D-1).
- Report S&S of superinfection or pseudomembranous colitis (see Appendix D-1).
- Monitor for seizures especially in those with renal insufficiency.

Patient & Family Education

- Learn S&S of hypersensitivity, superinfection, and pseudomembranous colitis (see Appendix D-1); report any of these to physician promptly.
- Do not breast feed while using this drug.

MESALAMINE

(me-sal′a-meen)
Asacol, Canasa, Rowasa, Salofalk ♣ , Pentasa
Classifications: SKIN AND MUCOUS MEMBRANE AGENT; ANTI-INFLAMMATORY; PROSTAGLANDIN INHIBITOR
Pregnancy Category: C

AVAILABILITY 250 mg controlled-release capsule (Pentasa); 400 mg delayed-release tablet (Asacol); 500 mg suppository, 4 g/60 mL rectal suspension (Rowasa); 500 mg suppositories (Canasa)

ACTIONS Thought to diminish inflammation by blocking cyclooxygenase and inhibiting prostaglandin synthesis in the colon.
THERAPEUTIC EFFECTS Provides topical anti-inflammatory action in the colon of patients with ulcerative colitis.

USES Indicated in active mild to moderate distal ulcerative colitis, proctosigmoiditis, or proctitis; maintenance of remission of ulcerative colitis.
UNLABELED USES Crohn's disease.

CONTRAINDICATIONS Hypersensitivity to mesalamine.
CAUTIOUS USE Renal impairment, pregnancy (category C). Sensitivity to sulfasalazine or salicylates. Not known if it is excreted in breast milk. Safe use in children <17 y is not established; has been used in some children when sulfasalazine therapy cannot be used.

ROUTE & DOSAGE

Ulcerative Colitis
Child: **PO** 50 mg/kg/day divided into doses given q6–12h
Adult: **Rectal** (Rowasa) 4 g once/day at bedtime, enema should be retained for about 8 h if possible or 1 suppository (500 mg) b.i.d.; (Canasa) 500 mg b.i.d., may increase up to 500 mg t.i.d. **PO** (Asacol) 800 mg t.i.d. times 3–6 wk; (Pentasa) 500 mg t.i.d. times 3–6 wk

STORAGE
Store at 15°–30° C (59°–86° F) away from heat and light.

ADMINISTRATION
Oral
- Ensure that controlled-release and enteric forms of the drug are not crushed or chewed.
- Shake the bottle well to make sure the suspension is mixed.

Rectal
- Use rectal suspension at bedtime with the objective of retaining it all night.

ADVERSE EFFECTS CNS: *Headache,* fatigue, asthenia, malaise, weakness, dizziness. **GI:** *Abdominal pain, cramps, or discomfort,* flatulence, nausea, diarrhea, constipation, hemorrhoids, rectal pain, hepatitis (rare). **CV:** Pericarditis. **Skin:** Sensitivity reactions, rash, pruritus, alopecia, psoriasis. **Body as a Whole:** Fever, anaphylaxis. **Hematologic:** Thrombocytopenia (rare), eosinophilia. **Urogenital:** Interstitial nephritis.

PHARMACOKINETICS Absorption: PR 5–35% absorbed from colon depending on retention time of enema or suppository. PO Asacol, approximately 28% absorbed; 80% of drug is released in colon 12 h after ingestion. PO Pentasa, 50% of drug is released in colon at a pH <6. **Peak:** 3–6 h. **Distribution:** Rectal administration may reach as high as the

Common adverse effects in *italic;* life-threatening effects underlined; generic names in **bold;** drug classifications in SMALL CAPS; ♣ Canadian drug name; ✪ Prototype drug.

785

ascending colon. Asacol is released in the ileum and colon; Pentasa is released in the jejunum, ileum, and colon. Low concentrations of mesalamine and higher concentrations of its metabolites are excreted in breast milk. **Metabolism:** Rapidly acetylated in the liver and colon wall. **Elimination:** Excreted primarily in feces; absorbed drug excreted in urine. **Half-Life:** 2–15 h (depending on formulation).

NURSING IMPLICATIONS

Assessment & Drug Effects

- Lab tests: Monitor carefully urinalysis, BUN, and creatinine, especially in patients with preexisting kidney disease. The kidney is the major target organ for toxicity.
- Assess for S&S of allergic-type reactions (e.g., hives, itching, wheezing, <u>anaphylaxis</u>). Suspension contains a sulfite that may cause reactions in asthmatics and some nonasthmatic persons.
- Expect response to therapy within 3–21 days; however, the usual course of therapy is from 3–6 wk depending on symptoms and sigmoidoscopic examinations.

Patient & Family Education

- Report to prescriber promptly: Cramping, abdominal pain, or bloody diarrhea, which are indications for immediate drug withdrawal.
- Check with prescriber if rectal irritation (e.g., bleeding, blistering, pain, burning, itching) occurs while using this drug.
- Check with prescriber before using any new medicine (prescription or OTC).
- Continue medication for full time of treatment even if you are feeling better.
- Do not breast feed while taking this drug without consulting physician.
- Store this medication out of reach of children.

MESNA

(mes′na)
Mesnex
Classifications: ANTIDOTE; DETOXIFYING AGENT
Pregnancy Category: B

AVAILABILITY 100 mg/mL injection

ACTIONS Detoxifying agent used to inhibit the hemorrhagic cystitis induced by ifosfamide. Analogous to the physiological cysteine-cystine system.

THERAPEUTIC EFFECTS In the kidney, thiol compound reacts chemically with urotoxic ifosfamide metabolites, resulting in their detoxification, and thus significantly decreases the incidence of hematuria.

USES Prophylaxis for ifosfamide-induced hemorrhagic cystitis. Not effective in preventing hematuria due to other pathologic conditions such as thrombocytopenia.

UNLABELED USES Reduces the incidence of cyclophosphamide-induced hemorrhagic cystitis.

CONTRAINDICATIONS Hypersensitivity to mesna or other thiol compounds; lactation.
CAUTIOUS USE Pregnancy (category B); only if the benefits clearly outweigh any possible risk to fetus.

ROUTE & DOSAGE

Use with Ifosfamide

Child/Adult: **IV** Dose = 20% of ifosfamide dose and is given at time of ifosfamide administration and 4 and 8 h after ifosfamide administration

STORAGE
Refrigerate diluted solutions or use within 6 h of mixing even though diluted solutions are chemically and physically stable for 24 h at 25° C (77° F). Store unopened ampule at 15°–30° C (59°–86° F) unless otherwise specified. Inspect solutions for precipitates and discoloration; do not use if these are seen. Discard any unused portion of the ampule because drug oxidizes on contact with air.

ADMINISTRATION
Note: To be effective, mesna must be administered with each dose of ifosfamide.

Intravenous

PREPARE **Direct:** Add 4 mL of D5W, NS, or RL for each 100 mg of mesna to yield 20 mg/mL.
ADMINISTER **Direct:** Give a single dose by direct IV over 60 sec or over 15–30 min.
INCOMPATIBILITIES **Solution/Additive: Carboplatin, cisplatin, ifosfamide with epirubicin. Y-Site: Amphotericin B cholesteryl complex.**

ADVERSE EFFECTS GI: *Bad taste in mouth, soft stools,* nausea, vomiting. **CV:** Hypotension.

DIAGNOSTIC TEST INTERFERENCE May produce a false-positive result in test for *urinary ketones.*

INTERACTIONS No clinically significant interactions established.

PHARMACOKINETICS Metabolism: Rapidly oxidized in liver to active metabolite dimesna; dimesna is further metabolized in kidney. **Elimination:** 65% excreted in urine within 24 h. **Half-Life:** Mesna 0.36 h, dimesna 1.17 h.

NURSING IMPLICATIONS

Assessment & Drug Effects
- Child: Must be given under care and direction of pediatric oncology specialist. Use recommended handling techniques for hazardous medications (see Part I).

- Monitor urine for hematuria.
- Be aware that a false-positive test for urinary ketones may arise in patients treated with mesna. In this test, a red-violet color develops that, with the addition of glacial acetic acid, will turn to violet.
- About 6% of patients treated with mesna along with ifosfamide still develop hematuria.

Patient & Family Education

- Mesna prevents ifosfamide-induced hemorrhagic cystitis; it will not prevent or alleviate other adverse reactions or toxicities associated with ifosfamide therapy.
- Report any unusual or allergic reactions to physician.
- Check with physician before using any new prescription or OTC medicine.
- Do not breast feed while using this drug.

METAPROTERENOL SULFATE

(met-a-proe-ter′e-nole)

Alupent, Metaprel

Classifications: AUTONOMIC NERVOUS SYSTEM AGENT; BETA-ADRENERGIC AGONIST; BRONCHODILATOR

Prototype: Albuterol

Pregnancy Category: C

AVAILABILITY 10 mg, 20 mg tablet; 10 mg/5 mL syrup; 75 mg, 150 mg metered-dose inhaler; 0.4%, 0.6%, 5% solution for inhalation

ACTIONS Potent synthetic sympathomimetic amine similar to isoproterenol in chemical structure and pharmacologic actions. Acts selectively on beta$_2$-adrenergic receptors to relax smooth muscle of bronchi, uterus, and blood vessels supplying skeletal muscles.

THERAPEUTIC EFFECTS Bronchodilator; controls bronchospasm in asthmatics.

USES Bronchodilator in symptomatic relief of asthma and reversible bronchospasm associated with bronchitis and emphysema.

UNLABELED USES Treatment and prophylaxis of heart block and to avert progress of premature labor (tocolytic action).

CONTRAINDICATIONS Sensitivity to other sympathomimetic agents; cardiac arrhythmias associated with tachycardia; narrow-angle glaucoma; hyperthyroidism; pregnancy (category C), lactation. Safety in children <12 y (for aerosol use) is not established.

CAUTIOUS USE Older adults; hypertension, cardiovascular disorders including coronary artery disease; hyperthyroidism; diabetes.

ROUTE & DOSAGE

Bronchospasm

Child: **PO** <2 y, 0.4 mg/kg/dose q6–8h; 2–6 y, 0.33–0.85 mg/kg/dose q6–8h; 6–9 y, 10 mg/dose q6–8h; >9 y, 20 mg/dose q6–8h

Common adverse effects in *italic*; life-threatening effects <u>underlined</u>; generic names in **bold**; drug classifications in SMALL CAPS; ✦ Canadian drug name; ✪ Prototype drug.

Adult: **PO** 20 mg q6–8h **Metered-Dose Inhaler** 2–3 inhalations q3–4h (max 12 inhalations/day) **Nebulizer** 5–10 inhalations of 5% solution diluted in 2.5 mL NS **IPPB** 2.5 mL of 0.4–0.6% solution q4–6h

Single-Dose Solution for Inhalation

Infant: 2.5 mL 0.4% q4–6 h
Child: 2.5 mL 0.6% q4–6 h

STORAGE
Store all forms at 15°–30° C (59°–86° F); protect from light and heat.

ADMINISTRATION
▪ Note: Patient may use tablets and aerosol concomitantly.

Oral
▪ Give with food to reduce GI distress.

Inhalation
▪ Instruct patient to shake metered-dose aerosol container, exhale through nose as completely as possible, administer aerosol while inhaling deeply through mouth, and to hold breath about 10 sec before exhaling slowly. Administer second inhalation 10 min after first.
▪ Spacers may be used for children (see Part I).

M

ADVERSE EFFECTS CNS: Nervousness, weakness, drowsiness, *tremor (particularly after PO administration),* headache, fatigue. **CV:** *Tachycardia,* hypertension, <u>cardiac arrest</u>, palpitation. **GI:** Nausea, vomiting, bad taste. **Urogenital:** Occasional difficulty in micturition and muscle cramps. **Respiratory:** Throat irritation, cough, exacerbation of asthma.

INTERACTIONS Drug: Epinephrine, other SYMPATHOMIMETIC BRONCHODILATORS may compound effects of metaproterenol; MAO INHIBITORS, TRICYCLIC ANTIDEPRESSANTS potentiate action of metaproterenol on vascular system; the effects of both metaproterenol and BETA-ADRENERGIC BLOCKERS are antagonized.

PHARMACOKINETICS Absorption: 40% of PO doses reach systemic circulation. **Onset:** 1 min inhaled; 15 min PO. **Peak:** 1 h all routes. **Duration:** 1–5 h inhaled; 4 h PO. **Metabolism:** Metabolized in liver. **Elimination:** Excreted in urine.

NURSING IMPLICATIONS

Assessment & Drug Effects
▪ Monitor respiratory status. Auscultate lungs before and after inhalation to determine efficacy of drug in decreasing airway resistance.
▪ Monitor cardiac status. Report tachycardia and hypotension.

Patient & Family Education
▪ Report failure to respond to usual dose. Drug may have shorter duration of action after long-term use.
▪ Do not increase dose or frequency unless ordered by prescriber; there is the possibility of serious adverse effects.

Common adverse effects in *italic;* life-threatening effects <u>underlined</u>; generic names in **bold;** drug classifications in SMALL CAPS; ♣ Canadian drug name; ⊘ Prototype drug.

789

- Anticipate tremor as a possible adverse effect. Report difficulty or changes in school performance.
- Work with school to plan access to medication for the child at school.
- Do not breast feed while taking this drug without consulting prescriber.
- Store this medication out of reach of children.

METHADONE HYDROCHLORIDE

(meth′a-done)

Dolophine, Methadone

Classifications: CENTRAL NERVOUS SYSTEM AGENT; NARCOTIC (OPIATE) AGONIST; ANALGESIC

Prototype: Morphine

Pregnancy Category: B (D for use of high doses at term)

Controlled Substance: Schedule II

AVAILABILITY 5 mg, 10 mg, 40 mg tablets; 5 mg/5 mL, 10 mg/5 mL, 10 mg/mL oral solution; 10 mg/mL injection

ACTIONS Synthetic derivative similar to morphine but is orally effective and has longer duration of action. A single oral dose produces less sedation and euphoria than does morphine, but repeated doses produce marked sedation. Causes less constipation than morphine, but respiratory depressant effect and antitussive actions are comparable. Highly addictive, with abuse potential that matches that of morphine; abstinence syndrome develops more slowly; withdrawal symptoms are less intense but more prolonged.

THERAPEUTIC EFFECTS Relieves severe pain and manages withdrawal therapy from narcotics.

USES To relieve severe pain; for detoxification and temporary maintenance treatment in hospital and in federally controlled maintenance programs for ambulatory patients with narcotic abstinence syndrome.

CONTRAINDICATIONS Obstetric analgesia. Safety during pregnancy (category B, category D for use of high doses, chronic use, or at term), lactation, or for treatment of narcotic addiction in patients <18 y is not established.

CAUTIOUS USE Liver, kidney, or cardiac dysfunction.

ROUTE & DOSAGE

Moderate to Severe Acute Pain

Child: **PO/IV** 0.1 mg/kg q4h times 2–3 doses, then q6–12h prn (max 10 mg/dose)
Adult: **PO/SC/IM** 2.5–10 mg q3–4h prn

Chronic Pain

Adult: **PO/SC/IM** 5–20 mg q6–8h

Detoxification Treatment

Neonate: **PO/IV** 0.05–0.2 mg/kg q12–24h or 0.5 mg/kg/day divided into doses given q8h; taper dose by 10–20%/wk over 1–1½ mo

---

Common adverse effects in *italic;* life-threatening effects <u>underlined;</u> generic names in **bold;** drug classifications in SMALL CAPS; ✦ Canadian drug name; ❂ Prototype drug.

Adult: **PO/SC/IM** 15–40 mg once/day, usually maintained at 20–120 mg/day

Note: Adjust dose downward in renal insufficiency.

STORAGE

Store at 15°–30° C (59°–86° F) in tight, light-resistant containers.

ADMINISTRATION

Oral

- Give for analgesic effect in the smallest effective dose to minimize the possible tolerance and physical and psychic dependence.
- Dilute dispersible tablets in 120 mL (8 oz) of water or fruit juice and allow at least 1 min for dispersion.

Subcutaneous/Intramuscular

- Note: IM route is preferred over SC when repeated parenteral administration is required (SC injections may cause local irritation and induration). Rotate injection sites.

Intravenous

- Verify correct IV concentration and rate of infusion for administration to neonates, infants, children with physician.
- IV route is used rarely. Get specific orders from physician.

INCOMPATIBILITIES **Solution/Additive: Aminophylline, ammonium chloride,** BARBITURATES, **chlorothiazide, heparin, methicillin, phenytoin, sodium bicarbonate.**

ADVERSE EFFECTS CNS: *Drowsiness,* light-headedness, dizziness, hallucinations, increased intracranial pressure. **GI:** Nausea, vomiting, dry mouth, *constipation.* **CV:** Bradycardia. **Body as a Whole:** Transient fall in BP, bone and muscle pain, sedation. **Urogenital:** Impotence. **Respiratory:** Respiratory depression.

INTERACTIONS Drug: Alcohol and other CNS DEPRESSANTS, **cimetidine** add to sedation and CNS depression; AMPHETAMINES may potentiate CNS stimulation; with MAO INHIBITORS, **selegiline, furazolidone** causes excessive and prolonged CNS depression, convulsions, cardiovascular collapse.

PHARMACOKINETICS Absorption: Well absorbed from GI tract. **Onset:** 30–60 min PO; 10–20 min IM/SC. **Peak:** 1–2 h. **Duration:** 6–8 h PO/IM/SC; may last 22–48 h with chronic dosing. **Distribution:** Crosses placenta; distributed into breast milk. **Metabolism:** Metabolized in liver. **Elimination:** Excreted in urine. **Half-Life:** Average of 15–25 h with adults about 35 h and children about 19 h.

NURSING IMPLICATIONS

Assessment & Drug Effects

- Evaluate patient's continued need for methadone for pain. Adjustment of dosage and lengthening of between-dose intervals may be possible.
- Monitor respiratory status. Principal danger of overdosage, as with morphine, is extreme respiratory depression.

- Be aware that because of the cumulative effects of methadone, abstinence symptoms may not appear for 36–72 h after last dose and may last 10–14 days. Symptoms are usually of mild intensity (e.g., anorexia, insomnia, anxiety, abdominal discomfort, weakness, headache, sweating, hot and cold flashes).
- Observe closely for recurrence of respiratory depression during use of narcotic antagonists such as naloxone, naltrexone, and levallorphan to terminate methadone intoxication. Because antagonist action is shorter (1–3 h) than that of methadone (36–48 h or more), repeated doses for 8–24 h may be required.
- Care by neonatologist and thorough nursing assessments are needed when used for treatment of drug addicted newborns.

Patient & Family Education

- Be aware that orthostatic hypotension, sweating, constipation, drowsiness, GI symptoms, and other transient adverse effects of therapeutic doses appear to be more prominent in ambulatory patients. Most adverse effects disappear over a period of several weeks.
- Make position changes slowly, particularly from lying down to upright position; sit or lie down if you feel dizzy or faint.
- Do not drive or engage in potentially hazardous activities until response to drug is known.
- Do not breast feed while taking this drug without consulting physician.
- Store this medication in locked area out of reach of children; this is a Schedule II drug.

METHAMPHETAMINE HYDROCHLORIDE

(meth-am-fet′a-meen)

Desoxyephedrine, Desoxyn

Classifications: CENTRAL NERVOUS SYSTEM AGENT; CEREBRAL STIMULANT; ANOREXIANT; AMPHETAMINE

Prototype: Amphetamine Sulfate

Pregnancy Category: C

Controlled Substance: Schedule II

AVAILABILITY 5 mg tablets; 5 mg, 10 mg, 15 mg long-acting tablets

ACTIONS Sympathomimetic amine chemically related to amphetamine. CNS stimulant actions approximately equal to those of amphetamine, but accompanied by less peripheral activity. However, larger doses produce increased cardiac output, possibly reflex slowing of heart rate, and sustained increase in BP, chiefly by cardiac stimulation.

THERAPEUTIC EFFECTS CNS stimulant actions approximately equal to those of amphetamine, but accompanied by less peripheral activity.

USES Short-term adjunct in management of exogenous obesity, as adjunctive therapy in attention deficit disorder (ADD), narcolepsy, epilepsy, and postencephalitic parkinsonism, and in treatment of certain depressive reactions, especially when characterized by apathy and psychomotor retardation.

CONTRAINDICATIONS During pregnancy, especially first trimester (category C), lactation; as anorexiant in children <12 y; patients receiving MAO INHIBITORS; arteriosclerotic parkinsonism.

CAUTIOUS USE Mild hypertension; psychopathic personalities; hyperexcitability states; history of suicide attempts; debilitated patients.

ROUTE & DOSAGE

Attention Deficit Disorder
Child: **PO** ≥6 y, 2.5–5 mg 1–2 times/day, may increase by 5 mg at weekly intervals up to 20–25 mg/day

Obesity
Adult: **PO** 2.5–5 mg 1–3 times/day 30 min before meals or 5–15 mg of long-acting form once daily

STORAGE
Preserve at 15°–30° C (59°–86° F) in tight, light-resistant containers.

ADMINISTRATION

Oral
- Give early in the day to avoid insomnia, if possible.
- Ensure that long-acting tablets are not chewed or crushed; these need to be swallowed whole.
- Give 30 min before each meal when used for treatment of obesity. If insomnia results, advise patient to inform physician.

ADVERSE EFFECTS CNS: Restlessness, tremor, hyperreflexia, insomnia, headache, nervousness, anxiety, dizziness, euphoria or dysphoria. **CV:** Palpitation, arrhythmias, hypertension, hypotension, <u>circulatory collapse</u>. **GI:** Dry mouth, unpleasant taste, nausea, vomiting, diarrhea, constipation. **Special Senses:** Increased intraocular pressure. **Body as a Whole:** Weight loss, decreased appetite.

INTERACTIONS Drug: Acetazolamide, sodium bicarbonate decreases methamphetamine elimination; **ammonium chloride, ascorbic acid** increases methamphetamine elimination; effects of both methamphetamine and BARBITURATES may be antagonized; **furazolidone** may increase BP effects of AMPHETAMINES—interaction may persist for several weeks after discontinuing furazolidone; antagonizes antihypertensive effects of **guanethidine, guanadrel;** MAO INHIBITORS, **selegiline** can cause hypertensive crisis (fatalities reported)—do not administer AMPHETAMINES during or within 14 days of administration of these drugs; PHENOTHIAZINES may inhibit mood-elevating effects of AMPHETAMINES; TRICYCLIC ANTIDEPRESSANTS enhance methamphetamine effects because they increase norepinephrine release; BETA-ADRENERGIC AGONISTS increase adverse cardiovascular effects of AMPHETAMINES.

PHARMACOKINETICS Absorption: Readily absorbed from the GI tract. **Duration:** 6–12 h. **Distribution:** All tissues especially the CNS; excreted in breast milk. **Metabolism:** Metabolized in liver. **Elimination:** Renal elimination.

NURSING IMPLICATIONS

Assessment & Drug Effects

- Monitor weight and record on growth grids throughout period of therapy. Report decrease in weight or height channel to prescriber.
- Be alert for paradoxic increase in depression or agitation in depressed patients. Report immediately; drug should be withdrawn.
- Do not exceed duration of a few weeks for treatment of obesity.

Patient & Family Education

- Do not take last dose after 3–4 p.m.
- Withdrawal after prolonged use is frequently followed by lethargy that may persist for several weeks.
- Weigh every other day under standard conditions and maintain and report weight loss.
- Be alert for development of tolerance; happens readily, and prolonged use may lead to drug dependence. Abuse potential is high. Methamphetamine is commonly known as "speed" or "crystal" among drug abusers.
- Be sure drug is adequately locked and out of reach of children both at home and in school if given in that setting.
- Do not breast feed while using this drug.

M

METHENAMINE HIPPURATE

(meth-en'a-meen hip'yoo-rate)
Hiprex, Urex

METHENAMINE MANDELATE

Mandelamine, Mandameth
Classifications: URINARY TRACT ANTI-INFECTIVE
Prototype: Trimethoprim
Pregnancy Category: C

AVAILABILITY Methenamine Hippurate 1 g tablets **Methenamine Mandelate** 0.5 g, 1 g tablets; 0.5 g/5 mL suspension

ACTIONS Tertiary amine liberates formaldehyde in an acid medium. Nonspecific antibiotic agent with bactericidal activity.
THERAPEUTIC EFFECTS Most bacteria and fungi are susceptible to formaldehyde; however, bacteria that are urease-positive (e.g., *Proteus* sp.) convert urea to ammonium hydroxide, which prevents the generation of formaldehyde from methenamine.

USES Prophylactic treatment of recurrent urinary tract infections (UTIs). Also long-term prophylaxis when residual urine is present (e.g., neurogenic bladder).

CONTRAINDICATIONS Renal insufficiency; liver disease; gout; severe dehydration; combined therapy with sulfonamides. Safety during pregnancy (category C) or lactation is not established.

CAUTIOUS USE Oral suspension for patients susceptible to lipoid pneumonia (e.g., infants, young children, older adults, debilitated patients).

ROUTE & DOSAGE

UTI Prophylaxis

Child: **PO** ≤6 y, (Mandelate) 18.4 mg/kg q.i.d.; *6–12 y,* (Hippurate) 0.5–1 g b.i.d.; (Mandelate) 500 mg q.i.d. or 50 mg/kg/day in 3 divided doses
Adult: **PO** (Hippurate) 1 g b.i.d.; (Mandelate) 1 g q.i.d.

STORAGE

- Store at 15°–30° C (59°–86° F) in tightly closed container; protect from excessive heat.

ADMINISTRATION

Oral

- Give after meals and at bedtime to minimize gastric distress.
- Give oral suspension with caution to debilitated patients because of the possibility of lipid (aspiration) pneumonia; it contains a vegetable oil base.

ADVERSE EFFECTS GI: Nausea, vomiting, diarrhea, abdominal cramps, anorexia. **Renal:** Bladder irritation, dysuria, frequency, albuminuria, hematuria, crystalluria.

DIAGNOSTIC TEST INTERFERENCE Methenamine (formaldehyde) may produce falsely elevated values for ***urinary catecholamines*** and ***urinary steroids (17-hydroxycorticosteroids)*** (by ***Reddy method***). Possibility of false ***urine glucose determinations*** with ***Benedict's*** test. Methenamine interferes with ***urobilinogen*** and possibly ***urinary VMA*** determinations.

INTERACTIONS Drug: Sulfamethoxazole forms insoluble precipitate in acid urine; **acetazolamide, sodium bicarbonate** may prevent hydrolysis to formaldehyde.

PHARMACOKINETICS Absorption: Readily absorbed from GI tract, although 10–30% of dose is hydrolyzed to formaldehyde in stomach. **Peak:** 2 h. **Duration:** Up to 6 h or until patient voids. **Distribution:** Crosses placenta; distributed into breast milk. **Metabolism:** Hydrolyzed in acid pH to formaldehyde. **Elimination:** Excreted in urine. **Half-Life:** 4 h.

NURSING IMPLICATIONS

Assessment & Drug Effects

- Monitor urine pH; value of 5.5 or less is required for optimum drug action.
- Monitor I&O ratio and pattern; drug most effective when fluid intake is maintained at 1500 or 2000 mL/day or amount appropriate for age of child.
- Do not force fluids with this drug; copious amounts may increase diuresis, elevate urine pH, and dilute formaldehyde concentration to subinhibitory levels.

- Consult physician about changing to enteric-coated tablet if patient complains of gastric distress.
- Supplemental acidification to maintain pH of 5.5 or below required for drug action may be necessary. Accomplish by drugs (ascorbic acid, ammonium chloride) or by foods.

Patient & Family Education

- Do not self-medicate with OTC antacids containing sodium bicarbonate or sodium carbonate (to prevent raising urine pH).
- Achieve supplementary acidification by limiting intake of foods that can increase urine pH (e.g., vegetables, fruits, and fruit juice [except cranberry, plum, prune]) and increasing intake of foods that can decrease urine pH (e.g., proteins, cranberry juice, plums, prunes).
- Do not breast feed while taking this drug without consulting prescriber.
- Store this medication out of reach of children.

METHIMAZOLE

(meth-im′a-zole)

Tapazole

Classifications: HORMONE AND SYNTHETIC SUBSTITUTE; ANTITHYROID AGENT
Prototype: Propylthiouracil
Pregnancy Category: D

AVAILABILITY 5 mg, 10 mg tablets

ACTIONS Thioamide with actions and uses similar to those of propylthiouracil but 10 times as potent. Actions are less consistent, but effects appear more promptly than with propylthiouracil. Inhibits synthesis of thyroid hormones as the drug accumulates in the thyroid gland. Does not affect existing T_3 or T_4 levels.

THERAPEUTIC EFFECTS Corrects hyperthyroidism by inhibiting synthesis of the thyroid hormone.

USES Hyperthyroidism and prior to surgery or radiotherapy of the thyroid; may be used cautiously to treat hyperthyroidism in pregnancy.

CONTRAINDICATIONS Pregnancy (category D), lactation.
CAUTIOUS USE Other drugs known to cause agranulocytosis.

ROUTE & DOSAGE

Hyperthyroidism

Child: **PO** Initial dose 0.4–0.7 mg/kg/day *or*
15–20 mg/m²/day divided into 3 doses; maintenance dose is ⅓–⅔ of initial dose divided into 3 daily doses (max 30 mg/day)
Adult: **PO** Initial dose may be 15–60 mg/day divided into 3 doses; maintenance dose is 5–15 mg/day divided into 3 doses (max 30 mg/day)

STORAGE

Store at 15°–30° C (59°–86° F) in light-resistant container.

Common adverse effects in *italic;* life-threatening effects <u>underlined</u>; generic names in **bold**; drug classifications in SMALL CAPS; ◆ Canadian drug name; ⦿ Prototype drug.

ADMINISTRATION

Oral

- Give at same time each day relative to meals.

ADVERSE EFFECTS GI: <u>Hepatotoxicity</u> (rare); weight gain. **Endocrine:** Hypothyroidism. **Hematologic:** *Leukopenia,* agranulocytosis, granulocytopenia, thrombocytopenia, pancytopenia, and aplastic anemia. **Musculoskeletal:** Arthralgia. **CNS:** Peripheral neuropathy, drowsiness, neuritis, paresthesias, vertigo. **Skin:** Rash, alopecia, skin hyperpigmentation, urticaria, and pruritus. **Urogenital:** Nephrotic syndrome.

INTERACTIONS Drug: Can reduce anticoagulant effects of **warfarin;** may increase serum levels of **digoxin;** may alter **theophylline** levels; may need to decrease dose of BETA-BLOCKERS.

PHARMACOKINETICS Absorption: Readily absorbed from GI tract. **Onset:** 30–40 min. **Peak:** 1 h. **Duration:** 2–4 h. **Distribution:** Crosses placenta; distributed into breast milk. **Elimination:** 12% excreted in urine within 24 h. **Half-Life:** 5–13 h.

NURSING IMPLICATIONS

Assessment & Drug Effects

- Lab tests: Periodic blood work, because agranulocytosis is a rare, but possible adverse effect.
- Closely monitor PT and INR in patients on oral anticoagulants. Anticoagulant activity may be potentiated.
- Monitor thyroid levels when euthyroid patient is changed to maintenance dose.

Patient & Family Education

- Adhere to established dosage regimen (i.e., not to double, decrease, or omit doses and not to alter the interval between doses).
- Be aware that skin rash or swelling of cervical lymph nodes may indicate need to discontinue drug and change to another antithyroid agent. Consult physician.
- Notify physician promptly if the following symptoms appear: Bruising, unexplained bleeding, sore throat, fever, jaundice.
- Drug-induced jaundice may persist up to 10 wk after withdrawal of drug.
- Methimazole does not induce hypothyroiditis.
- Do not breast feed while using this drug.
- Store this medication out of reach of children.

METHOCARBAMOL

(meth-oh-kar′ba-mole)
Marbaxin, Robaxin
Classifications: AUTONOMIC NERVOUS SYSTEM AGENT; CENTRAL-ACTING SKELETAL MUSCLE RELAXANT
Prototype: Cyclobenzaprine
Pregnancy Category: C

AVAILABILITY 500 mg, 750 mg tablet; 100 mg/mL injection

ACTIONS Similar to cyclobenzaprine, but it produces higher plasma levels more rapidly and for longer periods. Exerts skeletal muscle relaxant action by depressing multisynaptic pathways in the spinal cord and possibly by sedative effect.

THERAPEUTIC EFFECTS No direct action on skeletal muscles; just on multisynaptic pathways in spinal cord that control muscular spasm.

USES Adjunct to physical therapy and other measures in management of discomfort associated with acute musculoskeletal disorders. Also used intravenously as adjunct in management of neuromuscular manifestations of tetanus.

CONTRAINDICATIONS Comatose states; CNS depression; acidosis, kidney dysfunction (injectable methocarbamol contains polyethylene glycol 300 in vehicle, which may cause urea retention and acidotic problems).
CAUTIOUS USE Epilepsy. Safety during pregnancy (category C), lactation, or in children <12 y (except for tetanus) is not established.

ROUTE & DOSAGE

Acute Musculoskeletal Disorders
Adult: **PO** 1.5 g q.i.d. for 2–3 days, then 4–4.5 g/day in 3–6 divided doses **IM** 0.5–1 g q8h **IV** 1–3 g/day in divided doses (max rate of 300 mg/min)

Tetanus
Child: **PO** 15 mg/kg repeated q6h as needed up to 1.8 g/m^2/day for 3 consecutive days if necessary
Adult: **PO** Up to 24 g/day in divided doses crushed and suspended in saline, flushed down a nasogastric tube **IV** 1–2 g/day directly into IV tubing (max rate of 300 mg/min), may be repeated q6h until use of nasogastric tube is possible

STORAGE
Store at 15°–30° C (59°–86° F).

ADMINISTRATION
Intramuscular
- Do not exceed IM dose of 5 mL (0.5 g) into each gluteal region or location appropriate for the child (see Part I). Insert needle deep and carefully aspirate. Inject drug slowly. Rotate injection sites and observe daily for evidence of irritation.

Intravenous
PREPARE **Direct:** May be given undiluted or diluted in up to 250 mL of NS or D5W.
ADMINISTER **Direct:** Give at a rate of 300 mg or fraction thereof over 1 min or longer.
- Keep patient recumbent during and for at least 15 min after IV injection in order to reduce possibility of orthostatic hypotension and other adverse reactions.

Common adverse effects in *italic;* life-threatening effects <u>underlined;</u> generic names in **bold;** drug classifications in SMALL CAPS; ✦ Canadian drug name; ⊘ Prototype drug.

- Monitor IV flow rate.
- Take care to avoid extravasation of IV solution, which may result in thrombophlebitis and sloughing.

ADVERSE EFFECTS Body as a Whole: Fever, anaphylactic reaction, flushing, syncope, convulsions. **Skin:** Urticaria, pruritus, rash, thrombophlebitis, pain, sloughing (with extravasation). **Special Senses:** Conjunctivitis, blurred vision, nasal congestion. **CNS:** *Drowsiness, dizziness, light-headedness,* headache. **CV:** Hypotension, bradycardia. **GI:** Nausea, metallic taste. **Hematologic:** Slight reduction of white cell count with prolonged therapy.

DIAGNOSTIC TEST INTERFERENCE Methocarbamol may cause false increases in **urinary 5-HIAA** (with **nitrosonaphthol reagent**) and **VMA (Gitlow method).**

INTERACTIONS Drug: Alcohol and other CNS DEPRESSANTS enhance CNS depression.

PHARMACOKINETICS Absorption: Readily absorbed from GI tract. **Onset:** 30 min. **Peak:** 1–2 h. **Metabolism:** Metabolized in liver. **Elimination:** Excreted in urine. **Half-Life:** 1–2 h.

NURSING IMPLICATIONS

Assessment & Drug Effects
- Lab tests: Obtain periodic WBC counts during prolonged therapy.
- Monitor vital signs closely during IV infusion.
- Supervise ambulation following parenteral administration.

Patient & Family Education
- Make position changes slowly, particularly from lying down to upright position; dangle legs before standing.
- Be aware that adverse reactions after oral administration are usually mild and transient and subside with dosage reduction. Use caution regarding drowsiness and dizziness. Avoid activities requiring mental alertness and physical coordination until response to drug is known.
- Urine may darken to brown, black, or green on standing.
- Do not breast feed while taking this drug without consulting physician.
- Store this medication out of reach of children.

METHOHEXITAL SODIUM
(meth-oh-hex′i-tal)
Brevital Sodium
Classifications: CENTRAL NERVOUS SYSTEM AGENT; GENERAL ANESTHETIC; BARBITURATE
Prototype: Thiopental
Pregnancy Category: B
Controlled Substance: Schedule IV

AVAILABILITY 500 mg, 2.5 g, 5 g powder for injection

ACTIONS Rapid, ultra-short-acting barbiturate anesthetic agent. More potent than thiopental but has less cumulative effect and shorter duration of action, and recovery is more rapid.

THERAPEUTIC EFFECTS Induces brief general anesthesia without analgesia by depression of the CNS.

USES Induction of anesthesia, as supplement for other anesthetics, and as general anesthetic for brief operative procedures.

CONTRAINDICATIONS Hypersensitivity to methocarbamol.
CAUTIOUS USE Pregnancy (category B), lactation; hepatic impairment.

ROUTE & DOSAGE

Induction of Anesthesia

Child: **IV** 1–2 mg/kg **PR** 20–35 mg/kg as 10% solution (max 500 mg/dose)
Adult: **IV** 5–12 mL of 1% solution (50–120 mg) at a rate of 1 mL (5 mg) q5min, then 2–4 mL (20–40 mg) q4–7min prn

STORAGE

Store drug prepared in sterile water for injection at room temperature for at least 6 wk. Solutions prepared with isotonic NaCl injection or 5% dextrose injection are stable for ONLY about 24 h.

ADMINISTRATION

Intravenous

- Give to recumbent patient. Fall in BP may occur in susceptible patients receiving drug in upright position.

PREPARE **Direct:** Prepare a 1% solution (10 mg/mL) by diluting with sterile water for injection, D5W, or NS. Use only clear, colorless solutions. Do not allow contact with rubber stoppers or parts of syringes treated with silicone because solution is incompatible with acid solutions (see INCOMPATIBILITIES).

ADMINISTER **Direct:** Give 5 mg over 5–10 sec.

INCOMPATIBILITIES **Solution/Additive: Atropine, chlorpromazine, clindamycin, fentanyl, glycopyrrolate, hydralazine, kanamycin, lidocaine, methicillin, mechlorethamine, methyldopa, pentazocine, prochlorperazine, promazine, promethazine, streptomycin,** TETRACYCLINES.

ADVERSE EFFECTS CV: Hypotension, cardiac arrhythmias, cardiac arrest. **Musculoskeletal:** Muscle spasm. **CNS:** Postoperative psychomotor impairment that persists for 24 h, anxiety, drowsiness, emergence delirium, restlessness, and seizures. **Respiratory:** Bronchospasm, cough, hiccups, respiratory depression, apnea, dyspnea, <u>respiratory arrest</u>. **Skin:** Phlebitis and nerve injury adjacent to the injection site, local irritation, edema, ulceration, necrosis.

INTERACTIONS Drug: Alcohol and other CNS DEPRESSANTS enhance CNS depression.

PHARMACOKINETICS Absorption: 17% absorbed PR. **Distribution:** Crosses CNS, placenta and excreted in breast milk. **Metabolism:** Oxidized in liver. **Elimination:** Primarily excreted in urine.

NURSING IMPLICATIONS

Assessment & Drug Effects

- Hiccups are common, particularly with rapid injection; they sometimes persist after anesthesia.
- Keep facilities for assisting respiration and administration of oxygen readily available in the event of respiratory distress.

Patient & Family Education

- Do not breast feed when given this drug.

METHOTREXATE
(meth-oh-trex′ate)
Amethopterin, Mexate, MTX, Rheumatrex

METHOTREXATE SODIUM

Folex, Mexate
Classifications: ANTINEOPLASTIC; ANTIMETABOLITE; IMMUNOSUPPRESSANT
Prototype: Fluorouracil
Pregnancy Category: D

AVAILABILITY 2.5 mg tablets; 20 mg, 1 g powder for injection; 2.5 mg/mL, 25 mg/mL injection

ACTIONS Antimetabolite and folic acid antagonist. Blocks folic acid participation in nucleic acid synthesis, thereby interfering with mitotic process.
THERAPEUTIC EFFECTS Rapidly proliferating tissues (malignant cells, bone marrow) are sensitive to interference of the mitotic process by this drug. In psoriasis, reproductive rate of epithelial cells is higher than in normal cells. Induces remission slowly; use often preceded by other antineoplastic therapies.

USES Principally in combination regimens to maintain induced remissions in neoplastic diseases. Effective in treatment of gestational choriocarcinoma and hydatidiform mole and as immunosuppressant in kidney transplantation, for acute and subacute leukemias and leukemic meningitis, especially in children. Used in lymphosarcoma, in certain inoperable tumors of head, neck, and pelvis, and in mycosis fungoides. Also used to treat severe psoriasis nonresponsive to other forms of therapy, rheumatoid arthritis.
UNLABELED USES Psoriatic arthritis, SLE, polymyositis.

CONTRAINDICATIONS Pregnancy (category D), men and women during reproductive years; lactation; hepatic and renal insufficiency; concomitant administration of hepatotoxic drugs and hematopoietic depressants;

Common adverse effects in *italic;* life-threatening effects <u>underlined</u>; generic names in **bold;** drug classifications in SMALL CAPS; ♣ Canadian drug name; ⦿ Prototype drug.

801

alcohol; ultraviolet exposure to psoriatic lesions; preexisting blood dyscrasias.

CAUTIOUS USE Infections; peptic ulcer, ulcerative colitis; very young or old patients; cancer patients with preexisting bone marrow impairment; poor nutritional status.

ROUTE & DOSAGE

Trophoblastic Neoplasm

Adult: **PO** 15–30 mg/day for 5 days, repeat q12wk for 3–5 courses
IM/IV 15–30 mg/day for 5 days, repeat q12wk for 3–5 courses

Leukemia

Child: **PO/IM** 7.5–30 mg/m^2 q1–2wk **IT** <*1 y*, 6 mg; *1–2 y*, 8 mg;
2–3 y, 10 mg; *≥3 y*, 12 mg
Adult: **IM/IV Loading Dose** 3.3 mg/m^2/day **PO/IM/IV Maintenance
Dose** 20–30 mg/m^2 2 times/wk

Lymphoma

Adult: **PO** 12–25 mg/day for 4–8 days in several courses with 7–10
days rest intervals between courses of treatment, *or* 0.625–2.5
mg/kg/day for stage III lymphosarcoma

Psoriasis

Adult: **PO** 2.5–5 mg q12h for 3 doses each wk up to 25–30 mg/wk
IM/IV 10–25 mg/wk

Rheumatoid Arthritis

Child: **PO/IM** 5–15 mg/m^2/wk as single dose or in 3 divided doses
12 h apart
Adult: **PO** 2.5–5 mg q12h for 3 doses each wk or
7.5 mg once/wk

STORAGE

Preserve drug in tightly covered, light-resistant container.

ADMINISTRATION

Child: Must be given under care and direction of pediatric oncology specialist. Use recommended handling techniques for hazardous medications (see Part I).

Oral

- Give 1 h before or 2 h after meals.
- Use a test dose (5–10 mg parenterally) 1 wk before therapy for treatment of psoriasis.
- Avoid skin exposure and inhalation of drug particles.

Intravenous

- Note: Verify correct IV and IT concentration and rate of infusion for administration to children with physician.
- High dose given with leucovorin rescue (see leucovorin for details).

PREPARE Direct: Reconstitute powder vial by adding 2 mL of NS or D5W without preservatives to each 5 mg to yield 2.5 mg/mL. Reconstitute 1 g high-dose vial with 19.4 mL D5W or NS to yield 50 mg/mL. **IV Infusion:** Further dilute contents of high-dose vial in D5W or NS.

ADMINISTER **Direct:** Give at rate of 10 mg or fraction thereof over 60 sec. **IV Infusion:** Give over 1–4 h or as prescribed.

INCOMPATIBILITIES **Solution/Additive: Bleomycin, prednisolone, droperidol, heparin, metoclopramide, ranitidine. Y-Site: Chlorpromazine, droperidol, gemcitabine, idarubicin, ifosfamide, midazolam, nalbuphine, promethazine, propofol.**

ADVERSE EFFECTS CNS: *Headache,* drowsiness, blurred vision, dizziness, aphasia, hemiparesis; arachnoiditis, convulsions (after intrathecal administration); mental confusion, tremors, ataxia, coma. **GI:** <u>Hepatotoxicity</u>, GI ulcerations and hemorrhage, *ulcerative stomatitis, glossitis, gingivitis,* pharyngitis, nausea, vomiting, diarrhea, <u>hepatic cirrhosis</u>. **Urogenital:** Defective oogenesis or spermatogenesis, nephropathy, hematuria, menstrual dysfunction, infertility, abortion, fetal defects. **Hematologic:** *Leukopenia, thrombocytopenia,* anemia, <u>marked myelosuppression, aplastic bone marrow</u>, telangiectasis, thrombophlebitis at intraarterial catheter site, hypogammaglobulinemia, and hyperuricemia. **Skin:** Erythematous rashes, pruritus, urticaria, folliculitis, vasculitis, photosensitivity, depigmentation, hyperpigmentation, alopecia. **Body as a Whole:** Malaise, undue fatigue, systemic toxicity (after intrathecal and intraarterial administration), chills, fever, decreased resistance to infection, septicemia, osteoporosis, metabolic changes precipitating diabetes and <u>sudden death, pneumonitis, pulmonary fibrosis</u>.

DIAGNOSTIC TEST INTERFERENCE Severe reactions may occur when *live vaccines* are administered because of immunosuppressive activity of methotrexate.

INTERACTIONS Drug: Alcohol, azathioprine, sulfasalazine increase risk of hepatotoxicity; **chloramphenicol, etretinate,** SALICYLATES, NSAIDS, SULFONAMIDES, SULFONYLUREAS, **phenylbutazone, phenytoin,** TETRACYCLINES, **PABA, penicillin, probenecid** may increase methotrexate levels with increased toxicity; **folic acid** may alter response to methotrexate. May increase **theophylline** levels; **cholestyramine** enhances methotrexate clearance. **Herbal: Echinacea** may increase risk of hepatotoxicity.

PHARMACOKINETICS Absorption: Readily absorbed from GI tract. **Peak:** 0.5–2 h IM/IV; 1–4 h PO. **Distribution:** Widely distributed with highest concentrations in kidneys, gallbladder, spleen, liver, and skin; minimal passage across blood–brain barrier; crosses placenta; distributed into breast milk. **Metabolism:** Metabolized in liver. **Elimination:** Excreted primarily in urine. **Half-Life:** 2–4 h.

NURSING IMPLICATIONS

Assessment & Drug Effects

- Lab tests: Obtain baseline liver and kidney function, CBC with differential, platelet count, and chest x-rays. Repeat weekly during therapy.
- Prolonged treatment with small frequent doses may lead to hepatotoxicity, which is best diagnosed by liver biopsy.
- Monitor for and report ulcerative stomatitis with glossitis and gingivitis, often the first signs of toxicity. Inspect mouth daily; report patchy necrotic areas, bleeding and discomfort, or overgrowth (black, furry tongue).

Common adverse effects in *italic;* life-threatening effects <u>underlined</u>; generic names in **bold;** drug classifications in SMALL CAPS; ♣ Canadian drug name; ⊘ Prototype drug.

803

- Keep patient well hydrated (about 2000 mL/24 h or amount prescribed for child by physician).
- Monitor I&O ratio and pattern. Severe nephrotoxicity (hematuria, dysuria, azotemia, oliguria) fosters drug accumulation and kidney damage and requires dosage adjustment or discontinuation.
- Prevent exposure to infections or colds during leukopenia periods.
- Be alert for and report signs of infection such as respiratory infections, aching, rashes, and gastrointestinal distress.
- Assess immunization status prior to beginning therapy in order to be alert for diseases that pose risk.
- Be alert to onset of agranulocytosis (cough, extreme fatigue, sore throat, chills, fever) and report symptoms promptly. Therapy will be interrupted and appropriate antibiotic drugs prescribed.
- Be alert for and report symptoms of thrombocytopenia (e.g., ecchymoses, petechiae, epistaxis, melena, hematuria, vaginal bleeding, slow and protracted oozing following trauma).
- Report bloody diarrhea to physician; necessitates interruption of therapy to prevent perforation or hemorrhagic enteritis.
- Monitor blood glucose and HbAlc periodically in diabetics.

Patient & Family Education

- Be aware of dangers of drug and report promptly any abnormal symptoms to physician.
- Report signs of infections. Avoid exposure to persons with infectious diseases.
- Alcohol ingestion increases the incidence and severity of methotrexate hepatotoxicity.
- Practice fastidious mouth care to prevent infection, provide comfort, and maintain adequate nutritional status.
- Report joint pains to physician; drug may precipitate gouty arthritis.
- Do not self-medicate with vitamins. Some OTC compounds may include folic acid (or its derivatives), which alters methotrexate response.
- Use contraceptive measures if sexually active during and for at least 8 wk following therapy.
- Avoid exposure to sunlight and ultraviolet light. Wear sunglasses and sunscreen.
- Do not breast feed while using this drug.
- Store this medication out of reach of children.

METHOXAMINE HYDROCHLORIDE ⊘

(meth-ox′a meen)

Vasoxyl

Classifications: AUTONOMIC NERVOUS SYSTEM AGENT; ALPHA-ADRENERGIC AGONIST (SYMPATHOMIMETIC)

Pregnancy Category: C

AVAILABILITY 20 mg/mL ampules

ACTIONS Direct-acting sympathomimetic amine pharmacologically related to phenylephrine. Acts almost exclusively on alpha-adrenergic receptors. Pressor action is due primarily to direct peripheral vasoconstriction, which in turn causes rise in arterial BP. Has no direct effect on heart. Markedly reduces renal blood flow. Tends to slow ventricular rate by vagal stimulation in response to elevated BP.

THERAPEUTIC EFFECTS Terminates episodes of paroxysmal supraventricular tachycardia. Large doses may produce bradycardia. CNS stimulating action. True tachyphylaxis not reported.

USES To support, restore, or maintain BP during anesthesia and to terminate some episodes of paroxysmal supraventricular tachycardia.

CONTRAINDICATIONS Severe coronary or cardiovascular disease; hypovolemia, in combination with local anesthetics for tissue infiltration; within 2 wk of MAO inhibitors; pregnancy (category C).
CAUTIOUS USE History of hypertension or hyperthyroidism; following use of ergot alkaloids; lactation. Safety and effectiveness in children are not established.

ROUTE & DOSAGE

Hypotension During Anesthesia
Child: **IM** 0.25 mg/kg **IV** 0.08 mg/kg
Adult: **IM** 5–20 mg **IV** 3–5 mg
Paroxysmal Supraventricular Tachycardia
Adult: **IM** 10–20 mg **IV** 5–15 mg over 3–5 min

STORAGE
Store at 15°–30° C (59°–86° F) in light-resistant containers.

ADMINISTRATION
Intramuscular
- Give supplemental IM, as needed, after emergency IV infusion.

Intravenous
PREPARE **Direct:** Give undiluted. **IV Infusion:** May be diluted in 250 mL D5W.
ADMINISTER **Direct:** Give at a rate of 5 mg/min if systolic BP is less than 60 mm Hg. **IV Infusion:** Give at rate needed to maintain BP.
- Be alert for extravasation. Antidote: Infiltrate area as soon as possible with 10–15 mL NS saline solution containing 5–10 mg phentolamine.
- Protect drug from light.

ADVERSE EFFECTS Body as a Whole: Paresthesias, feeling of coldness (particularly with high dosage), restlessness, nervousness. **CV:** High BP, bradycardia. **GI:** Projectile vomiting. **CNS:** Severe headache, pilomotor erection (gooseflesh). **Urogenital:** Urinary urgency.

INTERACTIONS Drug: Phentolamine and PHENOTHIAZINES block vasopressor response. BETA-BLOCKERS may increase amount of methoxamine available to receptor sites. **Atropine** blocks reflex bradycardia and enhances vasopressor effects. MAO INHIBITORS, **vasopressin,** and ERGOT ALKALOIDS may cause hypertensive crisis.

Common adverse effects in *italic;* life-threatening effects <u>underlined</u>; generic names in **bold;** drug classifications in SMALL CAPS; ♣ Canadian drug name; ⊘ Prototype drug.

805

PHARMACOKINETICS Onset: Immediately after IV. **Peak:** 0.5–2 min IV; 15–20 min IM. **Duration:** 5–15 min IV; 60–90 min IM. **Metabolism:** Unknown. **Elimination:** Unknown.

NURSING IMPLICATIONS

Assessment & Drug Effects

- Supervise patients closely.
- Monitor vital signs continuously. Report any increase in BP above level prescribed by physician; report slowing of HR.
- Be alert for sudden changes in BP and pulse after drug has been discontinued.
- Monitor I&O. Urinary frequency with retention is a possibility. Report oliguria or change in I&O ratio.
- Methoxamine injection contains a bisulfite, an allergen for some patients.

Patient & Family Education

- Report headache to physician; it may be severe. This adverse effect may require analgesia for relief.
- Report nausea to physician; it may be accompanied by projectile vomiting.

METHYCLOTHIAZIDE
(meth-i-kloe-thye′a-zide)
Aquatensen, Duretic ♣, Enduron, Ethon
Classifications: ELECTROLYTIC AND WATER BALANCE AGENT; THIAZIDE DIURETIC; ANTIHYPERTENSIVE AGENT
Prototype: Hydrochlorothiazide
Pregnancy Category: C

AVAILABILITY 2.5 mg, 5 mg tablets

ACTIONS Thiazide diuretic that is similar to hydrochlorothiazide. Diuretic effect results from a drug-induced inhibition of the renal tubular reabsorption of electrolytes. The excretion of sodium and chloride is enhanced. There is also a loss of potassium ions via the kidney.
THERAPEUTIC EFFECTS BP is lowered, probably by the loss of sodium and water, and consequently blood volume. Edema is also decreased in CHF patients by the same mechanism.

USES Antihypertensive treatment and adjunctively in the management of edema associated with CHF, renal pathology, and hepatic cirrhosis.

CONTRAINDICATIONS Hypersensitivity to thiazides, and sulfonamide derivatives; anuria, hypokalemia, pregnancy (category C), lactation.
CAUTIOUS USE Impaired kidney or liver function; gout; SLE; hypercalcemia; diabetes mellitus.

ROUTE & DOSAGE

Edema
Adult: **PO** 2.5–10 mg once daily or 3–5 times/wk

Common adverse effects in *italic;* life-threatening effects <u>underlined;</u> generic names in **bold;** drug classifications in SMALL CAPS; ♣ Canadian drug name; ❷ Prototype drug.

Hypertension
Child: **PO** 0.05–0.2 mg/kg/day
Adult: **PO** 2.5–10 mg/day

STORAGE
Store at 15°–30° C (59°–86° F) unless otherwise instructed.

ADMINISTRATION
Oral
- Give early in a.m. after eating (reduces gastric irritation) to prevent sleep interruption because of diuresis. If 2 doses are ordered, administer second dose no later than 3 p.m.

ADVERSE EFFECTS Body as a Whole: Postural hypotension, sialadenitis, unusual fatigue, dizziness, paresthesias. **Skin:** Photosensitivity. **Special Senses:** Yellow vision. **Metabolic:** *Hypokalemia.* **Hematologic:** <u>Agranulocytosis.</u>

INTERACTIONS Drug: Amphotericin B, CORTICOSTEROIDS increase hypokalemic effects; may antagonize hypoglycemic effects of **insulin,** SULFONYLUREAS; **cholestyramine, colestipol** decrease thiazide absorption; intensifies hypoglycemic and hypotensive effects of **diazoxide;** increased potassium and magnesium loss may cause **digoxin** toxicity; decreases **lithium** excretion, increasing its toxicity; NSAIDS may attenuate diuresis, and risk of NSAID-induced kidney failure increased.

PHARMACOKINETICS Absorption: Incompletely absorbed. **Onset:** 2 h. **Peak:** 6 h. **Duration:** >24 h. **Distribution:** Distributed throughout extracellular tissue; concentrates in kidney; crosses placenta; distributed in breast milk. **Metabolism:** Does not appear to be metabolized. **Elimination:** Excreted in urine.

NURSING IMPLICATIONS

Assessment & Drug Effects
- Expect antihypertensive effects in 3–4 days; maximal effects may require 3–4 wk.
- Monitor BP and I&O ratio during first phase of antihypertensive therapy. Report a sudden fall in BP, which may initiate severe postural hypotension and potentially dangerous perfusion problems, especially in the extremities.
- Lab tests: Periodic serum electrolytes and CBC with differential.
- Monitor patient for S&S of hypokalemia (see Appendix D-1). Report promptly. Physician may change dose and institute replacement therapy.

Patient & Family Education
- Eat a balanced diet to protect against hypokalemia; generally not severe even with long-term therapy. Prevent onset by eating potassium-rich foods including a banana (about 370 mg potassium) and at least 180 mL (6 oz) orange juice (about 330 mg potassium) every day.
- Watch carefully for loss of glycemic control (diabetics) and early signs of hyperglycemia (see Appendix D-1). Symptoms are slow to develop.

- Avoid OTC drugs unless the physician approves them. Many preparations contain both potassium and sodium, and may induce electrolyte imbalance adverse effects.
- Orthostatic hypotension may be a problem; change positions slowly and in stages from lying down to upright positions; avoid hot baths or showers, extended exposure to sunlight, and standing still. Accept assistance as necessary to prevent falling.
- Do not drive or engage in potentially hazardous activities until adjustment to the hypotensive effects of drug has been made.
- Do not breast feed while taking this drug.
- Store this medication out of reach of children.

METHYLDOPA 🄿
(meth-ill-doe′pa)
Aldomet, Apo-Methyldopa ♣ , Dopamet ♣ , Novomedopa ♣

METHYLDOPATE HYDROCHLORIDE
(meth-ill-doe′pate)
Aldomet

Classifications: CARDIOVASCULAR AGENT; CENTRAL-ACTING ANTIHYPERTENSIVE; AUTONOMIC NERVOUS SYSTEM AGENT; ALPHA-ADRENERGIC AGONIST (SYMPATHOMIMETIC)
Pregnancy Category: C

AVAILABILITY 125 mg, 250 mg, 500 mg tablets; 50 mg/mL oral suspension; 50 mg/mL injection

ACTIONS Structurally related to catecholamines and their precursors. Has weak neurotransmitter properties; inhibits decarboxylation of dopa, thereby reducing concentration of dopamine, a precursor of norepinephrine. It also inhibits the precursor of serotonin.

THERAPEUTIC EFFECTS Lowers standing and supine BP, and unlike adrenergic blockers, is not so prone to produce orthostatic hypotension, diurnal BP variations, or exercise hypertension. Reduces renal vascular resistance; maintains cardiac output without acceleration, but may slow heart rate; tends to support sodium and water retention.

USES Treatment of sustained moderate to severe hypertension, particularly in patients with kidney dysfunction. Also used in selected patients with carcinoid disease. Parenteral form has been used for treatment of hypertensive crises but is not preferred because of its slow onset of action.

CONTRAINDICATIONS Active liver disease (hepatitis, cirrhosis); pheochromocytoma; blood dyscrasias. Safety during pregnancy (category C) is not established.

CAUTIOUS USE History of impaired liver or kidney function or disease angina pectoris; history of mental depression; lactation; young patients.

ROUTE & DOSAGE

Hypertension

Child: **PO** Initial dose 10 mg/kg/day in 2–4 equally divided doses; then every 2 days increase dose as need to (max dose 65 mg/kg/day or up to 3 g/day, whichever is less) **IV** Initial dose 2–4 mg/kg/dose then in 4–6 h increase dose to 5–10 mg/kg/dose every 6–8 h (max dose 65 mg/kg/day or 3 g/day, whichever is less)
Adult: **PO** 250 mg b.i.d. or t.i.d., may be increased up to 3 g/day in divided doses **IV** 250–500 mg q6h, may be increased up to 1 g q6h

STORAGE

Store at 15°–30° C (59°–86° F) in tightly closed, light-resistant containers. Store injectable form at <30° C and avoid freezing.

ADMINISTRATION

Oral

- Can give without regard to meals. Make dosage increases in evening to minimize daytime sedation. Some patients maintain adequate BP control with a single evening dose.

Intravenous

PREPARE **Intermittent:** Dilute in 100–200 mL of D5W, as needed, to yield 10 mg/mL
ADMINISTER **Intermittent:** Give over 30–60 min at a concentration of ≤10 mg/mL.
INCOMPATIBILITIES **Solution/Additive:** Poorly soluble in acidic media. **Amphotericin B, methohexital, verapamil. Y-Site: Fat emulsion.**

ADVERSE EFFECTS Body as a Whole: Hypersensitivity (*fever,* skin eruptions, ulcerations of soles of feet, flu-like symptoms, lymphadenopathy, eosinophilia). **CNS:** *Sedation, drowsiness,* sluggishness, headache, weakness, fatigue, dizziness, vertigo, *decrease in mental acuity,* inability to concentrate, amnesia-like syndrome, parkinsonism, mild psychoses, depression, nightmares. **CV:** Orthostatic hypotension, syncope, bradycardia, myocarditis, edema, weight gain *(sodium and water retention),* paradoxic hypertensive reaction (especially with IV administration). **GI:** Diarrhea, constipation, abdominal distension, malabsorption syndrome, nausea, vomiting, dry mouth, sore or black tongue, sialadenitis, abnormal liver function tests, jaundice, hepatitis, <u>hepatic necrosis</u> (rare). **Hematologic:** *Positive direct Coombs' test* (common especially in African-Americans), <u>granulocytopenia</u>. **Special Senses:** *Nasal stuffiness.* **Endocrine:** Gynecomastia, lactation, *decreased libido, impotence,* hypothermia (large doses), positive tests for lupus and rheumatoid factors. **Skin:** Granulomatous skin lesions.

DIAGNOSTIC TEST INTERFERENCE Methyldopa may interfere with *serum creatinine* measurements using *alkaline picrate method, AST* by *colorimetric methods,* and *uric acid* measurements by *phosphotungstate method* (with high methyldopa blood levels); it may produce false elevations of *urinary catecholamines* and increase in *serum amylase* in methyldopa-induced sialadenitis.

Common adverse effects in *italic;* life-threatening effects <u>underlined</u>; generic names in **bold**; drug classifications in SMALL CAPS; ♣ Canadian drug name; ☢ Prototype drug.

809

INTERACTIONS Drug: AMPHETAMINES, TRICYCLIC ANTIDEPRESSANTS, PHENO-THIAZINES may attenuate antihypertensive response; methyldopa may inhibit effectiveness of **ephedrine; haloperidol** may exacerbate psychiatric symptoms; with **levodopa,** additive hypotension, increased CNS toxicity, especially psychosis; increases risk of **lithium** toxicity; **methotrimeprazine** causes excessive hypotension; MAO INHIBITORS may cause hallucinations; oral iron preparations may decrease absorption of ORAL methyldopa; **phenoxybenzamine** may cause urinary incontinence. **Food:** Sodium and water retention and potassium loss occur when given with licorice.

PHARMACOKINETICS Absorption: About 50% absorbed from GI tract. **Peak:** 4–6 h. **Duration:** 24 h PO; 10–16 h IV. **Distribution:** Crosses placenta, distributed into breast milk. **Metabolism:** Metabolized in liver and GI tract. **Elimination:** Excreted primarily in urine. **Half-Life:** 1.7 h.

NURSING IMPLICATIONS

Assessment & Drug Effects
- Check BP and pulse at least q30 min until stabilized during IV infusion and observe for adequacy of urinary output.
- Take BP at regular intervals in lying, sitting, and standing positions during period of dosage adjustment.
- Be aware that transient sedation, drowsiness, mental depression, weakness, and headache commonly occur during first 24–72 h of therapy or whenever dosage is increased. Symptoms tend to disappear with continuation of therapy or dosage reduction.
- Supervision of ambulation in patients with impaired kidney function; both are particularly likely to manifest orthostatic hypotension with dizziness and light-headedness during period of dosage adjustment.
- Monitor fluid and electrolyte balance and I&O. Report oliguria and changes in I&O ratio. Weigh patient daily, and check for edema because methyldopa favors sodium and water retention.
- Lab tests: Schedule baseline and periodic blood counts and liver function tests especially during first 6–12 wk of therapy or if patient develops unexplained fever; periodic serum electrolytes.
- Be alert to and report symptoms of mental depression (e.g., anorexia, insomnia, inattention to personal hygiene, withdrawal). Drug-induced depression may persist after drug is withdrawn.
- Be alert that rising BP indicating tolerance to drug effect may occur during week 2 or 3 of therapy.

Patient & Family Education
- Exercise caution with hot baths and showers, prolonged standing in one position, and strenuous exercise that may enhance orthostatic hypotension. Make position changes slowly, particularly from lying down to upright posture; dangle legs a few minutes before standing.
- Avoid potentially hazardous tasks such as driving, biking, skateboarding, and sports until response to drug is known; drug may affect ability to perform activities requiring concentrated mental effort, especially during first few days of therapy or whenever dosage is increased.
- Do not ingest alcohol because it may potentiate sedation.

Common adverse effects in *italic;* life-threatening effects <u>underlined</u>; generic names in **bold**; drug classifications in SMALL CAPS; ♣ Canadian drug name; ⊘ Prototype drug.

- Do not to take OTC medications unless approved by physician.
- May cause urine to turn red to reddish brown color.
- Do not breast feed while taking this drug without consulting prescriber.
- Store this medication out of reach of children.

METHYLPHENIDATE HYDROCHLORIDE
(meth-ill-fen′i-date)
Concerta, Metadate CD, Metadate ER, Ritalin, Ritalin LA, Ritalin SR
Classifications: CENTRAL NERVOUS SYSTEM AGENT; CEREBRAL STIMULANT
Prototype: Amphetamine
Pregnancy Category: C
Controlled Substance: Schedule II

AVAILABILITY 5 mg, 10 mg, 20 mg tablets; 20 mg, 30 mg, 40 mg sustained-release capsules; 18 mg, 27 mg, 36 mg, 54 mg sustained-release tablets

ACTIONS Piperidine derivative with actions and abuse potential qualitatively similar to those of amphetamine. Acts mainly on cerebral cortex exerting a stimulant effect.
THERAPEUTIC EFFECTS Results in mild CNS and respiratory stimulation with potency intermediate between amphetamine and caffeine. More prominent on mental than on motor activities. Also believed to have an anorexiant effect.

USES Adjunctive therapy in hyperkinetic syndromes characterized by attention deficit disorder, narcolepsy, mild depression, and apathetic or withdrawn senile behavior.

CONTRAINDICATIONS Hypersensitivity to drug; history of marked anxiety, agitation; motor tics or Tourette's disease, within 14 days of MAO inhibitors. Safety in pregnancy (category C), lactation, or in children <6 y of age is not established.
CAUTIOUS USE Alcoholic; emotionally unstable patient; history of drug dependence; hypertension; history of seizures.

ROUTE & DOSAGE

Attention Deficit Disorder
Child: **PO** ≥6 y **Immediate-Release Tablets:** Initial 0.3 mg/dose or 2.5–5 mg/dose before breakfast and lunch, with a gradual increase of 0.1 mg/dose or by 5–10 mg/day weekly as needed (max dose 2 mg/kg/day or 60 mg/day) (some children may need an extra p.m. dose); **Sustained Release** (8-h duration) can be utilized after stabilizing dose is established with immediate release tablets. These tablets are substituted to the nearest equivalent total daily dosage and taken once a day. (Thus, if taking 20 mg twice daily, dosage would be 40 mg/daily); sustained release given daily before breakfast (max dose 60 mg/day); **Concerta** Initial 18 mg q.a.m. before breakfast, increased at weekly intervals by 18 mg increments (max dose 54 mg/day)

Common adverse effects in *italic;* life-threatening effects underlined; generic names in **bold;** drug classifications in SMALL CAPS; ♦ Canadian drug name; ❂ Prototype drug.

811

Narcolepsy

Adult: **PO** 10 mg b.i.d. or t.i.d. 30–45 min after meals (range: 20–40 mg/day)

STORAGE

Store at 15°–30° C (59°–86° F) in tightly closed, light-resistant containers.

ADMINISTRATION

Oral

- Give 30–45 min before meals. Immediate release given on empty stomach with water. Concerta and Metadate given with water, milk, or juice. Ritalin LA may be given without regard to food. To avoid insomnia, give last dose before 4 p.m.
- Ensure that sustained-release form is not chewed or crushed. It must be swallowed whole.
- Can open Metadate CD capsules or Ritalin LA capsules and sprinkle on cold food and take immediately.

ADVERSE EFFECTS CNS: Dizziness, drowsiness, *nervousness, insomnia.* **CV:** Palpitations, changes in BP and pulse rate, angina, cardiac arrhythmias. **Special Senses:** Difficulty with accommodation, blurred vision. **GI:** Dry throat, anorexia, nausea, <u>hepatotoxicity</u>, abdominal pain. **Body as a Whole:** Hypersensitivity reactions (rash, fever, arthralgia, urticaria, <u>exfoliative dermatitis</u>, erythema multiforme); growth suppression.

INTERACTIONS Drug: MAO INHIBITORS may cause hypertensive crisis; antagonizes hypotensive effects of **guanethidine, bretylium;** potentiates action of CNS STIMULANTS (e.g., **amphetamine, caffeine**); may inhibit metabolism and increase serum levels of **fosphenytoin, phenytoin, phenobarbital,** and **primidone, warfarin,** TRICYCLIC ANTIDEPRESSANTS. **Herb:** St. John's wort may cause serious side effects to be increased. **Food:** May increase oral absorption. High-fat meals delay absorption of Ritalin LA.

PHARMACOKINETICS Absorption: Readily absorbed from GI tract. **Peak:** 1.9 h; 4–7 h sustained release. **Duration:** 3–6 h; 8 h sustained release. **Elimination:** Excreted in urine. **Half-Life:** 2–4 h.

NURSING IMPLICATIONS

Assessment & Drug Effects

- Monitor BP and pulse monthly or with each well child visit.
- Lab tests: Obtain periodic CBC with differential and platelet counts during prolonged therapy.
- Chronic abusive use can lead to tolerance, psychic dependence, and psychoses.
- Assess patient's condition with periodic drug-free periods during prolonged therapy.
- Supervise drug withdrawal carefully following prolonged use. Abrupt withdrawal may result in severe depression and psychotic behavior.
- Drug is usually discontinued if no improvement seen in 1 mo.

Patient & Family Education

- Report adverse effects to prescriber, particularly nervousness and insomnia. These effects may diminish with time or require reduction of dosage or omission of afternoon or evening dose.
- Check weight weekly and report weight loss. Check height and weight in children; failure to gain in either should be reported to prescriber.
- Concerta tablet shell is usually expelled in the stool.
- Work with school personnel to ensure safe administration at school if dose is taken there.
- Do not breast feed while taking this drug without consulting prescriber.
- Store this medication in locked area out of reach of children; this is a Schedule II drug.

METHYLPREDNISOLONE
(meth-ill-pred-niss'oh-lone)

Medrol

METHYLPREDNISOLONE ACETATE

Depoject, Depo-Medrol, Depopred, Duralone, M-Prednisol, Rep-Pred

METHYLPREDNISOLONE SODIUM SUCCINATE

A-Methapred, Solu-Medrol

Classifications: HORMONE AND SYNTHETIC SUBSTITUTE; ADRENAL CORTICOSTEROID; GLUCOCORTICOID; ANTI-INFLAMMATORY

Prototype: Prednisone

Pregnancy Category: C

AVAILABILITY Methylprednisolone 2 mg, 4 mg, 8 mg, 16 mg, 24 mg, 32 mg tablets **Methylprednisolone Acetate** 20 mg/mL, 40 mg/mL, 80 mg/mL injection **Methylprednisolone Sodium Succinate** 40 mg, 125 mg, 500 mg, 1 g, 2 g powder for injection

ACTIONS Intermediate-acting synthetic adrenal corticosteroid with similar glucocorticoid activity; has considerably fewer sodium and water retention effects than hydrocortisone. Acetate has longer duration of action and more rapid onset of activity than parent compound. Sodium succinate form is characterized by rapid onset of action and is used for emergency therapy of short duration. It inhibits phagocytosis and release of allergic substances. Also modifies the immune response of the body to various stimuli.

THERAPEUTIC EFFECTS Anti-inflammatory and immunosuppressive properties.

USES An anti-inflammatory agent in the management of acute and chronic inflammatory diseases, for palliative management of neoplastic diseases, and for control of severe acute and chronic allergic processes. High-dose, short-term therapy: Management of acute bronchial asthma, prevention of fat embolism in patient with long bone fracture.

UNLABELED USES Acetate form used as a long-acting contraceptive and for spinal cord injury, lupus nephritis, multiple sclerosis.

CONTRAINDICATIONS Systemic fungal infections, live vaccine administration. Safety during pregnancy (category C) or lactation is not established.

CAUTIOUS USE Cushing's syndrome; GI ulceration; hypertension; varicella, vaccinia; diabetes mellitus; emotional instability or psychotic tendencies.

ROUTE & DOSAGE

Inflammation

Child: **PO/IM/IV** 0.5–1.7 mg/kg/day divided q6–12h
Adult: **PO** 2–60 mg/day in 1 or more divided doses **IM** (Acetate) 4–80 mg/wk for 1–4 wk; (Succinate) 10–250 mg q6h
IV 10–250 mg q6h

Status Asthmaticus

Child: **IM/IV** *Loading dose* 2 mg/kg/dose times one then 0.5–2 mg/kg/day q6h

Acute Spinal Cord Injury

Child/Adult: **IV** 30 mg/kg over 15 min, followed in 45 min by 5.4 mg/kg/h times 23 h

STORAGE
Store at 15°–30° C (59°–86° F). Do not freeze.

ADMINISTRATION

Oral

- Crush tablet before and give with fluid of patient's choice.
- Note: Preparation less irritating if given with food. Do not give with grapefruit juice.
- Use alternate day therapy when given over long period.

Intramuscular

- Give injection deep into large muscle (not deltoid). See Part I for safe IM site selection in children.

Intravenous

Note: Do not use methylprednisolone acetate for IV.
PREPARE **Direct/Intermittent:** Available in ACT-O-Vial from which the desired dose may be withdrawn after initial dilution with supplied diluent. May be further diluted according to prescribers orders.
ADMINISTER **Direct/Intermittent:** Give each 500 mg or fraction thereof over 2–3 min in adults. Children maximum concentration for low doses is 125 mg/mL given over 3–15 min and intermittent 2.5 mg/mL.
INCOMPATIBILITIES **Solution/Additive: Dextrose 5%/sodium chloride 0.45%, calcium gluconate, glycopyrrolate, metaraminol, nafcillin, penicillin G sodium, doxapram. Y-Site: Allopurinol, amsacrine, ciprofloxacin, cisatracurium (≥2 mg/mL concentration), diltiazem, etoposide, filgrastim, gemcitabine, ondansetron, paclitaxel, potassium chloride, propofol, sargramostim, vinorelbine.**

Common adverse effects in *italic;* life-threatening effects <u>underlined</u>; generic names in **bold;** drug classifications in SMALL CAPS; ♣ Canadian drug name; ● Prototype drug.

ADVERSE EFFECTS CNS: Euphoria, headache, insomnia, confusion, psychosis. **CV:** CHF, edema. **GI:** Nausea, vomiting, peptic ulcer. **Musculoskeletal:** Muscle weakness, delayed wound healing, muscle wasting, osteoporosis, aseptic necrosis of bone, spontaneous fractures. **Endocrine:** Cushingoid features, growth suppression in children, carbohydrate intolerance, hyperglycemia. **Special Senses:** Cataracts. **Hematologic:** Leukocytosis. **Metabolic:** Hypokalemia.

INTERACTIONS Drug: Amphotericin B, furosemide, THIAZIDE DIURETICS increase potassium loss; with ATTENUATED VIRUS VACCINES, may enhance virus replication or increase vaccine adverse effects; **isoniazid, phenytoin, phenobarbital, rifampin** decrease effectiveness of methylprednisolone because they increase metabolism of STEROIDS. **Food:** Grapefruit juice increases bioavailability of oral form of drug.

PHARMACOKINETICS Absorption: Readily absorbed from GI tract. **Peak:** 1–2 h PO; 4–8 day IM. **Duration:** 1.25–1.5 day PO; 1–5 wk IM. **Metabolism:** Metabolized in liver. **Half-Life:** >3.5 h; HPA suppression: 18–36 h.

NURSING IMPLICATIONS

Assessment & Drug Effects

- Lab tests: Monitor periodically kidney and liver function, thyroid function, CBC, serum electrolytes, weight, and total cholesterol.
- Monitor diabetics for loss of glycemic control.
- Monitor serum potassium and report S&S of hypokalemia (see Appendix D-1).
- Monitor for and report S&S of Cushing's syndrome (see Appendix D-1).

Patient & Family Education

- Consult prescriber for any of the following: Slow wound healing, significant insomnia or confusion, or unexplained bone pain.
- Do not alter established dosage regimen (i.e., not to stop, increase, decrease, or omit doses or change dose intervals). Withdrawal symptoms (rebound inflammation, fever) can be induced with sudden discontinuation of therapy.
- Report onset of signs of hypocorticism adrenal insufficiency immediately: Fatigue, nausea, anorexia, joint pain, muscular weakness, dizziness, fever.
- Do not breast feed while taking this drug without consulting physician.
- Store this medication out of reach of children.

METOCLOPRAMIDE HYDROCHLORIDE ℗

(met-oh-kloe-pra′mide)

Clopra, Emex ♣, Maxeran ♣, Maxolon, Reglan

Classifications: GASTROINTESTINAL AGENT; PROKINETIC AGENT (GI STIMULANT); AUTONOMIC NERVOUS SYSTEM AGENT; DIRECT-ACTING CHOLINERGIC (PARASYMPATHOMIMETIC); ANTIEMETIC

Pregnancy Category: B

Common adverse effects in *italic;* life-threatening effects underlined; generic names in **bold;** drug classifications in SMALL CAPS; ♣ Canadian drug name; ℗ Prototype drug.

AVAILABILITY 5 mg, 10 mg tablets; 5 mg/5 mL solution (sugar free); 5 mg/mL injection

ACTIONS Potent central dopamine receptor antagonist. Structurally related to procainamide but has little antiarrhythmic or anesthetic activity. Exact mechanism of action not clear but appears to sensitize GI smooth muscle to effects of acetylcholine by direct action.

THERAPEUTIC EFFECTS Increases resting tone of esophageal sphincter, and tone and amplitude of upper GI contractions. As a result, gastric emptying and intestinal transit are accelerated with little effect, if any, on gastric, biliary, or pancreatic secretions. Antiemetic action results from drug-induced elevation of CTZ threshold and enhanced gastric emptying. In diabetic gastroparesis, indicated by relief of anorexia, nausea, vomiting, persistent fullness after meals.

USES Management of diabetic gastric stasis (gastroparesis); to prevent nausea and vomiting associated with emetogenic cancer chemotherapy (e.g., cisplatin, dacarbazine); to facilitate intubation of small bowel; symptomatic treatment of gastroesophageal reflux.

CONTRAINDICATIONS Sensitivity or intolerance to metoclopramide; allergy to sulfiting agents; history of seizure disorders; concurrent use of drugs that can cause extrapyramidal symptoms; pheochromocytoma; mechanical GI obstruction or perforation; history of breast cancer. Safety during pregnancy (category B) or lactation is not established.

CAUTIOUS USE CHF; hypokalemia; kidney dysfunction; GI hemorrhage; history of intermittent porphyria.

ROUTE & DOSAGE

Gastroesophageal Reflux
Neonates/Infant/Child: **PO/IV/IM** 0.4–0.8 mg/kg/day in 4 equally divided doses (max dose 0.8 mg/kg/day)
Adult: **PO** 10–15 mg q.i.d. before meals and bedtime

Diabetic Gastroparesis
Adult: **PO** 10 mg q.i.d. before meals and bedtime for 2–8 wk

Small-Bowel Intubation
Child: **IM/IV** <6 y, 0.1 mg/kg administered over 1–2 min; 6–14 y, 2.5–5 mg administered over 1–2 min
Child/Adult: >14 y: **IM/IV** 10 mg administered over 1–2 min

Chemotherapy-Induced Emesis
Child/Adult: **PO** 1–2 mg/kg/dose 1 h before antineoplastic administration, may repeat q2h for 3 more doses if needed **IM/IV** 1–2 mg/kg/dose 30 min before antineoplastic administration, may repeat q2h for 2 doses, then q3h for 3 doses if needed. Medicating prior to treatment with diphenhydramine decreases extrapyramidal reactions. Reduce dosages with renal impairment.

STORAGE
Store at 15°–30° C (59°–86° F) in light-resistant bottle. Tablets are stable for 3 y; solutions and injections for 5 y. Discard open ampules; do not store for future use.

ADMINISTRATION

Oral

- Give 30 min before meals and at bedtime.

Intravenous

Note: Verify correct IV concentration and rate of infusion for administration to infants or children with physician.

PREPARE Direct: Doses of 10 mg or less may be given undiluted. **IV Infusion:** Doses >10 mg IV should be diluted in at least 50 mL of D5W, NS, D5/0.45% NaCl, RL or other compatible solution.

ADMINISTER Direct: Give over 1–2 min in adults; do not give push with children. **IV Infusion:** Give over 15 min. Note: In children dilute to 0.2 mg/mL (maximum 5 mg/mL) and infuse over 15–30 min. Bags of metoclopramide should be protected from light during IV infusion (use of aluminum foil or a thick cotton cover).

INCOMPATIBILITIES Solution/Additive: Ampicillin, calcium gluconate, cephalothin, chloramphenicol, cisplatin, erythromycin, floxacillin, fluorouracil, furosemide, methotrexate, penicillin G potassium, sodium bicarbonate, TETRACYCLINES, **Y-Site: Allopurinol, amphotericin B cholesteryl complex, amsacrine, cefepime, doxorubicin liposome, furosemide, propofol.**

M

ADVERSE EFFECTS CNS: *Mild sedation, fatigue, restlessness,* agitation, headache, insomnia, disorientation, *extrapyramidal symptoms* (acute dystonic type): **GI:** Nausea, constipation, *diarrhea,* dry mouth, altered drug absorption. **Skin:** Urticarial or maculopapular rash. **Body as a Whole:** Glossal or periorbital edema. **Hematologic:** Methemoglobinemia. **Endocrine:** Galactorrhea, gynecomastia, amenorrhea, impotence. **CV:** <u>Hypertensive crisis</u> (rare).

DIAGNOSTIC TEST INTERFERENCE Metoclopramide may interfere with gonadorelin test by increasing *serum prolactin* levels.

INTERACTIONS Drug: Alcohol and other CNS DEPRESSANTS add to sedation; ANTICHOLINERGICS, OPIATE ANALGESICS may antagonize effect on GI motility; PHENOTHIAZINES may potentiate extrapyramidal symptoms; may decrease absorption of **acetaminophen, aspirin, atovaquone, cimetidine, diazepam, digoxin, lithium, tetracycline;** may antagonize the effects of **amantadine, bromocriptine, levodopa, pergolide, ropinirole, pramipexole;** may cause increase in extrapyramidal and dystonic reactions with PHENOTHIAZINES, THIOXANTHENES, **droperidol, haloperidol, loxapine, metyrosine;** may prolong neuromuscular blocking effects of **succinylcholine.**

PHARMACOKINETICS Absorption: Readily absorbed from GI tract. **Onset:** 30–60 min PO; 10–15 min IM; 1–3 min IV. **Peak:** 1–2 h. **Duration:** 1–3 h. **Distribution:** Distributed to most body tissues including CNS; crosses placenta; distributed into breast milk. **Metabolism:** Minimally metabolized in liver. **Elimination:** 95% excreted in urine, 5% in feces. **Half-Life:** 2.5–6 h.

NURSING IMPLICATIONS

Assessment & Drug Effects

▪ Report immediately the onset of restlessness, involuntary movements, facial grimacing, rigidity, or tremors. Extrapyramidal symptoms are most likely to occur in children and young adults, with high-dose treatment of vomiting associated with cancer chemotherapy. Symptoms usually appear within 24–48 h of initiation of therapy. Symptoms can take months to regress.

▪ Be aware that during early treatment period, serum aldosterone may be elevated; after prolonged administration periods, it returns to pretreatment level.

▪ Lab tests: Periodic serum electrolyte.

▪ Monitor for possible hypernatremia and hypokalemia (see Appendix D-1), especially if patient has CHF or cirrhosis.

▪ Adverse reactions associated with increased serum prolactin concentration (galactorrhea, menstrual disorders, gynecomastia) usually disappear within a few weeks or months after drug treatment is stopped.

Patient & Family Education

▪ Avoid driving and other potentially hazardous activities (biking, skateboarding, and sports) for a few hours after drug administration.

▪ Avoid alcohol and other CNS depressants.

▪ Report S&S of acute dystonia, such as trembling hands and facial grimacing, (see Appendix D-1) immediately.

▪ Do not breast feed while taking this drug without consulting prescriber.

▪ Store this medication out of reach of children.

METOLAZONE

(me-tole′a-zone)

Diulo, Mykrox, Zaroxolyn

Classifications: ELECTROLYTIC AND WATER BALANCE AGENT; THIAZIDE-LIKE DIURETIC; ANTIHYPERTENSIVE

Prototype: Hydrochlorothiazide

Pregnancy Category: D

AVAILABILITY 0.5 mg, 2.5 mg, 5 mg, 10 mg tablets

ACTIONS Diuretic structurally and pharmacologically similar to hydrochlorothiazide. Diuretic action is associated with drug interference with transport of sodium ions across renal tubular epithelium. This enhances excretion of sodium, chloride, potassium, bicarbonate, and water. **THERAPEUTIC EFFECTS** Produces a decrease in the systolic and diastolic BPs, and reduces edema in CHF and kidney failure patients. Appears to be more effective as a diuretic than thiazides in patients with severe kidney failure.

USES Management of hypertension as sole agent or to enhance effectiveness of other antihypertensives in severe form of hypertension; also edema associated with CHF and kidney disease.

CONTRAINDICATIONS Anuria, hypokalemia; hepatic coma or precoma; hypersensitivity to metolazone and sulfonamides; pregnancy (category D), lactation.

CAUTIOUS USE History of gout; allergies; concomitant use of digitalis glycosides; kidney and liver dysfunction.

ROUTE & DOSAGE

Edema
Child: **PO** 0.2–0.4 mg/kg/day in equally divided q12–24h
Adult: **PO** 5–20 mg/day

Hypertension
Adult: **PO** 2.5–5 mg/day; (Mykrox) 0.5–1 mg/day

STORAGE
Store at 15°–30° C (59°–86° F) in tightly closed container.

ADMINISTRATION

Oral
- Do not interchange slow availability tablets and rapid availability tablets. They are not equivalent.
- Schedule doses to avoid nocturia and interrupted sleep. Give early in a.m. after eating to prevent gastric irritation (if given in 2 doses, schedule second dose no later than 3 p.m.).

ADVERSE EFFECTS GI: Cholestatic jaundice, **Body as a Whole:** Vertigo, orthostatic hypotension. **Hematologic:** Venous thrombosis, leukopenia. **Metabolic:** Dehydration, *hypokalemia, hyperuricemia, hyperglycemia.*

INTERACTIONS Drug: Amphotericin B, CORTICOSTEROIDS increase hypokalemic effects; may antagonize hypoglycemic effects of SULFONYLUREAS, **insulin; cholestyramine, colestipol** decrease thiazide absorption; intensifies hypoglycemic and hypotensive effects of **diazoxide;** because of increased **potassium** and **magnesium** loss, may cause **digoxin** toxicity; decreases **lithium** excretion, increasing its toxicity; NSAIDS may attenuate diuresis—increased risk of NSAID-induced kidney failure. **Food:** Licorice increases sodium and water retention and potassium loss.

PHARMACOKINETICS Absorption: Incompletely absorbed; Mykrox has greater absorption. **Onset:** 1 h. **Peak:** 2–8 h. **Duration:** 12–24 h. **Distribution:** Distributed throughout extracellular tissue; concentrates in kidney; crosses placenta; distributed in breast milk. **Metabolism:** Does not appear to be metabolized. **Elimination:** Excreted in urine. **Half-Life:** 14 h.

NURSING IMPLICATIONS

Assessment & Drug Effects
- Terminate therapy when adverse reactions are moderate to severe.
- Expect possible antihypertensive effects in 3 or 4 days, but 3–4 wks are required for maximum effect.

M

- Lab tests: Determine serum potassium at regular intervals. Prolonged treatment and inadequate potassium intake increase potential for hypokalemia (see Appendix D-1). Periodic plasma glucose and urinalysis determinations.

Patient & Family Education

- Do not drink alcohol; it potentiates orthostatic hypotension. Can cause dry mouth.
- Antihypertensive therapy may require as adjunct a high-potassium, low-sodium, and low-calorie diet.
- Include potassium-rich foods in the diet.
- Be aware that if hypokalemia develops, dietary potassium supplement of 1000–2000 mg (25–50 mEq) is usually adequate treatment.
- Do not breast feed while taking this drug.
- Store this medication out of reach of children.

METRONIDAZOLE ❻
(me-troe-ni′da-zole)
Flagyl, Flagyl ER, Flagyl IV RTU, Flagyl 375, Metizol, Metric 21, Metro I.V., MetroGel, MetroGel Vaginal, MetroLotion, Noritate, Protostat
Classifications: ANTI-INFECTIVE; ANTITRICHOMONAL; AMEBICIDE; ANTIBIOTIC
Pregnancy Category: B

AVAILABILITY 250 mg, 500 mg tablets; 375 mg capsules; 750 mg sustained-release tablets; 5 mg/mL injection; 0.75% lotion; 1% cream; 0.75% gel

ACTIONS Synthetic compound with direct trichomonacidal and amebicidal activity as well as antibacterial activity against anaerobic bacteria and some gram-negative bacteria.
THERAPEUTIC EFFECTS Effective against *Trichomonas vaginalis, Entamoeba histolytica,* and *Giardia lamblia.* Exhibits antibacterial activity against obligate anaerobic bacteria, gram-negative anaerobic bacilli, and *Clostridia.* Microaerophilic *Streptococci* and most aerobic bacteria are resistant.

USES Asymptomatic and symptomatic trichomoniasis in females and males; acute intestinal amebiasis and amebic liver abscess; preoperative prophylaxis in colorectal surgery, elective hysterectomy or vaginal repair, and emergency appendectomy. IV metronidazole is used for the treatment of serious infections caused by susceptible anaerobic bacteria in intra-abdominal infections, skin infections, gynecologic infections, septicemia, and for both pre- and postoperative prophylaxis, bacterial vaginosis. **Topical:** Rosacea.
UNLABELED USES Treatment of pseudomembranous colitis, Crohn's disease, *H. pylori* eradication.

CONTRAINDICATIONS Blood dyscrasias; active CNS disease; first trimester of pregnancy (category B), lactation.

CAUTIOUS USE Coexistent candidiasis; second and third trimesters of pregnancy (category B); alcoholism; liver disease.

ROUTE & DOSAGE

Trichomoniasis, Giardiasis, *Gardnerella*

Child: **PO** 15 mg/kg/day in equally 3 divided doses for 7–10 days
Adult: **PO** 2 g once or 250 mg t.i.d.; 375 mg b.i.d. or 500 mg b.i.d. for 7 days **Vaginal** Apply once or twice daily times 5 days

Amebiasis

Infant/Child: **PO** 35–50 mg/kg/day in 3 equally divided doses for 10 days
Adult: **PO** 500–750 mg t.i.d. for 10 days

Anaerobic Infections

Neonate: **PO/IV** *<7 days, <1.2 kg,* 7.5 mg/kg every 48 h; *1.2–2 kg,* 7.5 mg/kg every 24 h; *≥2 kg,* 15 mg/kg/day in 2 equally divided doses every 12 h; *≥7 days, <1.2 kg,* 7.5 mg/kg every 48 h; *1.2–2 kg,* 15 mg/kg/day in 2 equally divided doses every 12 h; *≥2 kg,* 30 mg/kg/day in 2 equally divided doses every 12 h
Child: **PO/IV** 30 mg/kg/day divided q6h (max 4 g/day)
Adult: **PO** 7.5 mg/kg q6h (max 4 g/day) **IV Loading Dose** 15 mg/kg **IV Maintenance Dose** 7.5 mg/kg q6h (max 4 g/day)

Pseudomembranous Colitis

Child: **PO** 30 mg/kg/day in equally divided dose q6h times 7 days
Adult: **PO** 250–500 mg t.i.d. **IV** 250–500 mg t.i.d. or q.i.d.

Bacterial Vaginosis

Adult: **PO** (Flagyl ER) 750 mg daily times 7 days

Rosacea

Adult: **Topical** Apply thin film to affected area b.i.d.
Reduce dosages required with renal impairment.

STORAGE

Store at 15°–30° C (59°–86° F); protect from light. Reconstituted Flagyl I.V. is chemically stable for 96 h when stored below 30° C (86° F) in room light. Diluted and neutralized IV solutions containing Flagyl I.V. should be used within 24 h of mixing.

ADMINISTRATION

Oral

- Crush tablets before ingestion if patient cannot swallow whole.
- Ensure that Flagyl ER (extendrelease form) is not chewed or crushed. It must be swallowed whole. Give on an empty stomach, 1 h before or 2 h after meals.
- Give immediately before, with, or immediately after meals or with food or milk to reduce GI distress.
- Give lower than normal doses in presence of liver disease.

Intravenous

Note: Verify correct IV concentration and rate of infusion for administration to neonates, infants, or children with physician.

PREPARE **Intermittent:** Sequence for preparing solution (important) consists of (1) reconstitution with 4.4 mL sterile water or NS, (2) dilution in IV solution to yield 8 mg/mL in NS, D5W, or RL, (3) pH neutralization with approximately 5 mEq sodium bicarbonate injection for each 500 mg of Flagyl I.V. used. Avoid use of aluminum-containing equipment when manipulating IV product (including syringes equipped with aluminum needles or hubs). Note: Flagyl IV RTU does not require mixing, diluting, or neutralizing. Each container contains 14 mEq of sodium.

ADMINISTER **Intermittent:** Give IV solution slowly at a rate of one dose per hour. In children maximum infusion concentrations 5–8 mg/mL given over at least 30–60 min.

INCOMPATIBILITIES **Solution/Additive:** TPN, **amoxicillin/clavulanate, aztreonam, dopamine, meropenem. Y-Site: Amphotericin B cholesteryl complex, aztreonam, filgrastim, meropenem, warfarin.**

- Note: Precipitation occurs if neutralized solution is refrigerated. Use diluted and neutralized solution within 24 h of preparation.

ADVERSE EFFECTS Body as a Whole: Hypersensitivity (rash, urticaria, pruritus, flushing), fever, fleeting joint pains, overgrowth of *Candida*. **CNS:** Vertigo, headache, ataxia, confusion, irritability, depression, restlessness, weakness, fatigue, drowsiness, insomnia, paresthesias, sensory neuropathy (rare). **GI:** *Nausea,* vomiting, anorexia, epigastric distress, abdominal cramps, diarrhea, constipation, dry mouth, metallic or bitter taste, proctitis. **Urogenital:** Polyuria, dysuria, pyuria, incontinence, cystitis, decreased libido, dyspareunia, dryness of vagina and vulva, sense of pelvic pressure. **Special Senses:** Nasal congestion. **CV:** ECG changes (flattening of T wave).

DIAGNOSTIC TEST INTERFERENCE Metronidazole may interfere with certain chemical analyses for *AST,* resulting in decreased values.

INTERACTIONS Drug: ORAL ANTICOAGULANTS potentiate hypoprothrombinemia; **alcohol** may elicit disulfiram reaction; oral solutions of **citalopram, ritonavir; lopinavir/ritonavir,** and IV formulations of **sulfamethoxazole; trimethoprim, SMX-TMP, nitroglycerin** may elicit disulfiram reaction due to the alcohol content of the dosage form; **disulfiram** causes acute psychosis; **phenobarbital** increases metronidazole metabolism; may increase **lithium** levels; **fluorouracil, azathioprine** may cause transient neutropenia.

PHARMACOKINETICS Absorption: 80% of dose absorbed from GI tract. **Peak:** 1–3 h. **Distribution:** Widely distributed to most body tissues, including CSF, bone, cerebral and hepatic abscesses; crosses placenta; distributed in breast milk. **Metabolism:** 30–60% metabolized in liver. **Elimination:** 77% excreted in urine; 14% excreted in feces within 24 h. **Half-Life:** 6–8 h.

NURSING IMPLICATIONS

Assessment & Drug Effects

- Discontinue therapy immediately if symptoms of CNS toxicity (see Appendix D-1) develop. Monitor especially for seizures and peripheral neuropathy (e.g., numbness and paresthesia of extremities).
- Lab tests: Obtain total and differential WBC counts before, during, and after therapy, especially if a second course is necessary.
- Monitor for S&S of sodium retention, especially in patients on corticosteroid therapy or with a history of CHF.
- Monitor patients on lithium for elevated lithium levels.
- Report appearance of candidiasis or its becoming more prominent with therapy to prescriber promptly.
- Repeat feces examinations, usually up to 3 mo, to ensure that amebae have been eliminated.

Patient & Family Education

- Adhere closely to the established regimen without schedule interruption or changing the dose.
- Refrain from intercourse during therapy for trichomoniasis unless male partner wears a condom to prevent reinfection.
- Have sexual partners receive concurrent treatment. Asymptomatic trichomoniasis in the male is a frequent source of reinfection of the female.
- Do not drink alcohol during therapy or for 48 h after discontinuing of metronidazole; may induce a disulfiram-type reaction (see Appendix D-1). Avoid alcohol-containing medications for at least 48 h after treatment is completed.
- Urine may appear dark or reddish brown (especially with higher than recommended doses). This appears to have no clinical significance.
- Report symptoms of candidal overgrowth: Furry tongue, color changes of tongue, glossitis, stomatitis; vaginitis, curd-like, milky vaginal discharge; proctitis. Treatment with a candidacidal agent may be indicated.
- Do not breast feed while taking this drug.
- Store this medication out of reach of children.

MEXILETINE

(mex-il′e-teen)

Mexitil

Classifications: CARDIOVASCULAR AGENT; ANTIARRHYTHMIC, CLASS IB

Prototype: Lidocaine

Pregnancy Category: C

AVAILABILITY 150 mg, 200 mg, 250 mg capsules

ACTIONS Analog of lidocaine with class IB electrophysiologic properties similar to those of procainamide. Shortens action potential refractory period duration and improves resting potential.

THERAPEUTIC EFFECTS Has little or no effect on atrial tissue and produces modest suppression of sinus node automatically and AV nodal conduction. Prolongs the His-to-ventricular interval (HQ) only if patient has preexisting conduction disturbance.

USES Acute and chronic ventricular arrhythmias; prevention of recurrent cardiac arrests; suppression of PVCs due to ventricular tachyarrhythmias.
UNLABELED USES Wolff-Parkinson-White syndrome and supraventricular arrhythmias.

CONTRAINDICATIONS Severe left ventricular failure, cardiogenic shock, severe bradyarrhythmias. Preexisting second- or third-degree heart block; pregnancy (category C), lactation; concurrent administration of drugs that alter urinary pH.
CAUTIOUS USE Patients with sinus node conduction irregularities, intraventricular conduction abnormalities; hypotension; severe congestive heart failure; liver dysfunction.

ROUTE & DOSAGE

Ventricular Arrhythmias

Child: **PO** 1.4–5 mg/kg/dose q8h
Adult: **PO** 200–300 mg q8h (max 1200 mg/day)
Reduced dosages required with renal impairment.

ADMINISTRATION

Oral

- Give with food or milk to reduce gastric distress.

ADVERSE EFFECTS CNS: *Dizziness, tremor, nervousness, incoordination,* headache, blurred vision, paresthesias, numbness. **CV:** <u>Exacerbated arrhythmias</u>, palpitations, chest pain, syncope, hypotension. **GI:** *Nausea, vomiting, heartburn,* diarrhea, constipation, dry mouth, abdominal pain. **Skin:** Rash. **Body as a Whole:** Dyspnea, edema, arthralgia, fever, malaise, hiccups. **Urogenital:** Impotence, urinary retention.

INTERACTIONS Drug: Phenytoin, phenobarbital, rifampin may decrease mexiletine levels; **cimetidine, fluvoxamine** may increase mexiletine levels; may increase **theophylline** levels; may increase proarrhythmic effects of **dofetilide** (separate administration by at least 1 wk). **Food:** Foods that alter urine pH can decrease the excretion of mexiletine. Caffeine decreases clearance of mexiletine.

PHARMACOKINETICS Absorption: Readily absorbed from GI tract. **Peak:** 2–3 h. **Distribution:** Distributed into breast milk. **Metabolism:** Metabolized in liver. **Elimination:** Excreted in urine; renal elimination increases with urinary acidification. **Half-Life:** 10–12 h.

NURSING IMPLICATIONS

Assessment & Drug Effects

- Check pulse and BP before administration; make sure both are stabilized.
- Effective **serum concentration range** is 0.5–2 mcg/mL.

Common adverse effects in *italic;* life-threatening effects <u>underlined</u>; generic names in **bold**; drug classifications in SMALL CAPS; ♣ Canadian drug name; ☻ Prototype drug.

Toxic Range: >2 mcg/mL.

- Lab tests: Baseline and periodic liver function tests.
- Supervise ambulation in the weak, debilitated patient during drug stabilization period. CNS adverse reactions predominate (e.g., intention tremors, nystagmus, blurred vision, dizziness, ataxia, confusion, nausea).
- Encourage drug compliance; affected particularly by the distressing adverse effects of tremor, ataxia, and eye symptoms.
- Check frequently with patient about adherence to drug regimen. If adverse effects are increasing, consult physician. Dose adjustment or discontinuation may be needed.

Patient & Family Education

- Learn about pulse parameters to be reported: Changes in rhythm and rate (bradycardia = pulse below 60 in adults; for children, check with physician for pulse parameters); symptomatic bradycardia (lightheadedness, syncope, dizziness), and postural hypotension.
- Do not breast feed while taking this drug.
- Store this medication out of reach of children.

MIDAZOLAM HYDROCHLORIDE

(mid'az-zoe-lam)
Versed
Classifications: CENTRAL NERVOUS SYSTEM AGENT; BENZODIAZEPINE ANXIOLYTIC; SEDATIVE-HYPNOTIC
Prototype: Lorazepam
Pregnancy Category: D
Controlled Substance: Schedule IV

AVAILABILITY 1 mg/mL, 5 mg/mL injection (contains 1% benzyl alcohol)

ACTIONS Short-acting parenteral benzodiazepine. Mechanism of action unclear. Intensifies activity of gamma-aminobenzoic acid (GABA), a major inhibitory neurotransmitter of the brain, by interfering with its reuptake and promoting its accumulation at neuronal synapses. This calms the patient, relaxes skeletal muscles, and in high doses produces sleep.
THERAPEUTIC EFFECTS CNS depressant with muscle relaxant, sedative-hypnotic, anticonvulsant, and amnestic properties.

USES Sedation before general anesthesia, induction of general anesthesia; to impair memory of perioperative events (anterograde amnesia); for conscious sedation prior to short diagnostic and endoscopic procedures; and as the hypnotic supplement to nitrous oxide and oxygen (balanced anesthesia) for short surgical procedures.

CONTRAINDICATIONS Intolerance to benzodiazepines; acute narrow-angle glaucoma; shock, coma; acute alcohol intoxication; intra-arterial injection. Safety in pregnancy (category D), labor and delivery, or lactation is not established.
CAUTIOUS USE Patient with COPD; chronic kidney failure; CHF; the premature neonates, neonates.

ROUTE & DOSAGE

Sedation for Diagnostic & Therapeutic Procedures with Mechanical Ventilation

Neonate: **IV Continous Infusions** *<32 wk,* 0.5 mcg/kg/min; *≥32 wk,* 1 mcg/kg/min
Infants/Child: **IV Intermittent Infusions** 1–2 mcg/kg/min
Infants/Child: 0.05–0.15 mg/kg/dose q1–2h as needed

Sedation for Diagnostic and Therapeutic Procedures

Infants/Child: IM child: 0.1–0.15 mg/kg, 30 to 60 min before proce-dure. (max dose 10 mg) **IV** *≥6 mo–5 y,* 0.05–0.1 mg/kg/dose infused over 2–3 min followed by careful titration of 0.05 mg/kg, q2–3min up to max dose of 6 mg; *6–12 y,* 0.025–0.05 mg/kg/dose infused over 2–3 min followed by careful titration of 0.05 mg/kg q2–3min to max dose of 10 mg; *12–16 y,* use adult dose (max dose 10 mg)
Intranasal 0.2–0.3 mg/kg/dose, may repeat in 15 min
Adult: **IM** 0.07–0.08 mg/kg 30–60 min before procedure **IV** 1–1.5 mg, may repeat in 2 min prn; *Intubated Patients,* 0.05–0.2 mg/kg/h by continuous infusion

Status Epilepticus

Child: **IV Loading Dose** *>2 mo,* 0.15 mg/kg times 1 **IV Maintenance Dose** 1 mcg/kg/min continuous infusion, may titrate upward as needed q5min

Preoperative Sedation

Child: **PO** *<5 y,* 0.5 mg/kg; *>5 y,* 0.4–0.5 mg/kg

STORAGE

Store at 15°–30° C (59°–86° F); therapeutic activity is retained for 2 y from date of manufacture.

ADMINISTRATION

Intramuscular

- Inject IM drug deep into a large muscle mass appropriate for age (see Part I).

Intranasal

- Use the 5 mg/mL injectable product. Using a syringe, without a needle give ½ of dose into each nares. Inject each dose over 15 sec.

Intravenous

PREPARE Direct: Dilute in D5W or NS to a concentration of 0.25 mg/mL (e.g., 1 mg in 4 mL or 5 mg in 20 mL) **IV Infusion:** Add 5 mL of the 5 mg/mL concentration to 45 mL of D5W or NS to yield 0.5 mg/mL.
ADMINISTER Direct: *Sedation,* Give over ≥2 min; *Induction of Anesthe-sia,* Give over 20–30 sec. **IV Infusion:** Give at a rate based on weight.
INCOMPATIBILITIES Solution/Additive: Ringers' lactated, dimenhy-drinate, pentobarbital, perphenazine, prochlorperazine, raniti-dine. **Y-Site:** Albumin, amoxicillin, amoxicillin/clavulanate, amphotericin B cholesteryl complex, ampicillin, bumetanide,

Common adverse effects in *italic;* life-threatening effects <u>underlined;</u> generic names in **bold;** drug classifications in SMALL CAPS; ✦ Canadian drug name; ✪ Prototype drug.

butorphanol, ceftazidime, cefuroxime, clonidine, dexamethasone, dimenhydrinate, floxacillin, foscarnet, fosphenytoin,
furosemide, hydrocortisone, imipenem/cilastatin, methotrexate,
nafcillin, omeprazole, pentobarbital, perphenazine, prochlorperazine, sodium bicarbonate, thiopental, TPN.

ADVERSE EFFECTS CNS: *Retrograde amnesia,* headache, euphoria,
drowsiness, excessive sedation, confusion. **CV:** Hypotension. **Special
Senses:** Blurred vision, diplopia, nystagmus, pinpoint pupils. **GI:** Nausea, vomiting. **Respiratory:** Coughing, <u>laryngospasm</u> (rare), <u>respiratory
arrest. Infant gasping syndrome</u> **Skin:** Hives, swelling, burning, pain, induration at injection site, tachypnea. **Body as a Whole:** Hiccups, chills,
weakness.

INTERACTIONS Drug: Alcohol, CNS DEPRESSANTS, ANTICONVULSANTS potentiate CNS depression; **cimetidine** increases midazolam plasma levels, increasing its toxicity; may decrease antiparkinsonism effects of **levodopa;**
may increase **phenytoin** levels; **smoking** decreases sedative and antianxiety effects. **Food:** Grapefruit juice increases bioavailability and delays absorption of midazolam. **Herbal: Kava-kava, valerian** may
potentiate sedation.

PHARMACOKINETICS Onset: 1–5 min IV; 5–15 min IM, 20–30 min PO.
Peak: 20–60 min. **Duration:** <2 h IV; 1–6 h IM. **Distribution:** Crosses
blood–brain barrier and placenta. **Metabolism:** Metabolized in liver.
Elimination: Excreted in urine. **Half-Life:** 1–4 h.

NURSING IMPLICATIONS

Assessment & Drug Effects

- Inspect insertion site for redness, pain, swelling, and other signs of extravasation during IV infusion.
- Monitor for hypotension, especially if the patient is premedicated with
  a narcotic agonist analgesic.
- Monitor vital signs for entire recovery period. In obese patient, half-life
  is prolonged during IV infusion; therefore, duration of effects is prolonged (i.e., amnesia, postoperative recovery).
- Be aware that overdose symptoms include somnolence, confusion, sedation, diminished reflexes, coma, and untoward effects on vital signs.
- Rapid IV infusion may cause severe hypotension and seizures especially in the neonate. Injection contains benzyl alcohol and large doses
  may cause "gasping syndrome" in neonates.

Patient & Family Education

- Do not drive or engage in potentially hazardous activity until response
  to drug is known. You may feel drowsy, weak, or tired for 1–2 days after drug has been given.
- Be prepared for amnesia to prevent an upsetting postoperative period.
- Review written instructions to assure future understanding and compliance. Patient teaching during amnestic period may not be remembered.
  Even if dose is small and depth of amnesia is unclear, repeat information.

Common adverse effects in *italic;* life-threatening effects <u>underlined;</u> generic names
in **bold;** drug classifications in SMALL CAPS; ♣ Canadian drug name; ⊙ Prototype drug.

827

MILRINONE LACTATE

(mil'ri-none)

Primacor

Classifications: CARDIOVASCULAR AGENT; INOTROPIC AGENT; VASODILATOR
Prototype: Inamrinone
Pregnancy Category: C

AVAILABILITY 1 mg/mL, 200 mcg/mL injection

ACTIONS Member of a new class of inotropic/vasodilator agents. Positive inotropic action and vasodilator, with little chronotropic activity; mode of action and structure are different from digitalis and catecholamines as well as beta-adrenergic agonists. Inhibitory action against cyclic-AMP phosphodiesterase in cardiac and smooth vascular muscle. Increases cardiac contractility.

THERAPEUTIC EFFECTS In therapeutic dose, increases myocardial contractility. Therefore, increases cardiac output and decreases pulmonary wedge pressure and vascular resistance, without increasing myocardial oxygen demand or significantly increasing heart rate.

USES Short-term management of CHF.
UNLABELED USES Short-term use to increase the cardiac index in patients with low cardiac output after surgery. To increase cardiac function prior to heart transplantation.

CONTRAINDICATIONS Hypersensitivity to milrinone; patients with acute MI, aortic or pulmonic valvular disease.
CAUTIOUS USE With atrial flutter or fibrillation; pregnancy (category C), lactation. Safety and efficacy in children not established.

ROUTE & DOSAGE

Neonate/Infant/Child: **(limited data with children) IV Loading Dose**
50 mcg/kg IV over 15 min, then continuous infusion of 0.25–0.75 mcg/kg/min to effect (max dose 1.13 mg/kg/day)
Adult: **IV Loading Dose** 50 mcg/kg IV over 10 min **IV Maintenance Dose** 0.375–0.75 mcg/kg/ min

STORAGE

Store according to manufacturer's directions.

ADMINISTRATION

Intravenous

Note: Correct preexisting hypokalemia before administering milrinone. See manufacturer's information for dosage reduction in the presence of renal impairment.

PREPARE **Loading Dose:** Give undiluted or dilute each 1 mg in 1 mL NS or 0.45% NaCl. **IV Infusion:** Dilute 20 mg of milrinone in D5W, NS, or 0.45% NaCl to yield 100 mcg/mL with 180 mL diluent; 150 mcg/mL with 113 mL diluent; 200 mcg/mL with 80 mL diluent.

ADMINISTER **Loading Dose:** Give 50 mcg/kg over 10 min in adults or over 15 min with children. **IV Infusion:** Give at a rate based on weight. Use a microdrip set and infusion pump.

INCOMPATIBILITIES **Solution/Additive: Furosemide, procainamide. Y-Site: Furosemide** (will cause precipitate)**, procainamide.**

ADVERSE EFFECTS CV: Increased ectopic activity, PVCs, ventricular tachycardia, ventricular fibrillation, supraventricular arrhythmias; possible increase in angina symptoms, hypotension.

INTERACTIONS Drug: Disopyramide may cause excessive hypotension.

PHARMACOKINETICS Peak: 2 min. **Duration:** 2 h. **Distribution:** 70% protein bound. **Elimination:** 80–85% excreted unchanged in urine within 24 h. Active renal tubular secretion is primary elimination pathway. **Half-Life:** 1.7–2.7 h.

NURSING IMPLICATIONS

Assessment & Drug Effects

- Monitor cardiac status closely during and for several hours following infusion. Supraventricular and ventricular arrhythmias have occurred.
- Monitor BP and promptly slow or stop infusion in presence of significant hypotension. Closely monitor those with recent aggressive diuretic therapy for decreasing blood pressure.
- Monitor fluid and electrolyte status. Hypokalemia should be corrected whenever it occurs during administration.
- In children the hemodynamtic effects can last up to 3–5 h after administration.

Patient & Family Education

- Report immediately angina that occurs during infusion to physician.
- Be aware that drug may cause a headache, which can be treated with analgesics.

M

MINERAL OIL

Agoral Plain, Heavy Mineral Oil, Kondremul Plain, Milkinol, Neo-Cultol, Zymenol
Classifications: GASTROINTESTINAL AGENT; STOOL SOFTENER
Prototype: Docusate
Pregnancy Category: C

AVAILABILITY Liquid and emulsion

ACTIONS Mixture of hydrocarbons obtained from petroleum. Aids passage of stool by lubricating it and by slowing the rate of water absorption from the feces while it is in the large intestine.
THERAPEUTIC EFFECTS Lubricates and softens feces, retards water absorption from fecal content, eases passage of stool.

USES Temporary relief of constipation, when straining at stool is contraindicated (e.g., hypertension, certain cardiac disorders, following anorectal surgery), and to relieve fecal impaction. Also used as pharmaceutical solvent and vehicle.

CONTRAINDICATIONS Nausea, vomiting, abdominal pain, intestinal obstruction; oral administration to dysphagic patients; use with emollients.
CAUTIOUS USE Oral use in debilitated patients or children <5 y; pregnancy (category C), lactation.

ROUTE & DOSAGE

Constipation
Child: **PO** ≥ 6 y, 5–15 mL once daily
Adult: **PO** 15–30 mL prn **PR** 90–120 mL

ADMINISTRATION

Oral

- Give preferably in the evening. Digestion and passage of food from stomach may be delayed if taken within 2 h of mealtime.
- Give cold with 30 mL of fruit juice or carbonated beverage to increase palatability. Emulsified preparation is more palatable.
- Give with patient in upright position and avoid giving just before patient retires. Potential of lipid pneumonia from aspiration is especially high in debilitated patients, children <5 y, or those who are uncooperative .
- Use as retention enema is generally followed by a cleansing enema in 30–60 min. Consult prescriber.

ADVERSE EFFECTS Body as a Whole: Anal seepage, pruritus ani; interference with postoperative anorectal wound healing. **Respiratory:** <u>With aspiration: pulmonary granuloma, lipid pneumonitis.</u> **GI:** Anorexia, nausea, vomiting. **Metabolic:** Nutritional deficiencies (with prolonged use). **Hematologic:** Hypoprothrombinemia (with prolonged use).

INTERACTIONS Drug: May potentiate effects of ORAL ANTICOAGULANTS by decreasing the absorption of Vitamin K; large doses may decrease the absorption of **warfarin;** STOOL SOFTENERS may form a concretion in the GI tract; may decrease absorption of oral contraceptives. **Food:** Interferes with absorption of fat-soluble vitamins (A, D, E, K), calcium, phosphorus.

PHARMACOKINETICS Absorption: Limited absorption from GI tract. **Distribution:** Distributes to mesenteric lymph nodes, intestinal mucosa, liver, and spleen. **Elimination:** Eliminated in stool in 6–10 h.

NURSING IMPLICATIONS

Assessment & Drug Effects
- Monitor bowel movements.

Patient & Family Education
- Be aware that prolonged use (>2 wk) can reduce absorption of fat-soluble vitamins A, D, E, and K, carotene, calcium, and phosphates.

Common adverse effects in *italic;* life-threatening effects <u>underlined;</u> generic names in **bold;** drug classifications in SMALL CAPS; ♣ Canadian drug name; ❶ Prototype drug.

- Frequent or prolonged use of mineral oil may result in dependence. In children, do not give longer than 1 wk.
- Do not breast feed while taking this drug without consulting physician.
- Store this medication out of reach of children.

MINOCYCLINE HYDROCHLORIDE
(mi-noe-sye′kleen)
Minocin, Dynacin, Vectrin
Classifications: ANTI-INFECTIVE; TETRACYCLINE ANTIBIOTIC
Prototype: Tetracycline
Pregnancy Category: D

AVAILABILITY 50 mg, 75 mg, 100 mg tablets; 50 mg, 100 mg capsules; 50 mg/5 mL suspension (contains 5% alcohol); 100 mg injection

ACTIONS Semisynthetic tetracycline derivative that appears to be active against strains of *Staphylococci* resistant to other tetracyclines; photosensitivity occurs only rarely. Reported to be more completely absorbed than other TETRACYCLINES because it is more lipid soluble.

THERAPEUTIC EFFECTS Effective against *Mycobacterium marinum* infections, *Urea plasma urealyticum, Neisseria gonorrhoeae.*

USES Treatment of mucopurulent cervicitis, granuloma inguinale, lymphogranuloma venereum, proctitis, bronchitis, lower respiratory tract infections caused by *Mycoplasma pneumoniae,* rickettsial infections, chlamydial infections, non-gonococcal urethritis, chlamydial conjunctivitis, plague, brucellosis, bartonellosis, tularemia, UTI, and prostatitis; acne vulgaris, gonorrhea, cholera, meningococcal carrier state.

CONTRAINDICATIONS Hypersensitivity to tetracyclines; oral administration in meningococcal infections; pregnancy (category D), lactation, children <8 y.

CAUTIOUS USE Renal and hepatic impairment.

ROUTE & DOSAGE

Anti-Infective
Child: **PO/IV** >8–12 y, 4 mg/kg/dose times 1 followed by 2 mg/kg/dose q12h (max dose 200 mg/day)
Adult: **PO/IV** 200 mg followed by 100 mg q12h

Acne
Adult: **PO** 50 mg 1–3 times/day

Meningococcal Carrier State
Child: **PO** >8 y, 4 mg/kg followed by 2 mg/kg q12h times 5 days (max 100 mg/dose)
Adult: **PO** 100 mg q12h times 5 days

STORAGE
Store at 15°–30° C (59°–86° F) in tightly closed, light-resistant containers. Protect from moisture. Reconstituted solution is stable at room

Common adverse effects in *italic;* life-threatening effects <u>underlined;</u> generic names in **bold;** drug classifications in SMALL CAPS; ♣ Canadian drug name; ● Prototype drug.

831

temperature for 24 h; further diluted solution should be used immediately.

ADMINISTRATION

Oral

- Shake suspension well before administration.
- Oral therapy is the preferred route; institute as soon as possible.
- May take with food but not with milk or dairy products.
- Check expiration date. Outdated medication can cause severe adverse effects.

Intravenous

PREPARE Intermittent: Reconstitute 100 mg with 5 mL of sterile water for injection; further dilute with 500–1000 mL of D5W, NS, D5/NS, or RL.

ADMINISTER Intermittent: Start infusion immediately after preparation. Avoid rapid infusion. Give at a rate determined by the total volume of solution.

INCOMPATIBILITIES Solution/Additive: Doxapram, rifampin. Y-Site: Allopurinol, amifostine, hydromorphone, meperidine, morphine, piperacillin/tazobactam, propofol, thiotepa, TPN.

ADVERSE EFFECTS CNS: *Weakness, light-headedness, ataxia, dizziness,* or *vertigo.* **GI:** Nausea, cramps, diarrhea, flatulence.

INTERACTIONS Drug: ANTACIDS, **iron, calcium, magnesium, zinc, kaolin and pectin, sodium bicarbonate, bismuth subsalicylate** can significantly decrease minocycline absorption; effects of both **desmopressin** and minocycline antagonized; increases **digoxin** absorption, increasing risk of **digoxin** toxicity; **methoxyflurane** increases risk of kidney failure. **Food:** Milk and dairy products significantly decrease minocycline absorption; food may also decrease its absorption.

PHARMACOKINETICS Absorption: 90–100% absorbed from GI tract. **Peak:** 2–3 h. **Distribution:** Tends to accumulate in adipose tissue; crosses placenta; distributed into breast milk. **Metabolism:** Partially metabolized. **Elimination:** 20–30% excreted in feces; about 12% excreted in urine. **Half-Life:** 11–26 h.

NURSING IMPLICATIONS

Assessment & Drug Effects

- Obtain history of hypersensitivity reactions prior to administration; drug is contraindicated with known tetracycline hypersensitivity.
- Lab: C&S should be drawn prior to initiation of therapy.
- Monitor IV infusion site carefully, since thrombophlebitis occurs relatively often (see Appendix D-1).
- Monitor carefully for signs of hypersensitivity response (see Appendix D-1), particularly in patients with history of allergies, especially to drugs.
- Monitor at-risk patients for S&S of superinfection (see Appendix D-1).
- Assess risk of toxic effects carefully; increases with renal and hepatic impairment.

- Determine serum drug level in patients receiving prolonged therapy.
- Supervise ambulation, since lightheadedness, dizziness, and vertigo occur frequently (30–90%).

Patient & Family Education

- Avoid hazardous activities or those requiring alertness (biking, skateboarding, and sports) while taking minocycline.
- Do not take within 2 h of antacids, calcium, or iron. Do not take with milk or dairy products.
- Use sunscreen when outdoors and otherwise protect yourself from direct sunlight because photosensitivity reaction may occur.
- Report vestibular adverse effects (e.g., dizziness), which usually occur during first week of therapy. Effects are reversible if drug is withdrawn.
- Report loose stools or diarrhea or other signs of superinfection promptly to prescriber.
- Use or add barrier contraceptive while they are taking drug if using hormonal contraceptive.
- Do not breast feed while taking this drug.
- Store this medication out of reach of children.

MINOXIDIL

(mi-nox'i-dill)
Loniten, Rogaine
Classifications: CARDIOVASCULAR AGENT; NONNITRATE VASODILATOR; ANTIHYPERTENSIVE
Prototype: Hydralazine
Pregnancy Category: C

AVAILABILITY 2.5 mg, 10 mg tablets; 2%, 5% solution

ACTIONS Direct-acting vasodilator similar to other drugs of this class, but hypotensive effect is more pronounced. Appears to act by blocking calcium uptake through cell membrane. Reduces elevated systolic and diastolic blood pressures in supine and standing positions, by decreasing peripheral vascular resistance.

THERAPEUTIC EFFECTS Hypotensive action accompanied by reflex activation of sympathetic, vagal inhibitory, and renal homeostatic mechanisms; increased sympathetic stimulation also activates the renin-angiotensin-aldosterone system. Net result is increased heart rate and cardiac output, sodium retention, and edema, which usually necessitates concomitant supportive drug therapy. Drug-induced hair growth with systemic minoxidil usually develops after 1 y of therapy: it is nonvirilizing, involving face and limbs of the female and generalized increase in body hair in men. Topical minoxidil reverses balding to some degree.

USES Treat severe hypertension that is symptomatic or associated with damage to target organs and is not manageable with maximum therapeutic doses of a diuretic plus two other antihypertensive drugs. Used with a diuretic to prevent fluid retention and a beta-adrenergic blocking agent (e.g., propranolol) or an alpha-adrenergic agonist (e.g., clonidine or

---

Common adverse effects in *italic*; life-threatening effects <u>underlined</u>; generic names in **bold**; drug classifications in SMALL CAPS; ♣ Canadian drug name; ☻ Prototype drug.

833

methyldopa) to prevent tachycardia. *Topical:* To treat alopecia areata and male pattern alopecia.

CONTRAINDICATIONS Pheochromocytoma; acute MI, dissecting aortic aneurysm, valvular dysfunction, heart failure. Safety during pregnancy (category C) or lactation is not established.
CAUTIOUS USE Severe renal impairment; recent MI (within preceding month); coronary artery disease, chronic CHF.

ROUTE & DOSAGE

Hypertension

Child: **PO** 0.2 mg/kg/day (max 5 mg/day) initially, gradually increased at 3 day intervals by 0.1–0.2 mg/kg/day up to range of 0.25–1 mg/kg/day given in 1–2 divided doses (max 50 mg/day)
Children >12 y/Adult: **PO** 5 mg/day, increased q3–5days up to 40 mg/day in single or divided doses as needed (max 100 mg/day)

Alopecia

Adult: **Topical** Apply 1 mL of 2% solution to affected area b.i.d.

STORAGE
Store at 15°–30° C (59°–86° F) in tightly covered container unless otherwise directed

ADMINISTRATION

Oral

- Dose increments are usually made at 3–5 day intervals. If more rapid adjustment is necessary, adjustments can be made q6h with careful monitoring.

Topical

- Do not apply topical product to an irritated scalp (e.g., sunburn, psoriasis).

ADVERSE EFFECTS CV: *Tachycardia,* angina pectoris, *ECG changes,* pericardial effusion and tamponade, rebound hypertension (following drug withdrawal); *edema,* including pulmonary edema; *CHF (salt and water retention).* **Skin:** *Hypertrichosis,* transient pruritus, darkening of skin, hypersensitivity rash, <u>Stevens-Johnson syndrome</u>. With topical use: itching, flushing, scaling, dermatitis, folliculitis. **Body as a Whole:** Fatigue.

DIAGNOSTIC TEST INTERFERENCE *Hct, Hgb,* and ***erythrocyte count*** usually decrease (about 7%) during early therapy; ***serum alkaline phosphatase, BUN,*** and ***creatinine*** may increase during early therapy.

INTERACTIONS Drug: Epinephrine, norepinephrine cause excessive cardiac stimulation; **guanethidine** causes profound orthostatic hypotension. **Food:** Licorice increases sodium and water retention and potassium loss.

PHARMACOKINETICS Absorption: Readily absorbed from GI tract. **Onset:** 30 min PO; at least 4 mo topical. **Peak:** 2–8 h PO. **Duration:** 2–5 day PO; new hair growth will remain 3–4 mo after withdrawal of topical. **Distribution:** Widely distributed including into breast milk. **Metabolism:** Metabolized in liver. **Elimination:** 97% excreted in urine and feces. **Half-Life:** 4.2 h.

NURSING IMPLICATIONS

Assessment & Drug Effects

- Take BP and apical pulse before administering medication and report significant changes. Consult physician for parameters.
- Lab tests: Periodic serum electrolytes.
- Do not stop drug abruptly. Abrupt reduction in BP can result in CVA and MI. Keep physician informed.
- Monitor fluid and electrolyte balance closely throughout therapy. Sodium and water retention commonly occur. Consult prescriber regarding sodium restriction. Monitor potassium intake and serum potassium levels in patient on diuretic therapy.
- Monitor I&O and daily weight. Report unusual changes in I&O ratio or daily weight gain, greater than 1 kg (2 lb) gain, or in children any sudden increase in body weight in relation to their age and baseline body weight.
- Observe patient daily for edema and auscultate lungs for rales. Be alert to signs and symptoms of CHF (see Appendix D-1).
- Observe for symptoms of pericardial effusion or tamponade. Symptoms are similar to those of CHF, but additionally patient may have paradoxical pulse (normal inspiratory reduction in systolic BP may fall as much as 10–20 mm Hg).

Patient & Family Education

- Learn about usual pulse rate and count radial pulse for one full minute before taking drug. Report an increase of 20 or more bpm.
- Notify physician promptly if the following S&S appear: Increase of 20 or more bpm in resting pulse; breathing difficulty; dizziness; lightheadedness; fainting; edema (tight shoes or rings, puffiness, pitting); weight gain, chest pain, arm or shoulder pain; easy bruising or bleeding.
- Change positions from lying to standing carefully because such movement may cause dizziness.
- Be aware of possibility of hypertrichosis: Elongation, thickening, and increased pigmentation of fine body hair, especially of face, arms, and back. Develops 3–9 wk after start of therapy and occurs in approximately 80% of patients; reversible within 1–6 mo after drug withdrawal.
- Report any dermatologic adverse effects or any other adverse effect promptly to physician.
- Schedule follow-up examinations for q4–6mo.
- Comply strictly with regular regimen; maximizes chance of at least some hair regrowth.
- Do not breast feed while taking this drug without consulting prescriber.
- Store this medication out of reach of children.

Common adverse effects in *italic*; life-threatening effects <u>underlined</u>; generic names in **bold**; drug classifications in SMALL CAPS; ♣ Canadian drug name; ⊘ Prototype drug.

MITOMYCIN

(mye-toe-mye′sin)

Mutamycin

Classifications: ANTINEOPLASTIC; ANTIBIOTIC
Prototype: Doxorubicin
Pregnancy Category: D

AVAILABILITY 5 mg, 20 mg, 40 mg injection

ACTIONS Potent antibiotic antineoplastic compound. Effective in certain tumors unresponsive to surgery, radiation, or other chemotherapeutic agents. Action mechanism unclear but reportedly combines with DNA, thereby interfering with cellular and enzymatic RNA and protein synthesis.

THERAPEUTIC EFFECTS Highly destructive to rapidly proliferating cells and slowly developing carcinomas.

USES In combination with other chemotherapeutic agents in palliative, adjunctive treatment of disseminated adenocarcinoma of breast, pancreas, or stomach, squamous cell carcinoma of head, neck, lung, and cervix. Not recommended to replace surgery or radiotherapy or as a single primary therapeutic agent.

CONTRAINDICATIONS Hypersensitivity or idiosyncrasy reaction; thrombocytopenia; coagulation disorders or bleeding tendencies; pregnancy (category D), lactation.

CAUTIOUS USE Renal impairment; myelosuppression.

ROUTE & DOSAGE

Cancer

Child/Adult: IV 10–20 mg/m^2/day as a single dose q6–8wk, additional doses based on hematologic response

STORAGE

Store at vials at 15°–30° C (59°–86° F), protect from light. Store drug reconstituted with sterile water for injection (0.5 mg/mL) for 14 days refrigerated or 7 days at room temperature. Drug diluted in D5W (20–40 mcg/mL) is stable at room temperature for 3 h.

ADMINISTRATION

Must be given under care and direction of Pediatric Oncology Specialist. Use recommended handling techniques for hazardous medications (see Part I).

Intravenous

Note: Verify correct IV concentration and rate of infusion/injection for administration to children with physician.

PREPARE IV Infusion: Dilute each 5 mg with 10 mL sterile water for injection. Shake to dissolve. If product does not clear immediately, allow

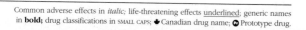

to stand at room temperature until solution is obtained. Reconstituted solution is purple.

***ADMINISTER* IV Infusion:** Give reconstituted solution over 5–10 min or longer as determined by total volume of solution. Usual final concentration is 20–40 mcg/mL. Monitor IV site closely. Avoid extravasation to prevent extreme tissue reaction (cellulitis) to the toxic drug.

***INCOMPATIBILITIES* Solution/Additive:** DEXTROSE-CONTAINING SOLUTIONS, **bleomycin. Y-Site: Aztreonam, cefepime, etoposide, filgrastim, gemcitabine, sargramostim, vinorelbine.**

ADVERSE EFFECTS CNS: Paresthesias. **GI:** Stomatitis, *nausea, vomiting,* anorexia, hematemesis, diarrhea. **Hematologic:** <u>Bone marrow toxicity (thrombocytopenia, leukopenia</u> occurring 4–8 wk after treatment onset), thrombophlebitis, anemia. **Respiratory:** <u>Acute bronchospasm</u>, hemoptysis, dyspnea, nonproductive cough, pneumonia, <u>interstitial pneumonitis</u>. **Skin:** Desquamation; induration, pain, necrosis, cellulitis at injection site; reversible alopecia, purple discoloration of nail beds **Body as a Whole:** Pain, headache, fatigue, edema. **Urogenital:** <u>Hemolytic uremic syndrome</u>, renal toxicity.

PHARMACOKINETICS Metabolism: Metabolized rapidly in liver. **Elimination:** Excreted in urine. **Half-Life:** 17 min.

M

NURSING IMPLICATIONS

Assessment & Drug Effects

- Lab tests: Perform WBC with differential, platelet count, PT, INR, aPTT, Hgb, Hct, and serum creatinine frequently during and for at least 7 wk after treatment.
- Do not administer if serum creatinine is >1.7 mg/dL or if platelet count falls below 150,000/mm^3 and WBC is down to 4000/mm^3 or if prothrombin or bleeding times are prolonged.
- Monitor I&O ratio and pattern. Report any sign of impaired kidney function: Change in ratio, dysuria, hematuria, oliguria, frequency, urgency. Keep patient well hydrated (at least 2000–2500 mL orally daily if tolerated). In children, maintain a fluid intake to produce an adequate urinary output in relationship to age. Drug is nephrotoxic.
- Observe closely for signs of infection, such as respiratory infection, aching, rashes, gastrointestinal distress, etc. Assess immunization status prior to beginning therapy in order to be alert for diseases that pose risk. Monitor body temperature frequently.
- Inspect oral cavity daily for signs of stomatitis or superinfection (see Appendix D-1).

Patient & Family Education

- Avoid exposure to persons with infectious diseases. Report signs of infection.
- Report respiratory distress to physician immediately.
- Report signs of common cold to physician immediately.
- Understand that hair loss is reversible after cessation of treatment.
- Do not breast feed while taking this drug.

Common adverse effects in *italic;* life-threatening effects <u>underlined</u>; generic names in **bold;** drug classifications in SMALL CAPS; ♣ Canadian drug name; ⊘ Prototype drug.

837

MITOXANTRONE HYDROCHLORIDE

(mi-tox′an-trone)
Novantrone
Classifications: ANTINEOPLASTIC; ANTIBIOTIC; IMMUNOSUPPRESSANT
Prototype: Doxorubicin
Pregnancy Category: D

AVAILABILITY 2 mg/mL injection

ACTIONS Non-cell-cycle specific antitumor agent with less cardiotoxicity than doxorubicin. Interferes with DNA synthesis by intercalating with the DNA double helix, blocking effective DNA and RNA transcription.
THERAPEUTIC EFFECTS Highly destructive to rapidly proliferating cells in all stages of cell division.

USES In combination with other drugs for the treatment of acute nonlymphocytic leukemia (ANLL) in adults, bone pain in advanced prostate cancer. Reducing neurologic disability and/or the frequency of clinical relapses in patients with secondary progressive, progressive relapsing, or worsening relapsing-remitting multiple sclerosis.
UNLABELED USES Breast cancer, refractory lymphomas.

CONTRAINDICATIONS Hypersensitivity to mitoxantrone; myelosuppression; pregnancy (category D), lactation.
CAUTIOUS USE Impaired cardiac function; impaired liver and kidney function; systemic infections.

ROUTE & DOSAGE

Combination Therapy for ANLL

Child: **IV** ≤2 y, 0.4 mg/kg/day once a day for 3–5 days; >2 y, 8–12 mg/m² /day once a day for 3–5 days.
Adult: **IV Induction Therapy:** 12 mg/m²/day on days 1–3, may need to repeat induction course. **IV Consolidation Therapy:** 12 mg/m² on days 1 and 2 (max lifetime dose 80–120 mg/m²)

Solid Tumors

Child: **IV** 5–8 mg/m² once a week or 18–20 mg/m² once q3–4wk

Multiple Sclerosis

Adult: **IV** 12 mg/m² over 5–15 min q3mo (max lifetime dose 140 mg/m²)
Reduce dosages required with hepatic impairment.

STORAGE

Discard unused portions of diluted solution. Once opened, multiple-use vials may be stored refrigerated at 2°–8° C (35°–46° F) for 14 days.

ADMINISTRATION

Intravenous

- Must be given under care and direction of pediatric oncology specialist. Use recommended handling techniques for hazardous medications (see Part I).

- If mitoxantrone touches skin, wash immediately with copious amounts of warm water.

PREPARE **IV Infusion:** Withdraw contents of vial and add to at least 50 mL of D5W or NS. Use goggles, gloves, and protective gown during drug preparation and administration.

ADMINISTER **IV Infusion:** Give into the tubing as a freely running IV of D5W or NS and infused over at least 3 min or longer (i.e., 30–60 min) depending on the total volume of IV solution. Continuous IV concentration should be 0.02–0.5 mg/mL. If extravasation occurs, stop infusion and immediately restart in another vein.

INCOMPATIBILITIES **Solution/Additive: Heparin, hydrocortisone, paclitaxel. Y-Site: Amphotericin B cholesteryl complex, aztreonam, doxorubicin liposome, paclitaxel, piperacillin/tazobactam, propofol, TPN.**

ADVERSE EFFECTS CV: Arrhythmias, decreased left ventricular function, *CHF,* tachycardia, ECG changes, <u>MI</u> (occurs with cumulative doses of >80–100 mg/m^2), edema. **GI:** *Nausea, vomiting,* diarrhea, <u>hepatotoxicity</u>. **Hematologic:** <u>*Leukopenia, thrombocytopenia*</u>. **Other:** Discolors urine and sclera a blue-green color. **Skin:** Mild phlebitis, blue skin discoloration, alopecia.

INTERACTIONS Drug: May impair immune response to VACCINES such as influenza and pneumococcal infections. May have increased risk of infection with **yellow fever vaccine.**

PHARMACOKINETICS Distribution: Rapidly taken up by tissues and slowly released into plasma, resulting in low renal, hepatic, and metabolic clearance rates; 95% protein bound. **Metabolism:** Metabolized in liver. **Elimination:** Excreted primarily in bile. **Half-Life:** 37 h.

NURSING IMPLICATIONS

Assessment & Drug Effects

- Monitor IV insertion site. Transient blue skin discoloration may occur at site if extravasation has occurred.
- Monitor cardiac functioning throughout course of therapy; report S&S of CHF or cardiac arrhythmias.
- Lab tests: Perform liver function tests prior to and during course of treatment. Monitor serum uric acid levels and initiate hypouricemic therapy before antileukemic therapy. Monitor carefully CBC with differential prior to and during therapy.
- Be alert for and report signs of infections such as respiratory infections, aching, rashes, gastrointestinal distress, etc. Assess immunization status prior to beginning therapy in order to be alert for diseases that pose risk.

Patient & Family Education

- Understand potential adverse effects of mitoxantrone therapy.
- Expect urine to turn blue-green for 24 h after drug administration; sclera, tears and skin may also take on a bluish color.
- Be aware that stomatitis/mucositis may occur within 1 wk of therapy.
- Do not to risk exposure to those with known infections during the periods of myelosuppression.

- Avoid exposure to persons with infectious diseases. Report signs of infection.
- Do not breast feed while taking this drug.

MIVACURIUM CHLORIDE

(miv-a-cur′i-um)

Mivacron

Classifications: AUTONOMIC NERVOUS SYSTEM AGENT; MUSCLE RELAXANT; NONDEPOLARIZING

Prototype: Tubocurarine

Pregnancy Category: C

AVAILABILITY 2 mg/mL injection (contains benzyl alcohol)

ACTIONS Short-acting, skeletal muscle relaxant that combines competitively to cholinergic receptors on the motor neuron end plate. Antagonizes action of acetylcholine, and blocks neuromuscular transmission. Neuromuscular blocking action is readily reversible with an anticholinesterase agent.

THERAPEUTIC EFFECTS Blocks nerve impulse transmission, which results in skeletal muscle relaxation and paralysis.

USES Adjunct to general anesthesia, to facilitate tracheal intubation, and to provide skeletal muscle relaxation during surgery or mechanical ventilation.

CONTRAINDICATIONS Allergic reactions to mivacurium or its ingredients.

CAUTIOUS USE Kidney function impairment, liver function impairment; older adult patients; pregnancy (category C), lactation.

ROUTE & DOSAGE

Tracheal Intubation and Mechanical Ventilation

Child: **IV Loading Dose** 2–12 y, 0.2 mg/kg given over 5–15 sec (range: 0.09–0.2 mg/kg) **IV Maintenance Dose** Same as adult **IV Continuous Infusion** 10–15 mcg/kg/min

Adult: **IV Loading Dose** 0.15 mg/kg given over 5–15 sec (over 60 sec in patients with cardiovascular disease)

IV Maintenance Dose: 0.1 mg/kg generally q15min **IV Continuous Infusion:** Initial infusion of 9–10 mcg/kg/min, reduce infusion to 4 mcg/kg/min if started with initial bolus

Renal Impairment

Cl_{cr} Decrease infusion rates by 50%

STORAGE

Store at 15°–30° C (59°–86° F) light-resistant containers. Store diluted solution at 5°–25° C (41°–77° F) for up to 24 h.

ADMINISTRATION

Intravenous

PREPARE **Direct:** Add 3 mL of D5W, NS, D5/NS, RL, or D5/RL to each 1 mL mivacurium to yield 0.5 mg/mL. **IV Infusion:** Available premixed (50 mL of 0.5 mg/mL).

ADMINISTER **Direct:** Give over 15–60 sec. Maximum concentration 0.5 mg/mL. **IV Infusion:** Refer to manufacturer's infusion rate tables. The use of a peripheral nerve stimulator permits optimal dosing and minimizes risks of overdose or underdose.

INCOMPATIBILITIES **Solution/Additive:** ALKALINE SOLUTIONS pH >8.5 (BARBITURATES).

ADVERSE EFFECTS CV: Transient decrease in arterial BP, hypotension, increases and decreases in heart rate. **Skin:** *Transient flushing about the face, neck, and/or chest* (especially with rapid administration).

INTERACTIONS Drug: GENERAL ANESTHETICS **(enflurane, halothane, isoflurane)** may enhance the degree of neuromuscular blockade produced by mivacurium. AMINOGLYCOSIDES, TETRACYCLINES, **amphotericin B, bacitracin, furosemide, thiazides** POLYMYXINS, **lincomycin, clindamycin, colistin, magnesium, vancomycin salts, lithium,** LOCAL ANESTHETICS, **procainamide,** and **quinidine** may enhance the neuromuscular blockade.

PHARMACOKINETICS Peak: 2–6 min. **Duration:** 25–30 min in adults, 8–16 min in children. **Distribution:** Limited tissue distribution. **Metabolism:** Rapidly hydrolyzed by plasma cholinesterase.

NURSING IMPLICATIONS

Assessment & Drug Effects

- Assess patients with neuromuscular disease carefully and adjust drug dosage using a peripheral nerve stimulator when they experience prolonged neuromuscular blocks.
- Monitor hemodynamic status carefully in patients with significant cardiovascular disease or those with potentially greater sensitivity to release of histamine-type mediators (e.g., asthma).
- Monitor for significant drop in BP because overdose may increase the risk of hemodynamic adverse effects. State of consciousness is not altered by this drug.

MOMETASONE FUROATE

(mo-met′-a-sone)

Elocon, Nasonex

Classifications: SKIN AND MUCOUS MEMBRANE AGENT; ANTI-INFLAMMATORY; HORMONES AND SYNTHETIC SUBSTITUTES; STEROID

Prototype: Hydrocortisone

Pregnancy Category: C

Common adverse effects in *italic;* life-threatening effects underlined; generic names in **bold;** drug classifications in SMALL CAPS; ◆ Canadian drug name; ❷ Prototype drug.

841

AVAILABILITY 50 mcg spray; 0.1% ointment; cream; lotion

ACTIONS Controls inflammation at the cellular level through stabilization of the lysosomal membrane.

THERAPEUTIC EFFECTS Relieves itching and puritus of the skin and decreases symptoms of seasonal allergic rhinitis.

USES Nasal inhalation for the management of symptoms of seasonal perennial rhinitis. Topical for treatment of dermatoses.

CONTRAINDICATIONS Hypersensitivity to mometasone furoate or its ingredients; pregnancy category C; safety and efficacy of nasal preparation in children <2 y not established.

CAUTIOUS USE Patients receiving systemic corticosteroids; use with extreme caution if at all in respiratory tuberculosis, untreated fungal, bacterial, or viral infections, and ocular herpes simplex; nasal inhalation therapy for nasal septal ulcers, nasal trauma, or surgery. Use caution in children because it may cause a reduction of growth velocity in children in high doses. During lactation.

ROUTE & DOSAGE

Allergic Rhinitis

Child: ≥2–11 y, **Intranasal** 1 spray in each nostril once daily
Adult: **Intranasal** 2 sprays (50 mcg each) in each nostril once daily

Topical Inflamation

Child/Adult: **Topical** apply cream or ointment sparingly once daily or b.i.d.

STORAGE

Store at 2°–30° C (36°–86° F) Topical preparations expire after 24 mo from manufactured date.

ADMINISTRATION

Intranasal

- **Nasal Inhaler:** Directions for use of nasal inhaler provided by manufacturer. Pump must be primed by actuating 10 times until fine spray is evident. If pump is not used in 1-wk period it must be primed prior to usage. Clear nares prior to usage. See ADMINISTRATION section on how to clear nares and for administration with children **Topical:** Apply in a thin film and rub into affected area. Do not use occlusive dressings.

ADVERSE EFFECTS Body as a Whole: Candidal infection of oropharynx and occasionally larynx, hoarseness, dry mouth, sore throat, sore mouth; transient nasal irritation, burning, sneezing, epistaxis, bloody mucus, nasopharyngeal itching, dryness, crusting, and ulceration, *headache*. **GI:** Nausea, vomiting (2–12 y). **Metabolic:** With excessive dosages, symptoms of hypercorticism, dysmenorrhea.

PHARMACOKINETICS Absorption: Topical varies.

NURSING IMPLICATIONS

Assessment & Drug Effects

- Use only as directed. Nasal form usually started 2–4 wk before onset of allergy season.
- Observe for symptoms of systemic corticosteroid effects (see Appendix D-1).

Patient & Family Education

- Use only as directed and do not increase dosage or take longer than prescribed.
- Gently blow nose to clear nostrils. Prime inhaler first before usage. If 2 sprays in each nostril are prescribed, direct one spray toward upper, and the other toward the lower part of the nostril.
- Wash cap and plastic nose piece daily with warm water; dry thoroughly.
- Inhaled steroids do not provide immediate symptomatic relief and are not prescribed for this purpose. Relief usually seen in 2 days but may take 1–2 wk for optimum effects.
- Observe nasopharyngeal area for signs of candidal infection.
- Topical usage use only as prescribed; do not share with others.
- Use thin applications of topical forms and do not cover with occlusive dressing.
- Avoid exposure to chickenpox or measles during usage. If exposed contact physician.
- Avoid use of OTC drugs containing hydrocortisones.
- Store this medication out of reach of children.

MONTELUKAST

(mon-te-lu'cast)
Singulair
Classifications: BRONCHODILATOR (RESPIRATORY SMOOTH MUSCLE RELAXANT); LEUKOTRIENE RECEPTOR ANTAGONIST
Prototype: Zafirlukast
Pregnancy Category: B

AVAILABILITY 5 mg, 10 mg tablets; 4 mg chewable tablets (contains phenylalanine)

ACTIONS Selective receptor antagonist of leukotriene D_4, thus inhibiting bronchoconstriction. Leukotrienes are considered more important than prostaglandins as inflammatory agents; they induce bronchoconstriction and mucus production. Elevated sputum and blood levels of leukotrienes have been documented during acute asthma attacks.

THERAPEUTIC EFFECTS Controls asthmatic attacks by inhibiting leukotriene release as well as inflammatory action associated with the attack. Indicated by improved pulmonary functions and better controlled asthmatic symptoms.

USES Prophylaxis and chronic treatment of asthma.

CONTRAINDICATIONS Hypersensitivity to montelukast; severe asthma attacks; bronchoconstriction due to asthma or NSAIDs; status asthmaticus; chewable tablets in phenylketonuria lactation.

CAUTIOUS USE Hypersensitivity to other leukotriene receptor antagonists (e.g., zafirlukast, zileuton); severe liver disease; severe asthma; pregnancy (category B); children <6 y.

ROUTE & DOSAGE

Asthma

Child: **PO** 2–5 y, 4 mg daily in evening; *6–14 y,* 5 mg/day in evening
Child/Adult >14 y: **PO** 10 mg daily in evening

STORAGE

Store at 15°–30° C (59°–86° F) in a tightly closed container, protect from light.

ADMINISTRATION

Oral

- Give in the evening for maximum effectiveness.
- Ensure chewable tablets for children are not swallowed whole.
- Chewable tablets contain phenylalanine; do not use for those with PKU.
- Granules may not be mixed in liquid, can give in applesauce or ice cream.

ADVERSE EFFECTS Body as a Whole: Asthenia, fever, trauma. **CNS:** Dizziness, *headache.* **GI:** Abdominal pain, dyspepsia, gastroenteritis, dental pain, abnormal liver function tests (ALT, AST), diarrhea, nausea. **Respiratory:** Nasal congestion, cough, influenza, laryngitis, pharyngitis, sinusitis. **Skin:** Rash. **Urogenital:** Pyuria.

INTERACTIONS Drug: Phenobarbital and **rifampin** may increase clearance of montelukast.

PHARMACOKINETICS Absorption: Rapidly absorbed from GI tract, bioavailability 64%. **Peak:** 3–4 h for oral tablet, 2–2.5 h for chewable tablet. **Distribution:** >99% protein bound. **Metabolism:** Extensively metabolized by cytochromes P450 3A4 and 2C9. **Elimination:** Excreted in feces. **Half-Life:** 2.7–5.5 h.

NURSING IMPLICATIONS

Assessment & Drug Effects

- Monitor effectiveness when used in combination with phenobarbital or other potent cytochrome P-450 enzyme inducers carefully.
- Lab test: Periodic liver function tests.

Patient & Family Education

- Do not use for reversal of an acute asthmatic attack. Take this drug only as prescribed.
- Inform prescriber if short-acting inhaled bronchodilators are needed more often than usual with montelukast.

- Use chewable tablets (contain phenylalanine) with caution with PKU.
- Do not breast feed while taking this drug.
- Store this medication out of reach of children.

MORPHINE SULFATE ℗

(mor′feen)

Astramorph PF, Avinza, Duramorph, Epimorph ✦, Kadian, MSIR, MS Contin, Oramorph SR, Roxanol, RMS, Statex ✦

Classifications: CENTRAL NERVOUS SYSTEM AGENT; ANALGESIC; NARCOTIC (OPIATE) AGONIST

Pregnancy Category: B (D in long-term use or high dose)

Controlled Substance: Schedule II

AVAILABILITY 10 mg, 15 mg, 30 mg tablets/capsules; 15 mg, 20 mg, 30 mg, 60 mg, 100 mg, 120 mg, 200 mg controlled-release tablets/capsules; 10 mg/2.5 mL, 10 mg/5 mL, 20 mg/mL, 20 mg/5 mL, 30 mg/1.5 mL, 100 mg/5 mL oral solution; 0.5 mg/mL, 1 mg/mL, 2 mg/mL, 4 mg/mL, 5 mg/mL, 8 mg/mL, 10 mg/mL, 15 mg/mL, 25 mg/mL, 50 mg/mL injection; 5 mg, 10 mg, 20 mg, 30 mg suppositories

ACTIONS Natural opium alkaloid with agonist activity by binding with the same receptors as endogenous opioid peptides. Narcotic agonist effects are identified with three types of receptors: Analgesia at supraspinal level, euphoria, respiratory depression and physical dependence; analgesia at spinal level, sedation and miosis; and dysphoric, hallucinogenic and cardiac stimulant effects.

THERAPEUTIC EFFECTS Controls severe pain; also used as an adjunct to anesthesia.

USES Symptomatic relief of severe acute and chronic pain after nonnarcotic analgesics have failed and as preanesthetic medication; also used to relieve dyspnea of acute left ventricular failure and pulmonary edema and pain of MI.

CONTRAINDICATIONS Hypersensitivity to opiates; increased intracranial pressure; convulsive disorders; acute alcoholism; acute bronchial asthma, chronic pulmonary diseases, severe respiratory depression; chemical-irritant induced pulmonary edema; prostatic hypertrophy; diarrhea caused by poisoning until the toxic material has been eliminated; undiagnosed acute abdominal conditions; following biliary tract surgery and surgical anastomosis; pancreatitis; acute ulcerative colitis; severe liver or renal insufficiency; Addison's disease; hypothyroidism; during labor for delivery of a premature infant, in premature infants; pregnancy (category B; D in long-term use or when high dose is used); lactation.

CAUTIOUS USE Toxic psychosis; cardiac arrhythmias, cardiovascular disease; emphysema; kyphoscoliosis; cor pulmonale; severe obesity; reduced blood volume; very young or debilitated patients; labor.

Common adverse effects in *italic;* life-threatening effects underlined; generic names in **bold;** drug classifications in SMALL CAPS; ✦ Canadian drug name; ℗ Prototype drug.

845

ROUTE & DOSAGE

Pain Relief

Neonate: **IV/IM/SC** (use only preservative-free preparations) 0.05 mg/kg q4–8h (max 0.1 mg/kg) *or* 0.01 mg/kg/h by continuous infusion (max rate 0.01–0.02 mg/kg/h)

Infant/Child: **PO** 0.2–0.5 mg/kg q4–6h; 0.3–0.6 mg/kg/dose sustained-release q12h **IV** 0.05–0.1 mg/kg q4h or 0.025–2.6 mg/kg/h by continuous infusion **IM/SC** 0.1–0.2 mg/kg q4h (max 15 mg/dose)

Adult: **PO** 10–30 mg q4h prn or 15–30 mg sustained-release q8–12h; (Kadian) dose q12–24h, increase dose prn for pain relief **IV** 2.5–15 mg q4h or 0.8–10 mg/h by continuous infusion, may increase prn to control pain or 5–10 mg given epidurally q24h **IM/SC** 5–20 mg q4h **PR** 10–20 mg q4h prn

STORAGE

Store at 15°–30° C (59°–86° F). Avoid freezing. Refrigerate suppositories. Protect all formulations from light.

ADMINISTRATION

Oral

- Use a fixed, individualized schedule when narcotic analgesic therapy is started to provide effective management; blood levels can be maintained and peaks of pain can be prevented (usually a 4-h interval is adequate).
- Use lower dosage for debilitated patients than for adults.
- Do not break in half, crush, or allow sustained-release tablet to be chewed. Sustained-release capsule's contents can be sprinkled over a small amount of applesauce immediately before giving; instruct patient not to chew particles. Have patient rinse mouth and swallow to ensure entire dosage has been consumed.
- Do not give patient sustained-release tablet within 24 h of surgery.
- Dilute oral solution in approximately 30 mL or more of fluid or semi-solid food. A calibrated dropper comes with the bottle. Read labels carefully when using liquid preparation; available solutions: 20 mg/mL; 100 mg/mL.
- Can be given sublingually; morphine oral solution has greater bioavailability than when swallowed (bypasses first-pass metabolism by the liver).

Intravenous

Note: Verify correct IV concentration and rate of infusion/injection for administration to neonates, infants, or children with physician.

***PREPARE* Direct:** Dilute 2–10 mg in at least 5 mL of sterile water for injection.

***ADMINISTER* Direct:** Give a single dose over at least 5 min at a concentration of 0.5–5 mg/mL. Avoid rapid administration.

***INCOMPATIBILITIES* Solution/Additive: Aminophylline, amobarbital, chlorothiazide, floxacillin, fluorouracil, haloperidol, heparin, meperidine, pentobarbital, phenobarbital, phenytoin, sodium bicarbonate, thiopental. Y-Site: Amphotericin B cholesteryl complex, cefepime, doxorubicin liposome, minocycline, sargramostim, tetracycline.**

ADVERSE EFFECTS Body as a Whole: Hypersensitivity (*pruritus,* rash, urticaria, edema, hemorrhagic urticaria [rare], <u>anaphylactoid reaction</u> [rare]), sweating, skeletal muscle flaccidity; cold, clammy skin, hypothermia. **CNS:** Euphoria, insomnia, disorientation, visual disturbances, dysphoria, paradoxic CNS stimulation (restlessness, tremor, delirium, insomnia), convulsions (infants and children); decreased cough reflex, drowsiness, dizziness, deep sleep, coma. **Special Senses:** Miosis. **CV:** Bradycardia, palpitations, syncope; flushing of face, neck, and upper thorax; orthostatic hypotension, cardiac arrest. **GI:** *Constipation,* anorexia, dry mouth, biliary colic, *nausea,* vomiting, elevated transaminase levels. **Urogenital:** Urinary retention or urgency, dysuria, oliguria, reduced libido or potency (prolonged use). **Other:** Prolonged labor and respiratory depression of newborn. **Hematologic:** Precipitation of porphyria. **Respiratory:** <u>Severe respiratory depression</u> (as low as 2–4/min) or arrest; pulmonary edema.

DIAGNOSTIC TEST INTERFERENCE False-positive ***urine glucose*** determinations may occur using ***Benedict's solution. Plasma amylase*** and ***lipase*** determinations may be falsely positive for 24 h after use of morphine; ***transaminase levels*** may be elevated.

INTERACTIONS Drug: CNS DEPRESSANTS, SEDATIVES, BARBITURATES, **alcohol,** BENZODIAZEPINES, and TRICYCLIC ANTIDEPRESSANTS potentiate CNS depressant effects. Use MAO INHIBITORS cautiously; they may precipitate hypertensive crisis. PHENOTHIAZINES may antagonize analgesia. **Herbal: Kava-kava, valerian, St. John's wort** may increase sedation.

M

PHARMACOKINETICS Absorption: Variably absorbed from GI tract. **Peak:** 60 min PO; 20–60 min PR; 50–90 min SC; 30–60 min IM; 20 min IV. **Duration:** Up to 7 h. **Distribution:** Crosses blood–brain barrier and placenta; distributed in breast milk. **Metabolism:** Metabolized primarily in liver. **Elimination:** 90% of drug and metabolites excreted in urine in 24 h; 7–10% excreted in bile.

NURSING IMPLICATIONS

Assessment & Drug Effects

- Obtain baseline respiratory rate, depth, and rhythm and size of pupils before administering the drug. Respirations of 12/min or below and miosis are signs of toxicity. Withhold drug and report to physician.
- Observe patient closely to be certain pain relief is achieved. Record relief of pain and duration of analgesia.
- Be alert to elevated pulse or respiratory rate, restlessness, anorexia, or drawn facial expression that may indicate need for analgesia.
- Differentiate among restlessness as a sign of pain and the need for medication, restlessness associated with hypoxia, and restlessness caused by morphine-induced CNS stimulation (a paradoxic reaction that is particularly common in women).
- Monitor for respiratory depression; it can be severe for as long as 24 h after epidural or intrathecal administration.
- Monitor carefully those at risk for severe respiratory depression after epidural or intrathecal injection: Debilitated patients or those with decreased respiratory reserve (e.g., emphysema, severe obesity, kyphoscoliosis).

- Continue monitoring for respiratory depression for at least 24 h after each epidural or intrathecal dose.
- Assess vital signs at regular intervals. Morphine-induced respiratory depression may occur even with small doses, and it increases progressively with higher doses (generally max: 90 min after SC, 30 min after IM, and 7 min after IV).
- Encourage changes in position, deep breathing, and coughing (unless contraindicated) at regularly scheduled intervals. Narcotic analgesics also depress cough and sigh reflexes and thus may induce atelectasis, especially in postoperative patients.
- Be alert for nausea and orthostatic hypotension (with light-headedness and dizziness) in ambulatory patients or when a supine patient assumes the head-up position or in patients not experiencing severe pain. Monitor level of sedation. Naloxane used to reverse effects of morphine.
- Monitor I&O ratio and pattern. Report oliguria or urinary retention. Morphine may dull perception of bladder stimuli; therefore, encourage the patient to void at least q4h. Palpate lower abdomen to detect bladder distention.
- Avoid bulk-forming laxatives due to increased risk of bowel impaction; use stimulant laxatives if necessary.

Patient & Family Education

- Avoid alcohol and other CNS depressants while receiving morphine.
- Do not use any OTC drug unless approved by physician.
- Do not smoke or ambulate without assistance after receiving drug. Bedside rails are advised.
- Use caution or avoid tasks requiring alertness (e.g., biking, skateboarding, sports, and driving a car) until response to drug is known since morphine may cause drowsiness, dizziness, or blurred vision.
- Do not breast feed while taking this drug.
- Store this medication in locked area out of reach of children; this is a Schedule II drug.

MUPIROCIN

(mu-pi-ro′sin)
Bactroban, Bactroban Nasal
Classifications: ANTI-INFECTIVE; PSEUDOMONIC ACID ANTIBIOTIC
Pregnancy Category: B

AVAILABILITY 2% ointment; cream

ACTIONS Topical antibacterial produced by fermentation of *Pseudomonas fluorescens*.
THERAPEUTIC EFFECTS Inhibits bacterial protein synthesis by binding with the bacterial transfer-RNA. Susceptible bacteria are *Staphylococcus aureus* (including methicillin-resistant and beta-lactamase-producing strains), *Staphylococcus epidermidis, Staphylococcus saprophyticus,* and *Streptococcus pyogenes*.

USES Impetigo due to *Staphylococcus aureus, beta-hemolytic Streptococci,* and *Streptococcus pyogenes;* nasal carriage of *S. aureus.*
UNLABELED USES Superficial skin infections.

CONTRAINDICATIONS Hypersensitivity to any of its components and for ophthalmic use.

CAUTIOUS USE Burn patients; impaired kidney function, pregnancy (category B) or lactation.

ROUTE & DOSAGE

Impetigo

Child/Adult: **Topical** Apply small amount to affected area t.i.d., if no response in 3–5 days, reevaluate (usually continue for 1–2 wk)

Elimination of Staphylococcal Nasal Carriage

Child: **Intranasal** Apply intranasally b.i.d. to q.i.d. for 5–14 days

ADMINISTRATION

Topical
- Apply thin layer of medication to affected area.
- Cover area being treated with a gauze dressing if desired.

ADVERSE EFFECTS Skin: Burning, stinging, pain, pruritus, rash, erythema, dry skin, tenderness, swelling. **Special Senses:** Intranasal, local stinging, soreness, dry skin, pruritus.

INTERACTIONS Drug: Incompatible with **salicylic acid 2%;** do not mix in HYDROPHILIC VEHICLES (e.g., **Aquaphor**) or COAL TAR SOLUTIONS; **chloramphenicol** may interfere with bactericidal action of mupirocin.

PHARMACOKINETICS Absorption: Not systemically absorbed.

NURSING IMPLICATIONS

Assessment & Drug Effects
- Watch for signs and symptoms of superinfection (see Appendix D-1). Prolonged or repeated therapy may result in superinfection by nonsusceptible organisms.
- Reevaluate drug use if patient does not show clinical response within 3–5 days.
- Discontinue the drug and notify physician if signs of contact dermatitis develop or if exudate production increases.

Patient & Family Education
- Discontinue drug and contact prescriber if a sensitivity reaction or chemical irritation occurs (e.g., increased redness, itching, burning).
- Do not breast feed while taking this drug without consulting prescriber.
- Store this medication out of reach of children.

MUROMONAB-CD₃

(myoo-roe-moe′nab)
Orthoclone OKT3
Classifications: IMMUNOSUPPRESSANT; MONOCLONAL ANTIBODY
Prototype: Cyclosporine
Pregnancy Category: C

Common adverse effects in *italic;* life-threatening effects <u>underlined;</u> generic names in **bold;** drug classifications in SMALL CAPS; ✦ Canadian drug name; ◐ Prototype drug.

849

AVAILABILITY 5 mg/mL injection

ACTIONS Murine monoclonal antibody (purified IgG_2). Specifically targets the T_3 (CD_3) molecule in the antigenic recognition site of the human T-cell membrane. Following this antigenic challenge, CD_3-positive T-cells are rapidly removed from circulation, and T-lymphocyte action leading to renal inflammation and destruction is blocked, thus reversing graft rejection. Lymphomas may follow immunosuppression therapy with muromonab-CD_3; incidence is related to intensity and duration of drug-induced immunosuppression.

THERAPEUTIC EFFECTS CD_3-positive T-lymphocytes immunosuppression results in reversing graft rejection of a transplanted kidney.

USES Acute allograft rejection in kidney transplant patients.
UNLABELED USES Acute allograft rejection in heart and liver transplant patients.

CONTRAINDICATIONS Intolerance to any product of murine origin; patient with fluid overload; weight gain of more than 3% within week prior to treatment; infection: Chickenpox (existing, recent, including recent exposure), herpes zoster. Safety during pregnancy (category C) or lactation is not established.
CAUTIOUS USE Repeated courses.

M

ROUTE & DOSAGE

Transplant Rejection

Child: **IV** <12 y, 0.1 mg/kg daily times 10–14 days *or* ≤30 kg, 2.5 mg daily; >30 kg, 5 mg daily for 10–14 days
Child Over 12 y/Adult: **IV** 5 mg/day administered in <1 min for 10–14 days

STORAGE
Store at 2°–8° C (36°–46° F) unless otherwise stipulated. Avoid freezing.

ADMINISTRATION
Note: Only persons experienced with immunosuppressive therapy and management of kidney transplant patients should administer Muromonab-CD_3 and only in an area equipped with staff and facilities to deal with cardiac resuscitation.

Intravenous
Note: Verify correct rate of IV injection for administration to infants or children with physician.
- Administer IV methylprednisolone sodium succinate before and IV hydrocortisone sodium succinate 30 min after muromonab-CD_3 to decrease incidence of first dose reaction. ■ Be aware that concomitant maintenance immunosuppressive therapy is reduced or discontinued during drug therapy with muromonab-CD_3 and resumed about 3 days prior to end of therapy.

***PREPARE* Direct:** Give undiluted. Do not shake ampule. Draw sterile solution into syringe through a low protein-binding 0.2- or 0.22-micron filter. Discard filter; attach syringe to an appropriate needle for IV bolus injection.

ADMINISTER Direct: Give by rapid (bolus) injection. Do not give by IV infusion or in conjunction with other drug solutions.

ADVERSE EFFECTS All: Especially during first 2 day of therapy. **GI:** _Nausea, vomiting, diarrhea._ **Respiratory:** <u>Severe pulmonary edema</u>, _dyspnea, chest pain, wheezing._ **Body as a Whole:** _Fever, chills,_ malaise, _tremor, increased susceptibility to cytomegalovirus, herpes simplex,_ Pneumocystis carinii, Legionella, Cryptococcus, Serratia organisms, and gram-negative bacteria. **CV:** Tachycardia, <u>anaphylaxis</u> rare.

PHARMACOKINETICS Onset: The number of circulating CD₃-positive T-cells decreases within minutes. **Peak:** 2–7 day. **Duration:** 7 day.

NURSING IMPLICATIONS

Assessment & Drug Effects

- Assess and monitor vital signs. If temperature rises above 37.8° C (100° F), suspect infection (commonly observed in first 45 days of therapy). Take temperature before treatment and several hours after drug administration to detect first signs of infection.
- Consult physician if patient has a fever exceeding 37.8° C (100° F) before treatment. Make immediate attempts to lower temperature to at least 37.8° C (100° F) with antipyretics before muromonab-CD₃ is administered.
- Be alert to susceptibility of patient with pretreatment fluid overload to acute pulmonary edema (may be fatal). Be prepared for prompt intubation, oxygenation, and corticosteroid drug administration should it occur.
- Monitor patient's response closely for 48 h for first dose reaction (occurs within 45–60 min after first dose and lasts several hours). It may occur (less severe) after second dose; then usually does not occur with subsequent doses. Symptoms: Chills, dyspnea, malaise, high fever.

Patient & Family Education

- Report any of the following to physician: Chest pain, difficulty breathing, wheezing, nausea and vomiting, significant weight gain, an infection, or fever.
- Use an effective method of birth control for 12 wk following the end of therapy.

MYCOPHENOLATE MOFETIL

(my-co-phen′o-late mo′fe-till)
CellCept
Classification: IMMUNOSUPPRESSANT
Prototype: Cyclosporine
Pregnancy Category: C

AVAILABILITY 250 mg capsules; 500 mg tablets; 200 mg/ml oral suspension (contains aspartame), 500 mg injection

ACTIONS Prodrug with immunosuppressant properties; inhibits T- and B-lymphocyte proliferation responses; inhibits antibody formation, and blocks the generation of cytotoxic T cells.
THERAPEUTIC EFFECTS Antirejection effects attributed to decreased number of activated lymphocytes in the graft site. Synergistic with cyclosporine.

USES Prophylaxis of organ rejection in patients receiving allogenic kidney transplants or heart transplants.
UNLABELED USES Rejection prophylaxis for liver transplants, treatment of rheumatoid arthritis and psoriasis.

CONTRAINDICATIONS Hypersensitivity to mycophenolate mofetil; pregnancy (category C), lactation.
CAUTIOUS USE Viral or bacterial infections; presence or history of carcinoma; bone marrow suppression; active peptic ulcer disease; severe diarrhea; malabsorption syndromes; renal impairment. Safety and efficacy in children are not established.

ROUTE & DOSAGE

Prophylaxis for Kidney Transplant Rejection
Child: **(limited use with children) PO** 600 mg/m^2/dose b.i.d. (max dose 2000 mg/day)
Adult: **PO/IV** Start within 24 h of transplant, 1 g b.i.d. in combination with corticosteroids and cyclosporine

Prophylaxis for Heart Transplant Rejection
Adult: **PO/IV** 1.5 g b.i.d. started within 24 h of transplant

STORAGE
Store at 15°–30° C (59°–86° F).

ADMINISTRATION
Note: Only persons experienced with immunosuppressive therapy and management of kidney transplant patients should manage administration of mycophenolate mofetil.

Oral
- Give oral drug on an empty stomach.
- Adjust dosage with severe chronic kidney failure.
- Do not open or crush capsules; avoid contact with powder in capsules, and wash thoroughly with soap and water if contact occurs.
- Contains phenylalanine; do not use in those with PKU.

Intravenous

***PREPARE* IV Infusion:** Reconstitute each vial with 14 mL D5W. Further dilute vial used in an additional 70 mL with D5W to yield 6 mg/mL.
***ADMINISTER* IV Infusion:** Slowly infuse over ≥2 h. Avoid rapid injection.
***INCOMPATIBILITIES* Solution/Additive & Y-Site:** Do not mix or infuse with other medications. ▪ Begin IV mycophenolate mofetil within 24 h of transplant and continued for up to 14 days. ▪ Switch patient to oral drug as soon as possible.

ADVERSE EFFECTS CNS: *Headache, tremor,* insomnia, dizziness, weakness. **CV:** *Hypertension.* **Endocrine:** Hyperglycemia, hypercholesterolemia, hypophosphatemia, hypokalemia, hyperkalemia, *peripheral edema*. **GI:** *Diarrhea, constipation, nausea,* anorexia, vomiting, *abdominal pain, dyspepsia.* **Urogenital:** *UTI, hematuria,* renal tubular necrosis, burning, frequency, vaginal burning or itching, vaginal bleeding, kidney stones. **Hematologic:** <u>*Leukopenia*</u>, *anemia, thrombocytopenia,* hypochromic anemia, leukocytosis. **Respiratory:** *Respiratory infection, dyspnea,* increased cough, pharyngitis. **Skin:** Rash. **Body as a Whole:** Leg or hand cramps, bone pain, myalgias, <u>*sepsis (bacterial, fungal, viral)*</u>.

INTERACTIONS Drug: Acyclovir, ganciclovir, salicylates may increase mycophenolate serum levels. ANTACIDS, **cholestyramine** decreases mycophenolate absorption. **Mycophenolate** may decrease protein binding of **phenytoin** or **theophylline,** causing increased serum levels.

PHARMACOKINETICS Absorption: Rapidly absorbed from GI tract; 94% reaches systemic circulation; absorption decreased by food. **Onset:** 4 wk. **Metabolism:** Metabolized in liver to active form, mycophenolic acid. **Elimination:** 87% excreted in urine. **Half-Life:** 11 h.

NURSING IMPLICATIONS

Assessment & Drug Effects

- Lab tests: Monitor CBC weekly for first month, biweekly for second and third months, then once per month for first year. If neutropenia develops (ANC $<1.3 \times 10^3$/mcL), withhold dose and notify physician. Periodically monitor and report abnormalities for any of the following: Kidney and liver function, serum electrolytes, lipase, and amylase; blood glucose; routine urinalysis.
- Monitor for and report any S&S of sepsis or infection.

Patient & Family Education

- Comply exactly with dosing regimen and scheduled laboratory tests.
- Report to physician immediately S&S of infection, such as UTI or respiratory infection.
- Report all troubling adverse reactions (e.g., blood in urine and swelling in arms and legs) to physician as soon as possible.
- Avoid taking OTC antacids simultaneously with mycophenolate mofetil. Separate the two drugs by 2 h.
- Childbearing age women should use two forms of contraception while on this drug and for 6 wk after drug is discontinued.
- Do not breast feed while taking this drug.
- Store this medication out of reach of children.

NAFARELIN ACETATE
(na-fa're-lin)
Synarel
Classifications: HORMONE AND SYNTHETIC SUBSTITUTE; GONADOTROPIN-RELEASING HORMONE ANALOG
Prototype: Leuprolide
Pregnancy Category: X

Common adverse effects in *italic;* life-threatening effects <u>underlined</u>; generic names in **bold;** drug classifications in SMALL CAPS; ✦ Canadian drug name; ◑ Prototype drug.

853

AVAILABILITY 200 mcg/metered spray

ACTIONS Potent agonist analog of gonadotropin-releasing hormone (GnRH). Inhibits pituitary gonadotropin secretion of LH and FSH.

THERAPEUTIC EFFECTS Decrease in serum estradiol or testosterone concentrations results in the quiescence of tissues and functions that depend on LH and FSH. Stops the development of secondary sex characteristics and slows linear skeletal growth and maturation in precocious puberty.

USES Endometriosis and precocious puberty.

CONTRAINDICATIONS Hypersensitivity to GnRH or GnRH agonist analog; undiagnosed abnormal vaginal bleeding; pregnancy (category X), lactation.

CAUTIOUS USE Polycystic ovarian disease.

ROUTE & DOSAGE

Precocious Puberty

Child: **Inhalation** 1600 mcg/day in two equally divided doses in the a.m. and in the p.m. Given as 2 sprays in each nostril (total of 4 sprays, 800 mcg each a.m.) and 2 sprays in each nostril (total 4 sprays), 800 mcg, each p.m. Therapy is continued until the resumption of puberty is indicated. May be increased to 1800 mcg/day in two equally divided doses in the a.m. and in the p.m. (3 sprays each nostril)

Endometriosis

Adults ≥18 y: **Inhalation** 2 inhalations/day (200 mcg/inhalation), one in each nostril, begin between days 2 and 4 of menstrual cycle; in patients with persistent regular menstruation after 2 mo of therapy, may increase to 800 mcg/day as 2 inhalations (one in each nostril) b.i.d.; continue therapy for 6 mo; retreatment is not advised because of lack of safety data

STORAGE

Store at 15°–30° C (59°–86° F); protect from light.

ADMINISTRATION

Inhalation

- Withhold any topical nasal decongestant, if being used, until at least 2 h after nafarelin administration.

ADVERSE EFFECTS GI: *Bloating, abdominal cramps,* weight gain, nausea. **Endocrine:** *Hot flashes, anovulation, amenorrhea, vaginal dryness,* galactorrhea. **Metabolic:** Decreased bone mineral content (reversible). **CNS:** Transient headache, inertia, mild depression, moodiness, fatigue. **Respiratory:** Nasal irritation. **Urogenital:** *Impotence, decreased libido, dyspareunia.*

DIAGNOSTIC TEST INTERFERENCE Increased *alkaline phosphatase;* marked increase in *estradiol* in first 2 wk, then decrease to below baseline; decreased *FSH* and *LH* levels; decreased *testosterone* levels.

INTERACTIONS Drug: No clinically significant interactions established.

PHARMACOKINETICS Absorption: 21% absorbed from nasal mucosa. **Onset:** 4 wk. **Peak:** 12 wk. **Duration:** 30–50 days after discontinuing drug. **Distribution:** 78–84% bound to plasma proteins; crosses placenta. **Metabolism:** Hydrolyzed in kidney. **Elimination:** 44–55% excreted in urine over 7 days, 19–44% in feces. **Half-Life:** 2.7 h.

NURSING IMPLICATIONS

Assessment & Drug Effects
- Make appropriate inquiries about breakthrough bleeding, which may indicate that patient has missed successive drug doses.
- Initial transient increases in puberty signs are possible.

Patient & Family Education
- Important: Instruct child not to blow nose or sneeze immediately after instillation.
- Read the information pamphlet provided with nafarelin.
- Inform prescriber if breakthrough bleeding occurs or menstruation persists.
- Use or add barrier contraceptive during treatment.
- Do not breast feed while taking this drug.
- Store this medication out of reach of children.

N

NAFCILLIN SODIUM

(naf-sill′in)
Nafcillin ♦ Nallpen ♦
Classifications: ANTI-INFECTIVE; BETA-LACTAM ANTIBIOTIC; PENICILLIN; ANTISTAPHYLOCOCCAL PENICILLIN
Prototype: Penicillin G potassium
Pregnancy Category: B

AVAILABILITY 1 g, 2 g injection; 20 mg/mL in 3.6% dextrose

ACTIONS Semisynthetic, acid-stable, penicillinase-resistant penicillin. Mechanism of bactericidal action is by interfering with synthesis of mucopeptides essential to formation and integrity of bacterial cell wall.
THERAPEUTIC EFFECTS Effective against both penicillin-sensitive and penicillin-resistant strains of *Staphylococcus aureus*. Also active against pneumococci and group A beta-hemolytic *Streptococci*. Highly active against penicillinase-producing *Staphylococci* but less potent than penicillin G against penicillin-sensitive microorganisms and generally ineffective against methicillin-resistant *Staphylococcus aureus* (MRSA).

USES Primarily, infections caused by penicillinase-producing *Staphylococci*. May also be used to initiate treatment in suspected staphylococcal infections pending culture and sensitivity test results. As with other penicillins, serum concentrations are considerably enhanced by concurrent use of probenecid.

CONTRAINDICATIONS Hypersensitivity to penicillins, cephalosporins, and other allergens; use of oral drug in severe infections, gastric dilatation, cardiospasm, or intestinal hypermotility; lactation. Safety during pregnancy (category B) is not established.
CAUTIOUS USE History of or suspected atopy or allergy (eczema, hives, hay fever, asthma).

ROUTE & DOSAGE

Staphylococcal Infections

Neonate: **IM/IV** ≤7 *days, <2 kg,* 50 mg/kg/day in 2 equally divided doses q12h; ≥2 *kg,* 75 mg/kg/day in 3 equally divided dose q8h; >7 *days, <1.2 kg,* 50 mg/kg/day in 2 equally divided doses q12h; *1.2–2 kg,* 75 mg/kg/day in 3 equally divided dose q8h; ≥2 *kg,* 100 mg/kg/day in 4 equally divided doses q6h
Infant/Child: **IM/IV** 50–200 mg/kg/day in equally divided q4–6h (max dose 12 g/24 h)
Adult: **IM/IV** 500 mg–2 g q4–6h up to 12 g/day

STORAGE

Label and date vials of reconstituted solution. Remains stable for 7 days under refrigeration and for 3 days at 15°–30° C (59°–86° F).

ADMINISTRATION

Intramuscular

- Reconstitute each 500 mg with 1.7 mL of sterile water for injection or NaCal injection to yield 250 mg/mL. Shake vigorously to dissolve.
- In adults: Make certain solution is clear. Select site carefully. Inject deeply into gluteal muscle. Rotate injection sites.
- In children: The preferred IM site in children <3 y is the midlateral or anterolateral thigh. Check agency policy. See Part I for site recommendations.

Intravenous

Note: Verify correct IV concentration and rate of infusion in neonates, infants, children with physician.
PREPARE **Direct:** Reconstitute as for IM injection. Further dilute with 15–30 mL of D5W, NS, or 0.45% NaCl. **Intermittent:** Dilute reconstituted solution in 100–150 mL of compatible IV solution. **Continuous:** Add desired dose to a volume of IV solution that maintains concentration of drug between 2–40 mg/mL.
ADMINISTER **Direct:** Give over at least 10 min. **Intermittent:** Give over 30–90 min. **Continuous:** Give at ordered rate.
INCOMPATIBILITIES **Solution/Additive: Aminophylline, ascorbic acid, aztreonam, bleomycin, cytarabine, hydrocortisone, methylprednisolone, promazine. Y-Site: Droperidol, innovar, labetalol, nalbuphine, pentazocine, verapamil.**
- Note: Usually, limit IV therapy to 24–48 h because of the possibility of thrombophlebitis (see Appendix D-1) ▪ Discard unused portions 24 h after reconstitution.

ADVERSE EFFECTS Body as a Whole: Drug fever, <u>anaphylaxis</u> (particularly following parenteral therapy). **GI:** Nausea, vomiting, *diarrhea,* increase in

Common adverse effects in *italic;* life-threatening effects <u>underlined</u>; generic names in **bold;** drug classifications in SMALL CAPS; ♣ Canadian drug name; ☉ Prototype drug.

serum transaminase activity (following IM). **Hematologic:** Eosinophilia, thrombophlebitis following IV; neutropenia (long-term therapy). **Metabolic:** Hypokalemia (with high IV doses). **Skin:** Urticaria, pruritus, rash, pain and tissue irritation. **Urogenital:** Allergic interstitial nephritis.

DIAGNOSTIC TEST INTERFERENCE Nafcillin in large doses can cause false-positive *urine protein* tests using *sulfosalicylic acid method.*

INTERACTIONS Drug: May antagonize hypoprothrombinemic effects of **warfarin.** Probenecid prolongs half-life of nafcillin.

PHARMACOKINETICS Absorption: Incompletely and erratically absorbed orally. **Peak:** 30–120 min IM; 15 min IV. **Duration:** 4 h PO; 4–6 h IM. **Distribution:** Distributes into CNS with inflamed meninges; crosses placenta; distributed into breast milk. **Metabolism:** Enters enterohepatic circulation. **Elimination:** Primarily excreted in bile; 10–30% excreted in urine. **Half-Life:** 1 h.

NURSING IMPLICATIONS

Assessment & Drug Effects

- Lab tests: Perform C&S prior to initiation of therapy and periodically thereafter. Obtain twice weekly differential WBC counts in patients receiving IV nafcillin therapy for longer than 2 wk.
- Obtain a careful history before therapy to determine any prior allergic reactions to penicillins, cephalosporins, and other allergens.
- Inspect IV site for inflammatory reaction. Also check IV site for leakage and extravasation.
- Note: Allergic reactions, principally rash, occur most commonly. Nausea, vomiting, and diarrhea may occur with oral therapy.
- Monitor neutrophil count. Nafcillin-induced neutropenia (agranulocytosis) occurs commonly during third week of therapy. It may be associated with malaise, fever, sore mouth, or throat. Perform periodic assessments of liver and kidney functions during prolonged therapy.
- Be alert for signs of bacterial or fungal superinfections (see Appendix D-1) in patients on prolonged therapy.
- Determine IV sodium intake for patients with sodium restriction. Nafcillin sodium contains approximately 3 mEq of sodium per gram.

Patient & Family Education

- Report promptly S&S of neutropenia (see Assessment & Drug Effects), superinfection, or hypokalemia (see Appendix D-1).
- Do not breast feed while taking this drug.

N

NALBUPHINE HYDROCHLORIDE

(nal'byoo-feen)

Nubain

Classifications: CENTRAL NERVOUS SYSTEM AGENT; ANALGESIC; NARCOTIC (OPIATE) PARTIAL AGONIST-ANTAGONIST

Prototype: Pentazocine

Pregnancy Category: C

AVAILABILITY 10 mg/mL, 20 mg/mL injection

ACTIONS Synthetic narcotic analgesic with agonist and weak antagonist properties. Analgesic potency is about 3 or 4 times greater than that of pentazocine and approximately equal to that produced by equivalent doses of morphine. On a weight basis, produces respiratory depression about equal to that of morphine; however, in contrast to morphine, doses >30 mg produce no further respiratory depression. Antagonistic potency is approximately one fourth that of naloxone and about 10 times greater than that of pentazocine.

THERAPEUTIC EFFECTS Analgesic action that relieves moderate to severe pain with apparently low potential for dependence.

USES Symptomatic relief of moderate to severe pain. Also preoperative sedation analgesia and as a supplement to surgical anesthesia.

CONTRAINDICATIONS History of hypersensitivity to drug. Safety during pregnancy (category C) or lactation is not established. Prolonged use during pregnancy could result in neonatal withdrawal syndrome.

CAUTIOUS USE History of emotional instability or drug abuse; head injury, increased intracranial pressure; impaired respirations; impaired kidney or liver function; biliary tract surgery.

ROUTE & DOSAGE

N

Moderate to Severe Pain

Child 1–14 y: **IV/IM/SC** 0.1–0.15 mg/kg q3–6h as needed
Adult >14 y: **IV/IM/SC** 10–20 mg q3–6h prn (max 160 mg/day)

STORAGE
Store at 15°–30° C (59°–86° F); avoid freezing.

ADMINISTRATION

Intramuscular/Subcutaneous
- Inject undiluted.

Intravenous

Note: Verify correct rate of IV injection in infants, children with physician.
PREPARE Direct: Give undiluted.
ADMINISTER Direct: Give at a rate of 10 mg or fraction thereof over 3–5 min. in adults. Children 5–15 min.
INCOMPATIBILITIES Solution/Additive: Diazepam, pentobarbital, promethazine, thiethylperazine. Y-Site: Nafcillin.

ADVERSE EFFECTS CV: Hypertension, hypotension, bradycardia, tachycardia, flushing. **GI:** Abdominal cramps, bitter taste, *nausea, vomiting,* dry mouth. **CNS:** *Sedation, dizziness,* nervousness, depression, restlessness, crying, euphoria, dysphoria, distortion of body image, unusual dreams, confusion, hallucinations; numbness and tingling sensations, headache, vertigo. **Respiratory:** Dyspnea, asthma, <u>respiratory depression</u>. **Skin:** Pruritus, urticaria, burning sensation, *sweaty, clammy skin.* **Special Senses:** Miosis, blurred vision, speech difficulty. **Urogenital:** Urinary urgency.

INTERACTIONS Drug: Alcohol and other CNS DEPRESSANTS add to CNS depression.

PHARMACOKINETICS Onset: 2–3 min IV; 15 min IM. **Peak:** 30 min IV. **Duration:** 3–6 h. **Distribution:** Crosses placenta. **Metabolism:** Metabolized in liver, 50% protein bound. **Elimination:** Eliminated primarily in feces and also in urine. **Half-Life:** 1–8 y, 0.9 h; adult, 3.5–5 h.

NURSING IMPLICATIONS

Assessment & Drug Effects

- Assess respiratory rate before drug administration. Withhold drug and notify physician if respiratory rate falls below 12 or pre-established rate for child.
- Watch for allergic response in persons with sulfite sensitivity.
- Administer with caution to patients with hepatic or renal impairment.
- Monitor ambulatory patients; nalbuphine may produce drowsiness.
- Watch for respiratory depression of newborn if drug is used during labor and delivery.
- Avoid abrupt termination of nalbuphine following prolonged use, which may result in symptoms similar to narcotic withdrawal: nausea, vomiting, abdominal cramps, lacrimation, nasal congestion, piloerection, fever, restlessness, anxiety.

Patient & Family Education

- Do not engage in potentially hazardous activities or drive until response to drug is known.
- Avoid alcohol and other CNS depressants.
- Tolerance and dependency may result with long-term use; if used for prolonged period do not discontinue abruptly.
- Do not take OTC medications while on this drug without consulting physician.
- Dry mouth may occur.
- Do not breast feed while taking this drug without consulting physician.

NALIDIXIC ACID

(nal-i-dix′ik)
NegGram
Classifications: URINARY TRACT ANTI-INFECTIVE; ANTIBIOTIC; QUINOLONE
Prototype: Ciprofloxacin
Pregnancy Category: B (second and third trimester)

AVAILABILITY 250 mg, 500 mg, 1 g tablets; 250 mg/5 mL suspension

ACTIONS Synthetic quinolone. Intracellular action (by unknown mechanism) inhibits microbial DNA replication and RNA synthesis.

THERAPEUTIC EFFECTS Marked bactericidal activity against most gram-negative urinary tract pathogens with the exception of strains of *Pseudomonas*. Also effective against some strains of *Shigella* and *Salmonella*. Gram-positive bacteria are relatively resistant to drug action.

Common adverse effects in *italic;* life-threatening effects <u>underlined</u>; generic names in **bold**; drug classifications in SMALL CAPS; ♣ Canadian drug name; ☯ Prototype drug.

859

USES Urinary tract infections caused by susceptible gram-negative organisms including most *Proteus* strains, *Klebsiella, Enterobacter,* and *Escherichia coli.*

UNLABELED USES GI tract infections caused by susceptible strains of *Shigella sonnei;* prophylaxis of bacteriuria and in bladder irrigation for low-grade cystitis.

CONTRAINDICATIONS History of convulsive disorders; first trimester of pregnancy; infants <3 mo; febrile infants with renal involvement.

CAUTIOUS USE Prepubertal child; second and third trimesters of pregnancy (category B); kidney or liver disease; epilepsy; respiratory insufficiency; patients and breast-feeding infants with G6PD deficiency.

ROUTE & DOSAGE

Urinary Tract Infections

Child: **PO** *>3 mo,* Acute therapy: 55 mg/kg/day in divided doses every 6 h; Chronic therapy: 30 mg/kg/day in equally divided doses every 12 h
>12 y/Adult: **PO** Acute therapy: 1 g q.i.d.; Chronic therapy: 500 mg q.i.d.

STORAGE
Store at 15°–30° C (59°–86° F) in tight container; avoid freezing.

ADMINISTRATION

Oral

- Give with food or milk if drug causes GI distress. Otherwise, give on an empty stomach 1 h before or 2 h after meals. Suspension: Shake well before administering. Raspberry-flavored tablet may be crushed and mixed with fluid or food.

ADVERSE EFFECTS Body as a Whole: Angioedema, fever, chills, arthralgia, hypersensitivity pneumonitis, <u>anaphylaxis</u> (rare). **CNS:** Drowsiness, headache, malaise, dizziness, vertigo, syncope, weakness, myalgia, peripheral neuritis, confusion, excitement, mental depression, seizures, insomnia. **GI:** Abdominal pain, *nausea, vomiting,* diarrhea, cholestasis, transient increase in AST. **Hematologic:** Eosinophilia, hemolytic anemia (especially in G6PD deficiency). **Skin:** Photosensitivity, pruritus, urticaria, rash. **Metabolic:** In premature infants, may cause metabolic acidosis.

DIAGNOSTIC TEST INTERFERENCE False-positive urine tests for *glucose* with *cupric sulfate reagent* (e.g., *Benedict's* or *Clinitest*) but not with *glucose oxidase methods* (e.g., *Clinistix, TesTape*). May cause elevation of *urinary 17-ketosteroids (Zimmerman method)* and *urine vanillylmandelic acid (VMA).*

INTERACTIONS Drug: ANTACIDS, **sucralfate, calcium, magnesium, didanosine,** MULTIVITAMINS (containing **iron** or **zinc**) may decrease absorption of nalidixic acid; may increase hypoprothrombinemic effects of **warfarin.**

PHARMACOKINETICS Absorption: Readily absorbed from GI tract. **Peak:** Urine: 3–4 h. **Distribution:** Crosses placenta; distributed into breast milk.

Metabolism: Partially metabolized in liver; some metabolism in kidneys. **Elimination:** Excreted in urine. **Half-Life:** 6–7 h.

NURSING IMPLICATIONS

Assessment & Drug Effects

- Lab tests: Perform C&S tests prior to initiation of treatment and periodically thereafter. Obtain blood counts and kidney or liver function tests if therapy is continued longer than 2 wk.
- Watch for CNS reactions, which tend to occur 30 min after initiation of treatment or after second or third dose. Infants and children are especially susceptible. Report immediately the onset of marked irritability, vomiting, bulging of anterior fontanelle, headache, excitement or drowsiness, papilledema, vertigo.

Patient & Family Education

- Use drug exactly as prescribed and do not change dosage. Omitted doses, especially in early days of therapy, may promote development of bacterial resistance. Take full amount of medication.
- Do not take nalidixic acid with highly-alkaline foods, dairy products, or antacids because they may decrease absorption of this drug.
- Contact physician immediately for unexplained behavior changes, severe headaches or seizures.
- Avoid exposure to direct sunlight or ultraviolet light while receiving drug. Contact physician if photosensitivity occurs. You may be photosensitive up to 3 mo after termination of drug.
- Contact your physician if you notice visual disturbances during first few days of therapy. Symptoms usually disappear promptly with reduction of dosage or discontinuation of therapy.
- Maintain adequate hydration according to age and weight during treatment period. Consult physician if you notice a change in your urination pattern.
- Do not breast feed while taking this drug without consulting physician.
- Store this medication out of reach of children.

NALOXONE HYDROCHLORIDE ℗

(nal-ox′one)

Narcan, Narcan Neonatal

Classifications: CENTRAL NERVOUS SYSTEM AGENT; NARCOTIC (OPIATE) ANTAGONIST

Pregnancy Category: B

AVAILABILITY 0.02 mg/mL, 0.4 mg/mL, 1 mg/mL injection

ACTIONS Analog of oxymorphone. A "pure" narcotic antagonist, essentially free of agonistic (morphine-like) properties. Thus, it produces no significant analgesia, respiratory depression, psychotomimetic effects, or miosis when administered in the absence of narcotics and possesses more potent narcotic antagonist action.

THERAPEUTIC EFFECTS Reverses the effects of opiates, including respiratory depression, sedation, and hypotension. Displaces narcotics at opiate receptor sites.

USES Narcotic overdosage; complete or partial reversal of narcotic depression including respiratory depression induced by natural and synthetic narcotics and by pentazocine and propoxyphene. Neonatal opiate depression. Drug of choice when nature of depressant drug is not known and for diagnosis of suspected acute opioid overdosage.
UNLABELED USES Shock and to reverse alcohol-induced or clonidine-induced coma or respiratory depression.

CONTRAINDICATIONS Respiratory depression due to nonopioid drugs. Safety during pregnancy (other than labor) (category B) or lactation is not established.
CAUTIOUS USE Neonates and children; known or suspected narcotic dependence; cardiac irritability.

ROUTE & DOSAGE

Asphyxia Neonatorum
Neonate: **IV** 0.01 mg/kg into umbilical vein or any IV site, may be repeated q2–3min until desired response up to 3 doses. Repeat dosage may be necessary at 1 to 2 h intervals. **Endotracheal (ET) dosing:** 2- to 10-fold higher than IV dosing

Opiate Overdose
Neonates: 5 y or ≤20 kg, **IV** 0.1 mg/kg, may be repeated q2–3min until desired response up to 10 mg if necessary; >5 y or >20 kg, **IV** 2 mg/dose, may be repeated q2–3min until desired response
Adult: **IV** 0.4–2 mg, may be repeated q2–3min up to 10 mg if necessary

Postoperative Opiate Depression
Child: **IV** 0.005–0.01 mg/kg, may be repeated q2–3min until desired response up to 3 doses. Repeat dosage may be necessary at 1 to 2 h intervals
Adult: **IV** 0.1–0.2 mg, may be repeated q2–3min for up to 3 doses until desired response

STORAGE
Use IV solutions diluted with NS, D5W (4 mcg/mL) within 24 h. Store at 15°–30° C (59°–86° F); protect from excessive light

ADMINISTRATION
Endotracheal
Dilute to 3–5 mL with NS. Follow with positive-pressure ventilation.
Intravenous

PREPARE Direct: May be given undiluted. **IV Infusion:** Dilute 2 mg in 500 mL of D5W or NS to yield 4 mcg/mL (0.004 mg/mL). Recommended that 0.02 mg/mL no longer be used in neonates due to potential for high fluid volume overload.

ADMINISTER Direct: Give 0.4 mg or fraction thereof over 10–15 sec adults and over 30 sec in children. **IV Infusion:** Adjust rate according to patient response.
INCOMPATIBILITIES *Do not mix with alkaline solutions.* **Y-Site: Amphotericin B cholesteryl complex.**

ADVERSE EFFECTS Body as a Whole: Reversal of analgesia, tremors, hyperventilation, slight drowsiness, sweating. **CV:** Increased BP, tachycardia. **GI:** Nausea, vomiting. **Hematologic:** Elevated partial thromboplastin time.

INTERACTIONS Drug: Reverses analgesic effects of NARCOTIC (OPIATE) AGONISTS and NARCOTIC (OPIATE) ANGONIST-ANTAGONISTS.

PHARMACOKINETICS Onset: 2 min. **Duration:** 45 min. **Distribution:** Crosses placenta. **Metabolism:** Metabolized in liver. **Elimination:** Excreted in urine. **Half-Life:** Neonate, 1.2–3 h; adult, 30–90 min.

NURSING IMPLICATIONS

Assessment & Drug Effects

- Observe patient closely; duration of action of some narcotics may exceed that of naloxone. Keep physician informed; repeat naloxone dose may be necessary.
- Note: Narcotic abstinence symptoms induced by naloxone generally start to diminish 20–40 min after administration and usually disappear within 90 min.
- Monitor respirations and other vital signs.
- Monitor for associated drug side effects in neonates whose mothers received this drug during labor and delivery.
- Monitor surgical and obstetric patients closely for bleeding. Naloxone has been associated with abnormal coagulation test results.
- Monitor for reversal of analgesia, which may be manifested by nausea, vomiting, sweating, tachycardia.

Patient & Family Education

- Report postoperative pain that emerges after administration of this drug to physician.

NANDROLONE DECANOATE

(nan'droe-lone)
Androlone-D, Deca-Durabolin, Hybolin Decaneate

NANDROLONE PHENPROPIONATE

Durabolin, Hybolin Improved, Nandrobolic
Classifications: HORMONE AND SYNTHETIC SUBSTITUTE; ANABOLIC/ANDROGEN STEROID
Prototype: Testosterone
Pregnancy Category: X
Controlled Substance Schedule III

AVAILABILITY 100 mg/mL, 200 mg/mL injection (in oil)

ACTIONS Synthetic steroid with high ratio of anabolic activity to androgenic activity. Both esters have same actions and uses but differ in duration of action. Decanoate actions last 3–4 wk; phenpropionate ester continues to exert anabolic effect for 1–3 wk.

THERAPEUTIC EFFECTS Increase hemoglobin and red cell mass and increase lean body mass in patients with cachexia (muscle wasting).

USES Control of metastatic breast cancer, management of anemia of renal insufficiency.

CONTRAINDICATIONS Males with prostate or breast cancer; women with breast cancer, liver dysfunction, nephrotic syndrome, hypercalcemia; pregnancy (category X), lactation.

CAUTIOUS USE History of MI, diabetes, epilepsy, or migraines; children.

ROUTE & DOSAGE

Anemia (Decanoate)
Child: **IM** 2–13 y, 25–50 mg q3–4wk
Adult: **IM** 50–200 mg/wk

ADMINISTRATION

Intramuscular

- Follow agency policy regarding IM injections in children. See Part I for description of administration of IM injections to children for safe site locations. Rotate sites.
- Inject drug deep IM.
- Intermittent therapy is usually recommended (4-mo course of treatment followed by 6–8-wk rest period).

ADVERSE EFFECTS Body as a Whole: Muscle cramps. **GI:** *Nausea, vomiting,* diarrhea, anorexia, abdominal fullness, cholestatic jaundice, <u>hepatic necrosis, hepatocellular neoplasms</u>. **Hematologic:** Leukopenia. **Metabolic:** Sodium, chloride, water, potassium, phosphate, and calcium retention, ankle edema, glucose intolerance, increased cholesterol. **CNS:** Excitation, insomnia, chills, toxic confusion. **Endocrine:** *Acne, virilization.*

INTERACTIONS Drug: May increase hypoprothrombinemic effects of **warfarin;** may decrease **insulin** and SULFONYLUREA requirements; CORTICOSTEROIDS may increase edema. **Herbal: Echinacea** may increase risk of hepatotoxicity.

PHARMACOKINETICS Absorption: Slowly absorbed from IM injection site over 4 days. **Peak:** 3–6 days. **Metabolism:** Metabolized in liver to active metabolite. **Half-Life:** 6–8 days.

NURSING IMPLICATIONS

Assessment & Drug Effects

- Lab tests: Obtain baseline and periodic liver function evaluations and electrolyte levels especially serum calcium.

- Monitor for S&S of hepatic toxicity (see Appendix D-1) and electrolyte imbalance, especially hyperkalemia and hypercalcemia (see Appendix D-1).
- Take bone maturation radiographs (wrist) prior to and monitor during treatment to assess for drug accelerating bone growth. Monitor for signs of precious puberty in males <7 y. Semen evaluations should be performed in adolescents every 3–4 mo.
- Monitor diabetics for loss of glycemic control.

Patient & Family Education

- Note: In women, the drug may cause virilization (e.g., increased facial and body hair, deepening of voice).
- Do not breast feed while taking this drug.

NAPHAZOLINE HYDROCHLORIDE 💿

(naf-az'oh-leen)

Ak-Con, Albalon, Allerest, Clear Eyes, Comfort, Degest-2, Muro's Opcon, Nafazair, Naphcon, Privine, VasoClear, Vasocon

Classifications: EYE, EAR, NOSE AND THROAT (EENT) PREPARATION; VASO-CONSTRICTOR; DECONGESTANT; AUTONOMIC NERVOUS SYSTEM AGENT; ALPHA-ADRENERGIC AGONIST (SYMPATHOMIMETIC)

Pregnancy Category: C

N

AVAILABILITY 0.012%, 0.02%, 0.03%, 0.1% ophthalmic solution; 0.05% nasal solution

ACTIONS Direct-acting imidazoline derivative with marked alpha-adrenergic activity. Differs from other sympathomimetic amines in that systemic absorption may cause CNS depression rather than stimulation.

THERAPEUTIC EFFECTS Produces rapid and prolonged vasoconstriction of arterioles, thereby decreasing fluid exudation and mucosal engorgement.

USES Nasal decongestant and ocular vasoconstrictor. For short-term use only (3–5 days).

CONTRAINDICATIONS Narrow-angle glaucoma; concomitant use with MAO inhibitors or tricyclic antidepressants. Safety during pregnancy (category C), lactation, or in infants is not established.

CAUTIOUS USE Hypertension, cardiac irregularities; diabetes; hyperthyroidism; children <6 y.

ROUTE & DOSAGE

Congestion

Child 6–12 y: **Intranasal** 1 drop or 1 spray of 0.05% solution q6h for no more than 3–5 days

Child >12 y/Adult: **Intranasal** 1–2 drops or 1–2 sprays of 0.05% solution in each nostril q3–6h for no more than 3–5 days.

Common adverse effects in *italic;* life-threatening effects underlined; generic names in **bold;** drug classifications in SMALL CAPS; ◆ Canadian drug name; 💿 Prototype drug.

Ophthalmic

Child >6 y/Adult: Instill 1–2 drops of a 0.01 to 0.1% solution q3–4h for no more than 3–4 days.

STORAGE

Store at 15°–30° C (59°–86° F); protect from freezing

ADMINISTRATION

Instillation Nasal

- Instill nasal spray with patient in upright position. If administered in reclining position, a stream rather than a spray may be ejected, with possibility of systemic reaction.
- Minimize amount of drug swallowed by taking care not to direct the flow toward nasopharynx and by positioning patient properly with the head tilted slightly downward.

Ophthalmic

See Part I of book for instillation. Apply pressure to the lacrimal sac for 1–2 min following drop instillation into the conjunctiva.

ADVERSE EFFECTS Body as a Whole: Hypersensitivity reactions, headache, nausea, weakness, sweating, drowsiness, hypothermia, <u>coma</u>. **CV:** Hypertension, bradycardia, <u>shock-like hypotension</u>. **CNS:** CNS depression, especially in infants and with large doses. **Special Senses:** Transient nasal stinging or burning, dryness of nasal mucosa, pupillary dilation, increased intraocular pressure, rebound redness of the eye.

INTERACTIONS Drug: TRICYCLIC ANTIDEPRESSANTS, **maprotiline** may potentiate pressor effects. Discontinue prior anesthetics because they may cause myocardial sensitization to sympathomimetics.

PHARMACOKINETICS Onset: Within 10 min. **Duration:** 2–6 h.

NURSING IMPLICATIONS

Assessment & Drug Effects

- Watch for rebound congestion and chemical rhinitis with frequent and continued use.
- Monitor BP periodically for development or worsening of hypertension, especially with ophthalmic route.
- Overdose: Bradycardia and hypotension can result. Report promptly.

Patient & Family Education

- Do not exceed prescribed regimen since it may cause rebound congestion. Systemic effects can result from swallowing excessive medication.
- Discontinue medication and contact prescriber if nasal congestion is not relieved after 5 days or if ocular pain, vision changes, or ocular symptoms are not improved in 4 days.
- Prevent contamination of eye solution by taking care not to touch eyelid or surrounding area with dropper tip.
- Do not share this medication with others or give to children under 6 y, especially infants.

- Contact prescriber if symptoms worsen.
- Do not breast feed while taking this drug without consulting physician.
- Store this medication out of reach of children.

NAPROXEN

(na-prox′en)

Apo-Naproxen ◆, EC-Naprosyn, Naprelan, Naprosyn, Naxen ◆, Novonaprox ◆

NAPROXEN SODIUM

Aleve, Anaprox, Anaprox DS

Classifications: CENTRAL NERVOUS SYSTEM AGENT; ANALGESIC; NSAID; ANTIPYRETIC
Prototype: Ibuprofen
Pregnancy Category: B

AVAILABILITY 200 mg, 250 mg, 375 mg, 500 mg tablets; 375 mg, 500 mg sustained-release tablets; 125 mg/5 mL suspension

ACTIONS Propionic acid derivative. NSAID with properties similar to those of other propionic acid derivatives, e.g., ibuprofen, fenoprofen, ketoprofen. Mechanism of action thought to be related to inhibition of prostaglandin synthesis.
THERAPEUTIC EFFECTS Analgesic, anti-inflammatory and antipyretic effects; also inhibits platelet aggregation and prolongs bleeding time but does not alter whole blood clotting, prothrombin time or platelet count. Cross-sensitivity with other NSAIDs has been reported.

USES Anti-inflammatory and analgesic effects in symptomatic treatment of acute and chronic rheumatoid arthritis, juvenile arthritis (naproxen only), and for treatment of primary dysmenorrhea. Also management of ankylosing spondylitis, osteoarthritis, and gout. Used for mild to moderate pain and fever.
UNLABELED USES Paget's disease of bone, Bartter's syndrome.

CONTRAINDICATIONS Active peptic ulcer; patients in whom asthma, rhinitis, urticaria, bronchospasm, or shock is precipitated by aspirin or other NSAIDS. Safety during pregnancy (category B), lactation, or in children <2 y is not established.
CAUTIOUS USE History of upper GI tract disorders; impaired kidney, liver, or cardiac function; patients on sodium restriction, low pretreatment Hgb concentration; fluid retention, hypertension, heart failure.

ROUTE & DOSAGE

Note: 275 mg naproxen sodium = 250 mg naproxen.

Inflammatory Disease

Child: **PO** >2 y, 10–15 mg/kg/day in 2 equally divided doses (max 1000 mg/day)
Adult: **PO** 250–500 mg b.i.d. (max 1000 mg/day naproxen; 1100 mg/day naproxen sodium); Naprelan is dosed daily

N

Mild to Moderate Pain, Dysmenorrhea

Child: **PO** >2 y, 5–7 mg/kg/dose q8–12h
Adult: **PO** 500 mg followed by 200–250 mg q6–8h prn up to 1250 mg/day

STORAGE

Store at 15°–30° C (59°–86° F) in tightly closed container; protect from freezing.

ADMINISTRATION

Oral

- For accurate dosing of child, use suspension. Shake suspension well before giving (orange, pineapple flavored).
- Ensure that sustained-release or enteric-coated form is not chewed or crushed. It must be swallowed whole.
- Give with food or an antacid (if prescribed) to reduce incidence of GI upset.

ADVERSE EFFECTS CNS: *Headache, drowsiness, dizziness,* lightheadedness, depression. **CV:** Palpitation, dyspnea, peripheral edema, CHF, tachycardia. **Special Senses:** Blurred vision, tinnitus, hearing loss. **GI:** *Anorexia, heartburn,* indigestion, *nausea,* vomiting, thirst, <u>GI bleeding</u>, elevated serum ALT, AST. **Hematologic:** Thrombocytopenia, leukopenia, eosinophilia, inhibited platelet aggregation, agranulocytosis (rare). **Skin:** Pruritus, rash, skin sensitivity, ecchymosis. **Urogenital:** Nephrotoxicity. **Respiratory:** Pulmonary edema.

DIAGNOSTIC TEST INTERFERENCE Transient elevations in ***BUN*** and serum ***alkaline phosphatase*** may occur. Naproxen may interfere with some urinary assays of ***5-HIAA*** and may cause falsely high ***urinary 17-KGS*** levels (using ***m-dinitrobenzene reagent***). Naproxen should be withdrawn 72 h before adrenal function tests.

INTERACTIONS Drug: Bleeding time effects of ORAL ANTICOAGULANTS, **heparin** may be prolonged; may increase **lithium** toxicity. Increases serum concentrations of methotrexate. **Herbal: Feverfew, garlic, ginger, ginkgo, ginseng, dong quai** may increase bleeding potential. Increased risk of photosensitivity with St. John's wort. **Food:** Alcohol increases risk of GI reactions.

PHARMACOKINETICS Absorption: Almost completely absorbed from GI tract when taken on empty stomach. **Peak:** 2–4 h naproxen; 1–2 h naproxen sodium. **Duration:** 7 h. **Metabolism:** Metabolized in liver. **Elimination:** Excreted primarily in urine; some biliary excretion (<1%). **Half-Life:** Child, 8–10 h; adult, 12–15 h.

NURSING IMPLICATIONS

Assessment & Drug Effects

- Take detailed drug history prior to initiation of therapy. Observe for signs of allergic response in those with aspirin or other NSAID sensitivity.

Common adverse effects in *italic;* life-threatening effects <u>underlined</u>; generic names in **bold;** drug classifications in SMALL CAPS; ♣ Canadian drug name; ⦿ Prototype drug.

- Lab tests: Obtain baseline and periodic evaluations of Hgb and kidney and liver function in patients receiving prolonged or high-dose therapy.
- Schedule baseline and periodic auditory and ophthalmic examinations in patients receiving prolonged or high dose therapy.
- Monitor therapeutic effectiveness. Patients with arthritis may experience symptomatic relief (reduction in joint pain, swelling, stiffness) within 24–48 h with naproxen sodium therapy and in 2–4 wk with naproxen.

Patient & Family Education
- Take with full glass of water or other fluids, or generous amount appropriate for age.
- Be aware that the therapeutic effect of naproxen may not be experienced for 3–4 wk.
- Do not take for management of minor discomfort.
- Do not drive or engage in potentially hazardous activities until response to drug is known.
- Avoid alcohol and aspirin (as well as other NSAIDS and OTC combination products containing NSAIDS) unless otherwise advised by a health care provider. Potential to increase risk of GI ulceration and bleeding.
- Tell your dentist or surgeon if you are taking naproxen before any treatment; it may prolong bleeding time.
- Do not take during pregnancy, especially close to term, unless under close supervision of care provider.
- Do not breast feed while taking this drug without consulting physician.
- Store this medication out of reach of children.

NEDOCROMIL SODIUM
(ned'o-cro-mil)
Tilade, Alocril
Classifications: ANTI-INFLAMMATORY; MAST CELL STABILIZER; ANTIASTHMATIC
Prototype: Cromolyn sodium
Pregnancy Category: B

AVAILABILITY 1.75 mg aerosol inhaler; 2% ophthalmic solution

ACTIONS Inhibits activation of and mediators release from inflammatory cell types associated with asthma (e.g., neutrophils, mast cells, monocytes).
THERAPEUTIC EFFECTS Inhibits release of inflammatory mediators including histamine and prostaglandin D$_2$. Has no intrinsic bronchodilator, antihistamine, or glucocorticoid effects.

USE Maintenance therapy for patients with mild to moderate asthma. Only used in conjunction with first- and second-line agents. Ocular use for allergic conjunctivitis.

CONTRAINDICATIONS Hypersensitivity to nedocromil; acute bronchospasm, particularly status asthmaticus.
CAUTIOUS USE Pregnancy (category B), lactation. Safety and effectiveness in children <6 y are not established.

ROUTE & DOSAGE

Asthma

Child >6 y/Adult: **Inhalation** 2 inhalations 2–4 times per day at regular intervals. **NOT** for acute asthma attacks

Allergic Conjunctivitis

Child >3 y/Adult: 1–2 drops in each eye twice a day during allergen exposure

ADMINISTRATION

Inhalation

- Shake inhaler prior to usage. Use correct administration technique to ensure maximum drug efficacy. Review instruction leaflet supplied by manufacturer.
- Reduce dosage in stages, with each lower dose maintained for several weeks of good control prior to further decreasing dose.

Opthmalic

See Part I for proper instillation technique.

ADVERSE EFFECTS GI: *Abnormal bitter taste,* nausea, vomiting. **CNS:** Headache, dizziness. **Respiratory:** Sore throat irritation, cough. **ENT:** Dry mouth with inhaled preparation; unpleasant taste and nasal congestion with ocular preparation. Conjunctivitis, photophobia, dryness, redness, and itching.

INTERACTIONS Drug: No clinically significant interactions established.

PHARMACOKINETICS Absorption: 90% of dose is deposited in throat and swallowed. Less than 7% is absorbed systemically in patients with asthma. **Onset:** 1 wk for therapeutic effect. **Peak:** 10–20 min. **Metabolism:** Does not appear to be metabolized. **Elimination:** 6% excreted in urine in 72 h. **Half-Life:** 2.3 h.

NURSING IMPLICATIONS

Assessment & Drug Effects

- Assess for coughing and bronchospasms induced by nedocromil. These are indications for discontinuation of drug and should be promptly reported.
- Monitor patients for whom systemic or inhaled steroid therapy has been reduced, because nedocromil may not fully substitute for the decrease in dose of steroid.

Patient & Family Education

- Learn to administer the drug properly. Review patient instruction leaflet.
- Clean oral inhaler at least twice a week. Do not immerse canister in water because it may block aerosol valve stem.
- Do not use it to treat acute bronchospasms because nedocromil is not a bronchodilator.

- May take up to 1 wk before therapeutic effects are achieved.
- May cause dry mouth.
- Continue regular nedocromil therapy even during symptom-free periods.
- Prevent contamination of eye solution by taking care not to touch eyelid or surrounding area with dropper tip.
- Use only as directed and do not share this medication with others.
- Do not breast feed while taking this drug without consulting physician.
- Store this medication out of reach of children.

NELFINAVIR MESYLATE

(nel-fin'a-vir)

Viracept

Classifications: ANTI-INFECTIVE AGENT; ANTIRETROVIRAL AGENT; PROTEASE INHIBITOR

Prototype: Saquinavir

Pregnancy Category: C

AVAILABILITY 250 mg tablets; 50 mg/g powder for oral suspension

ACTIONS Inhibits HIV-1 protease, which is responsible for the production of HIV-1 viral particles in an infected individual.

THERAPEUTIC EFFECTS Inhibition of the viral protease prevents the cleavage of the viral polypeptide, resulting in the production of an immature, noninfectious virus. Indicated by decreased viral load.

USE Treatment of HIV infection in combination with other antiviral agents (use of 3 antiviral drugs now recommended)

CONTRAINDICATIONS Hypersensitivity to nelfinavir; concurrent administration with terfenadine, astemizole, cisapride, amiodarone, quinidine, rifampin, triazolam, or midazolam; lactation.

CAUTIOUS USE Liver function impairment, hemophilia; phenylkentonuria, pregnancy (category C). Safety and effectiveness in children <2 y are not established.

ROUTE & DOSAGE

HIV Infection

Neonates: **PO** Investigational form PACTG 353: 40 mg/kg/dose b.i.d.
Child: **PO** 2–13 y (early puberty, Tanner Stages I to II) 20–30 mg/kg t.i.d. with food (max 750 mg/dose)
Adult: **PO** (late puberty, Tanner Stages IV and V) 750 mg t.i.d. or 1250 mg b.i.d. with food

STORAGE

Store at 15°–30° C (59°–86° F). Do not store mixed oral powders for longer than 6 h.

Common adverse effects in *italic;* life-threatening effects <u>underlined</u>; generic names in **bold;** drug classifications in SMALL CAPS; ✦ Canadian drug name; ⊘ Prototype drug.

871

ADMINISTRATION

Oral

- Give with a meal or light snack.
- Oral powder should be added to fluid and may be mixed with a small amount of water, milk, soy milk, or dietary supplements, pudding, or ice cream; liquid should be consumed immediately. Do not mix oral powder, crushed tablets, or tablet with acid food or juice (e.g., orange or apple juice, or applesauce), which can depart bitter taste to mixture.
- This drug contains 11.2 mg of phenylalanine per gram and will affect those with phenylketonuria.

ADVERSE EFFECTS Body as a Whole: Allergic reactions, back pain, fever, malaise, pain, asthenia, myalgia, arthralgia. **CNS:** Headache, anxiety, depression, dizziness, insomnia, seizures. **GI:** Abdominal pain, *diarrhea,* nausea, flatulence, anorexia, dyspepsia, <u>GI bleeding</u>, hepatitis, vomiting, pancreatitis, increased liver function tests. **Hematologic:** Anemia, leukopenia, thrombocytopenia. **Respiratory:** Dyspnea, pharyngitis, rhinitis. **Skin:** Rash (erythmatous with generalized maculopapules), pruritus, sweating, urticaria.

INTERACTIONS Drug: Other PROTEASE INHIBITORS, **ketoconazole** may increase nelfinavir levels; **rifabutin, rifampin** may decrease nelfinavir levels; nelfinavir may decrease methodone levels, nelfinavir will decrease ORAL CONTRACEPTIVE levels; may increase levels of **atorvastatin, simvastatin. Herbal: St. John's wort** may decrease antiretroviral activity. **Food:** Acidic juices and foods depart bitter taste.

PHARMACOKINETICS Absorption: Food increases the amount of drug absorbed. **Distribution:** >98% protein bound. **Metabolism:** Metabolized in the liver by CYP3A. **Elimination:** Primarily excreted in feces. **Half-Life:** 3.5–5 h.

NURSING IMPLICATIONS

Assessment & Drug Effects

- Monitor hemophiliacs (type A or B) closely for spontaneous bleeding.
- Monitor carefully patients with hepatic impairment for toxic drug effects.

Patient & Family Education

- Drug must be taken exactly as prescribed. Do not alter dose or discontinue drug without consulting physician.
- This drug is not a cure for HIV
- Use a barrier contraceptive even if using hormonal contraceptives.
- Be aware that diarrhea is a common adverse effect that can usually be controlled by OTC medications.
- May cause redistribution of body fat with loss from face arms and legs, and increase in fat in trunk, breasts, upper back, and neck.
- Do not breast feed while taking this drug.
- Store this medication out of reach of children.

Common adverse effects in *italic;* life-threatening effects <u>underlined</u>; generic names in **bold;** drug classifications in SMALL CAPS; ♣ Canadian drug name; ● Prototype drug.

NEOMYCIN SULFATE

(nee-oh-mye'sin)
Mycifradin, Myciguent, Neo-Tabs, Neo-Fradin
Classifications: ANTI-INFECTIVE; AMINOGLYCOSIDE ANTIBIOTIC
Prototype: Gentamicin
Pregnancy Category: D

AVAILABILITY 500 mg tablet; 125 mg/5 mL oral solution; 3.5 mg/g (0.5%) ointment, cream

ACTIONS Aminoglycoside antibiotic obtained from *Streptomyces fradiae;* reported to be the most potent in neuromuscular blocking action and the most toxic of this group.

THERAPEUTIC EFFECTS Active against a wide variety of gram-negative bacteria, including *Citrobacter, Escherichia coli, Enterobacter, Klebsiella, Proteus* (including indole-positive and indole-negative strains), *Pseudomonas aeruginosa,* and *Serratia* sp. Also effective against certain gram-positive organisms, particularly, penicillin-sensitive and some methicillin-resistant strains of *Staphylococcus aureus* (MRSA).

USES Severe diarrhea caused by enteropathogenic *Escherichia coli;* preoperative intestinal antisepsis; to inhibit nitrogen-forming bacteria of GI tract in patients with cirrhosis or hepatic coma and for urinary tract infections caused by susceptible organisms. Also topically for short-term treatment of eye, ear, and skin infections. Available in a variety of creams, ointments, and sprays in combination with other antibiotics and corticosteroids.

CONTRAINDICATIONS Use of oral drug in patients with intestinal obstruction; ulcerative bowel lesions; topical applications over large skin areas; parenteral use in patients with kidney disease or impaired hearing; gravis; pregnancy (category D), lactation.

CAUTIOUS USE Renal failure. Topical otic applications in patients with perforated eardrum, children.

ROUTE & DOSAGE

Infant/Child: **PO** 50–100 mg/kg/day in equally divided doses q6–8h
Adult: 4–12 g/day in equally divided doses q4–6h for 5–6 days

Intestinal Antisepsis

Child: **PO** 90 mg/kg/day in equally divided doses q4h for 2–3 days
Adult: **PO** 6 g/day in equally divided doses q4h for 2–3 days *or* 1 g every hour for 4 doses; then 1 g every 4 h for 5 doses

Hepatic Coma

Child: **PO** 2.5–7 g/m^2/day in equally divided doses q4–6h for 5–6 days (max dose 12 g/day)
Adult: **PO** 4–12 g/day in 4 divided doses for 5–6 days

Diarrhea

Neonates: 50 mg/kg/day in equally divided doses q6h
Child: **PO** 8.75 mg/kg q6h for 2–3 days

Adult: **PO** 50 mg/kg in 4 divided doses for 2–3 days **IM** 1.3–2.6 mg/kg q6h

Cutaneous Infections

Child/Adult: **Topical** Apply a thin layer 2–4 times/day

Otic Suspension or Solutions

Child: 3 drops to infected ear canal 3–4 times per day
Adult: 4 drops to infected ear canal 3–4 times per day

Opthalmic

Child/Adult: **Ointment** Instill a small strip into conjunctival sac of infected eye daily to 4 times per day **Suspension** Instill 1–2 drops 2–4 times per day into infected eye

---

STORAGE

Store at 15°–30° C (59°–86° F) in tight, light-resistant containers.

ADMINISTRATION

Oral

- Oral solution is cherry flavored.
- Preoperative bowel preparation: Saline laxative is generally given immediately before neomycin therapy is initiated.

Topical

- Consult prescriber about what to use for cleansing skin before each application.
- Make sure ear canal is intact, clean, and dry prior to instillation for topical therapy of external ear.

ADVERSE EFFECTS Body as a Whole: Neuromuscular blockade with muscular and respiratory paralysis; hypersensitivity reactions. **GI:** Mild laxative effect, diarrhea, nausea, vomiting; prolonged therapy: malabsorption-like syndrome including cyanocobalamin (vitamin B_{12}) deficiency, low serum cholesterol. **Urogenital:** Nephrotoxicity. **Special Senses:** Ototoxicity, ringing in the ears. **Skin:** *Redness,* scaling, pruritus, contact dermatitis.

INTERACTIONS Drug: May decrease absorption of **cyanocobalamin, digoxin, methotrexate,** nephrotoxicity increases with **acyclovir, amphotericin B, cephalothin, cisplatin, aminoglycosides,** and **vancomycin.** Loop diuretics increase risk of ototoxicity; dimenhydrinate can mask symptoms of ototoxicity. This drug may inhibit bacteria necessary for vitamin K synthesis; monitor for bleeding if anticoagulants are being used concurrently.

PHARMACOKINETICS Absorption: 3% absorbed from GI tract in adults; up to 10% absorbed in neonates, readily absorbed through abraded skin. **Peak:** 1–4 h. **Elimination:** 97% excreted unchanged in feces. **Half-Life:** 2–3 h. Dialyzable from 50 to 100%.

NURSING IMPLICATIONS

Assessment & Drug Effects

- Perform audiometric studies twice weekly in patients with kidney or liver dysfunction receiving extended oral therapy.

- Lab tests: Obtain baseline and daily urinalysis for albumin, casts, and cells, and BUN every other day. Also, serum drug levels (toxic levels reportedly range from 8 to 30 mcg/mL, although individual variations exist).
- Monitor I&O in patients receiving oral or parenteral therapy. Report oliguria or changes in I&O ratio. Inadequate neomycin excretion results in high serum drug levels and risk of nephrotoxicity and ototoxicity.
- Encourge adequate fluid intake for age and weight.

Patient & Family Education
- Stop treatment and consult your prescriber if irritation occurs when you are using topical neomycin. Allergic dermatitis is common.
- Report any unusual symptom related to ears or hearing (e.g., tinnitus, roaring sounds, loss of hearing acuity, dizziness).
- Do not exceed prescribed dosage or duration of therapy.
- Do not breast feed while taking this drug.
- Store this medication out of reach of children.

NEOSTIGMINE BROMIDE 💊
(nee-oh-stig′meen)
Prostigmin

NEOSTIGMINE METHYLSULFATE
Prostigmin
Classifications: AUTONOMIC NERVOUS SYSTEM AGENT; CHOLINERGIC (PARASYMPATHOMIMETIC) AGENT; CHOLINESTERASE INHIBITOR
Pregnancy Category: C

AVAILABILITY 15 mg tablets; 0.5 mg/mL, 1 mg/mL injection

ACTIONS Produces reversible cholinesterase inhibition or inactivation. Has direct stimulant action on voluntary muscle fibers and possibly on autonomic ganglia and CNS neurons.

THERAPEUTIC EFFECTS Allows intensified and prolonged effect of acetylcholine at cholinergic synapses (basis for use in myasthenia gravis). Also produces generalized cholinergic response including miosis, increased tonus of intestinal and skeletal muscles, constriction of bronchi and ureters, slower pulse rate, and stimulation of salivary and sweat glands.

USES To prevent and treat postoperative abdominal distention and urinary retention; for symptomatic control of and sometimes for differential diagnosis of myasthenia gravis; and to reverse the effects of nondepolarizing muscle relaxants (e.g., tubocurarine).

CONTRAINDICATIONS Hypersensitivity to neostigmine, cholinergics, or bromides; bradycardia, hypotension; mechanical obstruction of intestinal or urinary tract; peritonitis; administration with other cholinergic drugs; pregnancy (category C), lactation.
CAUTIOUS USE Recent ileorectal anastomoses; epilepsy; bronchial asthma; bradycardia, recent coronary occlusion; vagotonia; hyperthyroidism; cardiac arrhythmias; peptic ulcer.

ROUTE & DOSAGE

Diagnosis of Myasthenia Gravis

Discontinue all anticholinesterase drugs 8 h before giving this drug and atropine should be given (adult IM and child SC) 30 min before test or IV immediately before neostigmine).
Child: **SC** 0.025–0.04 mg/kg as a single dose
Adult: **IM** 0.022 mg/kg, as a single dose

Treatment of Myasthenia Gravis

Child: **PO** 2 mg/kg/day given 6–8 times/day (max dose 375 mg/day)
IM/IV/SC 0.01–0.04 mg/kg q2–4h
Adult: **PO** 15–375 mg/day in 3–6 divided doses **IM/IV/SC** 0.5–2.5 mg q1–3h

Reversal of Nondepolarizing Neuromuscular Blockade

Infant: **IV** 0.025–0.1 mg/kg/dose
Child: **IV** 0.025–0.08 mg/kg/dose
Adult: **IV** 0.5–2.5 mg/dose (max dose 5 mg)

Postoperative Distention and Urinary Retention

Adult: **IM/SC** 0.25 mg q4–6h for 2–3 days

STORAGE

Store at 15°–30° C (59°–86° F) protect neostigmine methylsulfate from light.

ADMINISTRATION

Note: Size of oral dose is considerably larger than that of parenteral dose because drug is poorly absorbed when taken orally (15 mg of oral drug is approximately equivalent to 0.5 mg of parenteral form).

Oral

■ Give with food or milk to reduce GI distress.

Intramuscular/Subcutaneous

■ Give undiluted. Note 1 mg = 1 mL of 1:1000 solution: 0.5 mg = 1 mL of the 1:2000 solution: 0.25 mg = 1 mL of the 1:4000 solution.

Intravenous

PREPARE Direct: Give undiluted.
ADMINISTER Direct: Give at a rate of 0.5 mg or a fraction thereof over 1 min.

ADVERSE EFFECTS Body as a Whole: Muscle cramps, *fasciculations,* twitching, pallor, fatigability, generalized weakness, paralysis, agitation, fear, <u>death</u>. **CV:** Tightness in chest, bradycardia, hypotension, elevated BP. **GI:** *Nausea,* vomiting, eructation, epigastric discomfort, abdominal cramps, diarrhea, involuntary or difficult defecation. **CNS:** CNS stimulation. **Respiratory:** *Increased salivation* and bronchial secretions, sneezing, cough, dyspnea, diaphoresis, respiratory depression. **Special Senses:** Lacrimation, miosis, blurred vision. **Urogenital:** Difficult micturition.

INTERACTIONS Drug: Succinylcholine decamethonium may prolong phase I block or reverse phase II block; neostigmine antagonizes effects of **tubocurarine; atracurium, vecuronium, pancuronium; procainamide, quinidine, atropine** antagonize effects of neostigmine.

PHARMACOKINETICS Absorption: Poorly absorbed from GI tract (1–2%). **Onset:** 10–30 min IM or IV; 2–4 h PO. **Peak:** 20–30 min IM or IV; 1–2 h PO. **Distribution:** Not reported to cross placenta or appear in breast milk. **Metabolism:** Hydrolyzed by cholinesterases; also metabolized in liver. **Elimination:** 80% of drug and metabolites excreted in urine within 24 h. **Half-Life:** 50–90 min.

NURSING IMPLICATIONS

Assessment & Drug Effects

- Check pulse before giving drug to bradycardic patients. If below 60/min or other established parameter for child, consult physician. Atropine will be ordered to restore heart rate.
- Monitor pulse, respiration, and BP during period of dosage adjustment in treatment of myasthenia gravis.
- Report promptly and record accurately the onset of myasthenic symptoms and drug adverse effects in relation to last dose in order to assist physician in determining lowest effective dosage schedule.
- Reduce possible GI (muscarinic) side effects, which occur especially during early therapy, by giving drug with milk or food. Physician may prescribe atropine or other anticholinergic agent to suppress side effects. (*Note:* these drugs may mask toxic symptoms of neostigmine.)
- Note time of muscular weakness onset carefully in myasthenic patients. It may indicate whether patient is in cholinergic or myasthenic crisis: Weakness that appears approximately 1 h after drug administration suggests cholinergic crisis (overdose) and is treated by prompt withdrawal of neostigmine and immediate administration of atropine. Weakness that occurs 3 h or more after drug administration is more likely due to myasthenic crisis (underdose or drug resistance) and is treated by more intensive anticholinesterase therapy.
- Record drug effect and duration of action. S&S of myasthenia gravis relieved by neostigmine include lid ptosis; diplopia; drooping facies; difficulty in chewing, swallowing, breathing, or coughing; and weakness of neck, limbs, and trunk muscles.
- Manifestations of neostigmine overdosage often appear first in muscles of neck and those involved in chewing and swallowing, with muscles of shoulder girdle and upper extremities affected next.
- Monitor respiration, maintain airway or assisted ventilation, and give oxygen as indicated, when used as antidote for tubocurarine or other nondepolarizing neuromuscular blocking agents (usually preceded by atropine). Respiratory assistance is continued until recovery of respiration and neuromuscular transmission is assured.
- Report to physician if patient does not urinate within 1 h after first dose when used to relieve urinary retention.

Patient & Family Education

- Be aware that regulation of dosage interval is extremely difficult; dosage must be adjusted for each patient to deal with unpredictable exacerbations and remissions.

- Be aware that drug therapy is often required both day and night. Larger portions of total dose are given at times of greater fatigue; late afternoon and at mealtimes.
- Keep a diary of "peaks and valleys" of muscle strength.
- Keep an accurate record for physician of your response to drug. Learn how to recognize adverse effects, how to modify dosage regimen according to your changing needs, or how to administer atropine if necessary.
- Be aware that certain factors may require an increase in size or frequency of dose (e.g., physical or emotional stress, infection, menstruation, surgery), whereas remission requires a decrease in dosage.
- Some patients become refractory to neostigmine after prolonged use and require change in dosage or medication.
- Do not breast feed while taking this drug.
- Store this medication out of reach of children.

NEVIRAPINE ⦿

(ne-vir′a-peen)

Viramune

Classifications: ANTI-INFECTIVE; ANTIRETROVIRAL; NONNUCLEOSIDE REVERSE TRANSCRIPTASE INHIBITOR (NNRTI)

Pregnancy Category: C

N

AVAILABILITY 200 mg tablets, 50 mg/5 mL suspension

ACTIONS Nonnucleoside reverse transcriptase inhibitor (NNRTI) of HIV-1. Binds directly to reverse transcriptase and blocks RNA- and DNA-dependent polymerase activities.

THERAPEUTIC EFFECTS Prevents replication of the HIV-1 virus. Does not inhibit HIV-2 reverse transcriptase and DNA polymerases such as alpha, beta, gamma, and delta polymerases. Resistant strains appear rapidly.

USE In combination with other antiviral agents. Three drugs are currently recommended for treatment of HIV.

CONTRAINDICATIONS Hypersensitivity to nevirapine; lactation.

CAUTIOUS USE Liver disease; CNS disorders; pregnancy (category C). Safety and efficacy in neonates and children <2 mo are not established.

ROUTE & DOSAGE

HIV

Neonates ≤3 mo: **PO (investigational study in PACTG 365)** 5 mg/kg/dose once daily for 14 days, then 120 mg/m^2/dose every 12 h for 14 days, then 200 mg/m^2/dose every 12 h

Infants >3 mo–8 y: **PO** 120 mg/m^2 daily for 14 days, then increase, if tolerated, to 120–200 mg/m^2 q12h (max 200 mg/dose every 12 h)

Child >8 y: **PO** 4 mg/kg daily for 14 days, then increase 4 mg/kg/dose q12h, if tolerated (max 200 mg/dose every 12 h)

Adult: **PO** 200 mg once daily for first 14 days, then increase to 200 mg b.i.d.

STORAGE
Store at 15°–30° C (59°–86° F) in a tightly closed container.

ADMINISTRATION

Oral
- Reinitiate with 200 mg/day for 14 days, then increase to b.i.d. dosing, when dosing is interrupted for >7 days.
- Shake suspension prior to giving.
- Can be given with food or antacids.

ADVERSE EFFECTS Body as a Whole: Fever, paresthesia, myalgia. **CNS:** Headache. **GI:** Nausea, diarrhea, abdominal pain, hepatitis, increased liver function tests. **Hematologic:** Anemia, neutropenia. **Skin:** *Rash,* Stevens-Johnson syndrome.

INTERACTIONS Drug: May decrease plasma concentrations of PROTEASE INHIBITORS, ORAL CONTRACEPTIVES, digoxin, phenytoin, and theophylline; may decrease **methadone** levels inducing opiate withdrawal. Do not give with ketaconazole. Nevirapine levels may be decreased with rifampin, rifabutin. The severity of rash increases when used with prednisone. **Herbal: St. John's wort** may decrease antiretroviral activity.

PHARMACOKINETICS Absorption: Rapidly absorbed from GI tract. **Peak:** 4 h. **Distribution:** 60% protein bound, crosses placenta, distributed into breast milk. **Metabolism:** Metabolized in liver by cytochrome P-450-3A (CYP3A). **Elimination:** Excreted primarily in urine. **Half-Life:** 25–40 h.

N

NURSING IMPLICATIONS

Assessment & Drug Effects
- Lab tests: Obtain baseline and periodic liver and kidney function tests, routine blood chemistry, and CBC.
- Monitor weight, temperature, respiratory status with chest x-ray throughout therapy.
- Monitor carefully, especially during first 6 wk of therapy, for severe rash (with or without fever, blistering, oral lesions, conjunctivitis, swelling, joint aches, or general malaise).
- Withhold drug and notify physician if rash develops or liver function tests are abnormal.

Patient & Family Education
- This drug is not a cure for HIV.
- May cause redistribution of body fat with loss from face, arms, and legs, and increase in fat in trunk, breasts, upper back, and neck.
- Withhold drug and notify physician if rash appears, malaise, fever, arthralgia.
- Do not drive or engage in potentially hazardous activities until response to drug is known. There is a high potential for drowsiness and fatigue.
- Use or add barrier contraceptive if using hormonal contraceptive.
- Do not take herbal medications (St. John's wort) while on this drug.
- Do not breast feed while taking this drug.
- Store this medication out of reach of children.

NIACIN (VITAMIN B$_3$, NICOTINIC ACID)
(nye'a-sin)
Niac, Nicobid, Nico-400, Nicolar, Nicotinex, Novoniacin ♣, Slo-Niacin, Tri-B3 ♣

NIACINAMIDE (NICOTINAMIDE)
Classifications: VITAMIN B$_3$; CARDIOVASCULAR AGENT; ANTILIPEMIC; LIPID-LOWERING AGENT
Pregnancy: Category C

AVAILABILITY 50 mg, 100 mg, 250 mg, 500 mg tablets; 125 mg, 250 mg, 400 mg, 500 mg, 750 mg sustained-release tablets, capsules, 50 mg/5 mL elixir

ACTIONS Water-soluble, heat-stable, B-complex vitamin (B$_3$) that functions with riboflavin as a control agent in coenzyme system that converts protein, carbohydrate, and fat to energy through oxidation-reduction. Niacinamide, an amide of niacin, is used as an alternative in the prevention and treatment of pellagra.

THERAPEUTIC EFFECTS Produces vasodilation by direct action on vascular smooth muscles. Inhibits hepatic synthesis of VLDL, cholesterol and triglyceride, and, indirectly, LDL. Large doses effectively reduce elevated serum cholesterol and total lipid levels in hypercholesterolemia and hyperlipidemic states.

USES In prophylaxis and treatment of pellagra, usually in combination with other B-complex vitamins, and in deficiency states accompanying carcinoid syndrome, isoniazid therapy, Hartnup's disease, and chronic alcoholism. Also in adjuvant treatment of hyperlipidemia (elevated cholesterol or triglycerides) in patients who do not respond adequately to diet or weight loss. Also as vasodilator in peripheral vascular disorders, Ménière's disease, and labyrinthine syndrome, as well as to counteract LSD toxicity and to distinguish between psychoses of dietary and nondietary origin.

CONTRAINDICATIONS Hypersensitivity to niacin; hepatic impairment; severe hypotension; hemorrhaging or arterial bleeding; active peptic ulcer; pregnancy (category C), lactation, and children <16 y.
CAUTIOUS USE History of gallbladder disease, liver disease, and peptic ulcer; glaucoma; angina; coronary artery disease; diabetes mellitus; predisposition to gout; allergy, heavy alcohol usage.

ROUTE & DOSAGE

Niacin Deficiency
Adult: **PO** 10–20 mg/day **IV/IM/SC** 25–100 mg 2–5 times/day
Pellagra
Child: **PO** 50–100 mg/dose 3–4 times/day (max dose 500 mg daily)
Adult: **PO** 300–500 mg/day in divided doses

Hyperlipidemia

Child: **PO** 100–250 mg/day in 3 divided doses, may increase by 250 mg/day q2–3wk as tolerated
Adult: **PO** 1.5–3 g/day in divided doses, may increase up to 6 g/day if necessary

STORAGE
Store at 15°–30° C (59°–86° F) in a light- and moisture-proof container.

ADMINISTRATION

Oral

- Give oral drug with meals to decrease GI distress. Give with cold water (not hot beverage) to facilitate swallowing.
- May premedicate with 325 mg aspirin to reduce flushing phenomenon.
- Ensure that sustained-release form is not chewed or crushed. It must be swallowed whole.
- Elixir has 14% alcohol.

Intravenous

PREPARE Intermittent: Dilute 50–100 mg in 500 mL of NS to yield concentrations of 0.1–0.2 mg/mL.
ADMINISTER Intermittent: Give over 12–24 h.

ADVERSE EFFECTS CNS: *Transient headache, tingling of extremities,* syncope. With chronic use: Nervousness, panic, toxic amblyopia, proptosis, blurred vision, loss of central vision. **CV:** *Generalized flushing with sensation of warmth,* postural hypotension, vasovagal attacks, arrhythmias (rare). **GI:** *Abnormalities of liver function tests; jaundice, bloating, flatulence, nausea,* vomiting, GI disorders, activation of peptic ulcer, xerostomia. **Skin:** *Increased sebaceous gland activity,* dry skin, skin rash, *pruritus,* keratitis nigricans. **Metabolic:** Hyperuricemia, hyperglycemia, glycosuria, hypoprothrombinemia, hypoalbuminemia.

DIAGNOSTIC TEST INTERFERENCE Niacin causes elevated serum *bilirubin, uric acid, alkaline phosphatase, AST, ALT, LDH* levels and may cause *glucose intolerance.* Decreases *serum cholesterol* 15–30% and may cause false elevations with certain *fluorometric methods* of determining *urinary catecholamines.* Niacin may cause false-positive *urine glucose* tests using *copper sulfate reagents,* e.g., *Benedict's* solution.

INTERACTIONS Drug: Potentiates hypotensive effects of ANTIHYPERTENSIVE AGENTS. **Food:** Avoid alcohol and hot drinks at time of administration because they can increase flushing and pruritus.

PHARMACOKINETICS Absorption: Readily absorbed from GI tract. **Peak:** 20–70 min. **Distribution:** Distributed into breast milk. **Metabolism:** Metabolized in liver. **Elimination:** Excreted primarily in urine. **Half-Life:** 45 min.

NURSING IMPLICATIONS

Assessment & Drug Effects

- Monitor therapeutic effectiveness and record effect of therapy on clinical manifestations of deficiency (fiery red tongue, excessive saliva secretion and infection of oral membranes, nausea, vomiting, diarrhea, confusion). Therapeutic response usually begins within 24 h.

- Lab tests: Obtain baseline and periodic tests of blood glucose and liver function in patients receiving prolonged high-dose therapy.
- Monitor diabetics and patients on high doses closely. Hyperglycemia, glycosuria, ketonuria, and increased insulin requirements have been reported.
- Observe patients closely for evidence of liver dysfunction (jaundice, dark urine, light-colored stools, pruritus) and hyperuricemia in patients predisposed to gout (flank, joint, or stomach pain; altered urine excretion pattern).
- Vasodilatation effects occur within 20 min of PO drug intake and lasts for 20–60 min. Prescriber may premedicate with 325 mg of asprin to reduce this effect.

Patient & Family Education

- Be aware that you may feel warm and flushed in face, neck, and ears within first 2 h after oral ingestion and immediately after parenteral administration and may last several hours; symptoms may reoccur several times per week when taking sustained-release tablets. Effects may subside as therapy continues.
- Sit or lie down and avoid sudden posture changes if you feel weak or dizzy. Report these symptoms and persistent flushing to your prescriber. Relief may be obtained by reduction of dosage, increasing subsequent doses in small increments.
- Be aware that alcohol and large doses of niacin cause increased flushing and sensation of warmth.
- Do not take vitamins and other OTC medications containing niacin.
- Avoid exposure to direct sunlight until lesions have entirely cleared if you have skin manifestations.
- Do not breast feed while taking this drug.
- Store this medication out of reach of children.

NIFEDIPINE ⊕

(nye-fed′i-peen)

Adalat, Adalat CC, Procardia, Procardia XL

Classifications: CARDIOVASCULAR AGENT; CALCIUM CHANNEL BLOCKER; ANTIARRHYTHMIC (CLASS IV); NONNITRATE VASODILATOR

Pregnancy Category: C

AVAILABILITY 10 mg, 20 mg capsules; 30 mg, 60 mg, 90 mg sustained-release tablets

ACTIONS Calcium channel blocking agent that selectively blocks calcium ion influx across cell membranes of cardiac muscle and vascular smooth muscle without changing serum calcium concentrations. Class IV antiarrhythmic.

THERAPEUTIC EFFECTS Reduces myocardial oxygen utilization and supply and relaxes and prevents coronary artery spasm; has little or no effect on SA and AV nodal conduction with therapeutic dosing. Decreases peripheral vascular resistance and increases cardiac output. Vasodilation of both coronary and peripheral vessels is greater than that produced by verapamil or diltiazem and frequently results in reflex tachycardia. Decreased peripheral vascular resistance also leads to a rise in peripheral blood flow, the basis for use of this drug in treatment of Raynaud's phenomenon. Minimal effect on myocardial contractility.

USES Vasospastic "variant" or Printzmetal's angina and chronic stable angina without vasospasm. Mild to moderate hypertension alone or in combination with a diuretic.
UNLABELED USES Esophageal disorders; vascular headaches; Raynaud's phenomenon; asthma; cardiomyopathy; primary pulmonary hypertension.

CONTRAINDICATIONS Known hypersensitivity to nifedipine. Safety during pregnancy (category C) or in children is not established.
CAUTIOUS USE Concomitant use with hypotensives; CHF; aortic stenosis lactation.

ROUTE & DOSAGE

Angina
Adult: **PO** 10–20 mg t.i.d. up to 180 mg/day

Hypertension
Adolescent/Adult: **PO** 10–20 mg t.i.d. up to 180 mg/day or 30–60 mg sustained release once daily

Hypertensive Emergencies
Child: **PO** 0.25–0.5 mg/kg/dose q4–6h as needed (max dose 10 mg/dose or 1–2 mg/kg/day)

STORAGE
Store at 15°–25° C (59°–77° F); protect from light and moisture.

ADMINISTRATION
Oral
- Do not give within the first 1–2 wk following an MI.
- Liquid filled capsules can be better than the fluid can be swallowed or taken sublingually.
- 10 mg capsule (liquid filled) = 10 mg/0.34 mL; 20 mg capsule (liquid filled) = 20 mg/0.45 mL.
- Use only the sustained-release form to treat chronic hypertension. Ensure that sustained-release form is not chewed or crushed. It must be swallowed whole. Do not give with grapefruit juice.
- Discontinue drug gradually, with close medical supervision to prevent severe hypertension and other adverse effects.

ADVERSE EFFECTS Body as a Whole: Sore throat, weakness, fever, sweating, chills, febrile reaction. **CNS:** *Dizziness, light-headedness,* nervousness, mood changes, weakness, jitteriness, sleep disturbances, blurred vision, retinal ischemia, difficulty in balance, *headache.* **CV:** Hypotension, *facial flushing, heat sensation,* palpitations, *peripheral edema,* MI (rare), prolonged systemic hypotension with overdose. **GI:** Nausea, heartburn, *diarrhea,* constipation, cramps, flatulence, gingival hyperplasia, <u>hepatotoxicity</u>. **Musculoskeletal:** Inflammation, joint stiffness, muscle cramps. **Respiratory:** Nasal congestion, dyspnea, cough, wheezing. **Skin:** Dermatitis, pruritus, urticaria. **Urogenital:** Sexual difficulties, possible male infertility.

DIAGNOSTIC TEST INTERFERENCE Nifedipine may cause mild to moderate increases of *alkaline phosphatase, CPK, LDH, AST, ALT.*

INTERACTIONS Drug: BETA-BLOCKERS may increase likelihood of CHF; may increase risk of **phenytoin, digoxin,** toxicity. **Herbal: Melatonin** may increase blood pressure and heart rate. **Food:** Grapefruit juice may decrease bioavailability of nifedipine.

PHARMACOKINETICS Absorption: Readily absorbed from GI tract; 45–75% reaches systemic circulation (first-pass metabolism). **Onset:** 10–30 min. **Peak:** 30 min. **Distribution:** Distributed into breast milk. **Metabolism:** Metabolized in liver. **Elimination:** 75–80% excreted in urine, 15% in feces. **Half-Life:** 2–5 h.

NURSING IMPLICATIONS

Assessment & Drug Effects
- Monitor BP carefully during titration period. Patient may become severely hypotensive, especially if also taking other drugs known to lower BP. Withhold drug and notify physician if systolic BP <90.
- Monitor blood sugar in diabetic patients. Nifedipine has diabetogenic properties.
- Monitor for gingival hyperplasia and report promptly. This is a rare but serious adverse effect (similar to phenytoin-induced hyperplasia).

Patient & Family Education
- Keep a record of nitroglycerin use and promptly report any changes in previous pattern. Occasionally, people develop increased frequency, duration, and severity of angina when they start treatment with this drug or when dosage is increased.
- Be aware that withdrawal symptoms may occur with abrupt discontinuation of the drug (chest pain, increase in anginal episodes, MI, dysrhythmias).
- Inspect gums visually every day. Changes in gingivae may be gradual, and bleeding may be exhibited only with probing.
- Seek prompt treatment for symptoms of gingival hyperplasia (easy bleeding of gingivae and gradual enlarging of gingival mass, especially on buccal side of lower anterior teeth). Drug will be discontinued if gingival hyperplasia occurs.
- Research shows that smoking decreases the efficacy of nifedipine and has direct and adverse effects on the heart in the patient on nifedipine treatment.
- Sustained-release outer shell may be passed in the stool.
- Do not breast feed while taking this drug without consulting physician.
- Store this medication out of reach of children.

NITAZOXANIDE

(nit-a-zox'-a-nide)
Alinia
Classifications: ANTI-INFECTIVE; ANTIPROTOZOAL
Prototype: Metronidazole
Pregnancy Category: B

AVAILABILITY 100 mg/5 mL powder for reconstitution

ACTIONS Antiprotozoal activity believed to be due to interference with an essential enzyme needed for anaerobic energy metabolism in protozoa. Interference with the enzyme may not be the only pathway by which nitazoxanide exhibits antiprotozoal activity.

THERAPEUTIC EFFECTS Inhibits growth of sporozoites and oocysts of *Cryptosporidium parvum* and trophozoites of *Giardia lamblia*.

USES Treatment of diarrhea caused by *Cryptosporidium parvum* and *Giardia lamblia* in children.

CONTRAINDICATIONS Prior hypersensitivity to nitazoxanide.
CAUTIOUS USE Hepatic and biliary disease, renal disease and combined renal and hepatic disease; safety and efficacy in children <1 y or >11 y have not been studied according to manufacturer; pregnancy (category B); lactation.

N

ROUTE & DOSAGE

Diarrhea
Child: **PO** *12–47 mo,* 100 mg q12h × 3 days; *4–11 y,* 200 mg q12h × 3 days

STORAGE
Suspension may be stored for 7 days at 15°–30° C (59°–86° F), after which any unused portion must be discarded.

ADMINISTRATION
Oral
- Prepare suspension as follows: Tap bottle until powder loosens. Draw up 48 mL of water, add half to bottle, shake to suspend powder, then add remaining 24 mL of water and shake vigorously.
- Give required dose with food.
- Keep container tightly closed, and shake well before each administration.

ADVERSE EFFECTS CNS: Headache. **GI:** Abdominal pain, diarrhea, vomiting.

INTERACTIONS Drug: No clinically significant interactions reported.

PHARMACOKINETICS Peak: 1–4 h. **Distribution:** 99% protein bound. **Metabolism:** Rapidly hydrolyzed to an active metabolite, tizoxanide

---

(desacetyl-nitazoxanide). Tizoxanide then undergoes conjugation, primarily by glucuronidation. Highly protein bound. **Elimination:** Excreted in urine and feces.

NURSING IMPLICATIONS

Assessment & Drug Effects

- Monitor for therapeutic effectiveness: No watery stools and ≤2 soft stools with no hematochezia within the past 24 h or no symptoms and no unformed stools within the past 48 h.
- Monitor closely patients with preexisting hepatic or biliary disease for adverse reactions.
- Assess appetite, level of abdominal discomfort, and extent of bloating.
- Assess frequency and quantity of diarrhea and monitor total hydration status.
- Weigh daily to aid in assessment of possible fluid loss from diarrhea.

Patient & Family Education

- Note that 5 mL of the oral suspension contains approximately 1.5 g of sucrose, which is an important consideration for children with diabetes.
- Report either no improvement in or worsening of diarrhea and abdominal discomfort.
- Do not give to others who have diarrhea.
- Store this medication out of reach of children.

N

NITROFURANTOIN

(nye-troe-fyoor′an-toyn)

Apo-Nitrofurantoin ◆ , Furadantin, Furalan, Furanite, Nephronex ◆ , Nitrofan, Novofuran ◆

NITROFURANTOIN MACROCRYSTALS

Macrobid, Macrodantin

Classification: URINARY TRACT ANTI-INFECTIVE; ANTIBIOTIC
Prototype: Trimethoprim
Pregnancy Category: B

AVAILABILITY 25 mg, 50 mg, 100 mg capsules; 25 mg/mL suspension

ACTIONS Synthetic nitrofuran derivative presumed to act by interfering with several bacterial enzyme systems. Highly soluble in urine and reportedly most active in acid urine. Antimicrobial concentrations in urine exceed those in blood.

THERAPEUTIC EFFECTS Active against wide variety of gram-negative and gram-positive microorganisms, including strains of *Escherichia coli, Staphylococcus aureus, Streptococcus faecalis, enterococci,* and *Klebsiella aerobacter. Pseudomonas aeruginosa* and many strains of *Proteus* are resistant.

USES Pyelonephritis, pyelitis, and cystitis caused by susceptible organisms.

CONTRAINDICATIONS Anuria, oliguria, significant impairment of kidney function (creatinine clearance <40 mL/min); G6PD deficiency; infants <1 mo. Nitrofurantoin dual-release capsules in children <12 y. Safety during pregnancy (category B), pregnancy at term, or lactation is not established. **CAUTIOUS USE** History of asthma, anemia, diabetes, vitamin B deficiency, electrolyte imbalance, G6PD, debilitating disease.

ROUTE & DOSAGE

Pyelonephritis, Cystitis
Child: PO *1 mo–12 y,* 5–7 mg/kg/day in equally divided doses every 6 h (max dose 400 mg/day)
Adult: PO 50–100 mg q.i.d. or Macrobid 100 mg b.i.d.

Chronic Suppressive Therapy
Child: PO *1 mo–12 y,* 1–2 mg/kg/day in 1 dose (max dose 100 mg/day)
Adult: PO 50–100 mg at hour of sleep

STORAGE
Store in tight, light-resistant container at 15°–30° C (59°–86° F).

ADMINISTRATION

Oral
- Give with food or milk to minimize gastric irritation.
- Avoid crushing tablets because of the possibility of tooth staining; rather dilute oral suspension in milk, water, or fruit juice, and rinse mouth thoroughly after taking drug.

ADVERSE EFFECTS CNS: Peripheral neuropathy, headache, nystagmus, drowsiness, vertigo. **GI:** *Anorexia, nausea, vomiting,* abdominal pain, diarrhea, cholestatic jaundice, <u>hepatic necrosis</u>. **Hematologic (rare):** Hemolytic or megaloblastic anemia (especially in patients with G6PD deficiency), granulocytosis, eosinophilia. **Body as a Whole:** Angioedema, <u>anaphylaxis</u>, drug fever, arthralgia. **Respiratory:** Allergic pneumonitis, asthmatic attack (patients with history of asthma), pulmonary sensitivity reactions (<u>interstitial pneumonitis or fibrosis</u>). **Skin:** Skin eruptions, pruritus, urticaria, <u>exfoliative dermatitis</u>, transient alopecia. **Urogenital:** Genitourinary superinfections (especially with *Pseudomonas*), crystalluria (older adult patients), dark yellow or brown urine. **Other:** Tooth staining from direct contact with oral suspension and crushed tablets (infants).

DIAGNOSTIC TEST INTERFERENCE Nitrofurantoin metabolite may produce false-positive *urine glucose* test results with Benedict's reagent.

INTERACTIONS Drug: ANTACIDS may decrease absorption of nitrofurantoin; **nalidixic acid,** other QUINOLONES may antagonize antimicrobial effects; **probenecid, sulfinpyrazone** increase risk of nitrofurantoin toxicity. **Food:** Cranberry juice and other acidifers of urine may increase rate of absorption of nitrofurantoin.

PHARMACOKINETICS Absorption: Readily absorbed from GI tract. **Peak:** Urine: 30 min. **Distribution:** Crosses placenta; distributed into breast milk.

Metabolism: Partially metabolized in liver. **Elimination:** Primarily excreted in urine. **Half-Life:** 20 min.

NURSING IMPLICATIONS

Assessment & Drug Effects

- Lab tests: Perform C&S prior to therapy; recommended in patients with recurrent infections.
- Monitor I&O. Report oliguria and any change in I&O ratio. Drug should be discontinued if oliguria or anuria develops or creatinine clearance falls below 40 mL/min.
- Be alert to signs of urinary tract superinfections (e.g., milky urine, foul-smelling urine, perineal irritation, dysuria).
- Assess for nausea (which occurs fairly frequently). May be relieved by using macrocrystalline preparation (Macrodantin) or by reducing dosage.
- Watch for acute pulmonary sensitivity reaction, usually within first week of therapy. May be manifested by mild to severe flu-like syndrome. Eosinophilia generally develops in a few days. Recovery usually occurs rapidly after drug is discontinued.
- With prolonged therapy, monitor for subacute or chronic pulmonary sensitivity reaction, commonly manifested by insidious onset of malaise, cough, dyspnea on exertion, altered ABGs.
- Be alert for and advise the patient to report onset of muscle weakness, tingling, numbness, or other sensations. Peripheral neuropathy can be severe and irreversible. Drug should be withdrawn immediately.

Patient & Family Education

- Nitrofurantoin may impart a harmless brown color to urine.
- Avoid ingestion of alcohol while on this drug.
- Consult physician regarding fluid intake. Generally, fluids are not increased; however, intake should be adequate for age and weight.
- Do not breast feed while taking this drug without consulting physician.
- Store this medication out of reach of children.

NITROGLYCERIN ℗ᵣ

(nye-troe-gli′ser-in)

Cellegesic, Deponit, Minitran, Nitro-Bid, Nitro-Bid IV, Nitrocap, Nitrodisc, Nitro-Dur, Nitrogard, Nitrogard-SR, Nitroglyn, Nitrol, Nitrolingual, Nitrong, Nitrong SR, Nitrospan, Nitrostat, Nitrostat I.V., Nitro-T.D., Transderm-Nitro, Tridil

Classifications: CARDIOVASCULAR AGENT; NITRATE VASODILATOR
Pregnancy Category: C

AVAILABILITY 0.5 mg/mL, 5 mg/mL, 10 mg/mL, injection; 0.3 mg, 0.4 mg, 0.6 mg sublingual tablets; 0.4 mg/spray translingual spray; 2 mg, 3 mg buccal tablets; 2.5 mg, 6.5 mg, 9 mg, 13 mg sustained-release tablets, capsules; 0.1 mg/h, 0.2 mg/h, 0.3 mg/h, 0.4 mg/h, 0.6 mg/h, 0.8 mg/h transdermal patch; 2% ointment

---

Common adverse effects in *italic*; life-threatening effects <u>underlined</u>; generic names in **bold**; drug classifications in SMALL CAPS; ♣ Canadian drug name; ❷ Prototype drug.

ACTIONS Organic nitrate and potent vasodilator that relaxes vascular smooth muscle by unknown mechanism, resulting in dose-related dilation of both venous and arterial blood vessels. Promotes peripheral pooling of blood, reduction of peripheral resistance, and decreased venous return to the heart. Both left ventricular preload and afterload are reduced and myocardial oxygen consumption or demand is decreased.

THERAPEUTIC EFFECTS Therapeutic doses may reduce systolic, diastolic, and mean BP; heart rate is usually slightly increased. Produces antianginal, anti-ischemic, and antihypertensive effects.

USES Prophylaxis, treatment, and management of angina pectoris. IV nitroglycerin is used to control BP in perioperative hypertension, CHF associated with acute MI; to produce controlled hypotension during surgical procedures, and to treat angina pectoris in patients who have not responded to nitrate or beta-blocker therapy.

UNLABELED USES Sublingual and topical to reduce cardiac workload in patients with acute MI and in CHF. Ointment for adjunctive treatment of Raynaud's disease; ointment also used for inifiltration injury caused by vasoconstrictive drugs.

CONTRAINDICATIONS Hypersensitivity, idiosyncrasy, or tolerance to nitrates; severe anemia; head trauma, increased ICP; glaucoma (sustained-release forms). Also (IV nitroglycerin) hypotension, uncorrected hypovolemia, constrictive pericarditis, pericardial tamponade; pregnancy (category C), lactation.

CAUTIOUS USE Severe liver or kidney disease, conditions that cause dry mouth, early MI.

ROUTE & DOSAGE

Angina

Child: **IV Continuous Infusion** 0.25–0.5 mcg/kg/min, then titrate by 0.5–1 mcg/kg/min q3–5min until desired effect (max dose 20 mcg/kg/min)
Adult: **Sublingual** 1–2 sprays (0.4–0.8 mg) or a 0.3–0.6 mg tablet q3–5min as needed (max 3 doses in 15 min) **PO** 1.3–9 mg q8–12h **IV** Start with 5 mcg/min and titrate q3–5min until desired response **Transdermal Unit** Apply once q24h or leave on for 10–12 h, then remove and have a 10–12 h nitrate-free interval **Topical** Apply 1.5–5 cm (½–2 inch) strip of ointment q4–6h

STORAGE

- Store sublingual tablets and patches at 15°–30° C (59°–86° F) in orginal containers; keep tightly closed. IV solutions should be stored and diluted in glass bottles because this drug migrates into many plastics.
- Keep ointment container tightly closed and store in cool place.

ADMINISTRATION

Note: Drug forms appropriate for angina prophylaxis include ointment, transdermal unit, translingual spray, transmucosal tablet, and oral sustained-release forms. Drug forms appropriate for acute angina include sublingual tablet, translingual spray, or transmucosal tablet.

Common adverse effects in *italic;* life-threatening effects <u>underlined;</u> generic names in **bold;** drug classifications in SMALL CAPS; ♣ Canadian drug name; ● Prototype drug.

889

Sublingual Tablet

- Give 1 tablet and if pain is not relieved, give additional tablets at 5-min intervals, but not more than 3 tablets in a 15-min period.
- Leave tablets at bedside only if older child is being treated and is competent in self management and if young children do not have access to these tablets. Instruct in correct use. Request patient to report all attacks. Count tablets daily to verify amount of use.
- Instruct to sit or lie down on first indication of oncoming anginal pain and to place tablet under tongue or in buccal pouch (hypotensive effect of drug is intensified in the upright position).

Sustained-Release Buccal Tablet

- Place tablet between lip and gum above incisors or between cheek and gum allowing slow dissolution over 3–5 h.
- Touching tongue to tablet or drinking hot fluids hastens tablet dissolution, which can lead to decreased duration of medication effect and onset of anginal pain.
- Ensure that tablet is not chewed or swallowed or crushed.

Sustained-Release Tablet or Capsule

- Give on an empty stomach (1 h before or 2 h after meals), with a full glass of water. Ensure it is swallowed whole.
- Be aware that sustained-release form helps to prevent anginal attacks; it is not intended for immediate relief of angina.
- Ensure that tablet is not crushed or chewed.

Translingual Spray

- Do not shake canister. Spray preferably on or under tongue. Do not inhale spray.
- Repeat spray if needed q5min for a maximum of 3 metered doses.
- Instruct to wait at least 10 sec before swallowing.

Transdermal Ointment

- Using dose-determining applicator (paper application patch) supplied with package, squeeze prescribed dose onto this applicator. Using applicator spread ointment in a thin, uniform layer to premarked 5.5 by 9 cm (2¼ by 3½ inch) square. Place patch with ointment side down onto nonhairy skin surface (areas commonly used: chest, abdomen, anterior thigh, forearm). Cover with transparent wrap and secure with tape. Avoid getting ointment on fingers or hands.
- Rotate application sites to prevent dermal inflammation and sensitization. Remove ointment from previously used sites before reapplication.

Transdermal Unit

- Apply transdermal unit (transdermal patch) at the same time each day, preferably to skin site free of hair with intact skin and not subject to excessive movement. Avoid abraded, irritated, or scarred skin. Clip hair if necessary.
- Change application site each time to prevent skin irritation and sensitization.

Intravenous

- Note: Verify correct IV concentration and rate of infusion in infants and children with physician. Note that dosage for children is mcg/kg/min whereas adults are mcg/min.

Common adverse effects in *italic;* life-threatening effects <u>underlined</u>; generic names in **bold;** drug classifications in SMALL CAPS; ♣ Canadian drug name; ● Prototype drug.

- Check to see if patient has transdermal patch or ointment in place before starting IV infusion. The patch (or ointment) is usually removed to prevent overdosage.
- Be aware that when switching from IV to transdermal nitroglycerin, the IV infusion rate is reduced by 50% with simultaneous application of 5 or 10 mg/24 h transdermal patch.

PREPARE IV Infusion: IV nitroglycerin is available in differing concentrations. Be attentive to the dilution, dosage, and directions for administration on each vial or ampule. Note that a number of nitroglycerin preparations are available prediluted. Other forms must be diluted in D5W or NS, usually to concentrations between 25–500 mcg/mL. Use only glass bottles and manufacturer-supplied IV tubing. Withdraw medication into syringe and inject immediately into the IV solution to minimize contact with plastic. Regular IV tubing can absorb 40–80% of nitroglycerin.

ADMINISTER IV Infusion: Give by continuous infusion regulated exactly by an infusion pump. IV dosage titration requires careful and continuous hemodynamic monitoring.

INCOMPATIBILITIES Solution/Additive: Hydralazine, phenytoin. Y-Site: Alteplase.

- Use only glass containers for storage of reconstituted IV solution. Polyvinyl chloride (PVC) plastic can absorb nitroglycerin and therefore should not be used. Non-polyvinyl-chloride (non-PVC) sets are recommended or provided by manufacturer.

ADVERSE EFFECTS CNS: *Headache,* apprehension, blurred vision, weakness, vertigo, dizziness, faintness. **CV:** *Postural hypotension,* palpitations, tachycardia (sometimes with paradoxical bradycardia), increase in angina, syncope, and circulatory collapse. **GI:** Nausea, vomiting, involuntary passing of urine and feces, abdominal pain, dry mouth. **Hematologic:** Methemoglobinemia (high doses). **Skin:** Cutaneous vasodilation with flushing, rash, exfoliative dermatitis, contact dermatitis with transdermal patch; topical allergic reactions with ointment: pruritic eczematous eruptions, anaphylactoid reaction characterized by oral mucosal and conjunctival edema. **Body as a Whole:** Muscle twitching, pallor, perspiration, cold sweat; local sensation in oral cavity at point of dissolution of sublingual forms.

DIAGNOSTIC TEST INTERFERENCE Nitroglycerin may cause increases in determinations of *urinary catecholamines* and *VMA;* may interfere with the *Zlatkis-Zak color reaction,* causing a false report of decreased *serum cholesterol.*

INTERACTIONS Drug: Alcohol, ANTIHYPERTENSIVE AGENTS compound hypotensive effects; IV nitroglycerin may antagonize **heparin** anticoagulation.

PHARMACOKINETICS Absorption: Significant loss to first-pass metabolism after oral dosing. **Onset:** 2 min SL; 3 min PO; 30 min ointment. **Duration:** 30 min SL; 3–5 h PO; 3–6 h ointment. **Distribution:** Widely distributed; not known if distributes to breast milk. **Metabolism:** Extensively metabolized in liver. **Elimination:** Inactive metabolites excreted in urine. **Half-Life:** 1–4 min.

Common adverse effects in *italic;* life-threatening effects underlined; generic names in **bold**; drug classifications in SMALL CAPS; ♣ Canadian drug name; ۞ Prototype drug.

891

NURSING IMPLICATIONS

Assessment & Drug Effects

- Administer IV nitroglycerin with extreme caution to patients with hypotension or hypovolemia because the IV drug may precipitate a severe hypotensive state.
- Monitor patient closely for change in levels of consciousness and for dysrhythmias. IV nitroglycerin solution contains a substantial amount of ethanol as diluent. Ethanol intoxication can develop with high doses of IV nitroglycerin (vomiting, lethargy, coma, breath smells of alcohol). If intoxication occurs, infusion should be stopped promptly; patient recovers immediately with discontinuation of drug administration.
- Be aware that moisture on sublingual tissue is required for dissolution of sublingual tablet. However, because chest pain typically leads to dry mouth, a patient may be unresponsive to sublingual nitroglycerin.
- Assess for headaches. Approximately 50% of all patients experience mild to severe headaches following nitroglycerin. Transient headache usually lasts about 5 min after sublingual administration and seldom longer than 20 min. Assess degree of severity and consult as needed with physician about analgesics and dosage adjustment.
- Supervise ambulation as needed, especially with older adult or debilitated patients. Postural hypotension may occur even with small doses of nitroglycerin. Patients may complain of dizziness or weakness due to postural hypotension.
- Take baseline BP and heart rate with patient in sitting position before initiation of treatment with transdermal preparations.
- One hour after transdermal (ointment or unit) medication has been applied, check BP and pulse again with patient in sitting position. Report measurements to physician.
- Assess for and report blurred vision or dry mouth.
- Assess for and report the following topical reactions. Contact dermatitis from the transdermal patch; pruritus and erythema from the ointment.
- Be aware that local burning or tingling from the sublingual form has no clinical significance.
- Be alert for overdose symptoms: Hypotension, tachycardia; warm, flushed skin becoming cold and cyanotic; headache, palpitations, confusion, nausea, vomiting, moderate fever, and paralysis. Tissue hypoxia leads to coma, convulsions, cardiovascular collapse. Death can occur from asphyxia.

Patient & Family Education

- Sit or lie down on first indication of oncoming anginal pain.
- Spit out the rest of your sublingual tablet as soon as pain is completely relieved, especially if you are experiencing unpleasant adverse effects such as headache. Relax for 15–20 min after taking tablet to prevent dizziness or faintness.
- Be aware that pain not relieved by 3 sublingual tablets over a 15-min period may indicate acute MI or severe coronary insufficiency. Contact physician immediately or go directly to emergency room.
- Note: Sublingual tablets may be taken prophylactically 5–10 min prior to exercise or other stimulus known to trigger angina (drug effect lasts 30–60 min).

- Keep record for physician of number of angina attacks, amount of medication required for relief of each attack, and possible precipitating factors.
- Be aware that contact with water (swimming, bathing) does not affect your transdermal unit.
- If faintness, dizziness, or flushing occurs following application of transdermal unit or ointment, remove transdermal unit or ointment immediately from skin and notify physician.
- You can use a sublingual formulation while transdermal unit or ointment is in place if prescribed by physician.
- Report blurred vision or dry mouth. Both warrant withdrawal of drug.
- Change position slowly and avoid prolonged standing. Dizziness, lightheadedness, and syncope (due to postural hypotension) occur.
- Do not drink alcohol after taking nitroglycerin. It may cause severe postural hypotension (sharp drop in BP), vertigo, flushing, or pallor.
- Report any increase in frequency, duration, or severity of anginal attack.
- Withdraw gradually after prolonged use to prevent precipitating anginal attack.
- Do not breast feed while taking this drug without consulting physician.
- Store this medication out of reach of children.

NITROPRUSSIDE SODIUM

(nye-troe-pruss'ide)

Nipride, Nitropress

Classifications: CARDIOVASCULAR AGENT; ANTIHYPERTENSIVE; NONNITRATE VASODILATOR

Prototype: Hydralazine

Pregnancy Category: C

AVAILABILITY 50 mg injection

ACTIONS Potent, rapid-acting hypotensive agent with effects similar to those of nitrates.

THERAPEUTIC EFFECTS Acts directly on vascular smooth muscle to produce peripheral vasodilation, with consequent marked lowering of arterial BP, associated with slight increase in heart rate, mild decrease in cardiac output, and moderate lowering of peripheral vascular resistance.

USES Short-term, rapid reduction of BP in hypertensive crises and for producing controlled hypotension during anesthesia to reduce bleeding.

UNLABELED USES Refractory CHF or acute MI.

CONTRAINDICATIONS Compensatory hypertension, as in atriovenous shunt or coarctation of aorta, and for control of hypotension in patients with inadequate cerebral circulation. Safety during pregnancy (category C) or lactation is not established.

CAUTIOUS USE Hepatic insufficiency, hypothyroidism, severe renal impairment, hyponatremia, increased intracranial pressure.

Common adverse effects in *italic;* life-threatening effects <u>underlined</u>; generic names in **bold;** drug classifications in SMALL CAPS; ✦ Canadian drug name; ✪ Prototype drug.

893

ROUTE & DOSAGE

Hypertensive Crisis

Child/Adult: **IV** Begin with 0.3–0.5 mcg/kg/min, titrate to 3 mcg/kg/min (max dose 8–10 mcg/kg/min)

STORAGE

Store reconstituted solutions protected from light; stable for 24 h.

ADMINISTRATION

Intravenous

Note: Solutions must be freshly prepared with D5W and used no later than 4 h after reconstitution.

PREPARE **Continuous:** Dissolve each 50 mg in 2–3 mL of D5W. Further dilute in 250 mL D5W to yield 200 mcg/mL or 500 mL D5W to yield 100 mcg/mL. Following reconstitution, solutions usually have faint brownish tint; if solution is highly colored, do not use it. Promptly wrap container with aluminum foil or other opaque material to protect drug from light.

ADMINISTER **Continuous:** Administer by infusion pump or similar device that will allow precise measurement of flow rate required to lower BP. Give at the rate required to lower BP but do not exceed the maximum dose of 10 mcg/kg/min.

INCOMPATIBILITIES **Y-Site: Cisatracurium, haloperidol.**

ADVERSE EFFECTS Body as a Whole: Diaphoresis, apprehension, restlessness, muscle twitching, retrosternal discomfort. <u>Thiocyanate toxicity</u> (profound hypotension, tinnitus, blurred vision, fatigue, metabolic acidosis, pink skin color, absence of reflexes, faint heart sounds, loss of consciousness). **CV:** Profound hypotension, palpitation, increase or transient lowering of pulse rate, bradycardia, tachycardia, ECG changes. **GI:** Nausea, retching, abdominal pain. **Metabolic:** Increase in serum creatinine, fall or rise in total plasma cobalamins. **CNS:** Headache, dizziness. **Special Senses:** Nasal stuffiness. **Other:** Irritation at infusion site.

INTERACTIONS No clinically significant interactions established.

PHARMACOKINETICS Onset: Within 2 min. **Duration:** 1–10 min after infusion is terminated. **Metabolism:** Rapidly converted to cyanogen in erythrocytes and tissue, which is metabolized to thiocyanate in liver. **Elimination:** Excreted in urine primarily as thiocyanate. **Half-Life:** (thiocyanate): 2.7–7 days.

NURSING IMPLICATIONS

Assessment & Drug Effects

- Monitor constantly to titrate IV infusion rate to BP response.
- Relieve adverse effects by slowing IV rate or by stopping drug; minimize them by keeping patient supine.
- Notify physician immediately if BP begins to rise after drug infusion rate is decreased or infusion is discontinued.
- Monitor I&O.

- Lab tests: Monitor blood thiocyanate level in patients receiving prolonged treatment or in patients with severe kidney dysfunction (levels usually are not allowed to exceed 10 mg/dL). Determine plasma cyanogen level following 1 or 2 days of therapy in patients with impaired liver function.
- Monitor for acidosis because it may be first signs of cyanide toxicity. Excessive amounts of nitroprusside may cause cyanide toxicity especially in patients with impaired liver function.

NOREPINEPHRINE BITARTRATE

(nor-ep-i-nef'rin)
Levarterenol, Levophed, Noradrenaline
Classifications: AUTONOMIC NERVOUS SYSTEM AGENT; ALPHA- AND BETA-ADRENERGIC AGONIST (SYMPATHOMIMETIC)
Prototype: Epinephrine
Pregnancy Category: D

AVAILABILITY 1 mg/mL injection

ACTIONS Direct-acting sympathomimetic amine identical to body catecholamine norepinephrine. Acts directly and predominantly on alpha-adrenergic receptors; little action on beta receptors except in heart (beta$_1$ receptors). Vasoconstriction and cardiac stimulation; also powerful constrictor action on resistance and capacitance blood vessels.

THERAPEUTIC EFFECTS Peripheral vasoconstriction and moderate inotropic stimulation of heart result in increased systolic and diastolic blood pressure, myocardial oxygenation, coronary artery blood flow, and work of heart. Cardiac output varies with systemic BP.

USES To restore BP in certain acute hypotensive states such as shock, sympathectomy, pheochromocytomectomy, spinal anesthesia, poliomyelitis, MI, septicemia, blood transfusion, and drug reactions. Also as adjunct in treatment of cardiac arrest.

CONTRAINDICATIONS Use as sole therapy in hypovolemic states, except as temporary emergency measure; mesenteric or peripheral vascular thrombosis; profound hypoxia or hypercarbia; use during cyclopropane or halothane anesthesia; pregnancy (category D), lactation.

CAUTIOUS USE Hypertension; hyperthyroidism; severe heart disease; within 14 days of MAOI therapy; patients receiving tricyclic antidepressants.

ROUTE & DOSAGE

Child: **IV** Start with 0.05–0.1 mcg/kg/min titrate to maintenance dose of 0.1 mcg/kg/min (max dose 2 mcg/kg/min)
Adult: **IV** Start with 8–12 mcg/min, titrate to maintenance dose of 2–4 mcg/min

STORAGE

Store at 15°–30° C (59°–86° F); protect from light and moisture. Drug readily oxidizes on exposure to light and air, causing discoloration of solution.

Common adverse effects in *italic;* life-threatening effects <u>underlined</u>; generic names in **bold;** drug classifications in SMALL CAPS; ♣ Canadian drug name; ⊘ Prototype drug.

895

ADMINISTRATION

Intravenous

***PREPARE* IV Infusion:** Dilute a 4-mL ampule in 1000 mL of D5W or D5/NS. Do not use solution if discoloration or precipitate is present. Protect from light.

***ADMINISTER* IV Infusion:** An infusion pump is used. Usually give at the slowest rate possible required to maintain BP. Constantly monitor flow rate. Check infusion site frequently and immediately report any evidence of extravasation: Blanching along course of infused vein (may occur without obvious extravasation), cold, hard swelling around injection site. Antidote for extravasation ischemia: Phentolamine, neonates, 2.5–5 mg in 10 mL NS (max dose 0.1 mg/kg or 2.5 mg total); infants, children, and adults: 5–10 mg in 10–15 mL NS (max dose 0.1–0.2 mg/kg or 5 mg total). This injection, is infiltrated throughout affected area (using syringe with fine hypodermic needle) as soon as possible. If therapy is to be prolonged, change infusion sites at intervals to allow effect of local vasoconstriction to subside. Avoid abrupt withdrawal; when therapy is discontinued, infusion rate is slowed gradually.

***INCOMPATIBILITIES* Solution/Additive: Aminophylline, amobarbital, cephapirin, chlorothiazide, chlorpheniramine, pentobarbital, phenobarbital, phenytoin, secobarbital, sodium bicarbonate, sodium iodide, streptomycin, thiopental, whole blood. Y-Site: Insulin, thiopental.**

ADVERSE EFFECTS Body as a Whole: Restlessness, anxiety, *tremors,* dizziness, weakness, insomnia, pallor, plasma volume depletion, edema, hemorrhage, <u>intestinal</u>, <u>hepatic</u>, or <u>renal necrosis</u>, retrosternal and pharyngeal pain, profuse sweating. **CV:** Palpitation, hypertension, reflex bradycardia, <u>fatal arrhythmias</u> (large doses), severe hypertension. **GI:** Vomiting. **Metabolic:** Hyperglycemia. **CNS:** Headache, violent headache, <u>cerebral hemorrhage</u>, convulsions. **Respiratory:** Respiratory difficulty. **Skin:** Tissue necrosis at injection site (with extravasation). **Special Senses:** Blurred vision, photophobia.

INTERACTIONS Drug: ALPHA- AND BETA-BLOCKERS antagonize pressor effects; ERGOT ALKALOIDS, **furazolidone, guanethidine, methyldopa,** TRICYCLIC ANTIDEPRESSANTS may potentiate pressor effects; **halothane, cyclopropane** increase risk of arrhythmias.

PHARMACOKINETICS Onset: Very rapid. **Duration:** 1–2 min after termination of infusion. **Distribution:** Localizes in sympathetic nerve endings; crosses placenta. **Metabolism:** Metabolized in liver and other tissues by catecholamine *o*-methyl transferase and monoamine oxidase. **Elimination:** Excreted in urine.

NURSING IMPLICATIONS

Assessment & Drug Effects

- Monitor constantly while patient is receiving norepinephrine. Take baseline BP and pulse before start of therapy, then q2min from initiation of drug until stabilization occurs at desired level, then every 5 min during drug administration.

Common adverse effects in *italic;* life-threatening effects <u>underlined</u>; generic names in **bold;** drug classifications in SMALL CAPS; ♣ Canadian drug name; ❷ Prototype drug.

- Adjust flow rate to maintain BP at low normal (according to age levels, adults usually 80–100 mm Hg systolic) in normotensive patients. In previously hypertensive patients, systolic is generally maintained no higher than 40 mm Hg below preexisting systolic level.
- Observe carefully and record mental status (index of cerebral circulation), skin temperature of extremities, and color (especially of earlobes, lips, nail beds) in addition to vital signs.
- Monitor I&O. Urinary retention and kidney shutdown are possibilities, especially in hypovolemic patients. Urinary output is a sensitive indicator of the degree of renal perfusion. Report decrease in urinary output or change in I&O ratio.
- Be alert to patient's complaints of headache, vomiting, palpitation, arrhythmias, chest pain, photophobia, and blurred vision as possible symptoms of overdosage. Reflex bradycardia may occur as a result of rise in BP.
- Continue to monitor vital signs and observe patient closely after cessation of therapy for clinical sign of circulatory inadequacy.

NORTRIPTYLINE HYDROCHLORIDE
(nor-trip′ti-leen)
Aventyl, Pamelor
Classifications: CENTRAL NERVOUS SYSTEM AGENT; PSYCHOTHERAPEUTIC; TRICYCLIC ANTIDEPRESSANT
Prototype: Imipramine
Pregnancy Category: D

AVAILABILITY 10 mg, 25 mg, 50 mg, 75 mg capsules; 10 mg/5 mL solution

ACTIONS Secondary amine derivative of amitriptyline. Action mechanism unclear. Tricyclic antidepressant (TCA) with less sedative and anticholinergic effects than imipramine.
THERAPEUTIC EFFECTS Mood elevation may be due to its inhibition of reuptake of norepinephrine at the presynaptic membrane.

USES Endogenous depression. Similar in actions, uses, limitations, and interactions to imipramine.
UNLABELED USES Nocturnal enuresis in children.

CONTRAINDICATIONS Acute recovery period after MI; during or within 14 days of MAO inhibitor therapy. Children <12 y, pregnancy (category D), lactation.
CAUTIOUS USE Narrow-angle glaucoma, hyperthyroidism, concurrent administration of thyroid medications, concurrent use with electroshock therapy, seizure disorders, history of urinary retention.

ROUTE & DOSAGE

Antidepressant
Child 6–12 y: 1–3 mg/kg/day or 10–20 mg/day in 3–4 divided doses
Adolescent: **PO** 1–3 mg/kg/day or 30–50 mg/day in 3–4 divided doses (max dosage 150 mg/day)
Adult: **PO** 25 mg t.i.d. or q.i.d., gradually increased to 100–150 mg/day

Nocturnal Enuresis

Child: (Given 30 min before hour of sleep) **PO** *6–7 y (20–25 kg),* 10 mg/day, *8–11 y (25–35 kg),* 10–20 mg/day, *>11 y (35–54 kg)* 25–35 mg/day

STORAGE\

Store at 15°–30° C (59°–86° F) in tightly closed container

ADMINISTRATION

Oral

- Give with food to decrease gastric distress.
- Do not diltute in grape juice or carbonated beverages.
- Be aware that solutions contain 4% alcohol.
- Supervise drug ingestion to be sure patient swallows medication.

ADVERSE EFFECTS Body as a Whole: Tremors, hyperhydrosis. **CV:** *Orthostatic hypotension.* **GI:** Paralytic ileus, *dry mouth.* **Hematologic:** Arrhythmia, <u>agranulocytosis</u> (rare). **CNS:** Drowsiness, confusional state (especially in older adults and with high dosage). **Skin:** Photosensitivity reaction. **Special Senses:** Blurred vision. **Urogenital:** *Urinary retention.*

INTERACTIONS Drug: May decrease some antihypertensive response to ANTIHYPERTENSIVES; CNS DEPRESSANTS, **alcohol,** HYPNOTICS, BARBITURATES, SEDATIVES potentiate CNS depression; may increase hypoprothrombinemic effect of ORAL ANTICOAGULANTS; **ethchlorvynol** may cause transient delirium; **levodopa,** SYMPATHOMIMETICS (e.g., **epinephrine, norepinephrine**) pose possibility of sympathetic hyperactivity with hypertension and hyperpyrexia; MAO INHIBITORS pose possibility of severe reactions: Toxic psychosis, cardiovascular instability; **methylphenidate** increases plasma TCA levels; THYROID DRUGS may increase possibility of arrhythmias; **cimetidine** may increase plasma TCA levels. **Herbal: Ginkgo** may decrease seizure threshold. **St. John's wort** may cause **serotonin** syndrome (headache, dizziness, sweating, agitation).

PHARMACOKINETICS Absorption: Rapidly absorbed from GI tract. **Peak:** 7–8.5 h. **Distribution:** Crosses placenta; distributed in breast milk. **Metabolism:** Metabolized in liver. **Elimination:** Primarily excreted in urine. **Half-Life:** Child, 4–18 h; adult, 16–90 h.

NURSING IMPLICATIONS

Assessment & Drug Effects

- Be aware that nortriptyline has a narrow therapeutic plasma level range, or "therapeutic window." Drug levels above or below the therapeutic window are associated with decreased rate of response.
- Therapeutic response may not occur for 2 wk or more.
- Monitor BP and pulse rate during adjustment period of TCA therapy. If systolic BP falls more than 20 mm Hg or if there is a sudden increase in pulse rate, withhold medication and notify the prescriber.
- Notify physician if psychotic signs increase. Because of the small therapeutic window, a substitute TCA may be prescribed rather than an increase in dosage.
- Inspect oral membranes daily if patient is on high doses of TCA. Urge outpatient to report stomatitis or dry mouth. Sore mouth can be a major

cause of poor nutrition and noncompliance. Consult prescriber about use of a saliva substitute (e.g., VA-Oralube, Moi-Stir).

■ Monitor bowel elimination pattern, I&O ratio and weight. Urinary retention and severe constipation are potential problems. Advise increased fluid intake; consult physician about stool softener.

■ Observe patient with history of glaucoma. Symptoms that may signal acute attack (severe headache, eye pain, dilated pupils, halos of light, nausea, vomiting) should be reported promptly.

■ Report reduction or alleviation of fine tremors.

■ Be aware that alcohol potentiation may increase the danger of overdosage or suicide attempt.

■ Antidepressants increase risk of suicidal thinking and behavior in children and adolescents with major depressive disorder, obsessive compulsive disorder, and other psychiatric disorders. Observe closely for worsening of condition, suicidality, and behavior changes. Instruct family and caregivers to monitor for these symptoms and discuss with prescriber. A MedGuide describing risks and stating whether the drug is approved for the child's/adolescent's condition should be provided for all families when antidepressants are prescribed.

Patient & Family Education

■ May take several weeks to achieve therapeutic effect.

■ Be aware that the ability to perform tasks requiring alertness and skill (i.e., bike riding, skateboarding, and sports) may be impaired.

■ Do not use OTC or herbal medications while on this drug without consulting physician.

■ Do not take alcohol because alcohol and nortriptyline both have increased effects when used together and for up to 2 wk after the TCA is discontinued.

■ Nortriptyline enhances the effects of barbiturates and other CNS depressants are enhanced.

■ May cause photosensity. Use sunscreen and protective clothing in sunlight and avoid tanning booths.

■ Take only as directed and follow-up with prescriber is important.

■ Causes dry mouth.

■ Do not stop medication without prescriber's approval.

■ Do not breast feed while taking this drug.

■ Store this medication out of reach of children.

NYSTATIN

(nye-stat′in)

Mycostatin, Bio-Statin, Nadostine ✦ , Nilstat, Nyaderm ✦ , Nystex, O-V Statin, Pedi-Dri

Classifications: ANTI-INFECTIVE; ANTIFUNGAL ANTIBIOTIC
Prototype: Fluconazole
Pregnancy Category: C

AVAILABILITY 500,000 unit tablets; 100,000 units/mL oral suspension; 200,000 troches; 100,000 units vaginal tablets; 100,000 units/g cream, ointment, powder.

Common adverse effects in *italic;* life-threatening effects <u>underlined</u>; generic names in **bold**; drug classifications in SMALL CAPS; ✦ Canadian drug name; ❂ Prototype drug.

899

ACTIONS Nontoxic, nonsensitizing antifungal antibiotic produced by *Streptomyces noursei*. Binds to sterols in fungal cell membrane, thereby changing membrane potential and allowing leakage of intracellular components.

THERAPEUTIC EFFECTS Fungistatic and fungicidal activity against a variety of yeasts and fungi; not appreciably active against bacteria, viruses, or protozoa.

USES Local infections of skin and mucous membranes caused by *Candida* sp. including *Candida albicans* (e.g., paronychia; cutaneous, oropharyngeal, vulvovaginal, and intestinal candidiasis).

CONTRAINDICATIONS Use of vaginal tablets during pregnancy (category C); vaginal infections caused by *Gardnerella vaginalis* or *Trichomonas* sp.

CAUTIOUS USE Lactation.

ROUTE & DOSAGE

Candida Infections (Oral Suspension)

Neonate: 100,000 units 4 times/day by placing 50,000 units to each side of mouth

Infant: 200,000 units 4 times/day by placing 100,000 units to each side of mouth

Child/Adult: **PO** 400,000–600,000 units 4 times/day, or use troches 200,000–400,000 units 4 times/day **Candidal Diaper Rash** In addition to topical therapy, oral suspension 100,000 units 4 times/day may be used **Topical** For cutaneous infections 100,000 units applied 2 to 4 times/day

Intravaginal

Child >13 y/Adult: 1 tablet daily at bedtime for 2 wk

STORAGE

Store vaginal tablets in refrigerator below 15° C (59° F). Store other products at 15°–30° C (59°–86° F) in tightly closed container; protect from freezing.

ADMINISTRATION

Oral

- Give reconstituted powder for oral suspension immediately after mixing.
- Rinse mouth with 1–2 tsp using oral suspension. Keep in mouth (swish) as long as possible (at least 2 min), then spit it out. (If you cannot keep the liquid in your mouth or cannot spit, or if you have been told to "swish and swallow," you may swallow the drug.) For children, infants: Apply drug with swab to each side of mouth. Avoid food or drink for 30 min after treatment.
- Troches should not be crushed or chewed but allowed to slowly dissolve in mouth. (Only use with children who can follow directions.)
- Treatment should be continued for at least 48 h after symptoms dissipate and cultures are normal.

Topical

- Use cautiously in children due to greater surface area to body ratio.

ADVERSE EFFECTS GI: Nausea, vomiting, epigastric distress, diarrhea (especially with high oral doses).

PHARMACOKINETICS Absorption: Poorly absorbed from GI tract. **Elimination:** Excreted in feces.

NURSING IMPLICATIONS

Assessment & Drug Effects

- Monitor oral cavity, especially the tongue, for signs of improvement.
- Avoid occlusive dressings or applications of ointment preparation to moist, dark areas of body because they favor growth of yeast.

Patient & Family Education

- This drug may cause contact dermatitis. Stop using the drug and report to prescriber if redness, swelling, or irritation develops.
- Take for oral candidiasis (thrush) treatment after meals and at bedtime.
- Dissolve troche in mouth (about 30 min). Do not chew or swallow. Avoid food and drink during period of dissolving and for 30 min after treatment.
- Oral infections: Consult dentist about use of retainers while using nystatin and for usage after infection. Keep dental care items separate from other children. Child should be supplied with a new toothbrush or current one should be disinfected.
- Dust shoes and stockings, as well as feet, with nystatin dusting powder.
- Your prescriber will probably prescribe cream instead of ointment for intertriginous areas. For very moist lesions, powder is usually prescribed. Gently clean infected areas with tepid water before each application.
- Be aware that treatment of cutaneous candidal infections is continued for at least 2 wk and discontinued only after two negative tests for *Candida*.
- Continue medication for vulvovaginal candidiasis during menstruation. In most cases, 2 wk of therapy are sufficient; however, some patients may require longer treatment.
- Use vaginal tablets up to 6 wk before term to prevent thrush in the newborn.
- Do not breast feed while taking this drug without consulting physician.
- Store this medication out of reach of children.

OCTREOTIDE ACETATE

(oc-tre'o-tide)
Sandostatin, Sandostatin LAR depot
Classifications: HORMONES AND SYNTHETIC SUBSTITUTES; ANTIDIARRHEAL
Pregnancy Category: B

AVAILABILITY 0.05 mg/mL, 0.1 mg/mL, 0.2 mg/mL, 0.5 mg/mL, 1 mg/mL injection; 10 mg/5 mL, 20 mg/5 mL, 30 mg/5 mL depot injection

ACTIONS A long-acting peptide that mimics the natural hormone somatostatin. Suppresses secretion of serotonin, pancreatic peptides, gastrin, vasoactive intestinal peptide, insulin, glucagon, secretin, and motilin.
THERAPEUTIC EFFECTS Stimulates fluid and electrolyte absorption from the GI tract, prolongs intestinal transit time, and also inhibits the growth hormone.

USES Symptomatic treatment of severe diarrhea and flushing episodes associated with metastatic carcinoid tumors. Also watery diarrhea associated with vasoactive intestinal peptide (VIP) tumors.

UNLABELED USES Acromegaly associated with pituitary tumors, fistula drainage, variceal bleeding, postoperative chylothorax.

CONTRAINDICATIONS Hypersensitivity to octreotide.

CAUTIOUS USE Cholelithiasis, renal impairment; pregnancy (category B); diabetes, and hypothyroidism. Long-term use in children, it is not known whether drug is excreted in breast milk.

ROUTE & DOSAGE

Limited use of this drug with children. Dosages are from reported cases.

Intractable Diarrhea

Child: **SC** 1–10 mcg/kg/day in divided doses every 12 h, titrate to response (max dose 1500 mcg/day)

Carcinoid Syndrome

Child: **SC** 1–10 mcg/kg/day in 2–4 equally divided doses, titrate to response (max dose 1500 mcg/day)
Adult: **SC** 100–600 mcg/day in 2–4 divided doses, titrate to response
IM May switch to depot injection after 2 wk at 20 mg q4wk times 2 mo

VIPoma

Child: **SC** 1–10 mcg/kg/day in 2–4 divided doses, titrate to response
Adult: **SC** 200–300 mcg/day in 2–4 divided doses, titrate to response
IM May switch to depot injection after 2 wk at 20 mg q4wk times 2 mo

Acromegaly

Adult: **SC** 50 mcg t.i.d., titrate up to 100–500 mcg t.i.d. **IM** May switch to depot injection after 2 wk at 20 mg q4wk times at least 3 mo, then reassess

STORAGE

Refrigerate. Sandostatin is stable at room temperature for 14 days if protected from light. Discard any unused portion of Sandostatin LAR after reconstitution.

ADMINISTRATION

Subcutaneous/Intramuscular

- Note: Subcutaneous is the preferred route.
- Minimize GI side effects by giving injections between meals and at bedtime.
- Avoid multiple injections into the same site. Rotate SC sites on abdomen, hip, and thigh.
- Give deep IM into a large muscle appropriate for age (see Part I). To reduce local irritation, allow solution to reach room temperature before injection and administer slowly.
- Use Sandostatin LAR for IM depot injection only; do not give IV or subcutaneously.

Intravenous

PREPARE Direct: Give undiluted. **Intermittent:** Dilute in 50–200 mL D5W.

ADMINISTER Direct: Given mcg/kg/min infusions and titrate to response Adults: Give a single dose over 3 min. In carcinoid syndrome,

Common adverse effects in *italic*; life-threatening effects underlined; generic names in **bold**; drug classifications in SMALL CAPS; ♣ Canadian drug name; ✪ Prototype drug.

give rapid IV bolus over 60 sec. **Intermittent:** Given mcg/kg/min infusions and titrate to response. Adults: Give over 15–30 min.

ADVERSE EFFECTS CNS: Headache, fatigue, dizziness. **GI:** *Nausea, diarrhea,* abdominal pain and discomfort. **Metabolic:** Hypoglycemia, hyperglycemia, increased liver transaminases, hypothyroidism (after long-term use). **Body as a Whole:** Flushing, edema, injection site pain.

INTERACTIONS Drug: May decrease **cyclosporine** levels; may alter other drug and nutrient absorption because of alterations in GI motility. May alter oral hypoglycemic and insulin requirements. **Food:** Can alter absorption of fats taken in diet.

PHARMACOKINETICS Absorption: Rapidly absorbed from SC injection site. **Peak:** 0.4 h. **Duration:** Up to 12 h. **Metabolism:** 68% metabolized in liver. **Elimination:** Excreted in urine. **Half-Life:** 1.5 h.

NURSING IMPLICATIONS

Assessment & Drug Effects
- Lab tests: Periodic blood glucose, liver function tests, and serum electrolytes.
- Monitor for hypoglycemia and hyperglycemia (see Appendix D-1), because octreotide may alter the balance between insulin, glucagon, and growth hormone.
- Monitor fluid and electrolyte balance, because octreotide stimulates fluid and electrolyte absorption from GI tract.
- Dietary fat absorption may be altered in some clients. Monitor fecal fat and serum carotene to aid in the assessment of possible drug-induced aggravation of fat malabsorption.

Patient & Family Education
- Learn proper technique for SC injection if self-medication is required.
- Note: Preferred sites for SC injections of octreotide are the hip, thigh, and abdomen. Multiple injections at the same SC injection site within short periods of time are not recommended. This is to avoid irritating the area.
- Stress importance of follow-up laboratory tests and prescriber visits.
- Store this medication out of reach of children and properly dispose of used needles and syringes.

OFLOXACIN
(o-flox′a-cin)
Floxin, Ocuflox
Classifications: ANTI-INFECTIVE; QUINOLONE ANTIBIOTIC
Prototype: Ciprofloxacin
Pregnancy Category: C

AVAILABILITY 200 mg, 300 mg, 400 mg tablets; 200 mg, 400 mg injection; 0.3% otic and ophthalmic solution

OFLOXACIN

ACTIONS A fluoroquinolone antibiotic with a broad spectrum of activity against gram-positive and gram-negative aerobic and anaerobic bacteria. Inhibits DNA gyrase, an enzyme necessary for bacterial DNA replication and some aspects of its transcription, repair, recombination, and transposition.

THERAPEUTIC EFFECTS Most effective against gram-negative organisms including *Citrobacter diversus, C. freundii, Enterobacter cloacae, E. aerogenes, Escherichia coli, Klebsiella* species, *Morganella morganii, Proteus* species, *Salmonella* species, *Shigella* species, and *Yersinia enterocolitica*. More potent against *Serratia* species than is norfloxacin, and it is equipotent against *Providencia* species; less active against *Pseudomonas aeruginosa* but more potent against *Xanthomonas maltophilia* than is ciprofloxacin.

USES *Chlamydia trachomatis* infection, uncomplicated gonorrhea, prostatitis, respiratory tract infections, skin and skin structure infections, urinary tract infections due to susceptible bacteria, superficial ocular infections, pelvic inflammatory disease. Otic: Otitis externa, otitis media with perforated tympanic membranes.

UNLABELED USES EENT infections, *Helicobacter pylori* infections, *Salmonella* gastroenteritis.

CONTRAINDICATIONS Hypersensitivity to ofloxacin or other quinolone antibacterial agents; pregnancy (category C); lactation.

CAUTIOUS USE Renal disease; patients with a history of epilepsy, psychosis, or increased intracranial pressure. Safety and effectiveness in children and adolescents <18 y are not established. Safety and effectiveness of ophthalmic solution in children <1 y has not been established. Safety and effectiveness of otic solutions in children <1 y for treatment of otitis externa or acute otitis not established and use in chronic otitis not established in those <12 y.

ROUTE & DOSAGE

Uncomplicated Gonorrhea
Adult: **PO** 400 mg for 1 dose

Urinary Tract, Respiratory Tract, and Skin and Skin Structure Infections
Adult: **PO** 200–400 mg q12h times 7–10 days **IV** 400 mg q12h times 7 days

Superficial Ocular Infections
Child >1 y: **Ophthalmic** Instill 1 drop q2–4h for first 2 days, then q.i.d. for up to 5 additional days
Adult: **Ophthalmic** Instill 1–2 drops q2–4h for first 2 days, then q.i.d. for up to 5 additional days

Otitis Media, Otitis Externa
Child: 1–12 y, 5 drops instilled into affected ear canal b.i.d. for 10 days; >12 y, 10 drops instilled into affected ear canal b.i.d. for 10 days

Acute Otitis Externa with Tympanostomy Tubes
Child 1–12 y: 5 drops instilled into affected ear canal b.i.d. for 10 days

Chronic Suppurative Otitis Media
Child >12 y: 10 drops instilled into affected ear canal b.i.d. for 14 days

STORAGE

Store at 15°–30° C (59°–86° F) in tight containers; protect from moisture. Opthamalic solutions expire within 24 mo from date of manufacture if stored as directed.

ADMINISTRATION

Oral

- Do not give with meals.
- Avoid administering mineral supplements, dairy products, tube feedings, or vitamins with iron or zinc within 2 h of drug.
- Do not give antacids with magnesium, aluminum, or sucralfate within 4 h before or 2 h after drug.

Instillation

- Do NOT allow tip of dropper for ocular preparation to contact any surface.

Intravenous

PREPARE **Intermittent:** Withdraw the required dose from a 10-mL (40 mg/mL) or 20-mL (20 mg/mL) vial and add to 100 mL D5W, NS, D5/NS or other compatible solution. Final concentration may range from 0.4 mg/mL to 4 mg/mL.

ADMINISTER **Intermittent:** Give a single dose over at least 60 min. Avoid rapid infusion.

INCOMPATIBILITIES **Y-Site: Amphotericin B cholesteryl sulfate complex, cefepime, doxorubicin liposome.**

ADVERSE EFFECTS CNS: *Headache, dizziness, insomnia,* hallucinations, nightmares. **GI:** Nausea, vomiting, diarrhea, GI discomfort. **Urogenital:** Pruritus, pain, irritation, burning, vaginitis, vaginal discharge, dysmenorrhea, menorrhagia, dysuria, urinary frequency. **Skin:** Pruritus, rash.

DIAGNOSTIC TEST INTERFERENCE May cause false positive on *opiate screening tests.*

INTERACTIONS Drug: Ofloxacin absorption decreased when it is administered with MAGNESIUM- or ALUMINUM-CONTAINING ANTACIDS. Other CATIONS, including **calcium, iron,** and **zinc,** also appear to interfere with ofloxacin absorption. **Food:** Decreases ofloxacin absorption; do not take with dairy.

PHARMACOKINETICS Absorption: 90–98% absorbed from GI tract. **Peak:** 1–2 h. **Distribution:** Distributes to most tissues; 50% crosses into CSF with inflamed meninges; 20–32% protein bound; crosses placenta; distributed into breast milk. **Metabolism:** Slightly metabolized in liver. **Elimination:** 72–98% excreted in urine within 48 h. **Half-Life:** 5–7.5 h.

NURSING IMPLICATIONS

Assessment & Drug Effects

- Lab tests: Do C&S tests prior to initial dose. Treatment may be implemented pending results.

Common adverse effects in *italic;* life-threatening effects <u>underlined</u>; generic names in **bold**; drug classifications in SMALL CAPS; ♣ Canadian drug name; ☺ Prototype drug.

905

- Determine history of hypersensitivity reactions to quinolones or other drugs before therapy is started.
- Withhold ofloxacin and notify prescriber at first sign of a skin rash or other allergic reaction.
- Monitor for seizures, especially in patients with known or suspected CNS disorders. Discontinue ofloxacin and notify prescriber immediately if seizure occurs.
- Assess for S&S of superinfection (see Appendix D-1).

Patient & Family Education
- Drink fluids liberally unless contraindicated.
- Be aware that dizziness or light-headedness may occur; use appropriate caution.
- Avoid excessive sunlight or artificial ultraviolet light because of the possibility of phototoxicity.
- Do not take with dairy products, antacids, or multivitamins.
- Teach proper instillation of ear and eye drops (see Administration section).
- Do not use this drug on child other than child for whom the drug was prescribed.
- Do not breast feed while taking this drug.
- Store this drug out of reach of children.

OMEPRAZOLE ☻

(o-me′pra-zole)
Losec ♣ , Prilosec
Classifications: GASTROINTESTINAL AGENT; PROTON PUMP INHIBITOR
Pregnancy Category: C

AVAILABILITY 10 mg, 20 mg, 40 mg capsules

ACTIONS An antisecretory compound that is a gastric acid pump inhibitor. Suppresses gastric acid secretion by inhibiting the H^+, K^+-ATPase enzyme system [the acid (proton H^+) pump] in the parietal cells.
THERAPEUTIC EFFECTS Suppresses gastric acid secretion, relieving gastrointestinal distress and promoting ulcer healing.

USES Duodenal and gastric ulcer. Gastroesophageal reflux disease including severe erosive esophagitis (4- to 8-wk treatment). Long-term treatment of pathologic hypersecretory conditions such as Zollinger-Ellison syndrome, multiple endocrine adenomas, and systemic mastocytosis. In combination with clarithromycin to treat duodenal ulcers associated with *Helicobacter pylori*.

CONTRAINDICATIONS Long-term use for gastroesophageal reflux disease, duodenal ulcers; lactation.
CAUTIOUS USE Pregnancy (category C). Safety and effectiveness in children are not established.

ROUTE & DOSAGE

Gastroesophageal Reflux, Erosive Esophagitis, Duodenal Ulcer
Child: **PO** ≥2 y, 1 mg/kg/day once or b.i.d. Effective dose ranges of

0.3–3.3 mg/kg/day have been reported; or manufacturer recommends: **PO** ≥2 y, ≤20 kg, 10 mg once/day >20 kg, 20 mg once/day
Adult: **PO** 20 mg once/day for 4–8 wk

Gastric Ulcer

Adult: **PO** 20 mg b.i.d./day for 4–8 wk

Hypersecretory Disease

Adult: **PO** 60 mg once/day up to 120 mg t.i.d.

Duodenal Ulcer Associated with *H. pylori*

Child: **PO** *15–30 kg,* 10 mg b.i.d.; *>30 kg,* 20 mg b.i.d.
Adult: **PO** 40 mg once/day for 14 days, then 20 mg/day for 14 days, in combination with clarithromycin 500 mg t.i.d. for 14 days

---

ADMINISTRATION

Oral

- Give before food, preferably breakfast; capsules must be swallowed whole (do not open, chew, or crush).
- Pharmacy can compound suspension for children who are unable to take tablets.
- Note: Antacids may be administered with omeprazole.

ADVERSE EFFECTS CNS: Headache, dizziness, fatigue. **GI:** Diarrhea, abdominal pain, nausea, mild transient increases in liver function tests. **Urogenital:** Hematuria, proteinuria. **Skin:** Rash.

DIAGNOSTIC TEST INTERFERENCE Omeprazole has been reported to significantly impair peak **cortisol** response to exogenous ACTH. This finding is undergoing further investigation.

INTERACTIONS Drug: Concomitant administration of **diazepam** and omeprazole may increase diazepam concentrations. Concomitant administration of **phenytoin** and omeprazole may increase **phenytoin** levels. Concomitant administration of **warfarin** and omeprazole may increase **warfarin** levels and increase absorption of digoxin.

PHARMACOKINETICS Absorption: Poorly absorbed from GI tract; 30–40% reaches systemic circulation. Onset: 0.5–3.5 h. **Peak:** Peak inhibition of gastric acid secretion: 5 days. **Metabolism:** Metabolized in liver. **Elimination:** 80% excreted in urine, 20% in feces. **Half-Life:** 0.5–1.5 h.

NURSING IMPLICATIONS

Assessment & Drug Effects

- Lab tests: Monitor urinalysis for hematuria and proteinuria. Periodic liver function tests with prolonged use.

Patient & Family Education

- Report any changes in urinary elimination such as pain or discomfort associated with urination, or blood in urine.
- Report severe diarrhea; drug may need to be discontinued.
- May cause dry mouth.
- Do not breast feed while taking this drug.
- Store this medication out of reach of children.

ONDANSETRON HYDROCHLORIDE ⓟ
(on-dan′si-tron)
Zofran, Zofran ODT
Classifications: GASTROINTESTINAL AGENT; ANTIEMETIC; 5-HT₃ ANTAGONIST
Pregnancy Category: B

AVAILABILITY 4 mg, 8 mg, 24 mg tablets; 4 mg, 8 mg orally disintegrating tablets; 4 mg/5 mL oral solution; 2 mg/mL injection (contains parabens)

ACTIONS Selective serotonin (5-HT₃) receptor antagonist. Serotonin receptors are located centrally in the chemoreceptor trigger zone (CTZ) and peripherally on the vagal nerve terminals. Serotonin is released from the wall of the small intestine and stimulates the vagal efferents through the serotonin receptors and initiates the vomiting reflex.
THERAPEUTIC EFFECTS Prevents nausea and vomiting associated with cancer chemotherapy and anesthesia.

USES Prevention of nausea and vomiting associated with initial and repeated courses of cancer chemotherapy, including high-dose cisplatin; postoperative nausea and vomiting.
UNLABELED USES Treatment of hyperemesis gravidarum.

CONTRAINDICATIONS Hypersensitivity to ondansetron.
CAUTIOUS USE Zofran ODT contains aspartame and will affect phenylketonuria. Pregnancy (category B), lactation, and children ≤2 y.

ROUTE & DOSAGE

Nausea and Vomiting Related to Chemotherapy & Radiotherapy

Child: PO *4–11 y,* 4 mg 30 min before chemotherapy, then q8h times 2 more doses; *≤12 y,* 8 mg 30 min before chemotherapy, then q8h times 2 more doses; IV *>4 y,* 0.15 mg/kg over 15 min beginning 30 min before start of chemotherapy, followed by 0.15 mg/kg 4 and 8 h after first dose of ondansetron, may also give 8 mg bolus, then 1 mg/h by continuous infusion (max 32 mg/day), or 32 mg as single dose
Adult: IV 0.15 mg/kg or 32 mg infused over 15 min beginning 30 min before start of chemotherapy, followed by 0.15 mg/kg 4 and 8 h after first dose of ondansetron, may also give 8 mg bolus, then 1 mg/h by continuous infusion (max 32 mg/day), or 32 mg as single dose

Nausea & Vomiting with Highly Emetogenic Chemotherapy

Adult: PO Single 24 mg dose 30 min before administration of single-day highly emetogenic chemotherapy

Postoperative Nausea and Vomiting

Child: IV *≥2 y or ≤40 kg,* 0.1 mg/kg/dose times one dose; *>40 kg,* 4 mg times one dose by slow IV push
Adult: PO 8–16 mg 1 h preoperatively IM 4 mg injected immediately prior to anesthesia induction or once postoperatively if patient experiences nausea/vomiting shortly after surgery IV 4 mg by slow IV push, may repeat q8h as needed

ADMINISTRATION

Oral

- Give tablets 30 min prior to chemotherapy and 1–2 h prior to radiation therapy.
- Do NOT push orally disintegrating tablet through blister foil. Peel foil back and remove tablet. Tablets will disintegrate with/without liquid.
- Tablets can be swallowed with liquid.
- Oral tablet has <0.03 mg aspartame.

Intravenous

PREPARE **Direct:** May be given undiluted. **IV Infusion:** Dilute a single dose in 50 mL of D5W or NS (maximum concentration 1 mg/mL). May be further diluted in selected IV solution.

ADMINISTER **Direct:** Give over at least 30 sec, 2–5 min preferred. **IV Infusion:** Give over 15 min. When three separate doses are administered, infuse each over 15 min.

INCOMPATIBILITIES **Solution/Additive:** Meropenem. **Y-Site:** Acyclovir, allopurinol, aminophylline, amphotericin B, ampicillin, ampicillin/sulbactam, amsacrine, cefepime, cefoperazone, fluorouracil, furosemide, ganciclovir, lorazepam, meropenem, methylprednisolone, piperacillin, sargramostim, sodium bicarbonate, TPN.

ADVERSE EFFECTS CNS: Dizziness and light-headedness, *headache, sedation.* **GI:** *Diarrhea,* constipation, dry mouth, transient increases in liver aminotransferases and bilirubin. **Body as a Whole:** Hypersensitivity reactions.

INTERACTIONS Drug: **Rifampin** may decrease ondansetron levels.

PHARMACOKINETICS Peak: 1–1.5 h. **Metabolism:** Metabolized in liver. Bioavailability of oral drug 50–70%. **Elimination:** 44–60% excreted in urine within 24 h; approximately 25% excreted in feces. **Half-Life:** Child 3–7 y, 2.6 h; 7–12 y, 3.1 h; adult 3 h.

NURSING IMPLICATIONS

Assessment & Drug Effects

- Monitor fluid and electrolyte status. Diarrhea, which may cause fluid and electrolyte imbalance, is a potential adverse effect of the drug.
- Monitor cardiovascular status, especially in patients with a history of coronary artery disease. Rare cases of tachycardia and angina have been reported.
- If patient does not have adequate control of postoperative nausea and vomiting following initial dose, second dosage may not improve condition.

Patient & Family Education

- Be aware that headache requiring an analgesic for relief is a common adverse effect.
- May cause dry mouth.
- Store this medication out of reach of children.

OPIUM, POWDERED OPIUM TINCTURE (LAUDANUM)

(oh'pee-um)

Deodorized Opium Tincture

Classifications: CENTRAL NERVOUS SYSTEM AGENT; NARCOTIC (OPIATE) AGONIST; NARCOTIC ANALGESIC; ANTIDIARRHEAL

Prototype: Morphine

Pregnancy Category: B

Controlled Substance Schedule II

AVAILABILITY 10%, 2 mg/5 mL liquid

ACTIONS Is obtained from the unripe capsules of <u>Papaver somniferum</u> or <u>P. album</u> and contains several natural alkaloids including morphine, codeine, papaverine.

THERAPEUTIC EFFECTS Antidiarrheal due to inhibition of GI motility and propulsion; leads to prolonged transit of intestinal contents, desiccation of feces, and constipation.

USES Symptomatic treatment of acute diarrhea and to treat severe withdrawal symptoms in neonates born to women addicted to opiates or on narcotics for chronic pain control.

CONTRAINDICATIONS Diarrhea caused by poisoning (until poison is completely eliminated); increased intercranial pressure, severe respiratory depression, severe renal or hepatic insufficiency. Pregnancy (category B), lactation.

CAUTIOUS USE History of opiate agonist dependence; asthma; severe prostatic hypertrophy; hepatic disease, infants <3 mo.

ROUTE & DOSAGE

Acute Diarrhea

Child: **PO** 0.005–0.01 mL/kg q3–4h (max 6 doses/24 h)
Adult: **PO** 0.6 mL q.i.d. up to 1 mL q.i.d. (max 6 mL/day)

Neonatal Withdrawal

Full-term neonate: **PO** Make a 1:25 aqueous dilution (final concentration 0.4 mg/mL), then give 3–6 drops q3–6h as needed or 0.2 mL q3h, may increase by 0.05 mL q3h until withdrawal symptoms are controlled, then gradually decrease dose after withdrawal symptoms have stabilized (max dose 0.7 mL/dose)

STORAGE

Store at 15°–30° C (59°–86° F) in tight, light-resistant container; protect from sunlight and excessive heat.

ADMINISTRATION

Oral

- Do not confuse this preparation with camphorated opium tincture (paregoric), which contains only 2 mg anhydrous morphine/5 mL, thus requiring a higher dose volume than that required for therapeutic dose of Deodorized Opium Tincture.

- Ensure that proper 1:25 dilution has been made prior to administration.
- Give drug diluted with about one-third glass of water to ensure passage of entire dose into stomach.
- May give with food to decrease GI upset.

ADVERSE EFFECTS GI: Nausea and other GI disturbances. **CNS:** Depression of CNS.

INTERACTIONS Drug: Alcohol and other CNS DEPRESSANTS add to CNS effects.

PHARMACOKINETICS Absorption: Variable absorption from GI tract. **Distribution:** Crosses placenta; distributed into breast milk. **Metabolism:** Metabolized in liver. **Elimination:** Excreted in urine.

NURSING IMPLICATIONS

Assessment & Drug Effects
- Withhold medication and report to physician if respirations are 12/min or below or have changed in character and rate.
- Discontinue as soon as diarrhea is controlled; note character and frequency of stools.
- Offer small amounts of fluid frequently but attempt to maintain adequate hydration for age for 24 h requirement.
- Monitor body weight, I&O ratio and pattern, and temperature. If patient develops fever of 38.8° C (102° F) or above, electrolyte and hydration levels may need to be evaluated. Consult physician.
- Monitor infant for withdrawal symptoms with abstinence scales per institutional policy. Infant withdrawal should be gradual; stopping drug abruptly may increase withdrawal symptoms.

Patient & Family Education
- Be aware that constipation may be a consequence of antidiarrheal therapy but that normal habit pattern usually is reestablished with resumption of normal dietary intake.
- Note: Addiction is possible with prolonged use or with drug abuse.
- Do not breast feed while taking this drug.
- Store this medication in locked area out of reach of children; this is a Scheduled II drug.

OSELTAMIVIR PHOSPHATE

(o-sel'ta-mi-vir)
Tamiflu
Classifications: ANTI-INFECTIVE; ANTIVIRAL
Prototype: Acyclovir
Pregnancy Category: C

AVAILABILITY 75 mg capsule; 12 mg/mL suspension

ACTIONS Inhibits influenza A and B viral neuroaminidase enzyme, preventing the release of newly formed virus from the surface of the infected cells.

THERAPEUTIC EFFECTS Indicated by relief of flu symptoms. Prevents viral spread across the mucous lining of the respiratory tract. Inhibits replication of the influenza A and B virus.

USES Treatment of uncomplicated acute influenza in adults symptomatic for no more than 2 days.

CONTRAINDICATIONS Hypersensitivity to oseltamivir; lactation.
CAUTIOUS USE Renal impairment; pregnancy (category C). Safety and efficacy in chronic cardiac/respiratory disease are not established. Safety and efficacy in children <1 y not established.

ROUTE & DOSAGE

Influenza

Child 1–12 y: **PO** *>1 y, ≤15 kg*, 30 mg b.i.d. × 5 days (max dose 30 mg); *>15–23 kg*, 45 mg b.i.d. × 5 days; *>23–40 kg*, 60 mg b.i.d. × 5 days; *>40 kg*, 75 mg b.i.d. × 5 days
Child >12 y/Adult: **PO** *75* mg b.i.d. × 5 days

Renal Impairment

Adult: Cl_{cr} <30 mL/min: *75* mg daily times 5 days

STORAGE
Store at 15°–30° C (59°–86° F); protect from moisture.

ADMINISTRATION

Oral
- Give with food to decrease the risk of GI upset.
- Start within 48 h of onset of flu symptoms.
- Take missed dose as soon as possible unless next dose is due within 2 h.

ADVERSE EFFECTS Body as a Whole: Fatigue. **CNS:** Dizziness, headache, insomnia, vertigo. **GI:** Nausea, vomiting, diarrhea, abdominal pain. **Respiratory:** Bronchitis, cough.

PHARMACOKINETICS Absorption: Readily absorbed, 75% bioavailable. **Distribution:** 42% protein bound. **Metabolism:** Extensively metabolized to active metabolite oseltamivir carboxylate by liver esterases. **Elimination:** Primarily excreted in urine. **Half-Life:** 1–2 h; oseltamivir carboxylate, 6–10 h.

NURSING IMPLICATIONS

Assessment & Drug Effects
- Monitor ambulation in frail patients due to potential for dizziness and vertigo.

Patient & Family Education
- Not a replacement for influenza vaccine.
- Do not breast feed while taking this drug.
- Store this medication out of reach of children.

OXACILLIN SODIUM

(ox-a-sill'in)

Bactocill, Prostaphlin

Classifications: ANTI-INFECTIVE; ANTIBIOTIC, PENICILLIN; ANTISTAPHYLOCOCCAL PENICILLIN

Prototype: Penicillin G

Pregnancy Category: B

AVAILABILITY 250 mg, 500 mg capsules; 250 mg/5 mL suspension; 250 mg, 500 mg, 1 g, 2 g injection

ACTIONS Semisynthetic, acid-stable, penicillinase-resistant isoxazolyl penicillin.

THERAPEUTIC EFFECTS In common with other isoxazolyl penicillins (cloxacillin, dicloxacillin), it is highly active against most penicillinase-producing *staphylococci*, is less potent than penicillin G against penicillin-sensitive microorganisms, and is generally ineffective against gram-negative bacteria and methicillin-resistant *staphylococci* (MRSA).

USES Primarily, infections caused by penicillinase-producing staphylococci and penicillin-resistant staphylococci. May be used to initiate therapy in suspected staphylococcal infections pending culture and sensitivity test results. As with other penicillins, serum concentrations are enhanced by concurrent use of probenecid.

CONTRAINDICATIONS Hypersensitivity to penicillins or cephalosporins. Safe use during pregnancy (category B) is not established.

CAUTIOUS USE History of or suspected atopy or allergy (hives, eczema, hay fever, asthma); premature infants, neonates, lactation (may cause infant diarrhea).

ROUTE & DOSAGE

Neonate <7 days: **IM/IV** ≤2 kg, 50 mg/kg/day in equally divided doses q12h; >2 kg, 75 mg/kg/day in equally divided doses q8h
Neonate >7 days: <1.2 kg, 50 mg/kg/day in equally divided doses q12h; 1.2–2 kg, 75 mg/kg/day in equally divided doses q8h; ≥2 kg, 100 mg/kg/day in equally divided doses q6h

Staphylococcal Infections

Child <40 kg: **PO** 50–100 mg/kg/day in 4 divided doses q6h **IM/IV** (mild to moderate infections) 50–100 mg/kg/day divided q6h; (severe infections) 100–200 mg/kg/day divided q4–6h (max dosage 12 g/day)
Child >40 kg/Adult: **PO** 250–1000 mg q4–6h **IM/IV** 250 mg–2 g q4–6h up to 12 g/day

STORAGE

Store powder at 15°–30° C (59°–86° F) after reconstitution. Discard unused portions after 3 days at room temperature or 7 days under refrigeration.

ADMINISTRATION

Note: The total sodium content (including that contributed by buffer) in each gram of oxacillin is approximately 3.1 mEq or 71 mg.

Oral

- Give with a full glass of water or generous amount appropriate for age on an empty stomach (either 1 h before meals or 2 h after meals). Food reduces absorption.
- Oral form no longer available in U.S.

Intramuscular

- Reconstitute each 250 mg with 1.4 mL sterile water for injection to yield 250 mg/1.5 mL. Shake vial vigorously until drug is completely dissolved.
- Administer deep IM to infants and children according to agency policy or see safe site selection in Part I. Adults by deep intragluteal injection. Rotate injection sites.

Intravascular

Note: Verify correct IV concentration and rate of infusion/injection with physician and pharmacy before IV administration to neonates, infants, children (maximum concentration for push is 100 mg/mL given over 10 min; intermittent give at ≤40 mg/mL over 15–30 min).

PREPARE Direct: Reconstitute each 500 mg or fraction thereof with 5 mL with sterile water for injection or NS to yield 250 mg/1.5 mL. **Intermittent:** Further dilute in 50–100 mL of D5W, NS, D5/NS, or RL. **Continuous:** Further dilute in up to 1000 mL of compatible IV solutions.

ADMINISTER Direct: Give at a rate of 1 g or fraction thereof over 10 min. **Intermittent:** Give over 15–30 min. **Continuous:** Give over 6 h.

INCOMPATIBILITIES Solution/Additive: Cytarabine. **Y-Site: Sodium bicarbonate, verapamil.**

ADVERSE EFFECTS Body as a Whole: Thrombophlebitis (IV therapy), superinfections, wheezing, sneezing, fever, anaphylaxis. **GI:** Nausea, vomiting, flatulence, *diarrhea*, hepatocellular dysfunction (elevated AST, ALT, hepatitis). **Hematologic:** Eosinophilia, leukopenia, thrombocytopenia, granulocytopenia, agranulocytosis; neutropenia (reported in children). **Skin:** Pruritus, rash, urticaria. **Urogenital:** Interstitial nephritis, transient hematuria, albuminuria, azotemia (newborns and infants on high doses).

DIAGNOSTIC TEST INTERFERENCE Oxacillin in large doses can cause false-positive ***urine protein tests*** using sulfosalicylic acid methods.

INTERACTIONS Drug: Probenecid decreases elimination of oxacillin.

PHARMACOKINETICS Absorption: Incompletely and erratically absorbed orally. **Peak:** 30–120 min IM; 15 min IV. **Duration:** 4 h PO; 4–6 h IM. **Distribution:** Distributes into CNS with inflamed meninges; crosses placenta; distributed into breast milk. **Metabolism:** Enters enterohepatic circulation. **Elimination:** Primarily excreted in urine, some in bile. **Half-Life:** Neonate <15 days, 1.6 h; >1 wk–2 y, 0.9–1.8 h; adult, 0.5–1 h.

NURSING IMPLICATIONS

Assessment & Drug Effects

- Ask patient prior to first dose about hypersensitivity reactions to penicillins, cephalosporins, and other allergens.

- Lab test: Periodic liver functions, CBC with differential, platelet count, and urinalysis.
- Hepatic dysfunction (possibly a hypersensitivity reaction) has been associated with IV oxacillin; it is reversible with discontinuation of drug. Symptoms may resemble viral hepatitis or general signs of hypersensitivity and should be reported promptly: Hives, rash, fever, nausea, vomiting, abdominal discomfort, anorexia, malaise, jaundice (with dark yellow to brown urine, light-colored or clay-colored stools, pruritus).
- Withhold drug and immediately report the onset of hypersensitivity reactions and superinfections (see Appendix D-1).

Patient & Family Education
- Take oral medication around the clock, do not to miss a dose. Take all of the medication prescribed even if you feel better, unless otherwise directed by physician. Maintain fluid intake for age group.
- Do not breast feed while taking this drug without consulting physician.
- Store this medication out of reach of children.

OXAMNIQUINE
(ox-am'ni-kwin)
Vansil
Classifications: ANTI-INFECTIVE; ANTHELMINTIC
Prototype: Mebendazole
Pregnancy Category: C

AVAILABILITY 250 mg capsules

ACTIONS Hydroquinone derivative prepared in the presence of *Aspergillus sclerotium*. Mechanism of action not fully explained, but it appears that drug-induced strong contractions and paralysis of worm musculature leads to immobilization of their suckers and dislodgment from their usual residence in mesenteric veins to the liver.

THERAPEUTIC EFFECTS Dislodgment of schistosomes begins about 2 days after single oral dose; movement is not complete until 6 days after treatment with the drug. After treatment, surviving unpaired females return to mesenteric vessels; however, oviposition (egg laying) seems to stop in 24–48 h after drug treatment, reducing egg load and removing principal cause of pathology associated with schistosomal infection.

USES All stages of Schistosoma mansoni infection, including acute and chronic phases with hepatosplenic involvement.

CONTRAINDICATIONS Safe use during pregnancy (category C), lactation, or in children is not established.
CAUTIOUS USE History of convulsant disorders.

ROUTE & DOSAGE

Schistosomiasis

Child: **PO** <30 kg, 10 mg/kg times 2 doses at 2–8 h intervals
Adult: **PO** 12–15 mg/kg as single dose

STORAGE
Store product in tightly closed container at controlled room temperature less than 30° C (86° F).

ADMINISTRATION
Oral
- Give on an empty stomach, if possible.
- Administer with food if necessary to reduce GI distress and improve tolerance.

ADVERSE EFFECTS CNS: *Transitory dizziness, drowsiness, headache;* persistent fever (in patients being treated in Egypt); EEG abnormalities, convulsions (rare). **GI:** Anorexia, nausea, vomiting, abdominal pain, elevated liver enzyme concentrations. **Hematologic:** Increased erythrocyte sedimentation rate, reticulocyte count, and increased or decreased leukocyte count. **Skin:** Urticaria. **Urogenital:** Red-orange urine.

INTERACTIONS Food: Rate and extent of absorption are decreased by food.

PHARMACOKINETICS Absorption: Readily absorbed from GI tract. **Peak:** 1–3 h. **Metabolism:** Extensively metabolized in GI mucosa. **Elimination:** Excreted in urine. **Half-Life:** 1–2.5 h.

NURSING IMPLICATIONS

Assessment & Drug Effects
- Supervise ambulation and use other safety precautions because >30% of patients experience dizziness or drowsiness.
- If patient has a history of seizures, the possibility of seizures is increased because of drug action (occurs within hours of drug administration).

Patient & Family Education
- Use caution while driving or performing other tasks requiring alertness because drug can cause dizziness or drowsiness.
- Be aware that drug may change the normal urine color to a harmless orange-red.
- Do not breast feed while taking this drug without consulting physician.
- Store this medication out of reach of children.

OXCARBAZEPINE
(oc-car′ba-ze-peen)
Trileptal
Classifications: CENTRAL NERVOUS SYSTEM AGENT; ANTICONVULSANT
Prototype: Carbamazepine
Pregnancy Category: C

AVAILABILITY 150 mg, 300 mg, 600 mg tablets; 300 mg/5 mL suspension

ACTIONS Structurally related to tricyclic antidepressants (TCAs) but lacks antidepressant properties. Anticonvulsant properties may result from blockage of voltage-sensitive sodium channels, which results in stabilization of hyperexcited neural membranes.

THERAPEUTIC EFFECTS Inhibits repetitive neuronal firing, and decreased propagation of neuronal impulses.

USES Monotherapy or adjunctive therapy in the treatment of partial seizures in adults and children age 4–16 years.

CONTRAINDICATIONS Hypersensitivity to oxcarbazepine; pregnancy (category C), lactation; children <4 y.

CAUTIOUS USE Renal impairment; children <8 y; infertility, hyponatremia, SIADH, and drugs associated with SIADH as an adverse effect.

ROUTE & DOSAGE

Partial Seizures

Child: **PO** *4–16 y,* Initiate with 8–10 mg/kg/day in equally divided doses b.i.d. (max 600 mg/day), gradually increase weekly to target dose (divided b.i.d.) daily dose based on weight: *20–29 kg,* 900 mg/day b.i.d.; *29.1–39 kg,* 1200 mg/day b.i.d.; *>39 kg,* 1800 mg/day b.i.d. *Adult:* **PO** Start with 300 mg b.i.d. and increase by 600 mg/day every week to 2400 mg/day in 2 divided doses for monotherapy or 1200 mg/day as adjunctive therapy

Renal Impairment

Adult: Cl_{cr} <30 mL/min: Initiate at ½ usual starting dose (300 mg b.i.d.)

STORAGE

Store preferably at 25° C (77° F), but room temperature permitted. Keep container tightly closed. Oral suspension comes with an oral measuring device, follow manufacturers instructions for usage. Discard any unused portion after 7 wk of opening suspension bottle.

ADMINISTRATION

Oral

- Initiate therapy at one-half the usual starting dose (300 mg/day) if creatinine clearance <30 mL/min.
- May be given without regard to food.
- Shake suspension well before using. Suspension contains saccharin and ethanol.
- Do not abruptly stop this medication; withdraw drug gradually when discontinued to minimize seizure potential.

ADVERSE EFFECTS Body as a Whole: *Fatigue,* asthenia, peripheral edema, generalized edema, chest pain, weight gain. **CV:** Hypotension. **GI:** *Nausea, vomiting, abdominal pain,* diarrhea, dyspepsia, constipation, gastritis, anorexia, dry mouth. **Hematologic:** Lymphadenopathy. **Metabolic:** Hyponatremia. **Musculoskeletal:** Muscle weakness. **CNS:** *Headache, dizziness, somnolence, ataxia, nystagmus, abnormal gait,* insomnia, tremor, nervousness, agitation, abnormal coordination, speech disorder, confusion, abnormal thinking, aggregate convulsions, emotional lability. **Respiratory:** Rhinitis, cough, bronchitis, pharyngitis.

Common adverse effects in *italic;* life-threatening effects <u>underlined</u>; generic names in **bold**; drug classifications in SMALL CAPS; ♣ Canadian drug name; ❽ Prototype drug.

917

Skin: Acne, hot flushes, purpura rash (rare, but may be severe), <u>Stevens-Johnson syndrome.</u> **Special Senses:** *Diplopia, vertigo, abnormal vision,* abnormal accommodation, taste perversion, ear ache. **Urogenital:** Urinary tract infection, micturition frequency, vaginitis.

INTERACTIONS Drug: Carbamazepine, phenobarbital, phenytoin, valproic acid, verapamil may decrease oxcarbazepine levels; may increase levels of **phenobarbital, phenytoin;** may decrease levels of **felodipine,** ORAL CONTRACEPTIVES. **Herbal: Ginkgo** may decrease anticonvulsant effectiveness.

PHARMACOKINETICS Absorption: Rapidly and completely absorbed from GI tract. **Peak:** Steady-state levels reached in 2–3 days. **Distribution:** 40% protein bound. **Metabolism:** Extensively metabolized in liver to active 10-monohydroxy metabolite (MHD). **Elimination:** 95% excreted in kidneys. **Half-Life:** 2 h; MHD, 9 h.

NURSING IMPLICATIONS

Assessment & Drug Effects

- Monitor for and report S&S of hyponatremia (e.g., nausea, malaise, headache, lethargy, confusion) especially during 1st 3 mo of therapy; CNS impairment (e.g., somnolence, excessive fatigue, cognitive deficits, speech or language problems, incoordination, gait disturbances).
- Monitor phenytoin levels when administered concurrently.
- Lab tests: Periodic serum sodium, T_4 level; when oxcarbazepine is used as adjunctive therapy, closely monitor plasma level of the concomitant antiepileptic drug during titration of the oxcarbazepine dose.

Patient & Family Education

- Notify physician of the following: Dizziness, excess drowsiness, frequent headaches, malaise, double vision, lack of coordination, or persistent nausea.
- Exercise special caution with concurrent use of alcohol or CNS depressants.
- Use caution with potentially hazardous activities such as bike riding, skateboarding, sports, and driving until response to drug is known.
- Use or add barrier contraceptive because drug may render hormonal methods ineffective.
- Monitor seizure activity in response to this drug.
- Do not breast feed while taking this drug.
- Store this medication out of reach of children.

OXYBUTYNIN CHLORIDE

(ox-i-byoo'ti-nin)

Ditropan, Ditropan XL

Classifications: AUTONOMIC NERVOUS SYSTEM AGENT; ANTICHOLINERGIC (PARASYMPATHOLYTIC); ANTIMUSCARINIC; ANTISPASMODIC

Prototype: Atropine

Pregnancy Category: C

AVAILABILITY 5 mg tablets; 5 mg, 10 mg, 15 mg sustained-release tablets; 5 mg/5 mL syrup

ACTIONS Synthetic tertiary amine that exerts direct antispasmodic action and inhibits muscarinic effects of acetylcholine on smooth muscle.
THERAPEUTIC EFFECTS Prominent antispasmodic activity.

USES To relieve symptoms associated with voiding in patients with uninhibited neurogenic bladder and reflex neurogenic bladder. Also has been used to relieve pain of bladder spasm following transurethral surgical procedures.

CONTRAINDICATIONS Glaucoma, myasthenia gravis, partial or complete GI obstruction, paralytic ileus, intestinal atony (especially debilitated patients), megacolon, severe colitis, GU obstruction, unstable cardiovascular status. Safe use during pregnancy (category C), lactation, or in children <5 y is not established.
CAUTIOUS USE Autonomic neuropathy, hiatus hernia with reflex esophagitis; hepatic or renal dysfunction; urinary infection; hyperthyroidism; CHF, coronary artery disease, hypertension.

ROUTE & DOSAGE

Neurogenic Bladder
Child: **PO** 1–5 y, 0.2 mg/kg/dose b.i.d.–q.i.d.; >5 y, 5 mg b.i.d. (max 15 mg/day)
Adult: **PO** 5 mg b.i.d. or t.i.d. (max 20 mg/day) or 5 mg sustained-release daily, may increase up to 30 mg/day

0

STORAGE
Store at 15°–30° C (59°–86° F) in tight containers; protect oral solution from light.

ADMINISTRATION
Oral
- Ensure that sustained-release form is not chewed or crushed. It must be swallowed whole.
- Can be administered with food or milk to decrease GI upset.

ADVERSE EFFECTS CNS: *Drowsiness,* dizziness, weakness, insomnia, restlessness, psychotic behavior (overdosage). **CV:** Palpitations, tachycardia, flushing. **Special Senses:** Mydriasis, *blurred vision,* cycloplegia, increased ocular tension. **GI:** *Dry mouth,* nausea, vomiting, *constipation,* bloated feeling. **Urogenital:** Urinary hesitancy or retention, impotence. **Body as a Whole:** <u>Severe allergic reactions</u> including urticaria, skin rashes, suppression of lactation, decreased sweating, fever.

PHARMACOKINETICS Onset: 0.5–1 h. **Peak:** 3–6 h. **Duration:** 6–10 h. **Metabolism:** Metabolized in liver. **Elimination:** Excreted primarily in urine. **Half-Life:** 2–5 h.

NURSING IMPLICATIONS

Assessment & Drug Effects

- Periodic interruptions of therapy are recommended to determine patient's need for continued treatment. Tolerance has occurred in some patients.
- Keep physician informed of expected responses to drug therapy (e.g., effect on urinary frequency, urgency, urge incontinence, nocturia, completeness of bladder emptying).
- Monitor patients with colostomy or ileostomy closely; abdominal distention and the onset of diarrhea in these patients may be early signs of intestinal obstruction or of toxic megacolon.

Patient & Family Education

- Do not engage in potentially hazardous such as biking, skateboarding, sports, and other activities until response to drug is known.
- Exercise caution in hot environments. By suppressing sweating, oxybutynin can cause fever and heat stroke.
- May cause dry mouth.
- Inert outer shell of Ditropan XL is excreted intact in feces.
- Do not breast feed while taking this drug without consulting physician.
- Store this medication out of reach of children.

OXYCODONE HYDROCHLORIDE

(ox-i-koe′done)

OxyContin, Percolone, Endocodone, OxyFAST, Roxicodone

Classifications: CENTRAL NERVOUS SYSTEM AGENT; NARCOTIC (OPIATE) AGONIST; ANALGESIC

Prototype: Morphine

Pregnancy Category: B (D for prolonged use or use of high doses at term)

Controlled Substance: Schedule II

AVAILABILITY 5 mg, 15 mg, 30 mg tablets **OxyContin** 10 mg, 20 mg, 40 mg, 80 mg, 160 mg sustained-release tablets; 5 mg/5 mL, 20 mg/mL oral solution

Combination Products: Available in combination form of Oxycdone HCl/Ocycodone Terephthalate/aspirin as Percodan, Percodan-Demi, Roxiprin. 2.5 mg oxycodone/325 mg acetaminophen, 5 mg oxycodone/325 mg acetaminophen, 5 mg oxycodone/500 mg acetaminophen, 7.5 mg oxycodone/325 mg acetaminophen, 7.5 mg oxycodone/500 mg acetaminophen, 10 mg oxycodone/325 mg acetaminophen tablets; 5 mg oxycodone/500 mg acetaminophen capsules, 5 mg oxycodone/325 mg acetaminophen/5 mL solution 4.5 mg oxycodone HCL, 0.38 mg oxycodone tereph/325 mg asprin; 225 mg oxycodone HCL, 0.19 oxycodone tereph/325 mg asprin.

ACTIONS Semisynthetic derivative of an opium alkaloid with actions qualitatively similar to those of morphine. Most prominent actions involve CNS and organs composed of smooth muscle. Binds with stereospecific receptors in various sites of CNS to alter both perception of pain

and emotional response to pain, but precise mechanism of action not clear. As potent as morphine and 10–12 times more potent than codeine.
THERAPEUTIC EFFECTS Active against moderate to moderately severe pain. Appears to be more effective in relief of acute than long-standing pain.

USES Relief of moderate to moderately severe pain such as may occur with bursitis, dislocations, simple fractures and other injuries, and neuralgia. Relieves postoperative, postextractional, postpartum, and cancer pain.

CONTRAINDICATIONS Hypersensitivity to oxycodone and principal drugs with which it is combined; during pregnancy (category B); for prolonged use or high doses at term (category D); lactation, and children <6 y.
CAUTIOUS USE Alcoholism; renal or hepatic disease; viral infections; Addison's disease; cardiac arrhythmias; chronic ulcerative colitis; history of drug abuse or dependency; gallbladder disease, acute abdominal conditions; head injury, intracranial lesions; hypothyroidism; prostatic hypertrophy; respiratory disease; urethral stricture; debilitated patients; peptic ulcer or coagulation abnormalities.

ROUTE & DOSAGE

Moderate to Severe Pain

Child: **PO** *6–12 y,* 0.05–0.15 mg/kg/dose q4–6h prn (up to 5 mg/dose)
Adult: **PO** 5–10 mg q6h prn; OxyContin can be dosed q8h

Combination of Oxycodone and Acetaminophen

Child: **PO** *6–12 y,* 0.05–0.15 mg/kg/dose q4–6h prn (dosage based on oxycodone component)
Adult: **PO** 1–2 tablets q6h prn (max dose of acetaminophen is 4 g/day)

O

STORAGE
Store at 15°–30° C (59°–86° F); protect from light.

ADMINISTRATION

Oral
- Ensure that sustained-release form is not chewed or crushed. It must be swallowed whole.
- Can be given with food to decrease GI upset.
- Combination form contains acetaminophen. Do not exceed recommend dosages for acetaminophen per day.
- Do not use combination form containing aspirin with children because of asprin link to Reye Syndrome.

ADVERSE EFFECTS CNS: Euphoria, dysphoria, light-headedness, dizziness, *sedation*. **GI:** Anorexia, nausea, vomiting, *constipation*, jaundice, hepatotoxicity (combinations containing acetaminophen). **Respiratory:** Shortness of breath, respiratory depression. **Skin:** Pruritus, skin rash. **CV:** Bradycardia. **Body as a Whole:** Unusual bleeding or bruising. **Urogenital:** Dysuria, frequency of urination, urinary retention.

DIAGNOSTIC TEST INTERFERENCE *Serum amylase* levels may be elevated because oxycodone causes spasm of sphincter of Oddi. *Blood glucose determinations:* False decrease (measured by *glucose oxidase-peroxidase method*). *5-HIAA determination:* False positive with use of *nitroisonaphthol reagent* (quantitative test is unaffected).

INTERACTIONS Drug: Alcohol and other CNS DEPRESSANTS add to CNS depressant activity. **Herbal: St. John's wort** may increase sedation. **Food:** High-fat meals may increase peak levels in sustained-release 160-mg tablets.

PHARMACOKINETICS Absorption: Readily absorbed from GI tract. **Onset:** 10–15 min. **Peak:** 30–60 min. **Duration:** 4–5 h. **Distribution:** Crosses placenta; distributed into breast milk. **Metabolism:** Metabolized in liver. **Elimination:** Excreted primarily in urine. **Half-Life:** 3–5 h.

NURSING IMPLICATIONS

Assessment & Drug Effects

- Monitor patient's response closely, especially to sustained release preparations.
- Consult physician if nausea continues after first few days of therapy.
- Note: Light-headedness, dizziness, sedation, or fainting appear to be more prominent in ambulatory than in nonambulatory patients and may be alleviated if patient lies down.
- Evaluate patient's continued need for oxycodone preparations. Psychic and physical dependence and tolerance may develop with repeated use. The potential for drug abuse is high.
- Lab tests: Check hepatic function and hematologic status periodically in patients on high doses.
- Be aware that serious overdosage of any oxycodone preparation presents problems associated with a narcotic overdose (respiratory depression, circulatory collapse, extreme somnolence progressing to stupor or coma).

Patient & Family Education

- Do not alter dosage regimen by increasing, decreasing, or shortening intervals between doses.
- Habit formation and liver damage may result.
- Avoid potentially hazardous activities such as biking, skateboarding, sports, driving a car, or operating machinery while using oxycodone preparation.
- Do not drink large amounts of alcoholic beverages while using oxycodone preparations; risk of liver damage is increased.
- Check with physician before taking OTC drugs for colds, stomach distress, allergies, insomnia, or pain (especially if using combination forms).
- Inform surgeon or dentist that you are taking an oxycodone preparation before any surgical procedure is undertaken.
- Do not breast feed while taking this drug.
- Store this medication in locked area out of reach of children; this is a Scheduled II drug.

Common adverse effects in *italic;* life-threatening effects underlined; generic names in **bold;** drug classifications in SMALL CAPS; ♣ Canadian drug name; ❷ Prototype drug.

OXYMETAZOLINE HYDROCHLORIDE

(ox-i-met-az′oh-leen)

Afrin, Dristan Long Lasting, Duramist Plus, Duration, Nafrine ♣, Neo-Synephrine 12 Hour, Nostrilla, Sinex Long Lasting

Classifications: EYE, EAR, NOSE, AND THROAT (EENT) PREPARATION; VASO-CONSTRICTOR, DECONGESTANT; SYMPATHOMIMETIC

Prototype: Naphazoline
Pregnancy Category: C

AVAILABILITY 0.025%, 0.05% solution

ACTIONS Sympathomimetic agent that acts directly on alpha receptors of sympathetic nervous system. No effect on beta receptors.
THERAPEUTIC EFFECTS Constricts smaller arterioles in nasal passages and has prolonged decongestant effect.

USES Short-term use only for relief of nasal congestion in a variety of allergic and infectious disorders of the upper respiratory tract; used as nasal tampon to facilitate intranasal examination or before nasal surgery. Also used as adjunct in treatment and prevention of middle ear infection by decreasing congestion of eustachian ostia. Used to stop epistaxis.

CONTRAINDICATIONS Use in children <2 y. Safe use during pregnancy (category C) or lactation is not established.
CAUTIOUS USE Within 14 days of use of MAO inhibitors; coronary artery disease, hypertension, hyperthyroidism, diabetes mellitus.

O

ROUTE & DOSAGE

Nasal Congestion

Child 2–5 y: **Intranasal** 2–3 drops of 0.025% solution into each nostril b.i.d. for up to 3–5 days
Child ≥6 y/Adult: **Intranasal** 2–3 drops or 2–3 sprays of 0.05% solution into each nostril b.i.d. for up to 3–5 days **Ophthalmic** Instill 1–2 drops in infected eye q6h

ADMINISTRATION

Intranasal

- Place spray nozzle in nostril without occluding it and tilt head slightly forward prior to instillation of spray; sniff briskly during administration.
- Rinse dropper or spray tip in hot water after each use to prevent contamination of solution by nasal secretions.
- Usually given in the morning and at bedtime. Effects appear within 30 min and last about 6–7 h.

Ophthalmic

Do NOT allow tip of dropper for ocular preparation to contact any surface.

ADVERSE EFFECTS Special Senses: *Burning,* stinging, dryness of nasal mucosa, *sneezing.* **Body as a Whole:** Headache, lightheadedness, drowsiness, insomnia, palpitations, *rebound congestion.*

Common adverse effects in *italic;* life-threatening effects <u>underlined</u>; generic names in **bold;** drug classifications in SMALL CAPS; ♣ Canadian drug name; ☻ Prototype drug.

923

INTERACTIONS Drug: No clinically significant interactions established.

PHARMACOKINETICS Onset: 5–10 min. **Duration:** 6–10 h.

NURSING IMPLICATIONS

Assessment & Drug Effects

- Monitor for S&S of excess use. If noted, discuss possibility of rebound congestion.

Patient & Family Education

- Wash hands carefully after handling oxymetazoline. Anisocoria (inequality of pupil size, blurred vision) can develop if eyes are rubbed with contaminated fingers.
- Do not exceed recommended dosage. Rebound congestion (chemical rhinitis) may occur with prolonged or excessive use.
- Systemic effects can result from swallowing excessive medication.
- Do not breast feed while using this drug without consulting physician.
- Store this medication out of reach of children.

PALIVIZUMAB

(pal-i-viz′u-mab)
Synagis
Classifications: IMMUNOMODULATOR; IMMUNOGLOBULIN; MONOCLONAL ANTIBODY
Prototype: Basiliximab
Pregnancy Category: C

AVAILABILITY 50 mg, 100 mg vial

ACTIONS Monoclonal antibody (IgG1$_k$ produced by recombinant DNA technology) to the respiratory syncytial virus (RSV).

THERAPEUTIC EFFECTS Provides passive immunity against respiratory syncytial virus. Indicated by prevention of lower respiratory tract infection.

USES Prevention of serious lower respiratory tract infections in children susceptible to RSV.

CONTRAINDICATIONS Hypersensitivity to palivizumab in pediatric patients; children with cyanotic congenital heart disease.

CAUTIOUS USE Hypersensitivity to other immunoglobulin preparations, blood products, or other medications; in thrombocytopenia, coagulation disorders, kidney or liver dysfunction; acute RSV infection. Safety in pregnancy (category C) or lactation is not established.

ROUTE & DOSAGE

RSV

Child: **IM** 15 mg/kg every month during RSV season

Common adverse effects in *italic;* life-threatening effects <u>underlined</u>; generic names in **bold;** drug classifications in SMALL CAPS; ♣ Canadian drug name; ☻ Prototype drug.

STORAGE

Store powder at 2°–8° C (36°–46° F), prevent freezing, use reconstituted solutions within 6 h and discard any unused portions (contains no preservatives).

ADMINISTRATION

Intramuscular

- Reconstitute solution by gently injecting 1 mL of sterile water for injection (without preservative) toward the sides of the vial. Gently swirl for 30 sec to dissolve (do not shake solution). Allow to stand at room temperature for at least 20 min until solution clears.
- Give IM **only** into the anterolateral aspect of the thigh (see Part I). Volumes >1 mL should be divided and given in different sites.

ADVERSE EFFECTS Body as a Whole: *Otitis media,* pain, hernia. **GI:** Increased AST, diarrhea, nausea, vomiting, gastroenteritis. **Respiratory:** *URI, rhinitis,* pharyngitis, cough, wheeze, bronchiolitis, asthma, croup, dyspnea, sinusitis, apnea. **Skin:** *Rash.*

INTERACTIONS Drug: No clinically significant interactions established.

PHARMACOKINETICS Half-Life: 20 days.

NURSING IMPLICATIONS

Assessment & Drug Effects

- RSV prophylaxis begins with onset of RSV season and is terminated when weather becomes warm. Times vary according to regions.
- Monitor for signs of allergic reaction or anaphylactic shock following injection.
- Lab tests: Periodic monitoring of liver functions may be warranted.
- Monitor carefully for and immediately report S&S of respiratory illness including fever, cough, wheezing, and retractions.
- Assess for and report erythema or indurations at injection site.

Patient & Family Education

- Contact physician if S&S of respiratory illness, vomiting, diarrhea, or redness develop at injection site.
- Do not breast feed while taking this drug without consulting physician.
- Encourage parents to keep children away from crowds.

PAMIDRONATE DISODIUM

(pa-mi′dro-nate)
Aredia
Classifications: REGULATOR, BONE METABOLISM; BIPHOSPHONATE
Prototype: Etidronate
Pregnancy Category: C

AVAILABILITY 30 mg, 60 mg, 90 mg injection

Common adverse effects in *italic;* life-threatening effects underlined; generic names in **bold;** drug classifications in SMALL CAPS; ♣ Canadian drug name; ☻ Prototype drug.

925

ACTIONS A bone-resorption inhibitor thought to absorb calcium phosphate crystals in bone. May also inhibit osteoclast activity, thus contributing to inhibition of bone resorption.
THERAPEUTIC EFFECTS Does not inhibit bone formation or mineralization. Reduces bone turnover and, when used in combination with adequate hydration, increases renal excretion of calcium and reduces serum calcium concentrations.

USES Hypercalcemia of malignancy and Paget's disease, bone metastases in multiple myeloma; osteogenesis imperfecta.
UNLABELED USES Primary hyperparathyroidism, osteoporosis.

CONTRAINDICATIONS Hypersensitivity to pamidronate; lactation.
CAUTIOUS USE Chronic kidney failure and pregnancy (category C). Safety and effectiveness in children are not established.

ROUTE & DOSAGE

Hypercalcemia in Children
Limited experience but these dosages have been used:
Child: **IV** 0.5–1 mg/kg/dose times 1

Osteogenesis Imperfecta in Children
Limited experience but these dosages have been used:
Child: **IV** 0.5–1 mg/kg/day for 3 days, may repeat in 4–6 mo intervals

Moderate Hypercalcemia of Malignancy (corrected calcium 12–13.5 mg/dL)
Adult: **IV** 15–90 mg infused over 4–24 h, may repeat in 7 days

Severe Hypercalcemia of Malignancy (corrected calcium > 13.5 mg/dL)
Adult: **IV** 90 mg infused over 4–24 h, may repeat in 7 days

Paget's Disease, Metastases in Multiple Myeloma
Adult: **IV** 30 mg once daily for 3 days (90 mg total)

STORAGE
Refrigerate reconstituted pamidronate solution at 2°–8° C (36°–46° F); the IV solution may be stored at room temperature. Both are stable for 24 h.

ADMINISTRATION

Intravenous

PREPARE **IV Infusion:** Add 10 mL sterile water for injection to reconstitute the 30, 60, or 90 mg vial to produce concentrations of 3, 6, and 9 mg/1 mL, respectively. Withdraw the recommended dose and further dilute with D5W, NS, or 0.45% NaCl.
ADMINISTER **IV Infusion: For hypercalcemia of malignancy:** Use 1000 mL of IV solution. **For Paget's disease or osteolytic lesions of multiple myeloma:** Use 500 mL of IV solution. Infusing over 2–24 h may reduce renal toxicity
INCOMPATIBILITIES **Solution/Additive:** CALCIUM-CONTAINING SOLUTIONS (including LACTATED RINGER'S).

Common adverse effects in *italic;* life-threatening effects <u>underlined;</u> generic names in **bold;** drug classifications in SMALL CAPS; ✦ Canadian drug name; ❷ Prototype drug.

ADVERSE EFFECTS Body as a Whole: *Fever with or without rigors* generally occurs within 48 h and subsides within 48 h despite continued therapy; *thrombophlebitis at injection site;* general malaise lasting for several weeks; transient increase in bone pain. **Metabolic:** *Hypocalcemia.* **GI:** Nausea, abdominal pain, *epigastric discomfort.* **CV:** Hypertension. **Skin:** Rash.

INTERACTIONS Drug: Concurrent use of **foscarnet** may further decrease serum levels of ionized calcium.

PHARMACOKINETICS Absorption: 50% of IV dose is retained in body. **Onset:** 24–48 h. **Peak:** 6 days. **Duration:** 2 wk–3 mo. **Distribution:** Accumulates in bone; once deposited, remains bound until bone is remodeled. **Metabolism:** Not metabolized. **Elimination:** 50% excreted in urine unchanged. **Half-Life:** 28 h.

NURSING IMPLICATIONS

Assessment & Drug Effects
- Assess IV injection site for thrombophlebitis.
- Lab tests: Monitor serum calcium and phosphate levels, CBC, throughout course of therapy. Monitor kidney function (creatinine) prior to each dose.
- Monitor for S&S of hypocalcemia, hypokalemia, hypomagnesemia, and hypophosphatemia.
- Monitor for seizures especially in those with a preexisting seizure disorder.
- Monitor vital signs. Be aware that drug fever, which may occur with pamidronate use, is self-limiting, usually subsiding in 48 h even with continued therapy.

Patient & Family Education
- Be aware that transient, self-limiting fever with/without chills may develop.
- Generalized malaise, which may last for several weeks following treatment, is an anticipated adverse effect.
- Report to physician immediately perioral tingling, numbness, and paresthesia. These are signs of hypocalcemia.
- Do not breast feed while taking this drug.

PANCRELIPASE
(pan-kre-li′pase)
Cotazym, Cotazym-S, Festal II, Ilozyme, Ku-Zyme-Hp, Pancrease, Ultrase, Viokase
Classifications: HORMONES AND SYNTHETIC SUBSTITUTES; ENZYME; DIGESTANT
Pregnancy Category: C

AVAILABILITY Tablets or capsules containing lipase, protease, and amylase

PANCRELIPASE

ACTIONS Pancreatic enzyme concentrate of porcine origin standardized for lipase content. Similar to pancreatin but on a weight basis has 12 times the lipolytic activity and at least 4 times the trypsin and amylase content of pancreatin.
THERAPEUTIC EFFECTS Facilitates the hydrolysis of fats into glycerol and fatty acids, starches into dextrins and sugars, and proteins into peptides for easier absorption.

USES Replacement therapy in symptomatic treatment of malabsorption syndrome due to cystic fibrosis and other conditions associated with exocrine pancreatic insufficiency.

CONTRAINDICATIONS History of allergy to hog protein or enzymes. Safety during pregnancy (category C) is not established.
CAUTIOUS USE Lactation.

ROUTE & DOSAGE

Pancreatic Insufficiency

Note: These are initial dosages; individual dosages based on stool fat content and maintance body weight and growth for age. 8000 USP units are given for each 17 g dietary fat.
Infant: **PO** 2000–4000 units lipase per 120 mL of formula or per feeding by breast
Child: **PO** <4 y, 1000 units lipase/kg/meal given just before or during, with ½ dose taken with any food eaten or snacks eaten between meals; ≥4 y, 400–500 units lipase/kg/meal given just before or during, with ½ dose taken with any food eaten or snacks eaten between meals (max dose 2500 units lipase/kg)
Adult: **PO** 1–3 capsules or tablets or 1–2 packets of powder 1–2 h before, during, or 1 h after meals, with an extra dose taken with any food eaten between meals

STORAGE
Store at 15°–25° C (59°–77° F) in tightly closed containers.

ADMINISTRATION
Oral
- Ensure that enteric-coated preparations are not crushed or chewed.
- Note: For children, powder form may be sprinkled on food. Avoid inhalation of any powder because it could precipitate asthma attack.
- Open capsule and sprinkled contents on soft food, which should be swallowed without chewing to prevent mucous membrane irritation. Do not allow child to retain medication in mouth because it may cause stomatities or oral mucosal irritation. Follow with a full glass of water or juice. Cimetidine, ranitidine, or an antacid may be prescribed to be given before pancrelipase to prevent drug's destruction by gastric pepsin and acid pH.

ADVERSE EFFECTS GI: Anorexia, nausea, vomiting, diarrhea, high doses associated with chlonic strictures in children <12 y. **Respiratory:**

Bronchospasms, peranal irritation, flatulence, mouth irritation. **Metabolic:** Hyperuricosuria.

INTERACTIONS Drug: Iron absorption may be decreased. **Food:** Avoid sprinkling on alkaline foods such as dairy products (ice cream, custard, milk).

PHARMACOKINETICS Absorption: Not absorbed. **Distribution:** Acts locally in GI tract. **Elimination:** Excreted in feces.

NURSING IMPLICATIONS

Assessment & Drug Effects

■ Monitor I&O and weight. Note appetite and quality of stools, weight loss, abdominal bloating, polyuria, thirst, hunger, itching. Pancreatic insufficiency is frequently associated with steatorrhea, bulky stools, and insulin-dependent diabetes.

Patient & Family Education

■ Learn proper timing of medication in relation to meals.
■ Recommend patient not use generic forms of drug due to their association with treatment failure.
■ Do not breast feed while taking this drug without consulting physician.
■ Store this medication out of reach of children.

PANCURONIUM BROMIDE

(pan-kyoo-roe′nee-um)
Pavulon
Classifications: AUTONOMIC NERVOUS SYSTEM AGENT; SKELETAL MUSCLE RELAXANT, DEPOLARIZING, NONDEPOLARIZING
Prototype: Tubocurarine
Pregnancy Category: C

AVAILABILITY 1 mg/mL, 2 mg/mL (contain 1% benzyl alcohol) injection

ACTIONS Synthetic curariform nondepolarizing neuromuscular blocking agent. Similar to tubocurarine chloride, however reported to be approximately five times as potent as tubocurarine but produces little or no histamine release or ganglionic blockade and thus does not cause bronchospasm or hypotension.

THERAPEUTIC EFFECTS Produces skeletal muscle relaxation or paralysis by competing with acetylcholine at cholinergic receptor sites on skeletal muscle end plate and thus blocks nerve impulse transmission. In high doses has direct blocking effect on acetylcholine receptors of heart and may increase heart rate, cardiac output, and arterial pressure.

USES Adjunct to anesthesia to induce skeletal muscle relaxation. Also to facilitate management of patients undergoing mechanical ventilation.

CONTRAINDICATIONS Hypersensitivity to the drug or bromides; tachycardia severe renal impairment. Safety during pregnancy (category C) or lactation is not established.

CAUTIOUS USE Debilitated patients (mechanical ventilation must be used if giving pancuronium); myasthenia gravis; pulmonary, liver or kidney disease; fluid or electrolyte imbalance.

ROUTE & DOSAGE

Skeletal Muscle Relaxation

Child >1 mo/Adult: **IV** 0.04–0.1 mg/kg initial dose, may give additional doses of 0.01 mg/kg at 30–60 min intervals

STORAGE

Refrigerate at 2°–8° C (36°–46° F); do not freeze.

ADMINISTRATION

Intravenous

- Plastic syringe may be used for administration, but drug may adsorb to plastic with prolonged storage.
- Use a test dose of 0.02 mg/kg in infants ≥1 mo.

PREPARE **Direct:** Give undiluted.
ADMINISTER **Direct:** Give over 30–90 sec.
INCOMPATIBILITIES **Y-Site: Diazepam, thiopental.**

ADVERSE EFFECTS CV: *Increased pulse rate and BP,* ventricular extrasystoles. **Skin:** Transient acneiform rash, burning sensation along course of vein. **Body as a Whole:** Salivation, skeletal muscle weakness, <u>respiratory depression</u>.

DIAGNOSTIC TEST INTERFERENCE Pancuronium may decrease *serum cholinesterase* concentrations.

INTERACTIONS Drug: GENERAL ANESTHETICS increase neuromuscular blocking and duration of action; AMINOGLYCOSIDES, **bacitracin, polymyxin B, clindamycin, lidocaine,** parenteral **magnesium, quinidine, quinine, trimethaphan, verapamil** increase neuromuscular blockade; DIURETICS may increase or decrease neuromuscular blockade; **lithium** prolongs duration of neuromuscular blockade; NARCOTIC ANALGESICS possibly add to respiratory depression; **succinylcholine** increases onset and depth of neuromuscular blockade; **phenytoin** may cause resistance to or reversal of neuromuscular blockade.

PHARMACOKINETICS Onset: 30–45 sec. **Peak:** 2–3 min. **Duration:** 60 min. **Distribution:** Well distributed to tissues and extracellular fluids; crosses placenta in small amounts. **Metabolism:** Small amount metabolized in liver. **Elimination:** Excreted primarily in urine. **Half-Life:** 2 h.

NURSING IMPLICATIONS

Assessment & Drug Effects

- Assess cardiovascular and respiratory status continuously.
- Observe patient closely for residual muscle weakness and signs of respiratory distress during recovery period. Monitor BP and vital signs.

Peripheral nerve stimulator may be used to assess the effects of pancuronium and to monitor restoration of neuromuscular function.
- Antidote is neostigmine.
- Note: Consciousness is not affected by pancuronium. Patient will be awake and alert but unable to speak.

PANTOPRAZOLE SODIUM
(pan-to'pra-zole)
Protonix
Classifications: GASTROINTESTINAL AGENT; PROTON PUMP INHIBITOR
Prototype: Omeprazole
Pregnancy Category: B

AVAILABILITY 40 mg enteric-coated tablets; 40 mg vial

ACTIONS Gastric acid pump inhibitor; belongs to a class of antisecretory compounds. Gastric acid secretion is decreased by inhibiting the H^+, K^+-ATPase enzyme system responsible for acid production.
THERAPEUTIC EFFECTS Specifically, suppresses gastric acid secretion by inhibiting the acid (proton H^+) pump in the parietal cells.

USES Short-term treatment of erosive esophagitis associated with gastroesophageal reflux disease (GERD).

CONTRAINDICATIONS Hypersensitivity to pantoprazole; severe hepatic insufficiency, cirrhosis.
CAUTIOUS USE Mild to moderate hepatic insufficiency; pregnancy (category B), lactation. Safety and effectiveness in children <18 y are not established.

ROUTE & DOSAGE

Erosive Esophagitis
Limited experience with children but these dosages have been used:
Child >6–13y: **PO** 20 mg/day (0.5–1 mg/kg/day) for 28 days
Adult: **PO** 40 mg/day times 8–16 wk **IV** 40 mg/day times 7–10 days

STORAGE
Store preferably at 20°–25° C (66°–77° F), but room temperature permitted.

ADMINISTRATION
Oral
- Do not crush or break in half. Must be swallowed whole.
- Note: Therapy beyond 16 wk is not recommended.

Intravenous

PREPARE Reconstitute with 10 mL with NS and further dilute with D5W to 40 mg/50 mL **Infuse** Infuse each 40 mg in 50 mL of NS or D5W over a period of 15 min using filter provided (1.2 micron). Do not exceed 6 mg/min. Use dedicated line if possible or flush tubing with compatible solution before and after dosage.

Common adverse effects in *italic;* life-threatening effects <u>underlined</u>; generic names in **bold**; drug classifications in SMALL CAPS; ♣ Canadian drug name; ☻ Prototype drug.

931

ADVERSE EFFECTS GI: Diarrhea, flatulence, abdominal pain. **CNS:** Headache, insomnia. **Skin:** Rash.

INTERACTIONS Drug: May decrease absorption of **ampicillin,** IRON SALTS, **itraconazole, ketoconazole.**

PHARMACOKINETICS Absorption: Well absorbed with 77% bioavailability. **Peak:** 2.4 h. **Distribution:** 98% protein bound. **Metabolism:** Metabolized in liver primarily by CYP2C19. **Elimination:** 71% excreted in urine, 18% in feces. **Half-Life:** 1 h.

NURSING IMPLICATIONS

Assessment & Drug Effects

- Monitor for and immediately report S&S of angioedema or a severe skin reaction.
- Lab tests: Urea breath test 4–6 wk after completion of therapy.

Patient & Family Education

- Contact physician promptly if any of the following occur: Peeling, blistering, or loosening of skin; skin rash, hives, or itching; swelling of the face, tongue, or lips; difficulty breathing or swallowing.
- Do not breast feed while taking this drug without consulting physician.
- May cause dry mouth.
- Store this medication out of reach of children.

PANTOTHENIC ACID (DEXPANTHENOL) Calcium Pantothenate

(pan-to-then'-at)

Dexol, Ilopan, Panthoderm

Classifications: AUTONOMIC NERVOUS SYSTEM AGENT; CHOLINERGIC, DIRECT ACTING

Prototype: Bethanechol

Pregnancy Category: C

AVAILABILITY 100, 200, 250, 500 mg tablets; 250 mg/mL injection; 2% topical cream.

ACTIONS Analog of the coenzyme vitamin pantothenic acid, to which it is readily converted. A member of the B-complex group and precursor of coenzyme A, which is essential to normal epithelial function and biosynthesis of fatty acids, amino acids, and acetylcholine.

THERAPEUTIC EFFECTS Increases GI peristalsis and intestinal tone by stimulating acetylcholine. Topical application reportedly relieves itching and may aid healing of skin lesions by stimulating epithelialization and granulation.

USES Prevention or treatment of postoperative abdominal distention, intestinal atony, and paralytic ileus, for treatment of vitamin deficiency states. Topically to relieve itching and to promote healing in minor skin lesions.

CONTRAINDICATIONS Hemophilia; ileus due to mechanical obstruction. Safe use during pregnancy (category C), lactation, or in children is not established.
CAUTIOUS USE Hypokalemia.

ROUTE & DOSAGE

Note: Each 10 mg of calcium pantothenate = 9.2 mg pantothenic acid.
Dietary Supplement
Adult: **PO** 5–10 mg daily
Postoperative Abdominal Distention, Intestinal Atony, Paralytic Ileus
Child: **IM** 11–12.5 mg/kg, repeat in 2 h, then repeat q4–12h prn
Adult: **IM** 250–500 mg dexpanthenol form, repeat in 2 h, then repeat q4–12h prn **IV** 500 mg by slow IV infusion
Itching
Adult: **Topical** Apply 2% pantothenic acid to affected area 1–2 times/day

STORAGE
Store at 15°–30° C (59°–86° F); protect from freezing and excessive heat.

ADMINISTRATION
Topical
■ Do not administer within 1 h of succinylcholine.

Intramuscular
■ Give deep IM into a large muscle mass appropriate for age (see Part I).

Intravenous
PREPARE **IV Infusion:** Dilute in at least 500 mL of D5W or RL.
ADMINISTER **IV Infusion:** Infuse slowly over 3–6 h.

ADVERSE EFFECTS All: Generally well tolerated.

INTERACTION Drug: Prolongs muscle relaxation effects of **succinylcholine.**

PHARMACOKINETICS Absorption: Readily absorbed from IM site. **Distribution:** Highest concentration in liver, adrenals, heart, and kidneys; small amount distributed into breast milk. **Metabolism:** Rapidly converted to pantothenic acid, the active moiety. **Elimination:** 70% excreted in urine, 30% in feces.

NURSING IMPLICATIONS
Assessment & Drug Effects
■ Monitor for therapeutic effectiveness: May not see results in patients with hypokalemia until potassium imbalance is corrected.
■ Observe for and report bleeding tendency. Pantothenic acid may prolong bleeding time in some patients.
■ Report immediately any evidence of a hypersensitivity reaction (see Appendix D-1); drug should be discontinued.

Patient & Family Education

- Report abdominal cramping or diarrhea to physician.
- Teach about natural sources of the vitamin in the deficient child (meats, whole grains, legumes, milk, fruits, vegetables).
- Do not breast feed while taking this drug without consulting physician.
- Store this medication out of reach of children.

PAPAVERINE HYDROCHLORIDE

(pa-pav'er-een)

Cerespan, Genabid, Pavabid, Pavased, Pavatyme, Paverolan

Classifications: CARDIOVASCULAR AGENT; NONNITRATE VASODILATOR

Prototype: Hydralazine

Pregnancy Category: C

AVAILABILITY 150 mg sustained-release capsule; 30 mg/mL injection

ACTIONS Exerts nonspecific direct spasmolytic effect on smooth muscles unrelated to innervation. Action is especially pronounced on coronary, cerebral, pulmonary, and peripheral arteries when spasm is present.

THERAPEUTIC EFFECTS Acts directly on myocardium, depresses conduction and irritability, and prolongs refractory period. Stimulates respiration by action on carotid and aortic body chemoreceptors.

USES Primarily for relief of cerebral and peripheral ischemia associated with arterial spasm and MI complicated by arrhythmias. Also visceral spasm as in ureteral, biliary, and GI colic.

UNLABELED USES Impotence, cardiac bypass surgery.

CONTRAINDICATIONS Parenteral use in complete AV block. Safe during pregnancy (category C) or lactation is not established. Not recommended for use in neonates.

CAUTIOUS USE Glaucoma; myocardial depression; angina pectoris; recent stroke.

ROUTE & DOSAGE

Cerebral and Peripheral Ischemia

Child: **IM/IV** 6 mg/kg/day equally divided into 4 doses
Adult: **PO** 100–300 mg 3–5 times/day; 150 mg sustained-release q8–12h **IM/IV** 30–120 mg q3h as needed

STORAGE

Store at 15°–30° C (59°–86° F); avoid freezing.

ADMINISTRATION

Oral

- Give with or following meals; give milk or prescribed antacid to reduce possibility of nausea.
- Ensure that sustained-release form is not chewed or crushed. Must be swallowed whole.

Intramuscular

- Aspirate carefully before injecting IM to avoid inadvertent entry into blood vessel, and administer slowly.

***PREPARE* Direct:** Give undiluted or diluted in an equal volume of sterile water for injection.

***ADMINISTER* Direct:** Give slowly over 1–2 min. AVOID rapid injection. Causes arrhythmias and apnea that is fatal.

INCOMPATIBILITIES Lactated Ringer's causes a precipitate.

ADVERSE EFFECTS Body as a Whole: General discomfort, facial flushing, sweating, weakness, coma. **CNS:** Dizziness, drowsiness, headache, sedation. **CV:** Slight rise in BP, paroxysmal tachycardia, transient ventricular ectopic rhythms, AV block, arrhythmias. **GI:** Nausea, anorexia, constipation, diarrhea, abdominal distress, dry mouth and throat, <u>hepatotoxicity</u> (jaundice, eosinophilia, abnormal liver function tests); with rapid IV administration. **Respiratory:** Increased depth of respiration, <u>respiratory depression, fatal apnea</u>. **Skin:** Pruritus, skin rash. **Special Senses:** Diplopia, nystagmus. **Urogenital:** Priapism.

INTERACTIONS Drug: May decrease **levodopa** effectiveness; **morphine** may antagonize smooth muscle relaxation effect of papaverine.

PHARMACOKINETICS Absorption: Readily absorbed from GI tract. **Peak:** 1–2 h. **Duration:** 6 h regular tablets; 12 h sustained release. **Metabolism:** Metabolized in liver. **Elimination:** Excreted in urine chiefly as metabolites. **Half-Life:** 90 min.

NURSING IMPLICATIONS

Assessment & Drug Effects

- Monitor pulse, respiration, and BP in patients receiving drug parenterally. If significant changes are noted, withhold medication and report promptly to physician.
- Lab tests: Perform liver function and blood tests periodically. Hepatotoxicity (thought to be a hypersensitivity reaction) is reversible with prompt drug withdrawal.

Patient & Family Education

- Notify physician if any adverse effect persists or if GI symptoms, jaundice, or skin rash appear. Liver function tests may be indicated.
- Do not drive or engage in potentially hazardous activities until response to drug is known. Alcohol may increase drowsiness and dizziness.
- Do not breast feed while taking this drug without consulting physician.
- Store this medication out of reach of children.

PAREGORIC (CAMPHORATED OPIUM TINCTURE)

(par-e-gor′ik)

Classifications: GASTROINTESTINAL AGENT; ANTIDIARRHEAL; CENTRAL NERVOUS SYSTEM AGENT; NARCOTIC (OPIATE) AGONIST ANALGESIC

Prototype: Diphenoxylate HCl with atropine sulfate

Pregnancy Category: B (D for prolonged use or high doses at term)

Controlled Substance: Schedule III

Common adverse effects in *italic;* life-threatening effects <u>underlined;</u> generic names in **bold;** drug classifications in SMALL CAPS; ♣ Canadian drug name; ⊘ Prototype drug.

935

PAREGORIC (CAMPHORATED OPIUM TINCTURE)

AVAILABILITY 2 mg/mL liquid

ACTIONS Contains 2 mg anhydrous morphine, 45% alcohol, benzoic acid, camphor, and anise oil (licorice flavored). Pharmacologic activity is due to morphine content.

THERAPEUTIC EFFECTS Increases smooth muscle tone of GI tract, decreases motility and effective propulsive peristalsis while diminishing digestive secretions. Delayed transit of intestinal contents results in desiccation of feces and constipation.

USES Short-term treatment for symptomatic relief of acute diarrhea and abdominal cramps.

CONTRAINDICATIONS Hypersensitivity to opium alkaloids; diarrhea caused by poisons (until eliminated); pregnancy [(category B), with prolonged use or high doses at term (category D)].

CAUTIOUS USE Asthma; liver disease; history of opiate agonist dependence; severe prostatic hypertrophy, infants 3 mo more susceptible to respiratory depression; lactation.

ROUTE & DOSAGE

Acute Diarrhea
Child: **PO** 0.25–0.5 mL/kg 1–4 times/day
Adult: **PO** 5–10 mL after loose bowel movement, may be administered q2h up to q.i.d. if needed

Neonatal Abstinence Syndrome
0.1 mL/kg with feedings q3–4h, may increase by 0.1 mL/kg q3–4h until symptoms are controlled, then taper down over 2–4 wk

STORAGE
Store at 15°–30° C (59°–86° F) in tight, light resistant containers.

ADMINISTRATION

Oral
- Give paregoric in sufficient water (2 or 3 swallows) to ensure its passage into the stomach (mixture will appear milky). Do not confuse this drug with opium tincture, which is 25 times more potent.
- May give with food to decrease GI upset.

ADVERSE EFFECTS GI: Anorexia, nausea, vomiting, *constipation,* abdominal pain. **Body as a Whole:** Dizziness, faintness, drowsiness, facial flushing, sweating, physical dependence.

INTERACTIONS Drug: Alcohol and other CNS DEPRESSANTS add to CNS effects.

PHARMACOKINETICS Absorption: Readily absorbed from GI tract. **Duration:** 4–5 h. **Distribution:** Crosses placenta; distributed into breast milk. **Metabolism:** Metabolized in liver. **Elimination:** Excreted in urine. **Half-Life:** 2–3 h.

Common adverse effects in *italic;* life-threatening effects <u>underlined;</u> generic names in **bold;** drug classifications in SMALL CAPS; ♣ Canadian drug name; ❶ Prototype drug.

NURSING IMPLICATIONS

Assessment & Drug Effects

- Paregoric may worsen the course of infection-associated diarrhea by delaying the elimination of pathogens.
- Be aware that adverse effects are primarily due to morphine content. Paregoric abuse results because of the narcotic content of the drug.
- Assess for fluid and electrolyte imbalance until diarrhea has stopped.
- Monitor neonatal abstinence scores if treating withdrawal according to agency policies.
- In neonatal opiate withdrawal: Monitor for symptoms of paregoric overdosage (lethargy, hypotonia, respiratory depression with irregular rates, bradycardia) and symptoms of withdrawal return (high-pitched cry, yawning, sneezing, irritability, sucking of fists, poor feeding).

Patient & Family Education

- Adhere strictly to prescribed dosage schedule.
- Maintain bed rest if diarrhea is severe with a high level of fluid loss.
- Replace fluids and electrolytes as needed for diarrhea. Drink warm clear liquids and avoid dairy products, concentrated sweets, and cold drinks until diarrhea stops.
- Observe character and frequency of stools. Discontinue drug as soon as diarrhea is controlled. Report promptly to physician if diarrhea persists more than 3 days, if fever is >38.8° C (102° F), if abdominal pain develops, or if mucus or blood is passed.
- Understand that constipation is often a consequence of antidiarrheal treatment and a normal elimination pattern is usually established as dietary intake increases.
- Do not breast feed while taking this drug without consulting physician.
- Store this medication out of reach of children.

P

PAROMOMYCIN SULFATE ℗

(par-oh-moe-mye′sin)

Humatin

Classifications: ANTI-INFECTIVE; AMINOGLYCOSIDE ANTIBIOTIC; AMEBICIDE

Pregnancy Category: C

AVAILABILITY 250 mg tablets

ACTIONS Aminoglycoside antibiotic produced by certain strains of *Streptomyces rimosus* with broad spectrum of antibacterial activity closely paralleling that of kanamycin and neomycin.

THERAPEUTIC EFFECTS Exerts direct bactericidal and amebicidal action, primarily in lumen of GI tract. Ineffective against extraintestinal amebiasis.

USES Acute and chronic intestinal amebiasis and to rid bowel of nitrogen-forming bacteria in patients with hepatic coma; used preoperatively to suppress intestinal flora. Also tapeworm infestation.

CONTRAINDICATIONS Intestinal obstruction; impaired kidney function; pregnancy (category C) and lactation.

CAUTIOUS USE GI ulceration.

ROUTE & DOSAGE

Intestinal Amebiasis
Child/Adult: **PO** 25–35 mg/kg/day divided in 3 doses for 5–10 days (7 days usual)
Cestode Tapeworm *(Diphyllobothrium, Diphylidium caninum)*
Child: **PO** 11 mg/kg/dose every 15 min for 4 doses
Adult: **PO** 1 g every 15 min for 4 doses
Cestode Tapeworm *(Hymenolepis nana)*
Child/Adult: **PO** 45 mg/kg/dose daily for 5–7 days

STORAGE
Store at 15°–25° C (59°–77° F) in tightly closed containers.

ADMINISTRATION

Oral
- Give after meals to prevent gastric distress.

ADVERSE EFFECTS CNS: Headache, vertigo. **GI:** *Diarrhea, abdominal cramps,* steatorrhea, *nausea, vomiting, heartburn,* secondary enterocolitis. **Skin:** Exanthema, rash, pruritus. **Special Senses:** Ototoxicity. **Urogenital:** Nephrotoxicity (in patients with GI inflammation or ulcerations). **Body as a Whole:** Eosinophilia, overgrowth of nonsusceptible organisms.

DIAGNOSTIC TEST INTERFERENCE Prolonged use of paromomycin may cause reduction in ***serum cholesterol.***

INTERACTIONS Drug: May decrease absorption of **cyanocobalamin;** may decrease digoxin level; increases oral coagulant effects. **Food:** This drug may cause malabsorption of fats, sucrose, and xylose.

PHARMACOKINETICS Absorption: Poorly absorbed from intact GI tract. **Elimination:** In feces.

NURSING IMPLICATIONS

Assessment & Drug Effects
- Monitor therapeutic effectiveness. Criterion of cure is absence of amoebae in stool specimens examined at weekly intervals for 6 wk after completion of treatment, and thereafter at monthly intervals for 2 y.
- Monitor for appearance of a superinfection during therapy (see Appendix D-1).
- Lab test: Baseline WBC with differential. Repeat if superinfection is suspected.
- Monitor closely patients with history of GI ulceration for nephrotoxicity and ototoxicity (see Appendix D-1). Drug absorption can take place through diseased mucosa.

Patient & Family Education

- Do not prepare, process, or serve food until treatment is complete when receiving drug for intestinal amebiasis. Isolation is not required.
- Practice strict personal hygiene, particularly hand washing after defecation and before eating food.
- Report any dizziness, ringing in the ears, or decrease of hearing to physician. Check child's response to hearing daily.
- Do not breast feed while taking this drug.
- Store this medication out of reach of children.

PAROXETINE

(par-ox'e-teen)

Asimia, Paxil, Paxil CR

Classifications: CENTRAL NERVOUS SYSTEM AGENT; PSYCHOTHERAPEUTIC; ANTIDEPRESSANT; SELECTIVE SEROTONIN REUPTAKE INHIBITOR (SSRI)

Prototype: Fluoxetine

Pregnancy Category: C

AVAILABILITY 10 mg, 20 mg, 30 mg, 40 mg tablets; 12.5 mg, 25 mg sustained-release tablets; 10 mg/5 mL suspension

ACTIONS Antidepressant structurally unrelated to other serotonin reuptake inhibitors. Potent and highly selective inhibitor of serotonin reuptake by neurons in CNS.

THERAPEUTIC EFFECTS Efficacious in depression resistant to other antidepressants and in depression complicated by anxiety.

USES Depression, obsessive-compulsive disorders, panic attacks, excessive social anxiety, generalized anxiety, post-traumatic stress disorder (PTSD).

UNLABELED USES Diabetic neuropathy, myoclonus, bipolar depression in conjunction with lithium, chronic headache, premature ejaculation, fibromyalgia.

CONTRAINDICATIONS Hypersensitivity to paxil; concomitant use of MAO inhibitors, pregnancy (category C); alcohol.

CAUTIOUS USE History of mania, suicidal ideation, renal/hepatic impairment; older adult; history of metabolic disorders; volume-deleted patients, lactation. Safety and efficacy are not established in children.

ROUTE & DOSAGE

Depression

Limited experience but these dosages have been used with small number of children:

Child: PO >14 y, initial 10 mg/day then adjusted upward; average doses of 16.2 mg/day for 8 mo

Adult: PO 10–50 mg/day (max 80 mg/day); 25 mg sustained-release every day in morning, may increase by 12.5 mg (max 62.5 mg/day); use lower starting doses for patients with renal or hepatic insufficiency

ADMINISTRATION

Oral

- Recommended initial dose with debilitated, or those with severe renal or hepatic impairment is 10 mg/day.
- Ensure that sustained-release form is not chewed or crushed. Must be swallowed whole.
- Be aware that at least 14 days should elapse when switching a patient from/to a MAO inhibitor to/from paroxetine.

ADVERSE EFFECTS CV: Postural hypotension. **CNS:** *Headache,* tremor, agitation or nervousness, anxiety, paresthesias, dizziness, insomnia, *sedation.* **GI:** *Nausea,* constipation, vomiting, anorexia, diarrhea, dyspepsia, flatulence, increased appetite, taste aversion, *dry mouth.* **Urogenital:** Urinary hesitancy or frequency. **Hepatic:** Isolated reports of elevated liver enzymes. **Psychological:** increase suicide ideation. **Special Senses:** Blurred vision. **Skin:** Diaphoresis, rash, pruritus. **Metabolic:** Hyponatremia.

INTERACTIONS Drug: Activated charcoal reduces absorption of paroxetine. **Cimetidine** increases paroxetine levels. MAO INHIBITORS **selegiline** may cause an increased vasopressor response leading to hypertensive crisis or death. **Phenytoin** can cause liver enzyme induction resulting in lower paroxetine levels and shorter half-life. **Warfarin** may increase risk of bleeding may increase **thioridazine** levels and prolong QTc interval leading to heart block; increase ergotamine toxicity with **dihydroergotamine, ergotamine. Herbal: St. John's wort** may cause **serotonin** syndrome (headache, dizziness, sweating, agitation).

PHARMACOKINETICS Absorption: 99% absorbed from GI tract. **Onset:** 2 wk. **Peak:** 5–8 h. **Distribution:** Very lipophilic. 95% protein bound. Distributes into breast milk. **Metabolism:** Extensively metabolized in the liver to inactive metabolites. **Elimination:** Less than 2% is excreted unchanged in urine. Approximately 65% of dose appears in urine as metabolites. Metabolites of paroxetine are also excreted in feces, presumably via bile. **Half-Life:** 24 h.

NURSING IMPLICATIONS

Assessment & Drug Effects

- Monitor for adverse effects, which include headache, weakness, sedation, dizziness, insomnia; nausea, constipation, or diarrhea; dry mouth; sweating; male ejaculatory disturbance. These occur in more than 10% of all patients and may result in poor compliance with drug regimen.
- Monitor all patients, but especially those <18 y for suicidal ideation.
- Antidepressants increase risk of suicidal thinking and behavior in children and adolescents with major depressive disorder, obsessive compulsive disorder, and other psychiatric disorders. Observe closely for worsening of condition, suicidality, and behavior changes. Instruct family and caregivers to monitor for these symptoms and discuss with prescriber. A MedGuide describing risks and stating whether the drug is approved for the child's/adolescent's condition should be provided for all families when antidepressants are prescribed.
- Monitor for significant weight loss.
- Monitor patients with history of mania for reactivation of condition.

- Monitor patients with preexisting cardiovascular disease carefully because paroxetine may adversely affect hemodynamic status.

Patient & Family Education
- Use caution when operating hazardous machinery or equipment until response to drug is known.
- Concurrent use of alcohol may increase risk of adverse CNS effects.
- Adaptation to some adverse effects (especially dizziness and nausea) may occur over a period of 4–6 wk.
- Do not stop drug therapy after improvement in emotional status occurs.
- Notify physician of any distressing adverse effects.
- Discuss with caretakers or guardians the potential for suicidal ideations especially in those younger than 18 y. Report any of these symptoms to physician immediately.
- Do not breast feed while taking this drug without consulting physician.
- Store this medication out of reach of children.

PEMOLINE
(pem'oh-leen)
Cylert
Classifications: CENTRAL NERVOUS SYSTEM AGENT; CEREBRAL STIMULANT
Prototype: Amphetamine
Pregnancy Category: B
Controlled Substance: Schedule IV

AVAILABILITY 18.75 mg, 37.5 mg, 75 mg tablets; 37.5 mg chewable tablets

ACTIONS Action qualitatively similar to those of amphetamine but with weak sympathomimetic activity.
THERAPEUTIC EFFECTS Capable of producing increased motor activity, mental alertness, diminished sense of fatigue, and mild euphoria. Also thought to have anorexigenic effect.

USES Adjunctive therapy to other remedial measures (psychologic, educational, social) in minimal brain dysfunction [attention deficit disorder (ADD)] in carefully selected children. Second-line agent when other stimulants have failed.
UNLABELED USES Mild stimulant for geriatric patients; narcolepsy.

CONTRAINDICATIONS Known hypersensitivity to pemoline; liver disease, Tourette's syndrome, children <6 y. Safety during pregnancy (category B) or lactation is not established.
CAUTIOUS USE Impaired kidney function; history of drug abuse; psychosis; emotional instability.

ROUTE & DOSAGE

Attention Deficit Disorder
Child: PO >6 y, initial dose of 37.5 mg/day, may be increased by 18.75 mg at weekly intervals maintance 0.5–3 mg/kg/day (max 112.5 mg/day)

STORAGE
Store at 15°–25° C (59°–77° F) in tightly closed, light-resistant containers.

ADMINISTRATION

Oral

- Give in morning to provide maximal effectiveness and to avoid insomnia.
- Chewable tablet should be chewed, not swallowed whole.

ADVERSE EFFECTS Body as a Whole: Malaise, irritability, fatigue, dyskinetic movements, hallucinations, excitement, agitation, restlessness. **CNS:** *Insomnia,* mild depression, dizziness, headache, drowsiness, convulsions, nervousness tics **CV:** Tachycardia. **GI:** *Anorexia,* abdominal discomfort, <u>liver failure</u>, nausea, diarrhea, elevated AST, ALT, and alkaline phosphatase (after several months of therapy); jaundice. **Skin:** Skin rash. **Special Senses:** Dyskinetic movements of eyes.

INTERACTIONS Drug: MONOAMINE OXIDASE INHIBITORS (e.g., **selegiline, Parnate**) should be stopped 14 days before **sertraline** is started because of serious problems with other SEROTONIN-REUPTAKE INHIBITORS (shivering, nausea, diplopia, confusion, anxiety). **Tolbutamide** and **diazepam** clearance may be reduced. Use cautiously with other centrally acting CNS drugs, may alter insulin requirements with diabetics **Herbal: St. John's wort** may cause serotonin syndrome.

PHARMACOKINETICS Absorption: Readily absorbed from GI tract. **Onset:** 2–3 wk. **Peak:** 2–4 h. **Duration:** 8 h. **Metabolism:** Metabolized in liver. **Elimination:** Excreted in urine. **Half-Life:** 9–14 h.

NURSING IMPLICATIONS

Assessment & Drug Effects

- Monitor therapeutic effectiveness. Drug should be withdrawn if substantial clinical benefit is not seen following 3 wk of therapy.
- Note: Insomnia and anorexia (most frequent adverse effects) appear to be dose related.
- Monitor weight and height (growth rate) throughout therapy. Anorexia is often accompanied by weight loss.
- Be aware that careful clinical evaluation and supervision of patient are essential.
- This drug may lower seizure threshold.
- Lab tests: Obtain baseline and biweekly liver function studies for patients receiving long-term therapy. Discontinue pemoline if significantly abnormal liver functions are noted. (Drug should be discontinued if ALT increases more than 2 times the upper limit.)

Patient & Family Education

- Report to physician immediately any sign of liver malfunction such as dark urine, jaundice, loss of appetite.
- Avoid potentially hazardous activities (bike riding, skateboarding, sports, driving) until response to drug is known.
- Significant benefits of drug therapy may not be evident until third week of drug administration.
- Abrupt withdrawal of the drug may cause seizures.

Common adverse effects in *italic;* life-threatening effects <u>underlined</u>; generic names in **bold;** drug classifications in SMALL CAPS; ♣ Canadian drug name; ● Prototype drug.

- Be aware that pemoline can produce tolerance and physical and psychologic dependence.
- Store this medication out of reach of children.

PENICILLAMINE
(pen-i-sill'a-meen)
Cuprimine, Depen
Classification: CHELATING AGENT
Pregnancy Category: D

AVAILABILITY 150 mg, 250 mg capsules; 250 mg tablets

ACTIONS Thiol compound prepared by hydrolysis of penicillin but lacking antibacterial activity. Also combines chemically with cystine to form a soluble disulfide complex that prevents stone formation and may even dissolve existing cystic stones. Mechanism of action in rheumatoid arthritis not known but appears to be related to inhibition of collagen formation. Cross-sensitivity between penicillin and penicillamine can occur.
THERAPEUTIC EFFECTS Forms stable soluble chelate with copper, zinc, iron, lead, mercury, and possibly other heavy metals and promotes their excretion in urine. With Wilson's disease, therapeutic effectiveness is indicated by improvement in psychiatric and neurologic symptoms, visual symptoms, and liver function. In some patients, neurologic symptoms become more prominent during initial therapy and then subside. With rheumatoid arthritis, improvement in grip strength, decrease in stiffness following immobility, reduction of pain, decrease in sedimentation rate and rheumatoid factor.

USES To promote renal excretion of excess copper in Wilson's disease (hepatolenticular degeneration). Active rheumatoid arthritis in patients who have failed to respond to conventional therapy. Cystinuria.
UNLABELED USES Scleroderma, primary biliary cirrhosis, porphyria catenae tarda, lead poisoning.

CONTRAINDICATIONS Hypersensitivity to penicillamine or to any penicillin; history of penicillamine-related aplastic anemia or agranulocytosis; patients with rheumatoid arthritis who have renal insufficiency or who are pregnant; pregnancy (category D), lactation; concomitant administration with drugs that can cause severe hematologic or renal reactions (e.g., antimalarials, gold salts, immunosuppressants, oxyphenbutazone, phenylbutazone).
CAUTIOUS USE Allergy-prone individuals.

ROUTE & DOSAGE

Wilson's Disease
Infant/Child: PO 20 mg/kg/day in 2–4 equally divided doses (max 1 g/day)
Adult: PO 250 mg q.i.d., with 3 doses 1 h a.c. and the last dose at least 2 h after the last meal

---

Cystinuria

Child: **PO** 30 mg/kg/day in 4 equally divided doses with doses adjusted to limit urinary excretion of cystine to 100–200 mg/day (max dose 4 g/day)
Adult: **PO** 250–500 mg q.i.d., with doses adjusted to limit urinary excretion of cystine to 100–200 mg/day

Rheumatoid Arthritis

Child: **PO** 3 mg/kg/day (≤250 mg/day) times 3 mo, then 6 mg/kg/day (≤500 mg/day) in 2 equally divided doses times 3 mo (max 10 mg/kg/day [≤1.5 g/day] in 3–4 divided doses)
Adult: **PO** 125–250 mg/day may increase at 1–3 mo intervals up to 1–1.5 g/day

Lead Poisoning

Child: **PO** 30–40 mg/kg/day in 3–4 equally divided doses (max 1.5 g/day); initiate at 25% target dose, gradually increase to full dose over 2–3 wk, continue until blood level of lead is <15 mcg/dL

STORAGE
Store at 15°–30° C (59°–86° F) in tight closed containers.

ADMINISTRATION

Oral

- Give on empty stomach (1 h before or 2 h after meals) to avoid absorption of metals in foods by penicillamine.
- Give contents in 15–30 mL of chilled fruit juice or pureed fruit (e.g., applesauce) if patient cannot swallow capsules or tablets.
- Pharmacy can compound a liquid preparation.

ADVERSE EFFECTS Body as a Whole: Fever, arthralgia, lymphadenopathy, thyroiditis, SLE-like syndrome, thrombophlebitis, hyperpyrexia, myasthenia gravis syndrome, tingling of feet, weakness, edema of face, feet and lower legs, **GI:** *Anorexia, nausea, vomiting,* epigastric pain, diarrhea, oral lesions, *reduction or loss of taste perception (particularly salt and sweet), metallic taste,* activation of peptic ulcer, pancreatitis. **Urogenital:** Membranous glomerulopathy, *proteinuria,* hematuria. **Hematologic:** Thrombocytopenia, leukopenia, <u>agranulocytosis</u>, thrombotic thrombocytopenic purpura, <u>hemolytic anemia, aplastic anemia</u>. **Metabolic:** Pyridoxine deficiency. **Skin:** *Generalized pruritus, uric* mammary hyperplasia, alveolitis, skin friability, excessive skin wrinkling, *aria, early and late occurring rashes,* pemphigus-like rash, alopecia. **Special Senses:** Tinnitus, optic neuritis, ptosis.

INTERACTIONS Drug: ANTIMALARIALS, CYTOTOXICS, **gold** therapy may potentiate hematologic and renal adverse effects; **iron, zinc and antacids** may decrease penicillamine absorption. Decreases digoxin serum levels **Food:** Do not administer with milk or food. Decreases pyridoxine.

PHARMACOKINETICS Absorption: Readily absorbed from GI tract. **Peak:** 1 h. **Distribution:** Crosses placenta. **Metabolism:** Metabolized in liver. **Elimination:** Excreted in urine and feces.

NURSING IMPLICATIONS

Assessment & Drug Effects

- Lab tests: Check WBC with differential, direct platelet counts, Hgb, and urinalyses prior to initiation of therapy and every 3 days during the first month of therapy, then every 2 wk thereafter. Perform liver function tests and eye examinations before start of therapy and at least twice yearly thereafter.
- Withhold drug and contact physician if the patient with rheumatoid arthritis develops proteinuria >1 g (some clinicians accept >2 g) or if platelet count drops to <100,000/mm³, or platelet count falls below 3500–4000/mm³, or neutropenia occurs.
- Monitor blood levels for heavy metals.

Patient & Family Education

- Note: Clinical evidence of therapeutic effectiveness may not be apparent until 1–3 mo of drug therapy.
- Take exactly as prescribed. Allergic reactions occur in about one-third of patients receiving penicillamine. Temporary interruptions of therapy increase possibility of sensitivity reactions.
- Take temperature nightly during first few months of therapy. Fever is a possible early sign of allergy.
- Observe skin over pressure sites: knees, elbows, shoulder blades, toes, buttocks. Penicillamine increases skin friability.
- Report unusual bruising or bleeding, sore mouth or throat, fever, skin rash, or any other unusual symptoms to physician.
- Loss of taste may occur.
- Take dosage only as directed.
- Do not breast feed while taking this drug.
- Store this medication out of reach of children.

P

PENICILLIN G BENZATHINE

(pen-i-sill'in)
Bicillin, Bicillin L-A, Permapen
Classifications: ANTI-INFECTIVE; BETA-LACTAM ANTIBIOTIC; NATURAL PENICILLIN
Prototype: Penicillin G potassium
Pregnancy Category: B

AVAILABILITY 300,000 units/mL, 600,000 units/mL, 1,2000,000/2 mL, 2,400,000 units/4 mL injection

ACTIONS Acid-stable, penicillinase-sensitive, **long-acting form** of penicillin G. Absorbed slowly in body because of extremely low water solubility. Produces lower blood concentrations than other penicillin G compounds but has the longest duration of antimicrobial activity of all other available parenteral or repository penicillins. Acts by inhibiting bacteria cell wall synthesis.

THERAPEUTIC EFFECTS Effective against many strains of *Staphylococcus aureus,* gram-positive cocci, gram-negative cocci. Also effective against gram-positive bacilli and gram-negative bacilli.

USES Infections highly susceptible to penicillin G, such as streptococcal, pneumococcal, and staphylococcal infections, venereal disease such as syphilis (including early, late, and congenital forms), and nonvenereal diseases (e.g., yaws, bejel, and pinta). Also used in prophylaxis of rheumatic fever.

CONTRAINDICATIONS Hypersensitivity to penicillins or cephalosporins; lactation; pregnancy (category B).

CAUTIOUS USE History of or suspected allergy (eczema, hives, hay fever, asthma), hypersensitivity to cephaplosporins.

ROUTE & DOSAGE

Mild to Moderate Infections

Child: **IM** <27 kg, 300,000–600,000 units as a single dose ≥27 kg, 900,000 units as a single dose
Adult: **IM** 1,200,000 units as a single dose

Syphilis

Neonate: **IM** Congenital: 50,000 units/kg as single dose
Child >1 mo: **IM** Congenital: 50,000 units/kg every week for 3 wk (max 2,400,000 units/dose)
Child >1 mo: **IM** >1 y duration: 50,000 units/kg every week for 3 wk (max 2,400,000 units/dose)
Adult: **IM** <1 y duration: 2,400,000 units as single dose; >1 y duration: 2,400,000 units/wk for 3 wk

Prophylaxis for Rheumatic Fever

Child: **IM** 25,000–50,000 units/kg once every 3–4 wk (max 1,200,000 units/dose)
Adult: **IM** 1,200,000 units once q4wk

STORAGE

Store in refrigerator at 2°–8° C (36°–45° F). Avoid freezing.

ADMINISTRATION

Intramuscular

- Do not confuse penicillin G benzathine with preparations containing procaine penicillin G (e.g., Bicillin C-R).
- Make IM injection deep into upper outer quadrant of buttock for adults and older children. In infants and small children, the preferred site is the midlateral aspect of the thigh (see Part I). Rotate sites; overuse of a site can cause quadriceps femoris fibrosis and subsequent muscle atrophy.
- Injection can be painful, use topical cream to numb area prior to injection.
- Shake multiple-dose vial vigorously before withdrawing desired IM dose. Shake prepared cartridge unit vigorously before injecting drug.
- Select IM site with care. Injection into or near a major peripheral nerve can result in nerve damage. Inadvertent IV administration has resulted in arterial occlusion and cardiac arrest.
- Make injections at a slow steady rate to prevent needle blockage and minimize pain.

Common adverse effects in *italic;* life-threatening effects <u>underlined</u>; generic names in **bold**; drug classifications in SMALL CAPS; ✦ Canadian drug name; ❶ Prototype drug.

ADVERSE EFFECTS Body as a Whole: *Local pain,* tenderness, and fever associated with IM injection, chills, fever, wheezing, <u>anaphylaxis</u>, neuropathy, <u>nephrotoxicity</u>; superinfections, Jarisch-Herxheimer reaction in patients with syphilis. **Skin:** Pruritus, urticaria and other skin eruptions. **Hematologic:** Eosinophilia, hemolytic anemia, and other blood abnormalities. Also see penicillin G.

INTERACTIONS Drug: Probenecid decreases renal elimination; may decrease efficacy of ORAL CONTRACEPTIVES. Erthromycin, tetracyclines, and chloramphenicol may antagonize penicillins' activity.

PHARMACOKINETICS Absorption: Slowly absorbed from IM site. **Peak:** 12–24 h. **Duration:** 26 days. **Distribution:** Crosses placenta; distributed into breast milk. **Metabolism:** Hydrolyzed to penicillin in body. **Elimination:** Excreted slowly by kidneys.

NURSING IMPLICATIONS

Note: See penicillin G potassium for numerous additional nursing implications.

Assessment & Drug Effects

- Determine history of hypersensitivity reactions to penicillins, cephalosporins, or other allergens prior to initiation of drug therapy.
- Lab tests: Perform C&S tests prior to initiation of therapy and periodically thereafter. Perform periodic renal function tests.

Patient & Family Education

- Report immediately to physician the onset of an allergic reaction. There is great risk of severe and prolonged reactions because drug is absorbed so slowly.
- If allergy occurs, child should carry identification to inform health care providers.
- Do not breast feed while taking this drug.

PENICILLIN G POTASSIUM ●

(pen-i-sill'in)
Megacillin ◆ , Pfizerpen

PENICILLIN G SODIUM

Classifications: ANTI-INFECTIVE; BETA-LACTAM ANTIBIOTIC; NATURAL PENICILLIN
Pregnancy Category: B

AVAILABILITY 1,000,000 unit, 5,000,000 unit, 10,000,000 unit, 20,000,000 unit vials; 1,000,000 units/50 mL, 2,000,000 units/50 mL 3,000,000 units/50 mL injection

ACTIONS Acid-labile, penicillinase-sensitive, natural penicillin derived from cultures of *Penicillium notatum* or related molds. Antimicrobial spectrum is relatively narrow compared to that of the semisynthetic penicillins. Bactericidal at therapeutic serum levels; bacteriostatic at lower concentrations. Acts by interfering with synthesis of mucopeptides essential to formation and integrity of bacterial cell wall. Action is inhibited by penicillinase; therefore, penicillin G is ineffective against many strains of *Staphylococcus aureus*.

THERAPEUTIC EFFECTS Highly active against gram-positive cocci (e.g., non-penicillinase-producing *Staphylococcus, Streptococcus* groups A, C, G, H, L, M, and *Streptococcus pneumoniae*); and gram-negative cocci (*Neisseria gonorrhoeae, N. meningitidis*). Also effective against gram-positive bacilli (*Bacillus anthracis, Clostridium* species including gas gangrene and tetanus, and certain species of *Corynebacterium, Erysipelothrix,* and *Listeria*); gram-negative bacilli (*Fusobacterium, Pasteurella, Streptobacillus,* and *Bacteroides* sp.). Parenteral penicillin G is effective against some strains of *Salmonella* and *Shigella* and spirochetes (*Treponema pallidum, T. pertenue, Leptospira*).

USES Moderate to severe systemic infections caused by penicillin-sensitive microorganisms: Actinomycosis, anthrax, diphtheria (carrier state), empyema, erysipelas, gas gangrene, gonorrheal infections, leptospirosis, mastoiditis, meningitis, acute osteomyelitis, otitis media, pinta, pneumonia, rat bite fever, sinus infections; certain staphylococcal infections; streptococcal infections, including scarlet fever; syphilis (all stages); tetanus, urinary tract infections, Vincent's gingivostomatitis, yaws. Also used as prophylaxis in patients with rheumatic or congenital heart disease. Since oral preparations are absorbed erratically and thus must be given in comparatively high doses, this route is generally used only for mild or stabilized infections or long-term prophylaxis.

CONTRAINDICATIONS Hypersensitivity to any of the penicillins or cephalosporins; administration of oral drug to patients with severe infections; nausea, vomiting, hypermotility, gastric dilatation; cardiospasm. Use of penicillin G sodium in patients on sodium restriction. Safety during pregnancy (category B) or lactation is not established.

CAUTIOUS USE History of or suspected allergy (asthma, eczema, hay fever, hives); history of allergy to cephalosporins; kidney or liver dysfunction, myasthenia gravis, epilepsy, neonates, young infants. Use during lactation may lead to sensitization of infants.

ROUTE & DOSAGE

Note: PO form of the drug no longer available in U.S.

Moderate to Severe Infections

Neonate ≤7 days Postnatal: **IV/IM** ≤2000 g, 50,000 units/kg/day in equally divided doses q12h; >2000 g, 75,000 units/kg/day in equally divided doses q8h
Neonate >7 days Postnatal: **IV/IM** <1200 g, 50,000 units/kg/day in equally divided doses q12h; 1200–2000 g, 75,000 units/kg/day in equally divided doses q8h; >2000 g, 100,000 units/kg/day in equally divided doses q6h
Infant/Child: **PO** 25,000–100,000 units/kg/day in equally divided doses q6h **IV/IM** 100,000–250,000 units/kg/day in equally divided doses q4–6h; (Severe infections) 250,000–400,000 units/kg/day in equally divided doses q4–6h (max dose 24 million units/day)
Adult: **PO** 1.6–3.2 million units in equally divided doses q6h **IV/IM** 1.2–24 million units in equally divided doses q4–6h

Meningitis

Neonate ≤7 days Postnatal: **IV/IM** *≤2000 g,* 100,000 units/kg/day in equally divided doses q12h; *>2000 g,* 150,000 units/kg/day in equally divided doses q8h

Neonates >7 days Postnatal: **IV/IM** *<1200 g,* 100,000 units/kg/day in equally divided doses q12h; *1200–2000 g,* 150,000 units/kg/day in equally divided doses q8h; *>2000 g,* 200,000 units/kg/day in equally divided doses q6h

Meningococcal Meningitis

Child: **IV** 25,000–300,000 units/kg/day in equally divided doses q4h
Adult: **IM** 1–2 million units q2h **IV** 200,000–300,000/kg/day in equally divided doses q2–4h or 2 million to 3 million units/day by continuous infusion

STORAGE

Store tablets at 15°–30° C (59°–86° F) in tightly closed containers. Avoid excessive heat. Store oral suspensions and syrups in refrigerator and discard unused portions after 14 days. Store dry powder (for parenteral use) at room temperature. After reconstitution (initial dilution), store solutions for 1 wk under refrigeration. Intravenous infusion solutions containing penicillin G are stable at room temperature for at least 24 h.

ADMINISTRATION

Note: Check whether physician has prescribed penicillin G potassium or sodium.

Oral

- Give on an empty stomach, at least 1 h before or 2 h after meals to reduce possibility of drug destruction by gastric acid and delay in absorption by food.
- Give with a full glass of water. Instruct patient to avoid acidic or carbonated beverages 1 h before and after taking oral penicillin G.

Intramuscular

- Do not use the 20,000,000-unit dosage form for IM injection.
- Reconstitute for IM: Loosen powder by shaking bottle before adding diluent (sterile water for injection or sterile NS). Keep the total volume to be injected small. Solutions containing up to 100,000 units/mL cause the least discomfort. Note: Adding 10 mL diluent to the 1,000,000 unit vial = 100,000 units/mL. Shake well to dissolve.
- Select IM site carefully. IM injection is made deep into a large muscle mass. Inject slowly. Rotate injection sites. In infants and small children, the preferred site is the midlateral aspect of the thigh (see Part I). Rotate sites.
- Injection can be painful; use topical creams to numb area prior to injection.

Intravenous

***PREPARE* Intermittent/Continuous:** Reconstitute as for IM injection then withdraw the required dose and add to 100–1000 mL of D5W or NS IV solution, depending on length of each infusion.

***ADMINISTER* Intermittent/Continuous:** Give intermittent infusion over at least 1 h and continuous infusion at a rate required to infuse the daily dose in 24 h. With high doses, IV penicillin G should be administered slowly to avoid electrolyte imbalance from potassium or sodium content. Physician should prescribe specific flow rate for infants and children.

INCOMPATIBILITIES **Solution/Additive: Dextran 40, fat emulsion, aminophylline, amphotericin B, cephalothin, chlorpromazine, dopamine, hydroxyzine, metaraminol, pentobarbital, prochlor-perazine, promazine, sodium bicarbonate,** TETRACYCLINES, **thiopental, metoclopramide.**

ADVERSE EFFECTS Body as a Whole: Coughing, sneezing, feeling of uneasiness; <u>systemic anaphylaxis</u>, fever, widespread increase in capillary permeability and vasodilation with <u>resulting edema (mouth, tongue, pharynx, larynx), laryngospasm</u>, malaise, serum sickness (fever, malaise, pruritus, urticaria, lymphadenopathy, arthralgia, angioedema of face and extremities, neuritis prostration, eosinophilia), SLE-like syndrome, injection site reactions (pain, inflammation, abscess, phlebitis), superinfections (especially with *Candida* and gram-negative bacteria), neuromuscular irritability (twitching, lethargy, confusion, stupor, hyperreflexia, multifocal myoclonus, localized or generalized seizures, <u>coma</u>). **CV:** Hypotension, <u>circulatory collapse</u>, cardiac arrhythmias, <u>cardiac arrest</u>. **GI:** Vomiting, diarrhea, severe abdominal cramps, nausea, epigastric distress, diarrhea, flatulence, dark discoloration of tongue, sore mouth or tongue. **Urogenital:** Interstitial nephritis, Loeffler's syndrome, vasculitis. **Hematologic:** Hemolytic anemia, thrombocytopenia. **Metabolic:** Hyperkalemia (penicillin G potassium); hypokalemia, alkalosis, hypernatremia, CHF (penicillin G sodium). **Respiratory:** Bronchospasm, asthma. **Skin:** Itchy palms or axilla, pruritus, *urticaria*, flushed skin, *delayed skin rashes* ranging from urticaria to exfoliative dermatitis, Stevens-Johnson syndrome, fixed-drug eruptions, contact dermatitis.

DIAGNOSTIC TEST INTERFERENCE Blood grouping and compatibility tests: Possible interference associated with penicillin doses greater than 20 million units daily. **Urine glucose:** Massive doses of penicillin may cause false-positive test results with ***Benedict's solution*** and possibly ***Clinitest*** but not with *glucose oxidase methods*, e.g., ***Clinistix, Diastix, TesTape***. **Urine protein:** Massive doses of penicillin can produce false-positive results when turbidity measures are used (e.g., ***acetic acid*** and *heat, sulfo-salicylic acid*); ***Ames reagent*** reportedly not affected. **Urinary PSP excretion tests:** False decrease in urinary excretion of PSP. **Urinary steroids:** Large IV doses of penicillin may interfere with accurate measurement of ***urinary 17-OHCS*** (*Glenn-Nelson technique* not affected).

INTERACTIONS Drug: Probenecid decreases renal elimination; penicillin G may decrease efficacy of ORAL CONTRACEPTIVES; **colestipol** decreases penicillin absorption; POTASSIUM-SPARING DIURETICS may cause hyperkalemia with penicillin G potassium. **Food:** Food increases breakdown in stomach.

PHARMACOKINETICS Absorption: 15–30% of PO dose absorbed; very acid labile. **Peak:** 30–60 min PO; 15–30 min IM. **Distribution:** Widely distributed; good CSF concentrations with inflammed meninges; crosses placenta; distributed in breast milk. **Metabolism:** 16–30% metabolized. **Elimination:** 60% excreted in urine within 6 h. **Half-Life:** Infant/child, 0.5–1.2 h; adult, 0.4–0.9 h.

NURSING IMPLICATIONS

Assessment & Drug Effects

- Obtain an exact history of patient's previous exposure and sensitivity to penicillins and cephalosporins and other allergic reactions of any kind prior to treatment with penicillin.
- Hypersensitivity reactions are more likely to occur with parenteral penicillin but may also occur with the oral drug. Skin rash is the most common type allergic reaction and should be reported promptly to physician.
- Lab tests: Perform C&S tests prior to initiation of therapy; treatment may be started before results are known. Evaluate renal, hepatic, and hematologic systems at regular intervals in patients on high dose therapy. Additionally, check electrolyte balance periodically in patients receiving high parenteral doses.
- Observe all patients closely for at least 30 min following administration of parenteral penicillin. The rapid appearance of a red flare or wheal at the IM or IV injection site is a possible sign of sensitivity. Also suspect an allergic reaction if patient becomes irritable, has nausea and vomiting, breathing difficulty, or sudden fever. Report any of the foregoing to physician immediately.
- Be aware that reactions to penicillin may be rapid in onset or may not appear for days or weeks. Symptoms usually disappear fairly quickly once drug is stopped, but in some patients may persist for 5 days or more and require hospitalization for treatment.
- Allergy to penicillin is unpredictable. It has occurred in patients with a negative history of penicillin allergy and also in patients with no known prior contact with penicillin (sensitization may have occurred from penicillin used commercially in foods and beverages).
- Be alert for neuromuscular irritability in patients receiving parenteral penicillin in excess of 20 million unit/day who have renal insufficiency, hyponatremia, or underlying CNS disease, notably myasthenia gravis or epilepsy. Seizure precautions are indicated. Symptoms usually begin with twitching, especially of face and extremities.
- Monitor I&O, particularly in patients receiving high parenteral doses. Report oliguria, hematuria, and changes in I&O ratio. Consult physician regarding optimum fluid intake. Dehydration increases the concentration of drug in kidneys and can cause renal irritation and damage.
- Observe closely for signs of toxicity: Neonates, young infants, and patients with impaired kidney function receiving high-dose penicillin therapy. Urinary excretion of penicillin is significantly delayed in these patients.
- Observe patients on high-dose therapy closely for evidence of bleeding, and bleeding time should be monitored. (In high doses, penicillin interferes with platelet aggregation.)

Patient & Family Education

- Understand that hypersensitivity reaction may be delayed. Report skin rashes, itching, fever, malaise, and other signs of a delayed reaction to physician immediately (see ADVERSE EFFECTS).
- Penicillin is to be taken around the clock (i.e., t.i.d. means q8h, q.i.d. means q6h, etc.) Do not miss any doses and continue taking medication until it is all gone, unless otherwise directed by the physician.

Common adverse effects in *italic;* life-threatening effects <u>underlined;</u> generic names in **bold;** drug classifications in SMALL CAPS; ♣ Canadian drug name; ✪ Prototype drug.

951

- Measure liquid dosage form with specially marked measuring device; household teaspoons vary in size and measure.
- Notify physician if following symptoms appear when taking penicillin for treatment of syphilis (i.e., Jarisch-Herxheimer reaction occurs 8–24 h after treatment): Headache, chills, fever, myalgia, arthralgia, malaise, and worsening of syphilitic skin lesions. Reaction is usually self-limiting. Check with physician if symptoms do not improve within a few days or get worse.
- Report S&S of superinfection (see Appendix D-1).
- Understand importance of medical follow-up; present evidence suggests that glomerulonephritis, a possible complication of streptococcal infection, may not be prevented by penicillin.
- If allergy occurs, child should carry identification to inform health care providers.
- Do not breast feed while taking this drug without consulting physician.

PENICILLIN G PROCAINE
(pen-i-sill′in)
Crysticillin A.S., Pfizerpen-AS, Procaine Benzylpenicillin, Wycillin
Classifications: ANTI-INFECTIVE; BETA-LACTAM ANTIBIOTIC; NATURAL PENICILLIN
Prototype: Penicillin G potassium
Pregnancy Category: B

AVAILABILITY 600,000 units/1 mL, 1,200,000 units/2 mL, 2,400,000 units/4 mL injection

ACTIONS Long-acting form of penicillin G. The procaine salt has low solubility and thus creates a tissue depot from which penicillin is slowly absorbed. Onset of action is slower and produces lower serum concentrations than equivalent doses of penicillin G potassium, but has longer duration of action. Acts by inhibiting cell wall synthesis in bacteria.
THERAPEUTIC EFFECTS Same actions and antibacterial activity as for penicillin G potassium and is similarly inactivated by penicillinase and gastric acid.

USES Moderately severe infections due to penicillin G-sensitive microorganisms that are susceptible to low but prolonged serum penicillin concentrations. Commonly, uncomplicated *Pneumococcal* pneumonia, 1-day treatment of uncomplicated gonorrheal infections, and all stages of syphilis. May be used concomitantly with penicillin G or probenecid when more rapid action and higher blood levels are indicated.

CONTRAINDICATIONS History of hypersensitivity to any of the penicillins, cephalosporins, or to procaine or any other "caine-type" local anesthetic; neonates; pregnancy (category B), lactation.
CAUTIOUS USE History of or suspected allergy, renal impairment, and history of seizures.

ROUTE & DOSAGE

Moderate to Severe Infections

Avoid use in neonates <1200 g due to increase in procaine toxicity and sterile abscess formation.

Infant >1 mo/Child: **IM** 25,000–50,000 units/kg/day in equally divided doses daily or q12h (max dose 4.8 million units/day)

Adult: **IM** 600,000–1,200,000 units once/day

Pneumococcal Pneumonia

Adult: **IM** 600,000 units q12h

Uncomplicated Gonorrhea

Adult: **IM** 4,800,000 units divided between 2 different injection sites at one visit preceded by 1 g of probenecid 30 min before injections

Syphilis

Child: **IM** 50,000 units/kg/day once/day for 10 days

Adult: **IM** Primary, secondary, latent: 600,000 units/day for 8 days; late latent, tertiary, neurosyphilis: 600,000 units/day for 10–15 days

STORAGE

Store in the refrigerator 2°–8° C (35°–46° F); avoid freezing.

ADMINISTRATION

Intramuscular

- Shake multiple-dose vial thoroughly before withdrawing medication to ensure uniform suspension of drug.
- Use 20-gauge needle to avoid clogging.
- Do not give this preparation SC or IV.
- Give IM deep into upper outer quadrant of gluteus muscle; in infants and small children midlateral aspect of thigh is generally preferred. Select IM site carefully. See Part I for appropriate sites and safe amounts/injection in children. Accidental injection into or near major peripheral nerves and blood vessels can cause neurovascular damage. Rotate sites; overuse of a site can cause quadriceps femoris fibrosis and subsequent muscle atrophy.
- Aspirate carefully before injecting drug to avoid entry into a blood vessel. Inadvertent IV administration reportedly has resulted in pulmonary infarcts and death.
- Inject drug at a slow, but steady rate to prevent needle blockage. Give in two sites if the dose is very large.
- Injection can be painful, use topical cream to numb area prior to injection. Rotate injection sites.

ADVERSE EFFECTS Body as a Whole: Procaine toxicity (e.g., mental disturbances [anxiety, confusion, depression, combativeness, hallucinations], expressed fear of impending death, weakness, dizziness, headache, tinnitus, unusual tastes, palpitation, changes in pulse rate and BP, seizures). Also see Penicillin G.

INTERACTIONS Drug: Probenecid decreases renal elimination; may decrease efficacy of ORAL CONTRACEPTIVES.

Common adverse effects in *italic;* life-threatening effects underlined; generic names in **bold;** drug classifications in SMALL CAPS; ♣ Canadian drug name; ● Prototype drug.

953

PHARMACOKINETICS Absorption: Slowly absorbed from IM site. **Peak:** 1–3 h. **Duration:** 15–20 h. **Distribution:** Crosses placenta; distributed into breast milk. **Metabolism:** Hydrolyzed to penicillin in body. **Elimination:** Excreted by kidneys within 24–36 h. Delayed in neonates and infants

NURSING IMPLICATIONS

Assessment & Drug Effects

- Obtain an exact history of patient's previous exposure and sensitivity to penicillins, cephalosporins, and to procaine, and other allergic reactions of any kind prior to treatment.
- Test patient by injecting 0.1 mL of 1–2% procaine hydrochloride intradermally if sensitivity is suspected. Appearance of a wheal, flare, or eruption indicates procaine sensitivity.
- Be alert to the possibility of a transient toxic reaction to procaine, particularly when large single doses are administered. The reaction manifested by mental disturbance and other symptoms (see ADVERSE EFFECTS) occurs almost immediately and usually subsides after 15–30 min.

Patient & Family Education

- Report any skin reaction at the site of injection.
- Report onset of rash, itching, fever, chills or other symptoms of an allergic reaction to physician.
- If allergy occurs, child should carry identification to inform health care providers.
- Do not breast feed while taking this drug.

P

PENICILLIN V

PENICILLIN V POTASSIUM

(pen-i-sill'in)
Apo-Pen-VK ♣ , Beepen VK, Betapen-VK, Ledercillin VK, Nadopen-V ♣ , Novopen-VK ♣ , Penicillin VK, Pen-V, Pen-Vee K, Robicillin VK, V-Cillin K, Veetids
Classifications: ANTI-INFECTIVE; BETA-LACTAM ANTIBIOTIC; NATURAL PENICILLIN
Prototype: Penicillin G potassium
Pregnancy Category: B

AVAILABILITY 250 mg, 500 mg tablets; 125 mg/5 mL, 250 mg/5 mL suspension (both contain aspartame, sodium benzoate)

ACTIONS Acid-stable analog of penicillin G with which it shares actions; it is bactericidal, and is inactivated by penicillinase. Acts by inhibiting bacteria cell wall synthesis.
THERAPEUTIC EFFECTS Less active than penicillin G against gonococci and other gram-negative microorganisms.

USES Mild to moderate infections caused by susceptible *Streptococci, Pneumococci,* and *Staphylococci.* Also Vincent's infection and as prophylaxis in rheumatic fever.

CONTRAINDICATIONS Hypersensitivity to any penicillin or cephalosporin or beta-lactamase inhibitors; pregnancy (category B), lactation.

CAUTIOUS USE History of or suspected allergy (hay fever, asthma, hives, eczema); cystic fibrosis; renal impairment, hepatic impairment; preparations with aspartame in those with phenylketonuria; children <12 y, newborns.

ROUTE & DOSAGE

Mild to Moderate Infections

Child ≤12 y: **PO** 25–50 mg/kg/day in equally divided doses q6–8h (max dose 3 g/day)
Child >12 y/Adult: **PO** 125–500 mg q6–8h

Rheumatic Fever/*Pneumococcal* Prophylaxis

Child: **PO** ≤5 y, 125 mg b.i.d.; >5 y, **PO** 250 mg b.i.d.
Adult: **PO** 250 mg b.i.d.

Acute Group A *Streptococcal* Pharyngitis

Child: **PO** 250 mg b.i.d.–t.i.d. for 10 days
Child >12 y/Adult: **PO** 500 mg b.i.d.–t.i.d. for 10 days

Endocarditis Prophylaxis

Child: **PO** <30 kg, 1 g 30–60 min before procedure, then 250 mg q6h for 8 doses
Adult: **PO** 2 g 30–60 min before procedure, then 500 mg q6h for 8 doses

STORAGE

Store tablets at 15°–30° C (59°–86° F) in tightly closed containers. Avoid excessive heat. Store oral suspensions and syrups in refrigerator and discard unused portions after 14 days.

ADMINISTRATION

Oral

- Give 1 h before meals or 2 h after a meal on an empty stomach. If GI distress is a problem with compliance, can give with small amount of food.
- Do not coadminister with neomycin if both drugs are being used; malabsorption of penicillin V may result.
- Shake suspensions well before pouring.

ADVERSE EFFECTS Body as a Whole: Nausea, vomiting, *diarrhea,* epigastric distress. *Hypersensitivity reactions* (e.g., flushing, pruritus, urticaria or other skin eruptions, eosinophilia, <u>anaphylaxis</u>; hemolytic anemia, leukopenia, thrombocytopenia, neuropathy, superinfections).

INTERACTIONS Drug: **Probenecid** decreases renal elimination; may decrease efficacy of ORAL CONTRACEPTIVES; **colestipol** decreases absorption; **Food:** Food or milk decreases absorption in stomach.

PHARMACOKINETICS Absorption: 60–73% absorbed from GI tract. **Peak:** 30–60 min. **Duration:** 6 h. **Distribution:** Highest levels in kidneys; crosses placenta; distributed into breast milk. **Elimination:** Excreted in urine. **Half-Life:** 30 min.

Common adverse effects in *italic;* life-threatening effects <u>underlined</u>; generic names in **bold;** drug classifications in SMALL CAPS; ♣ Canadian drug name; ☻ Prototype drug.

955

NURSING IMPLICATIONS

Note: See penicillin G potassium for numerous additional nursing implications.

Assessment & Drug Effects

- Obtain careful history concerning hypersensitivity reactions to penicillins, cephalosporins, and other allergens before therapy begins.
- Lab tests: Perform C&S tests prior to initiation and at regular intervals throughout therapy. Evaluate renal, hepatic, and hematologic systems at regular intervals in patients receiving prolonged therapy.

Patient & Family Education

- Take penicillin V around the clock at specific intervals to maintain a constant blood level.
- Do not miss any doses and continue taking medication until it is all gone unless otherwise directed by the prescriber.
- Discontinue medication and promptly report to physician the onset of hypersensitivity reactions and superinfections (see Appendix D-1).
- Use specially marked measuring device to ensure accurate doses of oral liquid preparation.
- If allergy occurs, child should carry identification to inform health care providers.
- Do not breast feed while taking this drug.
- Store this medication out of reach of children. (Refrigerated preparations must also be out of reach of children.)

PENTAMIDINE ISOETHIONATE

(pen-tam'i-deen)
NebuPent, Pentacarinat ♣ , Pentam 300
Classifications: ANTI-INFECTIVE; ANTIPROTOZOAL
Pregnancy Category: C

AVAILABILITY 300 mg injection; 300 mg aerosol

ACTIONS Aromatic diamide antiprotozoal drug. Action mechanism is unclear, but drug appears to block parasite reproduction by interfering with nucleotide (DNA, RNA), phospholipid, and protein synthesis. Effective against the *Sporozoan* parasite, *Pneumocystis carinii*. Pentamidine also has trypanosomicidal and leishmanicidal activity, but required doses for these conditions are quite toxic.

THERAPEUTIC EFFECTS The parasite *P. carinii* rarely causes infection in the general population, but if the patient is immunocompromised (e.g., AIDS) it can be fatal.

USES *P. carinii* pneumonia (PCP).

UNLABELED USES African trypanosomiasis and visceral leishmaniasis. (Drug supplied for the latter use is through the Centers for Disease Control and Prevention, Atlanta, GA.)

CONTRAINDICATIONS Pregnancy (category C) and lactation.

CAUTIOUS USE Hypertension, hypotension; hyperglycemia; hypoglycemia; hypocalcemia; blood dyscrasias; liver or kidney dysfunction; diabetes mellitus.

Common adverse effects in *italic;* life-threatening effects <u>underlined</u>; generic names in **bold**; drug classifications in SMALL CAPS; ♣ Canadian drug name; ⊘ Prototype drug.

ROUTE & DOSAGE

Treatment of *Pneumocystis carinii* Pneumonia

Child/Adult: **IM/IV** 4 mg/kg once/day for 14–21 days; infuse IV over 60 min

Prophylaxis of *Pneumocystis carinii* Pneumonia

Child/Adult: **IM/IV** 4 mg/kg/dose every 2–4 wk; infuse IV over 60 min
Child ≥5 y/Adult: **Inhaled** 300 mg per nebulizer q4wk

STORAGE
Store at 15°–25° C (59°–77° F); protect from light. Protect reconstituted solutions from light. IV solutions are stable at room temperature for up to 24 h.

ADMINISTRATION

Inhaled
- Reconstitute contents of one vial in 6 mL sterile water (not saline) and administer using nebulizer.
- Do not mix with any other drug.

Intramuscular
- Dissolve contents of 1 vial (300 mg) in 3 mL sterile water for injection.
- Give deep IM into a large muscle mass appropriate for age (see Part I).
- The IM injection is painful and frequently causes local reactions (pain, indurations, swelling). Select alternate sites for daily doses and institute local treatment if indicated.

Intravenous
- Preferred over IM route.

PREPARE **IV Infusion:** Dissolve contents of 1 vial in 3–5 mL sterile water for injection or D5W. Further dilute in 50–250 mL of D5W.

ADMINISTER **IV Infusion:** Give over 60 min. Can cause severe hypotension if given too fast. If this occurs, infuse over 1–2 h.

INCOMPATIBILITIES **Y-Site: Aldesleukin,** CEPHALOSPORINS, **foscarnet, fluconazole.**

ADVERSE EFFECTS CNS: Confusion, hallucinations, neuralgia, dizziness, sweating. **CV:** <u>Sudden, severe hypotension</u>, cardiac arrhythmias, ventricular tachycardia, phlebitis. **GI:** Anorexia, nausea, vomiting, pancreatitis, unpleasant taste. **Urogenital:** <u>Acute kidney failure</u>. **Hematologic:** Leukopenia, thrombocytopenia, anemia. **Metabolic:** <u>Hypoglycemia</u>, hypocalcemia, *hyperkalemia*. **Respiratory:** *Cough, bronchospasm,* laryngitis, shortness of breath, chest pain, <u>pneumothorax</u>. **Skin:** Stevens-Johnson syndrome, facial flush (with IV injection), *local reactions at injection site.*

INTERACTIONS Drug: AMINOGLYCOSIDES, **amphotericin B, cidofovir, cisplatin, ganciclovir, cyclosporine, vancomycin,** other nephrotoxic drugs increase risk of nephrotoxicity.

PHARMACOKINETICS Absorption: Readily absorbed after IM injection. **Distribution:** Leaves bloodstream rapidly to bind extensively to body tissues. **Elimination:** 50–66% excreted in urine within 6 h; small amounts found in urine for as long as 6–8 wk. **Half-Life:** 6.5–13.2 h.

Common adverse effects in *italic;* life-threatening effects <u>underlined;</u> generic names in **bold;** drug classifications in SMALL CAPS; ♣ Canadian drug name; ⊘ Prototype drug.

957

NURSING IMPLICATIONS

Assessment & Drug Effects

- Monitor BP closely. Sudden severe hypotension may develop after a single dose. Place patient in supine position while receiving the drug. Monitor BP and heart rate continuously during the infusion, every half hour for 2 h thereafter, and then every 4 h until BP stabilizes.
- Lab tests: Monitor periodically serum electrolytes, renal function, CBC with differential, platelet count, and blood glucose.
- Measure and record I&O ratio and pattern and check patient's pulse (to detect arrhythmia) at least twice daily.
- Be alert and report promptly S&S of impending kidney dysfunction (e.g., changed I&O ratio, oliguria, edema). Dosage adjustment is indicated in renal failure.
- Characteristics of pneumonia in the immunocompromised patient include constant fever, scanty (if any) sputum, dyspnea, tachypnea, and cyanosis.
- Monitor temperature changes and institute measures to lower the temperature as indicated. Fever is a constant symptom in *P. carinii* pneumonia, but may be rapidly elevated (as high as 40° C [104° F]) shortly after drug infusion.

Patient & Family Education

- Report promptly to physician increasing respiratory difficulty.
- Monitor blood glucose for loss of glycemic control if diabetic.
- Report any unusual bruising or bleeding. Avoid using aspirin or other NSAIDs.
- Increase fluid intake (if not contraindicated) to 2–3 quarts (liters) per day in adolescents and adults. For children, refer to recommended fluid intake for age groups in the Physiological Considerations section of Part I.
- Do not breast feed while taking this drug without consulting physician.
- Store this medication out of reach of children.

PENTOBARBITAL

(pen-toe-bar'bi-tal)
Nembutal

PENTOBARBITAL SODIUM

Nembutal Sodium, Novopentobarb ♣

Classifications: CENTRAL NERVOUS SYSTEM AGENT; ANXIOLYTIC; SEDATIVE-HYPNOTIC; BARBITURATE
Prototype: Secobarbital
Pregnancy Category: D
Controlled Substance: Schedule II

AVAILABILITY 50 mg, 100 mg capsules; 20 mg/5 mL liquid; 30 mg, 60 mg, 120 mg, 200 mg suppositories; 50 mg/mL injection (contains 40% propylene glycol and 10% alcohol)

ACTIONS Short-acting barbiturate. Potent respiratory depressant. Initially, barbiturates suppress REM sleep, but with chronic therapy REM sleep returns to normal. Has no analgesic properties, and small doses may increase reaction to painful stimuli.

THERAPEUTIC EFFECTS Effective as a sedative and hypnotic. CNS depression may range from mild sedation to coma, depending on dosage, route of administration, degree of nervous system excitability, and drug tolerance.

USES Sedative or hypnotic for preanesthetic medication, induction of general anesthesia, adjunct in manipulative or diagnostic procedures, and emergency control of acute convulsions, to induce coma in patients with high intracranial pressure.

CONTRAINDICATIONS Pregnancy (category D) or lactation. History of sensitivity to barbiturates; parturition, fetal immaturity, uncontrolled pain. Use of sterile injection containing polyethylene glycol vehicle in patients with renal insufficiency.

CAUTIOUS USE Pregnant women with toxemia or history of bleeding.

ROUTE & DOSAGE

Sedative

Child: **PO** 2–6 mg/kg/day in 3 divided doses (max dose 100 mg/day)
Adult: **PO** 20–30 mg b.i.d. to q.i.d.

Preoperative Sedation

Child: **PO/IM:** 2–6 mg/kg/dose **IV** 1–3 mg/kg/dose every 10 min until asleep (max 100 mg/day)
Adult: **PO** 150–200 mg in 2 divided doses **IM** 150–200 mg in 2 divided doses **IV** 100 mg; may increase to 500 mg if necessary

Hypnotic

Child: **PO** <4 y, 3–6 mg/kg/dose at bedtime; ≥4 y, 1.5–3 mg/kg/dose at bedtime **IM** 2–6 mg/kg/dose (max 100 mg/dose)
Adult: **PO** 120–200 mg/dose. **IM** 150–200 mg/dose

P

STORAGE

Store at 15°–25° C (59°–77° F) in tightly closed, light-resistant containers. Protect parenteral solutions from light and freezing. Store suppositories at 2°–8° C (36°–45° F).

ADMINISTRATION

Note: Do not give within 14 days of starting/stopping a MAO inhibitor.

Intramuscular

- Do not use parenteral solutions that appear cloudy or in which a precipitate has formed.
- Make IM injections deep into large muscle mass. In children midlateral aspect of thigh is generally preferred. Select IM site carefully to ensure an injection into deep muscle mass. See Part I for appropriate sites and safe amounts/injection site in children. Aspirate needle carefully before injecting it to prevent inadvertent entry into blood vessel.

Intravenous

- Use IV route ONLY when other routes are not feasible.

PREPARE Direct: Give undiluted or diluted (preferred) with sterile water, D5W, NS, or other compatible IV solutions.

ADMINISTER Direct: Give slowly. Do not exceed rate of 50 mg/min.

Common adverse effects in *italic*; life-threatening effects underlined; generic names in **bold;** drug classifications in SMALL CAPS; ♣ Canadian drug name; ◐ Prototype drug.

959

INCOMPATIBILITIES **Solution/Additive:** Chlorpheniramine, codeine, ephedrine, hydrocortisone, hydroxyzine, inulin, levorphanol, methadone, norepinephrine, penicillin G, pentazocine, phenytoin, promazine, promethazine, sodium bicarbonate, streptomycin, succinylcholine, TETRACYCLINES, triflubromazine, vancomycin, cimetidine, benzquinamide, butorphanol, chlorpromazine, dimenhydrinate, diphenhydramine, droperidol, fentanyl, glycopyrrolate, meperidine, midazolam, morphine, nalbuphine, perphenazine, prochlorperazine, ranitidine. **Y-Site:** Cimetidine, butorphanol, glycopyrrolate, midazolam, nalbuphine, perphenazine, ranitidine.

▪ Take extreme care to avoid extravasation. Necrosis may result because parenteral solution is highly alkaline. ▪ Do not use cloudy or precipitated solution. Do not add to acid solutions; precipitate may occur.

ADVERSE EFFECTS Body as a Whole: Drowsiness, lethargy, hangover, paradoxical excitement. **CV:** Hypotension with rapid IV. **Respiratory:** With rapid IV (<u>respiratory depression, laryngospasm</u>, bronchospasm, <u>apnea</u>).

INTERACTIONS Drug: Phenmetrazine antagonizes effects of pentobarbital; CNS DEPRESSANTS, **alcohol,** SEDATIVES add to CNS depression; MAO INHIBITORS cause excessive CNS depression; **methoxyflurane** creates risk of nephrotoxicity. **Herbal: Kava-kava, valerian** may potentiate sedation.

PHARMACOKINETICS Onset: 15–30 min PO; 10–15 min IM; 1 min IV. **Duration:** 1–4 h PO; 15 min IV. **Distribution:** Crosses placenta. **Metabolism:** Metabolized primarily in liver. **Elimination:** Excreted in urine. **Half-Life:** 4–50 h.

P

NURSING IMPLICATIONS

Assessment & Drug Effects

▪ Monitor BP, pulse, and respiration q3–5min during IV administration. Observe patient closely; maintain airway. Have equipment for artificial respiration immediately available.

▪ Observe patient closely for adverse effects for at least 30 min after IM administration of hypnotic dose. Have patient remain on bedrest with side rails up.

Patient & Family Education

▪ Exercise caution when driving or engaging in hazardous activity (biking, skateboarding, and sports) for the remainder of day after taking drug.

▪ Avoid alcohol and other CNS depressants for 24 h after receiving this drug.

▪ Store this medication in locked area out of reach of children; this is a Scheduled II drug.

PERMETHRIN ⓟ

(per-meth′rin)

Acticin, Nix, Elimite, Acticin, Kwellada-P

Classifications: SKIN AND MUCOUS MEMBRANE AGENT; PEDICULICIDE
Pregnancy Category: B

AVAILABILITY 5% cream; 1% liquid

ACTIONS Pediculicidal and ovicidal activity against *Pediculus humanus* var. *capitis* (head louse). Inhibits sodium ion influx through nerve cell membrane channels, resulting in delayed repolarization of the action potential and paralysis of the pest.
THERAPEUTIC EFFECTS Prevents burrowing into host's skin. Because lice are completely dependent on blood for survival, they die within 24–48 h. Also active against ticks, mites, and fleas.

USES *Pediculosis capitis.*

CONTRAINDICATIONS Hypersensitivity to pyrethrins, chrysanthemums, sulfites, or other preservatives or dyes; acute inflammation of the scalp; lactation.
CAUTIOUS USE Children <2 y (liquid); pregnancy (category B).

ROUTE & DOSAGE

Head Lice

Child >2 mo/Adult: **Topical** Apply 1% cream in sufficient volume to clean wet hair to saturate the hair and scalp; leave on 10 min, then rinse hair thoroughly, may repeat in 7–10 days

Scabies

Infant/Toddler >2 mo: **Topical** Apply to the head and neck to toes (avoid the eyes, nose, and mouth), leave on for 8–14 h then wash off with water, may repeat in 7 days
Child >2 mo/Adult: **Topical** Apply 5% cream from neck to toe; leave on for 8–14 h then wash off with water, may repeat in 7 days

P

STORAGE

Store drug away from heat at 15°–25° C (59°–77° F) and direct light; avoid freezing.

ADMINISTRATION

Topical

- Saturate scalp as well as hair with the lotion; this is not a shampoo but a cream rinse.
- Hair should be washed with regular shampoo before treatment with permethrin, thoroughly rinsed and dried.
- Shake lotion well before application. One container holds enough for at least one treatment, but two containers may be necessary if patient has long hair. Avoid getting rinse into eyes and mucous membranes. Make sure rinse comes in contact with areas behind the ears and nape of neck.
- Rinse hair and scalp thoroughly and dry with a clean towel following 10-min exposure to the medication. It may be necessary to use a fine-toothed comb to remove nits from hair. Head lice are usually eliminated with one treatment, but second treatment can be done in 7–10 days.

Common adverse effects in *italic;* life-threatening effects <u>underlined;</u> generic names in **bold;** drug classifications in SMALL CAPS; ♣ Canadian drug name; ⊘ Prototype drug.

961

- Notify prescriber if crawling bugs are noticed in hair following shampoo because resistance is likely.
- Scabies: Use gloves to apply thin layer of cream avoiding all mucous membranes. Leave cream on skin as directed.

ADVERSE EFFECTS Skin: *Pruritus, transient tingling,* burning, stinging, numbness; erythema, edema, rash.

INTERACTIONS Drug: No clinically significant interactions established.

PHARMACOKINETICS Absorption: <2% of amount applied is absorbed through intact skin. **Metabolism:** Rapidly hydrolyzed to inactive metabolites. **Elimination:** Excreted primarily in urine.

NURSING IMPLICATIONS

Assessment & Drug Effects

- Do not attempt therapy if patient is known to be sensitive to any pyrethrin or pyrethroid. Stop treatment if a reaction occurs.

Patient & Family Education

- Use shampoo according to directions. Child should remove clothing from waist up while hair is shampooed.
- Do not use creme rinse following shampoo.
- Check hair 8–12 h after shampoo and comb with a fine-toothed comb (furnished with medication) to remove dead lice and remaining nits or nit shells.
- Be aware that drug remains on hair shaft up to 14 days; therefore, recurrence of infestation rarely occurs (<1%).
- Inspect hair shafts every 2–3 days for at least 1 wk to determine drug effectiveness. Contact prescriber if live lice are observed after 7 days. A renewed prescription for a second treatment may be ordered. Signs of inadequate treatment: Itching, redness of skin, skin abrasion, infected scalp areas.
- Resume regular shampooing after treatment; residual deposit of drug on hair is not reduced.
- Be aware that drug is usually irritating to the eyes and mucosa. Flush well with water if medicine accidentally gets into eyes.
- All bedding, personal clothes, and hair care items need to be washed in hot water. Items that cannot be washed should be placed in a dryer for 20 minutes on hot setting or sealed in airtight plastic bags for 2 wk. Vacuum carpets and upholstered furniture. Floors should be damp mopped.
- Soak brushes and combs in rubbing alcohol for 1 h.
- All symptomatic members of the family should be treated for lice. All members of the family even if asymptomatic should be treated for scabies. If infants in the home, check with prescriber about recommended treatment.
- If itching is a problem for patient with scabies consult physician.
- Inform all day care centers and schools of infestation.
- Caution parents to use only as directed and store this medication out of reach of children.

Common adverse effects in *italic;* life-threatening effects <u>underlined</u>; generic names in **bold;** drug classifications in SMALL CAPS; ♣ Canadian drug name; ✪ Prototype drug.

PERPHENAZINE

(per-fen′a-zeen)
Phenazine, Trilafon
Classifications: CENTRAL NERVOUS SYSTEM AGENT; PSYCHOTHERAPEUTIC; PHENOTHIAZINE ANTIPSYCHOTIC; ANTIEMETIC
Prototype: Chlorpromazine
Pregnancy Category: C

AVAILABILITY 2 mg, 4 mg, 6 mg, 8 mg, 16 mg, tablets; 16 mg/5 mL liquid; 5 mg/mL injection

ACTIONS Affects all parts of CNS similar to chlorpromazine, particularly the hypothalamus. Antipsychotic effect: Antagonizes the neurotransmitter dopamine by action on dopamine receptors in the brain. Antiemetic action results from direct blockade of dopamine in the chemoreceptor trigger zone (CTZ) in the medulla.

THERAPEUTIC EFFECTS Has antipsychotic and antiemetic properties. Produces less sedation and hypotension, greater antiemetic effects, higher incidence of extrapyramidal effects, and lower levels of anticholinergic adverse effects than chlorpromazine.

USES Psychotic disorders, symptomatic control of severe nausea and vomiting, acute conditions such as violent retching during surgery, and intractable hiccups.

CONTRAINDICATIONS Hypersensitivity to perphenazine and other phenothiazines; preexisting liver damage; suspected or established subcortical brain damage, comatose states; bone marrow depression. Safety during pregnancy (category C), lactation, or in children <12 y is not established.

CAUTIOUS USE Previously diagnosed breast cancer; liver or kidney dysfunction; cardiovascular disorders; alcohol withdrawal, epilepsy, psychic depression, patients with suicidal tendency; glaucoma; history of intestinal or GU obstruction; or debilitated patients; patients who will be exposed to extremes of heat or cold, or to phosphorous insecticides.

ROUTE & DOSAGE

Psychotic Disorders

Child: **PO** >12 y, 4 mg b.i.d. to q.i.d.; 8 mg sustained-release b.i.d. (max 16 mg/day) **IM/IV** Same as adult
Adult: **PO** 4–16 mg b.i.d. to q.i.d.; 8–32 mg sustained-release b.i.d. (max 64 mg/day) **IM** 5 mg q6h (max 15–30 mg/day) **IV** Dilute to 0.5 mg/mL in NS, administer at not more than 1 mg q1–2min or 5 mg by slow infusion

Nausea

Adult: **PO** 8–16 mg b.i.d. to q.i.d. **IM** 5 mg q6h (max 15 mg/day)

STORAGE
Store at 15°–25° C (59°–77° F) in tightly closed, light-resistant containers.

Common adverse effects in *italic;* life-threatening effects <u>underlined</u>; generic names in **bold;** drug classifications in SMALL CAPS; ♣ Canadian drug name; ✺ Prototype drug.

963

ADMINISTRATION

Oral

- Ensure that sustained-release form is not chewed or crushed. Must be swallowed whole.
- Dilute oral concentrate before administration: Dilute each 5 mL (16 mg) to 60 mL water, milk, saline solution, 7-Up, or other compatible carbonated beverages. Do not use liquids that cause color changes or precipitate.

Intramuscular

- Give deep IM into a large muscle mass appropriate for age (see Part I) with patient in recumbent position. Advise patient to continue lying down for at least 1 h after injection. Injection may be painful. Observe daily for signs of inflammation.

Intravenous

PREPARE **Direct:** Dilute each 5 mg in 9 mL NS.
ADMINISTER **Direct:** Give at a rate of 0.5 mg (1 mL) over 60 sec.
INCOMPATIBILITIES **Solution/Additive: Midazolam, pentobarbital, thiethylperazine. Y-Site: Cefoperazone, midazolam, pentobarbital.**

- Do not use precipitated or darkened parenteral solution; however, slight yellowing does not alter potency or therapeutic effects.

ADVERSE EFFECTS CNS: *Extrapyramidal effects (dystonic reactions, akathisia, parkinsonian syndrome, tardive dyskinesia), sedation,* convulsions. **CV:** *Orthostatic hypotension,* tachycardia, bradycardia. **Special Senses:** Mydriasis, blurred vision, corneal and lenticular deposits. **GI:** Constipation, *dry mouth,* increased appetite, <u>adynamic ileus,</u> Abnormal liver function tests, cholestatic jaundice. **Urogenital:** *Urinary retention,* gynecomastia, menstrual irregularities, inhibited ejaculation. **Hematologic:** <u>Agranulocytosis,</u> thrombocytopenic purpura, <u>aplastic</u> or hemolytic <u>anemia.</u> **Body as a Whole:** Photosensitivity, itching, erythema, urticaria, angioneurotic edema, drug fever, <u>anaphylactoid reaction,</u> pain at injection site, sterile abscess. Nasal congestion, decreased sweating. **Metabolic:** Hyperprolactinemia, galactorrhea, weight gain.

DIAGNOSTIC TEST INTERFERENCE Perphenazine may cause falsely abnormal *thyroid function* tests because of elevations of *thyroid globulin.*

INTERACTIONS Drug: Alcohol and other CNS DEPRESSANTS enhance CNS depression; ANTACIDS, ANTIDIARRHEALS may decrease absorption of phenothiazines; ANTICHOLINERGIC AGENTS add to anticholinergic effects including fecal impaction and paralytic ileus; BARBITURATES, ANESTHETICS increase hypotension and excitation. **Herb: Kava-kava** increases risk and severity of dystonic reactions.

PHARMACOKINETICS Absorption: Poorly absorbed from GI tract; 20% reaches systemic circulation. **Onset:** 10 min IM. **Peak:** 1–2 h IM; 4–8 h PO. **Duration:** 6–12 h. **Distribution:** Crosses placenta. **Metabolism:** Metabolized in liver with some metabolism in GI tract. **Elimination:** Excreted in urine and feces. **Half-Life:** 9.5 h.

Common adverse effects in *italic;* life-threatening effects <u>underlined</u>; generic names in **bold**; drug classifications in SMALL CAPS; ♣ Canadian drug name; ⊘ Prototype drug.

NURSING IMPLICATIONS

Assessment & Drug Effects

- Establish baseline BP before initiation of drug therapy and check it at regular intervals, especially during early therapy.
- Monitor BP and pulse continuously during IV administration. Keep patient supine until assured that vital signs are stable. Observe patients carefully for hypotension and extrapyramidal reactions.
- Report restlessness, weakness of extremities, dystonic reactions (spasms of neck and shoulder muscles, rigidity of back, difficulty swallowing or talking); motor restlessness (akathisia: inability to be still); and parkinsonian syndrome (tremors, shuffling gait, drooling, slow speech). A high incidence of extrapyramidal effects accompanies use of perphenazine, particularly with high doses and parenteral administration.
- Withhold medication and report IMMEDIATELY to physician S&S of irreversible tardive dyskinesia (i.e., fine, wormlike movements or rapid protrusions of the tongue, chewing motions, lip smacking). Patients on long-term therapy are high risk. Teach patients and responsible family members about symptoms because early reporting is essential.
- Lab tests: Obtain differential blood cell counts and liver and kidney function studies.
- ECG and ophthalmologic examination are recommended prior to initiation and periodically during therapy.
- Suspect hypersensitivity, withhold drug, and report to physician if jaundice appears between weeks 2 and 4.
- Monitor I&O ratio and bowel elimination pattern.
- Be alert to potential for altered tolerance to environmental temperature changes. Be cautious with external heat devices. Conditioned avoidance behavior may be depressed, and a severe burn could result.

Patient & Family Education

- Make all position changes slowly and in stages, particularly from recumbent to upright posture, and to lie down or sit down if light-headedness or dizziness occurs.
- Do not drive or engage in potentially hazardous activities until response to drug is known. Drug may produce hypotension (dizziness, light-headedness), and sedation especially during early therapy.
- Discontinue drug and report to physician immediately if jaundice appears between weeks 2 and 4.
- Avoid long exposure to sunlight and to sunlamps. Photosensitivity results in skin color changes from brown to blue-gray.
- Adhere to dosage regimen strictly. Contact physician before changing it for any reason.
- Discontinue gradually over a period of several weeks following prolonged therapy.
- Do not take OTC drugs while on this drug unless physician prescribes them.
- Be aware that perphenazine may discolor urine reddish brown.
- Do not breast feed while taking this drug without consulting physician.
- Store this medication out of reach of children.

P

PHENAZOPYRIDINE HYDROCHLORIDE
(fen-az-oh-peer'i-deen)
Azo-Standard, Baridium, Geridium, Phenazo ♣, Phenazodine, Pyridiate, Pyridium, Pyronium ♣, Urodine, Urogesic
Classification: URINARY TRACT ANALGESIC
Pregnancy Category: B

AVAILABILITY 95 mg, 97 mg, 97.2 mg, 100 mg, 150 mg, 200 mg tablets

ACTIONS Azo dye. Precise mechanism of action not known.
THERAPEUTIC EFFECTS Local anesthetic action on urinary tract mucosa which imparts little or no antibacterial activity.

USES Symptomatic relief of pain, burning, frequency, and urgency arising from irritation of urinary tract mucosa, as from infection, trauma, surgery, or instrumentation.

CONTRAINDICATIONS Renal insufficiency, glomerulonephritis, pyelonephritis during pregnancy (category B); severe hepatitis.
CAUTIOUS USE GI disturbances; G6PD deficiency, lactation.

ROUTE & DOSAGE

Cystitis
Child: PO 6–12 y, 12 mg/kg/day in 3 divided doses for 2 days or until symptoms controlled
Adult: PO 200 mg t.i.d. for 2 days or until symptoms controlled

STORAGE
Store at 15°–25° C (59°–77° F) in tightly closed containers.

ADMINISTRATION
Oral
▪ Give with or after meals.

ADVERSE EFFECTS Body as a Whole: Headache, vertigo. **GI:** Mild GI disturbances. **Urogenital:** Discoloration of urine orange-red, kidney stones, transient acute <u>kidney failure</u>. **Metabolic:** Methemoglobinemia, hemolytic anemia. **Skin:** Skin pigmentation. **Special Senses:** May stain soft contact lenses.

DIAGNOSTIC TEST INTERFERENCE Phenazopyridine may interfere with any urinary test that is based on color reactions or spectrometry: *bromsulphalein* and *phenolsulfonphthalein* excretion tests; urinary *glucose* test using *Clinistix* or *TesTape* (*copper-reduction methods* such as *Clinitest* and *Benedict's test* reportedly not affected); *bilirubin* using "foam test" or *Ictotest; ketones* using *nitroprusside* (e.g., *Acetest, Ketostix,* or *Gerhardt ferric chloride*); urinary protein using *Albustix, Albutest,* or *nitric acid ring test;* urinary *steroids; urobilinogen; assays* for *porphyrins.*

INTERACTIONS Drug: No clinically significant interactions established.

Common adverse effects in *italic;* life-threatening effects <u>underlined;</u> generic names in **bold;** drug classifications in SMALL CAPS; ♣ Canadian drug name; ❂ Prototype drug.

PHARMACOKINETICS Absorption: Readily absorbed from GI tract. **Distribution:** Crosses placenta in trace amounts. **Metabolism:** Metabolized in liver and other tissues. **Elimination:** Primarily excreted in urine.

NURSING IMPLICATIONS

Assessment & Drug Effects
- Lab tests: Obtain periodic blood work and kidney function tests in patients on prolonged therapy or with impaired kidney function.

Patient & Family Education
- Be aware that drug will impart an orange to red color to urine and may stain fabric.
- Discontinue drug report to physician immediately the appearance of yellowish tinge to skin or sclerae may indicate drug accumulation due to renal impairment.
- Discontinue drug when pain and discomfort are relieved (usually 3–15 days). Keep physician informed.
- Do not breast feed while taking this drug without consulting physician.
- Store this medication out of reach of children.

PHENOBARBITAL 🅟
(fee-noe-bar′bi-tal)
Barbital, Luminal, Solfoton

PHENOBARBITAL SODIUM
Luminal Sodium
Classifications: CENTRAL NERVOUS SYSTEM AGENT; ANTICONVULSANT; SEDATIVE-HYPNOTIC; BARBITURATE
Pregnancy Category: D
Controlled Substance: Schedule IV

AVAILABILITY 15 mg, 16 mg, 16.2 mg, 30 mg, 60 mg, 90 mg, 100 mg tablets; 16 mg capsules; 15 mg/5 mL, 20 mg/5 mL elixir (contains alcohol); 30 mg/mL, 60 mg/mL, 65 mg/mL, 130 mg/mL injection

ACTIONS Long-acting barbiturate. Sedative and hypnotic effects of barbiturates appear to be due primarily to interference with impulse transmission of cerebral cortex by inhibition of reticular activating system. CNS depression may range from mild sedation to coma, depending on dosage, route of administration, degree of nervous system excitability, and drug tolerance. Initially, barbiturates suppress REM sleep, but with chronic therapy REM sleep returns to normal.
THERAPEUTIC EFFECTS Produces sedative and hypnotic effects with no analgesic properties, and small doses may increase reaction to painful stimuli. Phenobarbital limits spread of seizure activity by increasing threshold for motor cortex stimuli. Barbiturates are habit forming.

USES Long-term management of tonic-clonic (grand mal) seizures and partial seizures; status epilepticus, eclampsia, febrile convulsions in

---

Common adverse effects in *italic;* life-threatening effects <u>underlined</u>; generic names in **bold;** drug classifications in SMALL CAPS; ♣ Canadian drug name; 🅟 Prototype drug.

young children. Also used as a sedative in anxiety or tension states; in pediatrics as preoperative and postoperative sedation and to treat pylorospasm in infants.

UNLABELED USES Treatment and prevention of hyperbilirubinemia in neonates and in the management of chronic cholestasis; benzodiazepine withdrawal.

CONTRAINDICATIONS Sensitivity to barbiturates; manifest hepatic or familial history of porphyria; severe respiratory or kidney disease; history of previous addiction to sedative hypnotics; uncontrolled pain; preexisting CNS depression; pregnancy (particularly early pregnancy) (category D), lactation; sustained-release formulation for children <12 y of age.

CAUTIOUS USE Impaired liver, kidney, cardiac, or respiratory function; history of allergies; debilitated patients; patients with fever; hyperthyroidism; diabetes mellitus or severe anemia; during labor and delivery; patients with borderline hypoadrenal function.

ROUTE & DOSAGE

Status Epilepticus Loading Doses

Neonate: **IV** 15–20 mg/kg in single or equally divided doses (max loading dose 20 mg/kg)
Infant/Child/Adult: **IV** 15–18 mg/kg in single or equally divided doses (max 20 mg/kg); for certain patients, may give additional 5 m/kg/dose every 15–30 min until seizure control (max total dose 30 mg/kg)

Anticonvulsant Maintenance

Neonate: **PO/IV** 3–4 mg/kg/days (max 5 mg/kg/day)
Infant: **PO/IV** 5–6 mg/kg/day in 1–2 equally divided doses
Child: **PO/IV** 1–5 y, 6–8 mg/kg/day in 1–2 equally divided doses; 6–12 y, 4–6 mg/kg/day in 1–2 equally divided doses; >12 y, 1–3 mg/kg/day in 1–2 equally divided doses
Adult: **PO** 100–300 mg/day **IV/IM** 200–600 mg up to 20 mg/kg

Sedative

Child: **PO** 2 mg/kg/day in 3 equally divided doses (max dose 100 mg/day) **IV/IM** 3–5 mg/kg/day at bedtime
Adult: **PO** 30–120 mg/day **IV/IM** 100–200 mg/day

Hyperbilirubinema

Child: **PO** <12 y, 3–8 mg/kg/day in 2–3 divided doses (dosages up to 12 mg/kg/day have been used)

STORAGE

Store elixir at 15°–25° C (59°–77° F) in light-resistant container.

ADMINISTRATION

Oral

- Make sure patient actually swallows pill and does not "cheek" it.
- Give crushed and mixed with a fluid or with food if patient cannot swallow pill. Do not permit patient to swallow dry crushed drug.
- Due to alcohol content in elixir, give slowly in neonates, infants, and children to prevent choking. Follow elixir with fluids.

Intramuscular

- Give IM deep into large muscle mass appropriate for age. See Part I for site selection and maximum amounts to safely inject at any one site. Select IM site carefully.

Intravenous

Note: Verify correct IV concentration and rate of infusion for neonates, infants, children with physician. Use IV route ONLY if other routes are not feasible.

***PREPARE* Direct:** Slowly add at least 10 mL of sterile water for injection to ampule. Rotate ampule to dissolve (may take several minutes). If solution not clear in 5 min or if a precipitate remains, discard.

***ADMINISTER* Direct:** Give 60 mg or fraction thereof over at least 60 sec or 1 mg/kg/min. Infants and children: Infuse no faster than 30 mg/60 sec. Give within 30 min after preparation.

***INCOMPATIBILITIES* Solution/Additive:** **Benzquinamide, cephalothin, chlorpromazine, codeine phosphate, ephedrine, hydralazine, hydrocortisone sodium succinate, hydroxyzine, insulin, levorphanol, meperidine, methadone, morphine, norepinephrine, procaine, prochlorperazine, promazine, promethazine, ranitidine, streptomycin,** TETRACYCLINES, **vancomycin. Y-Site: Amphotericin B cholesteryl complex, hydromorphone, TPN with albumin.**

- Be aware that extravasation of IV phenobarbital may cause necrotic tissue changes that necessitate skin grafting. Check injection site frequently.

ADVERSE EFFECTS Body as a Whole: Myalgia, neuralgia, <u>CNS depression, coma, and death</u>. **CNS:** *Somnolence,* nightmares, insomnia, "hangover," headache, anxiety, thinking abnormalities, dizziness, nystagmus, irritability, paradoxic excitement and exacerbation of hyperkinetic behavior (in children); confusion or depression or marked excitement (debilitated patients); ataxia. **CV:** Bradycardia, syncope, hypotension. **GI:** Nausea, vomiting, constipation, diarrhea, epigastric pain, liver damage. **Hematologic:** Megaloblastic anemia, <u>agranulocytosis</u>, thrombocytopenia. **Metabolic:** Hypocalcemia, osteomalacia, rickets. **Musculoskeletal:** Folic acid deficiency, vitamin D deficiency. **Respiratory:** <u>Respiratory depression</u>. **Skin:** Mild maculopapular, morbilliform rash; erythema multiforme, <u>Stevens-Johnson syndrome, exfoliative dermatitis</u> (rare).

DIAGNOSTIC TEST INTERFERENCE BARBITURATES may affect ***bromsulphalein*** retention tests (by enhancing liver uptake and excretion of dye) and increase ***serum phosphatase.***

INTERACTIONS Drug: Alcohol, CNS DEPRESSANTS compound CNS depression; phenobarbital may decrease absorption and increase metabolism of ORAL ANTICOAGULANTS; increases metabolism of CORTICOSTEROIDS, ORAL CONTRACEPTIVES, ANTICONVULSANTS, **digitoxin,** possibly decreasing their effects; ANTIDEPRESSANTS potentiate adverse effects of phenobarbital; **griseofulvin** decreases absorption of phenobarbital. Valproic acid, methylphenidate, chloramphenicol, felbamate, and propoxyphene may inhibit the metabolism of phenobarbital. **Food:** This drug may increase the metabolism of vitamins K and D. Can decrease magnesium, folate levels and vitamin B_6 levels. **Herbal: Kava-kava, valerian** may potentiate sedation.

PHARMACOKINETICS Absorption: 70–90% absorbed slowly from GI tract. **Peak:** 8–12 h PO; 30 min IV. **Duration:** 4–6 h IV. **Distribution:** 20–45% protein bound; crosses placenta; enters breast milk. **Metabolism:** Oxidized in liver to inactivated metabolites. **Elimination:** Excreted in urine. **Half-Life:** 2–6 days. *Therapeutic range 15–40 mcg/mL. Toxicity may occur over 40 mcg/mL.*

NURSING IMPLICATIONS

Assessment & Drug Effects

- Observe patients receiving large doses closely for at least 30 min to ensure that sedation is not excessive.
- Keep patient under constant observation when drug is administered IV, and record vital signs at least every hour or more often if indicated.
- Lab tests: Obtain liver function and hematology tests and determinations of serum folate and vitamin D levels during prolonged therapy.
- Monitor serum drug levels. *Serum concentrations* >50 mcg/mL may cause coma. *Therapeutic serum concentrations* of 15–40 mcg/mL produce anticonvulsant activity in most patients. These values are usually attained after 2 or 3 wk of therapy with a dose of 100–200 mg/day in adults.
- Expect barbiturates to produce restlessness when given to patients in pain because these drugs do not have analgesic action.
- Be prepared for paradoxical responses and report promptly in debilitated patient and children (i.e., irritability, marked excitement [inappropriate tearfulness and aggression in children], depression, and confusion).
- Monitor for drug interactions. Barbiturates increase the metabolism of many drugs, leading to decreased pharmacologic effects of those drugs. Whenever a barbiturate is added to an established regimen of another drug, observe for changes in effectiveness of the first drug at least during early phase of barbiturate use.
- Monitor for and report chronic toxicity symptoms (e.g., ataxia, slurred speech, irritability, poor judgment, slight dysarthria, nystagmus on vertical gaze, confusion, insomnia, somatic complaints).

Patient & Family Education

- Be aware that anticonvulsant therapy may cause drowsiness during first few weeks of treatment, but this usually diminishes with continued use.
- Avoid potentially hazardous activities requiring mental alertness (biking, skateboarding, and sports) until response to drug is known.
- Do not consume alcohol in any amount when taking a barbiturate; it may severely impair judgment and abilities.
- Increase vitamin D-fortified foods (e.g., milk products) because drug increases vitamin D metabolism. A vitamin D supplement may be prescribed.
- Maintain adequate dietary folate intake: Fresh vegetables (especially green leafy), fresh fruits, whole grains, liver. Long-term therapy may result in nutritional folate (B_9) deficiency. A supplement of folic acid may be prescribed.
- Adhere to drug regimen (i.e., do not change intervals between doses or increase or decrease doses) without contacting physician.
- Do not stop taking drug abruptly because of danger of withdrawal symptoms (8–12 h after last dose), which can be fatal.

- Report to physician the onset of fever, sore throat or mouth, malaise, easy bruising or bleeding, petechiae, jaundice, rash when on prolonged therapy.
- Avoid pregnancy when receiving barbiturates. Use or add barrier device to hormonal contraceptive when taking prolonged therapy. Monitor response for seizure control.
- Do not breast feed while taking this drug.
- Store this medication out of reach of children.

PHENOXYBENZAMINE HYDROCHLORIDE

(fen-ox-ee-ben′za-meen)
Dibenzyline
Classifications: AUTONOMIC NERVOUS SYSTEM AGENT; ALPHA-ADRENERGIC ANTAGONIST (BLOCKING AGENT), SYMPATHOLYTIC; ANTIHYPERTENSIVE AGENT
Prototype: Prazosin
Pregnancy Category: C

AVAILABILITY 10 mg capsules

ACTIONS Long-acting alpha-adrenergic blocking agent. Apparently produces noncompetitive blockade of alpha-adrenergic receptor sites at postganglionic synapse. Alpha-receptor sites are thus unable to react to endogenous or exogenous sympathomimetic agents.

THERAPEUTIC EFFECTS Blocks excitatory effects of epinephrine, including vasoconstriction, but does not affect adrenergic cardiac inhibitory actions. It produces a "chemical sympathectomy" and it can maintain it. Causes orthostatic hypotension in both normotensive and hypertensive patients.

USES Management of pheochromocytoma.
UNLABELED USES To improve circulation in peripheral vasospastic conditions such as Raynaud's acrocyanosis and frostbite sequelae, for adjunctive treatment of shock, hypertensive crisis.

CONTRAINDICATIONS Instances when fall in BP would be dangerous; compensated congestive heart failure; pregnancy (category C), lactation.
CAUTIOUS USE Marked cerebral or coronary arteriosclerosis, CHF; renal insufficiency; respiratory infections.

ROUTE & DOSAGE

Management of Pheochromocytoma

Child: **PO** Initial 0.2 mg/kg/day in 1 dose (maximum initial dose is 10 mg), may increase by 0.2 mg/kg/day at 4-day intervals to desired response (usual maintenance range 0.4–1.2 mg/kg/day in equally divided doses q6–8h
Adult: **PO** 5–10 mg b.i.d., may increase by 10 mg/day at 4-day intervals to desired response (usual range 20–40 mg/day in 2–3 divided doses)

STORAGE
Store at 15°–25° C (59°–77° F) in tightly closed containers.

ADMINISTRATION

Oral

- Give with milk or in divided doses to reduce gastric irritation.
- Preserve in airtight containers protected from light.

ADVERSE EFFECTS Body as a Whole: *Dizziness,* fainting, drowsiness, sedation, tiredness, weakness, lethargy, confusion, headache, <u>shock</u>. **CNS:** CNS stimulation (large doses). **CV:** *Postural hypotension, tachycardia,* palpitation. **GI:** Dry mouth. **Urogenital:** Inhibition of ejaculation. **Respiratory:** *Nasal congestion.* **Skin:** Allergic contact dermatitis. **Special Senses:** *Miosis,* drooping of eyelids.

INTERACTIONS Drug: Inhibits effects of **methoxamine, norepinephrine, phenylephrine;** additive hypotensive effects with ANTIHYPERTENSIVES.

PHARMACOKINETICS Absorption: Variably absorbed (approximately 30%) from GI tract. **Onset:** 2 h. **Peak:** 4–6 h. **Duration:** 3–4 days. **Distribution:** Accumulates in adipose tissue. **Elimination:** 80% excreted in urine and bile within 24 h. **Half-Life:** 24 h.

NURSING IMPLICATIONS

Assessment & Drug Effects

- Monitor BP and note pulse quality, rate, and rhythm in recumbent and standing positions during period of dosage adjustment. Observe patient closely for at least 4 days from one dosage increment to the next; hypotension and tachycardia are most likely to occur in standing position.
- Drug has cumulative action, thus onset of therapeutic effects may not occur until after 2 wk of therapy, and full therapeutic effects may not be apparent for several more weeks.

Patient & Family Education

- Make position changes slowly, particularly from reclining to upright posture, and dangle legs and exercise ankles and feet for a few minutes before standing.
- Be aware that light-headedness, dizziness, and palpitations usually disappear with continued therapy but may reappear under conditions that promote vasodilation, such as strenuous exercise or ingestion of a large meal or alcohol.
- Pupil constriction, nasal stuffiness, and inhibition of ejaculation generally decrease with continued therapy.
- Do not take OTC medications for coughs, colds, or allergy while taking this drug without approval of physician. Many contain agents that cause BP elevation.
- Do not breast feed while taking this drug.
- Store this medication out of reach of children.

PHENSUXIMIDE

(fen-sux′i-mide)
Milontin
Classifications: CENTRAL NERVOUS SYSTEM AGENT; ANTICONVULSANT SUCCINIMIDE
Prototype: Ethosuximide
Pregnancy Category: D

AVAILABILITY 500 mg capsules

ACTIONS Succinimide derivative reportedly less potent and less effective than other drugs of this class. Reduces the frequency of epileptiform attacks. **THERAPEUTIC EFFECTS** Apparently depresses the motor cortex and elevates the threshold of CNS sensitivity to seizure activity, thus lessening the incidence of seizure activity.

USES Management of petit mal epilepsy (absence seizures) and with other anticonvulsants when other forms of epilepsy coexist with petit mal.

CONTRAINDICATIONS Intermittent porphyria; liver or kidney disease; pregnancy (category D), lactation.

ROUTE & DOSAGE

Absence Seizures
Child/Adult: **PO** 0.5–1 g b.i.d. or t.i.d.

STORAGE
Store at 15°–25° C (59°–77° F) in tightly closed, light-resistant containers.

ADMINISTRATION

Oral
- Give consistently with respect to time of day.

ADVERSE EFFECTS Body as a Whole: *Drowsiness, dizziness, ataxia,* muscle weakness, flushing, periorbital edema. **GI:** *Anorexia, nausea, vomiting.* **Urogenital:** Reversible nephropathy. **Hematologic:** Granulocytopenia. **Skin:** Alopecia, pruritus, skin rash.

INTERACTIONS Drug: Carbamazepine decreases phensuximide levels; **isoniazid** significantly increases phensuximide levels; levels of both **phenobarbital** and phensuximide may be altered with increased seizure frequency.

PHARMACOKINETICS Absorption: Readily absorbed from GI tract. **Peak:** 1–4 h. **Metabolism:** Metabolized in liver. **Elimination:** Excreted slowly in urine; small amounts excreted in bile and feces. **Half-Life:** 5–12 h.

NURSING IMPLICATIONS

Assessment & Drug Effects
- Monitor weight, especially in children, because anorexic effects of drug might cause weight loss.
- Lab tests: Perform baseline and periodic liver and kidney function tests. Perform periodic blood tests, especially with long-term therapy.

Patient & Family Education
- Report onset of skin rash or other unusual symptoms to physician.
- Be aware that phensuximide may color urine pink, red, or redbrown.
- Do not use OTC medications while taking this drug unless the physician approves; loss of seizure control can be induced by ingredients in some popular OTC drugs.

Common adverse effects in *italic;* life-threatening effects underlined; generic names in **bold;** drug classifications in SMALL CAPS; ♣ Canadian drug name; ♦ Prototype drug.

973

- Do not drive or engage in potentially hazardous activities until response to drug is known.
- Do not breast feed while taking this drug.
- Store this medication out of reach of children.

PHENTOLAMINE MESYLATE

(fen-tole′a-meen)
Regitine, Rogitine ♣
Classifications: AUTONOMIC NERVOUS SYSTEM AGENT; ALPHA-ADRENERGIC ANTAGONIST (BLOCKING AGENT), SYMPATHOLYTIC
Prototype: Prazosin
Pregnancy Category: C

AVAILABILITY 5 mg injection

ACTIONS Alpha-adrenergic blocking agent structurally related to tolazoline but with more potent blocking effects. Competitively blocks alpha-adrenergic receptors, but action is transient and incomplete. Prevents hypertension resulting from elevated levels of circulating epinephrine or norepinephrine.
THERAPEUTIC EFFECTS Causes vasodilation and decreases general vascular resistance and pulmonary arterial pressure, primarily by direct action on vascular smooth muscle. Through stimulation of beta-adrenergic receptors, produces positive inotropic and chronotropic cardiac effects and increases cardiac output.

USES Diagnosis of pheochromocytoma and to prevent or control hypertensive episodes prior to or during pheochromocytomectomy.
UNLABELED USES Prevention of dermal necrosis and sloughing following IV administration or extravasation of vasopressive agents norepinephrine, epinephrine, dopamine, phenylephrine, vasopressin.

CONTRAINDICATIONS MI (previous or present), coronary artery disease. Safety during pregnancy (category C) or lactation is not established.
CAUTIOUS USE Gastritis, peptic ulcer, history of cardiac arrhythmias.

ROUTE & DOSAGE

To Prevent Hypertensive Episode During Surgery
Child: **IV/IM** 0.05–0.1 mg/kg (max 5 mg/dose) 1–2 h preoperative, may repeat dose q2–4h as needed
Adult: **IV/IM** 2–5 mg 1–2 h preoperative, may repeat dose q2–4h as needed

To Test for Pheochromocytoma
Child: **IV/IM** 0.05–0.1 mg/kg (max dose 5 mg)
Adult: **IV/IM** 5 mg/dose

To Prevent Necrosis from Norepinephrine Infusions
Adult: **IV** 10 mg added to each liter of IV fluid containing norepinephrine

---

Common adverse effects in *italic;* life-threatening effects <u>underlined</u>; generic names in **bold;** drug classifications in SMALL CAPS; ♣ Canadian drug name; ❷ Prototype drug.

To Treat Alpha-Adrenegic Drug Extravasation

Neonate: **Intradermal** 0.25–0.5 mg diluted in 10 mL of normal saline. Inject 1 mL of solution in 5 doses of 0.2 mL subcutaneous around extravasation site. (max dose 0.1 mg/kg or 2.5 mg total)

Infant/Child/Adult: **Intradermal** 5–10 mg diluted in 10 mL of normal saline; inject 1–5 mL in 5 divided doses into affected area within 12 h of extravasation (max dose 0.1–0.2 mg/kg or 5 mg total)

STORAGE

Store at 15°–25° C (59°–77° F). Reconstitued solution with sterile water is stable for 48 h at 15°–25° C (59°–77° F) or for 1 wk at 2°–8° C (36°–45° F).

ADMINISTRATION

Note: Place patient in supine position when receiving drug parenterally. Monitor BP and pulse q2min until stabilized.

Intradermal

Dilute medication. Use a 27- to 30-gauge needle. Infuse extravasion area with properly diluted solution dose using multiple small (0.2-mL) injections.

Intramuscular

■ Reconstitute 5-mg vial with 1 mL sterile water for injection.

Intravenous

PREPARE **Direct:** Reconstitute as for IM. May be further diluted with up to 10 mL sterile water. Use immediately.

ADMINISTER **Direct:** Give a single dose over 60 sec.

ADVERSE EFFECTS Body as a Whole: Weakness, dizziness, flushing, *orthostatic hypotension.* **GI:** *Abdominal pain, nausea, vomiting, diarrhea, exacerbation of peptic ulcer.* **CV:** *Acute and prolonged hypotension, tachycardia, anginal pain,* cardiac arrhythmias, <u>MI, cerebrovascular spasm</u>, shock-like state. **Special Senses:** Nasal stuffiness, conjunctival infection.

INTERACTIONS Drug: May antagonize BP raising effects of **epinephrine, ephedrine.**

PHARMACOKINETICS Peak: 2 min IV; 15–20 min IM. **Duration:** 10–15 min IV; 3–4 h IM. **Elimination:** Excreted in urine. **Half-Life:** 19 min.

NURSING IMPLICATIONS

Assessment & Drug Effects

■ Extravasation of alpha-adrenergic drugs results in vasoconstriction of the site. It appears pale and hard necrosis of the area will occur. Giving phentolamine results in vasodilation, and a return to normal skin color should occur if given within 12 h of extravasation. Monitor site closely; repeat doses may be necessary.

■ Test for pheochromocytoma: (1) Withhold medications not deemed absolutely essential for at least 24 h, preferably 48–72 h; antihypertensive agents withheld until BP returns to pretreatment level (rauwolfia drugs withdrawn at least 4 wk prior to testing). (2) Keep patient at rest in supine position throughout test, preferably in quiet darkened room. (3) Take BP q10min for at least 30 min; when BP stabilizes, (4) IV administration: Record BP immediately after injection and at 30-sec intervals for first 3 min; then at 1-min intervals for next 7 min. IM administration: BP determinations at 5-min intervals for 30–45 min.

Patient & Family Education

- Avoid sudden changes in position, particularly from reclining to upright posture. Dangle legs and exercise ankles and toes for a few minutes before standing to walk.
- Lie down or sit down in head-low position immediately if lightheaded or dizzy.

PHENYLEPHRINE HYDROCHLORIDE

(fen-ill-ef'rin)

AK-Dilate Ophthalmic, Alconefrin, Isopto Frin, Mydfrin, Neo-Synephrine, Nostril, Prefrin Liquifilm, Rhinall, Sinarest Nasal, Sinex, Vacon

Classifications: AUTONOMIC NERVOUS SYSTEM AGENT; ALPHA-ADRENERGIC AGONIST; EYE AND NOSE PREPARATION; MYDRIATIC; DECONGESTANT

Prototype: Methoxamine

Pregnancy Category: C

AVAILABILITY 10 mg chewable tablet; 0.125%, 0.16%, 0.5%, 1% nasal solution; 0.12%, 2.5%, 10% ophthalmic solution; 10 mg/mL injection

ACTIONS Potent, synthetic, direct-acting sympathomimetic with strong alpha-adrenergic and weak beta-adrenergic cardiac stimulant actions.

THERAPEUTIC EFFECTS Produces little or no CNS stimulation. Elevates systolic and diastolic pressures through arteriolar constriction; also constricts capacitance vessels and increases venous return to heart. Rise in BP causes reflex bradycardia. Topical applications to eye produce vasoconstriction and prompt mydriasis of short duration, usually without causing cycloplegia. Reduces intraocular pressure by increasing outflow and decreasing rate of aqueous humor secretion. Nasal decongestant action qualitatively similar to that of epinephrine but more potent and has longer duration of action.

USES Parenterally to maintain BP during anesthesia, to treat vascular failure in shock, and to overcome paroxysmal supraventricular tachycardia. Used topically for rhinitis of common cold, allergic rhinitis, and sinusitis; in selected patients with wide-angle glaucoma; as mydriatic for ophthalmoscopic examination or surgery, and for relief of uveitis.

CONTRAINDICATIONS Severe coronary disease, severe hypertension, ventricular tachycardia; acute pancreatitis, hepatitis, narrow-angle glaucoma (ophthalmic preparations); pregnancy (category C), lactation.

CAUTIOUS USE Hyperthyroidism; diabetes mellitus; myocardial disease, cerebral arteriosclerosis, bradycardia; 21 days before or following termination of MAO inhibitor therapy. **Ophthalmic solution (10%):** Cardio-vascular disease; diabetes mellitus; hypertension; aneurysms; infants.

ROUTE & DOSAGE

Hypotension

Child: **IM/SC** 0.1 mg/kg/dose q1–2h as needed (max dose 5 mg)
IV 0.1–0.5 mcg/kg/min, titrate to effect
Adult: **IM/SC** 2–5 mg/dose q1–2h as needed (dose not to exceed 5 mg) **IV** 0.1–0.18 mg/min until BP stabilizes; then 0.04–0.06 mg/min for maintenance

Vasoconstrictor

Child/Adult: **Ophthalmic** Instill 1 drop of a 2.5% solution into each eye 15 min prior to eye exam
Child: **Intranasal (for 3 days)** *>6 mo–1 y,* 1–2 drops of 0.16% solution q3h as necessary; *1–6 y,* 2–3 drops or sprays of 0.125% solution q3–4h as necessary; *6–12 y,* 2–3 drops or sprays of 0.25% solution q3–4h as necessary
Adult: **Intranasal** Small amount of nasal jelly placed into each nostril q3–4h as necessary or 2–3 drops or sprays of 0.25–0.5% solution q3–4h as necessary

STORAGE

Store at 15°–25° C (59°–77° F). Protect from exposure to air, light, or heat, any of which can cause solutions to change color to brown, form a precipitate, and lose potency.

ADMINISTRATION

Instillation

- Nasal preparations: Instruct patient to blow nose gently (with both nostrils open) to clear nasal passages before administration of medication. To clear infant and small child nares, see Techniques of Administration section in Part I.
- **Instillation: Drops:** Tilt head back while sitting or standing up, or lie on bed and hang head over side. Stay in position a few minutes to permit medication to spread through nose. **Spray:** With head upright, squeeze bottle quickly and firmly to produce 1 or 2 sprays into each nostril; wait 3–5 min, blow nose, and repeat dose. **Jelly:** Place in each nostril and sniff it well back into nose.
- Clean tips and droppers of nasal solution dispensers with hot water after use to prevent contamination of solution. Droppers of ophthalmic solution bottles should not touch any surface including the eye.
- Ophthalmic preparations: To avoid excessive systemic absorption, apply pressure to lacrimal sac during and for 1–2 min after instillation of drops.

Subcutaneous/Intramuscular

- Give undiluted.

Intravenous

PREPARE Direct: Dilute each 1 mg in 9 mL of sterile water. **IV Infusion:** Further dilute each 10 mg in 500 mL D5W or NS (concentration: 0.02 mg/mL).

P

ADMINISTER **Direct:** Give a single dose over 60 sec. **IV Infusion:** Titrate to maintain BP.

INCOMPATIBILITIES **Y-Site: Thiopental.**

ADVERSE EFFECTS **Special Senses:** *Transient stinging,* lacrimation, brow ache, headache, blurred vision, allergy (pigmentary deposits on lids, conjunctiva, and cornea with prolonged use), increased sensitivity to light. *Rebound nasal congestion* (hyperemia and edema of mucosa), *nasal burning,* stinging, dryness, *sneezing.* **CV:** Palpitation, tachycardia, bradycardia (over dosage), extrasystoles, hypertension. **Body as a Whole:** Trembling, sweating, pallor, sense of fullness in head, tingling of extremities, sleeplessness, dizziness, light-headedness, weakness, restlessness, anxiety, precordial pain, *tremor,* <u>severe visceral or peripheral vasoconstriction,</u> necrosis if IV infiltrates.

INTERACTIONS **Drug:** ERGOT ALKALOIDS, **guanethidine, reserpine,** TRICYCLIC ANTIDEPRESSANTS increase pressor effects of phenylephrine; **halothane, digoxin** increase risk of arrhythmias; MAO INHIBITORS cause hypertensive crisis; **oxytocin** causes persistent hypertension; ALPHA-BLOCKERS, BETA-BLOCKERS antagonize effects of phenylephrine.

PHARMACOKINETICS **Onset:** Immediate IV; 10–15 min IM/SC. **Duration:** 15–20 min IV; 30–120 min IM/SC; 3–6 h topical. **Metabolism:** Metabolized in liver and tissues by monoamine oxidase.

NURSING IMPLICATIONS

Assessment & Drug Effects

- Monitor pulse, BP, and central venous pressure (q2–5min) during IV administration.
- Control flow rate and dosage to prevent excessive dosage. IV overdoses can induce ventricular dysrhythmias.
- Observe for congestion or rebound miosis after topical administration to eye.

Patient & Family Education

- Be aware that instillation of 2.5–10% strength ophthalmic solution can cause burning and stinging.
- Do not exceed recommended dosage regardless of formulation.
- Inform the physician if no relief is experienced from preparation in 3–5 days.
- Be aware that systemic absorption from nasal and conjunctival membranes can occur, though infrequently (see ADVERSE EFFECTS). Discontinue drug and report to the physician if adverse effects occur.
- Wear sunglasses in bright light because after instillation of ophthalmic drops, pupils will be large and eyes may be more sensitive to light than usual. Stop medication and notify physician if sensitivity persists beyond 12 h after drug has been discontinued.
- Be aware that some ophthalmic solutions may stain contact lenses.
- Do not take any OTC preparations containing phenylephrine found in many cold and cough preparations while on this drug.
- Do not breast feed while taking this drug.
- Store this medication out of reach of children.

PHENYTOIN ⚠

(fen′i-toy-in)

Dilantin-125, Dilantin-30 Pediatric, Dilantin Infatab

PHENYTOIN SODIUM EXTENDED

Dilantin Kapseals

PHENYTOIN SODIUM PROMPT

Dilantin

Classifications: CENTRAL NERVOUS SYSTEM AGENT; ANTICONVULSANT; HYDANTOIN
Pregnancy Category: D

AVAILABILITY 100 mg prompt-release capsule; 30 mg, 100 mg sustained-release capsule; 50 mg chewable tablet; 125 mg/5 mL suspension (contains ≤0.6% alcohol); 50 mg/mL injection (contains 10% alcohol)

ACTIONS Hydantoin derivative chemically related to phenobarbital. Precise mechanism of anticonvulsant action is not known, but drug use is accompanied by reduced voltage, frequency, and spread of electrical discharges within the motor cortex. Class IB antiarrhythmic properties similar to those of lidocaine and tocainide (also class IB agents). Has class IB antiarrhythmic properties.

THERAPEUTIC EFFECTS Inhibits seizure activity. In abnormal tissue causes slight increase in AV conduction velocity depressed by digitalis glycoside; prolongs effective refractory period, suppresses ventricular pacemaker automaticity, and may slow conduction or cause complete block in abnormal ventricular fibers.

USES To control tonic-clonic (grand mal) seizures, psychomotor and nonepileptic seizures (e.g., Reye syndrome, after head trauma). Also used to prevent or treat seizures occurring during or after neurosurgery. Is not effective for absence seizures.

UNLABELED USES Antiarrhythmic agent (phenytoin IV) especially in treatment of digitalis-induced arrhythmias; treatment of trigeminal neuralgia (tic douloureux). Prophylaxis for seizures when high-dose busulfan is used in conditioning regimens for bone marrow transplant.

CONTRAINDICATIONS Hypersensitivity to hydantoin products; rash; seizures due to hypoglycemia; sinus bradycardia, complete or incomplete heart block; Adams-Stokes syndrome; pregnancy (category D), lactation.

CAUTIOUS USE Impaired liver or kidney function; alcoholism; blood dyscrasias; hypotension, heart block, bradycardia, severe myocardial insufficiency, impending or frank heart failure; debilitated, gravely ill patients; pancreatic adenoma; diabetes mellitus, hyperglycemia; respiratory depression; acute intermittent porphyria.

ROUTE & DOSAGE

Anticonvulsant
Loading
Neonate: **PO/IV** 15–20 mg/kg/day loading dose, then 12 h later

---

start 5 mg/kg/day in 2–3 equally divided doses (usual range is
5–8 mg/kg/day)
Infant/Child: **PO/IV** 15–20 mg/kg/day loading dose, then 12 h later
5 mg/kg/day in 2–3 divided doses

Maintenance

6 mo–3 y, 8–10 mg/kg/day b.i.d.–t.i.d.; *4–6 y,* 7.5–9 mg/kg/day
b.i.d.–t.i.d.; *7–9 y,* 7–8 mg/kg/day b.i.d.–t.i.d.; *10–16 y,* 6–7
mg/kg/day b.i.d.–t.i.d.
Adult: **PO** 15–18 mg/kg/day or 1 g loading dose, then 300 mg/day in
1–3 divided doses, may be gradually increased by 100 mg/wk until
seizures are controlled **IV** 15–18 mg/kg loading dose, then 100 mg t.i.d.

STORAGE

Store at 15°–25° C (59°–77° F) in tightly closed, light-resistant containers.
Protect oral suspension from light and freezing. Protect injectable form
from freezing.

ADMINISTRATION

Oral

- Ensure that sustained-release form is not chewed or crushed. Must be
  swallowed whole.
- Do not give within 2–3 h of antacid ingestion.
- Shake suspension vigorously before pouring to ensure uniform distribution of drug. Vanilla-orange flavored.
- Note: Prompt-release capsules and chewable tablets are not intended
  for once-a-day dosage because drug is too quickly bioavailable and can
  therefore lead to toxic serum levels.
- Use sustained-release capsules ONLY for once-a-day dosage regimens.

Intravenous

Note: Verify correct rate of IV injection for administration to infants or
children with physician.
- Inspect solution prior to use. May use a slightly yellowed injectable
  solution safely. Precipitation may be caused by refrigeration, but
  slow warming to room temperature restores clarity.

PREPARE **Direct:** Give undiluted. Use only when clear without precipitate.

ADMINISTER **Direct:** Give 50 mg or fraction thereof over 1 min (do not
exceed 0.5 mg/kg/min in neonates; infants, and children 1–3
mg/kg/min or 25 mg/min when used as antiarrhythmic). Follow with
an injection of sterile saline through the same in-place catheter or needle to decrease vein irritation. Do not use with solutions containing
dextrose.

INCOMPATIBILITIES **Solution/Additive: 5% dextrose, amikacin,
aminophylline, bretylium, cephapirin, codeine phosphate,
dobutamine, hydromorphone, insulin, levorphanol, lidocaine,
lincomycin, meperidine, metaraminol, methadone, morphine, nitroglycerin, norepinephrine, pentobarbital, procaine,
secobarbital, streptomycin, sufentanil. Y-Site: Amikacin, amphotericin B cholesteryl complex, bretylium, ciprofloxacin,
clindamycin, diltiazem, dobutamine, enalaprilat, lidocaine,**

P

heparin, hydromorphone, potassium chloride, propofol, sufentanil, theophylline, TPN, vitamin B complex with C.

- Observe injection site frequently during administration to prevent infiltration. Local soft tissue irritation may be serious, leading to erosion of tissues.

ADVERSE EFFECTS CNS: Usually dose related: Nystagmus, *drowsiness,* ataxia, dizziness, mental confusion, tremors, insomnia, headache, seizures. **CV:** Bradycardia, hypotension, <u>cardiovascular collapse</u>, ventricular fibrillation, phlebitis. **Special Senses:** Photophobia, conjunctivitis, diplopia, blurred vision. **GI:** *Gingival hyperplasia,* nausea, vomiting, constipation, epigastric pain, dysphagia, loss of taste, weight loss, hepatitis, liver necrosis. **Hematologic:** <u>Thrombocytopenia,</u> leukopenia, leukocytosis, agranulocytosis, pancytopenia, eosinophilia; megaloblastic, hemolytic, or <u>aplastic anemias</u>. **Metabolic:** Fever, hyperglycemia, glycosuria, weight gain, edema, transient increase in serum thyrotropic (TSH) level, osteomalacia or rickets associated with hypocalcemia and elevated alkaline phosphatase activity. **Skin:** Alopecia, hirsutism (especially in young female); rash: Scarlatiniform, maculopapular, urticaria, morbilliform; <u>bullous, exfoliative, or purpuric dermatitis; Stevens-Johnson syndrome, toxic epidermal necrolysis,</u> keratosis, <u>neonatal hemorrhage</u>. **Urogenital:** Acute renal failure, Peyronie's disease. **Respiratory:** Acute pneumonitis, pulmonary fibrosis. **Body as a Whole:** Periarteritis nodosum, acute systemic lupus erythematosus, craniofacial abnormalities (with enlargement of lips); lymphadenopathy.

DIAGNOSTIC TEST INTERFERENCE Phenytoin (HYDANTOINS) may produce lower than normal values for *dexamethasone* or *metyrapone* tests; may increase serum levels of *glucose, BSP,* and *alkaline phosphatase* and may decrease *PBI* and *urinary steroid* levels.

INTERACTIONS Drug: Alcohol decreases phenytoin effects; OTHER ANTICONVULSANTS may increase or decrease phenytoin levels; phenytoin may decrease absorption and increase metabolism of ORAL ANTICOAGULANTS; phenytoin increases metabolism of CORTICOSTEROIDS, ORAL CONTRACEPTIVES, and **nisoldipine,** thus decreasing their effectiveness; **amiodarone, chloramphenicol, sufonamides, omeprazole,** and **ticlopidine** increase phenytoin levels; ANTITUBERCULOSIS AGENTS decrease phenytoin levels. Antacids given concurrently will decrease phenytoin levels. **Food: Folic acid, calcium,** and **vitamin D** absorption may be decreased by phenytoin; phenytoin absorption may be decreased by enteral nutrition supplements. **Herb: Ginkgo** may decrease anticonvulsant effectiveness.

PHARMACOKINETICS Absorption: Completely absorbed from GI tract. **Peak:** 1.5–3 h prompt release; 4–12 h sustained release. **Distribution:** 95% protein bound; crosses placenta; small amount in breast milk. **Metabolism:** Oxidized in liver to inactive metabolites. **Elimination:** Metabolites excreted by kidneys. **Half-Life:** 22 h. *Therapeutic serum levels: 10–20 mcg/mL.*

NURSING IMPLICATIONS

Assessment & Drug Effects

- Continuously monitor vital signs and symptoms during IV infusion and for an hour afterward. Watch for respiratory depression. Constant observation and a cardiac monitor are necessary with older adults or patients with cardiac disease. Margin between toxic and therapeutic IV doses is relatively small.
- Monitor therapeutic serum concentration regularly: *10–20 mcg/mL; toxic level: 30–50 mcg/mL; lethal level: 100 mcg/mL.* Steady-state therapeutic levels are not achieved for at least 7–10 days. Serum levels may be artificially low in hypoalbuminemic states.
- Lab tests: Periodic serum phenytoin concentration; CBC with differential, platelet count, and Hct and Hgb; serum glucose, serum calcium, and serum magnesium; and liver function tests.
- Observe patient closely for neurologic adverse effects following IV administration. Have on hand oxygen, atropine, vasopressor, assisted ventilation, seizure precaution equipment (mouth gag, nonmetal airway, suction apparatus).
- Be aware that gingival hyperplasia appears most commonly in children and adolescents and never occurs in patients without teeth.
- Make sure patients on prolonged therapy have adequate intake of vitamin D-containing foods and sufficient exposure to sunlight.
- Monitor diabetics for loss of glycemic control.
- Check periodically for decrease in serum calcium levels. Particularly susceptible are patients receiving other anticonvulsants concurrently, as well as those who are inactive, have limited exposure to sun, or whose dietary intake is inadequate.
- Observe for symptoms of folic acid deficiency: Neuropathy, mental dysfunction.
- Be alert to symptoms of hypomagnesemia (see Appendix D-1); neuromuscular symptoms: Tetany, positive Chvostek's and Trousseau's signs, seizures, tremors, ataxia, vertigo, nystagmus, muscular fasciculations.

Patient & Family Education

- Be aware that drug may make urine pink or red to red-brown.
- Report symptoms of fatigue, dry skin, deepening voice when receiving long-term therapy because phenytoin can unmask a low thyroid reserve.
- Do not alter prescribed drug regimen. Stopping drug abruptly may precipitate seizures and status epilepticus.
- Gingival hyperplasia in children: Use good daily dental care (brushing, flossing, and gum massage). Infants on this drug need good dental care as soon as teeth erupt. Frequent dental checkups and surgery may be required to remove hyperplasia.
- Do not request/accept change in drug brand when refilling prescription without consulting physician. (Different brands may deliver differing blood levels.)
- Understand the effects of alcohol: Alcohol intake may increase phenytoin serum levels, leading to phenytoin toxicity.
- Do not take OTC medications while on this drug without consulting physician.
- Discontinue drug immediately if a measles-like skin rash or jaundice appears and notify physician.

P

Common adverse effects in *italic*; life-threatening effects <u>underlined</u>; generic names in **bold**; drug classifications in SMALL CAPS; ♣ Canadian drug name; ❂ Prototype drug.

- Do not breast feed while taking this drug.
- Store this medication out of reach of children.

PHYSOSTIGMINE SALICYLATE
(fi-zoe-stig'meen)
Antilirium
Classifications: AUTONOMIC NERVOUS SYSTEM AGENT; CHOLINERGIC (PARASYMPATHOMIMETIC); CHOLINESTERASE INHIBITOR
Prototype: Neostigmine
Pregnancy Category: C

AVAILABILITY 1 mg/mL injection (contains 2% benzyl alcohol)

ACTIONS Reversible anticholinesterase and tertiary amine. Chief effect is increasing concentration of acetylcholine at cholinergic transmission sites, which prolongs and exaggerates its action.
THERAPEUTIC EFFECTS Similar to neostigmine in actions and adverse effects, but produces greater secretion of glands, constriction of pupils, and effect on BP and less action on skeletal muscle. Also has direct blocking action on autonomic ganglia. Parenteral physostigmine can produce transient decrease in manic symptoms as well as precipitate mental depression.

USES To reverse CNS and cardiac effects of tricyclic antidepressant overdose, to reverse CNS toxic effects of atropine, scopolamine, and similar anticholinergic drugs, and to antagonize CNS depressant effects of diazepam. **Orphan Drug:** For hereditary ataxias.

CONTRAINDICATIONS Asthma; diabetes mellitus; gangrene, cardiovascular disease; mechanical obstruction of intestinal or urogenital tract; any vagotonic state; secondary glaucoma; inflammatory disease of iris or ciliary body; concomitant use with choline esters (e.g., methacholine, bethanechol) or depolarizing neuromuscular blocking agents (e.g., decamethonium, succinylcholine). Safety during pregnancy (category C) or lactation is not established.
CAUTIOUS USE Epilepsy; parkinsonism; bradycardia; hyperthyroidism; narrow-angle glaucoma, peptic ulcer; hypotension.

ROUTE & DOSAGE

Reversal of Anticholinergic Effects
Child: IV 0.01–0.03 mg/kg/dose, may repeat q15–20min (max total dose of 2 mg)
Adult: **IM/IV** 0.5–3 mg (IV not faster than 1 mg/min), repeat as needed

STORAGE
Store at 15°–25° C (59°–77° F) in tightly closed, light-resistant container.

ADMINISTRATION
Intramuscular/Intravenous
- Give undiluted.

Common adverse effects in *italic;* life-threatening effects underlined; generic names in **bold;** drug classifications in SMALL CAPS; ◆ Canadian drug name; ❷ Prototype drug.

983

- Use only clear, colorless solutions. Red-tinted solution indicates oxidation, and such solutions should be discarded.

Intravenous

Note: Verify correct rate of IV injection for infants or children with physician. Used only in children for life-threating event.
PREPARE Direct: Give undiluted.
ADMINISTER Direct: Give at a slow rate, no more than maximum rate of 0.5 mg/min in children and 1 mg/min in adults. Rapid administration and overdosage can cause a cholinergic crisis.

ADVERSE EFFECTS Body as a Whole: *Sweating,* cholinergic crisis (acute toxicity), hyperactivity, respiratory distress, convulsions. **CNS:** Restlessness, hallucinations, twitching, tremors, *sweating,* weakness, ataxia, convulsions, collapse. **GI:** *Nausea, vomiting, epigastric pain, diarrhea, salivation.* **Urogenital:** Involuntary urination or defecation. **Special Senses:** Miosis, *lacrimation,* rhinorrhea. **Respiratory:** Dyspnea, bronchospasm, respiratory paralysis, pulmonary edema. **Cardiovascular:** Irregular pulse, palpitation, bradycardia, rise in BP.

INTERACTIONS Drug: Antagonizes effects of **echothiophate, isoflurophate.**

PHARMACOKINETICS Absorption: Readily absorbed from mucous membranes, muscle, subcutaneous tissue; 10–12% absorbed from GI tract. **Onset:** 3–8 min IM/IV. **Duration:** 0.5–5 h IM/IV. **Distribution:** Crosses blood–brain barrier. **Metabolism:** Metabolized in plasma by cholinesterase. **Elimination:** Excretion not fully understood; small amounts excreted in urine. **Half-Life:** 15–40 min.

P

NURSING IMPLICATIONS

Assessment & Drug Effects

- Monitor vital signs and state of consciousness closely in patients receiving drug for atropine poisoning. Because physostigmine is usually rapidly eliminated, patient can lapse into delirium and coma within 1–2 h; repeat doses may be required.
- Monitor closely for adverse effects related to CNS and for signs of sensitivity to physostigmine. Have atropine sulfate readily available for clinical emergency.
- Discontinue parenteral or oral drug if following symptoms arise: Excessive salivation, emesis, frequent urination, or diarrhea.
- Eliminate excessive sweating or nausea with dose reduction.

PHYTONADIONE (VITAMIN K₁)

(fye-toe-na-dye′one)
AquaMEPHYTON, Konakion, Mephyton, Phylloquinone
Classifications: HORMONES AND SYNTHETIC SUBSTITUTES; VITAMIN; ANTIDOTE
Pregnancy Category: C

AVAILABILITY 5 mg tablets; 2 mg/mL, 10 mg/mL injection

ACTIONS Fat-soluble naphthoquinone derivative chemically identical to and with similar activity as naturally occurring vitamin K. Vitamin K is essential for hepatic biosynthesis of blood clotting Factors II, VII, IX, and X. **THERAPEUTIC EFFECTS** Promotes liver synthesis of clotting factors by unknown mechanism. Does not reverse anticoagulant action of heparin. Reportedly demonstrates wide margin of safety when used in newborns.

USES Drug of choice as antidote for overdosage of coumarin and indandione oral anticoagulants. Also reverses hypoprothrombinemia secondary to administration of oral antibiotics, quinidine, quinine, salicylates, sulfonamides, excessive vitamin A, and secondary to inadequate absorption and synthesis of vitamin K (as in obstructive jaundice, biliary fistula, ulcerative colitis, intestinal resection, prolonged hyperalimentation). Also prophylaxis of and therapy for neonatal hemorrhagic disease.

CONTRAINDICATIONS Hypersensitivity to AquaMEPHYTON; severe liver disease.
CAUTIOUS USE Injectable form contains benzyl alcohol, avoid use of large amounts in neonates because it can cause "gasping syndrome." Pregnancy (category C); lactation. Effect on fertility and teratogenic potential is not known.

ROUTE & DOSAGE

Hemorrhagic Disease of Newborns
Neonate: **IM/SC** 0.5–1 mg immediately after delivery (IM route preferred), may repeat in 6–8 h if necessary; Treatment: **IM/SC/IV** 1–2 mg/day

Anticoagulant Overdose
Infant: **SC/IM/IV** 1–2 mg/dose q4–8h
Child/Adult: **PO/SC/IM/IV** 2.5–10 mg/dose (rarely up to 50 mg/day for adults), may repeat parenteral dose after 6–8 h if needed or PO dose after 12–24 h
Adults: **IV** Emergency only: 10–15 mg at a rate of ≤1 mg/min, may be repeated in 4 h if bleeding continues

Other Prothrombin Deficiencies
Infant/Child: **PO** 2.5–5 mg/day **IM/SC** 1–2 mg/dose given 1 time
Adult: **PO** 2–25 mg/day **IM/SC/IV** 10 mg/dose given 1 time

STORAGE
Store at 25° C (59° F) in tightly closed, light-resistant container. Protect infusion solution from light by wrapping container with aluminum foil or other opaque material. Discard unused solution and contents in open ampule.

ADMINISTRATION
Intramuscular
Note: Konakion, which contains a phenol preservative, is intended ONLY for IM use. AquaMEPHYTON may be given SC, IM, or IV as prescribed.
- Give IM injection in adults and older children in upper outer quadrant of buttocks. For neonates, infants, and young children, anterolateral aspect of thigh or deltoid region is preferred (see Part I).

- Aspirate carefully to avoid intravascular injection.
- Apply gentle pressure to site following injection. Swelling (internal bleeding) and pain sometimes occur with SC or IM administration.

Intravenous

Note: Reserve IV route only for emergencies.

PREPARE **Direct:** Do not give 10 mg/mL concentrate as an IV push. Dilute a single dose in 10 mL D5W, NS, or D5/NS (max concentration 10 mg/mL).

ADMINISTER **Direct:** Give solution immediately after dilution at a rate not to exceed 1 mg/min.

INCOMPATIBILITIES **Solution/Additive: Ranitidine. Y-Site: Dobutamine.**

ADVERSE EFFECTS Body as a Whole: Hypersensitivity or <u>anaphylaxis-like reaction</u>: Facial flushing, cramp-like pains, convulsive movements, chills, fever, diaphoresis, weakness, dizziness, shock, <u>cardiac arrest</u>. **CNS:** Headache (after oral dose), brain damage, <u>death</u>. **GI:** Gastric upset. **Hematologic:** Paradoxic hypoprothrombinemia (patients with severe liver disease), severe hemolytic anemia. **Metabolic:** Hyperbilirubinemia, kernicterus. **Respiratory:** <u>Bronchospasm</u>, dyspnea, sensation of chest constriction, <u>respiratory arrest</u>. **Skin:** Pain at injection site, hematoma, and nodule formation, erythematous skin eruptions (with repeated injections). **Special Senses:** Peculiar taste sensation.

DIAGNOSTIC TEST INTERFERENCE Falsely elevated ***urine steroids*** (by modifications of ***Reddy, Jenkins, Thorn procedure***).

INTERACTIONS Drug: Antagonizes effects of **warfarin; cholestyramine, colestipol, mineral oil** decrease absorption of oral phytonadione.

PHARMACOKINETICS Absorption: Readily absorbed from intestinal lymph only if bile is present. **Onset:** 6–12 h PO; 1–2 h IM/SC; 15 min IV. **Peak:** Hemorrhage usually controlled within 3–8 h; normal prothrombin time may be obtained in 12–14 h after administration. **Distribution:** Concentrates briefly in liver after absorption; crosses placenta; distributed into breast milk. **Metabolism:** Rapidly metabolized in liver. **Elimination:** Excreted in urine and bile.

NURSING IMPLICATIONS

Assessment & Drug Effects

- Monitor patient constantly. Severe reactions, including fatalities, have occurred during and immediately after IV injection (see ADVERSE EFFECTS).
- Lab tests: Baseline and frequent PT/INR.
- Frequency, dose, and therapy duration are guided by PT/INR clinical response.
- Monitor therapeutic effectiveness, which is indicated by shortened PT, INR, bleeding, and clotting times, as well as decreased hemorrhagic tendencies.
- Be aware that patients on large doses may develop temporary resistance to coumarin-type anticoagulants. If oral anticoagulant is reinstituted, larger than former doses may be needed. Some patients may require change to heparin.

Patient & Family Education

- Maintain consistency in diet and avoid significant increases in daily intake of vitamin K-rich foods when drug regimen is stabilized. Know sources rich in vitamin K: Asparagus, broccoli, cabbage, lettuce, turnip greens, pork or beef liver, green tea, spinach, watercress, and tomatoes.
- Store this medication out of reach of children.

PILOCARPINE HYDROCHLORIDE ℗

PILOCARPINE NITRATE

(pye-loe-kar'peen)

Adsorbocarpine, Isopto Carpine, Minims Pilocarpine♣, Miocarpine ♣, Ocusert, Pilo, Pilocar, Salagen

Classifications: EYE PREPARATION; MIOTIC (ANTIGLAUCOMA AGENT); AUTONOMIC NERVOUS SYSTEM AGENT; DIRECT-ACTING CHOLINERGIC (PARASYMPATHOMIMETIC)

Pregnancy Category: C

AVAILABILITY 0.25%, 0.5%, 1%, 2%, 3%, 4%, 5%, 6%, 8%, 10% ophthalmic solution; 4% ophthalmic gel; 20 mcg/h, 40 mcg/h ocular insert; 5 mg tablets

ACTIONS Tertiary amine that acts directly on cholinergic receptor sites, thus mimicking acetylcholine. Induces miosis, spasm of accommodation, and fall in intraocular pressure (IOP) that may be preceded by a transitory rise.

THERAPEUTIC EFFECTS Decrease in IOP results from stimulation of ciliary and papillary sphincter muscles, which pull iris away from filtration angle, thus facilitating outflow of aqueous humor. Also decreases production of aqueous humor.

USES Open-angle and angle-closure glaucomas; to reduce IOP and to protect the lens during surgery and laser iridotomy; to counteract effects of mydriatics and cycloplegics following surgery or ophthalmoscopic examination; to treat xerostomia.

CONTRAINDICATIONS Secondary glaucoma, acute iritis, acute inflammatory disease of anterior segment of eye; pregnancy (category C), lactation. **CAUTIOUS USE** Bronchial asthma; hypertension. **Ocular therapeutic system:** Not used in acute infectious conjunctivitis, keratitis, retinal detachment, or when intense miosis is required.

ROUTE & DOSAGE

Acute Glaucoma

Child/Adult: **Ophthalmic** 1 drop of 1–2% solution in affected eye q5–10min for 3–6 doses, then 1 drop q1–3h until IOP is reduced

Chronic Glaucoma

Child/Adult: **Ophthalmic** 1 drop of 0.5–4% solution in affected eye q4–12h
Adult: 1 ocular system (Ocusert) every 7 days

PILOCARPINE HYDROCHLORIDE

Miotic
Child/Adult: **Ophthalmic** 1 drop of 1% solution in affected eye
Xerostomia
Adult: **PO** 5 mg t.i.d., may increase up to 10 mg t.i.d.

STORAGE
Store at 15°–25° C (59°–77° F).

ADMINISTRATION
Instillation
- Note: During acute phase, physician may prescribe instillation of drug into unaffected eye to prevent bilateral attack of acute glaucoma.
- Apply gentle digital pressure to periphery of nasolacrimal drainage system for 1–2 min immediately after instillation of drops to prevent delivery of drug to nasal mucosa and general circulation.

ADVERSE EFFECTS CNS: Oral (asthenia, headaches, dizziness, chills). **Special Senses:** Ciliary spasm with brow ache, twitching of eyelids, eye pain with change in eye focus, miosis, *diminished vision in poorly illuminated areas,* blurred vision, reduced visual acuity, sensitivity, contact allergy, lacrimation, follicular conjunctivitis, conjunctival irritation, cataract, <u>retinal detachment</u>. **GI:** *Nausea,* vomiting, abdominal cramps, diarrhea, epigastric distress, *salivation.* **Respiratory:** Bronchospasm, rhinitis. **CV:** Tachycardia. **Body as a Whole:** Tremors, *increased sweating,* urinary frequency.

INTERACTIONS Drug: The actions of pilocarpine and **carbachol** are additive when used concomitantly. Oral form may cause conduction disturbances with BETA-BLOCKERS. Antagonizes the effects of concurrent ANTICHOLINERGIC DRUGS (e.g., **atropine, ipratropium**). **Food:** High-fat meal decreases absorption of pilocarpine.

PHARMACOKINETICS Absorption: Topical penetrates cornea rapidly; readily absorbed from GI tract. **Onset:** Miosis 10–30 min; IOP reduction 60 min; salivary stimulation 20 min. **Peak:** Miosis 30 min; IOP reduction 75 min; salivary stimulation 60 min. **Duration:** Miosis 4–8 h; IOP reduction 4–14 h (7 days with Ocusert); salivary stimulation 3–5 h. **Metabolism:** Inactivated at neuronal synapses and in plasma. **Elimination:** Excreted in urine. **Half-Life:** 0.76–1.35 h.

NURSING IMPLICATIONS
Assessment & Drug Effects
- Be aware that hourly tonometric tests may be done during early treatment because drug may cause an initial transitory increase in IOP.
- Monitor changes in visual acuity.
- Monitor for adverse effects. Brow pain and myopia tend to be more prominent in younger patients and generally disappear with continued use of drug.

Patient & Family Education
- Understand that therapy for glaucoma is prolonged and that adherence to established regimen is crucial to prevent blindness.

Common adverse effects in *italic;* life-threatening effects <u>underlined</u>; generic names in **bold;** drug classifications in SMALL CAPS; ♣ Canadian drug name; ⊙ Prototype drug.

- Do not drive or engage in potentially hazardous activities until vision clears. Drug causes blurred vision and difficulty in focusing.
- Discontinue medication if symptoms of irritation or sensitization persist and report to physician.
- Do not breast feed while taking this drug without consulting physician.

Ocular Therapeutic System (Ocusert)

- Review information/directions about inserting the ocular system included in the drug package with health care provider. Demonstrate to establish ability to adjust, insert, and remove the system.
- Unit is placed in the eye cul-de-sac, where it remains for a week. Slow release of drug provides a nonfluctuating concentration of pilocarpine in the ciliary body and iris.
- Induced myopia, miosis, and spasm of accommodation are less than that produced by eye drops. However, because transient blurring and dimness of vision may occur following Ocusert insertion, have patient do so at bedtime; myopia will be at a stable level in the a.m.
- Several hours after Ocusert insertion, induced myopia decreases to a low base level that persists for the life of the therapeutic system.
- Notify physician if following symptoms do not subside: Conjunctival irritation with mild erythema and increase in mucous secretion; generally accompany early use of Ocusert.
- Wash system with cool tap water before replacing it into cul-de-sac if it contacts an unclean surface.
- If retention of the system is a problem, the superior conjunctival cul-de-sac may be a preferred site for insertion. This location is also preferred during sleep.
- To change placement: Ocusert may be transferred from the lower conjunctival sac to the superior sac by closing eyelids, rolling the eye toward the nose and, with gentle digital pressure through the closed eyelid, directly moving the system. Avoid moving it over the colored part of the eye.
- Remove system and replace with a new one if an unexpected increase in drug action occurs (sudden miosis, ciliary spasm, decreased visual acuity).
- Store this medication out of reach of children.

PIPERACILLIN SODIUM

(pi-per'a-sill-in)
Pipracil
Classifications: ANTI-INFECTIVE; BETA-LACTAM ANTIBIOTIC; ANTIPSEUDOMONAL PENICILLIN
Prototype: Mezlocillin
Pregnancy Category: B

AVAILABILITY 2 g, 3 g, 4 g injection

ACTIONS Action is similar to that of other penicillins. Interference with bacterial cell wall synthesis promotes loss of membrane integrity and leads to death of the organism.

THERAPEUTIC EFFECTS Extended-spectrum parenteral penicillin with antibiotic activity against most gram-negative and many gram-positive anaerobic and aerobic organisms including members of *Clostridium, Bacteroides, Klebsiella, Enterobacter, Pseudomonas, Proteus,* and *Serratia* species and the anaerobic and aerobic cocci. Less active than penicillin G against *Pneumococci* and group A *Streptococci* but comparable to ampicillin against *Enterococci.* Penicillinase-producing *Staphylococci* are resistant to piperacillin.

USES Susceptible organisms that cause gynecologic, skin and skin structure, gonococcal, and streptococcal infections; lower respiratory tract, intra-abdominal, and bone and joint infections; septicemia, urinary tract infections. Also prophylactically prior to and during surgery and as empiric anti-infective therapy in granulocytopenic patients.

CONTRAINDICATIONS Hypersensitivity to penicillins, cephalosporins, or other drugs. Safety in children <12 y not established, but it is used in these age groups; pregnancy (category B), lactation.
CAUTIOUS USE Liver and kidney dysfunction; hypersensitivity to cephalosporins.

ROUTE & DOSAGE

Uncomplicated Urinary Tract Infection
Adult: **IV/IM** 8–16 g/day divided q6–8h
Mild to Moderate Infections
Neonate: **IV** ≤7 days, 150 mg/kg/day in equally divided doses q8h; >7 days, 200 mg/kg/day in equally divided doses q6h
Infant/Child: **IM/IV** 200–300 mg/kg/day in equally divided doses q4–6h (max 24 g/day)
Adult: **IM/IV** 2–4 g/dose q4–8h (max 24 g/day)
Cystic Fibrosis
Child: **IM/IV** 350–600 mg/kg/day in equally divided doses q4–6h (max 24 g/day)
Moderate to Severe Infections
Adult: **IM/IV** 4 g q6h (150–200 mg/kg/day)
Life-Threatening Infection, *Pseudomonas* Infections
Adult: **IM/IV** 3 g q4h (max 24 g/day)
Uncomplicated Gonococcal Infections
Adult: **IM** 2 g with 1 g probenecid given 30 min before piperacillin; reduced dosages required with renal impairment

STORAGE
Reconstituted solution stable for 24 h at 15°–25° C (59°–77° F) and 7 days under refrigeration.

ADMINISTRATION
Note: Patients undergoing hemodialysis usually receive a maximum dosage of 2 g piperacillin q8h and an additional 1 g dose after each

Common adverse effects in *italic;* life-threatening effects underlined; generic names in **bold;** drug classifications in SMALL CAPS; ♣ Canadian drug name; ⊘ Prototype drug.

dialysis period. Doses and frequency are usually modified if creatinine clearance is <40 mL/min.

Intramuscular

- Limit IM injections to 2 g/site in adults is red. See in Part I for safe IM site selection and safe amount per site in children. Use deltoid muscle in adults only if well developed.
- Diluents for reconstitution include sterile or bacteriostatic water for injection, bacteriostatic NaCl injection, and sterile lidocaine HCl injection 0.5–1.0% without epinephrine for IM. When reconstituted, solution contains 1 g/2.5 mL.

Intravenous

Note: Verify correct IV concentration and rate of infusion for administration to neonates, infants, or children with physician.

PREPARE **Direct** (Not preferred): Reconstitute by diluting 1 g with 5 mL sterile water or NS for injection. Shake well until dissolved. **Intermittent** (Preferred): Further dilute with 50–100 mL NS or D5W.

ADMINISTER **Direct** (Not preferred): Give over 3–5 min. Avoid rapid injection. **Intermittent** (Preferred): Give over 30 min. In children give over 30–60 min in concentration of ≤20 mg/mL.

INCOMPATIBILITIES **Solution/Additive:** AMINOGLYCOSIDES. **Y-Site:** AMINOGLYCOSIDES, **amphotericin B cholesteryl complex, cisatracurium, filgrastim, fluconazole, gemcitabine, ondansetron, sargramostim, vinorelbine.**

ADVERSE EFFECTS Body as a Whole: Coughing, sneezing, feeling of uneasiness; <u>systemic anaphylaxis</u>, fever, widespread increase in capillary permeability and vasodilation with <u>resulting edema (mouth, tongue, pharynx, larynx), laryngospasm</u>, malaise, serum sickness (fever, malaise, pruritus, urticaria, lymphadenopathy, arthralgia, angioedema of face and extremities, neuritis prostration, eosinophilia), SLE-like syndrome, injection site reactions (pain, inflammation, abscess, phlebitis), superinfections (especially with *Candida* and gram-negative bacteria), neuromuscular irritability (twitching, lethargy, confusion, stupor, hyperreflexia, multifocal myoclonus, localized or generalized seizures, <u>coma</u>). **CV:** Hypotension, <u>circulatory collapse</u>, cardiac arrhythmias, <u>cardiac arrest</u>. **GI:** Vomiting, diarrhea, severe abdominal cramps, nausea, epigastric distress, diarrhea, flatulence, dark discoloration of tongue, sore mouth or tongue. **Urogenital:** Interstitial nephritis, Loeffler's syndrome, vasculitis. **Hematologic:** Hemolytic anemia, thrombocytopenia. **Metabolic:** Hyperkalemia, hypokalemia, alkalosis, hypernatremia, CHF (penicillin G sodium). **Respiratory:** Bronchospasm, asthma. **Skin:** Itchy palms or axilla, pruritus, *urticaria,* flushed skin, *delayed skin rashes* ranging from urticaria to exfoliative dermatitis, <u>Stevens-Johnson syndrome</u>, fixed-drug eruptions, contact dermatitis.

INTERACTIONS Drug: May increase risk of bleeding with ANTICOAGULANTS; **probenecid** decreases elimination of piperacillin. Aminoglycosides increases serum levels of piperacillin.

PHARMACOKINETICS Peak: 45 min IM; 5 min IV. **Distribution:** Widely distributed with highest concentrations in urine and bile; adequate CSF penetration with inflamed meninges; crosses placenta; distributed into breast milk. **Metabolism:** Slightly metabolized in liver. **Elimination:** Primarily excreted in urine, partly in bile. **Half-Life:** 0.5–1.35 h.

NURSING IMPLICATIONS

Assessment & Drug Effects

- Obtain history of hypersensitivity to penicillins, cephalosporins, or other drugs prior to administration.
- Lab tests: C&S prior to first dose of the drug; start drug pending results. Periodic CBC with differential, platelet count, Hgb and Hct, and serum electrolytes.
- Monitor for hypersensitivity response; discontinue drug and notify physician if allergic response noted.
- If giving with an aminoglycoside therapy, give aminoglycoside and piperacillin dosages 30–60 min apart.
- Lab tests: Periodic CBC with differential, platelet count, Hgb and Hct, and serum electrolytes.
- Monitor for hemorrhagic manifestations because high doses may induce coagulation abnormalities.

Patient & Family Education

- Report significant, unexplained diarrhea.
- Withhold drug and report to physician if signs of an allergic reaction develop (e.g., itching, rash, hives).
- Do not breast feed while taking this drug without consulting physician.

PIPERACILLIN/TAZOBACTAM

(pi-per′a-cil-lin/taz-o-bac′tam)
Zosyn
Classifications: ANTI-INFECTIVE; BETA-LACTAM ANTIBIOTIC; ANTIPSEUDOMONAL PENICILLIN
Prototype: Mezlocillin
Pregnancy Category: B

AVAILABILITY 2 g piperacillin and 0.25 g taxobactam, 3 g piperacillin and 0.375 g taxobactam, 4 g piperacillin and 0.5 g taxobactam injection

ACTIONS Antibacterial combination product consisting of the semisynthetic piperacillin and the beta-lactamase inhibitor tazobactam. Tazobactam component does not decrease the activity of the piperacillin component against susceptible organisms.

THERAPEUTIC EFFECTS Tazobactam is an inhibitor of a wide variety of bacterial beta-lactamases. It has little antibacterial activity itself; however, in combination with piperacillin, it extends the spectrum of bacteria that are susceptible to piperacillin. Two-drug combination has antibiotic activity against an extremely broad spectrum of gram-positive, gram-negative and anaerobic bacteria.

USES Treatment of moderate to severe appendicitis, uncomplicated and complicated skin and skin structure infections, endometritis, pelvic inflammatory disease, or nosocomial or community-acquired pneumonia caused by piperacillin-resistant, piperacillin/tazobactam-susceptible, beta-lactamase-producing bacteria.

CONTRAINDICATIONS Hypersensitivity to piperacillin, tazobactam, penicillins, cephalosporins, or beta-lactamase inhibitors such as clavulanic acid and sulbactam.

CAUTIOUS USE Kidney failure; pregnancy (category B), lactation. Safety and efficacy in children <12 y are not established but it is used in these age groups.

ROUTE & DOSAGE

Note: Dosage is based on piperacillin
Infant/Child: **IV** *<6 mo,* 150–300 mg piperacillin/kg/day divided q6–8h; *≥6 mo,* 240 mg piperacillin component/kg/day divided q8h
Adult: **IV** 3.375 g q6h, infused over 30 min, for 7–10 days

Renal Insufficiency

Adult: Cl$_{cr}$ 20–40 mL/min: 2.25 g q6h; <20 mL/min: 2.25 g q8h

STORAGE

Reconstituted solution stable for 24 h at 15°–25° C (59°–77° F) and 2 days under refrigeration.

ADMINISTRATION

Note: Verify correct IV concentration and rate of infusion for administration to infants or children with physician.

Intravenous

- For hemodialysis patients, the maximum dose is 2.25 g q8h; give one extra 0.75-g dose after each dialysis period.

PREPARE Intermittent: Reconstitute powder with 5 mL of diluent (e.g., D5W, NS); shake well until dissolved. Further dilute to at least 50 mL of selected diluent. Use single-dose vials immediately after reconstitution.

ADMINISTER Intermittent: Give over at least 30 min in adults. In children give over 30–60 min in concentration of ≤20 mg/mL.

INCOMPATIBILITIES Solution/Additive: Aminoglycosides. Y-Site: Acyclovir, aminoglycosides, amphotericin B, amphotericin B cholesteryl complex, chlorpromazine, cisplatin, dacarbazine, daunorubicin, doxorubicin, doxycycline, droperidol, famotidine, ganciclovir, gemcitabine, hydroxyzine, idarubicin, minocycline, mitomycin, mitoxantrone, nalbuphine, prochlorperazine, promethazine, vancomycin.

ADVERSE EFFECTS CNS: Headache, insomnia, fever. **GI:** Diarrhea, constipation, nausea, vomiting, dyspepsia, <u>pseudomembranous colitis</u>. **Skin:** Rash, pruritus, hypersensitivity reactions. **Metabolic:** Hypokalemia, hypernatremia.

INTERACTIONS Drug: May increase risk of bleeding with ANTICOAGULANTS; **probenecid** decreases elimination of piperacillin. Aminoglycosides increase serum levels of piperacillin.

PHARMACOKINETICS Distribution: Distributes into many tissues, including lung, blister fluid, and bile; crosses placenta; distributed into breast milk. **Metabolism:** Metabolized in liver. **Elimination:** Piperacillin and tazobactam are excreted in urine. **Half-Life:** 0.7–1.2 h.

NURSING IMPLICATIONS

Assessment & Drug Effects

- Obtain history of hypersensitivity to penicillins, cephalosporins, or other drugs prior to administration.
- Lab tests: C&S prior to first dose of the drug; start drug pending results. Monitor hematologic status with prolonged therapy (Hct and Hgb, CBC with differential and platelet count).
- Monitor patient carefully during the first 30 min after initiation of the infusion for signs of hypersensitivity (see Appendix D-1).
- If giving with an aminoglycoside therapy, give aminoglycoside and piperacillin dosages 30–60 min apart.

Patient & Family Education

- Report rash, itching, or other signs of hypersensitivity immediately.
- Report loose stools or diarrhea as these may indicate pseudomembranous colitis.
- Do not breast feed while taking this drug without consulting physician.

PIPERAZINE CITRATE

(pi′per-a-zeen)
Vermizine, Piperazine Citrate Entacy
Classification: ANTHELMINTIC
Pregnancy Category: B

AVAILABILITY 250 mg tablet

ACTIONS Blocks the effects of acetylcholine in the roundworm musculature at the neuromuscular junction. This results in paralysis of the worm.
THERAPEUTIC EFFECTS Mechanism unknown; believed to paralyze the musculature of parasites, resulting in removal of the organism by intestinal peristalsis of the host.

USES Most effective against roundworm *Ascaris lumbricoides* and pinworm *Enterobius vermicularis*.

CONTRAINDICATIONS Hypersensitivity to drug or its salts, in seizure disorders, and with impaired renal or hepatic function.
CAUTIOUS USE In anemia, severe malnutrition. Avoid prolonged use in children.

ROUTE & DOSAGE

Pinworms

Child/Adult: **PO** 65 mg/kg/day once per day for 7 days; may repeat in 1 wk (max dose of 2.5 mg/day)

Common adverse effects in *italic;* life-threatening effects underlined; generic names in **bold**; drug classifications in SMALL CAPS; ♣ Canadian drug name; ⊙ Prototype drug.

Roundworms
Child: **PO** 75 mg/kg/day for 2 days (max dose 3.5 g/day), may repeat dose in 1 wk for severe infestations
Adult: **PO** 3.5 g/day for 2 days (max dose 3.5 g/day), may repeat dose in 1 wk for severe infestations

STORAGE
Store at 15°–30° C (59°–86° F) in tightly closed container.

ADMINISTRATION

Oral
- Tablet can be crushed and mixed with a small amount of food to administer. Can be given with food to reduce GI upset, but best to take on an empty stomach.
- If severe worm load (which can lead to partial or complete intestinal obstruction), give drug through NG tube.

ADVERSE EFFECTS Body as a Whole: Headache, dizziness, ataxia, tremors, choreiform movements, muscular weakness, hyporeflexia, paresthesia, nystagmus, sense of detachment, memory defect, convulsions, EEG changes, blurred vision, paralytic strabismus, cataracts. **GI:** *Nausea, vomiting, diarrhea, abdominal pain.* **Hemotologic:** Hemolytic anemia, **Hypersensitivity:** Urticaria, erythema multiform purpura, fever, productive cough, arthralgia, lacrimation, bronchospasm.

INTERACTIONS Drug: Use of **chlorpromazine** and this drug may cause seizures. **Pyrantel pamoate** and this drug can be pharmacologically antagonistic. May cause increase in serum uric acid.

PHARMACOKINETICS Absorption: Well absorbed from the GI track. **Metabolism:** About 25% metabolized. **Elimination:** Excreted in urine unchanged.

NURSING IMPLICATIONS

Assessment & Drug Effects
- Obtain pinworm test during night or when child is sleeping, when worms migrate to perianal area to deposit their eggs. Commercial test kit available or can use cellophane tape with sticky side to outside of tongue blade. Obtain test by carefully exposing buttocks and pressing tape into anal area. Wear gloves and wash hands well after test. Roundworm diagnosed through stool samples; follow your agency procedure for collection.

Patient & Family Education
- Pinworms: Highly contagious; a female can deposit 17,000 eggs a night; ova mature within 3–8 h. Ova also spread by hand-to-mouth contact and through inhalation.
- All members of the family should be treated. All bed linen, towels, undergarments, and personal clothes should be washed. Carpets should be vacuumed, floors damp mopped, toilets disinfected daily.
- Infected child should sleep alone with tight-fitting underwear or diapers. Cut nails and keep clean. Change linens, bedclothes, and underwear daily.

Common adverse effects in *italic;* life-threatening effects <u>underlined</u>; generic names in **bold;** drug classifications in SMALL CAPS; ♣ Canadian drug name; ⊕ Prototype drug.

995

- This disease does not indicate family has unclean home. However, good hand washing is important to prevent spread of the disease.
- Roundworm: Common where human wastes are used as fertilizer.
- Occasionally worm may migrate to mouth, nose, or rectum.
- Good hand washing and washing of raw vegetables and fruits important.
- If CNS, GI, side effects or hypersensitivity occurs, withhold drug and notify physician.
- Caution parents not to give more frequently that prescribed or to younger children because of neurotoxicity. With all infections teach parent how to obtain stool culture.
- Store this medication out of reach of children.

PIRBUTEROL ACETATE

(pir-bu′ter-ol)
Maxair
Classifications: AUTONOMIC NERVOUS SYSTEM AGENT; BETA-ADRENERGIC AGONIST (SYMPATHOMIMETIC); BRONCHODILATOR
Prototype: Albuterol
Pregnancy Category: C

AVAILABILITY 0.2 mg/inhalation aerosol

ACTIONS Exhibits preferential effect on beta$_2$-adrenergic receptors compared with isoproterenol and, consequently, a lengthened duration of action. Stimulation of beta$_2$-adrenoreceptors relaxes bronchospasm and increases ciliary motion. Activates adenyl cyclase, the enzyme that catalyzes the conversion of ATP to cyclic adenosine monophosphate (cAMP).

THERAPEUTIC EFFECTS Increased cAMP is associated with relaxation of bronchial smooth muscle and inhibition of the release of histamine and other mediators of hypersensitivity from mast cells.

USES Prevention and reversal of bronchospasm associated with asthma.

CONTRAINDICATIONS Hypersensitivity to pirbuterol or any other adrenergic agent such as epinephrine, albuterol, or isoproterenol. Pregnancy (category C), lactation.

CAUTIOUS USE Heart disease, irregular heartbeat; high blood pressure, history of stroke or seizures; diabetes; thyroid disease; glaucoma. Safety and effectiveness in children <12 y not established.

ROUTE & DOSAGE

Asthma

Child >12 y/Adult: **Inhaled** 1–2 inhalations (0.4 mg) q6h (max 12 inhalations/day)

STORAGE
Store at 15°–25° C (59°–77° F).

ADMINISTRATION

Inhalation

- Shake inhaler canister well immediately before using.
- Direct patient to exhale deeply, loosely close lips around mouthpiece, then inhale slowly and deeply through mouthpiece while pressing top of canister. Spacers may be used for those having difficulty with inhaler usage.

ADVERSE EFFECTS CNS: Nervousness, headache, dizziness, tremor. **Metabolic:** Hypokalemia. **CV:** Palpitations, tachycardia. **GI:** Dry mouth, nausea, glossitis, abdominal pain, cramps, anorexia, diarrhea, stomatitis. **Other:** Cough, tolerance.

INTERACTIONS Drug: Epinephrine and other SYMPATHOMIMETIC BRON-CHODILATORS may have additive effects. BETA-BLOCKERS may antagonize the effects.

PHARMACOKINETICS Onset: 5 min. **Peak:** 30 min. **Duration:** 3–4 h. **Metabolism:** Metabolized in liver. **Elimination:** Eliminated by kidneys. **Half-Life:** 2–3 h.

NURSING IMPLICATIONS

Assessment & Drug Effects

- Monitor arterial blood gases and pulmonary functions periodically.
- Monitor vital signs. Report tachycardia, palpitations, and hypertension or hypotension.

Patient & Family Education

- Learn proper technique for using the inhaler.
- A "rescue" inhaler should be used first in the event of an asthma attack.
- Report palpitations, chest pain, nervousness, tremors, or other bothersome adverse effects promptly to physician.
- Contact prescriber immediately if symptoms of asthma worsen or you do not respond to the usual dose.
- Adhere rigidly to dosing directions and contact prescriber if breathing difficulty persists.
- Do not breast feed while taking this drug.
- Work with school personnel to plan for child's access to drug during school hours.
- Store this medication out of reach of children.

PLASMA PROTEIN FRACTION

(plas´ma)

Plasmanate, Plasma-Plex; Plasmatein, PPF, Protenate

Classifications: BLOOD FORMERS, COAGULATORS, AND ANTICOAGULANTS; PLASMA VOLUME EXPANDER

Prototype: Normal serum albumin, human

Pregnancy Category: C

AVAILABILITY 5% injection

ACTIONS Oncotic action approximately equivalent to that of human plasma; does not provide coagulation factors or gamma globulins.

THERAPEUTIC EFFECTS Heat-treated to minimize hazard of transmitting serum hepatitis; risk of sensitization is reduced because it lacks cellular elements. Does not require cross-matching.

USES Emergency treatment of hypovolemic shock due to burns, trauma, surgery, infections; temporary measure in treatment of blood loss when whole blood is not available; to replenish plasma protein in patients with hypoproteinemia (if sodium restriction is not a problem).

CONTRAINDICATIONS Severe anemia; cardiac failure; patients undergoing cardiopulmonary bypass surgery; pregnancy (category C).
CAUTIOUS USE Patients with low cardiac reserve; absence of albumin deficiency; liver or kidney failure.

ROUTE & DOSAGE

Plasma Volume Expansion
Child: **IV** 6.6–33 mL/kg at a rate of 5–10 mL/min
Adult: **IV** 250–500 mL at a maximum rate of 10 mL/min

Hypoproteinemia
Adult: **IV** 1–1.5 L/day infused at a rate not to exceed 5–8 mL/min

STORAGE
Store at 15°–25° C (59°–77° F). Do not exceed 30° C. Discard if solution becomes turbid. Discard opened unused portion after 4 h.

ADMINISTRATION

Intravenous

- Do not use solutions that show a sediment or appear turbid.
- Do not use solutions that have been frozen.

PREPARE **IV Infusion:** Give undiluted. Once container is opened, solution should be used within 4 h because it contains no preservatives. Discard unused portions.

ADMINISTER **IV Infusion:** Rate of infusion and volume of total dose will depend on patient's age, diagnosis, degree of venous and pulmonary congestion, Hct, and Hgb determinations. As with any oncotically active solution, infusion rate should be relatively slow. Range may vary from 1–10 mL/min.

ADVERSE EFFECTS GI: Nausea, vomiting, hypersalivation, headache. **Body as a Whole:** Tingling, chills, fever, cyanosis, chest tightness, backache, urticaria, erythema, <u>shock (systemic anaphylaxis)</u>, circulatory overload, pulmonary edema.

INTERACTIONS Drug: No clinically significant interactions established.

PHARMACOKINETICS Not studied.

NURSING IMPLICATIONS

Assessment & Drug Effects
- Monitor vital signs (BP and pulse). Frequency depends on patient's condition. Flow rate adjustments are made according to clinical

response and BP. Slow or stop infusion if patient suddenly becomes hypotensive.
- Report a widening pulse pressure (difference between systolic and diastolic); it correlates with increase in cardiac output.
- Report changes in I&O ratio and pattern.
- Observe patient closely during and after infusion for signs of hypervolemia or circulatory overload (see Appendix D-1). Report these symptoms immediately to physician.
- Make careful observations of patient who has had either injury or surgery in order to detect bleeding points that failed to bleed at lower BP.

PNEUMOCOCCAL VACCINE

(noo'mo'kok'el)
Prevnar (7-Valent Vaccine)
Classifications: ANTI-INFECTIVE, VACCINE
Pregnancy Category: Not recommended

AVAILABILITY Single-dose vial

ACTIONS Stimulates body production of antibodies against *Streptococcus pneumoniae* serotypes 4m 6B, 9V, 14m 18C, 19F, 23F; these serotypes cause about 80% of pneumococcal disease.

THERAPEUTIC EFFECTS The recommended three-dose regimen provides protection against the specified serotypes of pneumococcal infection.

USES Used to provide active immunity in infants from 2–23 mo and in older children from 24–59 mo at high risk of the disease; protects against acute otitis media and invasive pneumococcal disease; recommended to prevent infections in 24–59 mo children with cochlear implants, sickle cell and other blood diseases, pulmonary disease, diabetes mellitus, CSF leaks, congenital immune diseases, malignancy, renal failure, nephritic syndrome, organ transplantation, immunosuppressive medication.

CONTRAINDICATIONS Anaphylaxis to previous doses of the vaccine or to any of its components such as diphtheria toxoid (a carrier for the vaccine but does not provide immunity to diphtheria); thrombocytopenia; serious acute illness; immunosuppression.

ROUTE & DOSAGE

Infant: **IM** 0.5 mL at 2, 4, and 6 mo
Prevention against *Streptococcus pneumonia*

STORAGE
Keep refrigerated at 2°–8° C (36°–45° F); do not freeze.

ADMINISTRATION
Intramuscular
- Shake vial well before drawing up; solution that has particulates or is discolored should not be used.

Common adverse effects in *italic;* life-threatening effects <u>underlined;</u> generic names in **bold;** drug classifications in SMALL CAPS; ♣ Canadian drug name; ☢ Prototype drug.

999

- Give IM to infants in lateral thigh muscle.
- Use needle at least ⅞ to 1 inch for normal sized babies ≥4 mo in order to reach muscle mass.
- May be given in deltoid for 4–6 y dose and older doses.
- Schedule varies for immune compromised children and those not immunized in infancy; see Appendix (H-2).
- May be given at same visit with other childhood immunizations with a different site for each IM medication administered.

ADVERSE EFFECTS Body as a Whole: Fever, irritability, <u>anaphylaxis</u> (rare). **Skin:** Urticarial rash, tenderness, erythema, swelling.

INTERACTIONS Drug: Efficacy of vaccine may be lessened when child is immunosuppressed.

PHARMACOKINETICS Immunity to each of the vaccine serotypes is 92–100% after the three-dose series; duration of immunity is unknown.

NURSING IMPLICATIONS

Assessment & Drug Effects

- Take careful history to rule out contraindications or lowered immunity. Instruct parents about risks and benefits of immunization. Teach side effects and to seek care immediately for those that are unexpected or serious. Obtain written parental consent for immunization.
- Teach comfort measures (acetaminophen, cool compress to injection site) for mild side effects.
- Provide information about clinics and other resources to receive immunizations.
- Keep epinephrine 1:1000 and doses for children available whenever giving immunizations.
- Another pneumococcal vaccine is available for use in children >24 mo at risk of pneumococcal vaccine and in adults. This 23-valent vaccine (Pneumovax) is not effective in children <24 mo.

Patient and Family Education

- No booster doses are currently recommended after initial series. Realize that only 7 types of meningococcal disease are available in vaccine; there are several other types.
- Review needs for immunizations and make appointments to obtain.

POLIOVIRUS VACCINE INACTIVATED
(po′leo′)
Ipol
Classifications: ANTI-INFECTIVE, VACCINE
Pregnancy Category: Not recommended unless traveling to area of high risk

AVAILABILITY Multiple-dose vials
Combination Products: Pediarix (with hepatitis B and diphtheria, tetanus and acellular pertussis)

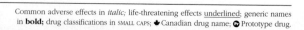
Common adverse effects in *italic;* life-threatening effects <u>underlined;</u> generic names in **bold;** drug classifications in SMALL CAPS; ♣ Canadian drug name; ⦿ Prototype drug.

ACTIONS Stimulates active immunity to poliovirus types 1, 2, 3
THERAPEUTIC EFFECTS The recommended four-dose regimen for infants or three-dose for older children provides protection against types 1, 2 and 3 poliovirus.

USES Used to provide active immunity against poliovirus in infants and children.

CONTRAINDICATIONS History of hypersensitivity to the vaccine or any of its components (phenoxyethanol, formaldehyde, neomycin, streptomycin, polymixin B); sever acute illness; safety and efficacy not established in children <6 mo.

ROUTE & DOSAGE

Prevention of Polio

Infant/Child: **IM/SC** 0.5 mL at 2, 4, 6, and 18 mo and 4–6 y

STORAGE
Keep refrigerated at 2°–8° C (36°–45° F); do not freeze.

ADMINISTRATION
Intramuscular/Subcutaneous
- Give to infants in lateral thigh muscle.
- May be given in deltoid for 4–6 y dose and older doses.
- Schedule varies for immune compromised children and those not immunized in infancy; see Appendix (H-2).

ADVERSE EFFECTS Skin: Tenderness, swelling, pain.

INTERACTIONS Drug: Efficacy of vaccine may be lessened when child is immunosuppressed.

PHARMACOKINETICS Primary immunization with 2–3 doses provides protection for diseases in 98–100% of children; immunity lasts about 6–12 y.

NURSING IMPLICATIONS
Assessment & Drug Effects
- Take careful history to rule out contraindications or lowered immunity. Instruct parents about risks and benefits of immunization. Teach side effects and to seek care immediately for those that are unexpected or serious. Obtain written parental consent for immunization.
- Teach comfort measures (acetaminophen, cool compress to injection site) for mild side effects.
- Provide information about clinics and other resources to receive immunizations.
- Keep epinephrine 1:1000 and doses for children available whenever giving immunizations.

Patient and Family Education
- Return as instructed for next immunization in the series. No booster doses are currently recommended after initial series unless traveling to an area with polio present.

Common adverse effects in *italic;* life-threatening effects <u>underlined</u>; generic names in **bold**; drug classifications in SMALL CAPS; ♣ Canadian drug name; ◐ Prototype drug.

1001

POLYCARBOPHIL

(pol-i-kar′boe-fil)

FiberCon, Mitrolan, Equalactin, FiberNorm

Classifications: GASTROINTESTINAL AGENT; BULK LAXATIVE; ANTIDIARRHEAL

Prototype: Psyllium

Pregnancy Category: C

AVAILABILITY 500 mg, 625 mg tablets; 500 mg, 625 mg chewable tablets

ACTIONS Hydrophilic agent that absorbs free water in intestinal tract and opposes dehydrating forces of bowel by forming a gelatinous mass.

THERAPEUTIC EFFECTS Restores more normal moisture level and motility in the lower GI tract; produces well-formed stool and reduces diarrhea.

USES Constipation or diarrhea associated with acute bowel syndrome, diverticulosis, irritable bowel and in patients who should not strain during defecation. Also choleretic diarrhea, diarrhea caused by small-bowel surgery or vagotomy, and disease of terminal ileum.

CONTRAINDICATIONS Partial or complete GI obstruction; fecal impaction; dysphagia; acute abdominal pain; rectal bleeding; undiagnosed abdominal pain, or other symptoms symptomatic of appendicitis; poisonings; before radiologic bowel examination; bowel surgery. Safety in children <3 y is not established.

CAUTIOUS USE Narcotic-associated constipation; pregnancy (category C), lactation.

ROUTE & DOSAGE

Constipation or Diarrhea

Child: **PO** *3–6 y,* 500 mg b.i.d. prn (max 1.5 g/day); *6–12 y,* 500 mg t.i.d. prn (max 3 g/day)

Adult: **PO** 1 g q.i.d. prn (max 6 g/day)

STORAGE

Store at 15°–30° C (59°–86° F) in tightly closed container unless otherwise directed.

ADMINISTRATION

Oral

- Chewable tablets should be chewed well before swallowing.
- Give each dose with a full glass (240 mL [8 oz]) of water or other liquid or generous amount for age group.
- Repeat dose every 30 min up to the maximum dose in 24 h with severe diarrhea.

ADVERSE EFFECTS GI: Esophageal blockage, intestinal impaction, *abdominal fullness.* **Metabolic:** Low serum potassium, elevated blood glucose levels (with extended use). **Respiratory:** Asthma. **Skin:** Skin rash.

INTERACTIONS Drug: May decrease absorption and clinical effects of ANTIBIOTICS, **warfarin, digoxin, nitrofurantoin,** SALICYLATES.

PHARMACOKINETICS Absorption: Not absorbed from GI tract. **Onset:** 12–24 h. **Peak:** 1–3 days.

NURSING IMPLICATIONS

Assessment & Drug Effects

- Determine duration and severity of diarrhea in order to anticipate signs of fluid-electrolyte losses.
- Monitor and record number and consistency of stools per day, presence and location of abdominal discomfort (i.e., tenderness, distention), and bowel sounds.
- Monitor and record I&O ratio and pattern. Dehydration is indicated if output is <30 mL/h for adolescents. For children (see Part I) for age appropriate output.
- Inspect oral cavity for dryness, and be alert to systemic signs of dehydration (e.g., thirst and fever). Dehydration from an episode of diarrhea appears rapidly in young children and older adults.

Patient & Family Education

- Consult physician if sudden changes in bowel habit persist more than 1 wk, action is minimal or ineffective for 1 wk, or if there is no antidiarrheal action within 2 days.
- Be aware that extended use of this drug may cause dependence for normal bowel function.
- Do not discontinue polycarbophil unless physician advises if also taking an oral anticoagulant, digoxin, salicylates, or nitrofurantoin.
- Do not breast feed while taking this drug without consulting physician.
- Store this medication out of reach of children.

POLYMYXIN B SULFATE

(pol-i-mix'in)
Aerosporin
Classifications: ANTI-INFECTIVE; ANTIBIOTIC
Pregnancy Category: B

AVAILABILITY 500,000 unit injection; 500,000 unit ophthalmic solution

ACTIONS Antibiotic derived from strains of *Bacillus polymyxa.* Binds to lipid phosphates in bacterial membranes and, through cationic detergent action, changes permeability to permit leakage of cytoplasm.
THERAPEUTIC EFFECTS Bactericidal against susceptible gram-negative organisms, particularly most strains of *Escherichia coli, Haemophilus influenzae, Enterobacter aerogenes,* and *Klebsiella pneumoniae.* Most species of *Proteus* and *Neisseria* are resistant, as are all gram-positive organisms and fungi.

USES Topically and in combination with other anti-infectives or corticosteroids for various superficial infections of eye, ear, mucous membrane, and skin. Concurrent systemic anti-infective therapy may be required for treatment of intraocular infection and severe progressive corneal ulcer. Used parenterally only in hospitalized patients for treatment of severe acute infections of urinary tract, bloodstream, and meninges; and in combination with Neosporin for continuous bladder irrigation to prevent bacteremia associated with use of indwelling catheter.

CONTRAINDICATIONS Hypersensitivity to polymyxin antibiotics; concurrent and sequential use of other nephrotoxic and neurotoxic drugs; concurrent use of skeletal muscle relaxants, ether, or sodium citrate. Safety during pregnancy (category B) or children <2 mo is not established.

CAUTIOUS USE Impaired kidney function; myasthenia gravis; lactation; IM route in infants and children because of severe pain at injection site.

ROUTE & DOSAGE

Infections

Child >2 mo–2 y: **IV** 15,000–45,000 units/kg/day divided q12h
IM 25,000–30,000 units/kg/day divided q6h
Child ≤2 y/Adult: **IV** 15,000–25,000 units/kg/day divided q12h
IM 25,000–30,000 units/kg/day divided q6h
Adult: **GU** 1 mL/L NS q24h **Topical** 1–2 drops in eye q1h

STORAGE

Protect unreconstituted product and reconstituted solution from light and freezing. Store in refrigerator at 2°–8° C (36°–46° F). Parenteral solutions are stable for 1 wk when refrigerated. Discard unused portion after 72 h.

ADMINISTRATION

Intramuscular

- Routine administration by IM route is not recommended because it causes intense discomfort, along the peripheral nerve distribution, 40–60 min after IM injection.
- Make IM injection in adults deep into upper outer quadrant of buttock. Select IM site carefully to avoid injection into nerves or blood vessels. Rotate injection sites. Follow agency policy for IM site used in children and see safe site selection in Techniques of Administration section in Part I.

Intravenous

PREPARE **Intermittent:** Reconstitute by dissolving 500,000 units in 5 mL sterile water for injection or NS to yield 100,000 units/mL. Withdraw a single dose and then further dilute in 300–500 mL of D5W.

ADMINISTER **Intermittent:** Infuse over period of 60–90 min. Inspect injection site for signs of phlebitis and irritation.

INCOMPATIBILITIES **Solution/Additive: Amphotericin B, cephalothin, chloramphenicol, chlorothiazide, heparin, magnesium sulfate, prednisolone, sodium phosphate, tetracycline.**

ADVERSE EFFECTS Body as a Whole: Irritability, facial flushing, ataxia, circumoral, lingual, and peripheral paresthesias (stocking glove distribution); severe pain (IM site), thrombophlebitis (IV site), superinfections, electrolyte disturbances (prolonged use; also reported in patients with acute leukemia); local irritation and burning (topical use), <u>anaphylactoid reactions</u> (rare). **CNS:** Drowsiness, dizziness, vertigo, convulsions, coma; <u>neuromuscular blockade (generalized muscle weakness, respiratory depression or arrest)</u>; meningeal irritation, increased protein and cell count in cerebrospinal fluid, fever, headache, stiff neck (intrathecal use). **Special Senses:** Blurred vision, nystagmus, slurred speech, dysphagia, ototoxicity (vestibular and auditory) with high doses. **GI:** GI disturbances. **Urogenital:** Albuminuria, cylindruria, <u>azotemia</u>, hematuria.

INTERACTIONS Drug: ANESTHETICS and NEUROMUSCULAR BLOCKING AGENTS may prolong skeletal muscle relaxation. AMINOGLYCOSIDES and **amphotericin B** have additive nephrotoxic potential.

PHARMACOKINETICS Absorption: Not absorbed from GI tract. **Peak:** 2 h IM. **Distribution:** Widely distributed except to CSF, synovial fluid, and eye; does not cross placenta. **Metabolism:** Unknown. **Elimination:** 60% Excreted unchanged in urine. **Half-Life:** 4.3–6 h.

NURSING IMPLICATIONS

Assessment & Drug Effects

- Lab tests: Obtain C&S tests prior to first dose and periodically thereafter to determine continuing sensitivity of causative organisms. Perform baseline serum electrolytes and kidney function tests before parenteral therapy. Frequent monitoring of kidney function and serum drug levels is advised during therapy. Monitor electrolytes at regular intervals during prolonged therapy.
- Review electrolyte results. Patients with low serum calcium and low intracellular potassium are particularly prone to develop neuromuscular blockade.
- Inspect tongue every day. Assess for S&S of superinfection (see Appendix D-1). Polymyxin therapy supports growth of opportunistic organisms. Report symptoms promptly.
- Monitor I&O. Maintain fluid intake sufficient to maintain daily urinary output of at least 1500 mL. Some degree of renal toxicity usually occurs within first 3 or 4 days of therapy even with therapeutic doses. Consult physician.
- Withhold drug and report findings to physician for any of the following: Decreases in urine output (change in I&O ratio), proteinuria, cellular casts, rising BUN, serum creatinine, or serum drug levels (not associated with dosage increase). All can be interpreted as signs of nephrotoxicity.
- Nephrotoxicity is generally reversible, but it may progress even after drug is discontinued. Therefore, close monitoring of kidney function is essential, even following termination of therapy.
- Be alert for respiratory arrest after the first dose and also as long as 45 days after initiation of therapy. It occurs most commonly in patients with kidney failure and high plasma drug levels and is often preceded by dyspnea and restlessness.

Patient & Family Education

- Report to physician immediately any muscle weakness, shortness of breath, dyspnea, depressed respiration. These symptoms are rapidly reversible if drug is withdrawn.

- Stop drug administration immediately and report to physician if you experience eyelid irritation, itching, and burning with ophthalmic drops.
- Report promptly to physician transient neurologic disturbances (burning or prickling sensations, numbness, dizziness). All occur commonly and usually respond to dosage reduction.
- Report promptly to physician the onset of stiff neck and headache (possible symptoms of neurotoxic reactions, including neuromuscular blockade). This response is usually associated with high serum drug levels or nephrotoxicity.
- Report promptly S&S of superinfection (see Appendix D-1).
- Do not breast feed while taking this drug without consulting physician.
- Store this medication out of reach of children.

POTASSIUM CHLORIDE
(poe-tass′ee-um)

Apo-K ♣, K-10, Kalium Durules ♣, Kaochlor, Kaochlor-20 Concentrate, Kaon-Cl, Kato, Kay Ciel, KCl 5% and 20%, K-Long ♣, Klor, Klor-10%, Klor-Con, Kloride, Klorvess, Klotrix, KDur, K-Lyte/Cl, K-tab, Micro-K Extentabs, Novolente K ♣, Roychlor 10% and 20% ♣, Rum-K, SK-Potassium Chloride, Slo-Pot, Slow-K

POTASSIUM GLUCONATE
Kaon, Kaylixir, K-G Elixir, Potassium Rougier ♣, Royonate ♣

Classifications: ELECTROLYTIC AND WATER BALANCE AGENT; REPLACEMENT SOLUTION
Pregnancy Category: A

P

AVAILABILITY Chloride 6.7 mEq, 8 mEq, 10 mEq, 20 mEq sustained-release tablets; 500 mg, 595 mg tablets; 20 mEq, 25 mEq, 50 mEq effervescent tablets; 20 mEq/15 mL, 40 mEq/15 mL, 45 mEq/15 mL liquid; 15 mEq, 20 mEq, 25 mEq powder; 2 mEq/mL injection; 10 mEq, 20 mEq, 30 mEq, 40 mEq, 60 mEq, 90 mEq vials **Gluconate** 20 mEq/15 mL liquid

ACTIONS Principal intracellular cation; essential for maintenance of intracellular isotonicity, transmission of nerve impulses, contraction of cardiac, skeletal, and smooth muscles, maintenance of normal kidney function, and for enzyme activity. Plays a prominent role in both formation and correction of imbalances in acid–base metabolism.

THERAPEUTIC EFFECTS Given special importance as therapeutic agents but are also dangerous if improperly prescribed and administered. Utilized for treatment of hypokalemia.

USES To prevent and treat potassium deficit secondary to diuretic or corticosteroid therapy. Also indicated when potassium is depleted by severe vomiting, diarrhea; intestinal drainage, fistulas, or malabsorption; prolonged diuresis, diabetic acidosis. Effective in the treatment of hypokalemic alkalosis (chloride, not the gluconate).

CONTRAINDICATIONS Severe renal impairment; severe hemolytic reactions; untreated Addison's disease; crush syndrome; early postoperative oliguria (except during GI drainage); adynamic ileus; acute dehydration;

heat cramps, hyperkalemia, patients receiving potassium-sparing diuretics, digitalis intoxication with AV conduction disturbance.

CAUTIOUS USE Cardiac or kidney disease; systemic acidosis; slow-release potassium preparations in presence of delayed GI transit or Meckel's diverticulum; extensive tissue breakdown (such as severe burns); pregnancy (category A); lactation.

ROUTE & DOSAGE

Normal Requirements
Neonate/Infant: 2–6 mEq/kg/day
Child: 2–3 mEq/kg/day
Adult: 40–80 mEq/kg/day

Hypokalemia
Neonate/Infant/Child: **PO** 1–4 mEq/kg/day in 1–2 equally divided doses (sustained-release tablets not recommended in children) **IV** 0.5–1 mEq/kg/dose (max dose 30 mEq) to infuse at 0.3–0.5 mEq/h (max dose 1 mEq/kg/h in critical situation); monitor closely
Adult: **PO** 10–100 mEq/day in divided doses **IV** 10–40 mEq/h diluted to at least 10–20 mEq/100 mL of solution (max 200–400 mEq/day monitor higher doses carefully)

STORAGE
Store at 15°–30° C (59°–86° F) in tightly closed, light-resistant container.

ADMINISTRATION

Oral
- Give while patient is sitting up or standing (never in recumbent position) to prevent drug-induced esophagitis. Some patients find it difficult to swallow the large sized KCl tablet.
- Do not crush or allow to chew any potassium salt tablets. Observe to make sure patient does not suck tablet (oral ulcerations have been reported if tablet is allowed to dissolve in mouth).
- Swallow whole tablet with a large glass of water or fruit juice (if allowed) to wash drug down and to start esophageal peristalsis.
- Dissolve effervescent tablets in water prior to giving.
- Follow directions for diluting various liquid forms of KCl exactly. In general, dilute each 20 mEq potassium in at least 90 mL water or juice and allowed to completely before administration.
- Dilute liquid forms as directed before giving it through nasogastric tube.

Intravenous

PREPARE **IV Infusion:** Add desired amount to 100–1000 mL IV solution (compatible with all standard solutions). Usual maximum is 80 mEq/1000 mL, however, 40 mEq/L is preferred to reduce irritation to veins. Higher concentrations for infusion are possible if infusing through a central venous line. Note: NEVER add KCl to an IV bag/bottle that is hanging. After adding KCl, invert bag/bottle several times to ensure even distribution.

***ADMINISTER* IV Infusion:** KCl is NEVER given IV push or in concentrated amounts by any route. Infuse at rate not to exceed 10 mEq/h. Adult patients with severe potassium depletion may be able to tolerate 20 mEq/h. Too rapid infusion may cause fatal hyperkalemia.

- Take extreme care to prevent extravasation and infiltration. At first sign, discontinue infusion and select another site.

***INCOMPATIBILITIES* Solution/Additive: Amphotericin B, dobutamine (potassium phosphate only). Y-Site: Amphotericin B cholesteryl complex, diazepam, ergotamine, methylprednisolone, phenytoin, promethazine.**

ADVERSE EFFECTS GI: *Nausea, vomiting,* diarrhea, abdominal distension. **Body as a Whole:** Pain, mental confusion, irritability, listlessness, paresthesias of extremities, muscle weakness and heaviness of limbs, difficulty in swallowing, <u>flaccid paralysis</u>. **Urogenital:** Oliguria, anuria. **Hematologic:** Hyperkalemia. **Respiratory:** <u>Respiratory distress</u>. **CV:** Hypotension, bradycardia; <u>cardiac depression, arrhythmias, or arrest</u>; altered sensitivity to digitalis glycosides. *ECG changes in hyperkalemia:* Tenting (peaking) of T wave (especially in right precordial leads), lowering of R with deepening of S waves and depression of RST; prolonged P-R interval, widened QRS complex, decreased amplitude and disappearance of P waves, prolonged Q-T interval, signs of right and left bundle block, <u>deterioration of QRS contour and finally ventricular fibrillation and death</u>.

INTERACTIONS Drug: POTASSIUM-SPARING DIURETICS, ANGIOTENSIN-CONVERTING ENZYME (ACE) INHIBITORS may cause hyperkalemia.

PHARMACOKINETICS Absorption: Readily absorbed from upper GI tract. **Elimination:** 90% excreted in urine, 10% in feces.

NURSING IMPLICATIONS

Assessment & Drug Effects

- Monitor I&O ratio and pattern in patients receiving the parenteral drug. Monitor infant and child output by mL/kg/h (see Physiological Considerations sections in Part I). If oliguria occurs, stop infusion promptly and notify physician.
- Lab test: Frequent serum electrolytes are warranted.
- Monitor for and report signs of GI ulceration (esophageal or epigastric pain or hematemesis).
- Monitor patients receiving parenteral potassium closely with cardiac monitor. Irregular heartbeat is usually the earliest clinical indication of hyperkalemia.
- Be alert for potassium intoxication (hyperkalemia, see S&S, Appendix D-1); may result from any therapeutic dosage, and the patient may be asymptomatic.
- The risk of hyperkalemia with potassium supplement increases (1) infants because of immature kidney function, (2) when dietary intake of potassium suddenly increases, and (3) when kidney function is significantly compromised.

Patient & Family Education

- Take only as instructed. Do not be alarmed when the tablet encasement appears in your stool. The sustained-release tablet (e.g., Slow-K)

Common adverse effects in *italic;* life-threatening effects <u>underlined;</u> generic names in **bold;** drug classifications in SMALL CAPS; ♣ Canadian drug name; ✪ Prototype drug.

utilizes a wax matrix as carrier for KCl crystals that passes through the digestive system.

- Learn about sources of potassium with special reference to foods and OTC drugs.
- Avoid licorice; large amounts can cause both hypokalemia and sodium retention.
- Do not use any salt substitute unless it is specifically ordered by the physician. These contain a substantial amount of potassium and electrolytes other than sodium.
- Do not self-prescribe laxatives. Chronic laxative use has been associated with diarrhea-induced potassium loss.
- Notify physician of persistent vomiting because losses of potassium can occur.
- Report continuing signs of potassium deficit to physician: Weakness, fatigue, polyuria, polydipsia.
- Advise dentist or new physician that a potassium drug has been prescribed as long-term maintenance therapy.
- Do not open foil-wrapped powders and tablets before use.
- Do not breast feed while taking this drug without consulting physician.
- Store this medication out of reach of children.

POTASSIUM IODIDE

(poe-tass'ee-um)
Pima, SSKI, Thyro-Block ♣
Classifications: EXPECTORANT; ANTITHYROID AGENT
Prototype: Guaifenesin
Pregnancy Category: D

P

AVAILABILITY 325 mg/5 mL syrup; 100 mg/mL (Lugol's solution) 1 g/mL solution

ACTIONS Pharmacologic use primarily related to iodide portion of molecule. Exact mechanism not clear but believed to increase secretion of respiratory fluids by direct action on bronchial tissue, thereby decreasing mucous viscosity. If patient is euthyroid, excess iodide ions causes minimal change in thyroid gland mass. Conversely, when the thyroid gland is hyperplastic, excess iodide ions temporarily inhibits secretion of thyroid hormone, fosters accumulation in thyroid follicles, and decreases vascularity of gland.

THERAPEUTIC EFFECTS Return of thyrotoxic symptoms may occur after 10–14 days of continuous treatment; consequently potassium iodide administration for hyperthyroidism is limited to short-term therapy. As an expectorant, the iodine ion portion of the molecule increases mucous secretion formation in the bronchi, and decreases viscosity of the mucous.

USES To facilitate bronchial drainage and cough in emphysema, asthma, chronic bronchitis, bronchiectasis, and respiratory tract allergies characterized by difficult-to-raise sputum. Also used alone for hyperthyroidism or in conjunction with antithyroid drugs and propranolol in treatment of

Common adverse effects in *italic*; life-threatening effects <u>underlined</u>; generic names in **bold**; drug classifications in SMALL CAPS; ♣ Canadian drug name; ❷ Prototype drug.

1009

thyrotoxic crisis; in immediate preoperative period for thyroidectomy to decrease vascularity, fragility, and size of thyroid gland and for treatment of persistent or recurring hyperthyroidism that occurs in Graves' disease patients. Used as a radiation protectant in patients receiving radioactive iodine and to shield the thyroid gland from radiation in the wake of a serious nuclear plant accident. (Use as an expectorant has been largely replaced by other agents.)

CONTRAINDICATIONS Hypersensitivity or idiosyncrasy to iodine; hyperthyroidism; hyperkalemia; acute bronchitis. Safety during pregnancy (category D), lactation, or in children <1 y is not established.
CAUTIOUS USE Renal impairment; cardiac disease; pulmonary tuberculosis; Addison's disease.

ROUTE & DOSAGE

To Reduce Thyroid Vascularity
Child/Adult: **PO** 50–250 mg t.i.d. for 10–14 days before surgery
Expectorant
Child: **PO** 60–250 mg p.c. b.i.d. or t.i.d.
Adult: **PO** 300–650 mg p.c. b.i.d. or t.i.d.
Thyroid Blocking in Radiation Emergency
Child: **PO** <1 y, 65 mg/day for 10 days; >1 y, 130 mg/day for 10 days
Adult: **PO** 130 mg/day for 10 days

STORAGE
Store in airtight, light-resistant container. Crystallization occurs at cold temperatures; warming and shaking will dissolve crystals.

ADMINISTRATION
Oral
- Use caution as several different strengths of KI exist.
- Give with meals in a full glass (240 mL) of water or fruit juice or generous amount of fluid appropriate for age and at bedtime with food or juice to disguise salty taste and minimize gastric distress.
- Avoid giving KI with milk; absorption of the drug may be decreased by dairy products.
- Adhere strictly to schedule and accurate dose measurements when iodide is administered to prepare thyroid gland for surgery, particularly at end of treatment period when possibility of "escape" (from iodide) effect on thyroid gland increases.
- Place container in warm water and gently agitating to dissolve if crystals are noted in the solution.
- Discard any solutions that has turned a brownish yellow on standing, especially if exposed to light (caused by liberated trace of free iodine).

ADVERSE EFFECTS GI: Diarrhea, nausea, vomiting, stomach pain, non-specific small bowel lesions (associated with enteric coated tablets).

Body as a Whole: <u>Angioneurotic edema</u>, cutaneous and mucosal hemorrhage, fever, arthralgias, lymph node enlargement, eosinophilia, paresthesias, periorbital edema, weakness. *Iodine poisoning (iodism):* Metallic taste, stomatitis, salivation, coryza, sneezing; swollen and tender salivary glands (sialadenitis), frontal headache, vomiting (blue vomitus if stomach contained starches, otherwise yellow vomitus), bloody diarrhea. **Metabolic:** Hyperthyroid adenoma, goiter, hypothyroidism, collagen disease–like syndromes. **CV:** Irregular heartbeat. **CNS:** Mental confusion. **Skin:** Acneiform skin lesions (prolonged use), flare-up of adolescent acne. **Respiratory:** Productive cough, pulmonary edema.

DIAGNOSTIC TEST INTERFERENCE Potassium iodide may alter ***thyroid function*** test results and may interfere with ***urinary 17-OHCS*** determinations.

INTERACTIONS Drug: ANTITHYROID DRUGS, **lithium** may potentiate hypothyroid and goitrogenic actions; POTASSIUM-SPARING DIURETICS, POTASSIUM SUPPLEMENTS, ACE INHIBITORS increase risk of hyperkalemia.

PHARMACOKINETICS Absorption: Adequately absorbed from GI tract. **Distribution:** Crosses placenta. **Elimination:** Cleared from plasma by renal excretion or thyroid uptake.

NURSING IMPLICATIONS

Assessment & Drug Effects

- Lab tests: Determine serum potassium levels before and periodically during therapy.
- Keep prescriber informed about characteristics of sputum: quantity, consistency, color.

Patient & Family Education

- Report to prescriber promptly the occurrence of GI bleeding, abdominal pain, distention, nausea, or vomiting.
- Report clinical S&S of iodism (see ADVERSE EFFECTS). Usually, symptoms will subside with dose reduction and lengthened intervals between doses.
- Avoid foods rich in iodine if iodism develops: Seafood, fish liver oils, and iodized salt.
- Be aware that sudden withdrawal following prolonged use may precipitate thyroid storm.
- Do not use OTC drugs while on this drug without consulting prescriber. Many preparations contain iodides and could augment prescribed dose (e.g., cough syrups, gargles, asthma medication, salt substitutes, cod liver oil, multiple vitamins [often suspended in iodide solutions]).
- Be aware that optimum hydration is the best expectorant when taking KI as an expectorant. Increase daily fluid intake.
- Caution parents to take drug as directed and not to use with other children without prescription.
- Do not breast feed while taking this drug without consulting physician.
- Store this medication out of reach of children.

PRALIDOXIME CHLORIDE
(pra-li-dox′eem)
2-PAM, Protopam Chloride
Classification: ANTIDOTE
Pregnancy Category: C

AVAILABILITY 1 g injection

ACTIONS Reactivates cholinesterase inhibited by phosphate esters by displacing the enzyme from its receptor sites; the free enzyme then can resume its function of degrading accumulated acetylcholine, thereby restoring normal neuromuscular transmission.

THERAPEUTIC EFFECTS Less effective against carbamate anticholinesterases (ambenonium, neostigmine, pyridostigmine). More active against effects of anticholinesterases at skeletal neuromuscular junction than at autonomic effector sites or in CNS respiratory center; therefore, atropine must be given concomitantly to block effects of acetylcholine and its accumulation in these sites.

USES As antidote in treatment of poisoning by organophosphate insecticides and pesticides with anticholinesterase activity (e.g., parathion, TEPP, sarin) by reversing the muscle paralysis and to control overdosage by anticholinesterase drugs used in treatment of myasthenia gravis (cholinergic crisis).
UNLABELED USES To reverse toxicity of echothiophate ophthalmic solution.

CONTRAINDICATIONS Use in poisoning by carbamate insecticide Sevin, inorganic phosphates, or organophosphates having no anticholinesterase activity; asthma, peptic ulcer, severe cardiac disease, patients receiving aminophylline, theophylline, morphine, succinylcholine, reserpine, or phenothiazines; pregnancy (category C).
CAUTIOUS USE Myasthenia gravis; renal insufficiency; concomitant use of barbiturates in organophosphorous poisoning; lactation, children.

ROUTE & DOSAGE

Organophosphate Poisoning
Note: Use with atropine.
Child: **IV** 20–40 mg/kg, repeat in 1–2 h if muscle weakness not relieved
Adult: **IV** 1–2 g in 100 mL NS infused over 15–30 min *or* 1–2 g as 5% solution in sterile water over not less than 5 min, may repeat after 1 h if muscle weakness not relieved **IM/SC** 1–2 g if IV route is not feasible
Anticholinesterase Overdose in Myasthenia Gravis
Adult: **IV** 1–2 g in 100 mL NS infused over 15–30 min, followed by increments of 250 mg q5min prn

ADMINISTRATION
Subcutaneous/Intramuscular
- Give only if unable to give IV; NOT preferred routes.
- Reconstitute as for direct IV injection (see following).

Intravenous

PREPARE Direct: Reconstitute 1-g vial by adding 20 mL NS (preservative free) to yield 50 mg/mL (a 5% solution). If pulmonary edema is present, give without further dilution. **IV Infusion:** Preferred method is to further dilute in 100 mL NS. Usually dilute to 20 mg/mL for child unless child is fluid restricted (maximum concentration is 50 mg/mL). In organophosphate poisonings, atropine is used in conjunction with this drug.

ADMINISTER Direct: In pulmonary edema, 1 g or fraction thereof over 5 min; do not exceed 200 mg/min. **IV Infusion:** Give over 15–30 min (preferred).

■ Stop infusion and reduce rate if hypertension occurs.

ADVERSE EFFECTS CNS: Dizziness, headache, drowsiness. **GI:** Nausea. **Special Senses:** Blurred vision, diplopia, impaired accommodation. **CV:** Tachycardia, hypertension (dose related). **Body as a Whole:** Hyperventilation, muscular weakness, <u>laryngospasm</u>, muscle rigidity.

INTERACTIONS Drug: May potentiate the effects of BARBITURATES.

PHARMACOKINETICS Peak: 5–15 min IV; 10–20 min IM. **Distribution:** Distributed throughout extracellular fluids; crosses blood–brain barrier slowly if at all. **Metabolism:** Probably metabolized in liver. **Elimination:** Rapidly excreted mostly unchanged in urine. **Half-Life:** 0.8–2.7 h.

NURSING IMPLICATIONS

Assessment & Drug Effects

■ Monitor BP, vital signs, and I&O. Report oliguria or changes in I&O ratio.
■ Monitor closely. It is difficult to differentiate toxic effects of organophosphates or atropine from toxic effects of pralidoxime.
■ Be alert for and report immediately: Reduction in muscle strength, onset of muscle twitching, changes in respiratory pattern, altered level of consciousness, increases or changes in heart rate and rhythm. Maintain patent airway, monitor secretions and remove as necessary.
■ Observe necessary safety precautions with unconscious patient because excitement and manic behavior reportedly may occur following recovery of consciousness.
■ Keep patient under close observation for 48–72 h, particularly when poison was ingested, because of likelihood of continued absorption of organophosphate from lower bowel.
■ In patients with myasthenia gravis, overdosage with pralidoxime may convert cholinergic crisis into myasthenic crisis.

PRAMOXINE HYDROCHLORIDE

(pra-mox′een)
Fleet Relief Anesthetic Hemorrhoidal, Prax, ProctoFoam, Tronolane, Tronothane ♣
Classifications: CENTRAL NERVOUS SYSTEM AGENT; LOCAL ANESTHETIC (MUCOSAL); ANTIPRURITIC
Prototype: Procaine
Pregnancy Category: C

AVAILABILITY 1% cream, gel, lotion, spray

ACTIONS Differs chemically from the amide- or ester-type anesthetics; therefore, it can be used in patients sensitive to these classes of drugs.
THERAPEUTIC EFFECTS Produces anesthesia by blocking conduction and propagation of sensory nerve impulses in skin and mucous membranes. Potency matches that of benzocaine as a topical anesthetic. Does not abolish gag reflex.

USES To relieve pain caused by minor burns and wounds; for temporary relief of pruritus secondary to dermatoses, hemorrhoids, and anal fissures; and to facilitate sigmoidoscopic examination.

CONTRAINDICATIONS Application to large areas of skin; prolonged use; preparation for laryngopharyngeal examination, bronchoscopy, or gastroscopy. Safety in children <2 y or during pregnancy (category C) is not established.
CAUTIOUS USE Extensive skin disorders; lactation.

ROUTE & DOSAGE

Relief of Minor Pain and Itching
Child >2 y/Adult: **Topical** Apply t.i.d. or q.i.d.

STORAGE
Store at 15°–30° C (59°–86° F) in tightly closed containers.

ADMINISTRATION

Topical

- Clean thoroughly and dry rectal area before use for temporary relief of hemorrhoidal pain and itching.
- Administer rectal preparations in the morning and evening and after bowel movement or as directed by physician.
- Apply lotion or cream to affected surfaces with a gloved hand. Wash hands thoroughly before and after treatment.
- Do not apply to eyes or nasal membranes.

ADVERSE EFFECTS Skin: Burning, stinging, sensitization.

INTERACTIONS No clinically significant interactions established.

PHARMACOKINETICS Onset: 3–5 min. **Duration:** Up to 5 h.

NURSING IMPLICATIONS

Patient & Family Education
- Drug is usually discontinued if condition being treated does not improve within 2–3 wk or if it worsens, or if rash or condition not present before treatment appears, or if treated area becomes inflamed or infected.
- Discontinue and consult prescriber if rectal bleeding and pain occur during hemorrhoid treatment.
- Do not breast feed while taking this drug without consulting physician.
- Store this medication out of reach of children.

PRAZIQUANTEL

(pray-zi-kwon′tel)
Biltricide
Classifications: ANTI-INFECTIVE; ANTHELMINTIC
Prototype: Mebendazole
Pregnancy Category: B

AVAILABILITY 600 mg tablets

ACTIONS Synthetic agent with broad-spectrum anthelmintic activity against all developmental stages of schistosomes and other trematodes (flukes) and against cestodes (tapeworm). Increases permeability of parasite cell membrane to calcium. Leads to immobilization of their suckers and dislodgment from their residence in blood vessel walls.

THERAPEUTIC EFFECTS Active against all developmental stages of schistosomes, including cercaria (free-swimming larvae). Activity against other trematodes (flukes) not fully understood; activity against cestodes (tapeworms) not clear but may be similar to that against schistosomes.

USES All stages of schistosomiasis (bilharziasis) caused by all schistosoma species pathogenic to humans. Other trematode infections caused by Chinese liver fluke.

UNLABELED USES Lung, sheep liver, and intestinal flukes and tapeworm infections.

CONTRAINDICATIONS Hypersensitivity to drug; ocular cysticercosis. Safety in children <4 y is not established; use during pregnancy (category B) only when clearly needed. Women should not breast feed on day of praziquantel therapy or for 72 h after last dose of drug.

ROUTE & DOSAGE

Schistosomiasis

Child >4 y/Adult: **PO** 20 mg/kg/dose in 2–3 doses at 4–6 h intervals on the same day, may repeat 2–3 mo after exposure

Other Trematodes

Child >4 y/Adult: **PO** 25 mg/kg/dose in 3 doses at 4–6 h intervals on the same day for 15 to 30 days

Cestodiasis (Adult or Intestinal Stage)

Adult: **PO** 10–20 mg/kg as single dose

Cestodiasis (Larval or Tissue Stage)

Adult: **PO** 50 mg/kg in 3 divided doses/day for 14 days

STORAGE
Store tablets in tight containers at <30° C (86° F).

Common adverse effects in *italic;* life-threatening effects <u>underlined;</u> generic names in **bold;** drug classifications in SMALL CAPS; ♦ Canadian drug name; ❷ Prototype drug.

1015

ADMINISTRATION

Oral

- Give dose with food and fluids. Tablets can be broken into quarters but should NOT be chewed.
- Advise patient to take sufficient fluid for age to wash down the medication. Tablets are soluble in water; gagging or vomiting because of bitter taste may result if tablets are retained in the mouth.
- Treatment for cestodiasis (tapeworm) is followed by gentle purgation 2 h after drug administration to facilitate rapid removal of tapeworms and ova.

ADVERSE EFFECTS CNS: *Dizziness, headache, malaise,* drowsiness, lassitude, CSF reaction syndrome (exacerbation of neurologic signs and symptoms such as seizures, increased CSF protein concentration, increased anticysticercal IgG levels, hyperthermia, intracranial hypertension) in patient treated for cerebral cysticercosis. **GI:** *Abdominal pain or discomfort with or without nausea;* vomiting, anorexia, diarrhea. **Hepatic:** *Increased AST, ALT (slight).* **Skin:** Pruritus, urticaria. **Body as a Whole:** Fever, sweating, symptoms of host-mediated immunologic response to antigen release from worms (fever, eosinophilia).

DIAGNOSTIC TEST INTERFERENCE Be mindful that selected drugs may interfere with stool studies for ova and parasites: ***iron, bismuth, oil*** (***mineral*** or ***castor***), ***Metamucil*** (if ingested within 1 wk of test), ***barium, antibiotics, antiamebic*** and ***antimalarial drugs,*** and ***gallbladder dye*** (if administered within 3 wk of test).

INTERACTIONS Drug: Phenytoin and **carbamazepine** can lead to therapeutic failure.

PHARMACOKINETICS Absorption: Rapidly absorbed, 80% reaches systemic circulation. **Peak:** 1–3 h. **Distribution:** Enters cerebrospinal fluid. **Metabolism:** Extensively metabolized to inactive metabolites. **Elimination:** Excreted primarily in urine. **Half-Life:** 0.8–1.5 h.

NURSING IMPLICATIONS

Assessment & Drug Effects

- Patient is reexamined in 2 or 3 mo to ensure complete eradication of the infections.

Patient & Family Education

- Do not drive or operate other hazardous machinery on day of treatment or the following day because of potential drug-induced dizziness and drowsiness.
- Do not take alcohol while taking this drug.
- Usually, all schistosomal worms are dead 7 days following treatment.
- Contact physician if you develop a sustained headache or high fever.
- Do not breast feed while taking this drug without consulting physician (see CONTRAINDICATIONS).
- Caution parents to take drug as directed and not to use for other children without prescription.
- Store this medication out of reach of children.

PRAZOSIN HYDROCHLORIDE ⊕

(pra'zoe-sin)

Minipress, Apo-Prazo ♣ , Novo-Parazin ♣

Classifications: AUTONOMIC NERVOUS SYSTEM AGENT; ALPHA-ADRENERGIC ANTAGONIST (BLOCKING AGENT, SYMPATHOLYTIC); CARDIOVASCULAR AGENT; ANTIHYPERTENSIVE; VASODILATOR

Pregnancy Category: C

AVAILABILITY 1 mg, 2 mg, 5 mg capsules

ACTIONS Selective inhibition of alpha$_1$-adrenoceptors; produces vasodilation in both resistance (arterioles) and capacitance (veins) vessels with the result that both peripheral vascular resistance and blood pressure are reduced.

THERAPEUTIC EFFECTS Lowers blood pressure in supine and standing positions with most pronounced effect on diastolic pressure. Minor effect on heart rate and cardiac output in the supine position and does not increase plasma renin activity. Tolerance to antihypertensive effect rarely occurs. Effective when used concomitantly with a beta-adrenergic blocking agent and a thiazide diuretic. Infrequently used in monotherapy because of tendency to support sodium and water retention resulting in increased plasma volume.

USES Treatment of hypertension.

UNLABELED USES Severe refractory congestive heart failure, Raynaud's disease or phenomenon, ergotamine-induced peripheral ischemia, pheochromocytoma.

CONTRAINDICATIONS Safety during pregnancy (category C) or lactation is not established.

CAUTIOUS USE Chronic kidney failure; hypertensive patient with cerebral thrombosis; men with sickle cell trait.

ROUTE & DOSAGE

Hypertension

Child: **PO** Start with 5 mcg/kg/dose q6h, gradually increase to 25 mcg/kg/dose q6h (max 15 mg/day or 0.4 mg/kg/day)
Adult: **PO** Start with 1 mg at bedtime, then 1 mg b.i.d. or t.i.d., may increase to 20 mg/day in divided doses

STORAGE

Store at 15°–30° C (59°–86° F) in tightly closed container away from strong light; do not freeze.

ADMINISTRATION

Oral

▪ Give initial dose at bedtime to reduce possibility of adverse effects such as postural hypotension and syncope. However, if first dose is taken during the day, advise patient not to drive a car for about 4 h after ingestion of drug.

- Give drug with food to reduce incidence of faintness and dizziness; food may delay absorption but does not affect extent of absorption.

ADVERSE EFFECTS CNS: *Dizziness, headache, drowsiness,* nervousness, vertigo, depression, paresthesia, insomnia. **CV:** Edema, dyspnea, syncope *first-dose phenomenon,* postural hypotension, *palpitations,* tachycardia, angina. **Special Senses:** Blurred vision, tinnitus, reddened sclerae. **GI:** Dry mouth, *nausea,* vomiting, diarrhea, constipation, abdominal discomfort, pain. **Urogenital:** Urinary frequency, incontinence, priapism (especially in men with sickle cell anemia), impotence. **Skin:** Rash, pruritus, alopecia, lichen planus. **Body as a Whole:** Diaphoresis, epistaxis, nasal congestion, arthralgia, transient leukopenia, increased serum uric acid, and BUN.

INTERACTIONS Drug: DIURETICS and other HYPOTENSIVE AGENTS increase hypotensive effects. **Food:** Licorice increases sodium and water retention.

PHARMACOKINETICS Absorption: Approximately 60% of oral dose reaches the systemic circulation. **Onset:** 2 h. **Peak:** 2–4 h. **Duration:** <24 h. **Distribution:** Widely distributed, including into breast milk. **Metabolism:** Extensively metabolized in liver. **Elimination:** 6–10% excreted in urine, the rest in bile and feces. **Half-Life:** 2–4 h.

NURSING IMPLICATIONS

Assessment & Drug Effects

- Be alert for first-dose phenomenon (rare adverse effect: 0.15% of patients); characterized by a precipitous decline in BP, bradycardia, and consciousness disturbances (syncope) within 90–120 min after the initial dose of prazosin. Recovery is usually within several hours. Preexisting low plasma volume (from diuretic therapy or salt restriction), beta-adrenergic therapy, and recent stroke appear to increase the risk of this phenomenon.
- Monitor blood pressure. If it falls precipitously with first dose, notify physician promptly.
- Full therapeutic effect may not be achieved until 4–6 wk of therapy.

Patient & Family Education

- Avoid situations that would result in injury if you should faint, particularly during early phase of treatment. In most cases, effect does not recur after initial period of therapy; however, it may occur during acute febrile episodes, when drug dose is increased, or when another antihypertensive drug is added to the medication regimen.
- Make position and direction changes slowly and in stages. Dangle legs and move ankles a minute or so before standing when arising in the morning or after a nap.
- Lie down immediately if you experience light-headedness, dizziness, a sense of impending loss of consciousness, or blurred vision. Attempting to stand or walk may result in a fall.

- Do not engage in other potentially hazardous activities such as biking, sports, or driving until response to drug is known.
- Take drug at same time(s) each day. Keep a daily record noting BP and time taken, when medication was taken, which arm was used, position (i.e., standing, sitting), and time of day. Take this record to physician for reference at checkup appointment.
- Report priapism or impotence. A change in the drug regimen usually reverses these difficulties. Because acute episodes of priapism followed by impotence spontaneously occur in men with sickle cell anemia, another antihypertensive should be selected. In these patients, drug-induced priapism is frequently irreversible.
- Do not take OTC medications, especially those that may contain an adrenergic agent (e.g., remedies for coughs, colds, allergy), while on this drug without consulting physician.
- Avoid alcohol with this drug.
- Be aware that adverse effects usually disappear with continuation of therapy, but dosage reduction may be necessary.
- Do not breast feed while taking this drug without consulting physician.
- Store this medication out of reach of children.

PREDNISOLONE

(pred-niss'oh-lone)
Delta-Cortef, Inflamase Forte, Prelone

PREDNISOLONE ACETATE

Econopred, Key-Pred, Pred Forte, Predcor

PREDNISOLONE SODIUM PHOSPHATE

AK-Pred, Hydeltrasol, Inflamase, Inflamase Mild, Orepred, Pred Mild, Pediapred

PREDNISOLONE TEBUTATE

Hydeltra-T.B.A., Prednisol TBA

Classifications: HORMONES AND SYNTHETIC SUBSTITUTES; ADRENAL CORTICOSTEROID; GLUCOCORTICOID
Prototype: Prednisone
Pregnancy Category: C

AVAILABILITY Prednisolone 5 mg tablet; 5 mg/5 mL, 15 mg/5 mL syrup; 0.12%, 0.125%, 1% ophthalmic suspension **Acetate** 25 mg/mL, 50 mg/mL injection **Sodium Phosphate** 5 mg/5 mL liquid; 20 mg/mL injection; 0.125%, 1% ophthalmic solution **Tebuate** 20 mg/mL injection

ACTIONS Analog of hydrocortisone with 3–5 times greater potency. Mineralocorticoid properties are minimal, and potential for sodium and water retention as well as potassium loss is reduced.
THERAPEUTIC EFFECTS Effective as an anti-inflammatory agent.

USES Principally as an anti-inflammatory and immunosuppressant agent.

CONTRAINDICATIONS Systemic fungal infection, varicella. Safety during pregnancy (category C) or lactation is not established.

ROUTE & DOSAGE

Anti-Inflammatory

Child: **PO** 0.1–2 mg/kg/day in single or divided doses *or* 4–60 mg/m^2 daily in 4 divided doses **IM** Acetate: 0.04–0.25 mg/kg 1–2 times/day
Adult: **PO** 5–60 mg/day in single or divided doses **IM** Acetate: 6–60 mg/day

Ophthalmic

Child/Adult: Instill 1–2 drops into affected eye hourly during day and q2h during night until desired response then 1 drop into affected eye q4h

STORAGE

Store at 15°–30° C (59°–86° F) in tightly closed, light-resistant container. Store oral solutions in light-resistant containers; Pediapred, store at 4°–25° C (39°–77° F) and may be refrigerated; Orapred, store in refrigerator 2°–8° C (36°–45° F).

ADMINISTRATION

Oral

- Give with meals or milk to reduce gastric irritation. If distress continues, consult physician about possible adjunctive antacid therapy.

Alternate-Day Therapy (ADT) for Patient on Long-Term Therapy

- With ADT, the 48-h requirement for steroids is administered as a single dose every other morning.
- Be aware that ADT minimizes adverse effects associated with long term treatment while maintaining the desired therapeutic effect.
- See **prednisone** for numerous additional nursing implications.

Intramuscular

- Note: Verify that drug supplied is appropriate for the ordered route. Prednisolone acetate is for IM use.
- Give deep IM into a large muscle mass administration in children or see Techniques of Administration section in Part I for appropriate site selections.

Intravenous

Note: Parenteral phosphate preparation is no longer available in the U.S.
PREPARE Direct: May be given undiluted. **IV Infusion:** May be added to 50–1000 mL of D5W or NS.
ADMINISTER Direct: Give at a rate of 10 mg or fraction thereof over 60 sec. **IV Infusion:** Do not exceed 10 mg/min.
INCOMPATIBILITIES Solution/Additive: Calcium glucceptate, metaraminol, methotrexate, polymyxin B.

Opthamalic

- Suspension requires shaking before instillation.

Common adverse effects in *italic;* life-threatening effects underlined; generic names in **bold**; drug classifications in SMALL CAPS; ♣ Canadian drug name; ◑ Prototype drug.

ADMINISTER Avoid touching the dropper to lashes or eye during instillation. Place pressure to lacramil sac for 1 to 2 min after instillation to prevent systemic absorption.

ADVERSE EFFECTS Endocrine: Hirsutism (occasional), adverse effects on growth and development of the individual and on sperm. **Special Senses:** Perforation of cornea; cataracts (with long-term use of topical drug). **Body as a Whole:** Sensitivity to heat; fat embolism, hypotension and shock-like reactions. **CNS:** Insomnia, psychosis. **GI:** Gastric irritation or ulceration. **Skin:** Ecchymotic skin lesions; vasomotor symptoms. Also see prednisone.

INTERACTIONS Drug: BARBITURATES, **phenytoin, rifampin** increase steroid metabolism; therefore, may need increased doses of prednisolone; **amphotericin B,** DIURETICS add to **potassium** loss; **ambenonium, neostigmine, pyridostigmine** may cause severe muscle weakness in patients with myasthenia gravis; VACCINES, TOXOIDS may inhibit antibody response.

PHARMACOKINETICS Absorption: Readily absorbed from GI tract. **Peak:** 1–2 h. **Duration:** 1–1.5 days. **Distribution:** Crosses placenta; distributed into breast milk. **Metabolism:** Metabolized in liver. **Elimination:** HPA suppression: 24–36 h; Excreted in urine. **Half-Life:** 3.5 h.

NURSING IMPLICATIONS

Assessment & Drug Effects

- Be alert to subclinical signs of lack of improvement such as continued drainage, low-grade fever, and interrupted healing. In diseases caused by microorganisms, infection may be masked, activated, or enhanced by corticosteroids. Observe and report exacerbation of symptoms after short period of therapeutic response.
- Monitor for fungal infection.
- Do not administer live vaccines (varicella, MMR) while on high-dose steroids.
- Be aware that temporary local discomfort may follow injection of prednisolone into bursa or joint.
- Do not use ophthalmic preparations if eye is infected.

Patient & Family Education

- Adhere to established dosage regimen (i.e., do not increase, decrease, or omit doses, change dose intervals or stop drug).
- Follow schedule to taper the drug as directed. Best to give one time daily dose before 9 a.m. because it will suppress the adrenal cortex activity less.
- Remove contact lens before ophthalmic dosing.
- Report gastric distress or any sign of peptic ulcer.
- Inform any other health care provider that you are taking this drug.
- Report any symptoms of infections.
- Do not use OTC medications while on this drug without contacting physician.
- Do not breast feed while taking this drug without consulting physician.
- Store this medication out of reach of children.

PREDNISONE ⚙
(pred′ni-sone)
Apo-Prednisone ✦, Deltasone, Meticorten, Orasone, Panasol, Prednicen-M, Sterapred, Winpred ✦
Classifications: HORMONES AND SYNTHETIC SUBSTITUTES; ADRENAL CORTICOSTEROID; GLUCOCORTICOID
Pregnancy Category: C

AVAILABILITY 1 mg, 2.5 mg, 5 mg, 10 mg, 20 mg, 50 mg tablets; 5 mg/5 mL, 5 mg/mL solution (contains 5% alcohol)

ACTIONS Immediate-acting synthetic analog of hydrocortisone. Effect depends on biotransformation to prednisolone, a conversion that may be impaired in patient with liver dysfunction. Less mineralocorticoid activity than hydrocortisone, but sodium retention and potassium depletion can occur.
THERAPEUTIC EFFECTS Has anti-inflammatory properties.

USES May be used as a single agent or conjunctively with antineoplastics in cancer therapy; also used in treatment of myasthenia gravis and inflammatory conditions and as an immunosuppressant.

CONTRAINDICATIONS Systemic fungal infections and known hypersensitivity.
CAUTIOUS USE Patients with infections; nonspecific ulcerative colitis; diverticulitis; active or latent peptic ulcer; renal insufficiency; hypertension; osteoporosis; myasthenia gravis. Safety during pregnancy (category C) or lactation is not established.

P

ROUTE & DOSAGE

Anti-Inflammatory
Child: **PO** 0.05–2 mg/kg/day in single or 4 divided doses (max dose 80 mg/day)
Adult: **PO** 5–60 mg/day in single or divided doses

Acute Asthma
Child: **PO** 1–2 mg/kg/day in 1–2 divided doses for 3–5 days *or <1 y,* 10 mg q12h; *1–4 y,* 20 mg q12h; *5–13 y,* 30 mg q12h; *>13 y,* 40 mg q12h times 3–5 days (max dosage 60 mg/day)

Asthma
Child: **PO** (long-term treatment) *<1 y,* 10 mg every other day; *1–4 y,* 20 mg every other day; *5–13 y,* 30 mg every other day; *>13 y,* 40 mg every other day

STORAGE
Store at 15°–30° C (59°–86° F) in tightly closed container.

ADMINISTRATION

Oral
- Crush tablet and give with fluid of patient's choice or place in nonessential food if unable to swallow whole. Tablet has an unpleasant taste so follow tablet with fluid of choice.

Common adverse effects in *italic;* life-threatening effects <u>underlined;</u> generic names in **bold;** drug classifications in SMALL CAPS; ✦ Canadian drug name; ⚙ Prototype drug.

- Liquid contains alcohol and is vanilla flavored.
- Give at meal times or with a snack to reduce gastric irritation.
- Best to give one time daily dose before 9 a.m. because it will suppress the adrenal cortex activity less.
- Dose adjustment may be required if patient is subjected to severe stress (serious infection, surgery, or injury) or if a remission or disease exacerbation occurs.
- Do not abruptly stop drug. Reduce dose gradually by scheduled decrements (various regimens) to prevent withdrawal symptoms and permit adrenals to recover from drug-induced partial atrophy.

Alternate-Day Therapy (ADT) for Patient on Long-Term Therapy

- With ADT, the 48-h requirement for steroids is administered as a single dose every other morning.
- Be aware that ADT minimizes adverse effects associated with long term treatment while maintaining the desired therapeutic effect.

ADVERSE EFFECTS CNS: Euphoria, headache, insomnia, confusion, psychosis. **CV:** CHF, edema. **GI:** Nausea, vomiting, peptic ulcer. **Musculoskeletal:** Muscle weakness, delayed wound healing, muscle wasting, osteoporosis, aseptic necrosis of bone, spontaneous fractures. **Endocrine:** Cushingoid features, growth suppression in children, carbohydrate intolerance, hyperglycemia. **Special Senses:** Cataracts. **Hematologic:** Leukocytosis. **Metabolic:** Hypokalemia.

INTERACTIONS Drug: BARBITURATES, **phenytoin, rifampin** increase steroid metabolism—increased doses of prednisone may be needed; **amphotericin B,** DIURETICS increase **potassium** loss; **ambenonium, neostigmine, pyridostigmine** may cause severe muscle weakness in patients with myasthenia gravis; may inhibit antibody response to VACCINES, TOXOIDS.

PHARMACOKINETICS Absorption: Readily absorbed from GI tract. **Peak:** 1–2 h. **Duration:** 1–1.5 days. **Distribution:** Crosses placenta; distributed into breast milk. **Metabolism:** Metabolized in liver. **Elimination:** Hypothalamus-pituitary axis suppression: 24–36 h; excreted in urine. **Half-Life:** 3.5 h.

NURSING IMPLICATIONS

Assessment & Drug Effects

- Establish baseline and continuing data regarding BP, I&O ratio and pattern, weight, and sleep pattern. Start flowchart as reference for planning individualized pharmacotherapeutic patient care.
- Check and record BP during dose stabilization period at least 2 times daily. Report an ascending pattern.
- Monitor patient for evidence of HPA axis suppression during long-term therapy by monitoring height and weight and determining plasma cortisol levels at weekly intervals.
- Lab tests: Obtain fasting blood glucose, serum electrolytes, and routine laboratory studies at regular intervals during long-term steroid therapy.

- Be aware that patients with low serum albumin are especially susceptible to adverse effects because of excess circulating free glucocorticoids.
- Be alert to signs of hypocalcemia (see Appendix D-1). Patients with hypocalcemia have increased requirements for pyridoxine (vitamin B_6), vitamins C and D, and folates.
- Be alert to possibility of masked infection and delayed healing (anti-inflammatory and immunosuppressive actions). Prednisone suppresses early classic signs of inflammation. When patient is on an extended therapy regimen, incidence of oral *Candida* infection is high. Inspect mouth daily for symptoms: White patches, black furry tongue, painful membranes and tongue.
- Monitor bone density. Compression and spontaneous fractures of long bones and vertebrae present hazards, particularly in long-term corticosteroid treatment of rheumatoid arthritis or diabetes, and in immobilized patients.
- Be aware of previous history of psychotic tendencies. Watch for changes in mood and behavior, emotional stability, sleep pattern, or psychomotor activity, especially with long-term therapy, that may signal onset of recurrence. Report symptoms to physician.
- If a patient is receiving aspirin concomitantly with a corticosteroid, salicylism may be induced when the corticosteroid dosage is decreased or discontinued.
- Be aware that long-term corticosteroid therapy is ordinarily not interrupted when patient undergoes major surgery, but dosage may be increased.
- Monitor for withdrawal syndrome (e.g., myalgia, fever, arthralgia, malaise) and hypocorticism (e.g., anorexia, vomiting, nausea, fatigue, dizziness, hypotension, hypoglycemia, myalgia, arthralgia) with abrupt discontinuation of corticosteroids after long-term therapy.
- Avoid live virus vaccines (varicella, MMR) in patients on high-dose corticosteroid therapy.

Patient & Family Education

- Take drug as prescribed and do not alter dosing regimen or stop medication without consulting physician.
- Be aware that a slight weight gain with improved appetite is expected, but after dosage is stabilized, a sudden slow but steady weight increase (2 kg [5 lb]/wk) should be reported to physician.
- Avoid or minimize alcohol and caffeine; may contribute to steroid-ulcer development in long-term therapy.
- Do not administer live vaccines (varicella, MMR) while on high dose steroids.
- Report symptoms of GI distress to physician and do not self-medicate to find relief.
- Do not use aspirin or other OTC drugs while on this drug unless they are prescribed specifically by the physician.
- Monitor for fungal infections.
- Report slow healing, any vague feeling of being sick, or return of pretreatment symptoms.
- Be fastidious about personal hygiene; give special attention to foot care, and be particularly cautious about bruising or abrading the skin.

Common adverse effects in *italic;* life-threatening effects <u>underlined</u>; generic names in **bold**; drug classifications in SMALL CAPS; ♣ Canadian drug name; ⊘ Prototype drug.

- Report persistent backache or chest pain (possible symptoms of vertebral or rib fracture) that may occur with long-term therapy.
- Tell dentist or new physician about prednisone therapy.
- Carry medical information at all times. It needs to indicate medical diagnosis, medication(s), physician's name(s), address(es), and telephone number(s).
- Do not breast feed while taking this drug without consulting physician.
- Store this medication out of reach of children.

PRIMAQUINE PHOSPHATE
(prim'a-kween)
Primaquine
Classifications: ANTI-INFECTIVE; ANTIMALARIAL
Prototype: Chloroquine
Pregnancy Category: C

AVAILABILITY 26.3 mg tablets (15 mg base)

ACTIONS Acts on primary exoerythrocytic forms of *Plasmodium vivax* and *Plasmodium falciparum* by an incompletely known mechanism. Destroys late tissue forms of *P. vivax* and thus effects radical cure (prevents relapse).

THERAPEUTIC EFFECTS Gametocidal activity against all species of plasmodia that infect man; interrupts transmission of malaria.

USES To prevent relapse ("radical" or "clinical" cure) of *P. vivax* and *P. ovale* malarias and to prevent attacks after departure from areas where *P. vivax* and *P. ovale* malarias are endemic. With clindamycin for the treatment of *Pneumocystis carinii* pneumonia (PCP) in AIDS.

CONTRAINDICATIONS Rheumatoid arthritis; lupus erythematosus (SLE); hemolytic drugs, concomitant or recent use of agents capable of bone marrow depression (e.g., quinacrine; patients with G6PD deficiency). NADH methemoglobin reductase deficiency; pregnancy (category C), lactation.

ROUTE & DOSAGE

Malaria Relapse Prevention
Child: **PO** 0.3 mg/kg/dose once/day for 14 days concomitantly or consecutively with chloroquine or hydroxychloroquine on first 3 days of acute attack (max dose 15 mg of base/day)
Adult: **PO** 15 mg once/day for 14 days concomitantly or consecutively with chloroquine or hydroxychloroquine on first 3 days of acute attack

Malaria Prophylaxis
Child: **PO** 0.3 mg/kg once/day for 14 days beginning immediately after leaving malarious area
Adult: **PO** 15 mg once/day for 14 days beginning immediately after leaving malarious area

STORAGE
Store at 25° C (77° F) in tight, light-resistant containers.

ADMINISTRATION

Oral

- Give drug at mealtime or with an antacid (prescribed); may prevent or relieve gastric irritation. Medication has a bitter taste. Notify prescriber if GI symptoms persist.

ADVERSE EFFECTS Hematologic: <u>Hematologic reactions including granulocytopenia and acute hemolytic anemia in patients with G6PD deficiency</u>, moderate leukocytosis or leukopenia, anemia, granulocytopenia, agranulocytosis. **GI:** Nausea, vomiting, epigastric distress, abdominal cramps. **Skin:** Pruritus. **Metabolic:** Methemoglobinemia (cyanosis). **Body as a Whole:** Headache, confusion, mental depression. **Special Senses:** Disturbances of visual accommodation. **CV:** Hypertension, arrhythmias (rare).

INTERACTIONS Drug: Toxicity of both **quinacrine** and primaquine increased.

PHARMACOKINETICS Absorption: Readily absorbed from GI tract. **Peak:** 6 h. **Metabolism:** Rapidly metabolized in liver to active metabolites. **Elimination:** Excreted in urine. **Half-Life:** 3.7–9.6 h.

NURSING IMPLICATIONS

Assessment & Drug Effects

- Be aware drug may precipitate acute hemolytic anemia in patients with G6PD deficiency, an inherited error of metabolism carried on the X chromosome, present in about 10% of American black males and certain white ethnic groups: Sardinians, Sephardic Jews, Greeks, and Iranians. Whites manifest more intense expression of hemolytic reaction than do blacks. Screen for prior to initiation of therapy.
- Lab tests: Perform repeated hematologic studies (particularly blood cell counts and Hgb) and urinalyses during therapy.

Patient & Family Education

- Examine urine after each voiding and to report to physician darkening of urine, red-tinged urine, and decrease in urine volume. Also report chills, fever, precordial pain, cyanosis (all suggest a hemolytic reaction). Sudden reductions in hemoglobin or erythrocyte count suggest an impending hemolytic reaction.
- Do not breast feed while taking this drug.
- Store this medication out of reach of children.

PRIMIDONE
(pri′mi-done)
Apo-Primidone ♣, Mysoline
Classifications: CENTRAL NERVOUS SYSTEM AGENT; BARBITURATE, ANTICONVULSANT
Prototype: Phenobarbital
Pregnancy Category: D

Common adverse effects in *italic*; life-threatening effects <u>underlined</u>; generic names in **bold**; drug classifications in SMALL CAPS; ♣ Canadian drug name; ✪ Prototype drug.

AVAILABILITY 50 mg, 250 mg tablets

ACTIONS Closely related chemically to barbiturates and with similar mechanism of action. Converted in body to phenobarbital. Impairs vitamin D, calcium, folic acid, and vitamin B_{12} metabolism and utilization.
THERAPEUTIC EFFECTS Antiepileptic properties result from raising the seizure threshold and changing seizure patterns.

USES Alone or concomitantly with other anticonvulsant agents in the prophylactic management of complex partial (psychomotor) and generalized tonic-clonic (grand mal) seizures.
UNLABELED USES Essential tremor.

CONTRAINDICATIONS Hypersensitivity to barbiturates, porphyria. Safety during pregnancy (category D) or lactation is not established.
CAUTIOUS USE Chronic lung disease; liver or kidney disease; hyperactive children.

ROUTE & DOSAGE

Seizures

Neonate: **PO** 12–20 mg/kg/day in 2–4 divided doses, initial dosing at lowest levels and titrate upward
Child <8 y: **PO** Usual dose 10–25 mg/kg/day in 3–4 divided doses or intial dose of 50–125 mg/day given at bedtime, increased by 50–125 mg/day increments every 3–7 days
Child ≥8 y/Adult: **PO** Initial dosing 125–250 mg/day given at bedtime, increased by 125–250 mg/day every 3–7 days (max 2 g/day) in 3–4 divided doses)

STORAGE
Store at 15°–30° C (59°–86° F) in tightly closed container.

ADMINISTRATION

Oral
- Give whole or crush with fluid of patient's choice.
- Give with food if drug causes GI distress.
- Note: Transition from another anticonvulsant to primidone normally requires at least 21 wk.

ADVERSE EFFECTS CNS: *Drowsiness, sedation, vertigo, ataxia, headache,* excitement (children), confusion, unusual fatigue, hyperirritability, emotional disturbances, acute psychoses (usually patients with psychomotor epilepsy). **Special Senses:** Diplopia, nystagmus, swelling of eyelids. **GI:** *Nausea, vomiting, anorexia.* **Hematologic:** Leukopenia, thrombocytopenia, eosinophilia, decreased serum folate levels, megaloblastic anemia (rare). **Skin:** Alopecia, maculopapular or morbilliform rash, edema, lupus erythematosus-like syndrome. **Urogenital:** Impotence. **Body as a Whole:** Lymphadenopathy, osteomalacia. Decreased levels of vitamin K, D, B_{12}, folate.

INTERACTIONS Drug: Alcohol, CNS DEPRESSANTS compound CNS depression; **phenobarbital** may decrease absorption and increase metabolism of ORAL ANTICOAGULANTS; increases metabolism of CORTICOSTEROIDS, ORAL CONTRACEPTIVES, ANTICONVULSANTS, **digitoxin,** possibly decreasing their

---

effects; ANTIDEPRESSANTS potentiate adverse effects of primidone; **griseofulvin** decreases absorption of primidone. **Valproic acid** increases active metabolite concentration **(phenobarbital). Phenytoin** decreases primidone concentration. **Herbal: Kava-kava, valerian** may potentiate sedation. **Food:** Metabolism of vitamins K and D may be increased by this drug.

PHARMACOKINETICS Absorption: Approximately 60–80% absorbed from GI tract. **Peak:** 4 h. **Distribution:** Distributed into breast milk. **Metabolism:** Metabolized in liver to phenobarbital and PEMA. **Elimination:** Excreted in urine. **Half-Life:** Primidone 3–24 h; PEMA 24–48 h; phenobarbital 72–144 h.

NURSING IMPLICATIONS

Assessment & Drug Effects

- Lab tests: Perform baseline and periodic CBC, complete blood chemistry (q6mo), and primidone blood levels. *(**Therapeutic blood level for primidone: 5–12 mcg/mL, toxic levels >15 mcg/mL.**)*
- Monitor primidone plasma levels (concentrations of primidone >10 mcg/mL are usually associated with significant ataxia and lethargy).
- Therapeutic response may not be evident for several weeks.
- Observe for S&S of folic acid deficiency: Mental dysfunction, psychiatric disorders, neuropathy, megaloblastic anemia. Determine serum folate levels if indicated.
- Be aware that presence of unusual drowsiness in breast-fed newborns of primidone-treated mothers is an indication to discontinue breast feeding.

Patient & Family Education

- Avoid driving and other potentially hazardous activities during beginning of treatment because drowsiness, dizziness, and ataxia may be severe. Symptoms tend to disappear with continued therapy; if they persist, dosage reduction or drug withdrawal may be necessary.
- Avoid alcohol and other CNS depressants unless otherwise directed by physician.
- Do not take OTC medications unless approved by physician.
- Pregnant women should receive prophylactic vitamin K therapy for 1 mo prior to and during delivery to prevent neonatal hemorrhage.
- Withdraw primidone gradually to avoid precipitating status epilepticus.
- Carry medical information at all times. It needs to indicate medical diagnosis, medication(s), physician's name(s), address(es), and telephone number(s).
- Do not breast feed while taking this drug without consulting physician.
- Store this medication out of reach of children.

PROBENECID

(proe-ben'e-sid)

Benemid, Benuryl ♣ , Probalan, SK-Probenecid

Classifications: ANTIGOUT AGENT; SULFONAMIDE; URICOSURIC AGENT
Prototype: Colchicine
Pregnancy Category: B

Common adverse effects in *italic;* life-threatening effects <u>underlined;</u> generic names in **bold;** drug classifications in SMALL CAPS; ♣ Canadian drug name; ❍ Prototype drug.

AVAILABILITY 0.5 g tablet

ACTIONS Sulfonamide-derivative renal tubular blocking agent. In sufficiently high doses, competitively inhibits renal tubular reabsorption of uric acid, thereby promoting its excretion and reducing serum urate levels.

THERAPEUTIC EFFECTS Prevents formation of new tophaceous deposits and causes gradual shrinking of old tophi by preventing uric acid buildup in the serum and tissues. As an additive to penicillin, it increases the serum concentration of the antibiotic, and also prolongs the serum concentration of the penicillins.

USES Hyperuricemia in chronic gouty arthritis and tophaceous gout.

UNLABELED USES Adjuvant to therapy with penicillin G and penicillin analogs to elevate and prolong plasma concentrations of these antibiotics; to promote uric acid excretion in hyperuricemia secondary to administration of thiazides and related diuretics, furosemide, ethacrynic acid, pyrazinamide.

CONTRAINDICATIONS Blood dyscrasias; uric acid kidney stones; during or within 2–3 wk of acute gouty attack; over excretion of uric acid (>1000 mg/day); patients with creatinine clearance <50 mg/min; use with penicillin in presence of known renal impairment; use for hyperuricemia secondary to cancer chemotherapy. Safety during pregnancy (category B), lactation, or in children <2 y is not established.

CAUTIOUS USE History of peptic ulcer.

ROUTE & DOSAGE

Gout

Adult: **PO** 250 mg b.i.d. for 1 wk, then 500 mg b.i.d. (max 3 g/day)

Adjunct for Penicillin or Cephalosporin Therapy

Child: **PO** 2–14 y or <50 kg, 25 mg/kg/times 1, then 40 mg/kg/day in 4 divided doses (max 500 mg/dose)

Child >50 kg/Adult: **PO** 500 mg q.i.d. or 1 g with single-dose therapy (e.g., gonorrhea)

STORAGE
Store at 15°–30° C (59°–86° F) in tightly closed container.

ADMINISTRATION

Oral

- Therapy is usually not initiated during an acute gouty attack. Consult prescriber.
- Minimize GI adverse effects by giving after meals, with food, milk, or antacid (prescribed). If symptoms persist, dosage reduction may be required.
- Give with a full glass of water or generous amount appropriate for age, if not contraindicated.
- Be aware that physician may prescribe concurrent prophylactic doses of colchicine for first 3–6 mo of therapy because frequency of acute gouty attacks may increase during first 6–12 mo of therapy.

ADVERSE EFFECTS Body as a Whole: Flushing, dizziness, fever, anaphylaxis. **CNS:** *Headache.* **GI:** *Nausea, vomiting, anorexia,* sore gums, hepatic necrosis (rare). **Urogenital:** Urinary frequency. **Hematologic:** Anemia, hemolytic anemia (possibly related to G6PD deficiency), aplastic anemia (rare). **Musculoskeletal:** Exacerbations of gout, uric acid kidney stones. **Skin:** Dermatitis, pruritus. **Respiratory:** Respiratory depression.

DIAGNOSTIC TEST INTERFERENCE False-positive results *urine glucose* tests are possible with *Benedict's solution* or *Clinitest* (*glucose oxidase methods* not affected, e.g., *Clinistix, TesTape*).

INTERACTIONS Drug: SALICYLATES may decrease uricosuric activity; may decrease **methotrexate** elimination, causing increased toxicity; decreases **nitrofurantoin** efficacy and increases its toxicity.

PHARMACOKINETICS Absorption: Readily absorbed from GI tract. **Onset:** 30 min. **Peak:** 2–4 h. **Duration:** 8 h. **Distribution:** Crosses placenta. **Metabolism:** Metabolized in liver. **Elimination:** Excreted in urine. **Half-Life:** 4–17 h.

NURSING IMPLICATIONS

Assessment & Drug Effects

- Decrease daily dosage with caution by 0.5 g q6mo to lowest effective dosage that maintains stable serum urate levels when gouty attacks have been absent for 6 mo or more and serum urate levels are controlled.
- Lab tests: Periodic serum urate levels, Hct and Hgb, and urinalysis. Determine acid–base balance periodically when urinary alkalinizers are used. Some prescribers prescribe acetazolamide at bedtime to keep urine alkaline and dilute throughout night.
- Patients taking sulfonylureas may require dosage adjustment. Probenecid enhances hypoglycemic actions of these drugs (see DIAGNOSTIC TEST INTERFERENCE).
- With gout expect urate tophaceous deposits to decrease in size. Classic locations are in cartilage of ear pinna and big toe, but they can occur in bursae, tendons, skin, kidneys, and other tissues.

Patient & Family Education

- Drink fluid liberally (approximately 3000 mL/day) to maintain daily urinary output of at least 2000 mL or more. Child should be hydrated according to age level and maintain normal urine outputs for that age group. This is important because increased uric acid excretion promoted by drug predisposes to renal calculi.
- Prescriber may advise restriction of high-purine foods during early therapy until uric acid level stabilizes. Foods high in purine include organ meats (sweetbreads, liver, kidney), meat extracts, meat soups, gravy, anchovies, and sardines. Moderate amounts are present in other meats, fish, seafood, asparagus, spinach, peas, dried legumes, wild game.
- Avoid alcohol because it may increase serum urate levels.

- Do not stop taking drug without consulting prescriber. Irregular dosage schedule may sharply elevate serum urate level and precipitate acute gout.
- Be aware that lifelong therapy is usually required in patients with symptomatic hyperuricemia. Keep scheduled appointments with physician and for kidney function and hematology lab work.
- Report symptoms of hypersensitivity to prescriber. Discontinuation of drug is indicated.
- Do not take aspirin or other OTC medications while on this drug without consulting prescriber. If a mild analgesic is required, acetaminophen is usually allowed.
- Do not breast feed while taking this drug without consulting prescriber.
- Store this medication out of reach of children.

PROCAINAMIDE HYDROCHLORIDE ⊕

(proe-kane-a′mide)
Procan, Procanbid, Pronestyl, Pronestyl SR
Classifications: CARDIOVASCULAR AGENT; ANTIARRHYTHMIC, CLASS IA
Pregnancy Category: C

AVAILABILITY 250 mg, 375 mg, 500 mg tablets, capsules; 250 mg, 500 mg, 750 mg, 1000 mg extended-release tablets; 100 mg/mL (contains benzyl alcohol and bisulfites), 500 mg/mL injection

ACTIONS Amide analog of procaine hydrochloride with cardiac actions similar to those of quinine. Class IA antiarrhythmic agent. Depresses excitability of myocardium to electrical stimulation, reduces conduction velocity in atria, ventricles, and His-Purkinje system. Increases duration of refractory period, especially in the atria.
THERAPEUTIC EFFECTS Produces slight change in contractility of cardiac muscle and cardiac output; suppresses automaticity of His-Purkinje ventricular muscle. Produces peripheral vasodilation and hypotension, especially with IV use.

USES Prophylactically to maintain normal sinus rhythm following conversion of atrial flutter or fibrillation by other methods. Also to prevent recurrence of paroxysmal atrial fibrillation and tachycardia, paroxysmal AV junctional rhythm, ventricular tachycardia, ventricular and atrial premature contractions. Also cardiac arrhythmias associated with surgery and anesthesia.
UNLABELED USES Malignant hyperthermia.

CONTRAINDICATIONS Myasthenia gravis; hypersensitivity to procainamide or procaine; blood dyscrasias; complete AV block, second- and third-degree AV block unassisted by pacemaker.
CAUTIOUS USE Patient who has undergone electrical conversion to sinus rhythm; hypotension, cardiac enlargement, CHF, MI, coronary occlusion, ventricular dysrhythmia from digitalis intoxication; hepatic or renal insufficiency; electrolyte imbalance; bronchial asthma; history of SLE. Safety during pregnancy (category C) or lactation is not established.

ROUTE & DOSAGE

Arrhythmias

Child: **PO** 15–50 mg/kg/day divided q3–6h (max dose 4g/day) **IM** 20–30 mg/kg/day divided q4–6h (max dose 4g/day) **IV Loading Dose** 3–6 mg/kg/dose over 5 min (max 100 mg/dose), then may repeat every 5–10 min as necessary to maximum dose of 15 mg/kg; do not exceed 500 mg in 30 min then maintenance IV of 0.02–0.08 mg/kg/min (20–80 mcg/kg/min) continuous infusion (max dose is 2 g/day)

Adult: **PO** 1 g followed by 250–500 mg q3h or 500 mg–1 g q6h sustained-release (b.i.d. for Procanbid) or 50 mg/kg/day in divided doses every 6 h **IM** 0.5–1 g q4–6h until able to take PO **IV** 50–100 mg/dose q5min at a rate of 25–50 mg/min until arrhythmia is controlled or 1 g given, then maintenance of 2–6 mg/min continous infusion

STORAGE

Store solution for up to 24 h at 15°–30° C (59°–86° F) and for 7 days under refrigeration at 2°–8° C (36°–46° F). Slight yellowing does not alter drug potency, but discard solution if it is markedly discolored or precipitated.

ADMINISTRATION

Oral

- Give first PO dose at least 4 h after last IV dose.
- Give oral preparation on empty stomach, 1 h before or 2 h after meals, with a full glass of water to enhance absorption. If drug causes gastric distress, give with food.
- Crush immediate-release (but NOT sustained-release) tablet if patient is unable to swallow it whole.
- Swallow sustained-release tablet whole. It has a wax matrix that is not absorbed but appears in the stool.
- Your pharmacy can compound liquid preparations from capsules.

Intramuscular

- Assess procainamide blood levels if more than three IM injections are required.

Intravenous

- Use IV route for emergency situations.

***PREPARE* Direct:** When given direct IV, dilute each 100 mg with 5–10 mL of D5W or sterile water for injection. **IV Infusion:** When given by IV infusion, add 1 g of procainamide to 250–500 mL of D5W solution to yield 4 mg/mL in 250 mL or 2 mg/mL in 500 mL. The 100 mg/mL preparation contains benzyl alcohol, which has been associated with neonatal "gasping syndrome" (see Physiological Considerations section in Part I for more information).

***ADMINISTER* Direct:** Usual rate 20 mg/min. Do not exceed 30 mg/min in children. Faster rates (up to 50 mg/min) in adults should be used with caution. Fast rates cause severe hypotension. **IV Infusion:** Child, maintenance of 0.02–0.08 mg/kg/min; adult, 2–6 mg/min.

***INCOMPATIBILITIES* Solution/Additive:** Bretylium, esmolol, ethacrynate, milrinone. **Y-Site:** Inamrinone (amrinone).

Common adverse effects in *italic*; life-threatening effects underlined; generic names in **bold**; drug classifications in SMALL CAPS; ♣ Canadian drug name; ◐ Prototype drug.

- Control IV administration over several hours by assessment of procainamide plasma levels. ■ Use an infusion pump with constant monitoring. Keep patient in supine position. Be alert to signs of too rapid administration of drug (speed shock: Irregular pulse, tight feeling in chest, flushed face, headache, loss of consciousness, shock, cardiac arrest).

ADVERSE EFFECTS CNS: Dizziness, psychosis. **CV:** Severe hypotension, pericarditis, <u>ventricular fibrillation</u>, AV block, tachycardia, flushing. **GI:** Bitter taste, nausea, vomiting, diarrhea, anorexia, (all mostly PO). **Hematologic:** <u>Agranulocytosis with repeated use</u>; thrombocytopenia. **Body as a Whole:** Fever, muscle and joint pain, angioneurotic edema, myalgia, *SLE-like syndrome (50% of patients on large doses for 1 y):* Polyarthralgias, pleuritic pain, pleural effusion. **Skin:** Maculopapular rash, pruritus, erythema, skin rash.

DIAGNOSTIC TEST INTERFERENCE Procainamide increases the plasma levels of ***alkaline phosphatase, bilirubin, lactic dehydrogenase*** and ***AST.*** It may also alter results of the ***edrophonium test.***

INTERACTIONS Drug: Other ANTIARRHYTHMICS add to therapeutic and toxic effects; ANTICHOLINERGIC AGENTS compound anticholinergic effects; ANTIHYPERTENSIVES add to hypotensive effects; **cimetidine** may increase procainamide and NAPA levels with increase in toxicity. **Food:** High-fat meals may increase absorption of extended release tablets.

PHARMACOKINETICS Absorption: 75–95% absorbed from GI tract. **Peak:** 15–60 min IM; 30–60 min PO. **Duration:** 3 h; 8 h with sustained release. **Distribution:** Distributed to CSF, liver, spleen, kidney, brain, and heart; crosses placenta; distributed into breast milk. **Metabolism:** Metabolized in liver to N-acetylprocainamide (NAPA), an active metabolite (30–60% metabolized to NAPA). **Elimination:** Excreted in urine. **Half-Life:** Procainamide 3 h; NAPA 6 h.

P

NURSING IMPLICATIONS

Assessment & Drug Effects

- Check apical radial pulses before each dose during period of adjustment to the oral route.
- Patients with severe heart, liver, or kidney disease and hypotension are at particular risk for adverse effects.
- Monitor the patient's ECG and BP continuously during IV drug administration.
- Discontinue IV drug temporarily when (1) arrhythmia is interrupted, (2) severe toxic effects are present, (3) QRS complex is excessively widened (greater than 50%), (4) PR interval is prolonged, or (5) BP drops 15 mm Hg or more. Obtain rhythm strip and notify physician.
- Ventricular dysrhythmias are usually abolished within a few minutes after IV dose and within an hour after PO or IM administration.
- Report promptly complaints of chest pain, dyspnea, and anxiety. Digitalization may have preceded procainamide in patients with atrial arrhythmias. Cardiotonic glycosides may induce sufficient increase in

atrial contraction to dislodge atrial mural emboli, with subsequent pulmonary embolism.

- Therapeutic procainamide blood levels are reached in approximately 24 h if kidney function is normal but are delayed in presence of renal impairment. ***Therapeutic Levels: 30–100 ng/mL.***

Patient & Family Education

- Keep a record of weekly weight. Notify physician if weight gain of 1 kg (2 lb) or more is accompanied by local edema. Consult physician for weight gain limits for infants and children.
- Record and report date, time, and duration of fibrillation episodes when taking maintenance doses: Light-headedness, giddiness, weakness, or faintness. Report any bruising or bleeding to physician.
- Keep a record of pulse rates. Report to physician changes in rate or quality.
- Report to physician signs of reduced procainamide control: Weakness, irregular pulse, unexplained fatigability, anxiety.
- Do not double dose or change an interval because a previous dose was missed. Take procainamide at evenly spaced intervals around the clock unless otherwise prescribed.
- Do not breast feed while taking this drug without consulting physician.
- Store this medication out of reach of children.

PROCARBAZINE HYDROCHLORIDE

(proe-kar′ba-zeen)
Matulane, Natulan ♣
Classifications: ANTINEOPLASTIC; ANTIMETABOLITE
Prototype: Fluorouracil
Pregnancy Category: D

AVAILABILITY 50 mg capsules

ACTIONS Hydrazine derivative with antimetabolite properties; cell-cycle specific for the S phase of cell division. Precise mechanism of action unknown. Suppresses mitosis at interphase, and causes chromatin derangement.

THERAPEUTIC EFFECTS Highly toxic to rapidly proliferating tissue. Has immunosuppressive properties and exhibits MAO inhibition activity. May delay myelosuppression. Reportedly does not affect survival time but may produce remissions of at least 1-mo duration.

USES Adjunct in palliative treatment of Hodgkin's disease.
UNLABELED USES Solid tumors.

CONTRAINDICATIONS Myelosuppression; alcohol ingestion; foods high in tyramine content; sympathomimetic drugs. MAO inhibitors should be discontinued 14 days prior to therapy; tricyclic antidepressants, 7 days before therapy. Safety during pregnancy (category D) or lactation is not established.
CAUTIOUS USE Concomitant administration with CNS depressants; hepatic or renal impairment; following radiation or chemotherapy before at least 1 mo has elapsed; hepatic and renal impairment; infection; diabetes mellitus.

ROUTE & DOSAGE

Adjunct for Hodgkin's Disease

Child: PO 50 mg/m^2/day in single or divided doses for 1 wk, then 100 mg/m^2/day until WBC is <4000/mm^3 or platelets are <100,000/mm^3 or maximum response obtained; drug is then discontinued until bone marrow recovery is satisfactory; treatment is started again at 50 mg/m^2/day

Adult: PO 2–4 mg/kg/day in single or divided doses for 1 wk, then 4–6 mg/kg/day until WBC <4000/mm^3 or platelets are <100,000/mm^3 or maximum response obtained; drug is then discontinued until bone marrow recovery is satisfactory; treatment is started again at 1–2 mg/kg/day

STORAGE

Store at 15°–30° C (59°–86° F) in tightly closed, light resistant-container. Protect from freezing, moisture, and light.

ADMINISTRATION

Oral

- Must be given under care and direction of pediatric oncology specialist. Use recommended handling techniques for hazardous medications (see Part I).
- Do not give if WBC count <4000/mm^3 or platelet count <100,000/mm^3. Consult physician.
- To decrease GI toxicity, give with meals or food.

ADVERSE EFFECTS CNS: Myalgia, arthralgia, paresthesias, weakness, fatigue, lethargy, drowsiness, neuropathies, mental depression, acute psychosis, hallucinations, dizziness, headache, ataxia, nervousness, insomnia, coma, confusion, seizures. **GI:** *Severe nausea and vomiting,* anorexia, stomatitis, dry mouth, dysphagia, diarrhea, constipation, jaundice, ascites. **Hematologic:** Bone marrow suppression (leukopenia, anemia, thrombocytopenia), hemolysis, bleeding tendencies. **Skin:** Dermatitis, pruritus, herpes, hyperpigmentation, flushing, alopecia. **Respiratory:** *Pleural effusion, cough,* hoarseness. **CV:** Hypotension, tachycardia. **Body as a Whole:** Chills, fever, sweating, photosensitivity; intercurrent infections. **Urogenital:** Gynecomastia, depressed spermatogenesis, atrophy of testes.

DIAGNOSTIC TEST INTERFERENCE Procarbazine may enhance the effects of ***CNS depressants.*** A disulfiram-like reaction may occur following ingestion of ***alcohol.***

INTERACTIONS Drug: **Alcohol,** PHENOTHIAZINES, and other **CNS depressants** add to CNS depression; TRICYCLIC ANTIDEPRESSANTS, MAO INHIBITORS, SYMPATHOMIMETICS, **ephedrine, phenylpropanolamine** may precipitate hypertensive crisis, hyperpyrexia; seizures, or death. **Food: Tyramine**-containing foods may precipitate hypertensive crisis [see **phenelzine sulfate** (MAO INHIBITOR)].

PHARMACOKINETICS Absorption: Readily absorbed from GI tract. **Peak:** 1 h. **Distribution:** Widely distributed with high concentrations in liver, kidneys, intestinal wall, and skin. **Metabolism:** Metabolized in liver. **Elimination:** Excreted in urine. **Half-Life:** 1 h.

NURSING IMPLICATIONS

Assessment & Drug Effects

- Start flow sheet and record baseline BP, weight, temperature, pulse, and I&O ratio and pattern.
- Be alert for and report signs of infection such as respiratory infections, aching, rashes, gastrointestinal distress, etc. Assess immunization status prior to beginning therapy in order to be alert for diseases that pose risk.
- Lab tests: Determine hematologic status (Hgb, Hct, WBC, differential, reticulocyte, and platelet counts) initially and at least every 3–4 days. Hepatic and renal studies (transaminase, alkaline phosphatase, BUN, urinalysis) are also indicated initially and at least weekly during therapy.
- Protect patient from exposure to infection and trauma when nadir of leukopenia (<4000/mm^3) is approached. Note and report changes in voiding pattern, hematuria, and dysuria (possible signs of urinary tract infection). Monitor I&O ratio and temperature closely.
- Withhold drug and notify physician of any of the following: CNS S&S (e.g., paresthesias, neuropathies, confusion); leukopenia (WBC count <4000/mm^3); thrombocytopenia (platelet count <100,000/mm^3); hypersensitivity reaction, the first small ulceration or persistent spot of soreness in oral cavity, diarrhea, and bleeding.
- Monitor for and report any of the following: Chills, fever, weakness, shortness of breath, productive cough, oral candiadiasis. Drug will be discontinued.
- Assess for signs of liver dysfunction: Jaundice (yellow skin, sclerae, and soft palate), frothy or dark urine, clay-colored stools.
- Tolerance to nausea and vomiting (most common adverse effects) usually develops by end of first week of treatment. Doses are kept at a minimum during this time. If vomiting persists, therapy will be interrupted.

Patient & Family Education

- Avoid exposure to persons with infectious diseases. Report signs of infection.
- Avoid OTC nose drops, cough medicines, and antiobesity preparations containing sympathomimetic drugs (e.g., ephedrine, amphetamine, epinephrine) and tricyclic antidepressants because they may cause hypertensive crises since procarbazine has MAO inhibitory activity. Do not use OTC preparations while on this drug without physician's approval.
- Report to physician any sign of impending infection.
- Do not eat foods high in tyramine content (e.g., aged cheese, beer, wine).
- Avoid alcohol; ingestion of any form of alcohol may precipitate a disulfiram-type reaction (see Appendix D-1).
- Report to physician immediately signs of hemorrhagic tendencies: Bleeding into skin and mucosa, epistaxis, hemoptysis, hematemesis, hematuria, melena, ecchymoses, petechiae. Bone marrow depression often occurs 2–8 wk after start of therapy.

Common adverse effects in *italic*; life-threatening effects underlined; generic names in **bold**; drug classifications in SMALL CAPS; ♣ Canadian drug name; ⊘ Prototype drug.

- Avoid excessive exposure to the sun because of potential photosensitivity reaction: Cover as much skin area as possible with clothing, and use sunscreen lotion (SPF >12) on all exposed skin surfaces.
- Use caution while driving or performing hazardous tasks until response to drug is known since drowsiness, dizziness, and blurred vision are possible adverse effects.
- Use contraceptive measures during procarbazine therapy.
- Do not breast feed while taking this drug without consulting physician.
- Store this medication out of reach of children.

PROCHLORPERAZINE 🅟
(proe-klor-per′a-zeen)
Compazine

PROCHLORPERAZINE EDISYLATE
Compazine

PROCHLORPERAZINE MALEATE
Compazine, Stemetil ♣

Classifications: PSYCHOTHERAPEUTIC; ANTIPSYCHOTIC PHENOTHIAZINE; GASTROINTESTINAL AGENT; ANTIEMETIC
Pregnancy Category: C

AVAILABILITY 5 mg, 10 mg, 25 mg tablets; 10 mg, 15 mg, 30 mg sustained-release capsule; 2.5 mg, 5 mg, 25 mg suppositories; 5 mg/mL injection **Edisylate** 5 mg/5 mL syrup, 5 mg/mL injection (contains benzyl alcohol)

ACTIONS Phenothiazine derivative similar to chlorpromazine. Mechanism that produces strong antipsychotic effects is unclear, but thought to be related to blockade of postsynaptic dopamine receptors in the brain. Action on the hypothalamus and reticular formation results in sedative effects. Antiemetic effect is produced by suppression of the chemoreceptor trigger zone (CTZ).
THERAPEUTIC EFFECTS Inhibits dopamine reuptake; may be basis for moderate extrapyramidal symptoms. Greater extrapyramidal effects and antiemetic potency but fewer sedative, hypotensive, and anticholinergic effects than chlorpromazine.

USES Management of manifestations of psychotic disorders, of excessive anxiety, tension, and agitation, and to control severe nausea and vomiting.

CONTRAINDICATIONS Hypersensitivity to phenothiazines (cross-sensitivity may exist); bone marrow depression; comatose or severely depressed states; children <9 kg (20 lb) or 2 y of age; pediatric surgery; short-term vomiting in children or vomiting of unknown etiology; Reye's syndrome or other encephalopathies; history of dyskinetic reactions or epilepsy; pregnancy (category C), lactation.
CAUTIOUS USE Patient with previously diagnosed breast cancer, children <5 y and those with acute illness or dehydration.

ROUTE & DOSAGE

Severe Nausea, Vomiting, Anxiety, Psychotic Disorders

Note: Use lowest possible doses in children.

Child: **PO/Rectal** >*10 kg,* 0.4 mg/kg/day in 3–4 equally divided doses or >*10 kg,* 2.5 mg q12–24h (max 7.5 mg/day); *15–18 kg,* 2.5 mg q8–12h (max 10 mg/day); *19–39 kg,* 2.5 mg q8h or 5 mg q12h (max 15 mg/day) **IM** 0.13 mg/kg/dose, switching to oral as soon as possible

Adult: **PO** 5–10 mg t.i.d. or q.i.d.; sustained release: 10 mg q12h or 15 mg daily **IM** 5–10 mg q3–4h up to 40 mg/day **IV** 2.5–10 mg q6–8h (max 10 mg/dose or 40 mg/day) **PR** 25 mg b.i.d.

STORAGE

Store at 15°–30° C (59°–86° F) in tightly closed, light-resistant container. Discard markedly discolored solutions; slight yellowing does not appear to alter potency.

ADMINISTRATION

Oral

- Dosages for emaciated patients and children should be increased slowly. Can give with food.
- Ensure that sustained-release form is not chewed or crushed. Must be swallowed whole.
- Do not give oral concentrate to children.
- Avoid skin contact with oral concentrate or injection solution because of possibility of contact dermatitis.

Intramuscular

- Do not inject drug SC.
- Make injection deep into the upper outer quadrant of the buttock in adults. Follow agency policy regarding IM injection site for children and see Techniques of Administration in Part I for site selections.

Intravenous

PREPARE Direct: Dilute each 5 mg (1 mL) in 4 mL of NS or other compatible solution to yield 1 mg/mL. **IV Infusion:** Dilute in 50–100 mL of D5W, NS, D5/0.45% NaCl, RL or other compatible solution.

ADMINISTER Direct: IV route not recommended for children. Do not exceed 10 mg for a single dose. Do not give a bolus dose. Give at a maximum rate of 5 mg/min. **IV Infusion:** Give over 15–30 min. Do not exceed direct IV rate.

INCOMPATIBILITIES Solution/Additive: Aminophylline, amphotericin B, ampicillin, calcium gluceptate, calcium gluconate, cephalothin, chloramphenicol, chlorothiazide, dimenhydrinate, furosemide, hydrocortisone, ketorolac, methohexital, midazolam, morphine, penicillin G sodium, pentobarbital, phenobarbital, sodium bicarbonate, dimenhydrinate, hydromorphone, thiopental. Y-Site: Aldesleukin, allopurinol, amifostine, amphotericin B cholesteryl complex, aztreonam, cefepime, etoposide, fludarabine, foscarnet, filgrastim, piperacillin-tazobactam.

ADVERSE EFFECTS CNS: *Drowsiness,* dizziness, *extrapyramidal reactions which are more common in children (akathisia, dystonia or parkinsonism),* persistent tardive dyskinesia, acute catatonia. **CV:** Hypotension. **GI:** Cholestatic jaundice. **Skin:** Contact dermatitis, photosensitivity. **Endocrine:** Galactorrhea, amenorrhea. **Special Senses:** Blurred vision. **Hematologic:** Leukopenia, agranulocytosis.

DIAGNOSTIC TEST INTERFERENCE Test for phenylketonuria gives false positive.

INTERACTIONS Drug: Alcohol, CNS DEPRESSANTS increase CNS depression; ANTACIDS, ANTIDIARRHEALS decrease absorption, therefore, administer 2 h apart; **phenobarbital** increases metabolism of prochlorperazine; GENERAL ANESTHETICS increase excitation and hypotension; antagonizes antihypertensive action of **guanethidine; phenylpropanolamine** poses possibility of sudden death; **propranolol** and chloroquine may increase concentrations. Inhibits the ability of bromocriptine to lower prolactin concentrations. Anticholinergics may decrease response to prochlorperazine; TRICYCLIC ANTIDEPRESSANTS intensify hypotensive and anticholinergic effects; decreases seizure threshold—ANTICONVULSANT dosage may need to be increased. **Herbal: Kava-kava** may increase risk and severity of dystonic reactions.

PHARMACOKINETICS Absorption: Readily absorbed from GI tract. **Onset:** 30–40 min PO; 60 min PR; 10–20 min IM. **Duration:** 3–4 h PO; 10–12 h sustained release PO; 3–4 h PR; up to 12 h IM. **Distribution:** Crosses placenta; distributed into breast milk. **Metabolism:** Metabolized in liver. **Elimination:** Excreted in urine.

NURSING IMPLICATIONS

Assessment & Drug Effects

- Position nauseated patients who have received prochlorperazine carefully to prevent aspiration of vomitus; may have depressed cough reflex.
- Most emaciated patients and children, especially those with dehydration or acute illness, appear to be particularly susceptible to extrapyramidal effects. Be alert to onset of symptoms: Early in therapy watch for pseudoparkinson's and acute dyskinesia. After 1–2 mo, be alert to akathisia.
- Keep in mind that the antiemetic effect may mask toxicity of other drugs or make it difficult to diagnose conditions with a primary symptom of nausea, such as intestinal obstruction and increased intracranial pressure.
- Lab tests: Periodic CBC with differential in long-term therapy.
- Be alert to signs of high core temperature: Red, dry, hot skin; full bounding pulse; dilated pupils; dyspnea; confusion; temperature over 40.6° C (105° F); elevated BP. Exposure to high environmental temperature, to sun's rays, or to a high fever associated with serious illness places this patient at risk for heat stroke. Inform physician and institute measures to reduce body temperature rapidly.

Patient & Family Education

- Take drug only as prescribed and do not alter dose or schedule. Consult prescriber before stopping the medication.

- Avoid hazardous activities such as biking, skating, sports, and driving a car until response to drug is known because drug may impair mental and physical abilities, especially during first few days of therapy.
- Be aware that drug may color urine reddish brown. It also may cause the sun-exposed skin to turn gray-blue.
- Protect skin from tanning booths, sunlamps and direct sun's rays and use a sunscreen lotion (SPF >12) to prevent photosensitivity reaction.
- Withhold dose and report to the prescriber if the following symptoms persist more than a few hours: Tremor, involuntary twitching, exaggerated restlessness. Other reportable symptoms include light-colored stools, changes in vision, sore throat, fever, rash.
- Do not breast feed while taking this drug.
- Store this medication out of reach of children.

PROMETHAZINE HYDROCHLORIDE
(proe-meth'a-zeen)
Histantil ✦, Pentazine, Phenazine, Phencen, Phenergan, Phenoject-50, Prometh, Prorex, Prothazine, V-Gan
Classifications: GASTROINTESTINAL AGENT; ANTIEMETIC; ANTIVERTIGO AGENT; PHENOTHIAZINE
Prototype: Prochlorperazine
Pregnancy Category: C

AVAILABILITY 12.5 mg, 25 mg, 50 mg tablets; 6.25 mg/5 mL (contains alcohol), 25 mg/5 mL syrup (contains alcohol); 12.5 mg, 25 mg, 50 mg suppositories; 25 mg/mL, 50 mg/mL injection

ACTIONS Long-acting derivative of phenothiazine with marked antihistamine activity and prominent sedative, amnesic, antiemetic, and anti-motion-sickness actions. Unlike other phenothiazine derivatives, relatively free of extrapyramidal adverse effects; however, in high doses it carries same potential for toxicity.
THERAPEUTIC EFFECTS In common with other antihistamines, exerts antiserotonin, anticholinergic, and local anesthetic action. Antiemetic action thought to be due to depression of CTZ in medulla.

USES Symptomatic relief of various allergic conditions, to ameliorate and prevent reactions to blood and plasma, and in prophylaxis and treatment of motion sickness, nausea, and vomiting. Preoperative, postoperative, and obstetric sedation and as adjunct to analgesics for control of pain.

CONTRAINDICATIONS Hypersensitivity to phenothiazines; narrow-angle glaucoma; stenosing peptic ulcer, pyloroduodenal obstruction; prostatic hypertrophy; bladder neck obstruction; epilepsy; bone marrow depression; comatose or severely depressed states; pregnancy (category C), lactation, neonates or premature infants, acutely ill or dehydrated children.
CAUTIOUS USE Impaired liver function; cardiovascular disease; asthma; acute or chronic respiratory impairment (particularly in children, asthma); hypertension; or debilitated patients; children with vomiting of unknown origin, acutely ill, dehydration, suspected Reye Syndrome, seizures, and family history of SIDS and sleep apnea.

ROUTE & DOSAGE

Motion Sickness

Child: **PO/PR** >2 y, 0.5 mg/kg 30 min–1 h before travel repeat q12h as needed (max dose 25 mg)
Adult: **PO/PR** 25 mg b.i.d. as needed, 30 min–1 h before travel

Nausea

Child: **PO/PR/IM/IV** >2 y, 0.25–0.5 mg/kg q4–6h prn (maximum dose 25 mg)
Adult: **PO/PR/IM/IV:** 12.5–25 mg q4–6h prn

Allergies

Child: **PO/PR/IM/IV** >2 y, 0.1 mg/kg/dose (max dose 12.5 mg) every 6 h and 0.5 mg/kg/dose at bedtime as needed (max dose 25 mg)
Adult: **PO/PR/IM/IV** 12.5 mg t.i.d. and 25 mg at bedtime

Sedation

Child: **PO/PR/IM/IV** >2 y, 0.5–1 mg/kg/dose (maximum dose 25 mg) preoperatively or bedtime
Adult: **PO/PR/IM/IV** 25–50 mg preoperatively or bedtime

STORAGE

Store at 15°–30° C (59°–86° F) in tightly closed, light resistant container.

ADMINISTRATION

Oral

- Giving with food, milk, or a full glass of water may minimize GI distress.
- Tablets may be crushed and mixed with water or food before swallowing.
- Oral doses for allergy are generally prescribed before meals and on retiring or as single dose at bedtime.

Intramuscular

- Give IM injection deep into large muscle mass appropriate for age (see Part I). Aspirate carefully before injecting drug. Intra-arterial injection can cause arterial or arteriolar spasm, with resultant gangrene. Subcutaneous injection (also contraindicated) can cause chemical irritation and necrosis. Rotate injection sites and observe daily.
- ***Incompatibilities*** when mixed in same syringe: Atropine, chlorpromazine, diphenhydramine, droperidol, fentanyl, glycopyrrolate, hydromorphone, hydroxyzine, hydrochloride, meperidine, midazolam, nalbuphine, pentazocine, prochlorperazine, scopolamine.

Intravenous

***PREPARE* Direct:** Concentrations of 25 mg/mL or less may be given undiluted. Dilute more concentrated preparations in NS to yield no more than 25 mg/mL (e.g., diluting the 50 mg/mL concentration in 9 mL yields 5 mg/mL). ■ Avoid IV administration in children. Inspect parenteral drug before preparation. Discard if it is darkened or contains precipitate.
***ADMINISTER* Direct:** Give each 25 mg over at least 1 min. Avoid extravasation; drug is a chemical irritant that can lead to necrosis.

Common adverse effects in *italic;* life-threatening effects <u>underlined</u>; generic names in **bold**; drug classifications in small caps; ♣ Canadian drug name; ❷ Prototype drug.

INCOMPATIBILITIES **Solution/Additive:** Aminophylline, carbenicillin, cefotetan, chloramphenicol, chlorothiazide, heparin, hydrocortisone, methicillin, methohexital, penicillin G sodium, pentobarbital, phenobarbital, thiopental, diatrizoate, dimenhydrinate, iodipamide, iothalamate, nalbuphine. **Y-Site:** Aldesleukin, allopurinol, amphotericin B cholesteryl complex, cefepime, cefoperazone, cefotetan, doxorubicin liposome, foscarnet, heparin, methotrexate.

ADVERSE EFFECTS Body as a Whole: Deep sleep, coma, convulsions, cardiorespiratory symptoms, extrapyramidal reactions, nightmares (in children), CNS stimulation, abnormal movements. **Respiratory:** Irregular respirations, <u>respiratory depression</u>. **CNS:** Sedation *drowsiness*, confusion, dizziness, disturbed coordination, restlessness, tremors. **CV:** Transient mild hypotension or hypertension. **GI:** Anorexia, nausea, vomiting, constipation. **Hematologic:** Leukopenia, <u>agranulocytosis</u>. **Special Senses:** *Blurred vision, dry mouth,* nose, or throat. **Skin:** Photosensitivity. **Urogenital:** Urinary retention.

DIAGNOSTIC TEST INTERFERENCE Promethazine may interfere with *blood grouping in ABO system* and may produce false results with *urinary pregnancy tests* (*Gravindex,* false-positive; *Prepurex* and *Dap tests,* false-negative). Promethazine can cause significant alterations of *flare response* in *intradermal allergen tests* if performed within 4 days of patient's receiving promethazine.

INTERACTIONS Drug: **Alcohol** and other CNS DEPRESSANTS add to CNS depression and anticholinergic effects.

PHARMACOKINETICS Absorption: Readily absorbed from GI tract. **Onset:** 20 min PO/PR/IM; 5 min IV. **Duration:** 2–8 h. **Distribution:** Crosses placenta. **Metabolism:** Metabolized in liver. **Elimination:** Slowly excreted in urine and feces.

NURSING IMPLICATIONS

Assessment & Drug Effects

- Supervise ambulation. Promethazine sometimes produces marked sedation and dizziness.
- Be aware that antiemetic action may mask symptoms of unrecognized disease and signs of drug overdosage as well as dizziness, vertigo, or tinnitus associated with toxic doses of aspirin or other ototoxic drugs.
- Patients in pain may develop involuntary (athetoid) movements of upper extremities following parenteral administration. These symptoms usually disappear after pain is controlled.
- Monitor respiratory function in patients with respiratory problems, particularly children. Drug may suppress cough reflex and cause thickening of bronchial secretions.

Patient & Family Education

- For motion sickness: Take initial dose 30–60 min before anticipated travel and repeat at 8–12 h intervals for adults and 12 h for children as necessary. For duration of journey, repeat dose on arising and again at

evening meal. In children, do not exceed dosage or take drug more frequently than prescribed.
- Do not drive or engage in other potentially hazardous activities (biking, skateboarding, and sports) requiring mental alertness and normal reaction time until response to drug is known.
- Avoid sunlamps, tanning booths, or prolonged exposure to sunlight. Use sunscreen lotion during initial drug therapy.
- Do not take OTC medications while on this drug without physician's approval.
- Children should only take this medication under physician's supervision.
- Avoid alcohol and other CNS depressants.
- Relieve dry mouth by frequent rinses with water or by increasing noncaloric fluid intake (if allowed), chewing sugarless gum, or sucking hard candy. If these measures fail, add a saliva substitute (e.g., Moi-Stir, Orex, Xero-Lube).
- Do not breast feed while taking this drug.
- Store this medication out of reach of children.

PROPOFOL
(pro'po-fol)
Diprivan
Classifications: CENTRAL NERVOUS SYSTEM AGENT; GENERAL ANESTHESIA; SEDATIVE-HYPNOTIC
Prototype: Thiopental
Pregnancy Category: B

AVAILABILITY 10 mg/mL injection

ACTIONS Sedative-hypnotic used in the induction and maintenance of anesthesia or sedation.
THERAPEUTIC EFFECTS Rapid onset (40 sec) and minimal excitation during induction of anesthesia.

USES Induction or maintenance of anesthesia as part of a balanced anesthesia technique; sedation in mechanically ventilated patients and procedures.

CONTRAINDICATIONS Hypersensitivity to propofol or propofol emulsion, which contains soybean oil and egg phosphatide; obstetrical procedures; patients with increased intracranial pressure, patients who are not intubated or mechanically ventilated or impaired cerebral circulation; pregnancy (category B), lactation. Do not use for sedation for procedures in children <3 y.
CAUTIOUS USE Patients with severe cardiac or respiratory disorders or history of epilepsy or seizures; in children with long-term usage.

ROUTE & DOSAGE

Induction of Anesthesia
Child: **IV** ≥3 y, 2.5–3.5 mg/kg over 20–30 sec
Adult: **IV** 2–2.5 mg/kg q10sec until induction onset

Maintenance of Anesthesia

Child: **IV** ≥3 y, 125–300 mcg/kg/min
Adult: **IV** 100–200 mcg/kg/min

Sedation for Procedures

Adult: **IV** 5 mcg/kg/min for at least 5 min, may increase by 5–10 mcg/kg/min q5–10min until desired level of sedation is achieved (may need maintenance rate of 5–50 mcg/kg/min)

STORAGE

Store unopened at 4°–22° C (40°–72° F). Refrigeration is not recommended. Protect from light.

ADMINISTRATION

- Use strict aseptic technique to prepare propofol for injection; drug emulsion supports rapid growth of microorganisms.
- Inspect ampuls and vials for particulate matter and discoloration. Discard if either is noted.
- Shake well before use. Inspect for separation of the emulsion. Do not use if there is evidence of separation of phases of the emulsion.

Intravenous

PREPARE **IV Infusion:** Give undiluted or diluted in D5W to a concentration not less than 2 mg/mL. Must draw up into a sterile syringe immediately after ampules or vials are opened. Begin drug administration immediately and completed within 6 h.

ADMINISTER **IV Infusion:** Use syringe or volumetric pump to control rate. Determine rate by weight. Administer immediately after spiking the vial. Complete infusion within 6 h.

INCOMPATIBILITIES **Y-Site:** Amikacin, amphotericin B, atracurium, bretylium, calcium chloride, ciprofloxacin, diazepam, digoxin, doxorubicin, gentamicin, methotrexate, methylprednisolone, metoclopramide, minocycline, mitoxantrone, netilmicin, phenytoin, tobramycin, verapamil.

ADVERSE EFFECTS CNS: Headache, dizziness, *twitching, bucking, jerking, thrashing, clonic/myoclonic movements.* **Special Senses:** Decreased intraocular pressure. **CV:** Hypotension, <u>ventricular asystole</u> (rare). **GI:** Vomiting, abdominal cramping. **Respiratory:** Cough, hiccups, apnea. **Other:** Pain at injection site.

DIAGNOSTIC TEST INTERFERENCE Propofol produces a temporary reduction in ***serum cortisol levels.*** However, propofol does not seem to inhibit adrenal responsiveness to ***ACTH.***

INTERACTIONS Drug: Concurrent continuous infusions of propofol and **alfentanil** produce higher plasma levels of **alfentanil** than expected. CNS DEPRESSANTS cause additive CNS depression.

PHARMACOKINETICS Onset: 9–36 sec. **Duration:** 6–10 min. **Distribution:** Highly lipophilic, crosses placenta, excreted in breast milk. **Metabolism:** Extensively metabolized in the liver. **Elimination:** Approximately 88% of the dose is recovered in the urine as metabolites. **Half-Life:** 5–12 h.

Common adverse effects in *italic;* life-threatening effects <u>underlined;</u> generic names in **bold;** drug classifications in SMALL CAPS; ♣ Canadian drug name; ❷ Prototype drug.

NURSING IMPLICATIONS

Assessment & Drug Effects

■ Monitor hemodynamic status and assess for dose-related hypotension.

■ Take seizure precautions. Tonic-clonic seizures have occurred following general anesthesia with propofol.

■ Metabolic acidosis with cardiac failure has occurred at an increased rate in propofol-treated patients compared with standard sedatives.

■ Be alert to the potential for drug induced excitation (e.g., twitching, tremor, hyperclonus) and take appropriate safety measures.

■ See Part I for monitoring during sedation for procedures.

■ Provide comfort measures; pain at the injection site is quite common especially when small veins are used.

■ May change color of urine to green.

PROPRANOLOL HYDROCHLORIDE ℗⁺
(proe-pran′oh-lole)
Apo-Propranolol ✦, Detensol ✦, Inderal, Inderal LA, Novopranol ✦
Classifications: AUTONOMIC NERVOUS SYSTEM AGENT; BETA-ADRENERGIC ANTAGONIST (BLOCKING AGENT, SYMPATHOLYTIC); ANTIHYPERTENSIVE; ANTIARRHYTHMIC, CLASS II
Pregnancy Category: C

AVAILABILITY 10 mg, 20 mg, 40 mg, 60 mg, 80 mg tablets; 60 mg, 80 mg, 120 mg, 160 mg sustained-release capsules; 20 mg/5 ml, 40 mg/mL, 80 mg/mL solution; 1 mg/mL injection

ACTIONS Nonselective beta-blocker of both cardiac and bronchial adrenoreceptors that competes with epinephrine and norepinephrine for available beta-receptor sites. In higher doses, exerts direct quinidine-like effects, which depresses cardiac function including contractility and arrhythmias. Lowers both supine and standing blood pressures in hypertensive patients. Mechanism of antimigraine action unknown but thought to be related to inhibition of cerebral vasodilation and arteriolar spasms.
THERAPEUTIC EFFECTS Blocks cardiac effects of beta-adrenergic stimulation; as a result, reduces heart rate, myocardial irritability (Class II antiarrhythmic) and force of contraction, depresses automaticity of sinus node and ectopic pacemaker, and decreases AV and intraventricular conduction velocity. Hypotensive effect is associated with decreased cardiac output, suppressed renin activity, as well as beta blockade. Also decreases platelet aggregability.

USES Management of cardiac arrhythmias, myocardial infarction, tachyarrhythmias associated with digitalis intoxication, anesthesia, and thyrotoxicosis, hypertrophic subaortic stenosis, angina pectoris due to coronary atherosclerosis, pheochromocytoma, hereditary essential tremor; also treatment of hypertension alone, but generally with a thiazide or other antihypertensives.
UNLABELED USES Anxiety states, migraine prophylaxis, essential tremors, schizophrenia, tardive dyskinesia, acute panic symptoms (e.g., stage fright), recurrent GI bleeding in cirrhotic patients, treatment of aggression and rage.

P

CONTRAINDICATIONS Greater than first-degree heart block; CHF, right ventricular failure secondary to pulmonary hypertension; sinus bradycardia, cardiogenic shock, significant aortic or mitral valvular disease; bronchial asthma or bronchospasm, severe COPD, allergic rhinitis during pollen season; concurrent use with adrenergic-augmenting psychotropic drugs or within 2 wk of MAO inhibition therapy. Safety during pregnancy (category C) or lactation is not established.

CAUTIOUS USE Peripheral arterial insufficiency; history of systemic insect sting reaction; patients prone to nonallergenic bronchospasm (e.g., chronic bronchitis, emphysema); major surgery; renal or hepatic impairment; diabetes mellitus; patients prone to hypoglycemia; myasthenia gravis; Wolff-Parkinson-White syndrome.

ROUTE & DOSAGE

Hypertension

Neonate: **PO** 0.25 mg/kg/dose q6–8h (max 5 mg/kg/day) **IV** 0.01 mg/kg slow IV push over 10 min q6–8h prn (max 0.15 mg/kg/dose q6–8h)
Child: **PO** 0.5–1 mg/kg/day in 2 divided doses (usual maintenance dose 1–5 mg/kg/day) (max dose 8 mg/kg/day)
Adult: **PO** 40 mg b.i.d., usually need 160–480 mg/day in divided doses

Angina

Adult: **PO** 10–20 mg b.i.d. or t.i.d., may need 160–320 mg/day in divided doses

Arrhythmias

Child: **PO** 1–4 mg/kg/day in 4 divided doses (max 16 mg/kg/day) **IV** 0.01–0.1 mg/kg/min over 10 min (max dose: infant, 1 mg; child, 3 mg)
Adult: **PO** 10–30 mg t.i.d. or q.i.d. **IV** 0.5–3 mg q4h prn

Migraine Prophylaxis

Child: **PO** 0.6–1.5 mg/kg/day every 8 h in divided doses (maximum dose 4 mg/kg/day or ≤35 kg, 10–20 mg t.i.d.; >35 kg, 20–40 mg t.i.d.)
Adult: **PO** 80 mg/day in divided doses, may need 160–240 mg/day

STORAGE

Store at 15°–30° C (59°–86° F) in tightly closed, light-resistant container.

ADMINISTRATION

- Do not give within 2 wk of a MAO inhibitor.
- Be consistent with regard to giving with food or on an empty stomach to minimize variations in absorption.
- Take apical pulse and BP before administering drug. Withhold drug if heart rate <60 bpm or systolic BP <90 mm Hg. For children consult normal age rates, see Physiological Considerations section in Part I. Consult physician for parameters.
- Ensure that sustained-release form is not chewed or crushed. Must be swallowed whole.
- Concentrated oral solutions must be mixed with water, fluids or juice before administering.

Common adverse effects in *italic;* life-threatening effects <u>underlined;</u> generic names in **bold;** drug classifications in SMALL CAPS; ♣ Canadian drug name; ● Prototype drug.

- Reduce dosage gradually over a period of 1–2 wk and monitor patient closely when discontinued.

Intravenous

Note: Verify correct IV concentration and rate of infusion for neonates with physician.
***PREPARE* Direct:** Give undiluted or dilute each 1 mg in 10 mL of D5W. **Intermittent:** Dilute a single dose in 50 mL of NS.
***ADMINISTER* Direct:** Give each 1 mg over 1 min. **Intermittent:** Give each dose over 15–20 min.
***INCOMPATIBILITIES* Y-Site: Amphotericin B cholesteryl complex, diazoxide.**

ADVERSE EFFECTS Body as a Whole: Fever; pharyngitis; respiratory distress, weight gain, LE-like reaction, cold extremities, leg fatigue, arthralgia. **Urogenital:** Impotence or decreased libido. **Skin:** Erythematous, psoriasis-like eruptions; pruritus. Reversible alopecia, hyperkeratoses of scalp, palms, feet; nail changes, dry skin. **CNS:** Drug-induced psychosis, sleep disturbances, depression, *confusion,* agitation, giddiness, lightheadedness, *fatigue,* vertigo, syncope, weakness, *drowsiness,* insomnia, vivid dreams, visual hallucinations, delusions, reversible organic brain syndrome. **CV:** Palpitation, profound *bradycardia,* <u>AV heart block, cardiac standstill</u>, hypotension, angina pectoris, <u>tachyarrhythmia</u>, acute CHF, peripheral arterial insufficiency resembling Raynaud's disease, myotonia, paresthesia of *hands.* **Special Senses:** Dry eyes (gritty sensation), visual disturbances, conjunctivitis, tinnitus, hearing loss, nasal stuffiness. **GI:** Dry mouth, cheilostomatitis, nausea, vomiting, heartburn, diarrhea, constipation, flatulence, abdominal cramps, <u>mesenteric arterial thrombosis, ischemic colitis</u>, pancreatitis. **Hematologic:** Transient eosinophilia, thrombocytopenic or nonthrombocytopenic purpura, <u>agranulocytosis</u>. **Metabolic:** Hypoglycemia, hyperglycemia, hypocalcemia (patients with hyperthyroidism). **Respiratory:** Dyspnea, <u>laryngospasm</u>, bronchospasm.

DIAGNOSTIC TEST INTERFERENCE BETA-ADRENERGIC BLOCKERS may produce false-negative test results in exercise tolerance ECG tests, and elevations in ***serum potassium, peripheral platelet count, serum uric acid, serum transaminase, alkaline phosphatase, lactate dehydrogenase, serum creatinine, BUN,*** and an increase or decrease in ***blood glucose*** levels in diabetic patients.

INTERACTIONS Drug: PHENOTHIAZINES have additive hypotensive effects. BETA-ADRENERGIC AGONISTS (e.g., **albuterol**) antagonize effects. **Atropine** and TRICYCLIC ANTIDEPRESSANTS block bradycardia. DIURETICS and other HYPOTENSIVE AGENTS increase hypotension. High doses of **tubocurarine** may potentiate neuromuscular blockade. **Cimetidine** decreases clearance, increases effects. ANTACIDS may decrease absorption. **Phenobarbital** and **rifampin** increase this drug's clearance. **Food:** Licorice increases potassium loss and retention of sodium and water.

PHARMACOKINETICS Absorption: Completely absorbed from GI tract but undergoes extensive first-pass metabolism. **Peak:** 60–90 min immediate release; 6 h sustained release; 5 min IV. **Distribution:** Widely distributed including CNS, placenta, and breast milk. **Metabolism:** Almost

P

completely metabolized in liver. **Elimination:** 90–95% excreted in urine as metabolites; 1–4% excreted in feces. **Half-Life:** Child, 3.9–6.4 h; adult, 2.3 h.

NURSING IMPLICATIONS

Assessment & Drug Effects

- Obtain careful medical history to rule out allergies, asthma, and obstructive pulmonary disease. Propranolol can cause bronchiolar constriction even in normal subjects.
- Monitor apical pulse, respiration, BP, and circulation to extremities closely throughout period of dosage adjustment. Consult physician for acceptable parameters.
- Evaluate adequate control or dosage interval for patients being treated for hypertension by checking blood pressure near end of dosage interval or before administration of next dose. *Theupeutic level: Child, 30–100 ng/mL.*
- Be aware that adverse reactions occur most frequently following IV administration soon after therapy is initiated; however, incidence is also high following oral use in patients with impaired kidney function. Reactions may or may not be dose related.
- Lab tests: Obtain periodic hematologic, kidney, liver, and cardiac functions when propranolol is given for prolonged periods.
- Monitor I&O ratio and daily weight as significant indexes for detecting fluid retention and developing heart failure.
- Consult physician regarding allowable salt intake. Drug plasma volume may increase with consequent risk of CHF if dietary sodium is not restricted in patients not receiving concomitant diuretic therapy.
- Fasting for more than 12 h may induce hypoglycemic effects fostered by propranolol.
- If patient complains of cold, painful, or tender feet or hands, examine carefully for evidence of impaired circulation. Peripheral pulses may still be present even though circulation is impaired. Caution patient to avoid prolonged exposure of extremities to cold.

Patient & Family Education

- Learn usual pulse rate and take apical pulse in children under 5 years and in those over 5 years take radial pulse before each dose. Report to physician if pulse is below the established parameter or becomes irregular.
- Be aware that propranolol suppresses clinical signs of hypoglycemia (e.g., BP changes, increased pulse rate) and may prolong hypoglycemia.
- Understand importance of compliance. Do not alter established regimen (i.e., do not stop, omit, increase, or decrease dosage or change dosage interval).
- Do not discontinue abruptly; can precipitate withdrawal syndrome (e.g., tremulousness, sweating, severe headache, malaise, palpitation, rebound hypertension, MI, and life-threatening arrhythmias in patients with angina pectoris).
- Be aware that drug may cause mild hypotension (experienced as dizziness or light-headedness) in normotensive patients on prolonged therapy. Make position changes slowly and avoid prolonged standing. Notify physician if symptoms persist.

Common adverse effects in *italic;* life-threatening effects <u>underlined;</u> generic names in **bold;** drug classifications in SMALL CAPS; ♣ Canadian drug name; ● Prototype drug.

- Do not drive or engage in potentially hazardous activities (biking, skateboarding, or sports) until response to drug is known.
- Consult physician before self-medicating with OTC drugs and avoid alcohol.
- Inform dentist, surgeon, or ophthalmologist that you are taking propranolol (drug lowers normal and elevated intraocular pressure).
- Do not breast feed while taking this drug without consulting physician.
- Store this medication out of reach of children.

PROPYLTHIOURACIL (PTU) ℗

(proe-pill-thye-oh-yoor′a-sill)
Propyl-Thyracil ♦
Classifications: HORMONES AND SYNTHETIC SUBSTITUTES; ANTITHYROID AGENT
Pregnancy Category: D

AVAILABILITY 50 mg tablets

ACTIONS Interferes with use of iodine and blocks synthesis of thyroxine (T_4) and triiodothyronine (T_3). Does not interfere with release and utilization of stored thyroid hormone; thus antithyroid action is delayed days and weeks until preformed T_3 and T_4 are degraded.

THERAPEUTIC EFFECTS Drug-induced hormone reduction results in compensatory release of thyrotropin (TSH), which causes marked hyperplasia and vascularization of thyroid gland. With good adherence to drug regimen, chemical euthyroidism can be achieved 6–12 wk after start of therapy.

USES Hyperthyroidism, iodine-induced thyrotoxicosis, and hyperthyroidism associated with thyroiditis; to establish euthyroidism prior to surgery or radioactive iodine treatment; palliative control of toxic nodular goiter.

CONTRAINDICATIONS Last trimester of pregnancy (category D), lactation; concurrent administration of sulfonamides or coal tar derivatives such as aminopyrine or antipyrine.

CAUTIOUS USE Infection; concomitant administration of anticoagulants or other drugs known to cause agranulocytosis; bone marrow depression; impaired liver function.

ROUTE & DOSAGE

Hyperthyroidism

Neonate: 5–10 mg/kg/day in divided doses every 8 h
Child: **PO** Initial dose 5–7 mg/kg/day in equally divided doses q8h, 6–10 y, then 50–150 mg/day in divided doses q8h; >10 y, 150–300 mg/day or 150 mg/m²/day in divided doses q8h; maintenance usually begins after 2 mo in the euthyroid child; dosage is usually ⅓ to ⅔ of initial doses
Adult: **PO** 300–450 mg/day divided q8h, may need 600–1200 mg/day initially; maintenance 100–150 mg/day in divided doses q8–12h

Thyrotoxic Crisis

Adult: **PO** 200 mg q4–6h until full control achieved

PROPYLTHIOURACIL (PTU)

STORAGE
Store drug at 15°–30° C (59°–86° F) in light-resistant container.

ADMINISTRATION
- Give at the same time each day with relation to meals. Food may alter drug response by changing absorption rate.
- Pharmacy can compound oral solution for infants. This can be mixed with breast milk or formula.
- If drug is being used to improve thyroid state before radioactive iodine (RAI) treatment, discontinued 3 or 4 days before treatment to prevent uptake interference. PTU therapy may be resumed if necessary 3–5 days after the RAI administration.

ADVERSE EFFECTS CNS: Paresthesias, headache, vertigo, drowsiness, neuritis. **GI:** Nausea, vomiting, diarrhea, dyspepsia, loss of taste, sialoadenitis, hepatitis. Jaundice **Hematologic:** Myelosuppression, lymphadenopathy, periarteritis, hypoprothrombinemia, thrombocytopenia, leukopenia, <u>agranulocytosis</u>. **Metabolic:** Hypothyroidism (goitrogenic): Enlarged thyroid, reduced GI motility, periorbital edema, puffy hands and feet, bradycardia, cool and pale skin, worsening of ophthalmopathy, sleepiness, fatigue, mental depression, dizziness, vertigo, sensitivity to cold, paresthesias, nocturnal muscle cramps, changes in menstrual periods, unusual weight gain. **Skin:** Skin rash, urticaria, pruritus, hyperpigmentation, lightening of hair color, abnormal hair loss. **Body as a Whole:** Drug fever, lupus-like syndrome, arthralgia, myalgia, hypersensitivity vasculitis, nephritis, lymphadenopathy.

DIAGNOSTIC TEST INTERFERENCE Propylthiouracil may elevate *prothrombin time* and serum *alkaline phosphatase, AST, ALT* levels.

INTERACTIONS Drug: Amiodarone, potassium iodide, sodium iodide, THYROID HORMONES can revere efficacy. Propylthiouracil may enhance anticogulant activity of anticogulants and may alter dispostion of beta-blockers.

PHARMACOKINETICS Absorption: Rapidly absorbed from GI tract. **Peak:** 1–1.5 h. **Distribution:** Appears to concentrate in thyroid gland; crosses placenta; some distribution into breast milk. **Metabolism:** Rapidly metabolized to inactive metabolites. **Elimination:** 35% excreted in urine within 24 h. **Half-Life:** 1–2 h.

NURSING IMPLICATIONS

Assessment & Drug Effects
- Be aware that about 10% of patients with hyperthyroidism have leukopenia <4000 cells/mm^3 and relative granulopenia.
- Observe for signs of clinical response to PTU (usually within 2 or 3 wk): Significant weight gain, reduced pulse rate, reduced serum T_4.
- Lab tests: Baseline and periodic T_3 and T_4; periodic CBC with differential and platelet count.
- Satisfactory euthyroid state may be delayed for several months when thyroid gland is greatly enlarged.

- Be alert to signs of hypoprothrombinemia: Ecchymoses, purpura, petechiae, unexplained bleeding. Warn ambulatory patients to report these signs promptly.
- Be alert for important diagnostic signs of excess dosage: Contraction of a muscle bundle when pricked, mental depression, hard and nonpitting edema, and need for high thermostat setting and extra blankets in winter (cold intolerance).
- Monitor for urticaria (occurs in 3–7% of patients during weeks 2–8 of treatment). Report severe rash.

Patient & Family Education

- Note that PTU treatment may be reinstituted if surgery fails to produce normal thyroid gland function.
- Be aware that thyroid hormone may be given concomitantly with PTU throughout pregnancy to prevent hypothyroidism in mother with little effect on fetus.
- Report severe skin rash or swelling of cervical lymph nodes. Therapy may be discontinued.
- Report to physician sore throat, fever, and rash immediately (most apt to occur in first few months of treatment). Drug will be discontinued and hematologic studies initiated.
- Avoid use of OTC drugs for asthma, or cough treatment without checking with the prescriber. Iodides sometimes included in such preparations are contraindicated.
- Learn how to take pulse accurately and check daily. Report to physician continued tachycardia.
- Report diarrhea, fever, irritability, listlessness, vomiting, weakness; these are signs of inadequate therapy or thyrotoxicosis.
- Chart weight 2 or 3 times weekly; clinical response is monitored through changes in weight and pulse.
- Continue monitoring and recording weight and pulse rate while in remission. Report onset of tremor, anxiety state, gradual ascending pulse rate, and loss of weight to prescriber (signs of hormone deficiency).
- Do not alter drug regimen (e.g., stop, increase, decrease, omit doses, change dosage intervals). Take dosage around the clock as prescribed.
- Check with prescriber about use of iodized salt and inclusion of seafood in the diet.
- Do not breast feed while taking this drug.
- Store this medication out of reach of children.

PROTAMINE SULFATE

(proe′ta-meen)
Protamine Sulfate
Classification: ANTIDOTE
Pregnancy Category: C

AVAILABILITY 10 mg/mL injection

ACTIONS Purified mixture of simple, low-molecular-weight proteins obtained from sperm or testes of suitable fish species. Anticoagulant effect when used alone.

THERAPEUTIC EFFECTS Because protamine is strongly basic, it combines with strongly acidic heparin to produce a stable complex; thus anticoagulant effect of both drugs is neutralized.

USES Antidote for heparin calcium or heparin sodium overdosage (after heparin has been discontinued).
UNLABELED USES Antidote for heparin administration during extracorporeal circulation.

CONTRAINDICATIONS Hemorrhage not induced by heparin overdosage; pregnancy (category C).
CAUTIOUS USE Cardiovascular disease; history of allergy to fish; vasectomized or infertile males; lactation; patients who have received protamine-containing insulin.

ROUTE & DOSAGE

Antidote for Heparin Overdose
Child/Adult: **IV** 1 mg for every 100 units of heparin to be neutralized (max 100 mg in a 2 h period), give the first 25–50 mg by slow direct IV and the rest over 2–3 h

STORAGE
Store protamine sulfate injection at 2°–8° C (36°–46° F); protamine powder for injection and reconstituted solution at 15°–30° C (59°–86° F). Solutions are stable for 72 h at this temperature.

ADMINISTRATION
Note: Titrate dose carefully to prevent excess anticoagulation because protamine has a longer half-life than heparin and also has some anticoagulant effect of its own.

Intravenous
Note: Verify correct IV concentration and rate of infusion for infants or children with physician.
PREPARE Direct: Reconstitute each 50 mg with 5 mL of sterile water for injection. Reconstitute with preservative free of sterile water for injection for use with neonates. Shake until dissolved. **Continuous:** Further dilute in 50 mL or more of NS or D5W.
ADMINISTER Direct: Give each 50 mg or fraction thereof slowly over 10–15 min. NEVER give more than 50 mg in any 10-min period or 100 mg in any 2-h period. **Continuous:** Do not exceed direct rate. Give over 2–3 h or longer as determined by coagulation studies.
INCOMPATIBILITIES Solution/Additive: RADIOCONTRAST MATERIALS.

ADVERSE EFFECTS CV: *Abrupt drop in BP* (with rapid IV infusion), bradycardia. **Body as a Whole:** Urticaria, angioedema, pulmonary edema, anaphylaxis, dyspnea, lassitude; transient flushing and feeling of warmth. **GI:** Nausea, vomiting. **Hematologic:** Protamine overdose or "heparin rebound" (hyperheparinemia).

INTERACTIONS No clinically significant interactions established.

PHARMACOKINETICS Onset: 5 min. **Duration:** 2 h.

NURSING IMPLICATIONS

Assessment & Drug Effects

- Do not use protamine if only minor bleeding occurs during heparin therapy because withdrawal of heparin will usually correct minor bleeding within a few hours.
- Monitor BP and pulse q15–30min, or more often if indicated. Continue for at least 2–3 h after each dose, or longer as dictated by patient's condition. Be prepared to treat patient for shock as well as hemorrhage.
- Lab tests: Monitor effect of protamine in neutralizing heparin by aPTT or ACT values. Coagulation tests are usually performed 5–15 min after administration of protamine, and again in 2–8 h if desirable.
- Observe patients undergoing extracorporeal dialysis or patients who have had cardiac surgery carefully for bleeding (heparin rebound). Even with apparent adequate neutralization of heparin by protamine, bleeding may occur 30 min to 18 h after surgery. Monitor vital signs closely. Additional protamine may be required in these patients.

PSEUDOEPHEDRINE HYDROCHLORIDE

(soo-doe-e-fed′rin)

Cenafed, Decongestant Syrup, Dimetapp Decongestant, Dorcol Children's Decongestant, Eltor ♣, Eltor 120 ♣, Halofed, Novafed, PediaCare, Pseudofrin ♣, Robidrine ♣, Sudafed, Sudrin

Classifications: AUTONOMIC NERVOUS SYSTEM AGENT; ALPHA- AND BETA-ADRENERGIC AGONIST (SYMPATHOMIMETIC); DECONGESTANT
Prototype: Epinephrine
Pregnancy Category: C

P

AVAILABILITY 30 mg, 60 mg tablets; 120 mg, 240 mg extended-release tablets; 15 mg chewable tablets (contains phenylalanine); 15 mg/5 mL, 30 mg/5 mL liquid; 7.5 mg/0.8 mL drops

ACTIONS Sympathomimetic amine that, like ephedrine, produces decongestion of respiratory tract mucosa by stimulating the sympathetic nerve endings including alpha, beta$_1$ and beta$_2$ receptors. Unlike ephedrine, also acts directly on smooth muscle and constricts renal and vertebral arteries. Has fewer adverse effects, less pressor action, and longer duration of effects than ephedrine.
THERAPEUTIC EFFECTS Effective as a nasal decongestant.

USES Symptomatic relief of nasal congestion associated with rhinitis, coryza, and sinusitis and for eustachian tube congestion.

CONTRAINDICATIONS Hypersensitivity to sympathomimetic amines; severe hypertension; coronary artery disease; use within 14 days of MAOIs; glaucoma; hyperthyroidism. Safety during pregnancy (category C), lactation, or extended release in children <12 y is not established.

CAUTIOUS USE Hypertension, heart disease, diabetes. Chewable tablet contains phenylalanine; avoid usage with phenyketonuria.

ROUTE & DOSAGE

Nasal Congestion

Child 2–5 y: **PO** 15 mg q4–6h (max 60 mg/day); *6–12 y,* 30 mg q4–6h (max 120 mg/day)
Child >12 y/Adult: **PO** 60 mg q4–6h or 120 mg extended-release q12h (max dose 240 mg/day)

STORAGE

Store at 15°–30° C (59°–86° F) in tightly closed, light-resistant container.

ADMINISTRATION

Oral

- Ensure that extended-release form is not chewed or crushed. Must be swallowed whole.
- Can administer with food or milk to reduce GI distress.

ADVERSE EFFECTS Body as a Whole: *Transient stimulation, weight loss* tremulousness, difficulty in voiding. **CV:** Arrhythmias, palpitation, hypertension, *tachycardia.* **CNS:** *Nervousness,* dizziness, headache, sleeplessness, numbness of extremities. **GI:** Anorexia, dry mouth, nausea, vomiting.

INTERACTIONS Drug: Other SYMPATHOMIMETICS increase pressor effects and toxicity; MAO INHIBITORS may precipitate hypertensive crisis; BETA-BLOCKERS may increase pressor effects; may decrease antihypertensive effects of **guanethidine, methyldopa, reserpine.**

PHARMACOKINETICS Absorption: Readily absorbed from GI tract. **Onset:** 15–30 min. **Duration:** 4–6 h (8–12 h sustained-release). **Distribution:** Crosses placenta; distributed into breast milk. **Metabolism:** Partially metabolized in liver. **Elimination:** Excreted in urine.

NURSING IMPLICATIONS

Assessment & Drug Effects

- Monitor HR and BP, especially in those with a history of cardiac disease. Report tachycardia or hypertension.

Patient & Family Education

- Avoid taking within 2 h of bedtime because drug may act as a stimulant.
- Discontinue medication and consult physician if extreme restlessness or signs of sensitivity occur.
- Consult prescriber before concomitant use of OTC medications while on this drug; many contain ephedrine or other sympathomimetic amines and might intensify action of pseudoephedrine.
- Do not breast feed while taking this drug without consulting prescriber.
- Store this medication out of reach of children.

Common adverse effects in *italic;* life-threatening effects <u>underlined</u>; generic names in **bold;** drug classifications in SMALL CAPS; ✦ Canadian drug name; ❷ Prototype drug.

PSYLLIUM HYDROPHILIC MUCILLOID ℗

(sill′ium)

Fiberall, Hydrocil, Instant, Karasil ♣, Konsyl, Metamucil, Modane Bulk, Perdiem Plain, Reguloid, Serutan, Siblin, Syllact, V-Lax

Classifications: GASTROINTESTINAL AGENT; BULK LAXATIVE
Pregnancy Category: C

AVAILABILITY 3.4 g/dose powder; 2.5 g, 3.4 g, 4.03 g/teaspoon granules; 3.4 g wafers; 1.7 g, 3.4 g chewable squares

ACTIONS Highly refined colloid of psyllium seed (*Plantago ovata*) with equal amount of dextrose added as dispersing agent.
THERAPEUTIC EFFECTS Bulk-producing laxative that promotes peristalsis and natural elimination.

USES Chronic atonic or spastic constipation and constipation associated with rectal disorders or anorectal surgery.

CONTRAINDICATIONS Esophageal and intestinal obstruction, nausea, vomiting, fecal impaction, undiagnosed abdominal pain, appendicitis; children <2 y.
CAUTIOUS USE Diabetics; constipation secondary to narcotic administration; pregnancy (category C), lactation. Some product forms contain phenylalamine, avoid usage with phenyketonuria.

ROUTE & DOSAGE

Constipation or Diarrhea

Note: 3.4 g psyllium hydrophilic mucilloid powder = 1 rounded tsp.
Child: **PO** >6–11 y, ½–1 tsp 1 to 3 times/day prn
Adult: **PO** 1–2 rounded tsp or 1 packet or 1 to 2 wafers, 1–3 times/day prn

STORAGE
Store at 15°–30° C (59°–86° F) in tightly closed, light-resistant container.

ADMINISTRATION

Oral
- Fill an 8-oz (240-mL) water glass with cool water, milk, fruit juice, or other liquid; sprinkle powder into liquid; stir briskly; and give immediately (if effervescent form is used, add liquid to powder). Granules should not be chewed.
- Follow each dose with an additional glass of liquid to obtain best results.
- Exercise caution with child patient who may aspirate the drug.

ADVERSE EFFECTS Hematologic: *Eosinophilia*. **GI:** *Nausea and vomiting*, *diarrhea* (with excessive use); GI tract strictures when drug used in dry form, abdominal cramps.

INTERACTIONS Drug: Psyllium may decrease absorption and clinical effects of ANTIBIOTICS, **warfarin, digoxin, nitrofurantoin,** SALICYLATES.

PHARMACOKINETICS Absorption: Not absorbed from GI tract. **Onset:** 12–24 h. **Peak:** 1–3 days.

NURSING IMPLICATIONS

Assessment & Drug Effects

- Report promptly to prescriber if patient complains of retrosternal pain after taking the drug. Drug may be lodged as a gelatinous mass (because of poor mixing) in the esophagus.
- Monitor therapeutic effectiveness. When psyllium is used as either a bulk laxative or to treat diarrhea, the expected effect is formed stools. Laxative effect usually occurs within 12–24 h. Administration for 2 or 3 days may be needed to establish regularity.
- Assess for complaints of abdominal fullness. Smaller, more frequent doses spaced throughout the day may be indicated to relieve discomfort of abdominal fullness.
- Monitor warfarin and digoxin levels closely if either is given concurrently.

Patient & Family Education

- Consult prescriber before use in children. Do not take more frequently then prescribed.
- Note sugar and sodium content of preparation if on low-sodium or low-calorie diet. Some preparations contain natural sugars, whereas others contain artificial sweeteners (phenylalanine); avoid usage with phenyketonuria.
- Understand that drug works to relieve both diarrhea and constipation by restoring a more normal moisture level to stool.
- Take only as directed, mixing with 8 oz of water, followed by fluids to ensure medication reaches stomach.
- Be aware that drug may reduce appetite if it is taken before meals.
- Do not breast feed while taking this drug without consulting physician.
- Store this medication out of reach of children.

PYRANTEL PAMOATE

(pi-ran′tel)

Antiminth, Pin-Rid

Classifications: ANTI-INFECTIVE; ANTHELMINTIC

Prototype: Mebendazole

Pregnancy Category: C

AVAILABILITY 180 mg capsules; 50 mg/mL suspension

ACTIONS Exerts selective depolarizing neuromuscular blocking action, which results in spastic paralysis of worm; also inhibits cholinesterase.

THERAPEUTIC EFFECTS Evacuation of worms from intestines.

Common adverse effects in *italic*; life-threatening effects underlined; generic names in **bold**; drug classifications in SMALL CAPS; ✦ Canadian drug name; ❂ Prototype drug.

USES *Enterobius vermicularis* (pinworm) and *Ascaris lumbricoides* (roundworm) infestations.
UNLABELED USES Hookworm infestations; trichostrongylosis.

CONTRAINDICATIONS Safety during pregnancy (category C), lactation, or in children <2 y is not established.
CAUTIOUS USE Liver dysfunction; malnutrition; dehydration; anemia.

ROUTE & DOSAGE

Pinworm or Roundworm
Child/Adult: **PO** 11 mg/kg as a single dose (max 1 g); dosage should be repeated after 2 wk with pinworm infections

Hookworm
Child/Adult: **PO** 11 mg/kg daily for 3 days (max 1 g/day)

STORAGE
Store below 30° C (86° F); protect from light.

ADMINISTRATION
Oral
- Shake suspension well before pouring it to ensure accurate dosage.
- Give with milk or fruit juices and without regard to prior ingestion of food or time of day.

ADVERSE EFFECTS CNS: Dizziness, headache, drowsiness, insomnia. **GI:** Anorexia, *nausea,* vomiting, abdominal distention, diarrhea, *tenesmus,* transient elevation of AST. **Skin:** Skin rashes.

INTERACTIONS Drug: Piperazine and pyrantel may be mutually antagonistic.

PHARMACOKINETICS Absorption: Poorly absorbed from GI tract. **Peak:** 1–3 h. **Metabolism:** Metabolized in liver. **Elimination:** >50% excreted in feces, 7% in urine.

NURSING IMPLICATIONS

Assessment & Drug Effects
- Lab tests: Monitor baseline and periodic AST/ALT in individuals with known liver dysfunction.

Patient & Family Education
- Do not drive or engage in other potentially hazardous activities until response to drug is known.
- To prevent pinworm reinfestations, bedding and clothing must be washed in hot water. Carefully remove bedding without shaking and clean or vacuum floors around bed. Disinfect toilets every day.
- Discourage children from scratching anal area.
- Use good hand washing techniques for all family members, especially after toileting.

- Monitor stools. Worms will be expelled in the stools; children may be frightened by this event and need to be prepared.
- Do not breast feed while taking this drug without consulting prescriber.
- Store this medication out of reach of children.

PYRAZINAMIDE
(peer-a-zin'a-mide)
PZA, Tebrazid ♣
Classifications: ANTI-INFECTIVE; ANTITUBERCULOSIS AGENT
Prototype: Isoniazid
Pregnancy Category: C

AVAILABILITY 500 mg tablets

ACTIONS Pyrazinoic acid amide, analog of nicotinamide, which is bacteriostatic against *Mycobacterium tuberculosis*. When employed alone, resistance may develop in 6–7 wk; therefore, administration with other effective agents is recommended. Appears to interfere with renal capacity to concentrate and excrete uric acid. Thus it may cause hyperuricemia.
THERAPEUTIC EFFECTS Bacteriostatic against *M. tuberculosis*. Not used as sole agent against TB infection.

USES Short-term therapy of advanced tuberculosis before surgery and to treat patients unresponsive to primary agents (e.g., isoniazid, streptomycin).

CONTRAINDICATIONS Severe liver damage. Safety during pregnancy (category C) or lactation is not established.
CAUTIOUS USE Presence or family history of gout or diabetes mellitus; impaired kidney function; history of peptic ulcer; acute intermittent porphyria; history of alcoholism.

ROUTE & DOSAGE

Tuberculosis
Child: **PO** 20–40 mg/kg/day in divided doses q12–24h (max 2 g/day)
Adult: **PO** 15–30 mg/kg/day in 3–4 divided doses (max 2 g/day)

STORAGE
Store at 15°–30° C (59°–86° F) in tightly closed container.

ADMINISTRATION
Oral
- Discontinue drug if hepatic reactions (jaundice, pruritus, icteric sclerae, yellow skin) or hyperuricemia with acute gout (severe pain in great toe and other joints) occurs.
- Suspension can be compounded by pharmacy.

ADVERSE EFFECTS Body as a Whole: *Active gout,* arthralgia, lymphadenopathy. **Urogenital:** Difficulty in urination. **CNS:** Headache. **Skin:**

Urticaria. **Hematologic:** Hemolytic anemia, decreased plasma prothrombin. **GI:** Splenomegaly, <u>fatal hemoptysis</u>, aggravation of peptic ulcer, *hepatotoxicity, abnormal liver function tests.* **Metabolic:** *Rise in serum uric acid.*

DIAGNOSTIC TEST INTERFERENCE Pyrazinamide may produce a temporary decrease in *17-ketosteroids* and an increase in *protein-bound iodine.*

INTERACTIONS Increase in fatal liver toxicity with **rifampin.** Decreases isoniazid levels

PHARMACOKINETICS Absorption: Readily absorbed from GI tract. **Peak:** 2 h. **Distribution:** Crosses blood–brain barrier. **Metabolism:** Metabolized in liver. **Elimination:** Excreted slowly in urine. **Half-Life:** 9–10 h.

NURSING IMPLICATIONS

Assessment & Drug Effect
- Observe and supervise closely. Patients should receive at least one other effective antituberculosis agent concurrently.
- Examine patients at regular intervals and question about possible signs of toxicity: Liver enlargement or tenderness, jaundice, fever, anorexia, malaise, impaired vascular integrity (ecchymoses, petechiae, abnormal bleeding).
- Hepatic reactions appear to occur more frequently in patients receiving high doses (doses >30 mg/kg/day).
- Lab tests: Obtain liver function tests (especially AST, ALT, serum bilirubin) prior to and at 2–4 wk intervals during therapy. Blood uric acid determinations are advised before, during, and following therapy.

Patient & Family Education
- Report to physician onset of difficulty in voiding. Keep fluid intake at 2000 mL/day if possible or appropriate for age.
- Monitor blood glucose (diabetics) for possible loss of glycemic control.
- Report any symptoms of fatigue, nausea, vomiting, joint pain, abdominal pain, or jaundice to physician immediately.
- Avoid direct sunlight, tanning beds, and sunlamps, which can lead to sunburn; wear appropriate protection and sunblock.
- Do not breast feed while taking this drug without consulting physician.
- Store this medication out of reach of children.

PYRIDOSTIGMINE BROMIDE

(peer-id-oh-stig'meen)
Mestinon, Regonol
Classifications: AUTONOMIC NERVOUS SYSTEM AGENT; CHOLINERGIC (PARASYMPATHOMIMETIC); CHOLINESTERASE INHIBITOR
Prototype: Neostigmine
Pregnancy Category: C

AVAILABILITY 60 mg/5 mL syrup (contains 5% alcohol); 60 mg tablet; 180 mg extended-release tablet; 5 mg/mL injection

ACTIONS Analog of neostigmine; indirect-acting cholinergic that inhibits cholinesterase activity. Drug facilitates transmission of impulses across myoneural junctions by blocking destruction of acetylcholine. Has fewer adverse effects and longer duration of action than neostigmine.

THERAPEUTIC EFFECTS Direct stimulant action on voluntary muscle fibers and possibly on autonomic ganglia and CNS neurons. Produces increased tone in skeletal muscles.

USES Myasthenia gravis and as an antagonist to nondepolarizing skeletal muscle relaxants (e.g., curariform drugs).

CONTRAINDICATIONS Hypersensitivity to anticholinesterase agents or to bromides. Mechanical obstruction of urinary or intestinal tract; bradycardia, hypotension. Safety during pregnancy (category C) or lactation is not established.

CAUTIOUS USE Bronchial asthma; epilepsy; vagotonia; hyperthyroidism; peptic ulcer; cardiac dysrhythmias.

ROUTE & DOSAGE

Myasthenia Gravis

Neonate: **PO** 5 mg q4–6h
Child: **PO** 7 mg/kg/day divided into 5–6 doses
IM/IV 0.05–0.15 mg/kg q4–6h (max dose 10 mg)
Adult: **PO** 60 mg–1.5 g/day spaced according to requirements and response of individual patient; sustained release: 180–540 mg 1–2 times/day at intervals of at least 6 h **IM/IV** Approximately ⅓₀th of PO dose

Reversal of Muscle Relaxants

Child: **IV** 0.1–0.25 mg/dose preceded by IV atropine
Adult: **IV** 10–20 mg immediately preceded by IV atropine

STORAGE

Store at 15°–30° C (59°–86° F). Protect from light and moisture.

ADMINISTRATION

Oral

- Give with food or fluid.
- Ensure that extended-release form is not chewed or crushed. Must be swallowed whole.
- Note: A syrup is available. Some patients may not like it because it is sweet; try to make it more palatable by giving it over ice chips. The syrup formulation contains 5% alcohol.

Intramuscular

- Note: Parenteral dose is about ⅓₀ the oral adult dose.
- Give deep IM into a large muscle. Follow agency policy for use with children and site selection (see Part I).

Intravenous

PREPARE Direct: Give undiluted. Do NOT add to IV solutions.
ADMINISTER Direct: Give at a rate of 0.5 mg over 1 min for myasthenia gravis; 5 mg over 1 min for reversal of muscle relaxants.

ADVERSE EFFECTS Skin: Acneiform rash. **Hematologic:** Thrombophlebitis (following IV administration). **GI:** *Nausea, vomiting, diarrhea.* **GU:** *Urinary frequency* **Special Senses:** *Miosis.* **Body as a Whole:** *Excessive, salivation and sweating,* weakness, fasciculation. **Respiratory:** Increased bronchial secretion, <u>bronchoconstriction</u>. **CV:** Bradycardia, hypotension.

INTERACTION Drug: Atropine NONDEPOLARIZING MUSCLE RELAXANTS antagonize effects of pyridostigmine.

PHARMACOKINETICS Absorption: Poorly absorbed from GI tract. **Onset:** 30–45 min PO; 15 min IM; 2–5 min IV. **Duration:** 3–6 h. **Distribution:** Crosses placenta. **Metabolism:** Metabolized in liver and in serum and tissue by cholinesterases. **Elimination:** Excreted in urine.

NURSING IMPLICATIONS

Assessment & Drug Effects

- Report increasing muscular weakness, cramps, or fasciculations. Failure of patient to show improvement may reflect either underdosage or overdosage.
- Observe patient closely if atropine is used to abolish GI adverse effects or other muscarinic adverse effects because it may mask signs of overdosage (cholinergic crisis): Increasing muscle weakness, which through involvement of respiratory muscles can lead to death.
- Monitor vital signs frequently, especially respiratory rate.
- Observe for signs of cholinergic reactions (see Appendix D-1), particularly when drug is administered IV.
- Observe neonates of myasthenic mothers who have received pyridostigmine closely for difficulty in breathing, swallowing, or sucking.
- Observe patient continuously when used as muscle relaxant antagonist. Airway and respiratory assistance must be maintained until full recovery of voluntary respiration and neuromuscular transmission is assured. Complete recovery usually occurs within 30 min.

Patient & Family Education

- Be aware that duration of drug action may vary with physical and emotional stress, as well as with severity of disease.
- Report onset of rash to physician. Drug may be discontinued.
- Sustained-release tablets may become mottled in appearance; this does not affect their potency.
- Do not breast feed while taking this drug without consulting physician.
- Store this medication out of reach of children.

PYRIDOXINE HYDROCHLORIDE (VITAMIN B₆)

(peer-i-dox´een)
Beesix, hexaBetalin, NesTrex
Classifications: HORMONES AND SYNTHETIC SUBSTITUTES; VITAMIN
Pregnancy Category: A (C if >RDA)

PYRIDOXINE HYDROCHLORIDE (VITAMIN B₆)

AVAILABILITY 25 mg, 50 mg, 100 mg, 250 mg, 500 mg tablets; 200 mg sustained release tablets; 100 mg/mL injection

ACTIONS Water-soluble complex of three closely related compounds with B_6 activity. Considered essential to human nutrition, although a deficiency syndrome is not well defined. Converted in body to pyridoxal, a coenzyme that functions in protein, fat, and carbohydrate metabolism and in facilitating release of glycogen from liver and muscle. In protein metabolism, participates in many enzymatic transformations of amino acids and conversion of tryptophan to niacin and serotonin. Aids in energy transformation in brain and nerve cells, and is thought to stimulate heme production.

THERAPEUTIC EFFECTS Evaluated by improvement of B_6 deficiency manifestations: Nausea, vomiting, skin lesions resembling those of riboflavin and niacin deficiency (seborrhea-like lesions about eyes, nose, and mouth, glossitis, stomatitis), edema, CNS symptoms (depression, irritability, peripheral neuritis, convulsions), hypochromic microcytic anemia.

USES Prophylaxis and treatment of pyridoxine deficiency, as seen with inadequate dietary intake, drug-induced deficiency (e.g., isoniazid, oral contraceptives), and inborn errors of metabolism (vitamin B_6-dependent convulsions or anemia). Also to prevent chloramphenicol-induced optic neuritis, to treat acute toxicity caused by overdosage of cycloserine, hydralzine, isoniazid (INH); alcoholic polyneuritis; sideroblastic anemia associated with high serum iron concentration. Has been used for management of many other conditions ranging from nausea and vomiting in radiation sickness and pregnancy to suppression of postpartum lactation.

CONTRAINDICATIONS Safety of large doses in pregnancy [category A (C if >RDA)] or lactation is not established.

ROUTE & DOSAGE

Dietary Deficiency

Child: **PO** 5–25 mg/day times 3 wk, then 1.5–2.5 mg/day
Adult: **PO/IM/IV** 2.5–10 mg/day times 3 wk, then may reduce to 2.5–5 mg/day

Pyridoxine Deficiency Syndrome

Adult: **PO/IM/IV** Initial dose up to 600 mg/day may be required
PO/IM/IV Maintenance Dose Up to 50 mg/day

Isoniazid-Induced Deficiency

Child: **PO** 10–50 mg/day times 3 wk, then 1–2 mg/kg/day
Adult: **PO/IM/IV** 100–200 mg/day times 3 wk, then 25–100 mg/day

Pyridoxine-Dependent Seizures

Neonate/Infant: **IM/IV** 50–100 mg/dose IM or rapid IV once
Maintenance PO 50–100 mg/day

STORAGE

Store at 15°–30° C (59°–86° F) in tight, light-resistant containers; avoid freezing.

ADMINISTRATION

Oral

- Ensure that sustained-release and enteric forms are not chewed or crushed. Must be swallowed whole.
- Give without regard to meals.

Intramuscular

- Give deep IM into a large muscle. Follow agency policy for and site selection in children or see Administration section in Part I.

Intravenous

PREPARE Direct: Give undiluted. **Continuous:** May be added to most standard IV solutions.
ADMINISTER Direct: Give at a rate of 50 mg or fraction thereof over 60 sec. **Continuous:** Give according to ordered rate for infusion.

ADVERSE EFFECTS Body as a Whole: Paresthesias, slight flushing or feeling of warmth, temporary burning or stinging pain in injection site. **CNS:** Somnolence, sensory neuropathy, seizures (particularly following large parenteral doses). **Metabolic:** Low folic acid levels.

INTERACTIONS Drug: Isoniazid, cycloserine, penicillamine, hydralazine, and ORAL CONTRACEPTIVES may increase pyridoxine requirements; may reverse or antagonize therapeutic effects of **levodopa.** Decreases serum levels of **phenobarbital** and **phenytoin.**

PHARMACOKINETICS Absorption: Readily absorbed from GI tract. **Distribution:** Stored in liver; crosses placenta. **Metabolism:** Metabolized in liver. **Elimination:** Excreted in urine.

NURSING IMPLICATIONS

Assessment & Drug Effects

- Monitor neurologic status to determine therapeutic effect in deficiency states.
- Record a complete dietary history so poor eating habits can be identified and corrected (a single vitamin deficiency is rare; patient can be expected to have multiple vitamin deficiencies).
- Lab tests: Periodic Hct and Hgb, and serum iron.

Patient & Family Education

- Learn rich dietary sources of vitamin B$_6$: Yeast, wheat germ, whole grain cereals, muscle and glandular meats (especially liver), legumes, green vegetables, bananas.
- Do not self-medicate with vitamin combinations (OTC) without first consulting physician.
- Do not breast feed while taking this drug without consulting physician.
- Store this medication out of reach of children.

PYRIMETHAMINE

(peer-i-meth'a-meen)
Daraprim
Classifications: ANTI-INFECTIVE; ANTIMALARIAL
Prototype: Chloroquine
Pregnancy Category: C

AVAILABILITY 25 mg tablets

ACTIONS Long-acting folic acid antagonist chemically related to metabolite of chloroguanide. Selectively inhibits action of dehydrofolic reductate in parasites with resulting blockade of folic acid metabolism.

THERAPEUTIC EFFECTS No gametocidal activity but prevents development of fertilized gametes in the mosquito and thus helps to prevent transmission of malaria. Exhibits little value as single agent in treatment of acute primary malarial attack because action against bloodborne schizonts is slow in onset. Cross-resistance with chloroguanide may occur.

USES Prophylaxis of malaria due to susceptible strains of plasmodia. May be used conjointly with fast-acting antimalarial (e.g., chloroquine, quinacrine, quinine) to initiate transmission control and suppressive cure. Used with a sulfonamide to provide synergistic action in treatment of toxoplasmosis.

CONTRAINDICATIONS Chloroguanide-resistant malaria; hypersensitivity to sulfonamides; megaloblastic anemia caused by folate deficiency; lactation; children <2 mo; pregnancy (category C).

CAUTIOUS USE Patients with convulsive disorders receiving high doses of an anticonvulsant (e.g., phenytoin).

ROUTE & DOSAGE

Malaria Chemoprophylaxis

Child: **PO** *<4 y, 6.25 mg once/wk; 4–10 y, 12.5 mg once/wk; >10 y, 25 mg once/wk*
Adult: **PO** *25 mg once/wk*

Toxoplasmosis

Infant ≥1 mo; Some clinicians recommend the following doses:
PO *2 mg/kg/day divided into 2 doses with a sulfonamide for 2 days then 1 mg/kg/day with a sulfonamide once daily for 6 mo, then for the following 6 mo 1 mg/kg/day once 3 times a week with a sulfonamide*
Child: **PO** *2 mg/kg/day divided into 2 doses for 3 days then 1 mg/kg/day (max dose 25 mg/day) divided into 2 doses for 4 wk; given concurrently with a sulfonamide*
Adult: **PO** *50–75 mg/day for 1–3 wk, then decrease dose by half and continue for 1 mo; given concurrently with a sulfonamide*

STORAGE

Store at 15°–30° C (59°–86° F) in tightly closed, light-resistant container.

ADMINISTRATION

Oral

- Minimize GI distress by giving with meals. If symptoms persist, dosage reduction may be necessary.
- Give on same day each week for malaria prophylaxis. Begin when individual enters endemic area and continue for 10 wk after leaving the area.
- This is not the drug of choice for malaria chemoprophylaxis due to development of resistant strains and adverse effects.
- In children usually given with folinic acid to prevent hematologic complications (folic acid deficiency).
- Oral form may be crushed and mixed by pharmacy into an oral suspension.

ADVERSE EFFECTS GI: Anorexia, vomiting, atrophic glossitis, abdominal cramps, diarrhea. **Skin:** Skin rashes, photosensitivity. **Hematologic:** *Folic acid deficiency (megaloblastic anemia, leukopenia, thrombocytopenia, pancytopenia, diarrhea).* **CNS:** CNS stimulation including convulsions, respiratory failure.

INTERACTIONS Drug: Folic acid, *para*-aminobenzoic acid (PABA) may decrease effectiveness against toxoplasmosis.

PHARMACOKINETICS Absorption: Readily absorbed from GI tract. **Peak:** 2 h. **Distribution:** Concentrates in kidneys, lungs, liver, and spleen; distributed into breast milk. **Elimination:** Excreted slowly in urine; excretion may extend over 30 days or longer. **Half-Life:** 54–148 h.

NURSING IMPLICATIONS

Assessment & Drug Effects

- Monitor patient response closely. Dosages required for treatment of toxoplasmosis approach toxic levels.
- Lab tests: Perform blood counts, including platelets, twice weekly during therapy.
- Withhold drug and notify physician if hematologic abnormalities appear.

Patient & Family Education

- Be aware that folic acid deficiency may occur with long-term use of pyrimethamine. Report to physician weakness, and pallor (from anemia), ulcerations of oral mucosa, sore throat, superinfections, glossitis; GI disturbances such as diarrhea and poor fat absorption, fever. Folate (folinic acid) replacement may be prescribed. Increase food sources of folates (if allowed) in diet. Avoid direct sunlight, tanning beds and sunlamps can lead to sunburn and increase in skin rashes.
- Do not breast feed while taking this drug.
- Store this medication out of reach of children.

QUINIDINE SULFATE
(kwin'i-deen sul-fate)
Apo-Quinidine ♣ , Novoquinidin ♣ , Quinidex Extentabs, Quinora

QUINIDINE GLUCONATE
Quinaglute Dura-Tabs

QUINIDINE POLYGALACTURONATE
Cardioquin
Classifications: CARDIOVASCULAR AGENT; ANTIARRHYTHMIC CLASS IA
Prototype: Procainamide
Pregnancy Category: C

AVAILABILITY Quinidine sulfate 200 mg, 300 mg tablets; 300 mg
sustained-release tablets **Quinidine gluconate** 324 mg sustained-
release tablets; 80 mg/mL injection **Quinidine polygalacturonate**
275 mg tablets (not available in U.S.)

ACTIONS Dextro-isomer of quinine and alkaloid of *Cinchona*. Class I-A
antiarrhythmic. Cardiac actions similar to those of procainamide. Depresses myocardial excitability, contractility, automaticity, and conduction velocity, and prolongs effective refractory period. Anticholinergic
action blocks vagal stimulation of AV node, thus tending to increase ventricular rate, particularly in larger doses.
THERAPEUTIC EFFECTS Depresses myocardial excitability, conduction
velocity, and irregularity of nerve impulse conduction.

USES Premature atrial, AV junctional, and ventricular contraction; paroxysmal atrial tachycardia, chronic ventricular tachycardia (when not associated with complete heart block); maintenance therapy after electrical
conversion of atrial fibrillation or flutter.
UNLABELED USES Quinidine gluconate for severe malaria.

CONTRAINDICATIONS Hypersensitivity or idiosyncrasy to quinine or
Cinchona derivatives; pregnancy (category C), lactation. Thrombocytopenic purpura resulting from prior use of quinidine; intraventricular
conduction defects, complete AV block, ectopic impulses and rhythms
due to escape mechanisms; thyrotoxicosis; acute rheumatic fever; subacute bacterial endocarditis, extensive myocardial damage, frank CHF, hypotensive states; myasthenia gravis; digitalis intoxication.
CAUTIOUS USE Incomplete heart block; impaired kidney or liver function; bronchial asthma or other respiratory disorders; myasthenia gravis;
potassium imbalance, G6PD deficiencies.

ROUTE & DOSAGE

Ectopic Beats *Sulfate*
Child: **PO Test dose** 2 mg/kg times 1 (max dose 200 mg)
6 mg/kg/dose q4–6h

Adult: **PO** 200–300 mg t.i.d. or q.i.d.

Arrhythmias *Gluconate*

Child: **IV Test dose** 2 mg/kg times 1 (max dose 200 mg)
2–10 mg/kg/dose q3–6h as needed

Ventricular Arrhythmias *Sulfate*

Adult: **PO** 400–600 mg q2–3h until arrhythmia terminates,
then 200–300 mg 3–4 times/day

Atrial Fibrillation or Flutter *Sulfate*

Adult: **PO** 200 mg q2–3h for 5–8 doses until sinus rhythm restored or
toxicity occurs (max 3–4 g), then 200–300 mg t.i.d. or q.i.d.

Acute Tachycardia *Gluconate*

Adult: **PO** 324–660 mg q8–12h **IM** 600 mg, then 400 mg q2h prn
IV 200–750 mg at a rate of 16 mg/min

STORAGE
Store at 15°–30° C (59°–86° F) in tight, light-resistant containers away
from excessive heat.

ADMINISTRATION
Note: Sulfate contains 83% anhydrous quinidine base; polygalacturonate,
80%; and gluconate, 62%. Examine parenteral solution before preparation; use only if clear and colorless.

Oral
- Note: Test dose is used by some physicians to determine idiosyncrasy
  before establishing full dosage schedule.
- Take with a full glass of water or generous amount of fluid appropriate for
  age on an empty stomach for optimum absorption (i.e., 1 h before or 2 h
  after meals). Administer drug with food if GI symptoms occur (nausea,
  vomiting, diarrhea are most common). Do not give with grapefruit juice.
- Reserve sustained-release tablets for maintenance and prophylactic
  therapy and do not chew or crush these tablets.
- Adjust dosage to maintain plasma concentration between 2–5 mcg/mL.
  Levels of 8 mcg/mL or more are associated with myocardial toxicity.

Intramuscular
- Aspirate carefully before injection to avoid inadvertent entry into blood
  vessel.

Intravenous
PREPARE **IV Infusion:** Dilute 800 mg (10 mL) in at least 40 mL D5W to
yield a maximum concentration of 16 mg/mL.
ADMINISTER **IV Infusion:** Give via infusion pump at a rate not to exceed
16 mg (1 mL)/min. Drug is absorbed through polyvinyl chloride tub-
ing, minimize tubing length.
INCOMPATIBILITIES **Solution/Additive: Amiodarone, atracurium.
Y-Site: Furosemide, heparin in dextrose.**
- Use supine position during drug administration; severe hypotension
  is most likely to occur in patients receiving drug via IV.
- Protect IV solutions from light and heat to prevent brownish discol-
  oration and possibly precipitation.

ADVERSE EFFECTS CNS: Headache, fever, tremors, apprehension, delirium, syncope with sudden loss of consciousness, seizures. **CV:** Hypotension, CHF, angioedema <u>widened QRS complex</u>, bradycardia, <u>heart block</u>, atrial flutter, <u>ventricular flutter, fibrillation</u> or tachycardia; quinidine syncope, <u>torsades de pointes</u>. **Special Senses:** Mydriasis, blurred vision, disturbed color perception, reduced visual field, photophobia, diplopia, night blindness, scotomas, optic neuritis, disturbed hearing (tinnitus, auditory acuity). **GI:** *Nausea, vomiting, diarrhea, abdominal pain,* hepatic dysfunction. **Hematologic:** <u>Acute hemolytic anemia</u> (especially in patients with G6PD deficiency), hypoprothrombinemia, leukopenia. Thrombocytopenia, <u>agranulocytosis</u> (both rare). **Body as a Whole:** Cinchonism (nausea, vomiting, headache, dizziness, fever, tremors, vertigo, tinnitus, visual disturbances), <u>angioedema</u>, acute asthma, <u>respiratory depression, vascular collapse</u>. **Skin:** Rash, urticaria, cutaneous flushing with intense pruritus, photosensitivity. **Metabolic:** SLE, hypokalemia.

INTERACTIONS Drug: May increase **digoxin** levels by 50%; **amiodarone** may increase quinidine levels, thus increasing its risk of heart block; other ANTIARRHYTHMICS, PHENOTHIAZINES, **reserpine** add to cardiac depressant effects; ANTICHOLINERGIC AGENTS add to vagolytic effects; CHOLINERGIC AGENTS may antagonize cardiac effects; ANTICONVULSANTS, BARBITURATES, **rifampin** increase the metabolism of quinidine, thus decreasing its efficacy; CARBONIC ANHYDRASE INHIBITORS, **sodium bicarbonate**, CHRONIC ANTACIDS decrease renal elimination of quinidine, thus increasing its toxicity; **verapamil** causes significant hypotension; may increase hypoprothrombinemic effects of **warfarin. Diltiazem** may increase levels and decrease elimination of quinidine. **Food:** Excessive intake of juices can alter urinary pH and increase clearance of quinidine. Grapefruit juice delays quinidine absorption. A diet high in alkaline ash foods (vegetables, citrus fruit, milk) may prolong half-life of quinidine by decreasing its excretion.

PHARMACOKINETICS Absorption: Almost completely absorbed from GI tract. **Onset:** 1–3 h. **Peak:** 0.5–1 h. **Duration:** 6–8 h. **Distribution:** Widely distributed to most body tissues except the brain; crosses placenta; distributed into breast milk. **Metabolism:** Metabolized in liver. **Elimination:** >95% excreted in urine, <5% in feces. **Half-Life:** 6–8 h.

NURSING IMPLICATIONS

Assessment & Drug Effects

- ▪ *Theraputic level: 2–5 mcg/mL. Toxicity level: 8 mcg/mL.*
- ▪ Observe cardiac monitor and report immediately the following indications for stopping quinidine: (1) sinus rhythm, (2) widening QRS complex in excess of 25% (i.e., >0.12 seconds), (3) changes in QT interval or refractory period, (4) disappearance of P waves, (5) sudden onset of or increase in ectopic ventricular beats (extrasystoles, PVCs), (6) decrease in heart rate to 120 bpm. Also report immediately any worsening of minor side effects.
- ▪ Continuous monitoring of ECG and BP is required. Observe patient closely (check sensorium and be alert for any sign of toxicity); determine plasma quinidine concentrations frequently when large doses

(more than 2 g/day) are used or when quinidine is given parenterally (i.e., quinidine gluconate).

- Observe patient closely following each parenteral dose. Amount of subsequent dose is gauged by response to preceding dose.
- Monitor vital signs q1–2h or more often as needed during acute treatment. Count apical pulse for a full minute. Report any change in pulse rate, rhythm, or quality or any fall in BP.
- Severe hypotension is most likely to occur in patients receiving high oral doses or parenteral quinidine (i.e., quinidine gluconate).
- Be aware: Reversion to sinus rhythm in long-standing fibrillation or when fibrillation is complicated by CHF involves some risk of embolization from dislodgment of atrial mural emboli.
- Quinidine can cause unpredictable rhythm abnormalities in the digitalized heart. Patients with atrial flutter or fibrillation may be pretreated with digitalis (until ventricular rate is 100 bpm) to increase AV nodal block and thus reduce possibility of paradoxic tachycardia.
- Lab tests: Periodic blood counts, serum electrolyte determinations, and kidney and liver function during long-term therapy.
- Monitor I&O. Diarrhea occurs commonly during early therapy; most patients become tolerant to this side effect. Evaluate serum electrolytes, acid–base, and fluid balance when symptoms become severe; dosage adjustment may be required.

Patient & Family Education

- Report feeling of faintness to physician. "Quinidine syncope" is caused by quinidine-induced changes in ventricular rhythm resulting in decreased cardiac output and syncope.
- Note: Hypersensitivity reactions usually appear 3–20 days after drug is started. Fever occurs commonly and may or may not be accompanied by other symptoms. Inform physician if these S&S occur.
- Eat a balanced diet with no excesses in fruit or fruit juices, milk, or a vegetarian diet. A diet high in alkaline ash foods (vegetables, citrus fruit, milk) may prolong half-life of quinidine by decreasing its excretion and increasing danger of toxicity.
- Do not self-medicate with OTC drugs without advice from physician.
- Do not increase, decrease, skip, or discontinue doses without consulting physician.
- Notify physician immediately of disturbances in vision, ringing in ears, sense of breathlessness, onset of palpitations, and unpleasant sensation in chest. Be sure to note the time of occurrence and duration of chest symptoms.
- Do not breast feed while taking this drug.
- Store this medication out of reach of children.

QUININE SULFATE

(kwye'nine)

Novoquinine ♣ , Quinamm, Quiphile

Classifications: ANTI-INFECTIVE; ANTIMALARIAL

Prototype: Chloroquine

Pregnancy Category: X

AVAILABILITY 200 mg, 260 mg, 325 mg capsules; 260 mg tablets

ACTIONS Chief alkaloid from bark of cinchona tree. Exact mechanism of antimalarial action uncertain. Inhibits protein synthesis and depresses many enzyme systems in malaria parasite. Has schizonticidal action and is gametocidal with *Plasmodium vivax* and *P. malariae,* but not *P. falciparum.* Resembles salicylates in analgesic and antipyretic properties and exerts curare-like skeletal muscle relaxant effect. Also has oxytocic action and hypoprothrombinemic effect. Qualitatively similar to quinidine in cardiovascular effects. Generally replaced by less toxic and more effective agents in treatment of malaria.

THERAPEUTIC EFFECTS Effective against *P. vivax* and *P. malariae,* but not *P. falciparum.* Generally replaced by less toxic and more effective agents in treatment of malaria.

USES Chloroquine-resistant falciparum malaria and in combination with other antimalarials for radical cure of relapsing vivax malaria; also relief of nocturnal recumbency leg cramps.

CONTRAINDICATIONS Tinnitus, optic neuritis; myasthenia gravis; G6PD deficiency; pregnancy (category X); avoid use during lactation.

CAUTIOUS USE Cardiac arrhythmias, myasthenia gravis and in hepatic impairment. Same precautions as for quinidine sulfate when used in patients with cardiovascular conditions.

ROUTE & DOSAGE

Acute Malaria

Child: **PO** 25 mg/kg/day in 3 divided doses q8h for 7 days (max dose 650 mg/dose)
Adult: **PO** 650 mg q8h for 3–7 days

Malaria Chemoprophylaxis

Adult: **PO** 325 mg b.i.d. for 6 wk following exposure

Nocturnal Leg Cramps

Adult: **PO** 200–300 mg at bedtime

STORAGE

Store at 15°–30° C (59°–86° F) in tightly closed, light-resistant containers.

ADMINISTRATION

Oral

- Give with or after meals or a snack to minimize gastric irritation. Quinine has potent local irritant effect on gastric mucosa. Do not crush capsule; drug is not only irritating but also extremely bitter.

ADVERSE EFFECTS Body as a Whole: Cinchonism (tinnitus, decreased auditory acuity, dizziness, vertigo, headache, visual impairment, *nausea, vomiting, diarrhea,* fever); hypersensitivity (Cutaneous flushing, visual impairment, pruritus, skin rash, fever, gastric distress, dyspnea, tinnitus); <u>hypothermia, coma.</u> **CNS:** Confusion, excitement, apprehension, syncope, delirium, convulsions, blackwater fever (extensive intravascular hemolysis with renal failure), <u>death</u>. **CV:** Angina, hypotension, tachycardia, <u>cardiovascular collapse</u>. **Hematologic:** Leukopenia, thrombocytopenia, <u>agranulocytosis</u>, hypoprothrombinemia, hemolytic anemia. **Respiratory:** Decrease respiration.

DIAGNOSTIC TEST INTERFERENCE Quinine may interfere with determinations of *urinary catecholamines* (*Sobel* and *Henry modification procedure*) and *urinary steroids (17-hydroxycorticosteroids)* (modification of *Reddy, Jenkins, Thorn* method).

INTERACTIONS Drug: May increase **digoxin** levels; ANTICHOLINERGIC AGENTS add to vagolytic effects; CHOLINERGIC AGENTS may antagonize cardiac effects; ANTICONVULSANTS, BARBITURATES, **rifampin** increases the metabolism of quinine, thus decreasing its efficacy; CARBONIC ANHYDRASE INHIBITORS, **sodium bicarbonate,** CHRONIC ANTACIDS decrease renal elimination of quinine, thus increasing its toxicity; **warfarin** may increase hypoprothrombinemic effects.

PHARMACOKINETICS Absorption: Well absorbed from GI tract. **Peak:** 1–3 h. **Duration:** 6–8 h. **Distribution:** Widely distributed to most body tissues except the brain; crosses placenta; distributed into breast milk. **Metabolism:** Metabolized in liver. **Elimination:** >95% excreted in urine, <5% in feces. **Half-Life:** 8–21 h.

NURSING IMPLICATIONS

Assessment & Drug Effects

- Be alert for S&S of rising plasma concentration of quinine marked by tinnitus and hearing impairment, which usually do not occur until concentration is 10 mcg/mL or more.
- Follow the same precautions with quinine as are used with quinidine in patients with atrial fibrillation; quinine may produce cardiotoxicity in these patients.

Patient & Family Education

- Learn possible adverse reactions and report onset of any unusual symptom promptly to physician.
- Do not breast feed while taking this drug.
- Store this medication out of reach of children.

RANITIDINE HYDROCHLORIDE

(ra-nye′te-deen)

Zantac, Zantac EFFERdose, Zantac GELdose, Zantac-75

Classifications: GASTROINTESTINAL AGENT; ANTISECRETORY (H$_2$-RECEPTOR ANTAGONIST)

Prototype: Cimetidine

Pregnancy Category: B

AVAILABILITY 75 mg, 150 mg, 300 mg tablets; 150 mg effervescent tablets (contains phenylalanine); 150 mg, 300 mg capsules; 15 mg/mL syrup (contains 7.5% benzyl alcohol); 0.5 mg/mL, 25 mg/mL injection

---

ACTIONS Potent anti-ulcer drug that competitively and reversibly inhibits histamine action at H_2-receptor sites on parietal cells, thus blocking gastric acid secretion. Indirectly reduces pepsin secretion but appears to have minimal effect on fasting and postprandial serum gastrin concentrations or secretion of gastric intrinsic factor or mucus.

THERAPEUTIC EFFECTS Blocks daytime and nocturnal basal gastric acid secretion stimulated by histamine and reduces gastric acid release in response to food, pentagastrin, and insulin. Shown to inhibit 50% of the stimulated gastric acid secretion.

USES Short-term treatment of active duodenal ulcer; maintenance therapy for duodenal ulcer patient after healing of acute ulcer; treatment of gastroesophageal reflux disease; short-term treatment of active, benign gastric ulcer; treatment of pathologic GI hypersecretory conditions (e.g., Zollinger-Ellison syndrome, systemic mastocytosis, and postoperative hypersecretion); heartburn.

CONTRAINDICATIONS Safe use during pregnancy (category B) or lactation is not established.

CAUTIOUS USE Hepatic and renal dysfunction, use of effervescent tablets in phenylketonuria.

ROUTE & DOSAGE

Duodenal Ulcer, Gastric Ulcer, Gastroesophageal Reflux

Premature/Term Infant: **PO** <2 wk, 2 mg/kg/day in equally divided q12h **IV** 1.5 mg/kg/dose as a loading dose then after 12 h start 1.5–2 mg/kg/day divided q12h *or* 0.04–0.08 mg/kg/h by continuous infusion

Child: **PO (GERD/erosive esophagitis)** 5–10 mg/kg/day in equally divided dose q12h (max 300 mg/day and in erosive esophagitis max dose 600 mg/day) **IM/IV** 2–4 mg/kg/day divided q6–8h (max dose 150 mg/day)

Adult: **PO** 150 mg b.i.d. or 300 mg at bedtime **IV** 50 mg/dose q6–8h; 150–300 mg/day by continuous infusion (max dose 400 mg/day)

Duodenal Ulcer

Child: **PO** 2–4 mg/kg/day in divided doses q12h (max dose 300 mg/day) **maintenance** 2–4 mg/kg/day in divided doses q12h (max dose 150 mg/day) **IV** 2–4 mg/kg/day in divided doses q6–8h (max dose 200 mg/day)

Adult: **PO** 150 mg at bedtime

Pathologic Hypersecretory Conditions

Adult: **PO** 150 mg b.i.d. up to 6.3 g/day **IV** 50 mg q6–8h

Heartburn

Adult: **PO** 75 mg b.i.d.
Reduced dosages required with renal impairment.

STORAGE

Store tablets in light-resistant, tightly capped container at 15°–30° C (59°–86° F) in a dry place.

ADMINISTRATION

Oral

- Give with or without food; simultaneous administration does not appear to reduce absorption or serum concentrations.
- Administer adjunctive antacid treatment 2 h before or after drug.
- Dilute effervescent tablet in 180 to 240 mL of water.

Intramuscular

- Note: Does not need to be diluted.

Intravenous

Note: Verify correct IV concentration and rate of infusion for infants and children with physician.

PREPARE **Direct:** Dilute 50 mg NS, D5W, RL, or other compatible IV solution to a total volume of 20 mL. **Intermittent:** Dilute 50 mg in 50–100 mL of NS, D5W, RL, or other compatible IV solution. **Continuous:** Dilute total daily dose in 250 mL of NS, D5W, RL, or other compatible IV solution. Final concentration should be ≤2.5 mg/mL.

ADMINISTER **Direct:** Give at a rate of 4 mL/min or 20 mL over not less than 5 min. **Intermittent:** Give over 15–30 min. **Continuous:** Give over 24 h.

INCOMPATIBILITIES **Solution/Additive: Amphotericin B, atracurium, cefamandole, cefazolin, cefoxitin, ceftazidime, cefuroxime, clindamycin, chlorpromazine, diazepam, ethacrynic acid, hydroxyzine, methotrimeprazine, midazolam, nalbuphine, pentobarbital, phenobarbital, phytonadione** OPIUM ALKALOIDS, **phenobarbital. Y-Site: Amphotericin B cholesteryl complex, methotrimeprazine, midazolam,** OPIUM ALKALOIDS, **phenobarbital.**

- Scheduled dose to coincide with end of treatment if patient is having hemodialysis.

ADVERSE EFFECTS CNS: Headache, malaise, dizziness, somnolence, insomnia, vertigo, mental confusion, agitation, depression, hallucinations. **CV:** Bradycardia (with rapid IV push). **GI:** Constipation, nausea, abdominal pain, diarrhea. **Skin:** Rash. **Hematologic:** Reversible decrease in WBC count, thrombocytopenia. **Body as a Whole:** Hypersensitivity reactions, anaphylaxis (rare).

DIAGNOSTIC TEST INTERFERENCE Ranitidine may produce slight elevations in *serum creatinine* (without concurrent increase in *BUN*); (rare) increases in *AST, ALT, alkaline phosphatase, LDH,* and total *bilirubin.* Produces false-positive tests for *urine protein* with *Multistix* (use *sulfosalicylic acid* instead).

INTERACTIONS Drug: May reduce absorption of **cefpodoxime, cefuroxime, delavirdine, ketoconazole, itraconazole.** Antacids reduce absorption of ranitidine.

PHARMACOKINETICS Absorption: Incompletely absorbed from GI tract (50% reaches systemic circulation). **Peak:** 2–3 h PO. **Duration:** 8–12 h. **Distribution:** Distributed into breast milk. **Metabolism:** Metabolized in liver. **Elimination:** Excreted in urine, with some excreted in feces. **Half-Life:** Infants, 3.5 h; child, 1.8–2 h; adult, 2–3 h.

R

Common adverse effects in *italic;* life-threatening effects underlined; generic names in **bold;** drug classifications in SMALL CAPS; ♣ Canadian drug name; ✿ Prototype drug.

1073

NURSING IMPLICATIONS

Assessment & Drug Effects

- Potential toxicity results from decreased clearance (elimination) and therefore prolonged action; greatest in those with hepatic or renal dysfunction.
- Lab tests: Periodic liver functions. Monitor creatinine clearance if renal dysfunction is present or suspected. When clearance is <50 mL/min, manufacturer recommends reduction of the dose to 150 mg once q24h with cautious and gradual reduction of the interval to q12h or less, if necessary.
- Be alert for early signs of hepatotoxicity (though low and thought to be a hypersensitivity reaction): jaundice (dark urine, pruritus, yellow sclera and skin), elevated transaminases (especially ALT) and LDH.
- Long-term therapy may lead to vitamin B_{12} deficiency.

Patient & Family Education

- Note: Long duration of action provides ulcer pain relief that is maintained through the night as well as the day.
- Be aware that even if symptomatic relief is provided by ranitidine, this should not be interpreted as absence of gastric malignancy. Follow-up examinations will be scheduled after therapy is discontinued.
- Adhere to scheduled periodic laboratory checkups during ranitidine treatment.
- Do not supplement therapy with OTC remedies for gastric distress or pain without prescriber's advice (e.g., Mylanta II reduces ranitidine absorption).
- Do not smoke; research shows smoking decreases ranitidine efficacy and adversely affects ulcer healing.
- Do not breast feed while taking this drug without consulting prescriber.
- Store this medication out of reach of children.

RASBURICASE

(ras-bur'i-case)
Elitek
Classifications: ANTIGOUT AGENT; ANTIMETABOLITE
Prototype: Colchicine
Pregnancy Category: C

AVAILABILITY 1.5 mg/vial powder for injection

ACTIONS A recombinant urate-oxidase enzyme produced by DNA technology from *Aspergillus flavus*. In humans, uric acid is the final step in the catabolic pathway of purines. Rasburicase catalyzes enzymatic oxidation of uric acid, thus it is only active at the end of the purine catabolic pathway. **THERAPEUTIC EFFECTS** Used to manage plasma uric acid levels in pediatric patients with leukemia, lymphoma, and solid tumor malignancies who are receiving anticancer therapy that results in tumor lysis and, therefore, elevates plasma uric acid.

USES Initial management of increased uric acid levels secondary to tumor lysis.

Common adverse effects in *italic;* life-threatening effects <u>underlined</u>; generic names in **bold**; drug classifications in SMALL CAPS; ◆ Canadian drug name; ◑ Prototype drug.

CONTRAINDICATIONS Deficiency in G6PD; history of anaphylaxis or hypersensitivity reactions; hypersensitivity to rasburicase; hemolytic reactions or methemoglobinemia reactions to rasburicase; pregnancy (category C); lactation; children <1 mo.

CAUTIOUS USE Safety and efficacy in adults is unknown.

ROUTE & DOSAGE

Hyperuricemia

Child: **IV** *>1 mo,* 0.15–0.2 mg/kg/dose once daily starting 4–24 h before chemotherapy × 5 days

STORAGE

Store drug and diluent in refrigerator; protect from light and freezing. Reconstituted solution stable for 24 h if refrigerated, then discard because it contains no preservatives.

ADMINISTRATION

Intravenous

PREPARE **IV Infusion:** Reconstitute each 1.5-mg vial of ELITEK with 1 mL of the provided diluent and mix by swirling very gently. **Do not shake.** Discard if particulate matter is visible or if product is discolored after reconstitution. Remove the predetermined dose from the reconstituted vials and inject into an infusion bag enough NS to achieve a final total volume of 50 mL.

ADMINISTER **IV Infusion:** Give over 30 min. **DO NOT GIVE BOLUS DOSE.** Infuse through an **unfiltered** line used for no other medications. If a separate line is not possible, flush the line with at least 15 mL of saline solution before/after infusion of rasburicase.

- Immediately discontinue IV infusion and institute emergency measures for S&S of anaphylaxis including chest pain, dyspnea, hypotension and/or urticaria.

INCOMPATIBILITIES **Solution/Additive/Y-Site:** Do not mix or infuse with other drugs.

ADVERSE EFFECTS Body as a Whole: *Fever,* sepsis, anaphylaxis **CNS:** *Headache.* **GI:** *Mucositis, vomiting, nausea, diarrhea, abdominal pain.* **Hematologic:** Neutropenia. **Skin:** *Rash.*

DIAGNOSTIC TEST INTERFERENCE May give false elevations for *uric acid* if blood sample is left at room temperature.

INTERACTIONS Drug: No clinically significant interactions established.

PHARMACOKINETICS Half-Life: 18 h.

NURSING IMPLICATIONS

Assessment & Drug Effects

- Lab tests: Patients at higher risk for G6PD deficiency (e.g., patients of African or Mediterranean ancestry) should be screened prior to starting therapy because this deficiency is a contraindication for this drug.

- Lab test special instructions: Blood for uric acid anaylsis must be collected into prechilled tubes containing heparin anticoagulant and **immediately immersed in an ice water bath.** Plasma samples must be prepared by centrifugation in a precooled centrifuge (4° C) 39° F and plasma must be maintained in an ice water bath and analyzed for uric acid within 4 h of collection.
- Monitor closely for S&S of hypersensitivity and be prepared to institute emergency measures for anaphylaxis.
- Monitor cardiovascular, respiratory, neurologic, and renal status throughout therapy.

Patient & Family Education
- Report immediately any distressing S&S to physician.

RESPIRATORY SYNCYTIAL VIRUS IMMUNE GLOBULIN (RSV-IVIG)
(res-pir′a-tory sin-cy′ti-al)
RespiGam
Classifications: IMMUNE GLOBULIN; IMMUNIZING AGENT; VACCINE
Pregnancy Category: C

AVAILABILITY 2500 mg/50 mL vial

ACTIONS Contains IgG immune globulin antibodies from human plasma.
THERAPEUTIC EFFECTS The preparation contains large amounts of RSV-neutralizing antibodies. Recipients should be high-risk premature infants and children.

USES Prevention of serious lower respiratory tract infection caused by RSV in children <24 mo with bronchopulmonary dysplasia or history of premature birth.

CONTRAINDICATIONS Previous severe reaction to RespiGam or other human immunoglobulin preparation, selective IgA deficiency, cyanotic heart disease.
CAUTIOUS USE Immunodeficiency, CHF, renal failure, volume depletion, sepsis, diabetes mellitus, pregnancy (category C).

ROUTE & DOSAGE

RSV

Neonate/Infant/Child: **IV** 750 mg/kg infused at 1.5 mL/kg/h for first 15 min, then 3 mL/kg/h for next 15 min, and to end of infusion; may repeat monthly during RSV season

STORAGE
Store vials at 2°–8° C (35°–46° F).

ADMINISTRATION

Intravenous

PREPARE **IV Infusion:** Give undiluted. Begin infusion within 6 h after vial is entered and complete within 12 h.

***ADMINISTER* IV Infusion:** Do not shake vial; infuse vial contents undiluted through a separate IV line if possible; if "piggyback" must be used, see manufacturer's directions. DO NOT EXCEED IV INFUSION RATES given in Route & Dosage section. Use a constant infusion pump. Maximum infusion rate is 3.6 mL/kg/h.

***INCOMPATIBILITY* Solution/Additive/Y-Site:** Do not mix with other drugs.

ADVERSE EFFECTS Body as a Whole: Fever, pyrexia, fluid overload. **CV:** Tachycardia, hypertension. **GI:** Vomiting, diarrhea, gastroenteritis. **Respiratory:** Respiratory distress, wheezing, rales, hypoxia, hypoxemia, tachypnea. **Skin:** Injection site inflammation.

INTERACTIONS Drug: May interfere with immune response to LIVE VIRUS VACCINES (mumps, rubella, measles); may need to repeat vaccine if given within 10 mo of RespiGam.

PHARMACOKINETICS Half-Life: 22–28 days.

NURSING IMPLICATIONS

Assessment & Drug Effects

- Monitor closely during and after each IV rate change.
- Assess vital signs and respiratory status prior to infusion, during and after each rate change, and at 30-min intervals until 30 min after infusion is completed, and periodically thereafter for 24 h.
- Slow infusion immediately if S&S of fluid overload appear and report to physician.
- Lab tests: Monitor routine blood chemistry, serum electrolytes, blood gases, osmolality.
- Monitor for aseptic meningitis syndrome, which may begin up to 2 days after infusion.

Patient & Family Education

- Be aware of the possibility of aseptic meningitis syndrome; learn S&S to report (headache, drowsiness, fever, photophobia, painful eye movements, muscle rigidity, nausea, vomiting).
- Avoid exposing child to those with URIs or crowds.
- Teach parents good handwashing techniques.

RIBAVIRIN

(rye-ba-vye′rin)
Virazole, Rebetol
Classifications: ANTI-INFECTIVE; ANTIVIRAL
Prototype: Acyclovir
Pregnancy Category: X

AVAILABILITY 6 g/100 mL vial

ACTIONS Synthetic nucleoside with broad-spectrum antiviral activity against DNA and RNA viruses. Exact mode of action is not fully understood but believed to involve multiple mechanisms including selective interference with viral ribonucleic protein synthesis. It does not influence interferon synthesis.

THERAPEUTIC EFFECTS Active against many RNA and DNA viruses, including respiratory syncytial virus (RSV), influenza A and B, parainfluenza, measles, mumps, Lassa fever, enterovirus 72 (formerly called hepatitis A), yellow fever, HIV, herpes simplex virus (HSV-1 and HSV-2), and vaccinia. Immune responses appear to depend on cellular drug concentrations. Low concentrations seem to stimulate immune responses while high concentrations appear to inhibit those responses. Generally not active against poliovirus and coxsackie viruses. Unlike other antiviral agents, virus resistance to ribavirin does not appear to develop.

USES Aerosol treatment of carefully selected hospitalized infants and young children with severe lower respiratory tract infection caused by respiratory syncytial virus (RSV). Oral used in combination with interferon-alfa to treat Hepatitis C.

UNLABELED USES Prophylaxis and treatment of influenza A and B, pneumonia caused by adenovirus; Lassa fever, measles, HSV-1, HSV-2, hepatitis A, herpes zoster, and for carefully selected patients with AIDS and AIDS-related complex (ARC).

CONTRAINDICATIONS Mild RSV infections of lower respiratory tract; infants requiring simultaneous assisted ventilation; severe cardiopulmonary disease; prolonged or multiple courses of ribavirin inhalation therapy. Safe use during pregnancy (category X) or exposure to those who are pregnant; lactation is not established.

CAUTIOUS USE COPD, asthma, renal impairment.

ROUTE & DOSAGE

RSV

Child: **Inhalation** 20 mg/mL via SPAG nebulizer administered over 12–18 h/day for a minimum of 3 days (max 7 days)
Hepatitis C (in combination with interferon-alfa)
Adult: **PO** 400 mg in a.m.; 600 mg in p.m. × 24–48 wk

Renal Impairment

Cl$_{cr}$ <50 mL/min, oral ribavirin should not be used

STORAGE

Store unopened vial in a dry place at 15°–25° C (59°–77° F) unless otherwise directed. Following reconstitution, store solution at 20°–30° C (68°–86° F) for 24 h.

ADMINISTRATION

Note: Aerosol solution is prepared with either sterile water for injection or sterile water for inhalation, without preservatives or any other added substance. See manufacturer's package insert for preparation directions. Inspect solution for discoloration or presence of particulate matter. Discard discolored or cloudy solutions.

Inhalation

- Administer only by SPAG-2 aerosol generator, following manufacturer's directions.

- Caution: Ribavirin has demonstrated teratogenicity in animals. Advise pregnant health care personnel or parent of the potential teratogenic risks associated with exposure during ribavirin administration to patients.
- Do not give other aerosol medication concomitantly with ribavirin.
- Discard solution in the SPAG-2 reservoir at least q24h and whenever liquid level is low before fresh reconstituted solution is added.

ADVERSE EFFECTS CV: Hypotension (faintness, light-headedness, unusual fatigue), <u>MI, cardiac arrest</u>. **Special Senses:** Conjunctivitis, erythema of eyelids. **Hematologic:** Reticulocytosis, <u>hemolytic anemia</u>. **Respiratory:** Deterioration of respiratory function, dyspnea, apnea, chest soreness, bacterial pneumonia, <u>ventilator dependence</u>. **GI:** Transient increases in AST, ALT, bilirubin; abdominal cramps, jaundice. **Skin:** Dermatologic: rash.

INTERACTION Drug: Ribavirin may antagonize the antiviral effects of **zalcitabine, zidovudine** against HIV.

PHARMACOKINETICS Absorption: Rapidly absorbed orally (44%) and systemically from lungs. **Peak:** Inhaled 60–90 min. PO 1.7–3 h. **Distribution:** Crosses placenta; distributed into breast milk. **Metabolism:** Metabolized in cells to an active metabolite. **Elimination:** 85% excreted in urine, 15% in feces. **Half-Life:** 24 h in plasma, 16–40 days in RBCs.

NURSING IMPLICATIONS

Assessment & Drug Effects

- Obtain specimens for rapid diagnosis of RSV infection before therapy is initiated or at least during the first 24 h of ribavirin therapy. Do not continue therapy without laboratory confirmation of RSV infection.
- Treatment efficacy in RSV infections appears greatest if initiated within the first 3 days.
- Monitor respiratory function and fluid status closely during therapy. Note baseline rate and character of respirations and pulse. Observe for signs of labored breathing: Dyspnea, apnea; rapid, shallow respirations, intercostal and substernal retraction, nasal flaring, limited excursion of lungs, cyanosis. Auscultate lungs for abnormal breath sounds.
- Observe patients requiring simultaneous assisted ventilation closely for S&S of worsening pulmonary function. Check equipment carefully every 2 h, including endotracheal tube, for malfunction. Precipitation of ribavirin and accumulation of fluid in tubing can obstruct the apparatus and cause inadequate ventilation and gas exchange. Monitor CBC, hemoglobin, and reticulocyte count.
- Consult physician about management of fluid and food intake and keep an accurate record of I&O.

R

RIBOFLAVIN (VITAMIN B₂)

(rye′bo-flay-vin)
Riboflavin (Vitamin B₂)
Classifications: HORMONE AND SYNTHETIC SUBSTITUTE; VITAMIN
Pregnancy Category: A (C if >RDA)

AVAILABILITY 25 mg, 50 mg, 100 mg tablets

ACTIONS Water-soluble vitamin and component of the flavoprotein enzymes, which work together with a wide variety of proteins to catalyze many cellular respiratory reactions by which the body derives its energy. **THERAPEUTIC EFFECTS** Evaluated by improvement of clinical manifestations of deficiency: Digestive disturbances, headache, burning sensation of skin (especially "burning" feet), cracking at corners of mouth (cheilosis), glossitis, seborrheic dermatitis (often at angle of nose and anogenital region) and other skin lesions, mental depression, corneal vascularization (with photophobia, burning and itchy eyes, lacrimation, roughness of eyelids), anemia, neuropathy.

USES To prevent riboflavin deficiency and to treat ariboflavinosis; also to treat microcytic anemia and as a supplement to other B vitamins in treatment of pellagra and beri-beri.

CONTRAINDICATIONS None.
CAUTIOUS USE Pregnancy (category A; category C if >RDA).

ROUTE & DOSAGE

Nutritional Deficiency
Child: **PO** 2.5–10 mg/day daily or b.i.d.
Adult: **PO** 5–30 mg/day in divided doses

STORAGE
Store at 15°–30° C (59°–86° F) in tightly closed, light-resistant containers.

ADMINISTRATION

Oral
- Give with food to enhance absorption.
- Store in airtight containers protected from light.

ADVERSE EFFECTS Urogenital: May discolor urine bright yellow.

DIAGNOSTIC TEST INTERFERENCE In large doses, riboflavin may produce yellow-green fluorescence in *urine* and thus cause false elevations in certain *fluorometric determinations* of *urinary catecholamines.*

INTERACTIONS Drug: No clinically significant interactions established.

PHARMACOKINETICS Absorption: Readily absorbed from GI tract. **Distribution:** Little is stored; excess amounts are excreted in urine. **Elimination:** Excreted in urine. **Half-Life:** 66–84 min.

NURSING IMPLICATIONS

Assessment & Drug Effects
- Collaborate with physician, dietitian, patient, and responsible family member in planning for diet. A complete dietary history is an essential part of vitamin replacement so that poor eating habits can be identified and corrected. Deficiency in one vitamin is usually associated with other vitamin deficiencies.

Patient & Family Education

- Be aware that large doses may cause an intense yellow discoloration of urine.
- Note: Rich dietary sources of riboflavin are found in liver, kidney, beef, pork, heart, eggs, milk and milk products, yeast, whole-grain cereals, vitamin A-enriched breakfast cereals, green vegetables, and mushrooms.
- Store this medication out of reach of children.

RIFABUTIN
(rif-a-bu′tin)
Ansamycin, Mycobutin
Classifications: ANTI-INFECTIVE; ANTITUBERCULOSIS AGENT
Prototype: Isoniazid
Pregnancy Category: B

AVAILABILITY 150 mg capsules

ACTIONS Semisynthetic bacteriostatic antibiotic. Mode of action may be to inhibit DNA-dependent RNA polymerase (an enzyme) in susceptible bacterial cells but not in human cells.
THERAPEUTIC EFFECTS Effective against *Mycobacterium avium complex* (MAC) (or *M. avium-intracellulare*) and many strains of *M. tuberculosis*.

USES The prevention of disseminated *M. avium* complex (MAC) disease in patients with advanced HIV infection. Preferred agent for multidrug treatment of tuberculosis in HIV patients on protease inhibitors.

CONTRAINDICATIONS Hypersensitivity to rifabutin or any other rifamycins; lactation.
CAUTIOUS USE Hepatic or renal impairments, pregnancy (category B).

ROUTE & DOSAGE

Prevention of MAC
Child <6 y: **PO** 5 mg/kg/day (max dose 300 mg/day)
Child >6 y/Adult: **PO** 300 mg daily, may give 150 mg b.i.d. if nausea is a problem
Reduced dosages required with renal impairment

STORAGE
Store at 15°–30° C (59°–86° F), unless otherwise directed.

ADMINISTRATION
Oral
- Give as usual dose of 300 mg/day or in two divided doses of 150 mg with food if needed to reduce GI upset.

ADVERSE EFFECTS CNS: *Headache.* **GI:** *Abdominal pain, dyspepsia, nausea, taste perversion, increased liver enzymes.* **Hematologic:** Thrombocytopenia, eosinophilia, leukopenia, <u>neutropenia</u>. **Skin:** Rash. **Body as a**

Whole: *Fever, arthralgia.* **Other:** *Turns urine, feces, saliva, sputum, perspiration, and tears orange. Soft contact lenses may be permanently discolored.*

INTERACTIONS Drug: May decrease levels of BENZODIAZEPINES, BETA-BLOCKERS, **clofibrate, dapsone,** NARCOTICS, ANTICOAGULANTS, CORTICO-STEROIDS, **cyclosporine, digoxin, quinidine,** ORAL CONTRACEPTIVES, PROGESTINS, SULFONYLUREAS, **ketoconazole, fluconazole,** BARBITURATES, **theophylline,** and ANTICONVULSANTS, resulting in therapeutic failure.

PHARMACOKINETICS Absorption: 12–20% of oral dose reaches the systemic circulation. **Peak:** 2–3 h. **Distribution:** 85% protein bound. Widely distributed, high concentrations in the lungs, liver, spleen, eyes, and kidney. Crosses placenta, distributed into breast milk. **Metabolism:** Metabolized in the liver. Causes induction of hepatic enzymes. **Elimination:** Approximately 53% of dose is excreted in urine as metabolites, 30% is excreted in feces. **Half-Life:** 16–96 h (average 45 h).

NURSING IMPLICATIONS

Assessment & Drug Effects

- Monitor patients for S&S of active TB. Report immediately.
- Lab tests: Monitor periodic blood work for neutropenia and thrombocytopenia, liver function tests.
- Evaluate patients on concurrent oral hypoglycemic therapy for loss of glycemic control.
- Review patient's complete drug regimen because dosage adjustment of a significant number of drugs may be needed when rifabutin is added to regimen.

Patient & Family Education

- Learn S&S of TB and MAC (e.g., persistent fever, progressive weight loss, anorexia, night sweats, diarrhea) and notify physician if any of these develop.
- Notify physician of following: Muscle or joint pain, eye pain or other discomfort, chest pain with dyspnea, rash, or a flu-like syndrome.
- Be aware that urine, feces, saliva, sputum, perspiration, tears, and skin may be colored brown-orange. Soft contact lens may be permanently discolored.
- Have frequent ophthalmologic examinations and notify physician of any eye problems.
- Rifabutin may reduce the activity of a wide variety of drugs. Provide a complete and accurate list of concurrent drugs to the physician for evaluation.
- Do not breast feed while taking this drug.
- Store this medication out of reach of children.

R

RIFAMPIN

(rif'am-pin)

Rifadin, Rimactane, Rofact ♣, Rifamate, Rifater

Classifications: ANTI-INFECTIVE; ANTIBIOTIC; ANTITUBERCULOSIS AGENT

Prototype: Isoniazid

Pregnancy Category: C

Common adverse effects in *italic;* life-threatening effects <u>underlined;</u> generic names in **bold;** drug classifications in SMALL CAPS; ♣ Canadian drug name; ❷ Prototype drug.

AVAILABILITY 150 mg, 300 mg capsules; 600 mg injection
Combination Products: 120 mg rifampin with 50 mg isoniazide and 300 mg pyrazinamide tablets; 300 mg rifampin with 150 mg isoniazide capsules

ACTIONS Semisynthetic derivative of rifamycin B, an antibiotic derived from *Streptococcus mediterranei,* with bacteriostatic and bactericidal actions. Inhibits DNA-dependent RNA polymerase activity in susceptible bacterial cells, thereby suppressing RNA synthesis.
THERAPEUTIC EFFECTS Active against *Mycobacterium tuberculosis, M. leprae, Neisseria meningitidis,* and a wide range of gram-negative and gram-positive organisms. It is used in conjunction with other antitubercular agents to treat tuberculosis because resistant strains emerge rapidly when it is employed alone.

USES Primarily as adjuvant with other antituberculosis agents in initial treatment and retreatment of clinical tuberculosis; as short-term therapy to eliminate meningococci from nasopharynx of asymptomatic carriers of *N. meningitidis* when risk of meningococcal meningitis is high.
UNLABELED USES Chemoprophylaxis synergy for contacts of patients with *Haemophilus influenzae* type B infection; alone or in combination with dapsone and other anti-infectives in treatment of leprosy (especially dapsone-resistant leprosy). Also infections caused by susceptible gram-negative and gram-positive bacteria that fail to respond to other anti-infectives; in combination with erythromycin or tetracycline for treatment of Legionnaire's disease. Use in combination with anti-infectives for synergy effect in *Staphylococcus aureus* infections.

CONTRAINDICATIONS Hypersensitivity to rifampin; obstructive biliary disease; meningococcal disease; intermittent rifampin therapy; lactation. Safe use during pregnancy (category C) or in children <5 y is not established.
CAUTIOUS USE Hepatic disease; history of alcoholism; concomitant use of other hepatotoxic agents and protease inhibitors.

ROUTE & DOSAGE

R

Pulmonary Tuberculosis

Child: **PO** 10–20 mg/kg/day in equally divided dose q12–24h (max 600 mg/day); according to CDC, after 1–2 mo uncomplicated case dosing can be 10–20 mg/kg/day (max dose 600 mg/day) twice weekly
Adult: **PO/IV** 10 mg/kg/day (max dose 600 mg/day) or 600 mg once/day in conjunction with other antituberculosis agents; according to CDC, after 1–2 mo treatmeat uncomplicated case dosing can be 10 mg/kg/day (max dose 600 mg/day) twice weekly

Meningococcal Carriers

Neonate ≤1 mo: **PO** 10 mg/kg/day b.i.d. for 2 consecutive days (max 600 mg/day)
Child >1 mo: **PO** 20 mg/kg/day b.i.d. for 2 consecutive days (max 600 mg/day)
Adult: **PO** 600 mg b.i.d. for 2 consecutive days

Prophylaxis for *H. influenzae* Type B

Neonate ≤1 mo: **PO** 10 mg/kg/day for 4 consecutive days (max 600 mg/day)

Child >1 mo: **PO** 20 mg/kg/day for 4 consecutive days (max 600 mg/day)
Adult: **PO** 600 mg/day for 4 days

Synergy for *Staphylococcus aureus* Infections

Neonate: **PO** 5–20 mg/kg/day equally divided dose q12h in conjunction with other antibiotics
Adult: **PO** 300–600 mg/day equally divided dose b.i.d. in conjunction with other antibiotics

Dapsone-Sensitive Multibacillary Leprosy

Adult: **PO** 600 mg once/mo with clofazimine and dapsone for a minimum of 2 y

STORAGE

Store at 15°–30° C (59°–86° F) in tight light resistant containers.

ADMINISTRATION

Oral

- Give 1 h before or 2 h after a meal. Peak serum levels are delayed and may be slightly lower when given with food; capsule contents may be emptied into fluid or mixed with food.
- Note: An oral suspension can be prepared from capsules for use with pediatric patients. Consult pharmacist for directions.
- Keep a desiccant in bottle containing capsules to prevent moisture causing instability.

Intravenous

***PREPARE* IV Infusion:** Dilute by adding 10 mL of sterile water for injection to each 600-mg vial to yield 60 mg/mL. Swirl to dissolve. Withdraw the ordered dose and further dilute in 500 mL (preferred) of D5W. If necessary, 100 mL of D5W may be used.
***ADMINISTER* IV Infusion:** Infuse 500 mL solution over 3 h and 100 mL solution over 30 min; maximum concentration 6 mg/mL. Note: A less concentrated solution infused over a longer period is preferred.
***INCOMPATIBILITIES* Solution/Additive:** Minocycline. **Y-Site:** Diltiazem.
- Use diluted solution within 4 h of preparation.

ADVERSE EFFECTS CNS: Fatigue, drowsiness, headache, ataxia, confusion, dizziness, inability to concentrate, generalized numbness, pain in extremities, muscular weakness. **Special Senses:** Visual disturbances, transient low-frequency hearing loss, conjunctivitis. **GI:** *Heartburn, epigastric distress, nausea, vomiting, anorexia, flatulence, cramps, diarrhea,* <u>pseudomembranous colitis,</u> *transient elevations in liver function tests* (bilirubin, BSP, alkaline phosphatase, ALT, AST), pancreatitis. **Hematologic:** Thrombocytopenia, transient leukopenia, anemia, including hemolytic anemia. **Body as a Whole:** Hypersensitivity (fever, pruritus, urticaria, skin eruptions, soreness of mouth and tongue, eosinophilia, hemolysis), flu-like syndrome. **Urogenital:** Interstitial nephritis, hemoglobinuria, hematuria, <u>acute renal failure,</u> light-chain proteinuria, menstrual disorders, <u>hepatorenal syndrome</u> (with intermittent therapy). **Respiratory:** Hemoptysis. **Other:** Increasing lethargy, liver enlargement and tenderness, jaundice, brownish-red or orange discoloration of skin, sweat, saliva, tears, and feces; unconsciousness.

DIAGNOSTIC TEST INTERFERENCE Rifampin interferes with contrast media used for **gallbladder study;** therefore, test should precede daily dose of rifampin. May also cause retention of **BSP.** Inhibits standard assays for **serum folate** and **vitamin B₁₂.**

INTERACTIONS Drug: Alcohol, isoniazid, pyrazinamide increase risk of hepatotoxicity; **p-aminosalicylic acid (PAS)** decreases concentrations of rifampin; decreases concentrations of **alfentanil, alosetron, alprazolam, amprenavir,** BARBITURATES, BENZODIAZEPINES, **carbamazepine, atovaquone, cevimeline, chloramphenicol, clofibrate,** CORTICOSTEROIDS, **cyclosporine, dapsone, delavirdine, diazepam, digoxin, diltiazem, disopyramide, estazolam, estramustine, fentanyl, fluconazole galantamine, fosphenytoin, indinavir, itraconazole, ketoconazole, lamotrigine, levobupivacaine, lopinavir, methadone, metoprolol, mexiletine, midazolam, nelfinavir,** ORAL SULFONYLUREAS, ORAL CONTRACEPTIVES, **phenytoin,** PROGESTINS, **propafenone, propranolol, quinidine, quinine, ritonavir, sirolimus, theophylline,** THYROID HORMONES, **tocainide, tramadol, verapamil, warfarin, zaleplon, and zonisamide,** leading to potential therapeutic failure. **Food:** May reduce the absorption of rifampin.

PHARMACOKINETICS Absorption: Readily absorbed from GI tract. **Peak:** 2–4 h. **Distribution:** Widely distributed, including CSF; crosses placenta; distributed into breast milk. **Metabolism:** Metabolized in liver to active and inactive metabolites; is enterohepatically cycled. **Elimination:** Up to 30% excreted in urine, 60–65% in feces. **Half-Life:** 3 h.

NURSING IMPLICATIONS

Assessment & Drug Effects

- Lab tests: Periodic liver function tests are advised. Closely monitor patients with hepatic disease.
- Check prothrombin times daily or as necessary to establish and maintain required anticoagulant activity when patient is also receiving an anticoagulant.

Patient & Family Education

- Do not interrupt prescribed dosage regimen. Hepatorenal reaction with flu-like syndrome has occurred when therapy has been resumed following interruption.
- Be aware that drug may impart a harmless red-orange color to urine, feces, sputum, sweat, and tears. Soft contact lens may be permanently stained.
- Report onset of jaundice, hypersensitivity reactions, and persistence of GI adverse effects to prescriber.
- Use or add barrier contraceptive if using hormonal contraception. Concomitant use of rifampin and oral contraceptives leads to decreased effectiveness of the contraceptive and to menstrual disturbances (spotting, breakthrough bleeding).
- Do not breast feed while taking this drug.
- Store this medication out of reach of children.

Common adverse effects in *italic;* life-threatening effects <u>underlined</u>; generic names in **bold;** drug classifications in SMALL CAPS; ♣ Canadian drug name; ⊘ Prototype drug.

1085

RIMANTADINE

(ri-man'ta-deen)
Flumadine
Classifications: ANTI-INFECTIVE; ANTIVIRAL
Prototype: Acyclovir
Pregnancy Category: C

AVAILABILITY 100 mg tablets; 50 mg/5 mL syrup

ACTIONS Antiviral agent for treatment and prophylaxis of influenza A infections. Thought to exert an inhibitory effect early in the viral replication cycle, probably by interfering with the viral uncoating procedure of the influenza A virus.

THERAPEUTIC EFFECTS Inhibits synthesis of both viral RNA and viral protein, thus preventing or interrupting influenza A infections.

USES Prophylaxis and treatment of influenza A in adults and prophylaxis of influenza A in children.

CONTRAINDICATIONS Hypersensitivity to rimantadine and amantadine; pregnancy (category C), lactation, children <1 y.

CAUTIOUS USE History of seizures, liver dysfunction, patients with uncontrolled psychosis. Safety and efficacy in treatment of symptomatic influenza infection in children are not established.

ROUTE & DOSAGE

Prophylaxis of Influenza A

Child <10 y: **PO** 5 mg/kg once daily (max 150 mg/day)
Child ≥10 y/Adult: **PO** 100 mg b.i.d.; reduce to 100 mg daily in patients with liver disease

Treatment of Influenza A

Child: **PO** *<10 y or <40 kg,* 5 mg/kg/day once daily or q12h (max 150 mg/day) for 5–7 days
Child ≥10 y or ≥40 kg/Adult: **PO** 100 mg b.i.d., reduce to 100 mg daily in patients with liver disease; initiate as soon as possible and preferably within 48 h of onset of symptoms and continue for about 5–7 days

STORAGE

Store at 15°–30° C (59°–86° F) in tightly closed, light-resistant containers.

ADMINISTRATION

Oral

May give without regard to food. Syrup is raspberry flavored.

ADVERSE EFFECTS CNS: Nervousness, dizziness, headache, sleep disturbances, fatigue or malaise, drowsiness, anticholinergic effects. **GI:** Nausea, vomiting, diarrhea, dyspepsia, dry mouth, anorexia, abdominal pain.

Common adverse effects in *italic;* life-threatening effects <u>underlined;</u> generic names in **bold;** drug classifications in SMALL CAPS; ♣ Canadian drug name; ♦ Prototype drug.

INTERACTIONS Drug: No clinically significant interactions established.

PHARMACOKINETICS Absorption: Readily absorbed from GI tract. **Peak:** Serum levels 3.2–4.3 h. **Distribution:** Concentrates in respiratory secretions. **Metabolism:** Extensively metabolized in liver. **Elimination:** Excreted by kidneys. **Half-Life:** 20–36 h.

NURSING IMPLICATIONS

Assessment & Drug Effects

- Monitor carefully for seizure activity in patients with a history of seizures. Seizures are an indication to discontinue the drug.
- Monitor cardiac, respiratory, and neurologic status while on drug. Report palpitations, hypertension, dyspnea, or pedal edema.

Patient & Family Education

- Report bothersome adverse effects to prescriber; especially hallucinations, palpitations, difficulty breathing, and swelling of legs.
- Use caution with hazardous activities (biking, skateboarding, sports, driving a car) until reaction to drug is known.
- Do not breast feed while taking this drug.
- Store this medication out of reach of children.

RISPERIDONE

(ris-per'i-done)

Risperdal, Risperdal M-TAB

Classifications: CENTRAL NERVOUS SYSTEM AGENT; ANTIPSYCHOTIC; ATYPICAL

Prototype: Clozapine

Pregnancy Category: C

AVAILABILITY 0.25 mg, 0.5 mg, 1 mg, 2 mg, 3 mg, 4 mg tablets; 0.5 mg, 1 mg, 2 mg quick-dissolving tablets 1 mg/mL solution

ACTIONS Mechanism is not well understood. Interferes with binding of dopamine to D_2-interlimbic region of the brain, serotonin (5-HT_2) receptors, and alpha-adrenergic receptors in the occipital cortex. It has low to moderate affinity for the other serotonin (5-HT) receptors and no affinity to nondopaminergic sites (e.g., cholinergic, muscarinic, or beta-adrenergic receptors).

THERAPEUTIC EFFECTS Effective in controlling symptoms of schizophrenia as well as other psychotic symptoms.

USES Reduction or elimination of psychotic symptoms in schizophrenia and related psychoses. Seems to improve negative symptoms such as apathy, blunted affect, and emotional withdrawal.

UNLABELED USES Bipolar disorder, management of patients with dementia-related psychotic symptoms. Adjunctive treatment of behavioral disturbances in patients with mental retardation.

CONTRAINDICATIONS Hypersensitivity to risperidone; pregnancy (category C), lactation.

CAUTIOUS USE Arrhythmias, hypotension, history of seizures, breast cancer, blood dyscrasia, cardiac disorders, renal or hepatic impairment. Safety and efficacy in children are not established.

ROUTE & DOSAGE

Behavior Problems Associated with Autism

Child: Limited use with children but these doses have been used.
>5–17 y **PO** 0.5–2.5 mg daily; start at 0.5 mg/day, and increase weekly by 0.5 per day to max of 8 mg/day

Psychosis

Adult: **PO** 1–6 mg b.i.d.; start with 1 mg b.i.d., increase by 1 mg b.i.d. daily to an initial target dose of 3 mg b.i.d. (max 8 mg/day)

Renal Impairment

Cl_{cr} <30 mL/min, start with 0.5 mg b.i.d., increase by 0.5 mg b.i.d. daily to an initial target of 1.5 mg b.i.d., may increase by 0.5 mg b.i.d. at weekly intervals (max 6 mg/day)

STORAGE

Store at 15°–30° C (59°–86° F).

ADMINISTRATION

Oral

- Note that quick-dissolving tablets dissolve rapidly when placed on tongue.
- Do not exceed increases/decreases of 1 mg b.i.d. in normal populations or 0.5 mg b.i.d. in the debilitated during dosage adjustments.
- Make further increases at 1-wk or longer intervals after the target dose of 3 mg b.i.d. in normal populations and 1.5 mg b.i.d. in debilitated patients are reached.

ADVERSE EFFECTS Body as a Whole: Orthostatic hypotension with initial doses, sweating, weakness, fatigue. **CNS:** *Sedation, drowsiness, headache,* transient blurred vision, *insomnia,* disinhibition, *agitation,* anxiety, increased dream activity, dizziness, catatonia, *extrapyramidal symptoms* (akathisia, dystonia, pseudoparkinsonism) especially with doses >10 mg/day, neuroleptic malignant syndrome (rare), increase risk of stroke in elderly. **CV:** Prolonged QTc interval, tachycardia. **GI:** Dry mouth, dyspepsia, nausea, vomiting, diarrhea constipation, abdominal pain, elevated liver function tests (AST, ALT). **Endocrine:** Galactorrhea. **Respiratory:** Rhinitis, cough, dyspnea. **Skin:** Photosensitivity. **Urogenital:** Urinary retention, menorrhagia, decreased sexual desire, erectile dysfunction, sexual dysfunction male and female.

DIAGNOSTIC TEST INTERFERENCE Liver function tests (AST, ALT) are elevated.

INTERACTIONS Drug: Risperidone may enhance the effects of certain ANTIHYPERTENSIVE AGENTS. May antagonize the antiparkinson effects of **bromocriptine, cabergoline, levodopa, pergolide, pramipexole,**

ropinirole. Carbamazepine may decrease risperidone levels. **Clozapine** may increase risperidone levels. **Cisapride** may cause dysrhythmias.

PHARMACOKINETICS Absorption: Rapidly absorbed; not affected by food. **Onset:** Therapeutic effect 1–2 wk. **Peak:** 1–2 h. **Distribution:** 0.7 L/kg; in animal studies, risperidone has been found in breast milk. **Metabolism:** Metabolized primarily in liver by cytochrome P-450 with an active metabolite, 9-hydroxyrisperidone. **Elimination:** 70% excreted in urine; 14% in feces. **Half-Life:** 20 h for slow metabolizers, 30 h for fast metabolizers.

NURSING IMPLICATIONS

Assessment & Drug Effects

- Reassess patients periodically and maintain on the lowest effective drug dose.
- Monitor cardiovascular status closely; assess for orthostatic hypotension, especially during initial dosage titration.
- Monitor closely those at risk for seizures.
- Assess degree of cognitive and motor impairment, and assess for environmental hazards.
- Lab tests: Monitor periodically serum electrolytes, liver function, and complete blood counts.
- Monitor responses in children carefully due to limited use with this population.

Patient & Family Education

- Do not or engage in potentially hazardous activities until the response to drug is known.
- Be aware of the risk of orthostatic hypotension.
- Learn adverse effects and report those that are bothersome to physician.
- Wear sunscreen and protective clothing to avoid photosensitivity.
- Notify physician if you intend to or become pregnant.
- Do not breast feed while taking this drug.
- Store this medication out of reach of children.

R

RITONAVIR

(ri-ton′a-vir)
Norvir
Classifications: ANTI-INFECTIVE; ANTIVIRAL; PROTEASE INHIBITOR
Prototype: Saquinavir
Pregnancy Category: B

AVAILABILITY 100 mg capsules; 80 mg/mL solution (contains 43% alcohol)

ACTIONS HIV protease is an enzyme required to produce the polyprotein procurers of functional proteins in infectious HIV. Protease inhibitors prevent cleavage of the viral polyproteins, resulting in the formation of immature noninfectious virus particles.

THERAPEUTIC EFFECTS Protease inhibitor of both HIV-1 and HIV-2 resulting in the formation of noninfectious viral particles.

USE Used in combination with three other antiretroviral agents or protease inhibitors for treatment of HIV infection.

CONTRAINDICATIONS Hypersensitivity to ritonavir; lactation.
CAUTIOUS USE Pregnancy (category B); hepatic impairment, renal insufficiency. Safety and efficacy in children <2 y are not established.

ROUTE & DOSAGE

HIV

Child: **PO** 2–12 y, 400 mg/m^2 b.i.d. (max 600 mg b.i.d.), start with 250 mg/m^2 b.i.d., increase by 50 mg/m^2 q2–3d
Adult: **PO** 600 mg b.i.d. 1 h before or 2 h after meal (may take with a light snack)

STORAGE

Store refrigerated at 2°–8° C (36°–46° F). Protect from light in tightly closed container.

ADMINISTRATION

Oral

- Give preferably with food; oral solution may be mixed with chocolate milk, pudding, or ice cream within 1 h of dosing to improve taste. Sucking on ice chips or frozen treats helps to dull taste buds. Offer strong-flavored food or fluids to remove taste from mouth following dosage.
- Do not give concurrently with any of the following drugs: Alprazolam, amiodarone, astemizole, bepridil, bupropion, cisapride, clozapine, clorazepate, diazepam, encainide, estazolam, flecainide, flurazepam, meperidine, midazolam, piroxicam, propafenone, propoxyphene, quinidine, rifabutin, triazolam, zolpidem.

ADVERSE EFFECTS CNS: *Asthenia,* fatigue, headache, fever, malaise, circumoral or peripheral paresthesia, insomnia, dizziness, somnolence, abnormal thinking, amnesia, agitation, anxiety, confusion, convulsions, aphasia, ataxia, diplopia, emotional lability, euphoria, hallucinations, decreased libido, nervousness, neuralgia, neuropathy, peripheral neuropathy, paralysis, tremor, vertigo. **CV:** Palpitations, vasodilation, hypotension, postural hypotension, syncope, tachycardia. **Hematologic:** Anemia, thrombocytopenia, lymphadenopathy. **GI:** *Nausea, diarrhea, vomiting,* abdominal pain, dyspepsia, stomatitis, anorexia, dry mouth, constipation, flatulence, cholecystitis, cholestasis, abnormal liver function tests, hepatitis. **Skin:** Rash, sweating, acne, contact dermatitis, pruritus, urticaria, skin ulceration, dry skin. **Body as a Whole:** Myalgia, allergic reaction, bronchitis, cough, rhinitis, taste alterations, visual disturbances, dysuria, hyperglycemia, diabetes.

INTERACTIONS Drug: **Carbamazepine, dexamethasone, phenobarbital, phenytoin, rifabutin, rifampin,** smoking can decrease ritonavir levels. **Ritonavir** may increase serum levels and toxicity of **clarithromycin,**

especially in patients with renal insufficiency (reduce **clarithromycin** dose in patients with Cl$_{cr}$ <60 ml/min); **desipramine; saquinavir, amiodarone, indinavir, astemizole, bepridil, bupropion, cisapride, clozapine, dihydroergotamine, flecainide, meperidine, pimozide, piroxicam, propoxyphene, quinidine, rifabutin. Ritonavir** decreases levels of ORAL CONTRACEPTIVES, **theophylline.** Liquid formulation may cause disulfiram-like reaction with **alcohol** or **metronidazole.** See the complete prescribing information for a comprehensive table of potential, but not studied, drug interactions. **Herbal: St. John's wort** may decrease antiretroviral activity.

PHARMACOKINETICS Absorption: Rapidly absorbed from GI tract. **Peak:** 2–4 h. **Distribution:** 98–99% protein bound. **Metabolism:** Metabolized in liver by cytochrome P-4503A4 (CYP3A4). **Elimination:** Excreted primarily in feces (>80%).

NURSING IMPLICATIONS

Assessment & Drug Effects

▪ Lab tests: Monitor periodically CBC with differential and platelet count, liver function, kidney function, serum albumin, lipid profile, CPK, serum amylase, electrolytes, blood glucose HbA$_{1C}$, and alkaline phosphatase. Contains 43% alcohol by volume—may pose a problem in overdosage situations.

▪ Withhold drug and notify physician in the presence of abnormal liver function.

▪ Assess for S&S of GI distress, peripheral neuropathy, and other potential adverse effects.

Patient & Family Education

▪ Learn potential adverse reactions and drug interactions; report to physician use of any OTC or prescription drugs.

▪ Alert patient that Ritonavir may change distribution of body fat increasing fat over, neck, back, and trunk while losing fat from face, arms, and legs.

▪ Do not breast feed while taking this drug.

▪ Take this drug exactly as prescribed. Do not skip doses. Take at same time each day.

▪ Store this medication out of reach of children.

SALMETEROL XINAFOATE

(sal-me′ter-ol xin′a-fo-ate)

Serevent

Classifications: AUTONOMIC NERVOUS SYSTEM AGENT; BETA-ADRENERGIC AGONIST (SYMPATHOMIMETIC); BRONCHODILATOR; RESPIRATORY SMOOTH MUSCLE RELAXANT

Prototype: Albuterol

Pregnancy Category: C

AVAILABILITY 25 mcg aerosol (no longer available in the U.S.); 50 mcg powder diskus for inhalation

---

ACTIONS Long-acting beta$_2$-adrenoreceptor agonist and an analog of albuterol. Stimulation of beta$_2$-adrenoreceptors relaxes bronchospasm and increases ciliary motility, thus facilitating expectoration. Inhibits the release of mediators (i.e., histamine) from mast cells, macrophages, and eosinophils.
THERAPEUTIC EFFECTS Relaxes bronchospasm and increases ciliary motility, thus facilitating expectoration of pulmonary secretions. Salmeterol also decreases airway reaction to allergens.

USES Maintenance therapy for asthma or bronchospasm. Third-line agent in conjunction with fast-acting bronchodilators and inhaled corticosteroids. Prevention of exercise-induced bronchospasm. Do not use to treat acute bronchospasm.

CONTRAINDICATIONS Hypersensitivity to salmeterol; primary treatment of status asthmaticus; pregnancy (category C), lactation. Safety and efficacy in children <4 y not established.
CAUTIOUS USE Cardiovascular disorders, cardiac arrhythmias, hypertension; history of seizures or thyrotoxicosis; liver and renal impairment, diabetes mellitus, sensitivity to other beta-adrenergic agonists; women in labor. Safety and efficacy in children <12 y are not established.

ROUTE & DOSAGE

Asthma or Bronchospasm

Child >12 y/Adult: **Inhalation** 2 inhalations of aerosol (42 mcg) or 1 powder diskus (50 mcg) b.i.d. approximately 12 h apart

Prevention of Exercise-Induced Bronchospasm

Child >12 y/Adult: **Inhaled** 2 inhalations of aerosol (42 mcg) or 1 powder diskus (50 mcg) 30–60 min before exercise 12 h apart

STORAGE
Store at room temperature, 15°–30° C (59°–86° F).

ADMINISTRATION

Inhalation

- Do not use to relieve symptoms of acute asthma.
- Shake canister well before using; close lips tightly around the mouthpiece; patient inhales deeply during each actuation. Use a spacer for children who have trouble following directions.

ADVERSE EFFECTS CNS: Dizziness, headache, tremor. **CV:** Palpitations, sinus tachycardia. **Respiratory:** <u>Respiratory arrest</u> (rare). **Skin:** Rash. **Body as a Whole:** Tolerance (tachyphylaxis).

INTERACTIONS Drug: Effects antagonized by BETA-BLOCKERS.

PHARMACOKINETICS Onset: 10–20 min. **Peak:** Effect 2 h. **Duration:** Up to 12 h. **Distribution:** 94–95% protein bound. **Metabolism:** Dissociates in solution; salmeterol base and xinafoate salt are metabolized, absorbed, distributed, and excreted independently; salmeterol is extensively metabolized by hydroxylation. **Elimination:** Eliminated primarily in feces. **Half-Life:** 3–4 h.

NURSING IMPLICATIONS

Assessment & Drug Effects

- Withhold drug and notify prescriber immediately if bronchospasms occur following its use.
- Monitor cardiovascular status; report tachycardia.
- Monitor liver enzymes periodically with long-term therapy.

Patient & Family Education

- Notify prescriber immediately of worsening asthma or failure to respond to the usual dose of salmeterol.
- Do not use an additional dose prior to exercise if taking twice-daily doses of salmeterol (Dosing should be 12 h apart).
- Take the preexercise dose 30–60 min before exercise and wait 12 h before an additional dose.
- Evaluate child's ability to use inhaler correctly.
- Daily rinse plastic cap and cap with warm water and dry.
- Do not breast feed while taking this drug.
- Work with school to arrange childs acess to medication during school hours.
- Canister and nozzle are to be stored in downward position.
- Store this medication out of reach of children.

SAQUINAVIR MESYLATE ⊙

(sa-quin'a-vir mes'y-late)
Fortovase, Invirase
Classifications: ANTIRETROVIRAL AGENT; PROTEASE INHIBITOR
Pregnancy Category: B

AVAILABILITY Invirase 200 mg capsules; **Fortovase** 200 mg soft gel capsules

ACTIONS Synthetic peptide that inhibits the activity of HIV protease and prevents the cleavage of viral polyproteins essential for the maturation of HIV.
THERAPEUTIC EFFECTS Indicated by reduced viral load (deceased number of RNA copies), and increased numbers of T-helper CD4 cells.

USE Advanced HIV infection, usually in combination with zidovudine or zalcitabine.

CONTRAINDICATIONS Significant hypersensitivity to saquinavir; concurrent administration with lovastatin, simvastatin; lactation.
CAUTIOUS USE Hepatic insufficiency; hepatitis B or C; pregnancy (category B). Safety and effectiveness in HIV-infected children <16 y are not established.

ROUTE & DOSAGE

Note: Invirase and Fortovase are **NOT** bioequivalent and **CANNOT** be interchanged.

HIV

Child: **PO safety and efficacy not established in those <16 y;** clinical study trial group protocol ACTG 397 in Pediatric AIDS 50 mg/kg/dose t.i.d. was used (max 1200 mg/dose t.i.d.)
Adult: **PO** >16 y, Invirase 600 mg (3 times 200 mg) t.i.d. taken 2 h after a full meal; Fortovase 1200 mg (6 times 200 mg) t.i.d. with meals

STORAGE

Store Invirase at 15°–30° C (59°–86° F) in tightly closed bottle. Store Fortovase in refrigerator. Capsules are stable for 3 mo at room temperature ≤25° C (≤77° F).

ADMINISTRATION

Oral

- Give with or up to 2 h after a full meal to ensure adequate absorption and bioavailability.
- Do not give with grapefruit juice.
- Do not administer to anyone taking rifampin or rifabutin because these drugs significantly decrease the plasma level of saquinavir.

ADVERSE EFFECTS CNS: Headache, paresthesia, numbness, dizziness, peripheral neuropathy, ataxia, confusion, convulsions, hyperreflexia, hyporeflexia, tremor, agitation, amnesia, anxiety, depression, excessive dreaming, hallucinations, euphoria, irritability, lethargy, somnolence. **CV:** Chest pain, hypertension, hypotension, syncope. **Endocrine:** Dehydration, hyperglycemia, diabetes, weight changes. **Hematologic:** Anemia, splenomegaly, thrombocytopenia, pancytopenia. **GI:** *Nausea, diarrhea, abdominal discomfort,* dyspepsia, mucosal damage, change in appetite, dry mouth. **Skin:** Rash, pruritus, acne, erythema, seborrhea, hair changes, photosensitivity, skin ulceration, dry skin. **Body as a Whole:** Myalgia, allergic reaction. **Respiratory:** Bronchitis, cough, dyspnea, epistaxis, hemoptysis, laryngitis, rhinitis. **Special Senses:** Xerophthalmia, earache, taste alterations, tinnitus, visual disturbances.

INTERACTIONS Drug: Rifampin, rifabutin significantly decrease **saquinavir** levels. **Phenobarbital, phenytoin, dexamethasone, carbamazepine** may also reduce **saquinavir** levels. **Saquinavir** levels may be increased by **delavirdine, ketoconazole, ritonavir, clarithromycin, indinavir.** May increase serum levels of **cisapride, triazolam, midazolam,** ERGOT DERIVATIVES, **nelfinavir, sildenafil.** May significantly increase **simvastatin** levels and toxicity. **Herbal: St. John's wort** may decrease antiretroviral activity. **Food:** Saquinavir levels are increased with grapefruit juice. Bioavailability of saquinavir is maximized by a high-fat meal.

PHARMACOKINETICS Absorption: Rapidly absorbed from GI tract; only 4% reaches systemic circulation; food significantly reduces absorption. **Distribution:** 98% protein bound. **Metabolism:** Metabolized in liver by cytochrome P-450. **Elimination:** Excreted primarily in feces (>70%).

Common adverse effects in *italic;* life-threatening effects underlined; generic names in **bold;** drug classifications in SMALL CAPS; ♣ Canadian drug name; ✪ Prototype drug.

NURSING IMPLICATIONS

Assessment & Drug Effects

- Lab tests: Monitor serum electrolytes, CBC with differential, liver function, blood glucose and HbA1c, CPK, and serum amylase prior to initiating therapy and periodically thereafter.
- Monitor for and report S&S of peripheral neuropathy.
- Assess for buccal mucosa ulceration or other distressing GI S&S.
- Monitor weight weekly.
- Monitor for toxicity if any of the following drugs is used concomitantly: Calcium channel blockers, clindamycin, dapsone, quinidine, triazolam, or simvastatin.

Patient & Family Education

- Take drug within 2 h of a full meal and do not take drug with grapefruit juice.
- Be aware of all drugs that should not be taken concurrently with saquinavir.
- Be aware that saquinavir is not a cure for HIV infection and that its long-term effects are unknown.
- Report any distressing adverse effects to physician.
- Do not take OTC drugs or the herbal medication St. John's wort while on this drug without physician's approval.
- Do not breast feed while taking this drug.
- Store this medication out of reach of children.

SARGRAMOSTIM (GM-CSF)

(sar-gra′mos-tim)

Leukine, Leukine Liquid, Prokine

Classifications: BLOOD FORMERS, COAGULATORS, AND ANTICOAGULANTS; HEMATOPOIETIC GROWTH FACTOR

Prototype: Epoetin alfa

Pregnancy Category: C

AVAILABILITY 250 mcg, 500 mcg injection

ACTIONS Recombinant human granulocyte macrophage colony stimulating factor (GM-CSF) produced by recombinant DNA technology in a yeast. GM-CSF is a hematopoietic growth factor that stimulates proliferation and differentiation of hematopoietic progenitor cells in the granulocyte-macrophage pathways.

THERAPEUTIC EFFECTS Increases the cytotoxicity of monocytes to certain neoplastic cell lines and activates polymorphonuclear neutrophils (PMNs) to inhibit the growth of tumor cells.

USES Myeloid reconstitution after autologous bone marrow transplantation for patients with non-Hodgkin's lymphoma (NHL), acute lymphoblastic leukemia (ALL), and Hodgkin's disease; mobilization of peripheral blood stem cells (PBSCs) for autologous transplantation.

SARGRAMOSTIM (GM-CSF)

UNLABELED USES To increase WBC counts in AIDS patients; to decrease leukopenia secondary to myelosuppressive chemotherapy; to correct neutropenia in aplastic anemia and in liver and kidney transplantations.

CONTRAINDICATIONS Excessive leukemic myeloid blasts in bone marrow or blood; history of idiopathic thrombocytopenia, purpura; known hypersensitivity to GM-CSF or yeast products.
CAUTIOUS USE History of cardiac arrhythmias, preexisting cardiac disease, hypoxia, CHF, pulmonary infiltrates; kidney and liver dysfunction; pregnancy (category C), lactation. Safety and efficacy in children are not established (no FDA approval for childhood dosing); however, adverse side effects have been comparable to those in adults.

ROUTE & DOSAGE

Autologous Bone Marrow Transplant
Child: **IV/SC** 250 mcg/m^2/day times 21 days, begin 2–4 h after bone marrow infusion or not less than 24 h after chemotherapy
Adult: **IV** 250 mcg/m^2/day infused over 2 h for 21 days, begin 2–4 h after bone marrow transfusion and not less than 24 h after last dose of chemotherapy or 12 h after last radiation therapy

Neutropenia
Child/Adult: **SC** 3–15 mcg/kg/day times one dose

STORAGE
Refrigerate the sterile powder, the reconstituted solution, and store diluted solution at 2°–8° C (36°–46° F). Reconstitute solutions with sterile water stable for 6 h at room temperature 15°–30° C (59°–86° F); discard after 6 h.

ADMINISTRATION
Note: Do not give within 24 h preceding or following chemotherapy or within 12 h preceding or following radiotherapy.

Subcutaneous
- Reconstitute each 250- or 500-mcg vial with 1 mL of sterile water for injection (without preservative). Direct sterile water against side of vial and swirl gently. Avoid excessive or vigorous agitation. Do not shake. Use without further dilution for SC injection.

Intravenous

Note: Verify correct IV concentration and rate of infusion administration in infants and children with physician.
PREPARE **IV Infusion:** Reconstitute as for SC, then further dilute reconstituted solution with NS. If the final concentration is <1 mcg/mL, add albumin (human) to NS before addition of sargramostim. Use 1 mg albumin per 1 mL of NS to give a final concentration of 0.1% albumin. Administer as soon as possible and within 6 h of reconstitution or dilution for IV infusion. Discard after 6 h. Sargramostim vials are single-dose vials; do not reenter or reuse. Discard unused portion.
ADMINISTER **IV Infusion:** Give over 2 h. Do not use an in-line membrane filter.

INCOMPATIBILITIES **Solution/Additive:** Hydrocortisone, hydroxyzine, haloperidol. **Y-Site:** Acyclovir, amphotericin B, ampicillin, ampicillin/sulbactam, amsacrine, cefonicid, cefoperazone, chlorpromazine, ganciclovir, haloperidol, hydrocortisone, hydromorphone, hydroxyzine, idarubicin, imipenem/cilastatin, lorazepam, methylprednisolone, mitomycin, morphine, nalbuphine, ondansetron, piperacillin, sodium bicarbonate, tobramycin.

- Interrupt administration and reduce the dose by 50% if absolute neutrophil count exceeds 20,000/mm^3 or if platelet count exceeds 500,000/mm^3. Notify physician.
- Reduce the IV rate 50% if patient experiences dyspnea during administration. Discontinue infusion if respiratory symptoms worsen. Notify physician.

ADVERSE EFFECTS CNS: Lethargy, malaise, headache, fatigue. **CV:** <u>Abnormal ST segment depression, supraventricular arrhythmias</u>, edema, *hypotension, tachycardia,* <u>pericardial effusion</u>, pericarditis. **Hematologic:** Anemia, *thrombocytopenia.* **GI:** Nausea, vomiting, diarrhea, anorexia. **Body as a Whole:** *Bone pain, myalgia, arthralgias,* weight gain, hyperuricemia, *fever.* **Respiratory:** Pleural effusion. **Skin:** *Rash, pruritus.* **Other:** *First-dose reaction* (some or all of the following symptoms: Hypotension, tachycardia, fever, rigors, flushing, nausea, vomiting, diaphoresis, back pain, leg spasms, and dyspnea).

INTERACTIONS Drug: CORTICOSTEROIDS should be used cautiously with sargramostim because the myeloproliferative effects may be potentiated. **Lithium** should be used with caution with sargramostim because it may potentiate the myeloproliferative effects.

PHARMACOKINETICS Absorption: Readily absorbed from SC site. **Onset:** 3–6 h. **Peak:** 1–2 h. **Duration:** 5–10 days SC. **Elimination:** Probably excreted in urine. **Half-Life:** 80–150 min.

NURSING IMPLICATIONS

Assessment & Drug Effects

- Lab tests: Obtain a CBC and platelet count prior to initiation of therapy. Monitor biweekly CBC with differential during therapy. Monitor kidney and liver function biweekly in patients with kidney or liver dysfunction prior to the initiation of therapy.
- Discontinue treatment if WBC more than 50,000/mm^3. Notify the physician.
- Occasional transient supraventricular arrhythmias have occurred during administration, particularly in those with a history of cardiac arrhythmias. Arrhythmias are reversed with discontinuation of drug.
- Give special attention to respiratory symptoms (dyspnea) during and immediately following infusion, especially in patients with preexisting pulmonary disease.
- Use drug with caution in patients with preexisting fluid retention, pulmonary infiltrates, or CHF. Peripheral edema, pleural or pericardial effusion has occurred after administration. It is reversible with dose reduction.

- Notify physician of any severe adverse reaction immediately.
- Discontinue therapy and notify physician if disease progression is detected. Potentially, drug can act as a growth factor for myeloid malignancies.

Patient & Family Education
- Notify nurse or physician immediately of any adverse effect (e.g., dyspnea, palpitations, peripheral edema, bone or muscle pain) during or after drug administration.
- Do not breast feed while taking this drug without consulting physician.

SCOPOLAMINE
(skoe-pol′a-meen)
Transderm-Scop, Transderm-V ✤

SCOPOLAMINE HYDROBROMIDE
Hyoscine, Isopto-Hyoscine, Murocoll, Triptone
Classifications: AUTONOMIC NERVOUS SYSTEM AGENT; ANTICHOLINERGIC (PARASYMPATHOLYTIC); ANTIMUSCARINIC; ANTISPASMODIC
Prototype: Atropine
Pregnancy Category: C

AVAILABILITY Scopolamine 0.4 mg tablets; 1.5 mg transdermal patch
Scopolamine HBr 0.4 mg tablets; 0.3 mg/mL, 0.4 mg/mL, 0.86 mg/mL, 1 mg/mL injection; 0.25% ophthalmic solution

ACTIONS Alkaloid of belladonna with peripheral actions resembling those of atropine. In contrast to atropine, produces CNS depression with marked sedative and tranquilizing effects, and is less effective in preventing reflex bradycardia during anesthesia. More potent in mydriatic and cycloplegic actions and in inhibiting secretions of salivary, bronchial, and sweat glands, but has less prominent effect on heart, intestines, and bronchial muscles.
THERAPEUTIC EFFECTS More potent than atropine in mydriatic and cycloplegic actions. Produces CNS depression with marked sedative and tranquilizing effects for use in anesthesia. Used as a preanesthetic agent to control bronchial, nasal, pharyngeal and salivary secretions.

USES In obstetrics with morphine to produce amnesia and sedation ("twilight sleep") and as preanesthetic medication. To control spasticity (and drooling) in postencephalitic parkinsonism, paralysis agitans, and other spastic states, as prophylactic agent for motion sickness and as mydriatic and cycloplegic in ophthalmology. Therapeutic system (Transderm-Scop) is used to prevent nausea and vomiting associated with motion sickness.

CONTRAINDICATIONS Hepatitis; asthma toxemia of pregnancy; hypersensitivity to anticholinergic drugs; hypersensitive to belladonna or barbiturates; narrow-angle glaucoma; GI or urogenital obstructive diseases; myasthenia gravis; pregnancy (category C), lactation.

S

CAUTIOUS USE Coronary heart disease, CHF, cardiac arrhythmias, tachycardia, hypertension; patients >40 y, pyloric obstruction, urinary bladder neck obstruction, angle-closure glaucoma, thyrotoxicosis, liver disease; paralytic ileus; hiatal hernia, ulcerative colitis, gastric ulcer; COPD, asthma or allergies; hyperthyroidism; brain damage, spastic paralysis; tartrazine or sulfite sensitivity; in infants and children.

ROUTE & DOSAGE

Preanesthetic
Child: **PO/IM/SC/IV** 0.006 mg/kg/dose (max dose 0.3 mg/dose)
Adult: **PO** 0.5–1 mg **IM/SC/IV** 0.3–0.6 mg

Motion Sickness
Child >12 y/Adult: **PO** 0.25–0.6 mg 1 h before anticipated travel
Topical: 1 patch starting 12 h before anticipated travel; remove in 72 h

Refraction
Adult: **Ophthalmic** 1–2 drops in eye 1 h before refraction

Uveitis
Adult: **Ophthalmic** 1–2 drops in eye up to q.i.d.

STORAGE
Preserve in tight, light-resistant containers at 15°–30° C (59°–86° F).

ADMINISTRATION

Instillation
- Minimize possibility of systemic absorption by applying pressure against lacrimal sac during and for 1 or 2 min following instillation of eye drops.

Transdermal
- Apply transdermal disc system (Transderm-Scop, a controlled-release system) to dry surface behind the ear.
- Replace with another disc on another site behind the ear if disc system becomes dislodged.

Subcutaneous or Intramuscular
- Give undiluted.

Intravenous
PREPARE **Direct:** Dilute required dose in 10 mL of sterile water for injection.
ADMINISTER **Direct:** Give a single dose over 1 min or in children over 2–3 min.

ADVERSE EFFECTS Body as a Whole: Fatigue, dizziness, *drowsiness,* disorientation, restlessness, hallucinations, toxic psychosis. **GI:** *Dry mouth and throat, constipation.* **Urogenital:** Urinary retention. **CV:** Decreased heart rate. **Special Senses:** Dilated pupils, photophobia, blurred vision, *local irritation,* follicular conjunctivitis. **Respiratory:** <u>Depressed respiration.</u> **Skin:** Local irritation from patch adhesive, rash.

Common adverse effects in *italic;* life-threatening effects <u>underlined;</u> generic names in **bold;** drug classifications in SMALL CAPS; ♣ Canadian drug name; ۞ Prototype drug.

1099

INTERACTIONS Drug: Amantadine, ANTIHISTAMINES, TRICYCLIC ANTIDEPRESSANTS, **quinidine, disopyramide, procainamide** add to anticholinergic effects; decreases **levodopa** effects; **methotrimeprazine** may precipitate extrapyramidal effects; decreases antipsychotic effects (decreased absorption) of PHENOTHIAZINES.

PHARMACOKINETICS Absorption: Readily absorbed from GI tract and percutaneously. **Peak:** 20–60 min. **Duration:** 5–7 days. **Distribution:** Crosses placenta; distributed to CNS. **Metabolism:** Metabolized in liver. **Elimination:** Excreted in urine.

NURSING IMPLICATIONS

Assessment & Drug Effects

- Observe patient closely; some patients manifest excitement, delirium, and disorientation shortly after drug is administered until sedative effect takes hold.
- Use of side rails is advisable because of amnesic effect of scopolamine.
- In the presence of pain, scopolamine may cause delirium, restlessness, and excitement unless given with an analgesic.
- Be aware that tolerance may develop with prolonged use.
- Terminate ophthalmic use if local irritation, edema, or conjunctivitis occur.

Patient & Family Education

- Vision may blur when used as mydriatic or cycloplegic; do not drive or engage in potentially hazardous activities (biking, skateboarding, and sports) until vision clears.
- Place disc on skin site the night before an expected trip or anticipated motion for best therapeutic effect.
- Wash hands carefully after handling scopolamine. Anisocoria (unequal size of pupils, blurred vision can develop by rubbing eye with drug-contaminated finger).
- Discard patches in a place inaccessible to children and pets.
- Store this medication out of reach of children.

S

SECOBARBITAL SODIUM ℗

(see-koe-bar'bi-tal)

Seconal Sodium

Classifications: CENTRAL NERVOUS SYSTEM AGENT; SEDATIVE-HYPNOTIC; BARBITURATE; ANXIOLYTIC

Pregnancy Category: D

Controlled Substance: Schedule II

AVAILABILITY 100 mg capsules

ACTIONS Short-acting barbiturate with CNS depressant effects as well as mood alteration from excitation to mild sedation, hypnosis, and deep coma. Depresses the sensory cortex, decreases motor activity, alters cerebellar function and produces drowsiness, sedation and hypnosis.

THERAPEUTIC EFFECTS Alters cerebellar function and produces drowsiness, sedation and hypnosis.

USES Hypnotic for simple insomnia and preoperatively to provide basal hypnosis for general, spinal, or regional anesthesia.

CONTRAINDICATIONS History of sensitivity to barbiturates; porphyria; severe liver function; severe respiratory disease; nephritic syndrome; pregnancy (category D), parturition, fetal immaturity; uncontrolled pain. Use of sterile injection containing polyethylene glycol vehicle in patients with renal insufficiency.

CAUTIOUS USE Pregnant women with toxemia or history of bleeding; labor and delivery, lactation; liver or kidney function impairment, debilitated individuals; children.

ROUTE & DOSAGE

Sedative

Child: **PO** 4–6 mg/kg/day in 3 divided doses every 8 h
Adult: **PO** 100–300 mg/day in 3 divided doses

Preoperative Sedative

Child: **PO** 2–6 mg/kg 1–2 h prior to surgery (max dose 100 mg/dose)
Adult: **PO** 100–300 mg 1–2 h before surgery

Hypnotic

Adult: **PO** 100–200 mg/dose at bedtime

STORAGE

Store at 15°–30° C (59°–86° F) in tightly closed containers

ADMINISTRATION

Oral

- Give hypnotic dose only after patient retires for the evening.
- Crush and mix with a fluid or with food if patient cannot swallow pill.

ADVERSE EFFECTS CNS: Drowsiness, lethargy, hangover, paradoxical excitement. **Respiratory:** <u>Respiratory depression, laryngospasm.</u>

INTERACTIONS Drug: Phenmetrazine antagonizes effects of secobarbital; CNS DEPRESSANTS, **alcohol,** SEDATIVES compound CNS depression; MAO INHIBITORS cause excessive CNS depression; **methoxyflurane** increases risk of nephrotoxicity. **Herbal: Kava-kava, valerian** may potentiate sedation. **Food:** May increase metabolism of vitamins D and K.

PHARMACOKINETICS Absorption: 90% absorbed from GI tract. **Onset:** 15–30 min. **Duration:** 1–4 h. **Distribution:** Crosses placenta; distributed into breast milk. **Metabolism:** Metabolized in liver. **Elimination:** Excreted in urine. **Half-Life:** 30 h.

NURSING IMPLICATIONS

Assessment & Drug Effects

- Be alert to unexpected responses and report promptly. Debilitated patients and children sometimes have paradoxical response to barbiturate therapy (i.e., irritability, marked excitement as inappropriate tearfulness and aggression in children, depression, and confusion). Protect patients from falling and monitor for irrational behavior, and effects of depression (anorexia, social withdrawal).

- Patient may become irritable, and uncooperative after a subhypnotic dose of a short-acting barbiturate (uncommon response).
- Be aware that barbiturates do not have analgesic action, and may produce restlessness when given to patients in pain.
- Long-term therapy may result in nutritional folate (B_9) and vitamin D deficiency.
- Lab tests: Obtain liver function and hematology tests, serum folate and vitamin D levels during prolonged therapy.
- Observe closely for changes in established drug regimen effectiveness whenever a barbiturate is added, at least during early phase of barbiturate use. Barbiturates increase the metabolism of many drugs, leading to decreased pharmacologic effects of those drugs.
- Be alert for acute toxicity (intoxication) characterized by profound CNS depression, respiratory depression that may progress to Cheyne-Stokes respirations, hypoventilation, cyanosis, cold clammy skin, hypothermia, constricted pupils (but may be dilated in severe intoxication), shock, oliguria, tachycardia, hypotension, respiration arrest, circulatory collapse, and death.

Patient & Family Education

- Do not drive or engage in potentially hazardous activities (biking, skateboarding, and sports) until response to drug is established.
- Store barbiturates in a safe place; not on the bedside table or other readily accessible places. It is possible to forget having taken the drug, and in half-wakened conditions take more and accidentally overdose.
- Barbiturates are reportedly teratogenic. Do not become pregnant. Use or add barrier contraception if using hormonal contraceptives.
- Report onset of fever, sore throat or mouth, malaise, easy bruising or bleeding, petechiae, jaundice, rash to physician during prolonged therapy.
- Do not consume alcohol in any amount when taking a barbiturate. It may severely impair judgment and abilities.
- Do not breast feed while taking this drug without consulting physician.
- Store this medication in locked area out of reach of children; this is a Schedule II drug.

SELENIUM SULFIDE

(se-lee′nee-um)

Exsel, Selsun, Selsun Blue

Classifications: SKIN AND MUCOUS MEMBRANE AGENT; ANTI-INFECTIVE; ANTIBIOTIC; ANTIFUNGAL

Pregnancy Category: C

AVAILABILITY 1% lotion, shampoo

ACTIONS Has antibacterial and mild antifungal activity, although mechanism of action and causal relationships are not established. Absorption of selenium sulfide into epithelial tissue cells is followed by degradation of compound to selenium and sulfide ions. Selenium ions block enzyme systems involved in epithelial cell growth. As a result, rate of turnover in cells with normal or higher than normal turnover rates is reduced.

THERAPEUTIC EFFECTS Active against *Pityrosporum ovale,* a yeast-like fungus found in the normal flora of the scalp. Also decreases rate of growth of the epithelial cells of the scalp and other epithelial layers of cells in the body. Utilized in treatment of seborrheic dermatitis and tinea versicolor.

USES Itching and flaking of the scalp associated with dandruff, seborrheic dermatitis of the scalp, and tinea versicolor.

CONTRAINDICATIONS Application to damaged or inflamed skin surfaces; as treatment of tinea versicolor during pregnancy. Use during pregnancy (category C) as antiseborrheic only when clearly needed; kidney failure or biliary tract obstruction, GI malfunction; Wilson's disease.

CAUTIOUS USE Prolonged skin contact; use in genital area or skin folds. Safe use in infants not established and use in children <2 y should be avoided

ROUTE & DOSAGE

Dandruff Control, Seborrheic Dermatitis

Child >2 y/Adult: **Topical** Massage 5–10 mL of a 1–2.5% solution into wet scalp and leave on for 2–3 min, rinse thoroughly, then repeat application and rinse well again (initially, shampoo 2 times/wk for 2 wk, then decrease to once q1–4wk prn)

Tinea Versicolor

Child >2 y/Adult: **Topical** Apply a 2.5% solution to affected area with a small amount of water to form a lather, leave on for 10 min, then rinse thoroughly, repeat daily for 7 days

STORAGE
Store at 15°–30° C (59°–86° F) in tight container; protected from heat. Avoid freezing.

ADMINISTRATION

Topical
- Wash hands thoroughly after application of selenium sulfide to affected areas. Remove jewelry before treatment; drug will damage it.
- Avoid contact with eyes or denuded skin.
- Rinse genital areas and skin folds well with water and dry thoroughly after treatment for tinea versicolor to prevent irritation.

ADVERSE EFFECTS Skin: *Skin irritation (stinging),* rebound oiliness of scalp, hair discoloration, diffuse hair loss (reversible), systemic toxicity (if applied to abraded, infected skin).

INTERACTIONS Drug: No clinically significant interactions established.

PHARMACOKINETICS Absorption: No percutaneous absorption if skin is intact.

Common adverse effects in *italic;* life-threatening effects underlined; generic names in **bold;** drug classifications in SMALL CAPS; ♣ Canadian drug name; ✪ Prototype drug.

1103

NURSING IMPLICATIONS

Assessment & Drug Effects

- Monitor therapeutic effectiveness.

Patient & Family Education

- Rinse thoroughly with water if lotion contacts eyes in order to prevent chemical conjunctivitis.
- Do not use drug more frequently than required to maintain control of dandruff.
- Hair loss is reversible, usually within 2–3 wk after treatment is discontinued.
- Discontinue use if skin is irritated or treatment fails. Systemic toxicity may result from application of lotion to damaged skin (percutaneous absorption) or from prolonged use (overdosage). Toxicity symptoms include: Tremors, anorexia, occasional vomiting, lethargy, weakness, severe perspiration, garlicky breath, lower abdominal pain. Symptoms disappear 10–12 days after treatment is stopped.
- Store this medication out of reach of children.

SENNA (SENNOSIDES)

(sen′na)

Black-Draught, Children's Senokot, Ex-Lax, Gentlax B, Senexon, Senokot, Senolax

Classifications: GASTROINTESTINAL AGENT; STIMULANT LAXATIVE
Prototype: Bisacodyl
Pregnancy Category: C

AVAILABILITY 8.6 mg, 15 mg, 25 mg tablets; 8.8 mg/5 mL, 15 mg/5 mL syrup

ACTIONS Prepared from dried leaflet of *Cassia acutifolia* or *Cassia angustifolia*. Similar to *cascara sagrada* but with more potent action. Senna glycosides are converted in colon to active aglycone, which stimulates peristalsis. Concentrate is purified and standardized for uniform action and is claimed to produce less colic than crude form.
THERAPEUTIC EFFECTS Peristalsis stimulated by conversion of drug to active chemical.

USES Acute constipation and preoperative and preradiographic bowel evacuation.

CONTRAINDICATIONS Hypersensitivity; appendicitis, fecal impaction, irritable colon, nausea, vomiting, undiagnosed abdominal pain, intestinal obstruction; pregnancy (category C), lactation; children <2 y.
CAUTIOUS USE Diabetes mellitus; fluid and electrolyte imbalances.

ROUTE & DOSAGE

Constipation

Child: **PO Standard Senna Concentrate** *>27 kg,* 1 tablet or ½ tsp bedtime **Syrup, Liquid** *1 mo–1 y,* 1.25–2.5 mL bedtime (max 5 mL); *1–5 y,* 2.5–5 mL bedtime; *5–15 y,* 5–10 mL bedtime

Common adverse effects in *italic;* life-threatening effects <u>underlined;</u> generic names in **bold;** drug classifications in SMALL CAPS; ◆ Canadian drug name; ● Prototype drug.

Adult: **PO Standard Senna Concentrate** 1–2 tablets or ½–1 tsp bedtime (max dose 4 tablets or 2 tsp b.i.d.) **Syrup, Liquid** 10–15 mL at bedtime (max 15 mL or 2 tsp b.i.d.)

STORAGE
Store at 15°–30° C (59°–86° F) in tightly closed light-resistant containers.

ADMINISTRATION

Oral

■ Give at bedtime, generally.
■ Avoid exposing drug to excessive heat; protect fluid extracts from light.

ADVERSE EFFECTS GI: Abdominal cramps, flatulence, nausea, watery diarrhea, excessive loss of water and electrolytes, weight loss, melanotic segmentation of colonic mucosa (reversible).

PHARMACOKINETICS Onset: 6–10 h; may take up to 24 h. **Metabolism:** Metabolized in liver. **Elimination:** Excreted in feces.

NURSING IMPLICATIONS

Assessment & Drug Effects

■ Reduce dose in patients who experience considerable abdominal cramping.

Patient & Family Education

■ Be aware that drug may alter urine and feces color; yellowish brown (acid), reddish brown (alkaline).
■ Continued use may lead to dependence (usage over 1 wk). Do not take more frequently or in amounts greater than prescribed. Consult prescriber if constipation persists.
■ See **bisacodyl** for additional nursing implications.
■ Do not breast feed while taking this drug.
■ Store this medication out of reach of children.

S

SERTRALINE HYDROCHLORIDE

(ser'tra-leen)
Zoloft
Classifications: CENTRAL NERVOUS SYSTEM AGENT; PSYCHOTHERAPEUTIC; ANTIDEPRESSANT; SELECTIVE SEROTONIN-REUPTAKE INHIBITOR (SSRI)
Prototype: Fluoxetine
Pregnancy Category: C

AVAILABILITY 25 mg, 50 mg, 100 mg tablets; 20 mg/mL liquid (contains 12% alcohol)

ACTIONS Potent inhibitor of serotonin (5 HT) reuptake in the brain, and chemically unrelated to TCA, tetracyclic, or other available antidepressants. Chronic administration of sertraline results in down regulation of

---

norepinephrine, a reaction found with other effective antidepressants. Sertraline does not inhibit MAO.

THERAPEUTIC EFFECTS Treats depression, obsessive-compulsive disorder, and panic disorder.

USES Major depression, obsessive-compulsive disorder, panic disorder, premenstrual dysphoric disorder, generalized anxiety, post-traumatic stress disorder.

CONTRAINDICATIONS Patients taking MAO inhibitors or within 14 days of discontinuing MAO inhibitor; antabuse.

CAUTIOUS USE Seizure disorders, major affective disorders, suicidal patients; may activate mania in the bipolar patient; liver dysfunction, renal impairment; pregnancy (category C). Unknown if sertraline is excreted in breast milk. Safety and effectiveness in children <6 y are not established.

ROUTE & DOSAGE

Depression, Anxiety

Child 6–12 y (Limited data with this age group): **PO** Begin with 25 mg/day, may increase by 25–50 mg/wk, as tolerated and needed, up to maximum dose 200 mg/day
Adolescent ≥13 y/Adult: **PO** Begin with 50 mg/day gradually increase every few weeks according to response (range: 50–200 mg) (maximum dose 200 mg/day)

Obsessive Compulsive Disorder

Child 6–12 y: **PO** Begin with 25 mg/day, may increase by 25–50 mg/wk, as tolerated and needed, up to maximum dose 200 mg/day
Adolescent ≥13 y/Adult: **PO** Begin with 50 mg/day may titrate at weekly intervals by 50 mg up to maximum dose 200 mg/day

STORAGE
Store at 15°–30° C (59°–86° F).

ADMINISTRATION

Oral

- Give in the morning or evening.
- May give with food but avoid giving with grapefruit juice.
- Oral concentrate must be mixed with at least 120 mL of water, lemon/lime soda, ginger ale, lemonade, or orange juice and consumed at once. The mixture will appear slightly hazy.
- Do not give concurrently with a MAO inhibitor or within 14 days of discontinuing a MAOI.

ADVERSE EFFECTS CV: Palpitations, chest pain, hypertension, hypotension, edema, syncope, tachycardia. **CNS:** *Agitation, insomnia, headache, dizziness, somnolence, fatigue,* ataxia, incoordination, vertigo, abnormal dreams, aggressive behavior, delusions, hallucinations, emotional lability, paranoia, suicidal ideation, depersonalization. **Endocrine:** Gynecomastia, male sexual dysfunction. **GI:** Nausea, vomiting, diarrhea, constipation, indigestion, anorexia, flatulence, abdominal pain, dry mouth.

Special Senses: Exophthalmos, blurred vision, dry eyes, diplopia, photophobia, tearing, conjunctivitis, mydriasis. **Skin:** Rash, urticaria, acne, alopecia. **Respiratory:** Rhinitis, pharyngitis, cough, dyspnea, bronchospasm. **Body as a Whole:** Myalgia, arthralgia, muscle weakness. **Metabolic:** Hyponatremia.

DIAGNOSTIC TEST INTERFERENCE May cause asymptomatic elevations in *liver function tests.* Slight decrease in *uric acid.*

INTERACTIONS Drug: MAOIS (e.g., **selegiline, phenelzine**) should be stopped 14 days before sertraline is started because of serious problems with other SEROTONIN-REUPTAKE INHIBITORS (shivering, nausea, diplopia, confusion, anxiety). **Sertraline** may increase levels and toxicity of **diazepam, pimozide, tolbutamide, warfarin**. Use cautiously with other centrally acting CNS drugs. **Herbal: St. John's wort** may cause **serotonin** syndrome (headache, dizziness, sweating, agitation). **Food:** Increased serum levels of sertraline can occur with grapfruit juice. Foods containing tryptophan may increase the side effects of sertraline.

PHARMACOKINETICS Absorption: Slowly absorbed from GI tract. **Onset:** 2–4 wk. **Distribution:** 99% protein bound; not known if distributed into breast milk. **Metabolism:** Extensive first-pass metabolism in liver to inactive metabolites. **Elimination:** 40–45% excreted in urine, 40–45% in feces. **Half-Life:** 24 h.

NURSING IMPLICATIONS

Assessment & Drug Effects
- Supervise patients especially adolescents at risk for suicide closely during initial therapy.
- Monitor for fluid and sodium imbalances.
- Monitor patients with a history of a seizure disorder closely.
- Lab tests: Monitor PT and INR with patients receiving concurrent warfarin therapy.
- Antidepressants increase risk of suicidal thinking and behavior in children and adolescents with major depressive disorder, obsessive compulsive disorder, and other psychiatric disorders. Observe closely for worsening of condition, suicidality, and behavior changes. Instruct family and caregivers to monitor for these symptoms and discuss with prescriber. A MedGuide describing risks and stating whether the drug is approved for the child's adolescent's condition should be provided for all families when antidepressants are prescribed.

Patient & Family Education
- Report diarrhea, nausea, dyspepsia, insomnia, drowsiness, dizziness, or persistent headache to physician.
- Avoid alcohol, tryptophan-containing foods, grapefruit juice, and St. John's wort while on sertraline.
- Report signs of bleeding promptly to physician when taking concomitant warfarin.
- Family members should be aware of need to supervise patients at risk for suicide closely during initial therapy.
- If insomnia occurs, take dose in morning.
- Do not breast feed while taking this drug without consulting prescriber.
- Store this medication out of reach of children.

SILVER SULFADIAZINE
(sul-fa-dye′a-zeen)
Silvadene, Thermazene
Classifications: ANTI-INFECTIVE; SULFONAMIDE
Prototype: Sulfisoxazole
Pregnancy Category: C

AVAILABILITY 1%, 10 mg/g cream

ACTIONS Produced by reaction of silver nitrate with sulfadiazine. Mechanism of action differs from that of either component. Silver salt is released slowly and exerts bactericidal effect only on bacterial cell membrane and wall, rather than by inhibiting folic acid synthesis; antibacterial activity is not inhibited by *p*-aminobenzoic acid (PABA). Contact with sodium chloride in body tissues and fluids results in slow release of sulfadiazine, which may be systemically absorbed from application site.
THERAPEUTIC EFFECTS Broad antimicrobial activity including many gram-negative and gram-positive bacteria and yeast.

USE Prevention and treatment of sepsis in second- and third-degree burns.

CONTRAINDICATIONS Hypersensitivity to other sulfonamides; G6PD deficiency; pregnancy (category C), pregnant women at term, lactation, premature infants and neonates <2 mo.
CAUTIOUS USE Impaired kidney or liver function; impaired respiratory function.

ROUTE & DOSAGE

Burn Wound Treatment
Child/Adult: **Topical** Apply 1% cream 1–2 times/day to thickness of approximately 1.5 mm (¹⁄₁₆ in)

STORAGE
Store at 15°–30° C (59°–86° F) away from heat.

ADMINISTRATION
Topical
- Do not use if cream darkens; it is water soluble and white.
- Apply with sterile, gloved hands to cleansed, debrided burned areas. Reapply cream to areas where it has been removed by patient activity; cover burn wounds with medication at all times.
- Clean wound according to physician's directions before reapplying drug.
- Note: Dressings are not required but may be used if necessary. Drug does not stain clothing.

ADVERSE EFFECTS Body as a Whole: Pain (occasionally), burning, itching, rash, reversible leukopenia. <u>Potential for toxicity</u> as for other sulfonamides if applied to extensive areas of the body surface.

INTERACTIONS Drug: PROTEOLYTIC ENZYMES are inactivated by silver in cream.

PHARMACOKINETICS Absorption: Not absorbed through intact skin, however, approximately 10% could be absorbed when applied to second- or third-degree burns. **Distribution:** Distributed into most body tissues. **Metabolism:** Metabolized in the liver. **Elimination:** Excreted in urine.

NURSING IMPLICATIONS

Assessment & Drug Effects
- Observe for and report hypersensitivity reaction: Rash, itching, or burning sensation in unburned areas.
- Lab tests: Obtain, urinalysis, and kidney function tests when drug is applied to extensive areas. Significant quantities of drug may be absorbed.
- Observe patient for reactions attributed to sulfonamides.
- Analgesic may be required. Occasionally, pain is experienced on application; intensity and duration depend on depth of burn.
- Continue treatment until satisfactory healing or burn site is ready for grafting, unless adverse reactions occur.

Patient & Family Education
- Do not apply more frequently than ordered or in thick quantities.
- Do not breast feed while taking this drug.
- Store this medication out of reach of children.

SIROLIMUS
(sir-o-li'mus)
Rapamune
Classifications: IMMUNOMODULATOR; IMMUNOSUPPRESSANT
Prototype: Cyclosporine
Pregnancy Category: C

AVAILABILITY 1 mg tablets; 1 mg/mL oral solution

ACTIONS Macrolide antibiotic structurally related to tacrolimus with immunosuppressive activity. Active in reducing a transplant rejection by inhibiting the response of helper T-lymphocytes and B-lymphocytes to cytokinesis (interleukin [IL]-2, IL-4, and IL-5).
THERAPEUTIC EFFECTS Inhibits antibody production and acute transplant rejection reaction in autoimmune disorders (e.g., systemic lupus erythematous [SLE]). Indicated by nonrejection of transplanted organ.

USES Prophylaxis of kidney transplant rejection.
UNLABELED USE Treatment of psoriasis.

CONTRAINDICATIONS Hypersensitivity to sirolimus; pregnancy (category C); lactation.
CAUTIOUS USE Hypersensitivity to or concurrent administration with tacrolimus; viral or bacterial infection; hyperlipidemia, diabetic patients; coronary artery disease; myelosuppression; liver disease.

ROUTE & DOSAGE

Kidney Transplant

Adolescent ≥ 13 y and <40 kg/Adult: **PO** 3 mg/m² loading dose immediately after transplant, then 1 mg/m²/day
Adult: **PO** 6 mg loading dose immediately after transplant, then 2 mg/day
Hepatic Impairment Reduce maintenance dose by 33%

STORAGE

Refrigerate oral solutions and pouches at 2°–8° C (36°–46° F). Protect from light. Contents must be used within 30 days if kept refrigerated.

ADMINISTRATION

Oral

- Give 4 h after oral cyclosporine.
- Add prescribed amount of sirolimus to a glass containing ≥2 oz (60 mL) of water or orange juice (do not use any other type of liquid). Stir vigorously and administer immediately. Refill glass with ≥4 oz (120 mL) of water or orange juice. Stir vigorously and administer immediately.
- Give consistently with respect to amount and type of food.
- Solution will get a slight haze upon refrigeration, bring to room temperature and agitate gently until haze disappears. Haze does not affect drugs potency.

ADVERSE EFFECTS Body as a Whole: *Asthenia, back pain, chest pain, fever, pain, arthralgia;* flu-like syndrome; generalized edema; infection; lymphocele; malaise, <u>sepsis</u>, arthrosis, bone necrosis, leg cramps, myalgia, osteoporosis, tetany, abscess, ascites, cellulitis, chills, face edema, hernia, pelvic pain, peritonitis. **CNS:** *Insomnia, tremor, headache,* anxiety, confusion, depression, dizziness, emotional lability, hypertonia, hyperesthesia, hypotonia, neuropathy, paresthesia, somnolence. **CV:** *Hypertension,* <u>atrial fibrillation</u>, CHF, hypervolemia, hypotension, palpitation, peripheral vascular disorder, postural hypotension, syncope, tachycardia, thrombophlebitis, thrombosis, vasodilation. **GI:** *Constipation, diarrhea, dyspepsia, nausea, vomiting, abdominal pain,* anorexia, dysphagia, eructation, esophagitis, flatulence, gastritis, gastroenteritis, gingivitis, gum hyperplasia, ileus, mouth ulceration, oral moniliasis, stomatitis, abnormal liver function tests. **Hematologic:** *Anemia,* <u>thrombocytopenia, leukopenia</u>, hemorrhage, ecchymosis, leukocytosis, lymphadenopathy, polycythemia, thrombotic, thrombocytopenic purpura. **Metabolic:** *Edema, hypercholesterolemia, hyperkalemia, hyperlipidemia, hypokalemia, hypophosphatemia, peripheral edema, weight gain,* Cushing's syndrome, diabetes, acidosis, hypercalcemia, hyperglycemia, hyperphosphatemia, hypocalcemia, hypoglycemia, hypomagnesemia, hyponatremia; increased LDH, alkaline phosphatase, BUN, creatine phosphokinase, ALT, or AST; weight loss. **Respiratory:** *Dyspnea, pharyngitis, upper respiratory tract infection,* asthma, atelectasis, bronchitis, cough, epistaxis, hypoxia, lung edema, pleural effusion, pneumonia, rhinitis, sinusitis. **Skin:** *Acne, rash,* fungal dermatitis, hirsutism, pruritus, skin hypertrophy, skin ulcer, sweating. **Urogenital:** *UTI,* albuminuria, bladder pain, dysuria, hematuria, hydronephrosis, impotence, kidney pain, nocturia, renal tubular necrosis, oliguria, pyuria, scrotal edema, incontinence, urinary retention, glycosuria. **Special Senses:** Abnormal vision, cataract, conjunctivitis, deafness, ear pain, otitis media, tinnitus.

INTERACTIONS Drug: Sirolimus concentrations increased by **cyclosporine, diltiazem, ketoconazole; sirolimus** concentrations decreased by **rifampin;** VACCINES may be less effective with **sirolimus. Food: Grapefruit juice** significantly decreases absorption of **sirolimus.**

PHARMACOKINETICS Absorption: Rapidly absorbed with 14% bioavailability. **Peak:** 2 h. **Distribution:** 92% protein bound, distributes in high concentrations to heart, intestines, kidneys, liver, lungs, muscle, spleen, and testes. **Metabolism:** Metabolized in liver by CYP3 A4. **Elimination:** 91% excreted in feces, 2.2% in urine. **Half-life:** 62 h.

NURSING IMPLICATIONS

Assessment & Drug Effects

- Monitor for S&S of graft rejection.
- Control hyperlipidemia prior to initiating drug.
- Draw trough whole-blood sirolimus levels 1 h before a scheduled dose.
- Lab tests: Obtain periodic lipid profile, CBC with differential, fasting plasma glucose, blood chemistry, BUN and creatinine (especially with other drugs known to cause renal impairment).

Patient & Family Education

- Avoid grapefruit juice within 2 h of taking sirolimus.
- Note: Decreased effectiveness possible for vaccines during therapy.
- Use or add barrier contraceptive before, during, and for 12 wk after discontinuing therapy.
- Do not breast feed while taking this drug.
- Store this medication out of reach of children.

SODIUM BICARBONATE (NAHCO₃)

(sod′i-um bi-car′bon-ate)
Sodium Bicarbonate
Classifications: GASTROINTESTINAL AGENT; ANTACID; FLUID AND ELECTROLYTE BALANCE AGENT
Pregnancy Category: C

AVAILABILITY 325 mg, 520 mg, 650 mg tablets; 4.2%, 5%, 7.5%, 8.4% injection

ACTIONS Short-acting, potent systemic antacid. Rapidly neutralizes gastric acid to form sodium chloride, carbon dioxide, and water. After absorption of sodium bicarbonate, plasma alkali reserve is increased and excess sodium and bicarbonate ions are excreted in urine, thus rendering urine less acid. Not suitable for treatment of peptic ulcer because it is short acting, high in sodium, and may cause gastric distention, systemic alkalosis, and possibly acid-rebound.

THERAPEUTIC EFFECTS Short-acting, potent systemic antacid; rapidly neutralizes gastric acid or systemic acidosis.

USES Systemic alkalizer to correct metabolic acidosis (as occurs in diabetes mellitus, shock, cardiac arrest, or vascular collapse), to minimize uric acid crystallization associated with uricosuric agents and tumor lysis syndrome, to increase the solubility of sulfonamides, and to enhance renal excretion of barbiturate and salicylate overdosage. Commonly used as home remedy for relief of occasional heartburn, indigestion, or sour stomach. Used topically as paste, bath, or soak to relieve itching and minor skin irritations such as sunburn, insect bites, prickly heat, poison ivy, sumac, or oak. Sterile solutions are used to buffer acidic parenteral solutions to prevent acidosis. Also as a buffering agent in many commercial products (e.g., mouthwashes, douches, enemas, ophthalmic solutions).

CONTRAINDICATIONS Prolonged therapy with sodium bicarbonate; patients losing chloride (as from vomiting, GI suction, diuresis); alkalosis, hypocalcemia, heart disease, hypertension; renal insufficiency; peptic ulcer; pregnancy (category C).
CAUTIOUS USE Edema, sodium retaining disorders; lactation.

ROUTE & DOSAGE

Urinary Alkalinizer

Child: **PO** 84–840 mg/kg/day in divided doses according to urinary pH titration
Adult: **PO** 4 g initially, then 1–2 g q4h according to urinary pH titration

Cardiac Arrest (must be adequately ventilated prior to dosage)

Child: **IV** 0.5–1 mEq/kg of a 4.2% solution q10min depending on arterial blood gas determinations, give over 1–2 min
Adult: **IV** 1 mEq/kg of a 7.5% or 8.4% solution initially, then 0.5 mEq/kg q10min depending on arterial blood gas determinations (8.4% solutions contain 50 mEq/50 mL), give over 1–2 min

Metabolic Acidosis

Neonate/Infant/Child: **IV** HCO_3^- (mEq) = 0.3 × weight in kg × base deficit (mEq/L) *or* HCO_3^- (mEq) = 0.5 × weight in kg × (24 - serum HCO_3^- [mEq/L])
Infant: **IV** 2–3 mEq/kg/day of a 4.2% solution over 4–8 h
Adult: **IV** HCO_3^- (mEq/L) = 0.2 × weight in kg × base deficit (mEq/L) *or* HCO_3^- (mEq/L) = 0.5 × wt (kg) × (24 - serum HCO_3^- [mEq/L])
Adult: **IV** 2–5 mEq/kg by IV infusion over 4–8 h

Antacid

Adult: **PO** 0.3–2 g 1–4 times/day or ½ tsp of powder in glass of water

STORAGE
Store in airtight containers. Note expiration date.

ADMINISTRATION

Oral

- Do not add oral preparation to calcium-containing solutions. Give 3 h after meals.

Topical

- Use manufacturer's directions: Bath or soak, ½ cup or more into tub of warm water; foot soak, 4 tbsp/L (qt) warm water; soak 5–10 min; paste, 3 parts sodium bicarbonate to 1 part water.
- Note: Solutions in water slowly decompose. Decomposition is accelerated by agitating or warming the solution.

Intravenous

PREPARE **IV Infusion:** May give 4.2% (0.5 mEq/mL) and 5% (0.595 mEq/mL) NaHCO₃ solutions undiluted. Dilute 7.5% (0.892 mEq/mL) and 8.4% (1 mEq/mL) solutions with compatible IV solutions. Dilute to at least 4.2% for infants and children.

ADMINISTER **IV Infusion:** Give a bolus dose only in emergency situations. Usually, the rate is 2–5 mEq/kg over 4–8 h; do not exceed 50 mEq/h. Maximum rate for neonates and infants is 10 mEq/min). Stop infusion immediately if extravasation occurs. Severe tissue damage has followed tissue infiltration.

INCOMPATIBILITIES **Solution/Additive: Alcohol 5%, lactated Ringer's, amoxicillin, ascorbic acid, bupivacaine, calcium salts, carboplatin, carmustine, cisplatin, codeine, corticotropin, dobutamine, dopamine, epinephrine, etidocaine, glycopyrrolate, hydromorphone, imipenem-cilastatin, insulin, isoproterenol, labetalol, levorphanol, lidocaine, magnesium sulfate, meperidine, mepivacaine, meropenem, methadone, methicillin, metoclopramide, morphine, norepinephrine, oxytetracycline, pentazocine, pentobarbital, phenobarbital, procaine, secobarbital, streptomycin, succinylcholine, tetracycline, thiopental, vancomycin, vitamin B complex with C. Y-Site: Allopurinol, amiodarone, amphotericin B cholesteryl complex, calcium chloride, diltiazem, doxorubicin liposome, idarubicin, imipenem-cilastatin, inamrinone, leucovorin, midazolam, nalbuphine, ondansetron, oxacillin, sargramostim, verapamil, vincristine, vindesine, vinorelbine.**

ADVERSE EFFECTS GI: *Belching, gastric distention,* flatulence. **Metabolic:** Metabolic alkalosis; electrolyte imbalance: <u>sodium overload (pulmonary edema)</u>, hypocalcemia (tetany), hypokalemia, milk-alkali syndrome, dehydration. **Other:** Rapid IV in neonates (Hypernatremia, reduction in CSF pressure, <u>intracranial hemorrhage</u>). **Skin:** Severe tissue damage following extravasation of IV solution. **Urogenital:** Renal calculi or crystals, impaired kidney function.

DIAGNOSTIC TEST INTERFERENCE Small increase in ***blood lactate*** levels (following IV infusion of sodium bicarbonate); false-positive ***urinary protein*** determinations (using ***Ames reagent, sulfacetic acid,*** heat and ***acetic acid*** or ***nitric acid ring method***); elevated ***urinary urobilinogen*** levels (***urobilinogen*** excretion increases in alkaline urine).

INTERACTIONS Drug: May decrease absorption of **ketoconazole;** may decrease elimination of **dextroamphetamine, ephedrine, pseudoephedrine, quinidine;** may increase elimination of **chlorpropamide, lithium, methotrexate,** SALICYLATES, TETRACYCLINES.

PHARMACOKINETICS Absorption: Readily absorbed from GI tract. **Onset:** 15 min. **Duration:** 1–2 h. **Elimination:** Excreted in urine within 3–4 h.

NURSING IMPLICATIONS

Assessment & Drug Effects

- Be aware that long-term use of oral preparation with milk or calcium can cause milk-alkali syndrome: Anorexia, nausea, vomiting, headache, mental confusion, hypercalcemia, hypophosphatemia, soft tissue calcification, renal and ureteral calculi, renal insufficiency, metabolic alkalosis.
- Lab tests: Urinary alkalinization: Monitor urinary pH as a guide to dosage (pH testing with nitrazine paper may be done at intervals throughout the day and dosage adjustments made accordingly).
- Lab tests: Metabolic acidosis: Monitor patient closely by observations of clinical condition; measurements of acid–base status (blood pH, P_{O_2}, P_{CO_2}, H_{CO_3}, and other electrolytes, are usually made several times daily during acute period). Observe for signs of alkalosis (over treatment) (see Appendix D-1).
- Observe for and report S&S of improvement or reversal of metabolic acidosis (see Appendix D-1).

Patient & Family Education

- Do not use sodium bicarbonate as antacid. A nonabsorbable OTC alternative for repeated use is safer.
- Do not take antacids longer than 2 wk except under advice and supervision of a physician. Self-medication with routine doses of sodium bicarbonate or soda mints may cause sodium retention and alkalosis, especially when kidney function is impaired.
- Be aware that commonly used OTC antacid products contain sodium bicarbonate: for example, Alka-Seltzer, Bromo-Seltzer, Gaviscon.
- Do not breast feed while taking this drug without consulting physician.
- Store this medication out of reach of children.

SODIUM POLYSTYRENE SULFONATE

(pol-ee-stye′reen)
Kayexalate, SPS Suspension
Classifications: ELECTROLYTE AND WATER BALANCE AGENT; CATION EXCHANGE
Pregnancy Category: C

AVAILABILITY 15 g/60 mL 1.25 g/5 mL, suspension; 100 mg/g powder

ACTIONS Sulfonic cation-exchange resin that removes potassium from body by exchanging sodium ion for potassium, particularly in large intestine; potassium-containing resin is then excreted. Small amounts of other cations such as calcium and magnesium may be lost during treatment.
THERAPEUTIC EFFECTS Removes potassium from body by exchanging sodium ion for potassium through the large intestine.

USE Hyperkalemia.

CONTRAINDICATIONS Patients with hypokalemia; hypersensitivity to Kayexalate.
CAUTIOUS USE Acute or chronic kidney failure; patients receiving digitalis preparations; patients who cannot tolerate even a small increase in sodium load (e.g., CHF, severe hypertension, and marked edema); pregnancy (category C), lactation.

ROUTE & DOSAGE

Hyperkalemia

Child: **PO** Calculate appropriate amount on exchange rate of 1 mEq of potassium per gram of resin and suspend in 70% sorbitol or other appropriate solution (usual dose: 1 g/kg/dose q6h) **PR** 1 g/kg/dose q2–6h
Adult: **PO** 15 g suspended in 70% sorbitol or 20–100 mL of other fluid 1–4 times/day **PR** 30–50 g/100 mL 70% sorbitol q6h as warm emulsion high into sigmoid colon

STORAGE
Store remainder of prepared solution for 24 h; then discard.

ADMINISTRATION

Oral
- Give as a suspension in a small quantity of water or in syrup. Usual amount of fluid ranges from 20–100 mL or approximately 3–4 mL/g of drug.

Rectal
- Use warm fluid (as prescribed) to prepare the emulsion for enema.
- Administer at body temperature and introduce by gravity, keeping suspension particles in solution by stirring. Flush suspension with 50–100 mL of fluid; then clamp tube and leave it in place.
- Urge patient to retain enema at least 30–60 min but as long as several hours if possible.
- Irrigate colon (after enema solution has been expelled) with 1 or 2 quarts flushing solution (nonsodium containing) or amount of solution appropriate for size and age. Drain returns constantly through a Y-tube connection.

S

ADVERSE EFFECTS GI: *Constipation, fecal impaction;* anorexia, gastric irritation, nausea, vomiting, diarrhea (with sorbitol emulsions). **Metabolic:** Sodium retention, hypocalcemia, hypokalemia, hypomagnesemia.

INTERACTIONS Drug: ANTACIDS, LAXATIVES containing **calcium** or **magnesium** may decrease potassium exchange capability of the resin.

PHARMACOKINETICS Absorption: Not absorbed systemically. **Onset:** Several hours to days. **Metabolism:** Not metabolized. **Elimination:** Excreted in feces.

NURSING IMPLICATIONS

Assessment & Drug Effects

▪ Lab tests: Determine serum potassium levels daily throughout therapy. Monitor acid–base balance, electrolytes, and minerals in patients receiving repeated doses.

▪ Serum potassium levels do not always reflect intracellular potassium deficiency. Observe patient closely for early clinical signs of severe hypokalemia (see Appendix D-1). ECGs are also recommended.

▪ Does not rapidly remove potassium from the body, if S&S of hyperkalemia are present, notify physician. May have to consider adjunctive therapy

▪ Consult physician about restricting sodium content from dietary and other sources because drug contains approximately 100 mg (4.1 mEq) of sodium per gram (1 tsp, 15 mEq sodium).

Patient & Family Education

▪ Check bowel function daily. Usually, a mild laxative is prescribed to prevent constipation (common adverse effect).

▪ Store this medication out of reach of children.

SOMATREM
(soe′ma-trem)
Protropin
Classifications: HORMONE AND SYNTHETIC SUBSTITUTE; GROWTH HORMONE
Prototype: Somatropin
Pregnancy Category: C

AVAILABILITY 5 mg (approximately 15 international units), 10 mg (approximately 30 international units) vials

ACTIONS Biosynthetic product of recombinant DNA technology. Contains exact sequence of 191 amino acids in pituitary-derived human growth hormone (GH) plus an amino-terminal methionyl group not found in natural GH. In presence of GH deficiency, promotes skeletal growth at epiphyseal plates of long bones by increasing levels of the mediator somatomedin-C and by increasing synthesis of protein, chondroitin sulfate, and collagen. Increases number and size of muscle cells. May induce GH antibody formation (IgG), but effect of antibodies on endogenous GH activity is unknown.

THERAPEUTIC EFFECTS Therapeutically equivalent to natural GH (somatropin) of pituitary origin. Affects metabolism and growth of most body tissues including red cell mass, with possible exception of eye and brain.

USE Long-term treatment of children with growth failure due to deficiency of endogenous GH.

CONTRAINDICATIONS Patient with closed epiphyses; underlying progressive intracranial tumor; pregnancy (category C).

CAUTIOUS USE Diabetes mellitus or family history of the disease; concomitant use of glucocorticoids; concomitant or prior use of thyroid or androgens in prepubertal male; hypothyroidism. Patient with known sensitivity to benzyl alcohol; lactation.

ROUTE & DOSAGE

Growth Hormone Deficiency
Child: **IM/SC** Doses up to 0.1 mg/kg (0.2 units/kg) 3 times/wk with a minimum of 48 h between doses, may be increased in older children if epiphyses have not closed

STORAGE
Store lyophilized powder and reconstituted solution at 2°–8° C (36°–46° F). Do not freeze. Expiration dates are on labels.

ADMINISTRATION
Intramuscular/Subcutaneous
- Reconstitute each vial (containing 5 mL lyophilized powder) with 1–5 mL bacteriostatic water for injection, aiming stream of water against vial wall. Swirl vial gently to mix contents. Do not shake.
- Note: pH of reconstituted solution is about 7.8.
- Do not use if reconstituted solution is cloudy or has crystals immediately after reconstitution or refrigeration.
- Reconstitute with sterile water for injection, USP, when administering to newborns; benzyl alcohol is the preservative in bacteriostatic water for injection and may be toxic to this age group (neonatal gasping syndrome).
- Use disposable syringe small enough to administer prescribed doses with accuracy and needle long enough to ensure injection into muscle layer. See Techniques of Administration section in Part I for safe IM site selection in children.
- Discard unused reconstituted solution within 7 days.

ADVERSE EFFECTS Body as a Whole: Allergic reactions, peripheral edema, headache, myalgia, weakness, organ enlargement, acromegalic features in children. **CV:** Hypertension, atherosclerosis. **Metabolic:** Glucose intolerance, ACTH deficiency, hypothyroidism, diabetes. **Other:** Recurrent intracranial tumor growth, persistent antibodies to GH; pain, swelling at injection site.

DIAGNOSTIC TEST INTERFERENCE Somatrem may reduce *glucose tolerance, serum T_4 (thyroxin) concentration, RAI uptake,* and *thyroxine-binding capacity.*

INTERACTIONS Drug: ANABOLIC STEROIDS, **thyroid hormone,** ANDROGENS, ESTROGENS may accelerate epiphyseal closure; **ACTH,** CORTICOSTEROIDS may inhibit growth response to somatrem.

PHARMACOKINETICS Metabolism: Metabolized in liver. **Elimination:** Excreted in urine. **Half-Life:** 3–5 h with chronic administration.

NURSING IMPLICATIONS

Assessment & Drug Effects
- Assess bone age annually in all patients and especially those also receiving thyroid, androgen, or estrogen replacement therapy, because

concurrent use of these agents may precipitate early epiphyseal closure. Urge parent to take child for growth assessment on appointed annual dates.

- Evaluate thyroid status at regular intervals. Untreated hypothyroidism may interfere with response to drug.
- Observe diabetics or those with family history of diabetes closely. Check blood or urine glucose and HbA$_{1C}$ regularly to recognize glucose intolerance.

Patient & Family Education

- Be aware that first-year growth of 17.5 cm (7 in) with somatrem has been reported, but average expectations are 7.5–12.5 cm (3–5 in), slightly less in second year, and after that, normal growth rate. Also, subcutaneous fat diminishes but returns to pretreatment level later.
- Record accurate height measurements at regular intervals and report to physician if rate is less than expected.
- Report child's complaints of hip or knee pain or a limp. Slipped capital femoral epiphysis may occur in patients with endocrine disorders.

SOMATROPIN 🅟ᵣ

(soe-ma-troe′pin)
Bio-Tropin, Genotropin, Humatrope, Norditropin, Nutropin, Nutropin AQ, Nutropin AQ Pen, Nutropin Depot, Serostim, Saizen
Classifications: HORMONE AND SYNTHETIC SUBSTITUTE; GROWTH HORMONE
Pregnancy Category: B

AVAILABILITY 1.5 mg, 4 mg, 5 mg, 5.8 mg, 6 mg, 8 mg, 10 mg injection; **Nutropin Depot** 13.5 mg, 18 mg, 22.5 mg vials

ACTIONS New recombinant growth hormone with the natural sequence of 191 amino acids characteristic of endogenous growth hormone (GH). Differs from somatrem by absence of an extra methionyl group in its structure. Somatropin appears to be less likely to produce serum antibodies to endogenous GH than somatrem.
THERAPEUTIC EFFECTS Induces growth responses similar to those produced in children treated with somatrem or with GH obtained from human pituitary glands.

USES Growth failure due to GH deficiency; replacement therapy prior to epiphyseal closure in patients with idiopathic GH deficiency; GH deficiency secondary to intracranial tumors or panhypopituitarism; inadequate GH secretion; short stature in girls with Turner's syndrome; AIDS wasting syndrome.

CONTRAINDICATIONS Patient with closed epiphyses; underlying progressive intracranial tumor; pregnancy (category B).
CAUTIOUS USE Diabetes mellitus or family history of the disease; lactation; concomitant or prior use of thyroid or androgens in prepubertal male; hypothyroidism.

ROUTE & DOSAGE

Growth Hormone Deficiency

Note: Dosing will vary with specific products.
Child: **SC Genotropin** 0.16–0.24 mg/kg/wk divided into 6–7 daily doses **Humatrope** 0.18 mg/kg/wk (0.54 international units/kg/wk) divided into equal doses given on either 3 alternate days or 6 times/wk **Norditropin** 0.024–0.034 mg/kg/day 6–7 times/wk **Nutropin, Nutropin AQ** 0.3 mg/kg/wk (0.9 international units/kg/wk) divided into 6–7 daily doses; **Nutropin Depot** 1.5 mg/kg every month or 0.75 mg/kg twice monthly
Adult: **SC Humatrope** 0.006 mg/kg (0.018 international units/kg) daily, may increase (max 0.0125 mg/kg/day [0.0375 international units/kg/day]) **Nutropin, Nutropin AQ** 0.006 mg/kg daily (max *<35 y*, 0.025 mg/kg/day; *>35 y*, 0.0125 mg/kg/day)

Inadequate Growth Hormone Secretion

Child: **SC Nutropin** 0.3 mg/kg every week

AIDS Wasting or Cachexia

Adults: **SC Serostim** *>55 kg*, 6 mg every night; *45–55 kg*, 5 mg every night; *35–45 kg*, 4 mg every night; *<35 kg*, 0.1 mg/kg every night

STORAGE

Store lyophilized powder at 2°–8° C (36°–46° F). After reconstitution most preparations are stable for at least 14 days under refrigeration. DO NOT FREEZE.

ADMINISTRATION

- Reconstitute each brand following its manufacturer's instructions (vary from brand to brand).
- Read and carefully follow directions for use supplied with the Nutropin AQ Pen™ Cartridge if this is the product being used.
- Rotate injection sites; abdomen and thighs are preferred sites. Do not use buttocks until the child has been walking for a year or more and the muscle is adequately developed. See Techniques of Administration section in Part I for safe IM site selection in children.

ADVERSE EFFECTS Body as a Whole:
Pain, swelling at injection site; myalgia. **Metabolic:** *Hypercalciuria;* oversaturation of bile with cholesterol, hyperglycemia, ketosis. **Endocrine:** High circulating GH antibodies with resulting treatment failure, accelerated growth of intracranial tumor.

INTERACTIONS Drug:
ANABOLIC STEROIDS, **thyroid hormone,** ANDROGENS, ESTROGENS may accelerate epiphyseal closure; **ACTH,** CORTICOSTEROIDS may inhibit growth response to somatropin.

PHARMACOKINETICS Metabolism:
Metabolized in liver. **Elimination:** Excreted in urine. **Half-Life:** 15–50 min.

NURSING IMPLICATIONS

Assessment & Drug Effects

- Assess bone age annually in all patients and especially those also receiving concurrent thyroid or androgen treatment, because these drugs may precipitate early epiphyseal closure. Urge parent to take child for bone age assessment on appointed annual dates.
- Lab test: Periodic serum and urine calcium and plasma glucose.
- Hypercalciuria, a frequent adverse effect in the first 2–3 mo of therapy, may be symptomless, however, it may be accompanied by renal calculi, with these reportable symptoms: Flank pain and colic, GI symptoms, urinary frequency, chills, fever, hematuria.
- Test for circulating GH antibodies (antisomatropin antibodies) in patients who respond initially but later fail to respond to therapy.
- Observe diabetics or those with family history of diabetes closely. Obtain regular urine for glycosuria or fasting blood glucose and HbA$_{1C}$.
- Examine patients with GH deficiency secondary to intracranial lesion frequently for progression or recurrence of underlying disease.

Patient & Family Education

- Be aware that during first 6 mo of successful treatment, linear growth rates may be increased 8–16 cm or more per year (average about 7 cm/y or approximately 3 in.). Additionally, SC fat diminishes but returns to pretreatment value later.
- Family needs to learn correct technique for administration if given at home.
- Report child's complaints of hip or knee pain or a limp. Slipped capital femoral epiphysis may occur in patients with endocrine disorders.
- Record accurate height measurements at regular intervals and report to physician if rate is less than expected.
- In general, growth response to somatropin is inversely proportional to duration of treatment.
- Discontinue treatment when patient has reached satisfactory adult height, when epiphyses have fused, or when patient fails to exhibit growth response.
- Store medication and syringes out of reach of children if given at home.

SPECTINOMYCIN HYDROCHLORIDE

(spek-ti-noe-mye'sin)
Trobicin
Classifications: ANTI-INFECTIVE; ANTIBIOTIC
Pregnancy Category: B

AVAILABILITY 400 mg/mL (contains 0.9% benzyl alcohol) injection

ACTIONS Antibiotic produced by *Streptomyces spectabilis*. Action is usually bacteriostatic. Variable activity against a wide variety of gram-negative and gram-positive organisms.

THERAPEUTIC EFFECTS Inhibits majority of *Neisseria gonorrhoeae* strains; effective for urethral and anorectal infections, but not pharyngeal. Not active against syphilis or chlamydial and mycoplasmal infections.

USES Only for treatment of uncomplicated gonorrhea in patients sensitized or resistant to penicillin or other effective drugs approved by U.S.

Centers for Disease Control and Prevention. American Academy of Pediatrics recommends use for treatment of gonococcal infections in children hypersensitive to cephalosporins.

UNLABELED USES Disseminated gonococcal infections caused by penicillinase-producing strains of *N. gonorrhoeae* (PPNG) and sexually transmitted epididymoorchitis.

CONTRAINDICATIONS Safety during pregnancy (category B), lactation, and in infants and children is not established.

CAUTIOUS USE History of allergies.

ROUTE & DOSAGE

Uncomplicated Gonorrhea

Child: IM <45 kg, 50 mg/kg as single dose
Child ≥8 y and ≥45 kg/Adult: **IM** 2 g as single dose

Disseminated Gonorrhea

Child ≥8 y and ≥45 kg/Adult: **IM** 2 g q12h for 7 days

STORAGE

Use solution within 24 h of reconstitution. Store at 15°–30° C (59°–86° F) unless otherwise directed.

ADMINISTRATION

Intramuscular

- Give IM injection deep into muscle mass. See Techniques of Administration section in Part I for safe IM site and volume/site selection in children. In adults give IM injection deep into upper outer quadrant of gluteus and give no more than 5 mL injected into single site (using 20-gauge needle). Injection may be painful.
- Reconstitute with supplied diluent (bacteriostatic water for injection with 0.9% benzyl alcohol). Shake vial vigorously immediately after adding diluent and before withdrawing drug.

ADVERSE EFFECTS Skin: *Pain and soreness at injection site,* urticaria, pruritus, transient rash **Body as a Whole:** Headache, dizziness, chills, fever, insomnia, nervousness. **GI:** Nausea, vomiting. **Metabolic:** Decrease in Hgb, Hct, Cl$_{cr}$, elevated serum alkaline phosphatase, ALT, BUN.

INTERACTIONS Drug: No clinically significant interactions established.

PHARMACOKINETICS Absorption: Readily absorbed from IM site. **Peak:** 1 h. **Metabolism:** Metabolized in liver. **Eliminations:** Excreted in urine. **Half-Life:** 1.2–2.8 h.

NURSING IMPLICATIONS

Assessment & Drug Effects

- Observe patient for 45–60 min after injection. Systemic anaphylaxis has been reported (apprehension, pruritus, hypertension, abdominal pain, collapse).
- Obtain serologic tests for syphilis at time of diagnosis in patients with gonorrhea and again after 3 mo.
- Monitor clinical effectiveness of drug to detect antibiotic resistance.

- Culture all gonococcal infection sites 3–7 days after spectinomycin therapy is completed to verify eradication of infection.
- Spectinomycin is not recommended for treatment of pharyngeal infections.
- Lab tests: Monitor Hgb and Hct when multiple doses are required.

Patient & Family Education
- Notify sexual partners of their risk of infection.
- Refrain from sexual intercourse until infection is resolved.
- Do not breast feed while taking this drug without consulting physician.

SPIRONOLACTONE ℗

(speer-on-oh-lak'tone)

Aldactone, Aldactazide, Novospiroton ♣

Classifications: ELECTROLYTIC AND WATER BALANCE AGENT; POTASSIUM-SPARING DIURETIC

Pregnancy Category: D

AVAILABILITY 25 mg, 50 mg, 100 mg tablets
Combination Products: 25 mg spironolactone and 25 mg hydrochlorothiazide, 50 mg spironolactone and 50 mg hydrochlorothiazide tablets

ACTIONS Steroidal compound and specific pharmacologic antagonist of aldosterone. Presumably acts by competing with aldosterone for cellular receptor sites in distal renal tubule. Promotes sodium and chloride excretion without concomitant loss of potassium. Diuretic effect reportedly not associated with hyperuricemia or hyperglycemia. Activity depends on presence of endogenous or exogenous aldosterone.

THERAPEUTIC EFFECTS A diuretic agent that promotes sodium and chloride excretion without concomitant loss of potassium. Lowers systolic and diastolic pressures in hypertensive patients.

USES Clinical conditions associated with augmented aldosterone production, as in essential hypertension, refractory edema due to CHF, hepatic cirrhosis, nephrotic syndrome, and idiopathic edema. May be used to potentiate actions of other diuretics and antihypertensive agents or for its potassium-sparing effect. Also used for treatment of (and as presumptive test for) primary aldosteronism.

UNLABELED USES Hirsutism in women with polycystic ovary syndrome or idiopathic hirsutism; adjunct in treatment of myasthenia gravis and familial periodic paralysis.

CONTRAINDICATIONS Anuria, acute renal insufficiency; progressing impairment of kidney function, hyperkalemia; pregnancy (category D), lactation.

CAUTIOUS USE BUN of 40 mg/dL or greater, liver disease.

ROUTE & DOSAGE

Edema

Neonate: **PO** 1–3 mg/kg/day divided q12–24h
Child: **PO** 1.5–3.3 mg/kg/day in single or divided doses daily or q.i.d., continued for at least 5 days (dose adjusted to optimal response)

Common adverse effects in *italic;* life-threatening effects underlined; generic names in **bold;** drug classifications in SMALL CAPS; ♣ Canadian drug name; ℗ Prototype drug.

Adult: **PO** 25–200 mg/day in divided doses daily or b.i.d., continued for at least 5 days (dose adjusted to optimal response; if no response, a thiazide or loop diuretic may be added)

Hypertension
Adult: **PO** 25–100 mg/day in single or divided doses, continued for at least 2 wk (dose adjusted to optimal response)

Primary Aldosteronism: Diagnosis
Child: **PO** Short Test: 125–375 mg/m^2/day in divided dose b.i.d. or q.i.d.
Adult: **PO** Short Test: 400 mg/day for 4 days; long test: 400 mg/day for 3–4 wk

Primary Aldosteronism: Treatment
Adult: **PO** 100–400 mg/day in divided doses

STORAGE
Store in tight, light-resistant containers. Suspension is stable for 1 mo under refrigeration.

ADMINISTRATION

Oral
- Give with food to enhance absorption.
- Crush tablets and give with fluid of patient's choice if unable to swallow whole.
- Oral suspensions can be compounded by pharmacy.

ADVERSE EFFECTS CNS: Lethargy, mental confusion, fatigue (with rapid weight loss), headache, drowsiness, ataxia. **Endocrine:** Gynecomastia (both sexes), inability to achieve or maintain erection, androgenic effects (hirsutism, irregular menses, deepening of voice); parathyroid changes, decreased glucose tolerance, SLE. **GI:** Abdominal cramps, nausea, vomiting, anorexia, diarrhea. **Skin:** Maculopapular or erythematous rash, urticaria. **Metabolic:** Fluid and electrolyte imbalance (particularly hyperkalemia and hyponatremia); elevated BUN, mild acidosis, hyperuricemia, gout. **Body as a Whole:** Drug fever. **Hematologic:** Agranulocytosis. **CV:** Hypertension (postsympathectomy patient).

DIAGNOSTIC TEST INTERFERENCE May produce marked increases in *plasma cortisol* determinations by *Mattingly fluorometric* method; these may persist for several days after termination of drug (spironolactone metabolite produces fluorescence). There is the possibility of false elevations in measurements of *digoxin serum levels* by *RIA* procedures.

INTERACTIONS Drug: Combinations of spironolactone and acidifying doses of **ammonium chloride** may produce systemic acidosis; use these combinations with caution. Diuretic effect of spironolactone may be antagonized by **aspirin** and other SALICYLATES. **Digoxin** should be monitored for decreased effect of CARDIAC GLYCOSIDE. Hyperkalemia may result with POTASSIUM SUPPLEMENTS, ACE INHIBITORS, ARBS, **heparin** may decrease **lithium** clearance resulting in increased tenacity; may alter anticoagulant response in **warfarin. Food: Salt substitutes** may increase risk of hyperkalemia. Licorice increases sodium and water retention and potassium loss. Avoid high-potassium foods.

PHARMACOKINETICS Absorption: Approximately 73% absorbed from GI tract. **Onset:** Gradual. **Peak:** 2–3 days; maximum effect may take up to 2 wk. **Duration:** 2–3 days or more. **Distribution:** Crosses placenta, distributed into breast milk. **Metabolism:** Metabolized in liver and kidneys to active metabolites. **Elimination:** 40–57% excreted in urine, 35–40% in bile. **Half-Life:** 1.3–2.4 h parent compound, 18–23 h metabolites.

NURSING IMPLICATIONS

Assessment & Drug Effects

- Check blood pressure before initiation of therapy and at regular intervals throughout therapy.
- Lab tests: Monitor serum electrolytes (sodium and potassium) especially during early therapy; monitor digoxin level when used concurrently.
- Assess for signs of fluid and electrolyte imbalance, and signs of digoxin toxicity.
- Monitor daily I&O and check for edema. Report lack of diuretic response or development of edema; both may indicate tolerance to drug.
- Weigh patient under standard conditions before therapy begins and daily throughout therapy. Weight is a useful index of need for dosage adjustment. For patients with ascites, physician may want measurements of abdominal girth.
- Observe for and report immediately the onset of mental changes, lethargy, or stupor in patients with liver disease.
- Adverse reactions are generally reversible with discontinuation of drug. Gynecomastia appears to be related to dosage level and duration of therapy; it may persist in some after drug is stopped.

Patient & Family Education

- Be aware that the maximal diuretic effect may not occur until third day of therapy and that diuresis may continue for 2–3 days after drug is withdrawn.
- Report signs of hyponatremia or hyperkalemia (see Appendix D-1), most likely to occur in patients with severe cirrhosis.
- Avoid replacing fluid losses with large amounts of free water (can result in dilutional hyponatremia).
- Weigh 2–3 times each week. Report gains/loss of ≥5 lb. Report in children any sudden increase in body weight in relation to their age or baseline body weight.
- Do not drive or engage in potentially hazardous activities until response to the drug is known.
- Avoid excessive intake of high potassium foods and salt substitutes.
- Do not breast feed while taking this drug.
- Store this medication out of reach of children.

STAVUDINE (D4T)

(sta'vu-deen)

Zerit

Classifications: ANTI-INFECTIVE; ANTIVIRAL

Prototype: Zidovudine (AZT)

Pregnancy Category: C

AVAILABILITY 15 mg, 20 mg, 30 mg, 40 mg capsules; 1 mg/mL solution

ACTIONS Synthetic analog of thymidine (a major nucleoside in DNA) with antiviral action against HIV, the causative agent of AIDS. Phosphorylated to stavudine triphosphate by endogenous thymidine kinase. Appears to act by being incorporated into the growing DNA chains by viral transcriptase, thus terminating viral replication.

THERAPEUTIC EFFECTS Inhibits the replication of HIV in human cells. Useful in patients with advanced disease, who are intolerant of other viral agents.

USES Treatment of adults with advanced HIV infection who are intolerant of other antiretroviral agents (zidovudine, didanosine, zalcitabine) or who have deteriorated on the other agents, as part of a 3-drug regiment.

CONTRAINDICATIONS Hypersensitivity to stavudine; pregnancy (category C), lactation.

CAUTIOUS USE Previous hypersensitivity to zidovudine, didanosine, or zalcitabine; folic acid or B_{12} deficiency; liver and renal insufficiency; peripheral neuropathy; history of pancreatitis.

ROUTE & DOSAGE

Advanced HIV Infection

Child: **PO** *<30 kg,* give 1 mg/kg/dose q12h; *≥30 kg,* same as adult dose

Adult: **PO** *<60 kg,* 30 mg q12h; *≥60 kg,* 40 mg q12h

Renal Impairment

Cl_{cr} 25–50 mL/min: Reduce dose by 50% (also in patients with peripheral neuropathy)

STORAGE

Store at 15°–30° C (59°–86° F).

ADMINISTRATION

Oral

- Adhere strictly to 12-h interval between doses. Can be given with food.
- Reconstitute powder by adding 202 mL of water to the container. Shake vigorously. Yields 200 mL of 1 mg/mL solution.

ADVERSE EFFECTS CNS: *Peripheral neuropathy,* paresthesias. **GI:** *Anorexia, nausea, vomiting, diarrhea,* cramping, pancreatitis, abdominal

Common adverse effects in *italic;* life-threatening effects <u>underlined;</u> generic names in **bold;** drug classifications in SMALL CAPS; ◆ Canadian drug name; ◑ Prototype drug.

1125

pain, elevated liver function tests. **Body as a Whole:** *Headache,* chills/fever, *myalgia.* **Hematologic:** Anemia, neutropenia. **Skin:** *Rash.* **Metabolic:** Lactic acidosis in pregnant women.

INTERACTIONS Drug: Didanosine may increase risk of pancreatitis and hepatotoxicity; **probenecid** can decrease elimination. Poor antiviral effect when given with zidovudine.

PHARMACOKINETICS Absorption: Readily absorbed from GI tract; 82% reaches systemic circulation. **Peak:** Effect 6 wk. **Distribution:** Distributes into CSF; excreted in breast milk of animals. **Metabolism:** Metabolized in liver; in addition to hepatic metabolism, some investigators suggest that degradation and salvage by other pyrimidine pathways may contribute to elimination; intracellularly, stavudine is phosphorylated by cellular enzymes to its active triphosphate form. **Elimination:** Excreted primarily in urine. **Half-Life:** 1–1.6 h.

NURSING IMPLICATIONS

Assessment & Drug Effects
- Monitor for peripheral neuropathy and report numbness, tingling, or pain, which may indicate a need to interrupt stavudine.
- Lab tests: Monitor liver enzymes, CBC with differential, PT and INR, and kidney function periodically.
- Monitor for development of opportunistic infection.

Patient & Family Education
- Take drug exactly as prescribed.
- Report to physician any adverse drug effects that are bothersome.
- Report symptoms of peripheral neuropathy to physician immediately. This drug is not a cure for HIV.
- Do not breast feed while taking this drug.
- Store this medication out of reach of children.

S | STREPTOMYCIN SULFATE

(strep-toe-mye′sin)
Streptomycin
Classifications: ANTI-INFECTIVE; AMINOGLYCOSIDE ANTIBIOTIC; ANTITUBERCULOSIS AGENT
Prototype: Gentamicin
Pregnancy Category: C

AVAILABILITY 400 mg/mL, 1 g injection

ACTIONS Aminoglycoside antibiotic derived from *Streptomyces griseus,* with bactericidal and bacteriostatic actions. Most commonly used concurrently with other antimicrobial agents because of rapid emergence of resistant strains when used alone.
THERAPEUTIC EFFECTS Active against a variety of gram-positive, gram-negative, and acid-fast organisms. Reportedly, it is the least nephrotoxic of the aminoglycosides.

USES Only in combination with other antitubercular drugs in treatment of all forms of active tuberculosis caused by susceptible organisms. Used alone or in conjunction with tetracycline for tularemia, plague, and brucellosis. Also used with other antibiotics in treatment of subacute bacterial endocarditis due to *Enterococci* and *Streptococci* (viridans group) and *Haemophilus influenzae* and in treatment of peritonitis, respiratory tract infections, granuloma inguinale, and chancroid when other drugs have failed.

CONTRAINDICATIONS History of toxic reaction or hypersensitivity to aminoglycosides; labyrinthine disease; myasthenia gravis; concurrent or sequential use of other neurotoxic or nephrotoxic agents; pregnancy (category C); lactation.

CAUTIOUS USE Impaired kidney function (given in reduced dosages); use in prematures, neonates, and children.

ROUTE & DOSAGE

Tuberculosis

Neonate: **IM** 10–20 mg/kg q24h
Infant: **IM** 20–30 mg/kg/day in equally divided doses q12h
Child: **IM** 20–40 mg/kg/day (max dose 1 g/day) or 20–40 mg/kg/dose given twice weekly (max dose 1.5 g/day)
Adult: **IM** 15 mg/kg up to 1 g/day as single dose or 25–30 mg/kg/dose given twice weekly (max dose 1.5 g/day)

Tularemia

Child: **IM** 20–40 mg/kg/day in equally divided q6–12h
Adult: **IM** 1–2 g/day in 1–2 in equally divided doses for 7–10 days

Plague

Child: **IM** 30 mg/kg/day in equally divided q8–12h
Adult: **IM** 2 g/day in 2–4 in equally divided doses
Reduced dosages required with renal impairment.

STORAGE

Store ampules at room temperature. Protect from light; exposure to light may slightly darken solution, with no apparent loss of potency

ADMINISTRATION

Intramuscular

- Give IM deep into large muscle mass to minimize possibility of irritation. Injections are painful. Use topical numbing creams prior to injection to decrease pain response. See Techniques of Administration section in Part I for safe IM site selection in children.
- Avoid direct contact with drug; sensitization can occur. Use gloves during preparation of drug.
- Use commercially prepared IM solution undiluted; intended only for IM injection (contains a preservative, and therefore is not suitable for other routes).

ADVERSE EFFECTS CNS: Paresthesias (peripheral, facial). **Body as a Whole:** Hypersensitivity angioedema, drug fever, enlarged lymph nodes,

<u>anaphylactic shock</u>, headache, inability to concentrate, lassitude, muscular weakness, *pain and irritation at IM site,* superinfections, neuromuscular blockade, arachnoiditis. **GI:** Stomatitis, hepatotoxicity. **Hematologic:** Blood dyscrasias (leukopenia, neutropenia, pancytopenia, hemolytic or aplastic anemia, eosinophilia). **Special Senses:** *Labyrinthine damage,* auditory damage, optic nerve toxicity (scotomas). **Urogenital:** Nephrotoxicity. **CNS:** Encephalopathy, CNS depression syndrome in infants (stupor, flaccidity, coma, paralysis, cardiac arrest). **Respiratory:** Respiratory depression. **Skin:** Skin rashes, pruritus, exfoliative dermatitis.

DIAGNOSTIC TEST INTERFERENCE Streptomycin reportedly produces false-positive *urinary glucose* tests using *copper sulfate methods (Benedict's solution, Clinitest)* but not with *glucose oxidase methods* (e.g., *Clinistix, TesTape*). False increases in protein content in *urine* and *CSF* using *Folin-Ciocalteau reaction* and decreased *BUN* readings with *Berthelot reaction* may occur from test interferences. *C&S* tests may be affected if patient is taking salts such as sodium and potassium chloride, sodium sulfate and tartrate, ammonium acetate, calcium and magnesium ions.

INTERACTION Drug: May potentiate anticoagulant effects of **warfarin;** additive nephrotoxicity with **acyclovir, amphotericin B,** AMINOGLYCOSIDES, **carboplatin, cidofovir, cisplatin, cyclosporine, foscarnet, ganciclovir,** SALICYLATES, **tacrolimus, vancomycin.** When used with **fursosemide, ethacrynic acid, urea,** and **mannitol,** increases ototoxicity.

PHARMACOKINETICS Peak: 1–2 h. **Distribution:** Diffuses into most body tissues and extracellular fluids; crosses placenta; distributed into breast milk. **Elimination:** Excreted in urine. **Half-Life:** Newborn, 4–10 h; adult, 2–3 h. Peak therapeutic serum range: 15–40 mcg/mL and trough <5 mcg/mL.

NURSING IMPLICATIONS

Assessment & Drug Effects

- Lab tests: Obtain C&S tests prior to and periodically during course of therapy. In patients with impaired kidney function, frequent determinations of serum drug concentrations and periodic kidney and liver function tests are advised (serum concentrations should not exceed 25 mcg/mL in these patients).
- Be alert for and report immediately symptoms of ototoxicity (see Appendix D-1). Symptoms are most likely to occur in patients with impaired kidney function, patients receiving high doses (1.8–2 g/day) or other ototoxic or neurotoxic drugs. Irreversible damage may occur if drug is not discontinued promptly.
- Early damage to vestibular portion of eighth cranial nerve (higher incidence than auditory toxicity) is initially manifested by moderately severe headache, nausea, vomiting, vertigo in upright position, difficulty in reading, unsteadiness, and positive Romberg sign.
- Be aware that auditory nerve damage is usually preceded by vestibular symptoms and high-pitched tinnitus, roaring noises, impaired hearing

(especially to high-pitched sounds), sense of fullness in ears. Audiometric test should be done if these symptoms appear, and drug should be discontinued. Hearing loss can be permanent if damage is extensive. Tinnitus may persist several days to weeks after drug is stopped.

- Monitor I&O. Report oliguria or changes in I&O ratio (possible signs of diminishing kidney function). Sufficient fluids to maintain urinary output of 1500 mL/24 h are generally advised. Output for child should be within parameters for age. Consult physician.
- Draw peak serum levels for streptomycin 1–2 h after dosage adminisration and trough just prior to dosing.

Patient & Family Education

- Report any unusual symptoms. Review adverse reactions with physician periodically, especially with prolonged therapy.
- Be aware of possibility of ototoxicity and its symptoms (see Appendix D-1).
- Report to physician immediately any of the following: Nausea, vomiting, vertigo, incoordination, tinnitus, fullness in ears, impaired hearing.
- Do not breast feed while taking this drug.

SUCCINYLCHOLINE CHLORIDE ℗

(suk-sin-ill-koe′leen)

Anectine, Quelicin, Sucostrin

Classifications: AUTONOMIC NERVOUS SYSTEM AGENT; DEPOLARIZING SKELETAL MUSCLE RELAXANT

Pregnancy Category: C

AVAILABILITY 20 mg/mL, 50 mg/mL, 100 mg/mL injection; 500 mg, 1 g vials

ACTIONS Synthetic, ultrashort-acting depolarizing neuromuscular blocking agent with high affinity for acetylcholine (ACh) receptor sites.

THERAPEUTIC EFFECTS Initial transient contractions and fasciculations are followed by sustained flaccid skeletal muscle paralysis, produced by state of accommodation that develops in adjacent excitable muscle membranes. Rapidly hydrolyzed by plasma pseudocholinesterase.

USES To produce skeletal muscle relaxation as adjunct to anesthesia; to facilitate intubation and endoscopy, to increase pulmonary compliance in assisted or controlled respiration, and to reduce intensity of muscle contractions in pharmacologically induced or electroshock convulsions.

CONTRAINDICATIONS Hypersensitivity to succinylcholine; family history of malignant hyperthermia, penetrating eye injuries. Safety in pregnancy (category C) is not established.

CAUTIOUS USE During delivery by cesarean section; lactation; kidney, liver, pulmonary, metabolic, or cardiovascular disorders; dehydration, electrolyte imbalance, patients taking digitalis, severe burns or trauma, fractures, spinal cord injuries, degenerative or dystrophic neuromuscular diseases (especially in children and adolescents with skeletal muscle myopathies), low plasma pseudocholinesterase levels (recessive genetic

---

trait, but often associated with severe liver disease, severe anemia, dehydration, marked changes in body temperature, exposure to neurotoxic insecticides, certain drugs); collagen diseases, porphyria, intraocular surgery, glaucoma.

ROUTE & DOSAGE

Surgical and Anesthetic Procedures

Child: **IV** 1–2 mg/kg administered over 10–30 sec, may give additional doses prn **IM** 2.5–4 mg/kg up to 150 mg maximum dose
Adult: **IV** 0.3–1.1 mg/kg administered over 10–30 sec, may give additional doses prn **IM** 2.5–4 mg/kg up to 150 mg

Prolonged Muscle Relaxation

Adult: **IV** 0.5–10 mg/min by continuous infusion

STORAGE

Store in refrigerator. Check each brand for specific storage instructions.

ADMINISTRATION

Intramuscular

- Give IM injections deeply, preferably high into deltoid muscle in adults. See Techniques of Administration section in Part I for safe IM site selection in children.

Intravenous

- Use only freshly prepared solutions; succinylcholine hydrolyzes rapidly with consequent loss of potency.
- Give initial small test dose (0.1 mg/kg) to determine individual drug sensitivity and recovery time.

PREPARE **Direct:** Give undiluted. **Intermittent or Continuous:** Dilute 1 g in 500–1000 mL of D5W or NS.

ADMINISTER **Direct:** Give a bolus dose over 30 sec. **Intermittent or Continuous:** Preferred. Give at a rate of 0.5–10 mg/min. Do not exceed 10 mg/min. Do not use continuous infusion in infants or children.

INCOMPATIBILITIES **Solution/Additive:** **Sodium bicarbonate, thiopental.**

- Note: Expiration date and storage before and after reconstitution vary with the manufacturer.

ADVERSE EFFECTS CNS: *Muscle fasciculations,* profound and prolonged muscle relaxation, muscle pain. **CV:** *Bradycardia,* tachycardia, hypotension, hypertension, arrhythmias, <u>sinus arrest</u>. **Respiratory:** <u>Respiratory depression,</u> bronchospasm, hypoxia, apnea. **Body as a Whole:** <u>Malignant hyperthermia,</u> increased IOP, excessive salivation, enlarged salivary glands. **Metabolic:** Myoglobinemia, hyperkalemia. **GI:** Decreased tone and motility of GI tract (large doses).

INTERACTIONS Drug: **Aminoglycosides, colistin, cyclophosphamide, cyclopropane, echothiophate iodide, halothane, lidocaine,** MAGNESIUM SALTS, **methotrimeprazine,** NARCOTIC ANALGESICS,

ORGANOPHOSPHAMIDE INSECTICIDES, MAO INHIBITORS, PHENOTHIAZINES, **procaine, procainamide, quinidine, quinine, propranolol** may prolong neuromuscular blockade; DIGITALIS GLYCOSIDES may increase risk of cardiac arrhythmias.

PHARMACOKINETICS Onset: 0.5–1 min IV; 2–3 min IM. **Duration:** 2–3 min IV; 10–30 min IM. **Distribution:** Crosses placenta in small amounts. **Metabolism:** Metabolized in plasma by pseudocholinesterases. **Elimination:** Excreted in urine.

NURSING IMPLICATIONS

Assessment & Drug Effects

- Lab tests: Obtain baseline serum electrolytes. Electrolyte imbalance (particularly potassium, calcium, magnesium) can potentiate effects of neuromuscular blocking agents.
- Be aware that transient apnea usually occurs at time of maximal drug effect (1–2 min); spontaneous respiration should return in a few seconds or, at most, 3 or 4 min.
- Have immediately available: Personnel and facilities for emergency endotracheal intubation, artificial respiration, and assisted or controlled respiration with oxygen.
- Monitor vital signs and keep airway clear of secretions.

Patient & Family Education

- Patient may experience postprocedural muscle stiffness and pain (caused by initial fasciculations following injection) for as long as 24–30 h.
- Be aware that hoarseness and sore throat are common even when pharyngeal airway has not been used.
- Report residual muscle weakness to physician.

SUCRALFATE

(soo-kral'fate)
Carafate, Sulcrate ♣
Classifications: GASTROINTESTINAL AGENT; ANTIULCER
Pregnancy Category: B

S

AVAILABILITY 1 g tablets; 1 g/10 mL suspension

ACTIONS A complex of aluminum hydroxide and sulfated sucrose structurally related to heparin that lacks its anticoagulant activity. Action is chemically unlike any other drug used for antiulcer therapy. Following oral administration, sucralfate and gastric acid react to form a viscous, adhesive, paste-like substance that resists further reaction with acid. This "paste" adheres to the GI mucosa with a major portion binding electrostatically to the positively charged protein molecules in the damaged mucosa of an ulcer crater or an acute gastric erosion caused by alcohol or other drugs.

THERAPEUTIC EFFECTS Absorbs bile, inhibits the enzyme pepsin, and blocks back-diffusion of H^+ ions. These actions plus adherence of the

---

paste-like complex protect damaged mucosa against further destruction from ulcerogenic secretions and drugs.

USES Short-term (up to 8-wk) treatment of duodenal ulcer.
UNLABELED USES Short-term treatment of gastric ulcer, aspirin-induced erosions, suspension for chemotherapy-induced mucositis.

CONTRAINDICATIONS Pregnancy (category B). Safety and efficacy in children are not established.
CAUTIOUS USE Chronic kidney failure or dialysis due to aluminum accumulation; lactation.

ROUTE & DOSAGE

Duodenal Ulcer

Child: **PO** Safety and efficacy in children is not established, but these doses have been used: 40–80 mg/kg/day q6h
Adult: **PO** 1 g q.i.d. 1 h before meals and at bedtime. **PO Maintenance** 1 g b.i.d.

STORAGE

Store in tight container at 15°–30° C (59°–86° F). Remains stable for 2 y after manufacture.

ADMINISTRATION

Oral

- Use drug solubilized in an appropriate diluent by a pharmacist when given through nasogastric tube.
- Tablet cannot be broken or dissolved in water before administration. Suspension should be shaken.
- Administer antacids prescribed for pain relief 30 min before or after sucralfate.
- Separate administration of QUINOLONES, digoxin, phenytoin, tetracycline from that of sucralfate by 2 h to prevent sucralfate from binding to these compounds in the intestinal tract and reducing their bioavailability.

ADVERSE EFFECTS GI: Nausea, gastric discomfort, *constipation,* diarrhea.

INTERACTIONS Drug: May decrease absorption of QUINOLONES (e.g., **ciprofloxacin, norfloxacin), digoxin, phenytoin, tetracycline.**

PHARMACOKINETICS Absorption: Minimally absorbed from GI tract (<5%). **Duration:** Up to 6 h (depends on contact time with ulcer crater). **Elimination:** 90% Excreted in feces.

NURSING IMPLICATIONS

Assessment & Drug Effects

- Be aware of drug interactions and schedule other medications accordingly.

Patient & Family Education

- Although healing has occurred within the first 2 wk of therapy, treatment is usually continued 4–8 wk.

- Be aware that constipation is a drug-related problem. Follow these measures unless contraindicated: Increase water intake to 8–10 glasses per day or with children appropriate intake for their age and weight; increase physical exercise, increase dietary bulk. Consult physician; a suppository or bulk laxative (e.g., Metamucil) may be prescribed.
- Do not breast feed while taking this drug without consulting physician.
- Store this medication out of reach of children.

SUFENTANIL CITRATE

(soo-fen′ta-nil)
Sufenta
Classifications: CENTRAL NERVOUS SYSTEM AGENT; NARCOTIC (OPIATE) AGONIST ANALGESIC; GENERAL ANESTHETIC
Prototype: Morphine
Pregnancy Category: C
Controlled Substance: Schedule II

AVAILABILITY 50 mcg/mL injection

ACTIONS Synthetic opioid related to fentanyl with similar pharmacologic actions, but about 7 times more potent. Onset of action and recovery from anesthesia occur more rapidly with sufentanil than with fentanyl. In common with other opiate agonists, sufentanil can cause respiratory depression and suppression of cough reflex.
THERAPEUTIC EFFECTS Effective agent for analgesia as a supplement or a primary anesthesia.

USES Analgesic supplement in maintenance of balanced general anesthesia and also as a primary anesthetic.

CONTRAINDICATIONS Pregnancy (category C), lactation.
CAUTIOUS USE Pulmonary disease, reduced respiratory reserve; impaired liver or kidney function.

ROUTE & DOSAGE

Adjunct to General Anesthesia
Adult: **IV** 1–8 mcg/kg, depending on duration of surgery, may give additional doses of 10–25 mcg if needed

As Primary Anesthetic
Child: **IV** <12 y, 10–25 mcg/kg administered with 100% oxygen and a muscle relaxant, may give additional doses of 25–50 mcg up to 1–2 mcg/kg/dose if needed
Adult: **IV** 1–30 mcg/kg administered with 100% oxygen and a muscle relaxant, may give additional doses of 10–25 mcg if needed

STORAGE
Store at 15°–30° C (59°–86° F) unless otherwise directed; protect from light.

ADMINISTRATION

Intravenous

- Administer only by qualified personnel, specifically trained in the use of IV anesthesia and in the management of respiratory depression.
- Have available a narcotic antagonist (e.g., naloxone) to reverse respiratory depression.

PREPARE **Direct:** Examine solution for particulate matter and discoloration (solution should be clear) before administration. Give undiluted.

ADMINISTER **Direct:** Give a bolus dose over 3–5 sec. **Epidural:** Give by slow injection and closely monitor respirations after each injection.

INCOMPATIBILITIES **Solution/Additive:** Diazepam, lorazepam, phenobarbital, phenytoin, sodium bicarbonate. **Y-Site:** Lorazepam, phenytoin, thiopental.

ADVERSE EFFECTS CV: Bradycardia, tachycardia, hypotension, hypertension, arrhythmias. **GI:** Nausea, vomiting, constipation. **Respiratory:** Bronchospasm, *respiratory depression, apnea.* **Body as a Whole:** *Skeletal muscle rigidity (especially of trunk),* chills, *itching,* spasms of sphincter of Oddi, urinary retention.

INTERACTIONS Drug: BETA-ADRENERGIC ANTAGONISTS increase incidence of bradycardia; **alcohol** and other CNS DEPRESSANTS such as BARBITURATES, TRANQUILIZERS, OPIATES and INHALATION GENERAL ANESTHETICS add to CNS depression; **cimetidine** increases risk of respiratory depression.

PHARMACOKINETICS Onset: 1.5–3 min. **Duration:** 40 min. **Distribution:** Crosses blood–brain barrier. **Metabolism:** Metabolized in liver and small intestine. **Elimination:** Excreted in urine and feces. **Half-Life:** 2–3 h.

NURSING IMPLICATIONS

Assessment & Drug Effects

- Monitor vital signs. Observe for skeletal muscle rigidity, especially of chest wall, and respiratory depression, particularly in patients who are obese, debilitated, or who have received high doses.
- Bear in mind that if naloxone is given to reverse respiratory depression, the duration of sufentanil-induced respiratory depression may exceed the duration of naloxone.

Patient & Family Education

- Avoid activities which require mental alertness for at least 24 h after receiving this drug.

SULFACETAMIDE SODIUM

(sul-fa-see′ta-mide)

AK-Sulf, Bleph 10, Cetamide, Isopto Cetamide, Ophthacet, Sebizon, Sodium Sulamyd, Sulf-10

Classifications: ANTI-INFECTIVE; SULFONAMIDE ANTIBIOTIC
Prototype: Sulfisoxazole
Pregnancy Category: C

AVAILABILITY 10% lotion; 1%, 10%, 15%, 30% solution; 10% ointment

ACTIONS Highly soluble sulfonamide that exerts bacteriostatic effect by interfering with bacterial utilization of PABA, thereby inhibiting folic acid biosynthesis required for bacterial growth.

THERAPEUTIC EFFECTS Effective against a wide range of gram-positive and gram-negative microorganisms.

USES Ophthalmic preparations are used for conjunctivitis, corneal ulcers, and other superficial ocular infections and as adjunct to systemic sulfonamide therapy for trachoma. The topical lotion is used for scaly dermatoses, seborrheic dermatitis, seborrhea sicca, and other bacterial skin infections.

CONTRAINDICATIONS Hypersensitivity to sulfonamides or to any ingredients in the formulation. Pregnancy (category C).

CAUTIOUS USE Application of lotion to denuded or debrided skin; lactation.

ROUTE & DOSAGE

Conjunctivitis

Child >2 y/Adult: **Ophthalmic** 1–2 drops of 10%, 15%, or 30% solution into lower conjunctival sac q2–3h, may increase interval as patient responds or use 1.5–2.5 cm (½–1 in) of 10% ointment q.i.d. and at bedtime

STORAGE
Store at 8°–15° C (46°–59° F) in tightly closed containers unless otherwise directed.

ADMINISTRATION
Instillation
- Be aware that ophthalmic preparations and skin lotion are not interchangeable.
- Check strength of medication prescribed (10% solution most frequently used).
- 30% solution used for severe infections.
- See Part I for instructions for instilling eye drops.
- Discard darkened solutions; results when left standing for a long time.

ADVERSE EFFECTS Special Senses: *Temporary stinging or burning sensation,* retardation of corneal healing associated with long-term use of ophthalmic ointment. **Body as a Whole:** Hypersensitivity reactions (<u>Stevens-Johnson syndrome</u>, lupus-like syndrome), superinfections with nonsusceptible organisms.

INTERACTIONS Drug: Tetracaine and other LOCAL ANESTHETICS DERIVED FROM PABA may antagonize the antibacterial effects of sulfonamides; SILVER PREPARATIONS may precipitate sulfacetamide from solution.

PHARMACOKINETICS Absorption: Minimal systemic absorption, but may be enough to cause sensitization. **Metabolism:** Metabolized in liver to inactive metabolites. **Elimination:** Excreted in urine.

NURSING IMPLICATIONS

Assessment & Drug Effects

▪ Discontinue if symptoms of hypersensitivity appear (erythema, skin rash, pruritus, urticaria).

Patient & Family Education

▪ Wash hands thoroughly with soap and running water (before and after instillation).
▪ Examine eye medication; discard if cloudy or dark in color.
▪ Avoid contaminating any part of eye dropper that is inserted in bottle.
▪ Tilt head back, pull down lower lid. At the same time, look up while drop is being instilled into conjunctival sac. Immediately apply gentle pressure just below the eyelid and next to nose for 1 min. Close eyes gently, so as not to squeeze out medication.
▪ Drops may cause burning, stinging, or sensitivity to light after instillation. If this continues report it to prescriber.
▪ Report purulent eye discharge to prescriber. Sulfacetamide sodium is inactivated by purulent exudates.
▪ Do not share medications with others and do not take more often than prescribed.
▪ Store this medication out of reach of children.

SULFADIAZINE
(sul-fa-dye′a-zeen)
Microsulfon
Classifications: ANTI-INFECTIVE; SULFONAMIDE ANTIBIOTIC
Prototype: Sulfisoxazole
Pregnancy Category: B

AVAILABILITY 500 mg tablets

ACTIONS Short-acting sulfonamide, slightly less soluble than sulfisoxazole. Exerts bacteriostatic effect by interfering with bacterial utilization of PABA, thereby inhibiting folic acid biosynthesis required for bacterial growth.
THERAPEUTIC EFFECTS Effective against a wide range of gram-positive and gram-negative microorganisms.

USES Used in combination with pyrimethamine for treatment of cerebral toxoplasmosis and chloroquine-resistant malaria.

CONTRAINDICATIONS Hypersensitivity to sulfonamides or to any ingredients in the formulation. Use in infants <2 mo of age due to displacement of bilirubin from albumin binding sites, which results in kernicterus; pregnancy (category C).
CAUTIOUS USE Multiple allergies; impaired renal or hepatic function, blood dyscrasias, G6PD deficiency, lactation.

ROUTE & DOSAGE

Mild to Moderate Infections

Child: **PO Loading Dose** *>2 mo,* 75 mg/kg/dose **PO Maintenance Dose** 150 mg/kg/day in 4–6 divided doses (max 6 g/day)
Adult: **PO Loading Dose** 2–4 g loading dose **PO Maintenance Dose** 2–4 g/day in 4–6 divided doses

Rheumatic Fever Prophylaxis

Child/Adult: **PO** *≤30 kg,* 500 mg/day *≥30 kg,* 1 g/day

Toxoplasmosis

Child: **PO** *>2 mo,* 100–200 mg/kg/day divided q6h for 3–4 wk
Adult: **PO** 2–8 g/day divided q6h

Congenital Toxoplasmosis

Neonate/Infant: **PO** 50 mg/kg q12h times 12 mo

STORAGE

Store at 15°–30° C (59°–86° F) in tight, light-resistant containers.

ADMINISTRATION

Oral

- Maintain sufficient fluid intake to produce urinary output of at least 3000–4000 mL/24 h for adults. In children maintain a fluid intake in relationship to their age to produce an adequate urinary output. Concomitant administration of urinary alkalinizer may be prescribed to reduce possibility of crystalluria and stone formation.

ADVERSE EFFECTS CNS: Headache, peripheral neuritis, peripheral neuropathy, tinnitus, hearing loss, vertigo, insomnia, drowsiness, mental depression, acute psychosis, ataxia, convulsions, <u>kernicterus</u> (newborns). **GI:** *Nausea, vomiting, diarrhea,* abdominal pains, hepatitis, jaundice, pancreatitis, stomatitis. **Hematologic:** <u>Acute hemolytic anemia</u> (especially in patients with G6PD deficiency), <u>aplastic anemia</u>, methemoglobinemia, <u>agranulocytosis</u>, thrombocytopenia, leukopenia, eosinophilia, hypoprothrombinemia. **Body as a Whole:** Headache, *fever,* chills, arthralgia, malaise, allergic myocarditis, serum sickness, <u>anaphylactoid reactions</u>, lymphadenopathy, local reaction following IM injection, fixed drug eruptions, diuresis, overgrowth of nonsusceptible organisms, LE phenomenon. **Skin:** Pruritus, urticaria, rash, erythema multiforme including <u>*Stevens-Johnson syndrome, exfoliative dermatitis*</u>, alopecia, photosensitivity, vascular lesions. **Urogenital:** *Crystalluria,* hematuria, proteinuria, <u>anuria, toxic nephrosis</u>, reduction in sperm count. **Metabolic:** Goiter, hypoglycemia. **Special Senses:** Conjunctivitis, conjunctival or scleral infection, retardation of corneal healing (ophthalmic ointment).

INTERACTIONS Drug: PABA-CONTAINING LOCAL ANESTHETICS may antagonize sulfa's effects; ORAL ANTICOAGULANTS potentiate hypoprothrombinemia; may potentiate SULFONYLUREA-induced hypoglycemia. May decrease concentrations of **cyclosporine;** may increase levels of **phenytoin. Herbal:** St. John's wort may increase the risk of photosensitivity. **Food:** Increased intake of acidifying juices or vitamin C may cause crystalluria.

PHARMACOKINETICS Absorption: Readily absorbed from GI tract. **Peak:** 3–6 h. **Distribution:** Distributed to most tissues, including CSF; crosses placenta. **Metabolism:** Metabolized in liver. **Elimination:** Excreted in urine.

NURSING IMPLICATIONS

Assessment & Drug Effects

- Lab tests: Baseline and periodic urine C&S to determine drug effectiveness; with long-term therapy, CBC, Hct and Hgb.
- Monitor hydration status.

Patient & Family Education

- Take drug exactly as prescribed. Do not alter schedule or dose; take total amount prescribed unless physician changes the regimen.
- Drink fluids liberally unless otherwise directed.
- Report early signs of blood dyscrasias (sore throat, pallor, fever) promptly to the physician.
- Do not breast feed while taking this drug without consulting physician.
- Sulfadiazine may cause photosensitivity so warn patients to avoid direct sunlight, tanning beds, and sun lamps.
- Store this medication out of reach of children.

SULFASALAZINE

(sul-fa-sal′a-zeen)
Azulfidine, PMS Sulfasalazine ♣ , PMS Sulfasalazine E.C. ♣ , Salazopyrin ♣ , SAS Enteric-500 ♣ , S.A.S.-500 ♣
Classifications: GASTROINTESTINAL AGENT; MUCOUS MEMBRANE AGENT; ANTI-INFLAMMATORY; SULFONAMIDE
Prototype: Mesalamine
Pregnancy Category: B (D if near term)

AVAILABILITY 500 mg tablets; 500 mg sustained-release tablets

ACTIONS Locally acting sulfonamide. Believed to be converted by intestinal microflora to sulfapyridine (provides antibacterial action) and 5-aminosalicylic acid (5-ASA) or mesalamine, which may exert an anti-inflammatory effect. Other proposed mechanisms of action include inhibition of prostaglandins known to cause diarrhea and affect mucosal transport, and interference with absorption of fluids and electrolytes from colon.
THERAPEUTIC EFFECTS Reduces *Clostridium* and *Escherichia coli* in the stools. Anti-inflammatory and immunomodulatory properties are effective in controlling the S&S of ulcerative colitis and rheumatoid arthritis.

USES Ulcerative colitis and relatively mild regional enteritis; rheumatoid arthritis.

UNLABELED USES Granulomatous colitis, Crohn's disease, scleroderma.

CONTRAINDICATIONS Sensitivity to sulfasalazine, other sulfonamides and salicylates; agranulocytosis; children <2 y; intestinal and urinary tract obstruction; pregnancy (category B, category D near term); porphyria.
CAUTIOUS USE Severe allergy, or bronchial asthma; blood dyscrasias; hepatic or renal impairment; lactation; children <6 y.

ROUTE & DOSAGE

Ulcerative Colitis, Rheumatoid Arthritis

Child: **PO** >2 y, *Mild:* 40–50 mg/kg/day in 4 divided doses q6h (max 75 mg/kg/day); maintenance dose is usually 30 mg/kg/day in 4 equally divided doses >2 y, *Moderate/severe:* 50–75 mg/kg/day in equally divided doses q4–6h (max 75 mg/kg/day or 6 g/day)
Adult: **PO** 1–2 g/day in equally divided doses q6–12h, may increase up to max dose of 6 g/day if needed

Juvenile Rheumatoid Arthritis

Child: **PO** >6 y, 10 mg/kg/day, increase weekly by 10 mg/kg/day (usual dose: 30–50 mg/kg/day in 2 equally divided doses q12h [max dose 2 g/day])

STORAGE
Store at 15°–30° C (59°–86° F) in tight, light-resistant containers.

ADMINISTRATION

Oral

- Give after eating to provide longer intestine transit time.
- Do not crush or chew sustained-release tablets; must be swallowed whole.
- Use evenly divided doses over each 24-h period; do not exceed 8-h intervals between doses.
- Consult physician if GI intolerance occurs after first few doses. Symptoms are probably due to irritation of stomach mucosa and may be relieved by spacing total daily dose more evenly over 24 h or by administration of enteric coated tablets.

ADVERSE EFFECTS Body as a Whole: *Nausea, vomiting, bloody diarrhea; anorexia,* arthralgia, rash, anemia, oligospermia (reversible), blood dyscrasias, <u>liver injury</u>, infectious mononucleosis–like reaction, <u>allergic reactions</u>.

INTERACTIONS Drug: Iron, ANTIBIOTICS may alter absorption of sulfasalazine; may decrease serum digoxin levels; increases anticoagulation effects. **Food:** Interferes with folic acid absorption from food.

PHARMACOKINETICS Absorption: 10–15% absorbed from GI tract unchanged; remaining drug is hydrolyzed in colon to sulfapyridine (most of which is absorbed) and 5-aminosalicylic acid (30% of which is absorbed). **Peak:** 1.5–6 h sulfasalazine; 6–24 h sulfapyridine. **Distribution:** Crosses placenta; distributed into breast milk. **Metabolism:** Metabolized in intestines and liver. **Elimination:** All metabolites are excreted in urine. **Half-Life:** 5–10 h.

NURSING IMPLICATIONS

Assessment & Drug Effects

- Monitor for GI distress. GI symptoms that develop after a few days of therapy may indicate need for dosage adjustment. If symptoms persist, prescriber may withhold drug for 5–7 days and restart it at a lower dosage level.
- Be aware that adverse reactions generally occur within a few days to 12 wk after start of therapy; most likely to occur in patients receiving high doses (4 g or more).
- Lab tests: Measure RBC folate in patients on high doses (more than 2 g/day); a daily supplement may be prescribed. Need to supplement dietary intake of iron, because sulfasalazine impairs folate absorption.

Patient & Family Education

- Need to supplement dietary intake of iron, because sulfasalazine impairs folate absorption.
- Examine stools and report to physician if enteric-coated tablets have passed intact in feces. Some patients lack enzymes capable of dissolving coating; conventional tablet will be ordered.
- Be aware that drug may color alkaline urine and skin orange-yellow.
- Remain under close medical supervision. Relapses occur in about 40% of patients after initial satisfactory response. Response to therapy and duration of treatment are governed by endoscopic examinations.
- Do not breast feed while taking this drug without consulting physician.
- Store this medication out of reach of children.

SULFISOXAZOLE ⊘

(sul-fi-sox′a-zole)

Gantrisin, Gantrison Pediatric Suspension

Classifications: ANTI-INFECTIVE; SULFONAMIDE
Pregnancy Category: B (D if near term)

S

AVAILABILITY 500 mg tablets; 500 mg/5 mL suspension (contains 0.3% alcohol)
Combination Products: 600 mg sulfisoxazole and 200 mg erthromycin ethylsuccinate/5 mL suspension

ACTIONS Short-acting derivative of sulfanilamide. Bacteriostatic action believed to be by competitive inhibition of *p*-aminobenzoic acid (PABA), thereby interfering with folic acid biosynthesis required for bacterial growth.
THERAPEUTIC EFFECTS Exhibits broad antimicrobial spectrum against both gram-positive and gram-negative organisms.

USES Acute, recurrent, and chronic urinary tract infections and chancroid; adjunctive therapy in trachoma, chloroquine-resistant strains of malaria, acute otitis media due to *Haemophilus influenzae,* and meningococcal and *H. influenzae* meningitis. Ophthalmic preparations used in treatment of conjunctivitis, corneal ulcer, and other superficial eye infections and as adjunct to systemic sulfonamide therapy for trachoma. Topical vaginal preparation used for *H. vaginalis* vaginitis.

CONTRAINDICATIONS History of hypersensitivity to sulfonamides, salicylates, or chemically related drugs; use in treatment of group A beta-hemolytic streptococcal infections; infants <2 mo of age (except in treatment of congenital toxoplasmosis); porphyria; advanced kidney or liver disease; intestinal and urinary obstruction; pregnancy (category B, category D if near term), lactation.

CAUTIOUS USE Impaired kidney or liver function; severe allergy; bronchial asthma; blood dyscrasias; patients with G6PD deficiency.

ROUTE & DOSAGE

Infection by Susceptible Organisms
Infant/Child: **PO** *>2 mo,* 75 mg/kg/dose initially, followed by 150 mg/kg/day q4–6h in equally divided doses (max 6 g/day)
Adult: **PO** 2–4 g initially, followed by 4–8 g/day q4–6h in equally divided doses **Vaginal** 1 applicator full 1–2 times/day

Infection
Otitis Media Prophylaxis
Child: **PO** *>2 mo,* 35–75 mg/kg/dose daily at bedtime

Rheumatic Fever Prophylaxis
Child: **PO** *<27 kg,* 500 mg/dose daily ≥*27 kg,* 1000 mg/dose daily

STORAGE
Store at 15°–30° C (59°–86° F) in tight, light-resistant containers.

ADMINISTRATION

Oral
- Give with full glass of water or other fluid or generous amount for age; tablet may be crushed.

ADVERSE EFFECTS CNS: Headache, peripheral neuritis, peripheral neuropathy, tinnitus, hearing loss, vertigo, insomnia, drowsiness, mental depression, acute psychosis, ataxia, convulsions, <u>kernicterus</u> (newborns). **GI:** *Nausea, vomiting, diarrhea,* abdominal pains, hepatitis, jaundice, pancreatitis, stomatitis. **Hematologic:** Acute hemolytic anemia (especially in patients with G6PD deficiency), <u>aplastic anemia</u>, methemoglobinemia, <u>agranulocytosis</u>, thrombocytopenia, leukopenia, eosinophilia, hypoprothrombinemia. **Body as a Whole:** Headache, *fever,* chills, arthralgia, malaise, allergic myocarditis, serum sickness, <u>anaphylactoid reactions</u>, lymphadenopathy, local reaction following IM injection, fixed drug eruptions, diuresis, overgrowth of nonsusceptible organisms, LE phenomenon. **Skin:** Pruritus, urticaria, rash, erythema multiforme including *<u>Stevens-Johnson syndrome, exfoliative dermatitis,</u>* alopecia, photosensitivity, vascular lesions. **Urogenital:** *Crystalluria,* hematuria, proteinuria, anuria, <u>toxic nephrosis</u>, reduction in sperm count. **Metabolic:** Goiter, hypoglycemia. **Special Senses:** Conjunctivitis, conjunctival or scleral infection, retardation of corneal healing (ophthalmic ointment).

DIAGNOSTIC TEST INTERFERENCE Sulfonamides may interfere with **BSP** retention and **PSP** excretion tests and may affect results of **thyroid function** tests (**I-131** may be decreased for about 7 days). Large doses of

SULFONAMIDES reportedly may produce false-positive **urine glucose** determinations with **copper reduction methods** (e.g., **Benedict's and Clinitest**). SULFONAMIDES may produce false-positive results for **urinary protein** (with **sulfosalicylic acid test**) and may interfere with **urine urobilinogen** determinations using **Ehrlich's reagent** or **Urobilistix.** Follow-up cultures are unreliable unless PABA is added to culture medium.

INTERACTIONS Drug: PABA-CONTAINING LOCAL ANESTHETICS may antagonize sulfa's effects; ORAL ANTICOAGULANTS potentiate hypoprothrombinemia; may potentiate SULFONYLUREA-induced hypoglycemia; may decrease concentrations of **cyclosporine;** may increase levels of **phenytoin. Herbal: St John's wort** may increase the risk of photosensitivity. **Food:** Interferes with folic acid absorption from food.

PHARMACOKINETICS Absorption: Readily absorbed from GI tract. **Peak:** 2–4 h. **Distribution:** Distributed in extracellular space; crosses blood–brain barrier and placenta; detected in breast milk. **Metabolism:** Metabolized in liver. **Elimination:** 95% excreted in urine in 24 h. **Half-Life:** 4.6–7.8 h.

NURSING IMPLICATIONS

Assessment & Drug Effects

- Lab tests: Obtain a specimen for C&S prior to initiation of therapy. Perform frequent kidney function tests and urinalyses; complete blood counts and liver function tests, especially during regimens longer than 2 wk.
- Monitor I&O. Report oliguria and changes in I&O ratio. Fluid intake should be adequate to support urinary output of at least 1500 mL/day to prevent crystalluria and stone formation in adults. In children, maintain fluid intake in relationship to their age to produce an adequate urinary output.
- Check urine pH daily with Nitrazine paper or Labstix; fall in urinary pH (more acidic) increases risk of crystalluria.
- Report increasing urine acidity. If urine is highly acidic, physician may prescribe a urinary alkalinizer.
- Monitor temperature. Sudden appearance of fever may signify sensitization (serum sickness) or hemolytic anemia (frequent in patients with G6PD deficiency, which is most common among black males and Mediterranean ethnic groups). Reactions generally develop within 10 days. Agranulocytosis may develop after 10 days to 6 wk of therapy.
- Report early manifestations of blood dyscrasias or hypersensitivity reactions immediately (fever with sore throat, malaise, unusual fatigue, joint pains, pallor, bleeding tendencies, rash, jaundice).
- Be alert for skin lesions, papular or vesiculobullous lesions, especially on sun-exposed areas, Stevens-Johnson syndrome (severe erythema multiforme) may be preceded by high fever, severe headache, stomatitis, conjunctivitis, rhinitis, urticaria, balanitis (inflammation of penis or clitoris). Termination of drug therapy is indicated.
- Observe patients with diabetes receiving oral hypoglycemic agents closely for hypoglycemic reactions. Obtain blood glucose and HbA$_{1C}$ levels before and shortly after initiation of therapy.

Patient & Family Education

- Do not take OTC medications without consulting prescriber. Many analgesic mixtures contain aspirin in combination with *p* aminobenzoic acid; avoid to prevent crystallization in urine.
- Use or add barrier contraceptives if using hormonal contraceptives, which may be unreliable while taking this drug.
- Avoid exposure to ultraviolet light and excessive sunlight to prevent photosensitivity reaction during therapy and for several months after treatment is discontinued.
- Inform dentist or new prescribers that you are taking a sulfonamide.
- Do not breast feed while taking this drug.
- Store this medication out of reach of children.

TACROLIMUS

(tac-rol'i-mus)
Prograf, Protopic
Classification: IMMUNOSUPPRESSANT
Prototype: Cyclosporine
Pregnancy Category: C

AVAILABILITY 0.5 mg, 1 mg, 5 mg capsules; 5 mg/mL injection; 0.1%, 0.03% ointment

ACTIONS Macrolide antibiotic produced by a soil fungus with immuno-suppressant activity more marked than that of cyclosporine. Inhibits helper T-lymphocytes by selectively inhibiting secretion of interleukin-2, interleukin-3, and interleukin-gamma; thus reduces transplant rejection.

THERAPEUTIC EFFECTS Inhibits antibody production (thus subduing immune response) by creating an imbalance in favor of suppressor T-lymphocytes.

USES Liver rejection prophylaxis; rejection prophylaxis for other organ transplants (kidney, heart, bone marrow, pancreas, small bowel), moderate to severe atopic dermatitis (e.g., eczema).

UNLABELED USES Acute organ transplant rejection, severe plaque-type psoriasis.

CONTRAINDICATIONS Hypersensitivity to tacrolimus or castor oil; pregnancy (category C), lactation.

CAUTIOUS USE Renal or hepatic insufficiency, hyperkalemia, diabetes mellitus, gout, history of seizures, hypertension.

ROUTE & DOSAGE

Rejection Prophylaxis

Child: **PO** Same as adult but start with upper end of dosage range
IV Same as adult but start with upper end of dosage range
Adult: **PO** 0.15–0.3 mg/kg/day in 2 divided doses q12h, start no sooner than 6 h after transplant; give first oral dose 8–12 h after discontinuing IV therapy **IV** 0.05–0.1 mg/kg/day as continuous IV infusion,

---

Common adverse effects in *italic;* life-threatening effects underlined; generic names in **bold;** drug classifications in SMALL CAPS; ◆ Canadian drug name; ☻ Prototype drug.

1143

start no sooner than 6 h after transplant, continue until patient can take oral therapy

Atopic Dermatitis

Child: **Topical** *2–15 y,* Apply thin layer of 0.03% ointment to affected area b.i.d., continue for 1 wk after clearing of symptoms; may increase to 0.1% if no response to 0.03%

Adult: **Topical** Apply thin layer of 0.03% or 0.1% ointment to affected area b.i.d., continue for 1 wk after clearing of symptoms

Severe Plaque-Type Psoriasis

Adult: **PO** Start with 0.05 mg/kg/day, increase to 0.1 mg/kg/day at week 3 and to 0.15 mg/kg/day at week 6 if necessary

STORAGE

Store ampules between 5°–25° C (41°–77° F); store capsules at 15°–30° C (59°–86° F). Store the diluted infusion in glass or polyethylene containers and discard after 24 h.

ADMINISTRATION

Oral

- Discontinue cyclosporine at least 24 h before the first dose of tacrolimus.
- Convert patient from IV to oral therapy as soon as possible.
- Give first oral dose 8–12 h after discontinuing IV infusion.
- Give on an empty stomach.
- Dispense dose in paper medication cup only.

Topical

- Ensure that skin is clean and completely dry before application.
- Apply a thin layer to the affected area and rub in gently and completely.
- Do not apply occlusive dressing over the site.

Intravenous

PREPARE **IV Infusion:** Dilute 5 mg/mL ampules with NS or D5W to a concentration of 0.004–0.02 mg/mL, or less for pediatric patients. Monitor patient continuously for the first 30 min of infusion for signs of respiratory difficulties and anaphylaxis.

ADMINISTER **IV Infusion:** Give as continuous IV. Use PVC free tubing to minimize drug absorption to the tubing.

INCOMPATIBILITIES **Y-Site: Phenytoin.**

ADVERSE EFFECTS CNS: *Headache, tremors, insomnia, paresthesia, hyperesthesia* and/or sensations of warmth, circumoral numbness. **CV:** *Mild to moderate hypertension.* **Endocrine:** Hirsutism, *hyperglycemia, hyperkalemia, hypokalemia, hypomagnesemia,* hyperuricemia, decreased serum cholesterol. **GI:** *Nausea, abdominal pain, gas,* appetite changes, *vomiting, anorexia, constipation,* diarrhea, ascites. **Hematologic:** Anemia, leukocytosis, thrombocytopenia purpura. **Urogenital:** UTI, oliguria, <u>nephrotoxicity</u>. **Respiratory:** *Pleural effusion, atelectasis, dyspnea.* **Special Senses:** Blurred vision, photophobia. **Skin:** *Flushing, rash, pruritus, skin irritation,* alopecia, erythema, folliculitis, hyperesthesia, <u>exfoliative dermatitis</u>, hirsutism, photosensitivity, skin discoloration, skin ulcer, sweating. **Body as a Whole:** *Pain, fever, peripheral edema.*

INTERACTIONS Drug: Use with AMINOGLYCOSIDES, **amphotericin B, cisplatin, cyclosporine,** increases risk of nephrotoxicity. **Cimetidine, clarithromycin, dilitazem, erythromycin, fluconazole, ketoconazole, methylprednisolone, metoclopramide, nifedipine, verapamil** may increase tacrolimus levels; **caspofungin, carbamazephine, phenobarbital, rifabutin, rifampin,** ANTACIDS, may decrease levels. NSAIDS may lead to oliguria or anuria. **Herbal: St. John's wort** decrease serum levels of tacrolimus. **Food:** Decreases absorption of tacrolimus. Tacrolimus drug levels may be increased with grapefruit juice.

PHARMACOKINETICS Absorption: Erratic and incompletely absorbed from GI tract; absolute bioavailability approximately 14–25%; absorption reduced by food. **Peak:** PO 1–4 h. **Duration:** 12 h IV. **Distribution:** Within plasma, tacrolimus is found primarily in lipoprotein-deficient fraction; 75–97% protein bound, mainly to albumin and alpha$_1$-acid glycoprotein; distributed into red blood cells; blood:plasma ratio reported >4; animal studies have demonstrated high concentrations of tacrolimus in lung, kidney, heart, and spleen, and similar tissue profile is to be expected in humans; distributed into breast milk. **Metabolism:** Extensively metabolized in liver. **Elimination:** Metabolites excreted primarily in bile. **Half-Life:** 8.7–11.3 h.

NURSING IMPLICATIONS

Assessment & Drug Effects

- Lab tests: Monitor serum electrolytes, blood glucose, uric acid, BUN, and creatinine clearance periodically.
- Monitor kidney function closely; report elevated serum creatinine or decreased urinary output.
- Monitor for neurotoxicity, and report tremors, changes in mental status, or other signs of toxicity.
- Monitor cardiovascular status and report hypertension.
- Monitor temperature and for signs of infection.

Patient & Family Education

- Learn complete dosing instructions.
- Be aware of potential adverse effects.
- Avoid others with infections, large crowds, and report any signs of infection to prescriber immediately.
- Minimize exposure to natural or artificial sunlight while using the ointment.
- Notify prescriber of S&S of neurotoxicity.
- Do not breast feed while taking this drug.
- Store this medication out of reach of children.

TERBUTALINE SULFATE

(ter-byoo′te-leen)
Brethaire, Brethine, Bricanyl
Classifications: AUTONOMIC NERVOUS SYSTEM AGENT; BETA-ADRENERGIC AGONIST; BRONCHODILATOR
Prototype: Albuterol
Pregnancy Category: B

AVAILABILITY 2.5 mg, 5 mg tablets; 0.2 mg aerosol; 1 mg/mL injection

ACTIONS Synthetic adrenergic stimulant with selective $beta_2$- and negligible $beta_1$-agonist (cardiac) activity. Exerts preferential effect on $beta_2$-receptors in bronchial smooth muscles, inhibits histamine release from mast cells, and increases ciliary motility.

THERAPEUTIC EFFECTS Relieves bronchospasm in chronic obstructive pulmonary disease (COPD) and significantly increases vital capacity. Promotes relaxation of vascular smooth muscle, contraction of GI and urinary sphincters, increase in renin, pancreatic beta-cell secretion, and serum HDL-cholesterol concentration. Increases uterine relaxation (thereby preventing or abolishing high intrauterine pressure).

USES Orally, subcutaneously, or intravenously as a bronchodilator in bronchial asthma and for reversible airway obstruction associated with bronchitis and emphysema.

UNLABELED USES To delay delivery in preterm labor.

CONTRAINDICATIONS Known hypersensitivity to sympathomimetic amines; severe hypertension and coronary artery disease; tachycardia with digitalis intoxication; within 14 days of MAO inhibitor therapy; angle-closure glaucoma. Used only after evaluation of risk-benefit ratio in pregnancy (category B) and lactation.

CAUTIOUS USE Angina, stroke, hypertension; diabetes mellitus; thyrotoxicosis; history of seizure disorders; cardiac arrhythmias; kidney and liver dysfunction.

ROUTE & DOSAGE

Bronchodilator

Child: **PO** *<12 y,* 0.05 mg/kg/dose q8h, gradually increase up to 0.15 mg/kg/dose q8h (max 5 mg/day) **SC** 0.005–0.01 mg/kg/dose (max 0.4 mg) q15–20min times 2 doses **Nebulization** *<2 y,* 0.5 mg in 2.5 mL normal saline q4–6h as needed; *2–9 y,* 1 mg in 2.5 mL normal saline q4–6h as needed; *>9 y,* 1.5–2.5 mg in 2.5 mL normal saline q4–6h as needed

Adolescent: **PO** *12–15 y,* 2.5 mg t.i.d. at 6 h intervals (max 7.5 mg/day) **SC** 0.25 mg q15–30min up to 0.5 mg in 4 h **IV** *Continuous infusion:* 0.08–0.4 mcg/kg/min **Inhaled** 2 inhalations separated by 60 sec q4–6h

Adult: **PO** 2.5–5 mg t.i.d. at 6 h intervals (max 15 mg/day) **SC** 0.25 mg q15–30min up to 0.5 mg in 4 h **Inhaled** 2 inhalations separated by 60 sec q4–6h

STORAGE
Store all forms at 15°–30° C (59°–86° F); protect from light. Do not freeze.

ADMINISTRATION

Oral

- Give with fluid of patient's choice; tablets may be crushed.
- Be certain about recommended doses: PO preparation, 2.5 mg; SC, 0.25 mg. A decimal point error can be fatal.
- Give with food if GI symptoms occur.

Subcutaneous
- Give SC injection into lateral upper arm.

Intravenous

PREPARE **IV Infusion:** For continuous infusion add to D5W or normal saline.
ADMINISTER **IV Infusion:** Give as continuous infusion. Dilute to maximum concentration of 1 mg/mL.
INCOMPATIBILITIES **Y-Site: Bleomycin. Nebulization:** IV solution of 1 mg/mL can be used for nebulization.

ADVERSE EFFECTS CNS: *Nervousness, tremor,* headache, *light-headedness,* drowsiness, fatigue, seizures. **CV:** *Tachycardia,* hypotension or hypertension, *palpitation,* maternal and fetal tachycardia. **GI:** Nausea, vomiting. **Body as a Whole:** Sweating, muscle cramps.

DIAGNOSTIC TEST INTERFERENCE Terbutaline may increase *blood glucose* and free *fatty acids.*

INTERACTIONS Drug: Epinephrine, other SYMPATHOMIMETIC BRONCHODILATORS may add to effects; MAO INHIBITORS, TRICYCLIC ANTIDEPRESSANTS potentiate action on vascular system; effects of both BETA-ADRENERGIC BLOCKERS and terbutaline antagonized.

PHARMACOKINETICS Absorption: 33–50% absorbed from GI tract. **Onset:** 30 min PO; <15 min SC; 5–30 min inhaled. **Peak:** 2–3 h PO; 30–60 min SC; 1–2 h inhaled. **Duration:** 4–8 h PO; 1.5–4 h SC; 3–4 h inhaled. **Distribution:** Distributed into breast milk. **Metabolism:** Metabolized in liver. **Elimination:** Excreted primarily in urine, 3% in feces. **Half-Life:** 3–4 h.

NURSING IMPLICATIONS

Assessment & Drug Effects
- Assess vital signs: Baseline pulse and BP and before each dose. If significantly altered from baseline level, consult physician. Cardiovascular adverse effects are more apt to occur when drug is given by SC route or it is used by a patient with cardiac arrhythmia.
- Most adverse effects are transient, however, rapid heart rate may persist for a relatively long time.
- Be aware that onset and degree of effect and incidence and severity of adverse effects of SC formulation resemble those of epinephrine.
- Aerosolized drug produces minimal cardiac stimulation or tremors.
- Be aware that muscle tremor is a fairly common adverse effect that appears to subside with continued use.
- Monitor for symptoms of hypoglycemia in neonates born of a mother who used terbutaline during pregnancy.
- Monitor patient being treated for premature labor for CV S&S for 12 h after drug is discontinued. Report tachycardia promptly.
- Monitor I&O ratio. Fluid restriction may be necessary. Consult physician.

Patient & Family Education
- Adhere to established dosage regimen (i.e., do not change dose intervals or omit, increase, or decrease the dose).

- Inhalator therapy: Review instructions for use of inhalator (included in the package).
- Learn how to take pulse and the limits of change that indicate need to notify the physician.
- Consult physician if breathing difficulty is not relieved or if it becomes worse within 30 min after an oral dose.
- Keep appointments with prescriber for evaluation of continued drug effectiveness and clinical condition. Terbutaline appears to have a short clinical period for sustained effectiveness. Plan with school personnel to ensure child's access to medication during school hours.
- Consult prescriber if symptomatic relief wanes; tolerance can develop with chronic use. Usually, a substitute agent will be prescribed.
- Do not self-dose this drug, particularly during long-term therapy. In the face of waning response, increasing the dose will not improve the clinical condition and may cause overdosage. Understand that decreasing relief with continued treatment indicates need for another bronchodilator, not an increase in dose.
- Do not puncture container, use or store it near heat or open flame, or expose to temperatures above 49° C (120° F), which may cause bursting. Contents of the aerosol (inhalator) are under pressure.
- Do not use any other aerosol bronchodilator while being treated with aerosol terbutaline. Do not self-medicate with an OTC aerosol.
- Do not use OTC drugs without physician approval. Many cold and allergy remedies, for example, contain a sympathomimetic agent that when combined with terbutaline may be cause harmful adverse effects.
- Do not breast feed while taking/using this drug.
- Store this medication out of reach of children.

TETRACYCLINE HYDROCHLORIDE

(tet-ra-sye′kleen)

Achromycin, Achromycin V, Nor-Tet, Novotetra ♣, Panmycin, Robitet, SK-Tetracycline, Sumycin, Tetracap, Tetracyn, Tetralan, Tetram, Topicycline

Classifications: ANTI-INFECTIVE; ANTIBIOTIC; TETRACYCLINE
Pregnancy Category: D

AVAILABILITY 100 mg, 250 mg, 500 mg capsules; 250 mg, 500 mg tablets; 125 mg/mL suspension; 2.2 mg/mL topical solution; 3% ointment

ACTIONS Broad-spectrum antibiotic derived from *Streptomyces aureofaciens* or produced semisynthetically from oxytetracycline. Tetracyclines usually are bacteriostatic but may be bactericidal in high concentrations. Exerts antiacne action by suppressing growth of *Propionibacterium acnes* within sebaceous follicles, thereby reducing free fatty acid content in sebum. Free fatty acids are thought to be produced by breakdown of triglycerides by lipases liberated from *P. acne* and are believed to be largely responsible for inflammatory skin lesions (papules, pustules, cysts) and comedones of acne. Evidence suggests that topical tetracycline may be as effective as the oral preparation for treatment of mild to moderate acne; moderate to severe acne may require oral and topical tetracycline.

THERAPEUTIC EFFECTS Effective against a variety of gram-positive and gram-negative bacteria and against most *chlamydiae, mycoplasmas, rickettsiae,* and certain protozoa (e.g., amebae). Exerts antiacne action by suppressing growth of *P. acnes* within sebaceous follicles.

USES Chlamydial infections (e.g., lymphogranuloma venereum, psittacosis, trachoma, inclusion conjunctivitis, nongonococcal urethritis); mycoplasmal infections (e.g., *Mycoplasma pneumoniae*); rickettsial infections (e.g., Q fever, Rocky Mt spotted fever, typhus); spirochetal infections: relapsing fever (*Borrelia*), leptospirosis, syphilis (penicillin-hypersensitive patients); amebiases; uncommon gram-negative bacterial infections (e.g., brucellosis, shigellosis, cholera, gonorrhea [penicillin-hypersensitive patients], granuloma inguinale, tularemia); gram-positive infections (e.g., tetanus). Also used orally and topically (solution) for inflammatory acne vulgaris; topical ointment is used for superficial skin infections. Ophthalmic preparation in combination formulation, used for trachoma and inclusion conjunctivitis.

UNLABELED USES Actinomycosis, acute exacerbations of chronic bronchitis; Lyme disease; pericardial effusion (metastatic); acute PID; sexually transmitted epididymoorchitis; with quinine for multidrug-resistant strains of *Plasmodium falciparum* malaria; anti-infective prophylaxis for rape victims; recurrent cystic thyroid nodules; melioidosis; and as fluorescence test for malignancy.

CONTRAINDICATIONS Hypersensitivity to tetracyclines or to any ingredient in the formulation; severe renal or hepatic impairment, common bile duct obstruction. Use during tooth development (last half of pregnancy [category D]), during infancy and childhood to the 8th year, or lactation. Safety of topical tetracycline preparations in children <11 y is not established.

CAUTIOUS USE History of kidney or liver dysfunction; myasthenia gravis; history of allergy, asthma, hay fever, urticaria; undernourished patients.

ROUTE & DOSAGE

Systemic Infection

Child: **PO** >8 y, 25–50 mg/kg/day in 4 equally divided doses q6h (max dose 3 g/day)
Adult: **PO** 250–500 mg q6–12h (1–2 g/day)

Acne

Child >8 y/Adult: **PO** 500–1000 mg/day in 4 divided doses
Topical Apply to cleansed areas twice daily

STORAGE

Store at 15°–30° C (59°–86° F) in tightly covered container in dry place. Protect from light.

ADMINISTRATION

Oral

■ Give with a full glass of water on an empty stomach at least 1 h before or 2 h after meals (food, milk, and milk products can reduce absorption by 50% or more).

- Do not give immediately before bed.
- Give with food if patient is having GI symptoms (e.g., nausea, vomiting, anorexia); do not give with foods high in calcium such as milk or milk products.
- Shake suspension well before pouring to ensure uniform distribution of drug. Use calibrated liquid measure to dispense.
- Consult prescriber about ordering the oral suspension formulation if patient cannot swallow pills.
- Check expiration date for all tetracyclines. Fanconi-like syndrome (renal tubular dysfunction) and also an LE-like syndrome have been attributed to outdated tetracycline preparations.
- Tetracycline decomposes with age, exposure to light, and when improperly stored under conditions of extreme humidity, heat, or cold. The resultant product may be toxic.

ADVERSE EFFECTS CNS: Headache, intracranial hypertension (rare). **Special Senses:** Pigmentation of conjunctiva due to drug deposit. **GI:** Reported mostly for oral administration, but also may occur with parenteral tetracycline (*nausea, vomiting,* epigastric distress, heartburn, *diarrhea,* bulky loose stools, steatorrhea, *abdominal discomfort, flatulence,* dry mouth); dysphagia, retrosternal pain, esophagitis, esophageal ulceration with oral administration, abnormally high liver function test values, decrease in serum cholesterol, fatty degeneration of liver (jaundice, increasing nitrogen retention [azotemia], hyperphosphatemia, acidosis, irreversible shock); foul-smelling stools or vaginal discharge, stomatitis, glossitis; black hairy tongue (lingua nigra), diarrhea; staphylococcal enterocolitis pseudomembranous colitis. **Body as a Whole:** Drug fever, angioedema, serum sickness, anaphylaxis. **Urogenital:** Particularly in patients with kidney disease; increase in BUN/serum creatinine, renal impairment even with therapeutic doses; Fanconi-like syndrome (outdated tetracycline) (characterized by polyuria, polydipsia, nausea, vomiting, glycosuria, proteinuria acidosis, aminoaciduria); vulvovaginitis, pruritus vulvae or ani (possibly hypersensitivity). **Skin:** Dermatitis, *phototoxicity:* discoloration of nails, onycholysis (loosening of nails); cheilosis; fixed drug eruptions particularly on genitalia; thrombocytopenic purpura; urticaria, rash, exfoliative dermatitis; with topical applications: skin irritation, dry scaly skin, transient stinging or burning sensation, slight yellowing of skin at application site, acute contact dermatitis. **Other:** Injury to growing bones and teeth (causes permanent discoloration of teeth); pancreatitis; local reactions: pain and irritation (IM site), Jarisch-Herxheimer reaction (see Nursing Implications).

DIAGNOSTIC TEST INTERFERENCE TETRACYCLINES may cause false increases in **urinary catecholamines** (by *fluorometric methods*), and false decreases in **urinary urobilinogen.** Parenteral TETRACYCLINES containing ascorbic acid reportedly may produce false-positive **urinary glucose** determinations by **copper reduction methods** (e.g., **Benedict's reagent, Clinitest**); TETRACYCLINES may cause false-negative results with **glucose oxidase methods** (e.g., **Clinistix, TesTape**).

INTERACTIONS Drug: ANTACIDS, **calcium,** and **magnesium** bind tetracycline in gut and decrease absorption. ORAL ANTICOAGULANTS potentiate hypoprothrombinemia. ANTIDIARRHEAL AGENTS with **kaolin** and pectin may

Common adverse effects in *italic;* life-threatening effects underlined; generic names in **bold;** drug classifications in SMALL CAPS; ◆ Canadian drug name; ❷ Prototype drug.

decrease absorption. Effectiveness of ORAL CONTRACEPTIVES decreased. **Methoxyflurane** may produce fatal nephrotoxicity. **Food:** Dairy products and iron supplements decrease tetracycline absorption.

PHARMACOKINETICS Absorption: 75–80% of dose absorbed orally. **Peak:** 2–4 h. **Distribution:** Widely distributed, preferentially binds to rapid growing tissues; crosses placenta; enters breast milk. **Metabolism:** Not metabolized; enterohepatic cycling. **Elimination:** 50–60% excreted in urine within 72 h. **Half-Life:** 6–12 h.

NURSING IMPLICATIONS

Assessment & Drug Effects

- Lab tests: Obtain baseline and periodic C&S tests to confirm susceptibility of infecting organism to tetracycline. Also, perform initial and periodic kidney, liver, and hematopoietic function tests, particularly during high-dose, long-term therapy. Determine serum tetracycline levels in patients at risk for hepatotoxicity (sometimes associated with pancreatitis and occurs most frequently in patients receiving other hepatotoxic drugs or with history of renal or hepatic impairment).
- Report GI symptoms (e.g., nausea, vomiting, diarrhea) to physician. These are generally dose dependent, occurring mostly with oral forms in patients receiving 2 g/day or more and during prolonged therapy. Frequently, symptoms are controlled by reducing dosage or administering with compatible foods.
- Be alert to evidence of superinfections (see Appendix D-1). Regularly inspect tongue and mucous membrane of mouth for candidiasis (thrush). Suspect superinfection if patient complains of irritation or soreness of mouth, tongue, throat, vagina, or anus, or persistent itching of any area, diarrhea, or foul-smelling excreta or discharge.
- Withhold drug and notify physician if superinfection develops. Superinfections occur most frequently in patients receiving prolonged therapy, the debilitated, or those who have diabetes, leukemia, systemic LE, or lymphoma. Women taking oral contraceptives reportedly are more susceptible to vaginal candidiasis.
- Obtain follow-up cultures from all gonococcal infection sites 3–7 days after completion of tetracycline therapy to verify eradication of infection.
- Monitor I&O in patients receiving parenteral tetracycline. Report oliguria or any changes in appearance of urine or in I&O.

Patient & Family Education

- Report onset of diarrhea to prescriber. It is important to determine whether diarrhea is due to irritating drug effect or superinfections or pseudomembranous colitis (caused by overgrowth of toxin-producing bacteria, *Clostridium difficile*) (see Appendix D-1). The latter two conditions can be **LIFE THREATENING** and require immediate withdrawal of tetracycline and prompt initiation of symptomatic and supportive therapy.
- Reduce incidence of superinfection (see Appendix D-1) by meticulous care of mouth, skin, and perineal area. Rinse mouth of food debris after eating; floss daily and use a soft-bristled toothbrush. Wash hands several times a day, particularly after each bowel movement and before eating.

- Avoid direct exposure to sunlight during and for several days after therapy is terminated to reduce possibility of photosensitivity reaction (appearing like an exaggerated sunburn, it begins a few minutes to hours following sun exposure, often with tingling, burning sensation).
- Report onset of severe headache or visual disturbances immediately. These are possible symptoms of increased intracranial pressure and necessitate prompt withdrawal of tetracycline to prevent irreversible loss of vision.
- Note: Tetracycline therapy for brucellosis or spirochetal infections may cause a Jarisch-Herxheimer reaction. The reaction is usually mild and appears abruptly within 6–24 h after initiation of therapy. It is manifested by malaise, fever, chills, headache, adenopathy, leukocytosis, exacerbation of skin lesions, arthralgia, transient hypotension. Treatment is symptomatic; recovery generally occurs within 24 h.
- Report immediately sudden onset of painful or difficult swallowing (dysphagia) to physician. Esophagitis and esophageal ulceration have been associated with bedtime administration of tetracycline capsules or tablets with insufficient fluid, particularly to patients with hiatal hernia or esophageal problems.
- Do not allow topical medication to contact eyes, nose, or mouth. Be aware that tetracycline may stain clothing.
- Clean affected skin area with soap and water; rinse and dry well before application of topical drug.
- Report a worsening infection or stinging and burning sensation with topical applications to prescriber if pronounced.
- Skin treated with topical drug will exhibit bright yellow to green fluorescence under ultraviolet light and "black light."
- Be aware that topicyline contains a sulfite that can cause an allergic reaction (itching, wheezing, anaphylaxis) in susceptible persons (e.g., asthmatics or allergic individuals).
- Response to acne therapy usually requires 2–8 wk, maximal results may not be apparent for up to 12 wk.
- Do not use in children under 8 y; causes permanent staining of teeth and adversely affects bone growth.
- Do not breast feed while taking/using this drug.
- Store this medication out of reach of children.

TETRAHYDROZOLINE HYDROCHLORIDE

(tet-ra-hye-drozz′a-leen)
Collyrium, Malazine, Murine Plus, Optigene, Soothe, Tyzine, Visine
Classifications: EYE, EAR, NOSE, AND THROAT PREPARATION; VASOCONSTRICTOR; DECONGESTANT
Prototype: Naphazoline
Pregnancy Category: C

AVAILABILITY 0.05% ophthalmic solution; 0.05%, 0.1% nasal solution

ACTIONS Related to naphazoline but shares more marked alpha-adrenergic than beta-adrenergic activity; large doses cause CNS depression rather than the stimulation produced by other sympathomimetic amines.

THERAPEUTIC EFFECTS Ophthalmic solution is effective for allergic reactions of the eye; nasal solution is anti-inflammatory and also decreases allergic congestion.

USES Symptomatic short-term relief of minor eye irritation and allergies and for nasopharyngeal congestion of allergic or inflammatory origin.

CONTRAINDICATIONS Hypersensitivity to any component; use of ophthalmic preparation in glaucoma or other serious eye diseases; use within 14 days of MAO inhibitor therapy. Use in children <2 y; use of 0.1% or higher strengths of nasal solution in children <6 y. Safety during pregnancy (category C) is not established.
CAUTIOUS USE Hypertension; cardiovascular disease; hyperthyroidism; diabetes mellitus; young children; lactation.

ROUTE & DOSAGE

Decongestant
Child: **Nasal** 2–6 y, 2–4 drops of 0.05% solution or spray in each nostril q3h prn
Child >6 y/Adult: **Nasal** 2–4 drops of 0.1% solution or spray in each nostril q3h prn
Adult: **Ophthalmic** Instill 1–2 drops of a 0.01–0.05% solution in conjuctiva of affected eye q.i.d.

STORAGE

ADMINISTRATION

Instillation

- Make sure interval between doses is at least 4–6 h because drug action lasts 4–8 h.
- Place patient in upright position when using nasal spray. (If patient is reclining, a stream rather than a spray may be ejected, with consequent overdosage.)
- Use lateral, head-low position to administer nasal drops.
- Opthamalmic: Do not touch dropper tip to eye or eyelashes during instillation. To decrease systemic absorption in, apply pressure to the inner canthus for 1–2 min after instillation.

ADVERSE EFFECTS Special Senses: *Transient stinging,* irritation, *sneezing,* dryness, headache, tremors, drowsiness, light-headedness, insomnia, palpitation. **Body as a Whole:** With overdose: Marked drowsiness, sweating, <u>coma</u>, hypotension, <u>shock</u>, bradycardia.

INTERACTIONS Drug: No clinically significant interactions established.

PHARMACOKINETICS Absorption: May be absorbed from nasal mucosa. **Duration:** 4–8 h.

NURSING IMPLICATIONS

Patient & Family Education

- Discontinue medication and consult prescriber if relief is not obtained within 48 h or if symptoms persist or increase.

- Do not exceed recommended dosage. Rebound congestion and rhinitis may occur with frequent or prolonged (>3 days) use of nasal preparation. Do not share this medication with others.
- Do not breast feed while using this drug without consulting physician.
- Store this medication out of reach of children.

THEOPHYLLINE 🅟
(thee-off'i-lin)
Bronkodyl, Elixophyllin, Lanophyllin, PMS Theophylline ◆, Pulmopylline ◆, Quibron-T, Respbid, Slo-Bid, Slo-Phyllin, Somophyllin, Somophyllin-12 ◆, Theo-Dur, Theo-24, Theolair, Theophylline Ethylenediamine, Theospan-SR, Uni-Dur, Uniphyl
Classifications: BRONCHODILATOR (RESPIRATORY SMOOTH MUSCLE RELAXANT); XANTHINE
Pregnancy Category: C

AVAILABILITY 100 mg, 125 mg, 200 mg, 250 mg, 300 mg tablets; 100 mg, 200 mg capsules; 80 mg/15 mL, 150 mg/15 mL liquid (some contain alcohol); 100 mg, 200 mg, 250 mg, 300 mg, 450 mg, 500 mg, 600 mg sustained-release tablets; 50 mg, 75 mg, 100 mg, 125 mg, 200 mg, 250 mg, 260 mg, 300 mg sustained-release capsules; 200 mg, 400 mg, 800 mg injection

ACTIONS Xanthine derivative that relaxes smooth muscle by direct action, particularly of bronchi and pulmonary vessels, and stimulates medullary respiratory center with resulting increase in vital capacity. Also relaxes smooth muscles of biliary and GI tracts. Stimulates myocardium, thereby increasing force of contractions and cardiac output, and stimulates all levels of CNS, but to a lesser degree than caffeine.
THERAPEUTIC EFFECTS Effective for relief of bronchospasm in asthmatics, chronic bronchitis, and emphysema.

USES Prophylaxis and symptomatic relief of bronchial asthma, as well as bronchospasm associated with chronic bronchitis and emphysema. Also used for emergency treatment of paroxysmal cardiac dyspnea and edema of CHF.
UNLABELED USES Treatment of apnea and bradycardia in prematurity and to reduce severe bronchospasm associated with cystic fibrosis and acute descending respiratory infection. Theophylline sodium glycinate is a mixture of sodium theophylline and aminoacetic (glycine). Contains 45–47% theophylline. Similar actions, uses, adverse reactions, and precautions as other theophylline derivatives but claimed to produce less gastric irritation.

CONTRAINDICATIONS Hypersensitivity to xanthines; coronary artery disease or angina pectoris when myocardial stimulation might be harmful; severe renal or liver impairment. Safety during pregnancy (category C) or lactation is not established.
CAUTIOUS USE Children and neonates; compromised cardiac or circulatory function, hypertension; hyperthyroidism; peptic ulcer; prostatic hypertrophy; seizure disorders, glaucoma; diabetes mellitus.

ROUTE & DOSAGE

Based on dosing therapeutic serum levels.

Bronchospasm

Infant: **PO/IV Maintenance Dose*** *2–6 mo,* 0.4 mg/kg/h; *6–11 mo,* 0.7 mg/kg/h
Child: **PO/IV Maintenance Dose*** *1–9 y,* 0.8 mg/kg/h; *10–12 y,* 0.6 mg/kg/h
Child/Adult: **PO/IV Loading Dose** 5 mg/kg/dose given once
Adult: **PO/IV Maintenance Dose*** *Nonsmoker,* 0.4 mg/kg/h; *Smoker,* 0.6 mg/kg/h; *With CHF or cirrhosis,* 0.2 mg/kg/h

Apnea of Prematurity

Neonate: **PO** 4–5 mg/kg/dose × 1 then **Maintenance** 3–6 mg/kg/24 h in equally divided doses q6–8h **IV Maintenance Dose*** 0.13 mg/kg/h or 4 mg/kg/day divided q12h

(***IV** by continuous infusion, **PO** divided q6h [immediate release] or q8–12h [sustained release])

ADMINISTRATION

Note: All doses based on ideal body weight.

Oral

- Wait 4–6 h after the last IV dose when switching from IV to oral dosing.
- Give with a full glass of water or generous amount of fluid per age, and after meals to minimize gastric irritation.
- Give sustained-release forms and enteric-coated tablets whole. Chewable tablets must be chewed thoroughly before swallowing. Sustained-release granules from capsules can be taken on an empty stomach or mixed with applesauce or water.
- Note: Timing of dose is critical. Be certain patient understands necessity of adhering to the correct intervals between doses.

Intravenous

- Give *prediluted solutions* at a rate not to exceed 20 mg/min.
PREPARE IV Infusion: Give IV theophylline ethylenediamine solution with a concentration of 25 mg/mL undiluted by direct IV or diluted (preferred) in up to 200 mL of D5W.
ADMINISTER IV Infusion: Give at a rate not to exceed 20 mg/min over 20 to 30 min.
INCOMPATIBILITIES Solution/Additive: Amikacin, ascorbic acid, bleomycin, CEPHALOSPORINS, chlorpromazine, clindamycin, codeine phosphate, dimenhydrinate, dobutamine, dopamine, doxapram, doxorubicin, epinephrine, hydralazine, hydroxyzine, insulin, isoproterenol, levorphanol, meperidine, methadone, methylprednisolone, morphine, nafcillin, norepinephrine, oxytetracycline, papaverine, penicillin G, pentazocine, procaine, prochlorperazine, promazine, promethazine, tetracycline, verapamil, vitamin B complex with C. **Y-Site:** Amiodarone, codeine phosphate, clindamycin, PHENOTHIAZINES (chlorpromazine, prochlorperazine), epinephrine, dobutamine, dopamine,

T

levorphanol, **meperidine, methadone, morphine, norepineph-rine, phenytoin, verapamil.**

ADVERSE EFFECTS CNS: Stimulation (irritability, restlessness, insomnia, dizziness, headache, tremor, hyperexcitability, muscle twitching, <u>drug-induced seizures</u>). **CV:** Palpitation, *tachycardia,* extrasystoles, flushing, marked hypotension, <u>circulatory failure</u>. **GI:** *Nausea,* vomiting, anorexia, epigastric or abdominal pain, diarrhea, activation of peptic ulcer. **Urogenital:** Transient urinary frequency, albuminuria, kidney irritation. **Respiratory:** Tachypnea, <u>respiratory arrest</u>. **Body as a Whole:** Fever, dehydration.

DIAGNOSTIC TEST INTERFERENCE False-positive elevations of ***serum uric acid*** (***Bittner*** or colorimetric methods). ***Probenecid*** may cause false high serum theophylline readings, and spectrophotometric methods of determining ***serum theophylline*** are affected by **furosemide, sulfathiazole,** phenylbutazone, **probenecid,** theobromine.

INTERACTIONS Drug: Increases **lithium** excretion, lowering lithium levels; **cimetidine,** high-dose **allopurinol** (600 mg/day), **tacrine,** QUINOLONES, MACROLIDE ANTIBIOTICS, and **zileuton** can significantly increase theophylline levels. **Herb: St. John's wort** may decrease theophylline efficacy.

PHARMACOKINETICS Absorption: Most products are 100% absorbed from GI tract. **Peak:** 30 min IV; uncoated tablet 1 h; sustained-release 4–6 h. **Duration:** 4–8 h; varies with age, smoking, and liver function. **Distribution:** Crosses placenta. **Metabolism:** Extensively metabolized in liver. **Elimination:** Parent drug and metabolites excreted by kidneys; excreted in breast milk.

NURSING IMPLICATIONS

Assessment & Drug Effects

- Lab tests: Monitor plasma level of theophylline. Be aware that ***therapeutic plasma level ranges from 10–20 mcg/mL*** (a narrow therapeutic range). ***Levels exceeding 20 mcg/mL are associated with toxicity.***
- Monitor drug levels in heavy smokers closely. Cigarette smoking induces hepatic microsomal enzyme activity, decreasing serum half-life and increasing body clearance of theophylline. An increase of dosage from 50–100% is usual in heavy smokers.
- Monitor plasma drug level closely in patients with heart failure, kidney or liver dysfunction, alcoholism, high fever. Plasma clearance of xanthines may be reduced.
- Take necessary safety precautions and forewarn patients of possible dizziness during early therapy.
- Monitor vital signs. Improvement in respiratory status is the expected outcome.
- Observe and report early signs of possible toxicity: Anorexia, nausea, vomiting, dizziness, shakiness, restlessness, abdominal discomfort, irritability, palpitation, tachycardia, marked hypotension, cardiac arrhythmias, seizures.
- Monitor for tachycardia which may be worse in patients with severe cardiac disease. Conversely, theophylline toxicity may be masked in patients with tachycardia.

T

Common adverse effects in *italic;* life-threatening effects <u>underlined</u>; generic names in **bold;** drug classifications in SMALL CAPS; ✦ Canadian drug name; ⦿ Prototype drug.

- Monitor patients on sustained release preparations for S&S of overdosage. Continued slow absorption leads to high plasma concentrations for a prolonged period.
- Note: Neonates of mothers using this drug have exhibited slight tachycardia, jitteriness, and apnea.
- Monitor CLOSELY for adverse effects in infants <6 mo and prematures; theophylline metabolism is prolonged as is the half-life in this age group.

Patient & Family Education

- Take medication at the same time every day.
- Avoid charcoal-broiled foods (high in polycyclic carbon content); may increase theophylline elimination and reduce the half-life as much as 50%.
- Limit caffeine intake because it may increase incidence of adverse effects.
- Cigarette smoking may significantly lower theophylline plasma concentration.
- Be aware that a low-carbohydrate, high-protein diet increases theophylline elimination, and a high-carbohydrate, low-protein diet decreases it.
- Drink fluids liberally (2000–3000 mL/day) or generous amounts appropriate for age if not contraindicated to decrease viscosity of airway secretions.
- Avoid self-dosing with OTC medications, especially cough suppressants, which may cause retention of secretions and CNS depression.
- Do not breast feed while taking this drug without consulting physician. Because theophylline is distributed into breast milk, it may be advisable to nurse the infant just before taking the drug.
- Store this medication out of reach of children.

THIABENDAZOLE

(thye-a-ben'da-zole)
Mintezol
Classifications: ANTI-INFECTIVE; ANTHELMINTIC
Prototype: Mebendazole
Pregnancy Category: C

T

AVAILABILITY 500 mg chewable tablets; 500 mg/5 mL suspension

ACTIONS Structurally related to mebendazole. Precise mechanism of action is not clear, however, it has a wide spectrum of anthelmintic activity. Inhibits helminth-specific enzyme fumarate reductase.

THERAPEUTIC EFFECTS Suppresses production of eggs or larvae by some parasites and may inhibit subsequent development of eggs or larvae passed in feces. Demonstrates anti-inflammatory, antipyretic, and analgesic effects.

USES Enterobiasis (pinworm infestation), ascariasis (roundworm), strongyloidiasis (threadworm), cutaneous larva migrans (creeping eruption), and hookworm infestations caused by *Ancyclostoma duodenale* or *Necator*

americanus. Used during invasive stage of trichinosis to relieve symptoms and for mixed helminthic infestations.

CONTRAINDICATIONS Safety during pregnancy (category C) or lactation is not established.

CAUTIOUS USE Liver or kidney dysfunction; when vomiting can be dangerous, severe dehydration or malnutrition; anemia; children weighing <15 kg.

ROUTE & DOSAGE

Enterobiasis, Ascariasis, Strongyloidiasis, Hookworm
Child: **PO** *14–70 kg,* 25 mg/kg b.i.d. times 2 days (max dose 3 g/day)
Adult: **PO** *<70 kg,* 25 mg/kg b.i.d. times 2 days; *>70 kg,* 1.5 g b.i.d. (max 3 g/day) times 2 days

STORAGE
Store in tight containers.

ADMINISTRATION
Oral
- Give after meals. Chewable tablets must be chewed thoroughly before swallowing.
- Shake suspension well before pouring.

ADVERSE EFFECTS CNS: Weariness, *dizziness,* drowsiness, headache. **CV:** Hypotension, bradycardia. **GI:** *Anorexia, nausea, vomiting,* epigastric distress, jaundice, cholestasis, parenchymal liver damage, diarrhea, perianal rash. **Urogenital:** Malodor of urine, crystalluria, hematuria, nephrotoxicity, enuresis. **Metabolic:** Transient rise in AST, transient leukopenia, hypersensitivity, hyperglycemia. **Skin:** Pruritus, rash, Stevens-Johnson syndrome.

PHARMACOKINETICS Absorption: Readily absorbed from GI tract. **Peak:** 1–2 h. **Metabolism:** Metabolized in liver. **Elimination:** >90% excreted in urine; 5% in feces.

NURSING IMPLICATIONS

Assessment & Drug Effects
- Provide supportive treatment prior to therapy if patient is anemic, dehydrated, or malnourished.
- Adverse effects generally occur 3–4 h after administration, are mild, and last for 2–8 h. Incidence tends to be related to dose and duration of treatment.
- Discontinued immediately with S&S of hypersensitivity: Fever, facial flush, chills, conjunctival infection, skin rashes, or erythema multiforme (including Stevens-Johnson syndrome), which can be fatal.

Patient & Family Education
- Chew tablet well before swallowing, shake suspension well before use.

- Do not drive or engage in potentially hazardous activities until response to drug is known. CNS adverse effects occur frequently.
- Do not breast feed while taking this drug without consulting physician.
- Store this medication out of reach of children.

THIAMINE HYDROCHLORIDE (VITAMIN B₁)

(thye′a-min)
Betalins, Bewon ♣, Biamine
Classification: VITAMIN B
Pregnancy Category: A

AVAILABILITY 50 mg, 100 mg, 250 mg tablets; 20 mg enteric-coated tablet; 100 mg/mL injection

ACTIONS Water-soluble B_1 vitamin and member of B-complex group used for thiamine replacement therapy.

THERAPEUTIC EFFECTS Functions as an essential coenzyme in carbohydrate metabolism. Also has role in conversion of tryptophan to nicotinamide. Effectiveness is evidenced by improvement of clinical manifestations of thiamine deficiency: Anorexia, gastric distress, depression, irritability, insomnia, palpitations, tachycardia, loss of memory, paresthesias, muscle weakness and pain, elevated blood pyruvic acid level (diagnostic test for thiamine deficiency), and elevated lactic acid level.

USES Treatment and prophylaxis of beriberi, to correct anorexia due to thiamine deficiency states, and in treatment of neuritis associated with pregnancy, pellagra, and alcoholism, including Wernicke-Korsakoff syndrome. Therapy generally includes other members of vitamin B complex, because thiamine deficiency rarely occurs alone. Severe deficiency is characterized by ophthalmoplegia, polyneuropathy, muscle wasting ("dry" beriberi), edema, serous effusions, and CHF ("wet" beriberi).

CONTRAINDICATIONS None.

ROUTE & DOSAGE

Thiamine Deficiency
Child: **IV/IM** 10–25 mg t.i.d.
Adult: **IV/IM** 50–100 mg t.i.d.

Beriberi
Child: **IV/IM** 10–25 mg/dose daily (if critical illness) *or* **PO** 10–50 mg every day for 2 wk then 5–10 mg/dose/day for 1 mo
Adult: **IV/IM** 5–30 mg t.i.d. for 2 wk, then **PO** 5–30 mg/day t.i.d. for 1 mo

Dietary Supplement
Infant: **PO** 0.3–0.5 mg/day
Child: **PO** 0.5–1 mg/day
Adult: **PO** 1–2 mg/day

T

STORAGE

Store at 15°–30° C (59°–86° F) in tightly closed, light resistant containers.

ADMINISTRATION

Oral

- Do not crush or chew enteric-coated tablets. These must be swallowed whole.
- Large oral dosages should be divided to increase absorption.

Intramuscular

- Give deep IM into a large muscle; may be painful. See Techniques of Administration section in Part I for safe IM site selection in children. Rotate sites and apply cold compresses to area if necessary for relief of discomfort.

Intravenous

Note: Intradermal test dose is recommended prior to administration in suspected thiamine sensitivity. Deaths have occurred following IV use.

PREPARE Direct: Give undiluted. **IV Infusion:** Diluted in 1000 mL of most IV solutions.

ADMINISTER Direct: Give at a rate of 100 mg over 5 min. **IV Infusion:** Give at the ordered rate.

INCOMPATIBILITIES Solution/Additive: Amobarbital, diazepam, erythromycin, furosemide, phenobarbital.

- Preserve in tight, light-resistant, nonmetallic containers. Thiamine is unstable in alkaline solutions (e.g., solutions of acetates, barbiturates, bicarbonates, carbonates, citrates) and neutral solutions.

ADVERSE EFFECTS Body as a Whole: Feeling of warmth, weakness, sweating, restlessness, tightness of throat, angioneurotic edema, <u>anaphylaxis</u>. **Respiratory:** Cyanosis, pulmonary edema. **CV:** <u>Cardiovascular collapse</u>, slight fall in BP following rapid IV administration. **GI:** GI hemorrhage, nausea. **Skin:** Urticaria, pruritus.

INTERACTIONS Drug: No clinically significant interactions established. **Food:** High carbohydrate intake increases thiamine requirement.

PHARMACOKINETICS Absorption: Limited absorption from GI tract. **Distribution:** Widely distributed, including into breast milk. **Elimination:** Excreted in urine.

NURSING IMPLICATIONS

Assessment & Drug Effects

- Record patient's dietary history carefully as an essential part of vitamin replacement therapy. Collaborate with physician, dietitian, patient, and responsible family member in developing a diet teaching plan that can be sustained by patient.
- Note: Body requirement of thiamine is directly proportional to carbohydrate intake and metabolic rate; requirement increases when diet consists predominantly of carbohydrates. Total absence of dietary thiamine produce deficiency state in about 3 wks.

Patient & Family Education

- Food–drug relationships: Learn about rich dietary sources of thiamine (e.g., yeast, pork, beef, liver, wheat and other whole grains, nutrient-added breakfast cereals, fresh vegetables, especially peas and dried beans).
- Store this medication out of reach of children.

THIOPENTAL SODIUM ⊕
(thye-oh-pen′tal)
Pentothal
Classifications: CENTRAL NERVOUS SYSTEM AGENT; GENERAL ANESTHETIC; SEDATIVE-HYPNOTIC; BARBITURATE
Pregnancy Category: C
Controlled Substance: Schedule III

AVAILABILITY 20 mg/mL, 25 mg/mL injection

ACTIONS Ultrashort-acting barbiturate; induces brief general anesthesia without analgesia by depression of CNS. Loss of consciousness is rapid. Reduction in cardiac output and peripheral vasodilation frequently accompany anesthesia. Rapid redistribution of agent out of brain reduces anesthesia level and increases reflex airway hyperactivity to mechanical stimulation. Muscle relaxation is slight, and reflexes are poorly controlled.
THERAPEUTIC EFFECTS Because analgesia is slight, thiopental is seldom used alone except for brief minor procedures. It does not act as an analgesic when given as an analgesic.

USES To induce hypnosis and anesthesia prior to or as supplement to other anesthetic agents or as sole agent for brief (15-min) operative procedures. Also used as an anticonvulsant and sedative-hypnotic and for narcoanalysis and narcosynthesis in psychiatric disorders.

CONTRAINDICATIONS Hypersensitivity to barbiturates; history of paradoxic excitation; absence of suitable veins for IV administration; status asthmaticus; acute intermittent or other hepatic porphyrias. Safety during pregnancy (category C), lactation, or children is not established.
CAUTIOUS USE Coronary artery disease, hypotension, shock; conditions that may potentiate or prolong hypnotic effect including excessive premedication, liver or kidney dysfunction, asthma, myxedema, Addison's disease, severe anemia, increased BUN; increased intracranial pressure; myasthenia gravis; asthma and other respiratory diseases.

ROUTE & DOSAGE

Induction of Anesthesia

Neonate: **IV** 3–4 mg/kg
Infant: **IV** 5–8 mg/kg
Child: **IV** 1–12 y, 5–6 mg/kg; >12 y, 3–5 mg/kg initially, followed by 1 mg/kg if needed
Adult: **IV Test Dose** 25–75 mg, then 50–75 mg at 20–40 sec intervals, an additional 50 mg may be given if needed

---

Convulsions

Child: **IV** 2–3 mg/kg/dose, repeat as needed
Adult: **IV** 75–125 mg/dose, repeat as needed

ICP

Child: **IV** 1.5–5 mg/kg/dose (given as intermittent infusion over 10–60 min); repeat as needed to lower intracranial pressure

Narcoanalysis

Adult: **IV** 100 mg/min until confusion occurs

STORAGE
Store at 15°–30° C (59°–86° F). Avoid excessive heat; protect from freezing.

ADMINISTRATION
Note: Verify correct IV concentration and rate of infusion to neonates, infants, children with physician.

Intravenous

Test dose: May be given to assess unusual sensitivity to drug. Following administration, observe patient for at least 1 min for unexpected deep anesthesia or respiratory depression.

PREPARE **Direct:** Reconstitute each 500 mg of powder by adding at least 20 mL of sterile water for injection to yield a 2.5% solution (25 mg/1 mL). Add 20 mL of reconstituted solution to at least 100 mL of NS or D5W. Prepare solution freshly and use promptly. If a precipitate is present, discard solution. Unused portions should be discarded within 24 h.

ADMINISTER **Direct:** Infuse each 25 mg over 1 min or more. Do not infuse solution with a concentration <2.5% (concentration <2% causes hemolysis). In children infuse over 10–60 min as an intermittent infusion (50 mg/mL maximum concentration).

INCOMPATIBILITIES **Solution/Additive:** DEXTROSE RINGER'S COMBINATIONS, **Ringer's lactate, 10% dextrose, amikacin, benzquinamide, cephapirin, chlorpromazine, codeine phosphate, dimenhydrinate, diphenhydramine, doxapram, ephedrine, fibrinolysin, glycopyrrolate, hydromorphone, insulin, levorphanol, meperidine, metaraminol, methadone, morphine, norepinephrine, penicillin G, prochlorperazine, promazine, promethazine, sodium bicarbonate, succinylcholine, tetracycline.** **Y-Site:** **Alfentanil, ascorbic acid, atracurium, atropine, cisatracurium, diltiazem, dobutamine, dopamine, ephedrine, epinephrine, furosemide, hydromorphone, labetalol, lidocaine, lorazepam, midazolam, morphine, nicardipine, norepinephrine, pancuronium, phenylephrine, succinylcholine, sufentanil, vecuronium.**

■ Consult physician if intra-arterial injection or extravasation occurs. The site will require particular attention to prevent arteritis, neuritis, and skin slough. An intra-arterial injection usually causes extreme pain before patient loses consciousness.

ADVERSE EFFECTS CNS: Headache, retrograde amnesia, emergence delirium, prolonged somnolence and recovery. **CV:** Myocardial depression, arrhythmias, circulatory depression. **GI:** Nausea, vomiting, regurgitation of gastric contents, rectal irritation, cramping, rectal bleeding, diarrhea. **Respiratory:** Respiratory depression with apnea; hiccups, sneezing, coughing, bronchospasm, laryngospasm. **Body as a Whole:** Hypersensitivity reactions, anaphylaxis (rare), hypothermia, thrombosis and sloughing (with extravasation); salivation, shivering, skeletal muscle hyperactivity.

DIAGNOSTIC TEST INTERFERENCE *Thiopental* may cause decrease in *I-123 and I-131 thyroidal uptake* test results.

INTERACTIONS Drug: CNS DEPRESSANTS potentiate CNS and respiratory depression. PHENOTHIAZINES increase risk of hypotension. **Probenecid** may prolong anesthesia. **Herbal: Kava-kava, valerian** may potentiate sedation.

PHARMACOKINETICS Onset: 30–60 sec. **Duration:** 10–30 min. **Distribution:** Distributed into muscle and liver; crosses placenta. **Metabolism:** Metabolized in liver. **Elimination:** Excreted in urine. **Half-Life:** 12 min.

NURSING IMPLICATIONS

Assessment & Drug Effects

- Monitor vital signs q3–5min before, during, and after anesthetic administration until recovery and into postoperative period, if necessary.
- Report increases in pulse rate or drop in blood pressure. Hypovolemia, cranial trauma, or premedication with opioids increases potential for apnea and symptoms of myocardial depression (decreased cardiac output and arterial pressure).
- Shivering, excitement, muscle twitching may develop during recovery period if patient is in pain.
- Assess for preexisting heart condition or asthma and notify physician.

Patient & Family Education

- Onset of drug effect is rapid, with loss of consciousness within 30–60 sec.

T

THIORIDAZINE HYDROCHLORIDE

(thye-or-rid′a-zeen)
Mellaril, Novoridazine ♣
Classifications: CENTRAL NERVOUS SYSTEM AGENT; PSYCHOTHERAPEUTIC; PHENOTHIAZINE ANTIPSYCHOTIC
Prototype: Chlorpromazine
Pregnancy Category: C

AVAILABILITY 10 mg, 15 mg, 25 mg, 50 mg, 100 mg, 150 mg, 200 mg tablets; 30 mg/mL, 100 mg/mL solution; 25 mg/5 mL suspension

ACTIONS Phenothiazine similar to chlorpromazine. Rarely produces extrapyramidal effects. Has weak antiemetic but strong anticholinergic and alpha-adrenergic agonist activity and potent sedative action.

THERAPEUTIC EFFECTS Effective in reducing excitement, hypermotility, abnormal initiative, affective tension, and agitation by inhibiting psychomotor functions. Also effective as an antipsychotic agent, and for behavioral disorders in children.

USES Psychotic disorder (used in treatment-resistant schizophrenia).

CONTRAINDICATIONS Hypersensitivity to phenothiazines. Severe CNS depression; CV disease; QTc prolongation syndrome (>450 msec); children <2 y. Safety during pregnancy (category C) or lactation is not established.
CAUTIOUS USE Premature ventricular contractions; previously diagnosed breast cancer; patients exposed to extremes in heat or to organophosphorus insecticides; respiratory disorders, seizure disorders.

ROUTE & DOSAGE

Psychotic Disorders
Child: **PO** >2 y, 0.5–3 mg/kg/day in divided doses; severe psychosis, may start at 25 mg t.i.d. (max dose 3 mg/kg/day)
Child >12 y/Adult: **PO** >12 y, 50–100 mg t.i.d., may increase up to 800 mg/day 2–4 times a day as needed or tolerated
Moderate to Marked Depression
Adult: **PO** 25 mg t.i.d., may increase up to 200 mg/day in divided doses

STORAGE
Store at 15°–30° C (59°–86° F) in tightly covered, light-resistant containers unless otherwise indicated.

ADMINISTRATION
Oral
- Give with fluid of patient's choice; tablet may be crushed.
- Schedule phenothiazine at least 1 h before or 1 h after an antacid or antidiarrheal medication.
- Dilute liquid concentrate just prior to administration with ½ glass of fruit juice, milk, water, carbonated beverage, or soup. Do not mix with enteric formulas.
- Add increases in dose to the first dose of the day to prevent sleep disturbance.

ADVERSE EFFECTS CNS: *Sedation,* dizziness, drowsiness, lethargy, extrapyramidal syndrome, nocturnal confusion, hyperactivity. **Special Senses:** Nasal congestion, blurred vision, pigmentary retinopathy. **GI:** Xerostomia, *constipation,* paralytic ileus. **Urogenital:** Amenorrhea, breast engorgement, gynecomastia, galactorrhea, *urinary retention.* **CV:** Ventricular dysrhythmias, hypotension, prolonged QTc interval.

INTERACTIONS Drug: Alcohol, ANXIOLYTICS, SEDATIVE-HYPNOTICS, other CNS DEPRESSANTS add to CNS depression; additive adverse effects with other PHENOTHIAZINES; **amiodarone, amoxapine, arsenic trioxide, astemizole, bepridil, cisapride, clarithromycin, daunorubicin, diltiazem, disopyramide, dofetilide, dolasetron, doxorubicin, encainide, erythromycin, flecainide, fluoxetine, fluvoxamine, gatifloxacin, grepafloxacin, haloperidol, ibutilide, indapamide, local anesthetics,**

maprotiline, moxifloxacin, octreotide, paroxetine, pentamidine, pimozide, procainamide, pindolol, propranolol, probucol, quinidine, risperidone, sotalol, sertraline, sparfloxacin, terfenadine, terodiline, tocainide, tricyclic antidepressants, venlafaxine, verapamil, ziprasidone can prolong QTc interval resulting in arrhythmias. **Herbal: Kava-kava** may increase risk and severity of dystonic reactions. **Food:** Use with enteric formulas, may cause liquid thioridazine preparations to precipitate.

PHARMACOKINETICS Absorption: Well absorbed from GI tract. **Onset:** Days to weeks. **Distribution:** Crosses placenta; distributed into breast milk. **Metabolism:** Metabolized in liver. **Elimination:** Excreted in urine. **Half-Life:** 26–36 h.

NURSING IMPLICATIONS

Assessment & Drug Effects

- Orthostatic hypotension may occur in early therapy. Female patients appear to be more susceptible than males.
- Be aware that patients may be unable to adjust to extremes of temperature because drug effects heat regulatory center in the hypothalamus. Patient may complain of being cold even at average room temperature.
- Monitor I&O ratio and bowel elimination pattern. Check for abdominal distention and pain. Encourage adequate fluid intake as prophylaxis for constipation and xerostomia. The depressed patient may not seek help for either symptom or for urinary retention.
- Lab tests: Obtain periodic CBC and liver function tests during therapy.
- Supervise patient closely during early course of therapy. Suicide is an inherent risk with any depressed patient (monitor adolescents carefully) and may remain a problem until there is significant clinical improvement.

Patient & Family Education

- Exercise care not to spill drug on skin because of danger of contact dermatitis. Wash skin well in soap and water if liquid drug is spilled.
- Take drug as prescribed and do not alter dosing regimen or stop medication without consulting physician.
- Avoid alcohol during phenothiazine therapy. Concomitant use enhances CNS depression effects.
- Be aware that marked drowsiness generally subsides with continued therapy or reduction in dosage.
- Do not drive or engage in potentially hazardous activities until response to drug is known.
- Make position changes slowly, particularly from lying down to upright posture; dangle legs a few minutes before standing.
- Vasodilation produced by hot showers or baths or by long exposure to environmental heat may accentuate hypotensive effect.
- Do not apply heating pad or hot water bottles to the body for external heat. Because of depressed conditioned avoidance behaviors, a severe burn may result.
- Report the onset of any change in visual acuity, brownish coloring of vision, or impairment of night vision to prescriber. Symptoms suggest pigmentary retinopathy (observed primarily in patients receiving extremely high doses). An ophthalmic consultation may be indicated.

T

- Note: Thioridazine may color urine pink-red to reddish brown.
- Do not use any OTC medications while on this drug unless approved by prescriber.
- Do not breast feed while taking this drug without consulting prescriber.
- Inform parents or guardians to carefully monitor for suicide thought or behavior.
- Store this medication out of reach of children.

THROMBIN
(throm'bin)
Thrombinar, Thrombostat
Classifications: BLOOD FORMERS, COAGULATORS, AND ANTICOAGULANTS; HEMOSTATIC
Prototype: Aminocaproic acid
Pregnancy Category: C

AVAILABILITY 1,000 unit, 5,000 unit, 10,000 unit, 20,000 unit, 50,000 unit vials

ACTIONS Sterile plasma protein prepared from prothrombin of bovine origin. Induces clotting of whole blood or fibrinogen solution without addition of other substances.
THERAPEUTIC EFFECTS Facilitates conversion of fibrinogen to fibrin, resulting in clotting of whole blood.

USES When oozing of blood from capillaries and small venules is accessible, as in dental extraction, plastic surgery, grafting procedures, and epistaxis; also to shorten bleeding time at puncture sites in heparinized patient (i.e., following hemodialysis).

CONTRAINDICATIONS Known hypersensitivity to any of drug components or to material of bovine origin; parenteral use; entry or infiltration into large blood vessels.
CAUTIOUS USE Pregnancy (category C).

T **ROUTE & DOSAGE**

Oozing Blood
Child/Adult: **Topical** 100–2000 NIH units/mL, depending on extent of bleeding, may be used as solution, in dry form, by mixing thrombin with blood plasma to form a fibrin "glue," or in conjunction with absorbable gelatin sponge

STORAGE
Store lyophilized preparation at 2°–8° C (36°–46° F).

ADMINISTRATION
Topical
- Ensure that sponge recipient area is free of blood before applying thrombin.

- Prepare solutions in sterile distilled water or isotonic saline.
- Use solutions within a few hours of preparation. If several hours are to elapse between time of preparation and use, solution should be refrigerated, or preferably frozen, and used within 48 h.
- Never inject as can result in intravascular clotting.

ADVERSE EFFECTS Body as a Whole: Sensitivity, allergic and febrile reactions, <u>intravascular clotting and death when thrombin is allowed to enter large blood vessels.</u>

INTERACTIONS Drug: No clinically significant interactions established.

PHARMACOKINETICS Not applicable.

THYROID
(thye′roid)
Armour Thyroid, Thyrar
Classifications: HORMONE AND SYNTHETIC SUBSTITUTE; THYROID AGENT
Prototype: Levothyroxine sodium
Pregnancy Category: A

AVAILABILITY 15 mg (¼ grain), 30 mg (½ grain), 60 mg (1 grain), 90 mg (1 ½ grain), 120 mg (2 grain), 180 mg (3 grain), 240 mg (4 grain), 300 mg (5 grain) tablets

ACTIONS Preparation of desiccated animal thyroid gland containing active thyroid hormones, l-thyroxine (T_4) and l-triiodothyronine (T_3). Action mechanism unknown; T_4 is largely converted to T_3, which exerts the principal effects.

THERAPEUTIC EFFECTS Influences growth and maturation of various tissues (including skeletal and CNS) at critical periods. Promotes a generalized increase in metabolic rate of body tissues. Indicated by diuresis, accompanied by loss of weight and puffiness, followed by sense of well-being, increased pulse rate, increased pulse pressure, increased appetite, increased psychomotor activity, loss of constipation, normalization of skin texture and hair, and increased T_3 and T_4 serum levels.

USES Replacement or substitution therapy in primary hypothyroidism (cretinism, myxedema, simple goiter, deficiency states in pregnancy) and secondary hypothyroidism caused by surgery, excess radiation, or antithyroid drug therapy. May be given as adjunct to antithyroid agents when it is desirable to limit release of thyrotropic hormones and to prevent goitrogenesis and hypothyroidism.

CONTRAINDICATIONS Thyrotoxicosis; acute MI uncomplicated by hypothyroidism, cardiovascular disease; morphologic hypogonadism; nephrosis; uncorrected hypoadrenalism.

CAUTIOUS USE Angina pectoris, hypertension, renal insufficiency; concomitant administration of catecholamines; diabetes mellitus; hyperthyroidism (history of); malabsorption states; pregnancy (category A), lactation.

T

ROUTE & DOSAGE

Mild to Moderate Hypothyroidism

Child: 0–6 mo, 4.8–6 mg/kg/day *or* 15–30 mg/day; 6–12 mo, 3.6–4.8 mg/kg/day *or* 30–45 mg/day; 1–5 y, 3–3.6 mg/kg/day *or* 45 to 60 mg/day; 6–12 y, 2.4–3 mg/kg/day *or* 60–90 mg/day; >12 y, 1.2–1.8 mg/kg/day *or* >90 mg/day
Adult: **PO** 60 mg/day, may increase q30days to 60–180 mg/day

Severe Hypothyroidism

Child: **PO** 15 mg/day, may increase by 15 mg q2wk if needed
Adult: **PO** 15 mg/day, increased q2wk to 60 mg/day, then may increase q30day if needed

STORAGE

Store at 15°–30° C (59°–86° F) in tightly closed, light-resistant containers.

ADMINISTRATION

Oral

- Give as a single dose, preferably on an empty stomach.
- Initiate dosage generally at low level and systematically increase in small increments to desired maintenance dose.
- Store in dark bottle to minimize spontaneous deiodination. Keep desiccated thyroid dry.

ADVERSE EFFECTS Endocrine: Hyperthyroidism, <u>thyroid storm</u>: High temperature (as high as 41° C [106° F]), tachycardia, vomiting, <u>shock, coma</u>. **Special Senses:** Staring expression in eyes. **CV:** CHF, angina, <u>cardiac arrhythmias</u>, palpitation, tachycardia. **Body as a Whole:** Weight loss, tremors, headache, nervousness, fever, insomnia, warm and moist skin, heat intolerance, leg cramps, menstrual irregularities, <u>shock</u>, changes in appetite. **GI:** Diarrhea or abdominal cramps. **Metabolic:** Hyperglycemia (usually offset by increased tissue oxidation of sugar).

DIAGNOSTIC TEST INTERFERENCE Thyroid increases *basal metabolic rate;* may increase *blood glucose levels, creatine phosphokinase, AST, LDH, PBI.* It may decrease *serum uric acid, cholesterol, thyroid-stimulating hormone (TSH), I-131* uptake. Many medications may produce false results in *thyroid function tests.*

INTERACTIONS Drug: ORAL ANTICOAGULANTS potentiate hypoprothrombinemia; may increase requirements for **insulin,** SULFONYLUREAS; **epinephrine** may precipitate coronary insufficiency; **cholestyramine** may decrease thyroid absorption.

PHARMACOKINETICS Absorption: Variably absorbed from GI tract. **Peak:** 1–3 wk. **Distribution:** Does not readily cross placenta; minimal amounts in breast milk. **Metabolism:** Deiodination in thyroid gland. **Elimination:** Excreted in urine and feces. **Half-Life:** T_3, 1–2 days; T_4, 6–7 days.

NURSING IMPLICATIONS

Assessment & Drug Effects

- Observe patient carefully during initial treatment for untoward reactions such as angina, palpitations, cardiac pain.
- Be alert for symptoms of overdosage (see ADVERSE EFFECTS) that may occur 1–3 wk after therapy is started. If they develop, interrupt treatment for several days and restart with reduced dosage.
- Monitor response until regimen is stabilized to prevent iatrogenic hyperthyroidism. In drug-induced hyperthyroidism, there may also be increased bone loss. Such a patient is vulnerable to pathologic fractures.
- Monitor vital signs: Pulse rate is an important clue to drug effectiveness. Assess pulse before each dose during period of dosage adjustment. Consult physician if rate is 100 or more or change in rate related range for childs age or if there has been a marked change in rate or rhythm.
- Lab tests: Monitor thyroid function q3mo during dose adjustment period. Monitor prothrombin time closely if patient is receiving concurrent anticoagulant therapy. A decrease in requirement usually develops within 1–4 wk after starting treatment with thyroid.
- Be aware that toxic effects of thyroid develop slowly and disappear gradually. T_4 effects require up to 3–6 wk to dissipate; T_3 effects last 6–14 days after drug withdrawal.
- Use serial height and weight measurement to monitor growth in juvenile undergoing treatment.

Patient & Family Education

- Adhere to established dosage regimen; do not change dose intervals without approval of the prescriber.
- Be aware that replacement therapy for hypothyroidism is lifelong; continued follow-up care is important.
- Do not change brands of thyroid unless prescriber approves. Hormone content varies among brands.
- Monitor pulse rate and report increases greater than parameter set by prescriber.
- Report onset of chest pain or other signs of aggravated CV disease (dyspnea, tachycardia) to physician promptly.
- Report evidence of any unexplained bleeding to physician when taking concomitant anticoagulant.
- Do not breast feed while taking this drug without consulting physician.
- Store this medication out of reach of children.

TIAGABINE HYDROCHLORIDE

(ti-a′ga-been)

Gabitril Filmtabs

Classifications: CENTRAL NERVOUS SYSTEM AGENT; ANTICONVULSANT; GABA INHIBITOR

Prototype: Valproic acid sodium (sodium valproate)

Pregnancy Category: C

AVAILABILITY 2 mg, 4 mg, 12 mg, 16 mg, 20 mg tablets

ACTIONS GABA inhibitor for the treatment of partial epilepsy. Potent and selective inhibitor of GABA uptake into presynaptic neurons; allows more GABA to bind to the surfaces of postsynaptic neurons in the CNS.
THERAPEUTIC EFFECTS Effectiveness indicated by reduction in seizure activity.

USES Adjunctive therapy for partial seizures.

CONTRAINDICATIONS Hypersensitivity to tiagabine; pregnancy (category C).
CAUTIOUS USE Liver function impairment; lactation; history of spike and wave discharge on EEG; status epilepticus.

ROUTE & DOSAGE

Seizures
Adolescent: **PO** *12–18 y,* start with 4 mg every day for 1 wk, then may increase dose by 4–8 mg/day every week (max 32 mg/day) in 2–4 divided doses
Adult: **PO** Start with 4 mg every day, may increase dose by 4–8 mg/day every week (max 56 mg/day) in 2–4 divided doses

STORAGE
Store at 15°–30° C (59°–86° F) in a tightly closed container; protect from light.

ADMINISTRATION
Oral
- Give with food to prevent the rapid absorption and possible increase in CNS side effects. When given on empty stomach, rapid absorption occurs, which can cause rapid elevation of plasma levels of tiagabine.
- Make dosage increases, when needed, at weekly intervals.

ADVERSE EFFECTS Body as a Whole: Infection, flu-like syndrome, pain, myasthenia, allergic reactions, chills, malaise, arthralgia. **CNS:** *Dizziness, asthenia, tremor, somnolence, nervousness,* difficulty concentrating, ataxia, depression, insomnia, abnormal gait, hostility, confusion, speech disorder, difficulty with memory, paresthesias, emotional lability, agitation, dysarthria, euphoria, hallucinations, <u>hyperkinesia, hypertonia,</u> hypotonia, myoclonus, twitching, vertigo. **CV:** Vasodilation, hypertension, palpitations, <u>tachycardia,</u> syncope, edema, peripheral edema. **GI:** Abdominal pain, diarrhea, nausea, vomiting, increased appetite, mouth ulcers. **Respiratory:** Pharyngitis, cough, bronchitis, dyspnea, epistaxis, pneumonia. **Skin:** Rash, pruritus, alopecia, dry skin, sweating, ecchymoses. **Special Senses:** Amblyopia, nystagmus, tinnitus. **Urogenital:** Dysmenorrhea, dysuria, metrorrhagia, incontinence, vaginitis, UTI.

INTERACTIONS Drug: Carbamazepine, phenytoin, phenobarbital decrease levels of tiagabine. Valproic acid levels may be decreased when used with tiagabine. **Herbal: Ginkgo** may decrease anticonvulsant effectiveness.

PHARMACOKINETICS Absorption: Rapidly absorbed; 90% bioavailability. **Peak:** 45 min. **Distribution:** 96% protein bound. **Metabolism:** Metabolized in liver, probably by cytochrome P-450 3A isoform. **Elimination:** 25% excreted in urine, 63% excreted in feces. **Half-Life:** 7–9 h (4–7 h with other enzyme-inducing drugs).

NURSING IMPLICATIONS

Assessment & Drug Effects

- Lab tests: Measure plasma levels of tiagabine before and after changes are made in the drug regimen.
- Be aware that concurrent use of other anticonvulsants may decrease effectiveness of tiagabine or increase the potential for adverse effects.
- Monitor carefully for S&S of CNS depression.

Patient & Family Education

- Do not stop taking drug abruptly; may cause sudden onset of seizures.
- Exercise caution while engaging in potentially hazardous activities (biking, skateboarding, driving, sports, etc.) because drug may cause dizziness.
- Use caution when taking other prescription or OTC drugs that can cause drowsiness.
- Record and track any seizure activity and inform physician if seizure activity increases.
- Report any of the following to the physician: Rash or hives; red, peeling skin; dizziness; drowsiness; depression; GI distress; nervousness or tremors; difficulty concentrating or talking.
- Do not breast feed while taking this drug without consulting physician.
- Store this medication out of reach of children.

TICARCILLIN DISODIUM

(ti-car-sill′in)
Ticar
Classifications: ANTI-INFECTIVE; ANTIBIOTIC; ANTIPSEUDOMONAL PENICILLIN
Prototype: Mezlocillin
Pregnancy Category: C

AVAILABILITY 1 g, 3 g, 6 g injection

ACTIONS Semisynthetic injectable penicillin that is bactericidal against gram-positive and gram-negative organisms.
THERAPEUTIC EFFECTS Susceptible organisms include *Pseudomonas aeruginosa, Escherichia coli, Proteus mirabilis, Proteus vulgaris, Enterobacter species, Haemophilus influenzae, Staphylococcus pneumoniae.*

USES Primarily for gram-negative bacterial infections, bacterial septicemia, skin and soft-tissue infections, acute and chronic respiratory infections, genitourinary tract infection by susceptible organisms, intraabdominal infections and infections of the female pelvis and reproductive system.

CONTRAINDICATIONS History of allergic reaction to any penicillin.
CAUTIOUS USE Allergy to cephalosporins; pregnancy (category C), lactation; renal or hepatic impairment.

ROUTE & DOSAGE

Urinary Tract Infections

Child: **IM/IV** 50–200 mg/kg/day in 4 divided doses
Adult: **IM/IV** 200 mg/kg/day in 4 divided doses or 1–2 g q6h

Systemic Infections

Neonate: **IV** ≤7 days, ≤2 kg, 150 mg/kg/day in equally divided doses q12h; ≥2 kg, 225 mg/kg/day in equally divided doses q8h; >7 days, <1.2 kg, 150 mg/kg/day in equally divided doses q12h; 1.2–2 kg, 225 mg/kg/day in equally divided doses q8h; >2 kg, 300 mg/kg/day in equally divided doses q6–8h
Infant/Child: **IM** 100–300 mg/kg/day in 4–6 divided doses (max 24 g/day)
Adult: **IM** 1–4 g/day in 6 divided doses (max 24 g/day)

Cystic Fibrosis

Child: **IM/IV** 300–400 mg/kg/day in 4–6 equally divided (max 24 g/day)
Reduced dosages required with renal impairment.

STORAGE

Do not use solutions refrigerated longer than 72 h for multidose purposes. Store dry powder at 15°–30° C (59°–86° F) or colder.

ADMINISTRATION

Intramuscular

- Do not exceed 2 g/per injection.
- Reconstitute each 1 g of ticarcillin with 2 mL of sterile water for injection or NS injection and use promptly. May also reconstitute with lidocaine hydrochloride injection (1%) without epinephrine to decrease the pain of the injection. Resulting concentration is 1 g/2.6 mL. In children IM site usually only used for urinary tract infections. Injection should be given deep into mucle mass. See Techniques of Administration section in Part I for safe IM site selection in children.

Intravenous

Note: Verify correct IV concentration and rate of infusion for administration to neonates, infants, children with physician.
PREPARE **Direct:** Reconstitute each 1 g of ticarcillin with 4 mL of sterile water for injection. Further dilute with at least 20 mL of D5W, NS, or other compatible IV solution. **Intermittent:** May dilute further in 50–100 mL of additional compatible IV solution.
ADMINISTER **Direct:** Give slowly at a rate of 1 g over 5 min or longer. In children, give over 10–20 min. **Intermittent:** Give 1 g over 30–120 min, maximum concentration is 100 mg/mL.
INCOMPATIBILITIES **Solution/Additive:** AMINOGLYCOSIDES, **amphotericin B, bleomycin, chloramphenicol, cytarabine, doxapram,**

lincomycin, TETRACYCLINES, **vitamin B complex with C. Y-Site:** AMINOGLYCOSIDES, **amphotericin B cholesteryl complex, fluconazole, promethazine, vancomycin.**

ADVERSE EFFECTS Body as a Whole: <u>Hypersensitivity reactions</u>, pain, burning, swelling at injection site; phlebitis, thrombophlebitis; <u>superinfections</u>. **CNS:** Headache, blurred vision, mental deterioration, convulsions, hallucinations, giddiness, neuromuscular hyperirritability. **GI:** *Diarrhea, nausea,* vomiting, disturbances of taste or smell, stomatitis, flatulence. **Hematologic:** Eosinophilia, thrombocytopenia, leukopenia, <u>neutropenia, hemolytic anemia</u>. **Metabolic** Hypernatremia, transient increases in serum AST, ALT, BUN, and alkaline phosphatase; increases in serum LDH, bilirubin, and creatinine and decreased serum uric acid.

PHARMACOKINETICS Peak: 1–2 h IM. **Distribution:** Low concentrations in CSF unless meninges are inflamed; crosses placenta; distributed into breast milk. **Elimination:** 80–90% excreted unchanged in urine within 24 h. **Half-Life:** 67 min.

NURSING IMPLICATIONS

Assessment & Drug Effects

- Obtain baseline C&S tests before initiating therapy; drug may be started pending results.
- Be aware that serious and sometimes fatal anaphylactoid reactions have been reported in patients with penicillin hypersensitivity or history of sensitivity to multiple allergens.
- Assess IV access site frequently for vein irritation and phlebitis.
- Discontinue ticarcillin if bleeding manifestations occur. (Some patients on high doses may develop hemorrhagic manifestations associated with abnormalities of coagulation.)
- Lab tests: Monitor kidney and liver functions, CBC, platelet counts, and serum electrolytes during prolonged treatment.
- Monitor cardiac status because of the high sodium content in drug. (Contains 6 mEq sodium per 1 g of drug, about 400 mg.)
- Monitor for and report hypokalemia (see Appendix D-1).

Patient & Family Education

- Report urticaria, rashes, or pruritus to physician immediately.
- Report frequent loose stools, diarrhea, or other possible signs of pseudomembranous colitis (see Appendix D-1) to physician.
- Do not breast feed while taking this drug without consulting physician.

TICARCILLIN DISODIUM/CLAVULANATE POTASSIUM

(tye-kar-sill'in/clav-yoo'la-nate)
Timentin
Classifications: ANTI-INFECTIVE; ANTIBIOTIC; ANTIPSEUDOMONAL PENICILLIN
Prototype: Mezlocillin
Pregnancy Category: B

TICARCILLIN DISODIUM/CLAVULANATE POTASSIUM

AVAILABILITY 3.1 g injection

ACTIONS Injectable extended-spectrum penicillin and fixed combination of ticarcillin disodium with the potassium salt of clavulanic acid, a beta-lactamase inhibitor produced by fermentation of *Streptomyces clavuligerus*. Used alone, clavulanic acid antibacterial activity is weak but in combination with ticarcillin prevents degradation by beta-lactamase and extends ticarcillin spectrum of activity against many strains of beta-lactamase-producing bacteria (synergistic effect). Synergism between the two drugs does not occur against organisms susceptible to ticarcillin alone.

THERAPEUTIC EFFECTS Susceptible strains of organisms include beta-lactamase strains of *Klebsiella* sp., *Escherichia coli, Staphylococcus aureus, Pseudomonas aeruginosa, Haemophilus influenzae, Citrobacter* sp., *Enterobacter cloacae, Serratia marcescens.*

USES Infections of lower respiratory tract and urinary tract and skin and skin structures, infections of bone and joint, and septicemia caused by susceptible organisms. Also mixed infections and as presumptive therapy before identification of causative organism.

CONTRAINDICATIONS Hypersensitivity to penicillins or to cephalosporins, clavulanate. Safety during pregnancy (category B) is not established.
CAUTIOUS USE Lactation; renal impairment.

ROUTE & DOSAGE

Moderate to Severe Infections

Term Neonate/Infant: **IV** *<3 mo*, 200–300 mg/kg/day divided q6–8h (based on ticarcillin)
Infant/Child: **IV** *>3 mo*, 200–300 mg/kg/day divided q4–6h (based on ticarcillin) (max dose 18–24 g/day)
Adult: **IV** *>60 kg*, 3.1 g q4–6h (max dose 18–24 g/day)
Reduced dosages required with renal impairment.

STORAGE
Store vial with sterile powder at 21°–24° C (69°–75° F) or colder. If exposed to higher temperature, powder will darken, indicating degradation of clavulanate potassium and loss of potency. Discard vial. See package insert for information about storage and stability of reconstituted and diluted IV solutions of drug.

ADMINISTRATION
Intravenous

Note: Verify correct IV concentration and rate of infusion for administration to infants and children with physician.
PREPARE **Intermittent:** Reconstitute by adding to 3.1 g of powder 13 mL sterile water for injection or NS injection to yield 200 mg/mL ticarcillin with 6.7 mg/mL clavulanic acid. Shake until dissolved. Further dilute with NS, D5W, or RL. Do not use if discoloration or particulate matter is present.

ADMINISTER **Intermittent:** Give over 30 min, maximum concentration is 100 mg/mL.

INCOMPATIBILITIES **Solution/Additive:** AMINOGLYCOSIDES, **doxapram.** **Y-Site:** AMINOGLYCOSIDES, **amphotericin B cholesteryl complex, vancomycin.**

ADVERSE EFFECTS Body as a Whole: <u>Hypersensitivity reactions</u>, pain, burning, swelling at injection site; phlebitis, thrombophlebitis; superinfections. **CNS:** Headache, blurred vision, mental deterioration, convulsions, hallucinations, giddiness, neuromuscular hyperirritability. **GI:** *Diarrhea, nausea,* vomiting, disturbances of taste or smell, stomatitis, flatulence. **Hematologic:** Eosinophilia, <u>thrombocytopenia</u>, leukopenia, <u>neutropenia, hemolytic anemia</u>. **Metabolic** Hypernatremia, transient increases in serum AST, ALT, BUN, and alkaline phosphatase; increases in serum LDH, bilirubin, and creatinine and decreased serum uric acid.

DIAGNOSTIC TEST INTERFERENCE May interfere with test methods used to determine ***urinary proteins*** except for tests for urinary protein that use ***bromphenol blue. Positive direct antiglobulin (Coombs') test*** results, apparently caused by clavulanic acid, have been reported. This test may interfere with ***transfusion cross-matching procedures.***

INTERACTIONS Drugs: May increase risk of bleeding with ANTICOAGU-LANTS; **probenecid** decreases elimination of ticarcillin.

PHARMACOKINETICS Distribution: Widely distributed with highest concentrations in urine and bile; crosses placenta; distributed into breast milk. **Metabolism:** Slightly metabolized in liver. **Elimination:** Excreted in urine. **Half-Life:** Ticarcillin, 1.1–1.2 h; clavulanate, 1.1–1.5 h.

NURSING IMPLICATIONS

Assessment & Drug Effects

- Lab tests: Obtain baseline C&S tests before initiating therapy; drug may be started pending results. Monitor kidney and liver functions, CBC, platelet count, and serum electrolytes during prolonged treatment.
- Be aware that serious and sometimes fatal anaphylactoid reactions have been reported in patient with penicillin hypersensitivity or history of sensitivity to multiple allergens. Reported incidence is low with this combination drug.
- Separate ticarcillin administration by 30–60 min from administration of an aminoglycoside.
- Monitor cardiac status because of high sodium content of drug. (Contains about 400 mg sodium per 1 g drug.)
- Overdose symptoms: This drug may cause neuromuscular hyperirritability or seizures.

Patient & Family Education

- Report urticaria, rashes, or pruritus to physician immediately.
- Report frequent loose stools, diarrhea, or other possible signs of pseudomembranous colitis (see Appendix D-1) to physician.
- Do not breast feed while taking this drug without consulting physician.

TOBRAMYCIN SULFATE
(toe-bra-mye'sin)
Nebcin, Tobrex, TOBI, Tomycine
Classifications: ANTI-INFECTIVE; AMINOGLYCOSIDE ANTIBIOTIC
Prototype: Gentamicin sulfate
Pregnancy Category: D

AVAILABILITY 10 mg/mL, 40 mg/mL injection; 300 mg/5 mL inhalation solution; 0.3% ophthalmic solution; 3 mg/g ophthalmic ointment

ACTIONS Broad-spectrum, aminoglycoside antibiotic derived from *Streptomyces tenebrarius*. Closely related to gentamicin in spectrum of antibacterial activity and pharmacologic properties. Reportedly causes less nephrotoxicity than gentamicin, but incidence of ototoxicity is similar. Cross-allergenicity and some cross-resistance among aminoglycosides have been demonstrated.

THERAPEUTIC EFFECTS Exhibits greater antibiotic activity against *Pseudomonas aeruginosa* than other aminoglycosides.

USE Treatment of severe infections caused by susceptible organisms.

CONTRAINDICATIONS History of hypersensitivity to tobramycin and other aminoglycoside antibiotics. Safety during pregnancy (category D) or lactation is not established.

CAUTIOUS USE Impaired kidney function; premature and neonatal infants; neuromuscular disorders, concurrent use with other neurotoxic or nephrotoxic agents or potent diuretics.

ROUTE & DOSAGE

Moderate to Severe Infections

Neonate: **IM/IV** ≤7 days, 1200–2000 g, 2.5 mg/kg/dose q12h; >2000 g, 2.5 mg/kg/dose q12h; >7 days, 1200–2000 g, 2.5 mg/kg/dose q8–12h; >2000 g, 2.5 mg/kg/dose q8h
Child: **IM/IV** <5 y, 2.5 mg/kg/dose q8h **IV** ≥5 y, 3 mg/kg/day divided q8h up to 5 mg/kg/day infused over 20–60 min **IM** ≥5 y, 2.5 mg/kg/dose q8h up to 5 mg/kg/day **Topical** 1–2 drops in affected eye q4h or 0.5 inch ribbon of ointment b.i.d. or t.i.d.
Adult: **IV** 3 mg/kg/day divided q8h up to 5 mg/kg/day infused over 20–60 min **IM** 3 mg/kg/day divided q8h up to 5 mg/kg/day; alternatively, 5–7 mg/kg/dose is used as part of an extended interval regimen using the Hartford nomogram for dosing frequency **Topical** 1–2 drops in affected eye q1–4h

Cystic Fibrosis

Child ≥5 y/Adult: **IM/IV** 2.5–3.5 mg/kg/dose q6–8h **Nebulized** ≥6 y, 300 mg inhaled b.i.d. times 28 days, may repeat after 28-day drug-free period

Common adverse effects in *italic;* life-threatening effects <u>underlined;</u> generic names in **bold;** drug classifications in SMALL CAPS; ♣ Canadian drug name; ☻ Prototype drug.

STORAGE

Store at 15°–30° C (59°–86° F) prior to reconstitution. After reconstitution, solution may be refrigerated and used within 96 h. If kept at room temperature, use within 24 h.

ADMINISTRATION

Note: All doses based on ideal body weight.

Ophthalmic Instillation

- Wash hands before and after instillation of eye medication. Apply gentle finger pressure to lacrimal sac (under inside of eyelid) for 1 min after drug has been instilled in eye. Do not touch dropper tip to lashes or eye.

Intramuscular

- Give deep IM into a large muscle mass. See Part I for safe IM site selection in children. Rotate injection sites.

Intravenous

Note: Verify correct IV concentration and rate of infusion to neonates, infants, or children with physician.

PREPARE **Intermittent:** Dilute each dose in 50–100 mL or more of D5W, NS or D5/NS. Final concentration should not exceed 10 mg/mL.

ADMINISTER **Intermittent:** Infuse diluted solution over 20–60 min in adults and 30–60 min in children. If giving penicillins or cephalosporins with this drug, seperate doses by 1 h from tobramycin.

INCOMPATIBILITIES **Solution/Additive: Alcohol 5% in dextrose,** CEPHALOSPORINS, PENICILLINS, **clindamycin, heparin. Y-Site: Allopurinol, amphotericin B cholesteryl complex,** CEPHALOSPORINS, **clindamycin, penicillins, heparin hetastarch, indomethacin, propofol, sargramostim.**

ADVERSE EFFECTS CNS: <u>Neurotoxicity</u> (including ototoxicity), *nephrotoxicity,* increased AST, ALT, LDH, serum bilirubin; anemia, fever, rash, pruritus, urticaria, nausea, vomiting, headache, lethargy, <u>superinfections; hypersensitivity.</u> **Special Senses:** *Burning, stinging of eye after drug instillation;* lid itching and edema.

INTERACTIONS Drug: ANESTHETICS, SKELETAL MUSCLE RELAXANTS add to neuromuscular blocking effects; **acyclovir, amphotericin B, bacitracin, capreomycin,** CEPHALOSPORINS, **colistin, cisplatin, carboplatin, methoxyflurane, polymyxin B, vancomycin, furosemide, ethacrynic acid** increase risk of ototoxicity, nephrotoxicity.

PHARMACOKINETICS Peak: 30–90 min IM. **Duration:** Up to 8 h. **Distribution:** Crosses placenta; accumulates in renal cortex. **Elimination:** Excreted in urine. **Half-Life:** Child, 1–1.5 h; adult, 2–3 h. **Peak level:** 4–12 mcg/mL. **Trough level:** 0.5–2 mcg/mL.

NURSING IMPLICATIONS

Assessment & Drug Effects

- Weigh patient before treatment for calculation of dosage.
- Obtain bacterial C&S tests prior to and during therapy.

- Observe patient receiving tobramycin closely because of the high potential for toxicity, even in conventional doses.
- Lab tests: Baseline and periodic kidney function; monitor serum drug concentrations to minimize rise of toxicity. Draw peak level 30 min after end of infusion and trough level just before beginning the infusion. These are usually done after 3rd dose, except in neonates or others with kidney immaturity or impairment. Prolonged peak serum concentrations >10 mcg/mL or trough concentrations >2 mcg/mL are not recommended.
- Monitor auditory, and vestibular functions closely, particularly in patients with known or suspected renal impairment and patients receiving high doses.
- Be aware that drug-induced auditory changes are irreversible (partial or total); usually bilateral. In cochlear damage, patient may be asymptomatic, and partial or bilateral deafness may continue to develop even after therapy discontinued.
- Evidence of renal insufficiency, ototoxicity (see Appendix D-1), or vestibular damage indicates need for dosage adjustment or withdrawal of drug.
- Monitor I&O. Report oliguria, changes in I&O ratio, and cloudy or frothy urine (may indicate proteinuria). Keep patient well hydrated to prevent chemical irritation in renal tubules; in those susceptible to renal toxicity.
- Monitor patient with neuromuscular disorder (e.g., myasthenia gravis) for muscular weakness. Observe ambulation and assist if necessary.
- Be aware that prolonged use of ophthalmic solution may encourage superinfection with nonsusceptible organisms including fungi.
- Report overdose symptoms for eye medication: Increased lacrimation, keratitis, edema and itching of eyelids.

Patient & Family Education

- Report symptoms of superinfections (see Appendix D-1) to physician. Prompt treatment with an antibiotic or antifungal medication may be necessary.
- Report S&S of hearing loss, tinnitus, or vertigo to physician.
- Do not breast feed while taking this drug without consulting physician.
- Store this medication out of reach of children.

TOLMETIN SODIUM

(tole'met-in)
Tolectin, Tolectin DS
Classifications: CENTRAL NERVOUS SYSTEM AGENT; ANALGESIC; NSAID; ANTIPYRETIC
Prototype: Ibuprofen
Pregnancy Category: B (D in third trimester)

AVAILABILITY 200 mg, 600 mg tablets; 400 mg capsules

ACTIONS Related to indomethacin. Exact mode of anti-inflammatory action not known. Inhibition of platelet aggregation is less than that produced by equal therapeutic doses of aspirin. Comparable to aspirin and indomethacin in antirheumatic activity, but incidence of GI symptoms and tinnitus is less than in aspirin-treated patients, and CNS effects are less than in patients receiving indomethacin.

THERAPEUTIC EFFECTS Possesses analgesic, anti-inflammatory, and antipyretic activity.

USES In acute flares and management of chronic rheumatoid arthritis. May be used alone or in combination with gold or corticosteroids.

CONTRAINDICATIONS History of intolerance or hypersensitivity to tolmetin, aspirin, and other NSAIDs; active peptic ulcer, patients with asthma, nasal polyps, rhinitis, "aspirin triad," in patients with functional class IV rheumatoid arthritis (severely incapacitated, bedridden, or confined to a wheelchair). Safety during pregnancy (category B, category D in third trimester), lactation, or children <2 y is not established.

CAUTIOUS USE History of upper GI tract disease; impaired kidney function; compromised cardiac function and anticoagulants.

ROUTE & DOSAGE

Anti-Inflammatory

Child: **PO** ≥2 y, 20 mg/kg/day in 3–4 equally divided doses, then increase by 5 mg/kg/day (max 30 mg/kg/day or 2 g/day)
Adult: **PO** 400 mg t.i.d. (max 2 g/day)

Analgesic

Child: **PO** ≥2 y, 5–7 mg/kg/dose q6–8h (max 30 mg/kg/day or 2 g/day)

STORAGE

Store at 15°–30° C (59°–86° F) in tightly capped, light-resistant container unless otherwise instructed.

ADMINISTRATION

Oral

- Schedule treatment (preferred) to include a morning dose (on arising) and a bedtime dose.
- Can give with milk or food to decrease GI upset.
- Give with fluid of patient's choice; crush tablet or empty capsule to mix with water or food if patient cannot swallow tablet/capsule.

ADVERSE EFFECTS CNS: *Headache, dizziness, vertigo, lightheadedness,* mood elevation or depression, tension, nervousness, weakness, drowsiness, insomnia, tinnitus. **CV:** Mild edema (about 7% patients), sodium and water retention, mild to moderate hypertension. **GI:** Epigastric or abdominal pain, dyspepsia, *nausea,* vomiting, heartburn, constipation, peptic ulcer, GI bleeding. **Hematologic:** Transient and small decreases in hemoglobin and hematocrit, purpura, petechiae, granulocytopenia, leukopenia. **Urogenital:** Hematuria, proteinuria, increased BUN. **Skin:** Toxic epidermal necrolysis, morbilliform eruptions, urticaria, pruritus. **Body as a Whole:** Anaphylaxis (especially after drug is discontinued and then reinstituted).

DIAGNOSTIC TEST INTERFERENCE Tolmetin prolongs *bleeding time,* inhibits *platelet aggregation,* elevates *BUN, alkaline phosphatase,* and *AST* levels; may decrease *hemoglobin* and *hematocrit* values. Metabolites may produce false-positive results for *proteinuria* (with tests that rely on acid precipitation, e.g., *sulfosalicylic acid*).

INTERACTIONS Drug: ORAL ANTICOAGULANTS, **heparin** may prolong bleeding time; may increase **lithium** toxicity; **aspirin,** other NSAIDS add to ulcerogenic effects; may increase **methotrexate** toxicity. **Herbal: Feverfew, garlic, ginger, ginkgo** may increase bleeding potential.

PHARMACOKINETICS Absorption: Rapidly absorbed from GI tract. **Peak:** 30–60 min. **Distribution:** Crosses blood–brain barrier and placenta; distributed into breast milk. **Metabolism:** Metabolized in liver. **Elimination:** Excreted in urine. **Half-Life:** 60–90 min.

NURSING IMPLICATIONS

Assessment & Drug Effects

- Monitor therapeutic effect. Therapeutic response for rheumatoid arthritis or osteoarthritis generally occurs within 1 wk with progressive improvement in succeeding week: Reduced joint pain and swelling, reduction in duration of morning stiffness, improved functional capacity (increase in grip strength, delayed onset of fatigue).
- Monitor patients with kidney damage closely. Evaluate I&O ratio and encourage adult or adolescent patient to increase fluid intake to at least 8 full glasses per day. In children, maintain a fluid intake in relationship to age to produce an adequate urinary output.
- Lab tests: Obtain periodic kidney function tests (routine urinalysis, creatinine clearance, and serum creatinine) for patient on long-term therapy.
- Check self-medicating habits of the patient. Sodium bicarbonate alkalinizes the urine, which increases urinary excretion of tolmetin and may reduce degree and duration of effectiveness.

Patient & Family Education

- Take drug with meals or milk if GI disturbances occur. Notify physician if symptoms persist; dosage reduction may be necessary, or antacid added.
- Monitor weight and report an increase >2 kg (4 lb)/wk an increase in childs weight in relation to age and size. With impaired kidney or cardiac function; check for swelling in ankles, tibiae, hands, and feet.
- Inform surgeon or dentist before treatment if you are taking tolmetin because of possible enhanced bleeding.
- Report promptly signs of abnormal bleeding (ecchymosis, epistaxis, melena, petechiae), itching, skin rash, persistent headache, edema.
- Avoid potentially hazardous activities (biking, skateboarding, driving, sports, etc.) until response to drug is known because dizziness and drowsiness are common adverse effects.
- Do not breast feed while taking this drug without consulting physician.
- Store this medication out of reach of children.

T

TOLNAFTATE

(tole-naf'tate)

Aftate, Pitrex ✦ , Tinactin

Classifications: SKIN AND MUCOUS MEMBRANE AGENT; ANTI-INFECTIVE; ANTI-FUNGAL ANTIBIOTIC

Prototype: Fluconazole

Pregnancy Category: C

AVAILABILITY 1% cream, solution, gel, powder, spray

ACTIONS Synthetic topical antifungal agent. Action mechanism not clear, but has been shown that tolnaftate distorts hyphae and stunts mycelial growth on susceptible fungi.
THERAPEUTIC EFFECTS Fungistatic or fungicidal to Microsporum, specifically *M. gypseum, M. canis, M. audouinii, M. japonicum, Trichophyton, T. rubrum, T. schoenleinii, T. tonsurans,* and *Epidermophyton floccosum,* but ineffective against *Candida albicans, Cryptococcus neoformans, Aspergillus fumigatus,* bacteria, protozoa, and viruses.

USES Tinea pedis (athlete's foot), tinea cruris (jock itch), tinea corporis (body ringworm); also tinea capitis and tinea unguium if infection is superficial, plantar or palmar lesions adjunctively with keratolytic agents, and tinea versicolor (caused by *Malassezia furfur*).

CONTRAINDICATIONS Skin irritations prior to therapy, nail and scalp infections. Safety during pregnancy (category C), lactation, or by children <2 y is not established.
CAUTIOUS USE Excoriated skin.

ROUTE & DOSAGE

Tinea Infestations

Child/Adult: **Topical** Apply 0.5–1 cm (¼–½ in.) of cream or 3 drops of solution b.i.d. in morning and evening; powder may be used prophylactically in normally moist areas

STORAGE

Store cream, gel, powder, and topical solution in light-resistant containers at 15°–30° C (59°–86° F); store aerosol container at 2°–30° C (38°–86° F). Avoid freezing and exposure to light.

ADMINISTRATION

Topical

- Cleanse site thoroughly with water and dry completely before applying. Massage thin layer gently into skin. Make sure area is not wet from excess drug after application.
- Shake aerosol powder container well before use.
- Note: Cream and powder are not recommended for nail or scalp infection.
- Use liquids (solutions) for scalp infection or to treat hairy areas.

ADVERSE EFFECTS Skin: Local irritation, stinging of skin from aerosol formulation.

INTERACTIONS Drug: No clinically significant interactions established.

PHARMACOKINETICS Not studied.

NURSING IMPLICATIONS

Patient & Family Education

- Expect relief from pruritus, soreness, and burning within 24–72 h after start of treatment.

- Continue treatment for 2–3 wk after disappearance of all symptoms to prevent recurrence.
- Return to prescriber for reevaluation in absence of improvement within 4 wk.
- Report rash, stinging, and burning if it results from medicine.
- Note: If skin has thickened as a result of the infection, desired clinical response may be delayed for 4–6 wk.
- Avoid contact with eyes of all drug forms.
- Place container in warm water to liquefy contents if solution solidifies. Potency is unaffected.
- Do not breast feed while using this drug without consulting prescriber.
- Store this medication out of reach of children.

TOPIRAMATE
(to-pir'a-mate)
Topamax
Classifications: CENTRAL NERVOUS SYSTEM AGENT; ANTICONVULSANT
Pregnancy Category: C

AVAILABILITY 25 mg, 50 mg, 100 mg, 200 mg tablets; 15 mg, 25 mg, capsules

ACTIONS Sulfamate-substituted monosaccharide with a broad spectrum of anticonvulsant activity. Its precise mechanism of action is unknown. Exhibits sodium channel blocking action, as well as enhancing the ability of GABA to induce a flux of chloride ions into the neurons, thus potentiating the activity of this inhibitory neurotransmitter (GABA).

THERAPEUTIC EFFECTS Indicated by a decrease in seizure activity. Effectively controls partial-onset seizures in adults and children by inhibiting GABA.

USES Adjunctive therapy for partial-onset seizures in adults and children age 2–16 y.

CONTRAINDICATIONS Hypersensitivity to topiramate. Effect on labor and delivery is unknown.

CAUTIOUS USE Renal impairment, hepatic impairment; pregnancy (category C), lactation. Although topiramate has been studied in patients 2–17 y of age, safety and effectiveness in children are not established.

ROUTE & DOSAGE

Partial-Onset Seizures

Child: **PO** 2–16 y, initiate with 1–3 mg/kg/day given at bedtime (max dose 25 mg/dose) times 1 wk, then increase by 1–3 mg/kg/day in 2 divided doses q1–2wk to a target range of 5–9 mg/kg/day
Adult: **PO** Initiate with 25–50 mg/day b.i.d., increase by 25–50 mg/wk to efficacy **PO Maintenance Dose** 200–400 mg/day divided b.i.d. (max 1600 mg/day)

Renal Impairment

Cl_{cr} <70 mL/min: Decrease dose by 50%

Common adverse effects in *italic;* life-threatening effects <u>underlined;</u> generic names in **bold;** drug classifications in SMALL CAPS; ♣ Canadian drug name; ◐ Prototype drug.

STORAGE
Store at 15°–30° C (59°–86° F) in a tightly closed container. Protect from light and moisture.

ADMINISTRATION

Oral
- Make dosage increments of 50 mg at weekly intervals to the recommended maintenance dose, usually 400 mg/day.
- Do not break tablets unless absolutely necessary because of bitter taste.
- Capsule contents may be sprinkled on teaspoon of food and taken immediately. Instruct patient to swallow without chewing. Follow dosage with fluids of choice.

ADVERSE EFFECTS Body as a Whole: *Fatigue, speech problems,* weight loss, *increased incidence of hyperthermia associated with oligohydrosis.* **CNS:** *Somnolence, dizziness, ataxia, psychomotor slowing, confusion, nystagmus, paresthesia, memory difficulty, difficulty concentrating, nervousness,* depression, anxiety, tremor. **GI:** Anorexia. **Renal:** Nephrolithiasis. **Special Senses:** Angle-closure glaucoma (rare).

INTERACTIONS Drug: Increased CNS depression with **alcohol** and other CNS DEPRESSANTS; may increase **phenytoin** concentrations; may decrease ORAL CONTRACEPTIVE, **digoxin, valproate** concentrations; may increase risk of kidney stone formation with other CARBONIC ANHYDRASE INHIBITORS. **Carbamazepine, phenytoin, valproate** may decrease topiramate concentrations. **Herb: Ginkgo** may decrease anticonvulsant effectiveness.

PHARMACOKINETICS Absorption: Rapidly absorbed from GI tract; 80% bioavailability. **Peak:** 2 h. **Distribution:** 13–17% protein bound. **Metabolism:** Minimally metabolized in the liver. **Elimination:** Excreted primarily in urine. **Half-Life:** 21 h.

NURSING IMPLICATIONS

Assessment & Drug Effects
- Monitor mental status and report significant cognitive impairment.
- Lab tests: Periodically monitor CBC with Hgb and Hct.

Patient & Family Education
- Do not stop drug abruptly; discontinue gradually to minimize seizures.
- Minimize risk of kidney stones, drink at least 6–8 full glasses of water each day. In children, maintain a fluid intake in relationship to age to produce an adequate urinary output.
- May cause photosensitivity so warn patients to avoid direct sunlight, tanning beds, and sun lamps.
- Exercise caution with potentially hazardous activities. Sedation is common, especially with concurrent use of alcohol or other CNS depressants.
- Use or add barrier contraceptive if using hormonal contraceptives.

T

- Be aware that psychomotor slowing and speech/language problems may develop while on topiramate therapy.
- Report adverse effects that interfere with activities of daily living.
- Do not breast feed while taking this drug without consulting physician.
- Store this medication out of reach of children.

TRAZODONE HYDROCHLORIDE
(tray'zoe-done)
Desyrel, Desyrel Dividose
Classifications: CENTRAL NERVOUS SYSTEM AGENT; PSYCHOTHERAPEUTIC; ANTIDEPRESSANT
Prototype: Imipramine
Pregnancy Category: C

AVAILABILITY 50 mg, 100 mg, 150 mg, 300 mg tablets

ACTIONS Centrally acting triazolopyridine derivative antidepressant chemically and structurally unrelated to tricyclic, tetracyclic, or other antidepressants. Potentiates serotonin effects by selectively blocking its reuptake at presynaptic membranes in CNS. Does not stimulate CNS and causes fewer anticholinergic genitourinary and neurologic effects as compared with other antidepressants. Produces varying degrees of sedation in normal and mentally depressed patient.
THERAPEUTIC EFFECTS Increases total sleep time, decreases number and duration of awakenings in depressed patient, and decreases REM sleep. Has anxiolytic effect in severely depressed patient.

USES Both inpatient and outpatient with major depression with or without prominent anxiety.
UNLABELED USES Adjunctive treatment of alcohol dependence, anxiety neuroses, drug-induced dyskinesias.

CONTRAINDICATIONS Initial recovery phase of MI; ventricular ectopy; electroshock therapy. Safety during pregnancy (category C) or in children <8 y is not established.
CAUTIOUS USE Patient with suicidal ideation; cardiac arrhythmias or disease; lactation.

ROUTE & DOSAGE

Depression (these doses have been used with children)
Child: **PO** 6–18 y, 1.5–2 mg/kg/day in divided doses b.i.d.–t.i.d., increase q3–4 day prn (max 6 mg/kg/day)
Adult: **PO** 150 mg/day in divided doses t.i.d., may increase by 50 mg/day q3–7days (max 400–600 mg/day)

STORAGE
Store in tightly closed, light-resistant container at 15°–30° C (59°–86° F).

ADMINISTRATION

Oral

- Give drug with food; increases amount of absorption by 20% and appears to decrease incidence of dizziness or light-headedness. Maintain the same schedule for food–drug intake throughout treatment period to prevent variations in serum concentration.

ADVERSE EFFECTS CNS: *Drowsiness,* light-headedness, tiredness, dizziness, insomnia, headache, agitation, impaired memory and speech, disorientation. **CV:** *Hypotension (including orthostatic hypotension),* hypertension, syncope, shortness of breath, chest pain, tachycardia, palpitations, bradycardia, <u>PVCs, ventricular tachycardia</u> (short episodes of 3–4 beats). **Special Senses:** Nasal and sinus congestion, blurred vision, eye irritation, sweating or clamminess, tinnitus. **GI:** *Dry mouth,* anorexia, constipation, abdominal distress, nausea, vomiting, dysgeusia, flatulence, diarrhea. **Urogenital:** Hematuria, increased frequency, delayed urine flow, early or absent menses, male priapism, ejaculation inhibition. **Hematologic:** Anemia. **Musculoskeletal:** Skeletal aches and pains, muscle twitches. **Skin:** Skin eruptions, rash, pruritus, acne, photosensitivity. **Body as a Whole:** Weight gain or loss.

INTERACTIONS Drug: ANTIHYPERTENSIVE AGENTS may potentiate hypotensive effects; **alcohol** and other CNS DEPRESSANTS add to depressant effects; may increase **digoxin** or **phenytoin** levels; MAO INHIBITORS may precipitate hypertensive crisis.

PHARMACOKINETICS Absorption: Readily absorbed from GI tract. **Onset:** 1–2 wk. **Peak:** 1–2 h. **Distribution:** Distributed into breast milk. **Metabolism:** Metabolized in liver. **Elimination:** 75% excreted in urine, 25% in feces. **Half-Life:** 5–9 h.

NURSING IMPLICATIONS

Assessment & Drug Effects

- Monitor pulse rate and regularity before administration if patient has preexisting cardiac disease.
- Note: Adverse effects generally are mild and tend to decrease and disappear after the first few weeks of treatment.
- Observe patient's level of activity. If it appears to be increasing toward sleeplessness and agitation with changes in reality orientation, report to physician. Manic episodes have been reported.
- Check patient for symptoms of hypotension. If orthostatic hypotension is troublesome, suggest measures to reduce danger of falling and help patient to tolerate the effects. Discuss with physician; reduction of dose or discontinuation of the drug may be prescribed.
- Male patient should report inappropriate or prolonged penile erections. The drug may be discontinued.
- Monitor patients especially adolescents for suicidal ideation.
- Antidepressants increase risk of suicidal thinking and behavior in children and adolescents with major depressive disorder, obsessive compulsive disorder, and other psychiatric disorders. Observe closely for worsening of condition, suicidality, and behavior changes. Instruct

T

Common adverse effects in *italic;* life-threatening effects <u>underlined</u>; generic names in **bold;** drug classifications in SMALL CAPS; ♣ Canadian drug name; ♦ Prototype drug.

1185

family and caregivers to monitor for these symptoms and discuss with prescriber. A MedGuide describing risks and stating whether the drug is approved for the child's/adolescent's condition should be provided for all families when antidepressants are prescribed.

- Be aware that overdose is characterized by an extension of common adverse effects: Vomiting, lethargy, drowsiness, and exaggerated anticholinergic effects. Seizures or arrhythmias are unusual.

Patient & Family Education

- Expect therapeutic response to begin in 1 wk; may require 2–4 wk to reach maximum levels. Adhere to regimen.
- Do not alter dose or intervals between doses.
- Consult physician if drowsiness becomes a distressing adverse effect. Dose regimen may be changed so that largest dose is at bedtime.
- Limit or abstain from alcohol use. The depressant effects of CNS depressants and alcohol may be potentiated by this drug.
- Do not self-medicate with OTC drugs for colds, allergy, or insomnia treatment without advice of physician. Many of these drugs contain CNS depressants.
- Keep follow-up appointments to permit dose adjustment or discontinuation, as indicated.
- Alert dentist, surgeon, or emergency personnel that drug is being used. Trazodone is discontinued as long as possible prior to elective surgery.
- Exercise caution while engaging in potentially hazardous activities (biking, skateboarding, driving, sports, etc.).
- Do not breast feed while taking this drug without consulting physician.
- Advise parents and guardians to monitor for and report signs of suicidal ideation.
- Store this medication out of reach of children.

TRIAMCINOLONE
(trye-am-sin'oh-lone)
Aristocort, Atolone, Kenacort, Kenalog-E

TRIAMCINOLONE ACETONIDE

Azmacort, Cenocort A$_2$, Kenalog, Triam-A, Triamonide, Trikort, Trilog, Tri-Nasal

TRIAMCINOLONE DIACETATE

Amcort, Aristocort Forte, Articulose LA, Cenocort Forte, Kenacort, Triam-Forte, Trilone, Tristoject

TRIAMCINOLONE HEXACETONIDE

Aristospan

Classifications: HORMONES AND SYNTHETIC SUBSTITUTES; ADRENAL CORTICOSTEROID; ANTI-INFLAMMATORY
Prototype: Hydrocortisone
Pregnancy Category: C

Common adverse effects in *italic;* life-threatening effects <u>underlined</u>; generic names in **bold**; drug classifications in SMALL CAPS; ♣ Canadian drug name; ✪ Prototype drug.

AVAILABILITY Triamcinolone 4 mg, 8 mg tablets; 4 mg/5 mL syrup
Triamcinolone acetonide 3 mg/mL, 10 mg/mL (contains benzyl alcohol), 40 mg/mL (contains benzyl alcohol) injection; 100 mcg aerosol; 55 mcg inhaler; 55 mcg spray; 0.5 mg/mL nasal spray; 0.025%, 0.1%, 0.5% cream, ointment, lotion; 10.3% topical spray **Triamcinolone diacetate** 25 mg/mL (contains benzyl alcohol), 40 mg/mL (contains benzyl alcohol) injection **Triamcinolone hexacetonide** 5 mg/mL (contains benzyl alcohol), 20 mg/mL (contains benzyl alcohol) injection

ACTIONS Immediate-acting synthetic fluorinated adrenal corticosteroid with glucocorticoid and antirheumatic activity 7–13 times more potent than that of hydrocortisone. Possesses minimal sodium and water retention properties in therapeutic doses.
THERAPEUTIC EFFECTS Anti-inflammatory and immunosuppressant drug that is effective in the treatment of bronchial asthma.

USES An inflammatory or immunosuppressant agent. Orally inhaled: Bronchial asthma in patient as a conventional inhalation treatment. Used in conjunction with a short-acting bronchodilator. Therapeutic doses do not appear to suppress HPA (hypothalamic–pituitary–adrenal) axis.

CONTRAINDICATIONS Safety during pregnancy (category C), lactation, or in children <6 y is not established. Kidney dysfunction, systemic fungal infections. Also see hydrocortisone.

ROUTE & DOSAGE

Inflammation, Immunosuppression

Child: **IM** 6–12 y, 0.03–0.02 mg/kg at 1–7 days dosing intervals
Intra-Articular 6–12 y, 2.5–15 mg, repeat as needed
Adult: **PO/IM/SC** 4–48 mg/day in divided doses **Intra-Articular** 2.5–40 mg/day repeat as needed **Inhaled** 2–4 inhalations q.i.d.
Topical Apply sparingly b.i.d.–t.i.d.

Acetonide

Child: **IM** 6–12 y, 0.03–0.2 mg q1–7days **Intranasal** 6–12 y, 2 sprays in each nostril daily (110 mcg/2 sprays) **Aqueous Spray Pump** 6–12 y, initial dose is 1 spray each nostril once/day (max dose for inhalations is 220 mcg/day)
Adult: **IM** 60 mg, may repeat with 20–100 mg q6wk **Intra-Articular** 2.5–4.0 mg **Intranasal** >12 y, 4 sprays in each nostril daily (110 mcg/2 sprays) **Aqueous Spray Pump** >12 y, initial dose is 2 sprays each nostril once/day (max dose for inhalations is 220 mcg/day)

Diacetate

Child: **PO** 0.117–1.66 mg/kg/day in 4 equally divided doses
Adult: **PO** 4–48 mg/day in 1–4 divided doses **IM** 40 mg once/wk **Intradermal** 5–48 mg (max 75 mg/wk), may repeat q1–2wk if needed **Intra-Articular** 2–40 mg q1–8wk

Hexacetonide

Adult: **Intralesional** Up to 0.5 mg/in.^{2} of skin **Intra-Articular** 2–20 mg q3–4wk

STORAGE
Store at 15°–30° C (59°–86° F). Protect from light.

ADMINISTRATION

Oral
▪ Give with fluid of patient's choice; tablet may be crushed.

Inhaled
Give after bronchodilator to ensure maximum drug exposure in the lower airways.

Subcutaneous or Intramuscular
▪ Do not give triamcinolone injection IV.
▪ See hydrocortisone for additional administration information.

ADVERSE EFFECTS CNS: Euphoria, headache, insomnia, confusion, psychosis. **CV:** CHF, edema. **GI:** Nausea, vomiting, peptic ulcer. **Musculoskeletal:** Muscle weakness, delayed wound healing, muscle wasting, osteoporosis, aseptic necrosis of bone, spontaneous fractures. **Endocrine:** Cushingoid features, growth suppression in children, carbohydrate intolerance, hyperglycemia. **Special Senses:** Cataracts. **Hematologic:** Leukocytosis. **Metabolic:** Hypokalemia. **Skin:** Burning, itching, folliculitis, hypertrichosis, hypopigmentation.

INTERACTIONS Drug: BARBITURATES, **phenytoin, rifampin** increase steroid metabolism—may need increased doses of triamcinolone; **amphotericin B,** DIURETICS add to potassium loss; **ambenonium, neostigmine, pyridostigmine** may cause severe muscle weakness in patients with myasthenia gravis; may inhibit antibody response to VACCINES, TOXOIDS.

PHARMACOKINETICS Absorption: Readily absorbed from all routes. **Onset:** 24–48 h PO, IM. **Peak:** 1–2 h PO; 8–10 h IM. **Duration:** 2.25 days PO; 1–6 wk IM. **Metabolism:** Metabolized in liver. **Elimination:** Excreted in urine. **Half-Life:** 2–5 h; HPA suppression, 18–36 h.

NURSING IMPLICATIONS

Assessment & Drug Effects
▪ Discuss adequate diet with dietitian, patient, and physician to counter natriuresis, negative nitrogen balance, with weight loss in most patients (along with headache, fatigue, and dizziness) and sodium retention with weight gain and moon facies in others. High-protein, high-potassium diet is often needed. Calcium supplements may need to be given to counter osteoporosis.
▪ Lab tests: Periodic serum electrolytes and blood glucose.
▪ Discontinue occlusive dressing and start appropriate antimicrobial treatment if a local infection develops at site of application. Consult physician.
▪ Report symptoms of hypercortisolism or Cushing's syndrome (see Appendix D-1), hyperglycemia (see Appendix D-1), and glucosuria (e.g., polyuria). These may arise from systemic absorption after topical application, especially in children and if used over extensive areas for prolonged periods or if occlusive dressings are used.

Patient & Family Education

- Be aware that postural hypotension may accompany sodium loss and weight loss.
- Adhere to drug regimen; do not increase or decrease established regimen and do not discontinue abruptly.
- Do not breast feed while using or taking this drug without consulting physician.
- Store this medication out of reach of children.

TRIAMTERENE

(trye-am′ter-een)
Dyrenium
Classifications: FLUID AND WATER BALANCE AGENT; POTASSIUM-SPARING DIURETIC
Prototype: Spironolactone
Pregnancy Category: B

AVAILABILITY 50 mg, 100 mg capsules

ACTIONS Structurally related to folic acid. Like spironolactone, has weak diuretic action and a potassium-sparing effect. Promotes excretion of sodium, chloride (to lesser extent), and carbonate. Unlike spironolactone, blocks potassium excretion by direct action on distal renal tubule rather than by inhibiting aldosterone. Decreased glomerular filtration rate and elevated BUN are associated with daily administration.
THERAPEUTIC EFFECTS Weak diuretic action and a potassium-sparing effect.

USES Adjunct in the management of edema associated with CHF, hepatic cirrhosis, nephrotic syndrome, idiopathic edema, steroid-induced edema, and edema due to secondary hyperaldosteronism. Also alone or in conjunction with a thiazide or loop diuretic in patients with hypertension because of its potassium-sparing activity.

CONTRAINDICATIONS Hypersensitivity to drug; anuria, severe or progressive kidney disease or dysfunction; severe liver disease; elevated serum potassium. Safety during pregnancy (category B) or lactation is not established.
CAUTIOUS USE Impaired kidney or liver function; history of gouty arthritis; diabetes mellitus, history of kidney stones.

ROUTE & DOSAGE

Edema

Child: **PO** 2–4 mg/kg/day in 1–2 divided doses (max 6 mg/kg/day or 300 mg/day)
Adult: **PO** 100 mg/day b.i.d. (max 300 mg/day), may be able to decrease to 100 mg/day

---

STORAGE

Store in tight, light-resistant containers at 15°–30° C (59°–86° F) unless otherwise directed.

ADMINISTRATION

Oral

- Empty capsule and give with fluid or mix with food, if patient cannot swallow capsule.
- Give drug with or after meals to prevent or minimize nausea.
- Schedule doses to prevent interruption of sleep from diuresis (e.g., with or after breakfast if a single dose is taken, or no later than 6 p.m. if more than one dose is prescribed). Consult physician.
- Withdraw drug gradually in patients on prolonged or high-dose therapy in order to prevent rebound increased urinary excretion of potassium.

ADVERSE EFFECTS GI: Diarrhea, nausea, vomiting, and other GI disturbances. **CNS:** Dizziness, headache, dry mouth, <u>anaphylaxis</u>, weakness, muscle cramps. **Skin:** Pruritus, rash, photosensitivity. **CV:** Hypotension (large doses). **Metabolic:** *Hyperkalemia* and other electrolyte imbalances, elevated BUN, elevated uric acid (patients predisposed to gouty arthritis), hyperchloremic acidosis. **Hematologic:** Blood dyscrasias: Granulocytopenia, eosinophilia, megaloblastic anemia in patients with reduced folic acid stores (e.g., hepatic cirrhosis).

DIAGNOSTIC TEST INTERFERENCE Pale blue fluorescence in urine interferes with *fluorometric assay* of *quinidine* and *lactic dehydrogenase activity.* Triamterene may cause increases in *blood glucose* levels (diabetic patients), *BUN, serum potassium, magnesium,* and *uric acid* and *urinary calcium excretion.*

INTERACTIONS Drug: May increase **lithium** levels, thus increasing its toxicity; **indomethacin** may decrease renal elimination of triamterene; ANGIOTENSIN-CONVERTING ENZYME (ACE) INHIBITORS, other POTASSIUM-SPARING DIURETICS may cause hyperkalemia. **Food:** Avoid increase in potassium-containing foods, potassium substitutes, or salt substitutes.

PHARMACOKINETICS Absorption: Rapidly but variably absorbed from GI tract. **Onset:** 2–4 h. **Duration:** 7–9 h. **Metabolism:** Metabolized in liver to active and inactive metabolites. **Elimination:** Excreted in urine. **Half-Life:** 100–150 min.

NURSING IMPLICATIONS

Assessment & Drug Effect

- Monitor BP during periods of dosage adjustment. Hypotensive reactions, although rare, have been reported. Take care with ambulation.
- Weigh patient under standard conditions, prior to drug initiation and daily during therapy.
- Diuretic response usually occurs on first day of therapy; maximum effect may not occur for several days.
- Monitor and report oliguria and unusual changes in I&O ratio. Consult physician regarding allowable fluid intake.

- Be alert for S&S of kidney stone formation; reported in patients taking high doses or who have low urine volume and increased urine acidity.
- Lab tests: Obtain baseline and periodic determinations of serum potassium and other electrolytes. Obtain periodic kidney function (BUN, serum creatinine) in patients with known or suspected renal insufficiency. Obtain periodic blood studies in patients on prolonged therapy or with cirrhosis since both are prone to develop megaloblastic anemia.
- Observe for S&S of hyperkalemia (see Appendix D-1), particularly in patients with renal insufficiency, on high-dose or prolonged therapy, and those with diabetes.
- Do not give to a diabetic patient unless blood glucose is controlled because triamterene may increase blood glucose. Monitor patients closely.

Patient & Family Education
- Do not take potassium supplements, potassium-rich diet, and salt substitutes; unlike most diuretics, triamterene promotes potassium retention.
- Do not restrict salt; there is a possibility of low-salt syndrome (hyponatremia). Consult physician.
- Report overpowering fatigue or weakness, malaise, fever, sore throat, or mouth (possible symptoms of granulocytopenia) and unusual bleeding or bruising (thrombocytopenia) to physician.
- Be aware that drug may cause photosensitivity; avoid exposure to sun and sunlamps.
- Drug may impart a harmless pale blue fluorescence to urine.
- Do not breast feed while taking this drug without consulting physician.
- Store this medication out of reach of children.

TRIFLUOPERAZINE HYDROCHLORIDE

(trye-floo-oh-per′a-zeen)
Novoflurazine ♣, Solazine ♣, Stelazine, Terfluzine ♣
Classifications: CENTRAL NERVOUS SYSTEM AGENT; PSYCHOTHERAPEUTIC; ANTIPSYCHOTIC PHENOTHIAZINE
Prototype: Chlorpromazine
Pregnancy Category: C

AVAILABILITY 1 mg, 2 mg, 5 mg, 10 mg tablets; 10 mg/mL liquid; 2 mg/mL injection

ACTIONS Phenothiazine similar to chlorpromazine. Produces less sedative, cardiovascular, and anticholinergic effects and more prominent antiemetic and extrapyramidal effects than other phenothiazines. Antipsychotic effects thought related to blockade of postsynaptic dopamine receptors in the brain.
THERAPEUTIC EFFECTS Indicated by increase in mental and physical activity. Strong antipsychotic drug with more prolonged pharmacologic effects than that of chlorpromazine.

USES Management of manifestations of psychotic disorders; "possibly effective" control of excessive anxiety and tension associated with neuroses or somatic conditions.

CONTRAINDICATIONS Hypersensitivity to phenothiazines; comatose states; CNS depression; blood dyscrasias; bone marrow depression; pre-existing liver disease; pregnancy (category C), lactation; children <6 y.
CAUTIOUS USE Previously detected breast cancer; compromised respiratory function; seizure disorders.

ROUTE & DOSAGE

Psychotic Disorders

Child: **PO** *6–12 y,* 1 mg 1–2 times/day, may increase up to 15 mg/day in hospitalized patients **IM** *6–12 y,* 1 mg 1–2 times/day, at least 4 h apart
Adult: **PO** 1–2 mg b.i.d., may increase up to 20 mg/day in hospitalized patients **IM** 1–2 mg q4–6h (max 10 mg/day)

STORAGE

Store in light-resistant container at 15°–30° C (59°–86° F) unless otherwise directed.

ADMINISTRATION

Oral

- Separate antacid and phenothiazine doses by at least 2 h.
- Dilute oral concentrate just before administration with about 60–120 mL suitable diluent (e.g., water, fruit juices, carbonated beverage, milk, soups, puddings). Avoid coffee or tea near time of taking oral preparation. Explain dosage and dilution to patient if drug is to be self-administered.
- Crush tablet and give with small amount of fluid or food if patient will not or cannot swallow pill.
- Monitor ingestion of tablet to ensure that patient does not hoard medication.

Intramuscular

- Give IM injection deep into muscle mass appropriate for age. See Techniques of Administration section in Part I for safe IM site selection in children.
- Note: Slight yellow discoloration of injectable drug reportedly does not alter potency. If color is markedly changed, discard solution.
- Wash hands if undiluted concentrate is spilled on skin to prevent contact dermatosis.

ADVERSE EFFECTS CNS: *Drowsiness,* insomnia, dizziness, agitation, *extrapyramidal effects,* <u>neuroleptic malignant syndrome</u>. **Special Senses:** Nasal congestion, *dry mouth,* blurred vision, pigmentary retinopathy. **Hematologic:** <u>Agranulocytosis</u>. **Skin:** Photosensitivity, skin rash, sweating. **GI:** Constipation. **CV:** Tachycardia, *hypotension*. **Respiratory:** Depressed cough reflex. **Endocrine:** Gynecomastia, galactorrhea.

INTERACTIONS Drug: Alcohol and other CNS DEPRESSANTS add to CNS depression. **Herbal: Kava-kava** may increase risk and severity of dystonic reactions.

PHARMACOKINETICS Absorption: Well absorbed from GI tract. **Onset:** Rapid onset. **Peak:** 2–3 h. **Duration:** Up to 12 h. **Metabolism:** Metabolized in liver. **Elimination:** Excreted in bile and feces.

NURSING IMPLICATIONS

Assessment & Drug Effects

- Monitor HR and BP. Hypotension is a common adverse effect.
- Hypotension and extrapyramidal effects (especially akathisia and dystonia) are most likely to occur in patients receiving high doses or parenteral administration. Withhold drug and notify physician if patient has dysphagia, neck muscle spasm, or if tongue protrusion occurs.
- Monitor I&O ratio and bowel elimination pattern. Check for abdominal distention and pain. Encourage adequate fluid intake as prophylaxis for constipation and xerostomia. The depressed patient may not seek help for either symptom or for urinary retention.
- Be aware that because trifluoperazine potentiates analgesics, its use may reduce amount of narcotic required in painful long-term illness such as cancer.
- Agitation, jitteriness, and sometimes insomnia may simulate original neurotic or psychotic symptoms. These adverse effects may disappear spontaneously.
- Expect maximum therapeutic response within 2–3 wk after initiation of therapy.

Patient & Family Education

- Take drug as prescribed; do not alter dosing regimen or stop medication without consulting physician.
- Consult physician about use of any OTC drugs during therapy.
- Do not take alcohol and other depressants during therapy.
- Avoid potentially hazardous activities such as biking, skateboarding, sports, driving, or operating machinery, until response to drug is known. Drowsiness and dizziness may be prominent during this time.
- Cover as much skin surface as possible with clothing when you must be in direct sunlight. Use a SPF >12 sunscreen on exposed skin.
- Urine may be discolored or reddish brown and is harmless.
- Do not breast feed while taking this drug.
- Store this medication out of reach of children.

TRIMETHOBENZAMIDE HYDROCHLORIDE

(trye-meth-oh-ben′za-mide)

Arrestin, Tebamide Pediatric Suppositories, Ticon, Tigan, T-Gen

Classifications: GASTROINTESTINAL AGENT; ANTIEMETIC

Prototype: Prochlorperazine

Pregnancy Category: C

AVAILABILITY 100 mg (no longer available in U.S.), 250 mg, 300 mg capsules; 100 mg, 200 mg suppositories; 100 mg/mL injection

ACTIONS Structurally related to ethanolamine antihistamines, but in therapeutic doses antihistamine activity is weak. Sedative and antiemetic actions; less effective than phenothiazine antiemetics but produces fewer adverse effects. Must be used with other agents when vomiting is severe. Primary locus of action is thought to be the chemoreceptor trigger zone (CTZ) in medulla.

TRIMETHOBENZAMIDE HYDROCHLORIDE

THERAPEUTIC EFFECTS Less effective than phenothiazine antiemetics but produces fewer adverse effects.

USES Control of nausea and vomiting.

CONTRAINDICATIONS Uncomplicated vomiting in viral illness; parenteral use in children; rectal administration in prematures and newborns; known sensitivity to benzocaine (in suppository) or to similar local anesthetics. Safety during pregnancy (category C) or lactation is not established.

CAUTIOUS USE Patients who have recently received other centrally acting drugs; in presence of high fever, dehydration, electrolyte imbalance.

ROUTE & DOSAGE

Nausea and Vomiting

Child (do not use in premature infant or neonate): **PO/Rectal** *<13.6 kg,* 100 mg t.i.d. or q.i.d.; *13.6–45 kg,* 100–200 mg t.i.d. or q.i.d. *Adult:* **PO** 250–300 mg t.i.d. or q.i.d. **Rectal/IM** 200 mg t.i.d. or q.i.d.

STORAGE

Store at 25° C (77° F). Avoid freezing of parenteral form.

ADMINISTRATION

Oral

- Empty capsule and give with water or mix with food if patient cannot swallow capsule. May give without regard to food or meals.

Intramuscular

- Give IM deep into upper outer quadrant of buttock in adults. Do not use IM form with children.
- Minimize possibility of irritation and pain by avoiding escape of solution along needle track. Use Z-track technique. Rotate injection sites.

ADVERSE EFFECTS Body as a Whole: Hypersensitivity reactions (including allergic skin eruptions), muscle cramps, pain, stinging, burning, redness, irritation at IM site; local irritation following rectal administration. **CNS:** Drowsiness, sedation, pseudoparkinsonism. **CV:** Hypotension. **GI:** Diarrhea, exaggeration of nausea, acute hepatitis, jaundice. **Special Senses:** Blurred vision.

INTERACTIONS Drug: Alcohol and other CNS DEPRESSANTS add to depressant activity; BELLADONNA ALKALOIDS may intensify anticholinergic effects; PHENOTHIAZINES may precipitate extrapyramidal syndrome.

PHARMACOKINETICS Onset: 10–40 min PO; 15 min IM. **Duration:** 3–4 h PO; 2–3 h IM. **Elimination:** 30–50% of dose excreted unchanged in urine within 48–72 h.

NURSING IMPLICATIONS

Assessment & Drug Effects

- Monitor BP. Hypotension may occur particularly in surgical patients receiving drug parenterally.

Common adverse effects in *italic;* life-threatening effects <u>underlined</u>; generic names in **bold;** drug classifications in SMALL CAPS; ♣ Canadian drug name; ● Prototype drug.

- Report promptly and stop drug therapy if an acute febrile illness accompanies or begins during therapy.
- Antiemetic effect of drug may obscure diagnoses of GI, Reye's syndrome in children, or other pathologic conditions or signs of toxicity from other drugs.
- Extrapyramidal symptoms, confusions, dizziness, sedation, and drowsiness more common in children.

Patient & Family Education

- Report promptly to physician onset of rash or other signs of hypersensitivity (see Appendix D-1). Discontinue drug immediately.
- Do not drive or engage in potentially hazardous activities (biking, skateboarding, etc.) until response to drug is known.
- Do not drink alcohol or alcoholic beverages during therapy with this drug.
- Do not breast feed while taking this drug without consulting physician.
- Store this medication out of reach of children.

TRIMETHOPRIM 🅿️

(trye-meth'oh-prim)
Primsol, Proloprim, Trimpex
Classifications: ANTI-INFECTIVE; URINARY TRACT
Pregnancy Category: C

AVAILABILITY 100 mg, 200 mg tablets; 50 mg/5 mL liquid

ACTIONS Anti-infective and folic acid antagonist with slow bactericidal action. Binding and interference with cell growth is 1000 times stronger in bacterial than in mammalian cells. Most pathogens causing urinary tract infection (UTI) are in normal vaginal and fecal flora.

THERAPEUTIC EFFECTS Effective against most common UTI pathogens, including *Escherichia coli, Enterobacter* sp., *Klebsiella pneumoniae, Proteus mirabilis,* most strains of *Haemophilus influenzae, Streptococcus pneumoniae, Streptococcus pyogenes, Staphylococcus organisms* (including *S. saprophyticus*). Not effective against *Bacteroides, Lactobacillus* sp., *Chlamydia* or *Pneumocystis carinii, Pseudomonas aeruginosa.* Resistant strains of Enterobacteriaceae (*E. coli* and *Klebsiella* and *Proteus* sp.) may develop during therapy.

USES Initial episodes of acute uncomplicated UTIs, acute otitis media in children.

UNLABELED USES Treatment and prophylaxis of chronic and recurrent UTI in both men and women; treatment in conjunction with dapsone of initial episodes of *Pneumocystis carinii* pneumonia; treatment of travelers' diarrhea.

CONTRAINDICATIONS Megaloblastic anemia secondary to folate deficiency; creatinine clearance <15 mL/min, impaired kidney or liver function; possible folate deficiency; pregnancy (category C), lactation, or in children with fragile X chromosome associated with mental retardation. Safety in infants <2 mo, treatment of otitis media <6 mo, and efficacy in children <12 y are not established.

ROUTE & DOSAGE

Urinary Tract Infection
Child: **PO** <12 y, 4–6 mg/kg q12h times 10 days
Adult: **PO** ≥12 y, 100 mg b.i.d. or 200 mg once/day

Acute Otitis Media
Child: **PO** ≥6 mo, 10 mg/kg/day divided q12h times 10 days

Travelers' Diarrhea
Adult: **PO** 200 mg b.i.d.

STORAGE
Store at 15°–30° C (59°–86° F) in dry, light-protected place.

ADMINISTRATION

Oral
- Give with as much fluid as appropriate for child's age and in older child give 240 mL (8 oz) of fluid if not contraindicated.

ADVERSE EFFECTS GI: Epigastric discomfort, nausea, vomiting, glossitis, abnormal taste sensation. **Hematologic:** Neutropenia, *megaloblastic anemia*, methemoglobinemia, leukopenia, thrombocytopenia (rare). **Skin:** *Rash, pruritus,* <u>exfoliative dermatitis</u>, photosensitivity. **Body as a Whole:** Fever. **Metabolic:** Increased serum transaminases (ALT, AST), bilirubin, creatinine, BUN.

DIAGNOSTIC TEST INTERFERENCE Interferes with serum ***methotrexate assays*** that use a competitive binding protein technique with a bacterial dihydrofolate reductase as the binding protein. May cause falsely elevated creatinine values when ***Jaffe reaction*** is used.

INTERACTION Drug: May inhibit **phenytoin** metabolism causing increased levels.

PHARMACOKINETICS Absorption: Almost completely absorbed from GI tract. **Peak:** 1–4 h. **Distribution:** Widely distributed, including lung, saliva, middle ear fluid, bile, bone, CSF; crosses placenta; appears in breast milk. **Metabolism:** Metabolized in liver. **Elimination:** 80% excreted in urine unchanged. **Half-Life:** 8–11 h.

NURSING IMPLICATIONS

Assessment & Drug Effects
- Lab tests: Obtain C&S tests before trimethoprim therapy is initiated; therapy may be started before results are received. Obtain periodic urine cultures, BUN, creatinine clearance, CBC, Hgb, and Hct. Follow-up cultures may be ordered at end of treatment to verify elimination of causative organism.
- Reinforce necessity to adhere to established drug regimen. Recurrent infection after terminating prophylactic treatment of UTI may occur even after 6 mo of therapy.

- Assess urinary pattern during treatment. Altered pattern (frequency, urgency, nocturia, retention, polyuria) may reflect emerging drug resistance, necessitating change of drug regimen. Periodically check for bladder distention.
- Be alert for toxic effects on bone marrow, particularly in malnourished, alcoholic, pregnant, or debilitated patients. Recognize and report signs of infection or anemia.
- Drug-induced rash, a common adverse effect, is usually maculopapular, pruritic, or morbilliform and appears 7–14 days after start of therapy with daily doses of 200 mg or less.
- Watch for overdose symptoms: nausea, vomiting, diarrhea, mental depression, confusion, facial swelling, elevated serum transaminases.

Patient & Family Education

- Take all prescribed medication; uncomplicated UTIs usually respond to treatment.
- Drink fluids liberally (2000–3000 mL/day, if not contraindicated) or in younger children maintain a fluid intake in relationship to their age to produce an adequate urinary output. This will help flush out urinary bacteria.
- Take urinary analgesic for pain and discomfort with voiding before full drug effects are experienced. Report pain and hematuria to prescriber immediately.
- Do not postpone voiding even though increases in fluid intake may cause more frequent urination.
- Change diapers immediately after child voids. Teach parent to wipe female child from front to back after voiding.
- Do not use douches or sprays during treatment periods; practice careful perineal hygiene to prevent reinfection.
- Report to prescriber promptly any symptoms of a hematologic disorder (fever, sore throat, pallor, purpura, ecchymosis).
- Consult prescriber if severe traveler's diarrhea does not respond to 3–5 days of therapy (i.e., persistence of symptoms of severe nausea, abdominal pain, diarrhea with mucus or blood, and dehydration).
- Do not breast feed while taking this drug.
- Store this medication out of reach of children.

TRIMETHOPRIM and SULFAMETHOXAZOLE (TMP-SMZ)

(tri-meth'o-prim, sul-fa-meth'ox-azole)
Bactrim, Co-Trimoxazole, Septra, Sulfatrim
Classifications: ANTI-INFECTIVE, URINARY TRACT AGENT; SULFONAMIDE
Prototype: Trimethoprim
Pregnancy Category: C

AVAILABILITY 80 mg trimethoprim/400 mg sulfamethoxazole, 160 mg trimethoprim/800 mg sulfamethoxazole tablets; 40 mg trimethoprim/200 mg sulfamethoxazole/5 mL suspension (contains 0.26% alcohol); 16 mg trimethoprim/80 mg sulfamethoxazole/5 mL injection

ACTIONS Fixed combination of sulfamethoxazole (SMZ), an intermediate acting anti-infective sulfonamide, and trimethoprim (TMP), a synthetic anti-infective. Both components of the combination are synthetic folate antagonist anti-infectives. Mechanism of action is principally enzyme inhibition, which prevents bacterial synthesis of essential nucleic acids and proteins.

THERAPEUTIC EFFECTS Effective against *Pneumocystis carinii* pneumonitis, *Shigellosis enteritis,* and severe complicated UTIs due to most strains of the Enterobacteriaceae. Bacterial resistance to the combined drugs develops more slowly than to either of the drugs alone.

USES *Pneumocystis carinii* pneumonitis, *Shigellosis* enteritis, and severe complicated UTIs due to most strains of the Enterobacteriaceae. Also children with acute otitis media due to susceptible strains of *Haemophilus influenzae,* and acute episodes of chronic bronchitis in adults.

UNLABELED USES Isosporiasis; prevention of traveler's diarrhea; cholera; treatment of infections caused by *Nocardia, Legionella micdadei,* and *Legionella pneumophila* and genital ulcers caused by *Haemophilus ducreyi;* prophylaxis for *P. carinii* pneumonia in neutropenic patients.

CONTRAINDICATIONS Hypersensitivity to TMP, SMZ, sulfonamides, or bisulfites; group A beta-hemolytic streptococcal pharyngitis; megaloblastic anemia due to folate deficiency; porphyria; creatinine clearance <15 mL/min; pregnancy (category C), lactation.

CAUTIOUS USE Impaired kidney or liver function; possible folate deficiency; severe allergy or bronchial asthma; G6PD deficiency, hypersensitivity to sulfonamide derivative drugs (e.g., acetazolamide, thiazides, tolbutamide). Not recommended for infants <2 mo.

ROUTE & DOSAGE

Systemic Infections

Child: **PO** >2 mo & <40 kg, 6–12 mg/kg/day TMP q12h; >40 kg, 160 mg TMP/800 mg SMZ (1 double-strength [DS] tablet) q12h **IV** >2 mo, 8–10 mg/kg/day TMP divided q6–12h infused over 60–90 min (max dose 960 mg TMP)
Adult: **PO** 160 mg TMP/800 mg SMZ (1 DS tablet) q12h **IV** 8–10 mg/kg/day TMP divided q6–12h infused over 60–90 min

Pneumocystis carinii Pneumonia

Adult: **IV** 20 mg/kg/day TMP divided q6h infused over 60–90 min

Prophylaxis for Pneumocystis carinii Pneumonia

Child: **PO** 150 mg/m^2/day TMP/750 mg/m^2 SMZ b.i.d. 3 consecutive day/wk (max 320 mg TMP/day)
Adult: **PO** 160 mg TMP/800 mg SMZ q24h

Renal Impairment

Cl$_{cr}$ 10–30 mL/min: reduce dose by 50%; <10 mL/min: reduce dose by 75%

STORAGE

Store at 15°–30° C (59°–86° F) in dry place protected from light. Avoid freezing.

ADMINISTRATION

Oral

- Give with a full glass of desired fluid or with appropriate fluid intake for child's age on an empty stomach. Suspension must be shaken before administration.
- Maintain adequate fluid intake (at least 1500 mL/day) during therapy. In children maintain a fluid intake in relationship to age to produce an adequate urinary output.

Intravenous

PREPARE **Intermittent:** Add contents of 5-mL ampule to 125 mL D5W. Use within 6 h. If less fluid is desired, dilute in 75 or 100 mL and use within 2 h or 4 h, respectively. Do not refrigerate.

ADMINISTER **Intermittent:** Give over 60–90 min. Avoid bolus or rapid injection. Do not mix other drugs or solutions with IV infusion. Discard solution if cloudy or if crystallization appears after mixing.

INCOMPATIBILITIES **Solution/Additive:** Stability in **dextrose** and **normal saline** is concentration dependent; **fluconazole, verapamil. Y-Site: Fluconazole, foscarnet, midazolam, vinorelbine.**

ADVERSE EFFECTS Skin: *Mild to moderate rashes (including fixed-drug eruptions),* toxic epidermal necrolysis. **GI:** *Nausea, vomiting,* diarrhea, *anorexia,* hepatitis, pseudomembranous enterocolitis, stomatitis, glossitis, abdominal pain. **Urogenital:** Kidney failure, oliguria, anuria, crystalluria. **Hematologic:** Agranulocytosis (rare), aplastic anemia (rare), megaloblastic anemia, hypoprothrombinemia, thrombocytopenia (rare). **Body as a Whole:** Weakness, arthralgia, myalgia, photosensitivity, allergic myocarditis.

DIAGNOSTIC TEST INTERFERENCE May elevate levels of serum creatinine, transaminase, bilirubin, alkaline phosphatase.

INTERACTIONS Drug: May enhance hypoprothrombinemic effects of ORAL ANTICOAGULANTS; may increase **methotrexate** toxicity.

PHARMACOKINETICS Absorption: Readily absorbed from GI tract. **Peak:** 1–4 h PO. **Distribution:** Widely distributed, including CNS; crosses placenta; distributed into breast milk. **Metabolism:** Metabolized in liver. **Elimination:** Excreted in urine. **Half-Life:** 8–10 h TMP, 10–13 h SMZ.

NURSING IMPLICATIONS

Assessment & Drug Effects

- Be aware that IV Septra contains sodium metabisulfite, which produces allergic-type reactions in susceptible patients: Hives, itching, wheezing, anaphylaxis. Susceptibility (low in general population) is seen most frequently in asthmatics or atopic nonasthmatic persons.
- Lab tests: Baseline and followup urinalysis; CBC with differential, platelet count, BUN and creatinine clearance with prolonged therapy.
- Monitor coagulation tests and prothrombin times in patient also receiving warfarin. Change in warfarin dosage may be indicated.
- Monitor I&O volume and pattern. Report significant changes to forestall renal calculi formation. Also report failure of treatment (i.e., continued

UTI symptoms). Thrombocytopenia (with concurrent thiazide diuretics); severe decrease in platelets (with or without purpura); bone marrow suppression; severe skin reactions.
- Be alert for overdose symptoms (no extensive experience has been reported): Nausea, vomiting, anorexia, headache, dizziness, mental depression, confusion, and bone marrow depression.

Patient & Family Education
- Report immediately to physician if rash appears. Other reportable symptoms are sore throat, fever, purpura, jaundice; all are early signs of serious reactions.
- Monitor for and report fixed eruptions to physician. This drug can cause fixed eruptions at the same site each time the drug is administered. Every contact with drug may not result in eruptions; therefore, patient may overlook the relationship.
- Offer generous amounts of fluid daily, unless otherwise directed. In children maintain a fluid intake to produce an adequate urinary output in relationship to age.
- May cause photosensitivity so warn patients to avoid direct sunlight, tanning beds, and sunlamps (sulfamethoxazole increases sun sensitivity).
- Do not breast feed while taking this drug.
- Store this medication out of reach of children.

TROLEANDOMYCIN

(troe-lee-an-doe-mye′sin)
Tao
Classifications: ANTI-INFECTIVE; MACROLIDE ANTIBIOTIC
Prototype: Erythromycin
Pregnancy Category: C

AVAILABILITY 250 mg capsules

ACTIONS Derivative of oleandomycin, a macrolide antibiotic prepared from cultures of *Streptomyces antibioticus*. Chemically related to erythromycin and has similar range of antibacterial activity, but reportedly less effective; has high potential for toxicity.
THERAPEUTIC EFFECTS Effective against susceptible strains of pneumococci and group A beta-hemolytic streptococci. Cross-sensitivity with erythromycin reported.

USES Acute, severe infections of upper respiratory tract caused by susceptible strains of pneumococci and group A beta-hemolytic streptococci.

CONTRAINDICATIONS History of hypersensitivity to any of the macrolide antibiotics; bacteremia; patients receiving astemizide, cisapride, pimozide, or terfenadine; use for prophylaxis or for minor infections; pregnancy (category C); porphyria.
CAUTIOUS USE Impaired liver function; lactation.

ROUTE & DOSAGE

Upper Respiratory Tract Infections
Child: **PO** 6.6–11 mg/kg/dose (usual dose 125–250 mg) q6h
Adult: **PO** 250–500 mg q6h

ADMINISTRATION

Oral

- Give on an empty stomach (1 h before or 2 h after meals). If GI discomfort develops, give with food.
- Give in evenly spaced intervals throughout the day, preferably around the clock, in order to maintain effective blood levels.

ADVERSE EFFECTS GI: *Abdominal cramps and discomfort, nausea,* vomiting, diarrhea, cholestatic jaundice. **Body as a Whole:** Allergic reactions (urticaria, skin rash, <u>anaphylaxis</u>); superinfections.

DIAGNOSTIC TEST INTERFERENCE Troleandomycin may cause false elevations of ***urinary 17-ketosteroids (Drekter),*** and ***17-hydroxycorticosteroids (Porter-Silver method).***

INTERACTIONS Drug: May increase levels of **carbamazepine, cispride,** CYCLOSPORINES, and **theophylline** and their toxicity; ORAL CONTRACEPTIVES may cause cholestatic jaundice; **warfarin** may increase **prothrombin time (PT); ergotamine** may induce ischemia and peripheral vasospasm.

PHARMACOKINETICS Absorption: Incompletely absorbed from GI tract. **Peak:** 2 h. **Distribution:** Distributed throughout body fluids; diffusion into CSF is poor unless meninges are inflamed. **Metabolism:** Metabolized in liver. **Elimination:** Excreted in bile and urine.

NURSING IMPLICATIONS

Assessment & Drug Effects

- Lab tests: Obtain periodic liver function tests in patients receiving drug longer than 10 days or in repeated courses.
- Some patients develop an allergic type of hepatitis with right upper quadrant pain, fever, nausea, vomiting, jaundice, eosinophilia, and leukocytosis. Liver changes are reversible if drug is discontinued immediately.
- Be aware that superinfections are most likely to occur in patients on prolonged or repeated therapy. Withdraw if symptoms present (see Appendix D-1), and start appropriate therapy.

Patient & Family Education

- Report signs of jaundice: Clay-colored stools, pruritus, yellow sclerae.
- Do not stop drug before full course of therapy is completed. Do not interrupt and then restart therapy or increase or decrease dose or interval.
- Do not breast feed while taking this drug without consulting physician.
- Store this medication out of reach of children

TROMETHAMINE

(troe-meth′a-meen)
Tham, Tham-E
Classifications: FLUID AND ELECTROLYTIC BALANCE AGENT; SYSTEMIC ALKALINIZER
Pregnancy Category: C

AVAILABILITY 18 g/500 mL injection

ACTIONS Sodium-free organic amine that acts as a proton acceptor in the body buffering system, thus preventing or correcting acidosis. As a weak base, it combines with hydrogen ions from carbonic, lactic, pyruvic, and other metabolic acids, and penetrates the cell membrane to combine with intracellular acid.

THERAPEUTIC EFFECTS Acts as a weak osmotic diuretic increasing urine pH and excretion of fixed acids, CO_2, and electrolytes. Used to correct or prevent metabolic acidosis. May be preferable to sodium bicarbonate in treatment of severe metabolic acidosis when sodium or CO_2 elimination is restricted.

USES To prevent or correct metabolic acidosis associated with cardiac bypass surgery and cardiac arrest and to correct excess acidity of stored blood (preserved with acid citrate dextrose) and used in cardiac bypass surgery. (Stored blood has a pH range of 6.8–6.22.)

UNLABELED USES Metabolic acidosis of status asthmaticus and neonatal respiratory distress syndrome.

CONTRAINDICATIONS Anuria, uremia; chronic respiratory acidosis; pregnancy (category C), children, neonates.

CAUTIOUS USE Renal impairment; >1 day of therapy.

ROUTE & DOSAGE

Note: Dosage may be estimated from buffer base deficit of extracellular fluid using the following formula as a guide: mL of 0.3-M tromethamine solution = body weight (kg) × base deficit (mEq/L).

Metabolic Acidosis Associated with Cardiac Arrest

Infant/Child/Adult: **IV** 3.5–6 mL/kg/dose (126–216 mg/kg) of a 0.3-M solution into large peripheral vein (max dose 500 mg/kg/dose); if chest is open, 55–165 mL (2–6 g) 0.3-M solution into ventricular cavity

Systemic Acidosis During Cardiac Bypass Surgery

Adult: **IV** 9 mL/kg or approximately 500 mL (18 g) 0.3-M solution; a single dose of up to 1000 mL (36 g) may be necessary in severe acidosis

Excess Acidity of ACD Priming Blood

Infant/Child/Adult: **IV** 14–70 mL (0.5–2.5 g) 0.3-M solution added to each 500 mL blood

STORAGE

Store drug (available as solution or powder) away from extreme heat. Do not freeze.

ADMINISTRATION

Intravenous

PREPARE **IV Infusion:** Maximum allowable concentration is 0.3 M. Available premixed as a 0.3-M solution or may be prepared by adding 36 g to 1 L of sterile water.

ADMINISTER **IV Infusion:** Give undiluted by slow IV infusion or added to pump-oxygenator blood or other priming fluid. Give over a period of no less than 1 h. ▪ Observe entry site carefully. Perivascular infiltration of the highly alkaline solution may lead to vasospasm, necrosis, and tissue sloughing. Stop infusion if extravasation occurs. ▪ Treat extravasation with a procaine and hyaluronidase infiltration to reduce vasospasm and to dilute tromethamine remaining in tissues. If necessary, local infiltration of an alpha-adrenergic blocking agent (e.g., phentolamine) into the area may be ordered. ▪ Concentrations ≥1.2 M administered through umbilical vein of infant can lead to hemorrhagic hepatic necrosis. ▪ Discard solution 24 h after reconstitution; solution is highly alkaline and can erode glass.

ADVERSE EFFECTS Body as a Whole: *Local irritation,* tissue inflammation, *chemical phlebitis,* extravasation. **Respiratory:** <u>Respiratory depression</u>. **Metabolic:** Transient decrease in blood glucose, hypervolemia, hyperkalemia (with depressed kidney function). **Other:** Hemorrhagic hepatic necrosis.

PHARMACOKINETICS Metabolism: No appreciable metabolism. **Elimination:** Rapidly and preferentially excreted by kidneys; 75% excreted within 8 h.

NURSING IMPLICATIONS

Assessment & Drug Effects

- Watch for signs of hypoxia (see Appendix D-1). Hypoxia and hypoventilation may result from drug-induced reduction of CO_2 tension (a potent stimulus to breathing), particularly if respiratory acidosis is also present.
- Drug-induced hypoxia is a particular risk when concomitant use of other respiratory depressants or with COPD or impaired kidney function.
- Lab tests: Monitor blood pH, P_{CO_2}, P_{O_2}, bicarbonate, glucose, and electrolytes before, during, and after treatment. Dosage is controlled to raise blood pH to normal limits (arterial: 7.35–7.45) and to correct acid–base imbalance.
- Monitor ECG and serum potassium if drug is given to patient with impaired kidney function (reduced drug elimination). Since hyperkalemia is often associated with metabolic acidosis, be alert to early signs (see Appendix D-1).
- Be alert for overdose symptoms (from total drug or too rapid administration): Alkalosis, overhydration, prolonged hypoglycemia, solute overload.

T

UREA

(yoor-ee'a)

Aquacare, Carbamide, Carmol, Nutraplus, Ureacin, Ureaphil

Classifications: ELECTROLYTIC AND WATER BALANCE AGENT; OSMOTIC DIURETIC; OXYTOCIC

Prototype: Mannitol

Pregnancy: Category C

AVAILABILITY 40 g/150 mL injection; 10%, 20%, 40% cream; 10%, 25% lotion

ACTIONS When present in high concentrations in blood, induces diuresis by elevating osmotic pressure of glomerular filtrate, with subsequent decrease in sodium and water reabsorption and promotion of chloride and potassium excretion.

THERAPEUTIC EFFECTS Volume and rate of urine flow is increased. Increased blood toxicity results in transudation of fluid from tissue, including brain, cerebrospinal, and intraocular fluid into the blood. When used as an abortifacient, urea (in dextrose) is injected into amniotic sac, followed by IV oxytocin at a rate of about 400 milliunits/min or prostaglandin F_2.

USES To reduce or prevent intracranial pressure (cerebral edema) and intraocular pressure and to prevent acute kidney failure during prolonged surgery or trauma. Also transabdominally for aborting second trimester of pregnancy. Topical preparation promotes hydration and removal of excess keratin in dry skin and hyperkeratotic conditions.

UNLABELED USES Severe migraine attacks; acute sickle cell crisis.

CONTRAINDICATIONS Severely impaired liver or kidney function; CHF; active intracranial bleeding; marked dehydration; IV injection into lower extremities; topical use for viral skin diseases or impaired circulation. (Contraindications for intra-amniotic urea: impaired kidney function, frank liver failure, active intracranial bleeding; marked dehydration, diabetes mellitus, sickle cell anemia).

CAUTIOUS USE Safe use in pregnancy (category C), lactation, or in children is not established. Use on face or broken skin.

ROUTE & DOSAGE

Reduction of Intracranial or Intraocular Pressure, Diuresis

Child: **IV** *<2 y,* 0.1–0.5 g/kg of 30% solution infused slowly over 1–2.5 h at a rate not to exceed 4 mL/min; *>2 y,* 0.5–1.5 g/kg of 30% solution infused slowly over 1–2.5 h at a rate not to exceed 4 mL/min
Adult: **IV** 1–1.5 g/kg of 30% solution infused slowly over 1–2.5 h at a rate not to exceed 4 mL/min (max 120 g/24 h)

Hydration of Dry Skin

Adult: **Topical** Apply 2–40% cream or lotion to affected area 1–3 times/day

STORAGE

Follow manufacturer's directions. Keep topical form in tightly closed containers.

ADMINISTRATION

Topical

- Prepare fresh solution for each patient; discard unused portion. Urea may be reconstituted with 5% or 10% dextrose injection or 10% invert sugar in water.
- Action of topical preparation is enhanced by applying it to skin that is still moist following washing or bathing.

Intravenous

PREPARE **IV Infusion:** Reconstitute (for 30%) by adding 105 mL D5W, 10% dextrose, or 10% invert sugar to a 40-g vial; yields 135 mL of 30% solution containing 300 mg urea/mL. Reconstituted solution should be used immediately. Discard unused portions.

ADMINISTER **IV Infusion:** Give (30% solution) at a rate no greater than 4 mL/min. Infusion flow rate will be prescribed by physician. Rapid administration may be associated with increased capillary bleeding and hemolysis. ▪ Use extreme care to avoid extravasation; thrombosis and tissue necrosis can occur. Urea has the potential for causing tissue damage because of its osmotic properties. Inspect injection site frequently. If extravasation is suspected, discontinue the IV line **STAT.** Institute local treatment (according to institution protocol or physician's instructions); elevate body part even if extravasation is minor. Do not infuse with blood or blood derivatives using same infusion sets.

ADVERSE EFFECTS CNS: Somnolence (prolonged use in patients with kidney dysfunction), *headache,* acute psychosis, confusion, disorientation, nervousness. **CV:** Tachycardia, hypotension, syncope. **GI:** *Nausea, vomiting,* increased thirst. **Metabolic:** Fluid and electrolyte imbalance, dehydration. **Special Senses:** Intraocular hemorrhage (rapid IV). **Skin:** Skin rash, pain, irritation, sloughing, venous thrombosis, chemical phlebitis at injection site. **Body as a Whole:** Hyperthermia. **Hematologic:** Hemolysis (rapid IV).

INTERACTION Drug: May increase rate of **lithium** excretion, decreasing its effectiveness.

PHARMACOKINETICS Peak: 1–2 h. **Duration:** 3–10 h for diuresis and intracranial pressure reduction; 5–6 h for intraocular pressure. **Distribution:** 10% of intra-amniotic instillation diffuses into maternal blood; distributed widely; good ocular penetration; crosses placenta; distributed into breast milk. **Elimination:** Excreted in urine; 50% may be reabsorbed. **Half-Life:** 1 h.

NURSING IMPLICATIONS

Assessment & Drug Effects

- Monitor I&O. If diuresis does not occur within 6–12 h following administration or if BUN exceeds 75 mg/dL, withhold drug and notify physician so that kidney function may be evaluated.
- Monitor vital signs and mental status; promptly report any changes.
- Observe postoperative patients closely for signs of hemorrhage. Urea reportedly may increase prothrombin time and promote internal oozing at suture sites.

- Withhold oral fluids and consult physician for hydration parameters if patient complains of a headache.
- Lab tests: Serum electrolytes and urinary sodium q12h. Frequent kidney function studies are advised, particularly in patients suspected of having kidney dysfunction.
- Watch for S&S of hyponatremia, hypokalemia, dehydration, or transient overhydration (due to hyperosmotic activity) (see Appendix D-1).
- Monitor for complaints of lower abdominal pain following intra-amniotic instillation. If patient complains of lower abdominal pain, it may be that drug is going into abdomen rather than into the amniotic sac.
- See mannitol for additional nursing implications.

Patient & Family Education
- Drink fluids to hasten excretion of urea. However, if a headache develops, stop drinking because the fluid intake may be counteracting the effects of the drug. Alert physician.
- Do not breast feed while taking this drug without consulting physician.
- Store this medication out of reach of children.

VALPROIC ACID (DIVALPROEX SODIUM, SODIUM VALPROATE)
(val-proe'ic)
Depacon, Depakene, Depakote, Depakote ER, Depakote Sprinkle, Epival ♣
Classifications: CENTRAL NERVOUS SYSTEM AGENT; ANTICONVULSANT; GABA INHIBITOR
Pregnancy Category: D

AVAILABILITY 250 mg capsules; 125 mg sprinkle capsules; 125 mg, 250 mg, 500 mg delayed-release tablets; 500 mg sustained-release tablets; 250 mg/5 mL syrup; 100 mg/mL injection

ACTIONS Anticonvulsant unrelated chemically to other drugs used to treat seizure disorders. Mechanism of action unknown; may be related to increased bioavailability of the inhibitory neurotransmitter gamma-aminobutyric acid (GABA) to brain neurons. Inhibits secondary phase of platelet aggregation.
THERAPEUTIC EFFECTS Depresses abnormal neuron discharges in the CNS, thus decreasing seizure activity.

USES Alone or with other anticonvulsants in management of absence (petit mal) and mixed seizures; mania; migraine headache prophylaxis.
UNLABELED USES Status epilepticus refractory to IV diazepam, petit mal variant seizures, febrile seizures in children, other types of seizures including psychomotor (temporal lobe), myoclonic, akinetic and tonic-clonic seizures, photosensitivity seizures, and those refractory to other anticonvulsants.

CONTRAINDICATIONS Patient with bleeding disorders or liver dysfunction or disease, pregnancy (category D), lactation.
CAUTIOUS USE History of kidney disease; adjunctive treatment with other anticonvulsants.

ROUTE & DOSAGE

Management of Seizures, Mania

Adult/Child: **PO/IV** 10–15 mg/kg/day in equally divided doses daily or t.i.d. when total daily dose >250 mg, increase at 1 wk intervals by 5–10 mg/kg/day until seizures are controlled or adverse effects develop (max 60 mg/kg/day) maintenance usually 30–60 mg/kg/day b.i.d.–t.i.d.

Migraine Headache Prophylaxis

Adult: **PO** 250 mg b.i.d. (max 1000 mg/day) or **Depakote ER** 500 mg daily times 1 wk, may increase to 1000 mg daily

Mania

Adult: **PO** 250 mg t.i.d. (max 60 mg/kg/day)

STORAGE

Most preparations can be stored at 15°–30° C (59°–86° F) in tightly closed containers. See manufacturer's recommendations. Injection form does not contain preservative; discard any unused portions after opening.

ADMINISTRATION

Oral

- Give tablets and capsules whole; instruct patient to swallow whole & not to chew. Instruct to swallow capsules whole or sprinkle entire contents on teaspoonful of soft food, and instruct to not chew food.
- Do not administer with milk.
- Avoid using a carbonated drink as diluent for the syrup because it will release drug from delivery vehicle; free drug painfully irritates oral and pharyngeal membranes.
- Reduce gastric irritation by administering drug with food because serious GI adverse effects can lead to discontinuation of therapy. Enteric-coated tablet or syrup formulation is usually well tolerated.
- Do not use Depakote-ER with children.

Intravenous

***PREPARE* IV Infusion:** Dilute each dose in 50 mL or more of D5W, NS, or RL.

***ADMINISTER* IV Infusion:** Give a single dose over at least 60 min (≤20 mg/min). Avoid rapid infusion.

***INCOMPATIBILITIES* Solution/Additive:** No compatibility data available. Should avoid mixing with other drugs.

ADVERSE EFFECTS CNS: Breakthrough seizures, *sedation, drowsiness,* dizziness, increased alertness, hallucinations, emotional upset, aggression; <u>deep coma, death (with overdose)</u>. **GI:** *Nausea, vomiting, indigestion (transient),* hypersalivation, anorexia with weight loss, increased appetite with weight gain, abdominal cramps, diarrhea, constipation, <u>liver failure, pancreatitis</u>. **Hematologic:** *Prolonged bleeding time,* leukopenia, lymphocytosis, thrombocytopenia, hypofibrinogenemia, <u>bone marrow depression</u>, anemia. **Skin:** Skin rash, photosensitivity, transient hair loss, curliness or waviness of hair. **Endocrine:** Irregular menses,

Common adverse effects in *italic;* life-threatening effects <u>underlined;</u> generic names in **bold;** drug classifications in SMALL CAPS; ♣ Canadian drug name; ● Prototype drug.

1207

V

secondary amenorrhea. **Metabolic:** Hyperammonemia (usually asympto-matic), hyperammonemic encephalopathy in patients with urea cycle disorders. **Respiratory:** Pulmonary edema (with overdose).

DIAGNOSTIC TEST INTERFERENCE Valproic acid produces false-positive results for *urine ketones,* elevated *AST, ALT, LDH,* and *serum alkaline phosphatase,* prolonged *bleeding time,* altered *thyroid function tests.*

INTERACTIONS Drug: Alcohol and other CNS DEPRESSANTS potentiate de-pressant effects; other ANTICONVULSANTS, phenytoin, and phenobarbital may decrease valproic acid levels and valproic acid increases phenobar-bital concentrations; BARBITURATES increase or decrease anticonvulsant and BARBITURATE levels; **haloperidol, loxapine, maprotiline,** MAOIS, PHENOTHIAZINES, THIOXANTHENES, TRICYCLIC ANTIDEPRESSANTS can increase CNS depression or lower seizure threshold; **aspirin, dipyridamole, warfarin** increase risk of spontaneous bleed and decrease clotting; **clonazepam** may precipitate absence seizures; SALICYLATES, **cimetidine** may increase valproic acid levels and toxicity. **Mefloquine** can decrease valproic acid levels; **isoniazid** may increase valproic acid levels and hepatotoxicity; **meropenem** may decrease valproic acid levels; **cholestyramine** may decrease absorption. **Herbal: Ginkgo** may de-crease anticonvulsant effectiveness.

PHARMACOKINETICS Absorption: Readily absorbed from GI tract. **Peak:** 1–4 h valproic acid; 3–5 h divalproex. **Therapeutic range:** 50–100 g/mL. **Distribution:** Crosses placenta; distributed into breast milk. **Metabolism:** Metabolized in liver. **Elimination:** Excreted primarily in urine; small amount excreted in feces and expired air. **Half-Life:** 5–20 h.

NURSING IMPLICATIONS

Assessment & Drug Effects
- Monitor for therapeutic effectiveness. *Therapeutic level: 50–100 mcg/mL; toxic level: >100–150 mcg/mL.*
- Monitor patient alertness especially with multiple drug therapy for seizure control. Evaluate plasma levels of the adjunctive anticonvul-sants periodically as indicators for possible neurologic toxicity.
- Monitor patient carefully during dose adjustments and promptly report presence of adverse effects. Increased dosage is associated with fre-quency of adverse effects.
- Lab tests: Perform baseline platelet counts, bleeding time, and serum liver enzyme levels, and periodically ammonia levels, then repeat all at least q2mo, especially during the first 6 mo of therapy.
- Multiple drugs for seizure control increase the risk of hyperammone-mia, marked by lethargy, anorexia, asterixis, increased seizure fre-quency, and vomiting. Report such symptoms promptly to physician. If they persist with decreased dosage, the drug will be discontinued.

Patient & Family Education
- Do not discontinue therapy abruptly; such action could result in loss of seizure control. Consult physician before you stop or alter dosage regimen.

Common adverse effects in *italic;* life-threatening effects <u>underlined;</u> generic names in **bold;** drug classifications in SMALL CAPS; ♣ Canadian drug name; ⊘ Prototype drug.

- Note to diabetic patients: Drug may cause a false-positive test for urine ketones. Notify physician if this occurs; a differential diagnostic blood test may be indicated.
- Notify physician promptly if spontaneous bleeding or bruising occurs (e.g., petechiae, ecchymotic areas, otorrhagia, epistaxis, melena).
- Withhold dose and notify physician for following symptoms: Visual disturbances, rash, jaundice, light-colored stools, protracted vomiting, diarrhea. Fatal liver failure has occurred in patients receiving this drug.
- Avoid alcohol and self-medication with other depressants during therapy.
- Consult physician before using any OTC drugs during anticonvulsant therapy. Combination drugs containing aspirin, sedatives, and medications for hay fever or other allergies are particularly UNSAFE.
- Do not drive or engage in potentially hazardous activities (biking, skateboarding, sports, etc.) until response to drug is known.
- Inform prescribers or dentist before any kind of surgery that you are taking valproic acid.
- Carry medical identification card at all times. It needs to indicate medical diagnosis, medication(s), physician's name, address, and telephone number.
- Do not breast feed while taking this drug.
- Store this medication out of reach of children.

VANCOMYCIN HYDROCHLORIDE
(van-koe-mye′sin)
Vancocin, Vancoled
Classifications: ANTI-INFECTIVE; ANTIBIOTIC
Pregnancy Category: C

AVAILABILITY 125 mg, 250 mg capsules; 1 g, 10 g oral powder; 500 mg, 1 g injection

ACTIONS Prepared from *Streptomyces orientalis,* with bactericidal and bacteriostatic actions. Acts by interfering with cell membrane synthesis in multiplying organisms.
THERAPEUTIC EFFECTS Active against many gram-positive organisms, including group A *beta-hemolytic Streptococci, Staphylococci, Pneumococci, Enterococci, Clostridia,* and *Corynebacteria.* Gram-negative organisms, mycobacteria, and fungi are highly resistant.

USES Parenterally for potentially life-threatening infections in patients allergic, nonsensitive, or resistant to other less toxic antimicrobial drugs. Used orally only in *Clostridium difficile* colitis (not effective by oral route for treatment of systemic infections).

CONTRAINDICATIONS Known hypersensitivity to vancomycin, previous hearing loss, IM administration; lactation. Safe use during pregnancy (category C) is not established.
CAUTIOUS USE Neonates; impaired kidney function; concurrent or sequential use of other ototoxic or nephrotoxic agents.

Common adverse effects in *italic;* life-threatening effects underlined; generic names in **bold;** drug classifications in SMALL CAPS; ✦ Canadian drug name; ❷ Prototype drug.

1209

VANCOMYCIN HYDROCHLORIDE

ROUTE & DOSAGE

Systemic Infections

Neonate: **IV Postnatal** ≤*7 days, <1200 g:* 15 mg/kg/day q24h; *1200–2000 g,* 10–15 mg/kg/dose q12–18h; *>2000 g,* 10–15 mg/kg /dose q8–12h; *>7 days, <1200 g:* 15 mg/kg/day q24h; *1200–2000 g,* 10–15 mg/kg/dose q8–12h; *>2000 g,* 15–20 mg/kg/dose q8h; infuse over 60–90 min
Infant/Child: **IV** *>1 mo,* 40 mg/kg/day in equally divided doses q6–8h, infuse over 60–90 min
Adult: **IV** 500 mg q6h or 1 g q12h (max dose 4 g/day), infuse over 60–90 min

Clostridium difficile Colitis

Child: **PO** 40–50 mg/kg/day in equally divided doses q6h (max 500 mg/day) for 7–10 days
Adult: **PO** 125–500 mg q6h for 7–10 days
Reduced dosages required with renal impairment.

STORAGE

Store oral and parenteral solutions in refrigerator for up to 14 days; after further dilution, parenteral solution is stable 24 h at room temperature 15° to 30° C (59°–86° F).

ADMINISTRATION

Oral

- Oral solution is prepared by adding to 10 g oral powder 115 mL of distilled water. The solution may be further diluted in 10 g of water.

Intravenous

***PREPARE* Intermittent:** Reconstitute 500 mg vial or 1 g vial with 10 mL or 20 mL, respectively, of sterile water for injection to yield 50 mg/mL. Further dilute each 1 g with at least by 200 mL of D5W, NS, or RL.
***ADMINISTER* Intermittent:** Give a single dose at a rate of 10 mg/min or over NOT LESS than 60 min. Avoid rapid infusion, which may cause sudden hypotension and "red-neck syndrome." Monitor IV site closely; necrosis and tissue sloughing will result from extravasation.
***INCOMPATIBILITIES* Solution/Additive: Aminophylline,** BARBITURATES, **cefotaxime, chloramphenicol, chlorothiazide, dexamethasone, heparin, sodium bicarbonate, warfarin. Y-Site: Albumin, aztreonam, cefepime, cefotaxime, cefotetan, cefoxitin, ceftazidime, ceftriaxone, cefuroxime, foscarnet, heparin, idarubicin, nafcillin, omeprazole, piperacillin/tazobactam, ticarcillin, ticarcillin/clavulanate, warfarin.**

ADVERSE EFFECTS Special Senses: Ototoxicity (auditory portion of eighth cranial nerve). **Urogenital:** <u>Nephrotoxicity leading to uremia</u>. **Body as a Whole:** Hypersensitivity reactions (chills, fever, skin rash, urticaria, <u>shock-like state</u>), <u>anaphylactoid reaction with vascular collapse</u>, superinfections, severe pain, thrombophlebitis at injection site, generalized tingling following rapid IV infusion. **Hematologic:** Transient leukopenia,

Common adverse effects in *italic;* life-threatening effects <u>underlined;</u> generic names in **bold;** drug classifications in SMALL CAPS; ✦ Canadian drug name; ❂ Prototype drug.

eosinophilia. **GI:** Nausea, warmth. **Other:** Injection reaction that includes *hypotension accompanied by flushing and erythematous rash on face and upper body* ("red-neck syndrome") following rapid IV infusion.

INTERACTIONS Drug: Adds to toxicity of OTOTOXIC and NEPHRO-TOXIC DRUGS (AMINOGLYCOSIDES, **amphotericin B, bumetanide, capreomycin, cidofovir, cisplatin, colistin, cyclosporine, foscarnet, furosemide, ganciclovir, IV pentamidine, polymyxin B, streptozocin, tacrolimus). Cholestyramine, colestipol** can decrease absorption of oral vancomycin; may increase risk of lactic acidosis with **metformin.**

PHARMACOKINETICS Absorption: Not absorbed from GI tract. **Peak:** 30 min after end of infusion. **Distribution:** Diffuses into pleural, ascitic, pericardial, and synovial fluids; small amount penetrates CSF if meninges are inflamed; crosses placenta. **Elimination:** 80–90% of IV dose excreted in urine within 24 h; PO dose excreted in feces. **Half-Life:** 4–8 h.

NURSING IMPLICATIONS

Assessment & Drug Effects

- Monitor BP and heart rate continuously through period of drug administration.
- If "red-neck syndrome"occurs with vancomycin, further dilute the infusion and slow rate of infusion to 90–120 min. "Red-neck syndrome" may be avoided in individuals by pretreating with IV diphenhydramine 1 mg/kg (max 50 mg). Give 30 min prior to vancomycin dose.
- Lab tests: Monitor urinalysis, kidney, & liver functions, and hematologic studies periodically.
- Monitor serial tests of vancomycin blood levels (peak and trough) in patients with borderline kidney function, in infants and neonates.
- Draw peak levels 1 h after administration of third consecutive dose (peak level 25–40 mg/L). Trough level should be obtained 30 min prior to the third consecutive dose (trough level <10 mg/L).
- Assess hearing daily. Drug may cause damage to auditory branch (not vestibular branch) of eighth cranial nerve, with consequent deafness, which may be permanent.
- Be aware that serum levels of 60–80 mcg/mL are associated with ototoxicity. Tinnitus and high-tone hearing loss may precede deafness, which may progress even after drug is withdrawn. Those on high doses are especially susceptible.
- Monitor I&O: Report changes in I&O ratio and pattern. Oliguria or cloudy or pink urine may be a sign of nephrotoxicity (also manifested by transient elevations in BUN, albumin, and hyaline and granular casts in urine).

Patient & Family Education

- Notify physician promptly of ringing in ears.
- Adhere to drug regimen. Do not increase, decrease, or interrupt dosage. The full course of prescribed drug therapy must be completed.
- Do not breast feed while taking this drug.
- Store this medication out of reach of children.

VARICELLA VACCINE
(var-i-cel′la)
Varivax
Classifications: ANTI-INFECTIVE; VACCINE; VIRAL
Prototype: Hepatitis B
Pregnancy Category: C

AVAILABILITY 1350 PFU/vial

ACTIONS A live attenuated vaccine that acts against both chickenpox and shingles, both of which are caused by *Varicella zoster* infection.
THERAPEUTIC EFFECTS Protects healthy children and adults from varicella effectively.

USES Vaccination against varicella in individuals ≥12 mo.

CONTRAINDICATIONS Hypersensitivity to any component of the vaccine; history of anaphylactoid reaction to neomycin; individuals with blood dyscrasia, leukemia, lymphomas, bone marrow or lymphatic system malignancies, concomitant immunosuppression therapy; individuals with primary or acquired immunodeficient states; active untreated tuberculosis; any febrile respiratory illness or other febrile infections; lactation; pregnancy (category C); children <1 y.
CAUTIOUS USE Acute lymphoblastic leukemia in remission.

ROUTE & DOSAGE

Varicella Protection
Child: **SC** *12 mo–12 y,* single dose of 0.5 mL
Adult: **SC** Primary immunization of 0.5 mL followed by 0.5 mL 4–8 wk after first dose, may need to revaccinate 3 mo after initial series if patient fails to seroconvert

STORAGE
Store powder vaccine in frost-free freezer at 15° C (+5° F) or colder. Store diluent separately at room temperature or in the refrigerator. After reconstitution keep refrigerated in dark until administration. If not administered in 30 minutes, dose must be discarded.

V ADMINISTRATION
Subcutaneous
- Reconstitute vaccine with 0.7 mL of supplied diluent; gently agitate the vial to mix. Withdraw entire contents of vial into syringe for injection. Change needle on syringe and administer immediately or within 30 min of reconstitution.
- Give SC into the outer aspect of the upper arm. Exercise caution not to inject IV.

ADVERSE EFFECTS CNS: Headache, fever. **Hematologic:** Mild thrombocytopenia. **Skin:** *Redness, swelling, or rash at injection site.* **Other:** Herpes zoster infection (rare).

INTERACTIONS Drug: Acyclovir decreases vaccine's effectiveness. It is recommended that **yellow fever vaccine** be given at least 1 mo apart from varicella or any other live virus vaccine. Measles (or MMR vaccine) must be given on same day as varicella or 6 weeks must separate the two vaccines. Avoid **salicylates** for 6 wk after vaccination to decrease risk of developing Reye's syndrome. Blood products interfer with immune response. Ninety days needed after blood products before giving varicella vaccine.

PHARMACOKINETICS Onset: Seroconversion approximately 42 days after vaccination. **Duration:** 5–10 y in healthy children. **Distribution:** Crosses placenta; distributed into breast milk.

NURSING IMPLICATIONS

Assessment & Drug Effects

- Withhold vaccine and notify prescriber if patient has a history of hypersensitivity to neomycin or a current febrile infection.
- Monitor for signs and symptoms of hypersensitivity (see Appendix D-1) and administer epinephrine 1:1000 if an anaphylactoid reaction occurs.

Patient & Family Education

- Avoid use of aspirin or any OTC products containing aspirin for 6 wk after vaccination, especially with children and adolescents.
- Notify prescriber about all adverse reactions (i.e., fever, rash, respiratory illness).
- Review need for future immunizations and make appointments.

VASOPRESSIN INJECTION ⊘
(vay-soe-press′in)
Pitressin
Classifications: HORMONES AND SYNTHETIC SUBSTITUTES; PITUITARY (ANTIDIURETIC)
Pregnancy Category: X

AVAILABILITY 20 pressor units/mL injection

ACTIONS Polypeptide hormone extracted from animal posterior pituitaries. Possesses pressor and antidiuretic (ADH) properties, but is relatively free of oxytocic properties. Produces concentrated urine by increasing tubular reabsorption of water (ADH activity), thus preserving up to 90% of water.

THERAPEUTIC EFFECTS May increase sodium and decrease potassium reabsorption but plays no causative role in edema formation. Small doses may produce anginal pain; large doses may precipitate MI, decrease heart rate and cardiac output, and increase pulmonary arterial pressure and BP. The tannate (in peanut oil) is preferred for chronic therapy; intranasal aqueous vasopressin is effective for daily maintenance of mild diabetes insipidus. Effective in the treatment of antidiuresis caused by diabetes insipidus.

USES Antidiuretic to treat diabetes insipidus, to dispel gas shadows in abdominal roentgenography, and as prevention and treatment of postoperative abdominal distention. Treat ventricular fibrillation or tachycardia refractory, to initial defibrillation in the adult ACLS algorithm, Also given to treat transient polyuria due to ADH deficiency (related to head injuries or to neurosurgery).

UNLABELED USES Test for differential diagnosis of nephrogenic, psychogenic, and neurohypophyseal diabetes insipidus; test to elevate ability of kidney to concentrate urine, and provocative test for pituitary release of corticotropin and growth hormone; emergency and adjunct pressor agent in the control of massive GI hemorrhage (e.g., esophageal varices).

CONTRAINDICATIONS Chronic nephritis accompanied by nitrogen retention; ischemic heart disease, PVCs, advanced arteriosclerosis; pregnancy (category X); during first stage of labor.

CAUTIOUS USE Epilepsy; migraine; asthma; heart failure, angina pectoris; any state in which rapid addition to extracellular fluid may be hazardous; vascular disease; preoperative and postoperative polyuric patients, kidney disease; goiter with cardiac complications; older adult patients, children, lactation.

ROUTE & DOSAGE

Diabetes Insipidus

Child: **IM/SC** 2.5–10 units aqueous solution 2–4 times/day **IV** continuous infusion: Start with 0.5 milliunits/kg/h (0.0005 units/kg/h) and double dosage every 30 min as necessary (max dose 10 milliunits/kg/h)
Adult: **IM/SC** 5–10 units aqueous solution 2–4 times/day (5–60 units/day) *or* 1.25–2.5 units in oil q2–3days **Intranasal** Apply to cotton pledget or intranasal spray.

Abdominal Distention, Abdominal Radiographic Procedures

Adult: **IM/SC** 5 units with 5–10 units q3–4h prn or 5–15 units q2h and 30 min prior to procedure

GI Hemorrhage

Child: **IV** 0.002–0.005 units/kg/min, then adjust dose as needed to max 0.01 units/kg/min
Adult: **IV** 0.1–1 units/mL at 0.2–0.4 units/min up to 0.9 units/min

STORAGE

Store at 15°–30° C (59°–86° F); prevent freezing.

ADMINISTRATION

Intramuscular/Subcutaneous

- Give 1–2 glasses of water or generous amount of fluid for age, with vasopressin to reduce adverse effects of tannate and improve therapeutic response.
- Do NOT administer **vasopressin tannate via IV.** Warm ampule to body temperature and shake vigorously to disperse active principle before withdrawing drug for IM administration.
- The tannate injection is often painful, and allergic reactions may develop. It is preferred for use in chronic therapy because of its longer duration of action.

Intravenous

PREPARE **IV Infusion:** Give vasopressin aqueous injection by continuous IV. Dilute with NS or D5W to a concentration of 0.1–1 units/mL. *ADMINISTER* **IV Infusion:** Titrate dose and rate to patient's response.

ADVERSE EFFECTS Skin: Rash, urticaria. **Body as a Whole:** <u>Anaphylaxis</u>; *tremor,* sweating, bronchoconstriction, *circumoral and facial pallor,* angioneurotic edema, *pounding in head, water intoxication* (especially with tannate), gangrene at injection site with intraarterial infusion. **GI:** *Eructations, passage of gas, nausea, vomiting,* heartburn, abdominal cramps, increased bowel movements secondary to excessive use. **CV:** Angina (in patient with coronary vascular disease); <u>cardiac arrest</u>, hypertension, bradycardia, minor arrhythmias, <u>premature atrial contraction</u>, <u>heart block</u>, <u>peripheral vascular collapse</u>, coronary insufficiency, <u>MI</u>; cardiac arrhythmia, pulmonary edema, bradycardia (with intraarterial infusion). **Urogenital:** Uterine cramps. **Respiratory:** Congestion, rhinorrhea, irritation, mucosal ulceration and pruritus, postnasal drip. **Special Senses:** Conjunctivitis.

DIAGNOSTIC TEST INTERFERENCE Vasopressin increases *plasma cortisol* levels.

INTERACTIONS Drug: Alcohol, demeclocycline, epinephrine, heparin, lithium, phenytoin may decrease antidiuretic effects of vasopressin; **guanethidine, neostigmine** increase vasopressor actions; **chlorpropamide, clofibrate, carbamazepine,** THIAZIDE DIURETICS may increase antidiuretic activity.

PHARMACOKINETICS Duration: 2–8 h in aqueous solution, 48–72 h in oil, 30–60 min IV infusion. **Distribution:** Extracellular fluid. **Metabolism:** Metabolized in liver and kidneys. **Elimination:** Excreted in urine. **Half-Life:** 10–20 min.

NURSING IMPLICATIONS

Assessment & Drug Effects

- Monitor infants and children closely. They are more susceptible to volume disturbances (such as sudden reversal of polyuria) than adults.
- Establish baseline data of BP, weight, I&O pattern and ratio. Monitor BP and weight throughout therapy. (Dose used to stimulate diuresis has little effect on BP.) Report sudden changes in pattern to physician.
- Be alert to the fact that even small doses of vasopressin may precipitate MI or coronary insufficiency. Keep emergency equipment and drugs (antiarrhythmics) readily available.
- Check patient's alertness and orientation frequently during therapy. Lethargy and confusion associated with headache may signal onset of water intoxication, which, although insidious in rate of development, can lead to convulsions and terminal coma.
- Monitor urine output, specific gravity, and serum osmolality while patient is hospitalized.
- Withhold vasopression, restrict fluid intake, and notify physician if urine-specific gravity is <1.015.

Patient & Family Education

- Be prepared for possibility of anginal attack and have coronary vasodilator available (e.g., nitroglycerin) if there is a history of coronary artery disease. Report to physician.
- Measure and record data related to polydipsia and polyuria. Learn how to determine specific gravity and how to keep an accurate record of output. Understand that treatment should diminish intense thirst and restore undisturbed normal sleep.
- Avoid concentrated fluids (e.g., undiluted syrups), since these increase urine volume.
- Do not breast feed while taking this drug without consulting physician.

VECURONIUM

(vek-yoo-roe′nee-um)
Norcuron
Classifications: AUTONOMIC NERVOUS SYSTEM AGENT; NONDEPOLARIZING SKELETAL MUSCLE RELAXANT
Prototype: Tubocurarine
Pregnancy Category: C

AVAILABILITY 10 mg, 20 mg vials

ACTIONS Intermediate-acting nondepolarizing skeletal muscle relaxant structurally similar to pancuronium. Demonstrates negligible histamine release and therefore has minimal direct effect on cardiovascular system, unlike older neuromuscular blocking agents.

THERAPEUTIC EFFECTS Inhibits neuromuscular transmission by competitively binding with acetylcholine to motor end plate receptors (common also with other drugs of this class). Results in skeletal muscular relaxation. Given ONLY after induction of general anesthesia.

USES Adjunct for general anesthesia to produce skeletal muscle relaxation during surgery. Especially useful for patients with severe kidney disease, limited cardiac reserve, and history of asthma or allergy. Also to facilitate endotracheal intubation.

UNLABELED USES Continuous infusion for facilitation of mechanical ventilation.

CONTRAINDICATIONS Safe use during pregnancy (category C), lactation, is not established; lack of proper personnel and equipment to ensure intubation.

CAUTIOUS USE Severe liver disease; impaired acid–base, fluid and electrolyte balance; severe obesity; adrenal or neuromuscular disease (myasthenia gravis, Eaton-Lambert syndrome); patients with slow circulation time (cardiovascular disease, old age, edematous states); malignant hyperthermia.

Common adverse effects in *italic;* life-threatening effects <u>underlined;</u> generic names in **bold;** drug classifications in SMALL CAPS; ✦ Canadian drug name; ❷ Prototype drug.

ROUTE & DOSAGE

Skeletal Muscle Relaxation

Neonate: **IV** 0.1 mg/kg/dose, followed by 0.03–0.15 mg/kg/dose q1–2h as necessary

Infant: **IV** >7 wk–1 y, 0.08–0.1 mg/kg/dose initially, then 0.05–0.1 mg/kg/dose every 1 h as necessary

Child/Adult: **IV** >1 y, 0.08–0.1 mg/kg/dose initially, then after 1 h, 0.05–0.1 mg/kg/dose every hour or 0.001 mg/kg/min by continuous infusion

STORAGE

Refrigerate after reconstitution below 30° C (86° F), unless otherwise directed. Discard solution after 24 h.

ADMINISTRATION

Note: Vecuronium is administered only by qualified clinicians.

Intravenous

PREPARE **Direct:** Dilute 10–20 mg with 50 mL sterile water for injection (supplied). If neonate dilute with SWI; the supplied dilute has benzyl alcohol which could cause "gasping syndrome." **Continuous:** Further dilute with up to 100 mL D5W, NS, or RL to yield 0.1–0.2 mg/mL.

ADMINISTER **Direct:** Give a bolus dose over 30 sec. **Continuous:** Give at the required rate.

INCOMPATIBILITIES **Y-Site: Amphotericin B cholesteryl complex, diazepam, etomidate, furosemide, thiopental.**

ADVERSE EFFECTS (≥1%) Body as a Whole: Skeletal muscle weakness, malignant hyperthermia. **Respiratory:** Apnea, respiratory depression.

INTERACTIONS Drug: GENERAL ANESTHETICS increase neuromuscular blockade and duration of action; AMINOGLYCOSIDES, **bacitracin, clindamycin, corticosteroids, lidocaine, parenteral magnesium, polymyxin B, quinidine, quinine, trimethaphan** may prolong neuromuscular blockade; **verapamil** increases neuromuscular blockade; DIURETICS may increase or decrease neuromuscular blockade; **lithium** prolongs duration of neuromuscular blockade; NARCOTIC ANALGESICS increase possibility of additive respiratory depression; **succinylcholine** increases onset and depth of neuromuscular blockade; **phenytoin** may cause resistance to or reversal of neuromuscular blockade.

PHARMACOKINETICS Onset: <1 min. **Peak:** 3–5 min. **Duration:** 25–40 min. **Distribution:** Well distributed to tissues and extracellular fluids; crosses placenta; distribution into breast milk unknown. **Metabolism:** Rapid nonenzymatic degradation in bloodstream. **Elimination:** 30–35% excreted in urine, 30–35% in bile. **Half-Life:** Infant, 65 min; child, 41 min, adult, 30–80 min.

NURSING IMPLICATIONS

Assessment & Drug Effects

- Lab tests: Baseline serum electrolytes, acid–base balance, and kidney & liver functions.
- Use peripheral nerve stimulator during and following drug administration to avoid risk of overdosage and to identify residual paralysis during recovery period. This is especially indicated when cautious use of drug is specified.
- Monitor vital signs at least q15min until stable, then every 30 min for the next 2 h. Also monitor airway patency until assured that patient has fully recovered from drug effects. Note rate, depth, and pattern of respirations. Obese patients and patients with myasthenia gravis or other neuromuscular disease may have ventilation problems.
- Evaluate patients for recovery from neuromuscular blocking (curare-like) effects as evidenced by ability to breathe naturally or take deep breaths and cough, to keep eyes open, and to lift head keeping mouth closed and by adequacy of hand grip strength. Notify physician if recovery is delayed.
- Note: Recovery time may be delayed in patients with cardiovascular disease, edematous states, and infants (over seven weeks to 1 year).
- Children 1–10 y may require more frequent dosing and higher doses.
- Antidotes are neostigmine, pyridostigmine, or edrophonium.

VERAPAMIL HYDROCHLORIDE

(ver-ap′a-mill)

Calan, Calan SR, Covera-HS, Isoptin, Isoptin SR, Verelan, Verelan PM

Classifications: CARDIOVASCULAR AGENT; CALCIUM CHANNEL BLOCKER; ANTIARRHYTHMIC

Prototype: Nifedipine
Pregnancy Category: C

AVAILABILITY 40 mg, 80 mg, 120 mg tablets; 120 mg, 180 mg, 240 mg sustained-release tablets; 100 mg, 120 mg, 180 mg, 200 mg, 240 mg, 300 mg sustained-release capsules; 5 mg/2 mL injection

ACTIONS Inhibits calcium ion influx through slow channels into cells of myocardial and arterial smooth muscle. Dilates coronary arteries and arterioles and inhibits coronary artery spasm. Decreases and slows SA and AV node conduction without affecting normal arterial action potential or intraventricular conduction. Associated vasodilation of arterioles decreases total peripheral vascular resistance and reduces arterial BP at rest. May slightly decrease heart rate.

THERAPEUTIC EFFECTS Dilates coronary arteries and inhibits coronary artery spasm, which increases myocardial oxygen delivery and produces an antianginal effect. Also decreases nodal conduction, which results in an antiarrhythmic effect.

V

USES Supraventricular tachyarrhythmias; Prinzmetal's (variant) angina, chronic stable angina; unstable, crescendo or preinfarctive angina and essential hypertension.

UNLABELED USES Paroxysmal supraventricular tachycardia, atrial fibrillation; prophylaxis of migraine headache; and as alternate therapy in manic depression.

CONTRAINDICATIONS Severe hypotension (diastolic <90 mm Hg), cardiogenic shock, cardiomegaly, digitalis toxicity, second- or third-degree AV block; Wolff-Parkinson-White syndrome including atrial flutter and fibrillation; accessory AV pathway, left ventricular dysfunction, severe CHF, sinus node disease, sick sinus syndrome (except in patients with functioning ventricular pacemaker). Safe use during pregnancy (category C), lactation, or in children (oral) is not established.

CAUTIOUS USE Duchenne's muscular dystrophy, myasthenia gravis; hepatic and renal impairment; MI followed by coronary occlusion, aortic stenosis, with digoxin or beta-blockers, in neonates and infants.

ROUTE & DOSAGE

Angina

Adult: **PO** 80 mg q6–8h, may increase up to 320–480 mg/day in divided doses (max dose 480 mg/day). (Note: Covera-HS must be given once daily at bedtime.)

Hypertension

Child: **PO** (dose not well established) 4–8 mg/kd/day t.i.d.
Adult: **PO** 40–80 mg t.i.d. or 90–240 mg sustained-release 1–2 times/day up to 480 mg/day (Note: Covera-HS must be given once daily at bedtime.)

Supraventricular Tachycardia, Atrial Fibrillation

Child: **IV** *<1 y,* 0.1–0.2 mg/kg/dose (not recommended in neonates and infants; if used must have continuous ECG monitor and IV calcium at bedside); *1–15 y,* 0.1–0.3 mg/kg/dose (max dose 5 mg first dose and 10 mg second dose)
Adult: **PO** 240–480 mg/day in divided doses **IV** 5–10 mg IV direct, may repeat in 15–30 min if needed

STORAGE

Store at 15°–30° C (59°–86° F); protect from light.

ADMINISTRATION

Oral

- Give with food to reduce gastric irritation. Do not give with grapefruit juice.
- Capsules can be opened and contents sprinkled on food. Do NOT dissolve or chew capsule contents.
- Give Covera-HS once a day in the evening.
- Do not withdraw abruptly; may increase and extend duration of pain in the angina patient.
- An oral suspension can be compounded by pharmacy.

Intravenous

PREPARE **IV Direct:** Given undiluted or diluted in 5 mL of sterile water for injection. Inspect parenteral drug preparation before administration. Make sure solution is clear and colorless.

ADMINISTER **Direct:** Give a single dose over 2–3 min. If child has low normal BP, give over 3–4 min. Maximum concentration 2.5 mg/mL.

INCOMPATIBILITIES **Solution/Additive: Albumin, aminophylline, amphotericin B, cotrimoxazole, hydralazine. Y-Site: Albumin, amphotericin B cholesteryl complex, ampicillin, mezlocillin, nafcillin, oxacillin, propofol, sodium bicarbonate.**

ADVERSE EFFECTS CNS: Dizziness, vertigo, *headache,* fatigue, sleep disturbances, depression, syncope. **CV:** *Hypotension,* congestive heart failure, bradycardia, severe tachycardia, peripheral edema, <u>AV block</u>. **GI:** Nausea, abdominal discomfort, *constipation,* elevated liver enzymes. **Body as a Whole:** Flushing, pulmonary edema, muscle fatigue, diaphoresis. **Skin:** Pruritus.

DIAGNOSTIC TEST INTERFERENCE Verapamil may cause elevations of serum *AST, ALT, alkaline phosphatase.*

INTERACTIONS Drug: BETA-BLOCKERS increase risk of CHF, bradycardia, or heart block; significantly increased levels of **digoxin** and **carbamazepine** and toxicity; potentiates hypotensive effects of HYPOTENSIVE AGENTS; levels of **lithium** and **cyclosporine** may be increased, increasing their toxicity; **calcium salts** (IV) may antagonize verapamil effects. **Herbal: Hawthorne** may have additive hypotensive effects. **Food: Grapefruit juice** may increase verapamil levels.

PHARMACOKINETICS Absorption: 90% absorbed, but only 25–30% reaches systemic circulation (first-pass metabolism). **Peak:** 1–2 h PO, 4–8 h sustained-release, 5 min IV. **Distribution:** Widely distributed, including CNS; crosses placenta; present in breast milk. **Metabolism:** Metabolized in liver. **Elimination:** 70% excreted in urine; 16% in feces. **Half-Life:** Infant, 4–6.9 h; adult, 2–8 h.

NURSING IMPLICATIONS

Assessment & Drug Effects

- Monitor therapeutic effectiveness. Drug should decrease angina frequency, nitroglycerin consumption, and episodes of ST segment deviation.
- Establish baseline data and periodically monitor: BP and pulse.
- Lab tests: Baseline and periodic liver and kidney functions.
- Instruct patient to remain in recumbent position for at least 1 h after dose is given to diminish subjective effects of transient asymptomatic hypotension that may accompany infusion.
- Monitor for AV block or excessive bradycardia when infusion is given concurrently with digitalis.
- Monitor I&O ratio during IV and early oral maintenance therapy. Renal impairment prolongs duration of action, increasing potential for toxicity and incidence of adverse effects. Advise patient to report gradual weight gain and evidence of edema.

- Monitor ECG continuously during IV administration. Essential because drug action may be prolonged and incidence of adverse reactions is highest during IV administration in patients with impaired kidney function, and patients of small stature.
- Check BP shortly before administration of next dose to evaluate degree of control during early treatment for hypertension.

Patient & Family Education

- Monitor apical pulse in those under 5 and radial pulse before each dose, notify physician of an irregular pulse or one slower than established guideline.
- Adhere to established guidelines for exercise program.
- Do not drive or engage in potentially hazardous activities (biking, skateboarding, sports, etc.) until response to drug is known.
- Decrease intake of caffeine-containing beverage (i.e., cola, coffee, tea, chocolate).
- Change positions slowly from lying down to standing to prevent falls because of drug-related vertigo until tolerance to reduced BP is established.
- Notify physician of easy bruising, petechiae, unexplained bleeding.
- Do not use OTC drugs, especially aspirin, unless they are specifically prescribed by physician.
- Do not breast feed while taking this drug without consulting physician.
- Store this medication out of reach of children.

VINBLASTINE SULFATE

(vin-blast'een)
Velban, Velbe A, VLB
Classifications: ANTINEOPLASTIC; MITOTIC INHIBITOR
Prototype: Vincristine
Pregnancy Category: D

AVAILABILITY 10 mg powder for injection; 1 mg/mL (contains benzyl alcohol) vial

ACTIONS Cell-cycle-specific alkaloid, extracted from periwinkle plant *Vinca rosea*. Arrests mitosis in metaphase by combining with microtubule proteins; may also interfere with other microtubular functions such as phagocytosis and cell mobility. Spectrum of activity is not completely established.
THERAPEUTIC EFFECTS Interferes with nucleic acid synthesis by arresting proliferating cells in metaphase. Exhibits potent myelosuppressive and immunosuppressive properties, but produces less neurotoxicity, in contrast to vincristine.

USES Palliative treatment of Hodgkin's disease and non-Hodgkin's lymphomas, choriocarcinoma, lymphosarcoma, neuroblastoma, mycosis fungoides, advanced testicular germinal cell cancer, histiocytosis, and other malignancies resistant to other chemotherapy. Used singly or in combination with other chemotherapeutic drugs.

CONTRAINDICATIONS Leukopenia, bacterial infection, pregnancy (category D), lactation, men and women of childbearing potential, patients with cachexia or skin ulcers.

CAUTIOUS USE Malignant cell infiltration of bone marrow; obstructive jaundice, hepatic impairment; history of gout; use of small amount of drug for long periods; use in eyes, neonates (contains benzyl alcohol).

ROUTE & DOSAGE

Antineoplastic

Child: IV 2.5 mg/m^2 infused over 1 min every week, may increase up to 12.5 mg/m^2 if tolerated

Hodgkin's Disease

Child: IV 2.5–6 mg/m^2/day once every 1–2 wk for 3–6 wk (max dose 12.5 mg/m^2)

Histocytosis

Child: IV Histocytosis 0.4 mg/kg once every 7–10 days

Germ Cell Tumor

Child: IV 0.2 mg/kg on days 1 and 2 every 3 wk cycle × 4 cycles
Adult: IV 3.7 mg/m^2 infused over 1 min every week, may increase up to 18.5 mg/m^2 if tolerated
Reduced dosages required with hepatic impairment.

STORAGE

Store in refrigerator. Refrigerate reconstituted solution in tight, light-resistant containers up to 30 days without loss of potency.

ADMINISTRATION

Intravenous

Must be given under care and direction of pediatric oncology specialist. Use recommended handling techniques for hazardous medications (see Part I).

PREPARE **Direct:** Add 10 mL NS to 10 mg of drug (yields 1 mg/mL). Do not use other diluents. Avoid contact with eyes. Severe irritation and persisting corneal changes may occur. Flush immediately and thoroughly with copious amounts of water. Wash both eyes; do not assume one eye escaped contamination.

ADMINISTER **Direct:** Drug is usually injected into tubing of running IV infusion of NS or D5W over period of 1 min at concentration of 1 mg/mL. Stop injection promptly if extravasation occurs. Use applications of moderate heat and local injection of hyaluronidase to help disperse extravasated drug. Restart infusion in another vein. Observe injection site for sloughing.

INCOMPATIBILITIES **Solution/Additive: Furosemide, heparin. Y-Site: Cefepime, furosemide.**

ADVERSE EFFECTS Body as a Whole: Fever, weight loss, muscular pains, weakness, parotid gland pain and tenderness, tumor site pain,

V

Raynaud's phenomenon. **CNS:** Mental depression, peripheral neuritis, numbness and paresthesias of tongue and extremities, loss of deep tendon reflexes, headache, convulsions. **GI:** Vesiculation of mouth, stomatitis, pharyngitis, anorexia, *nausea, vomiting,* diarrhea, ileus, abdominal pain, constipation, rectal bleeding, hemorrhagic enterocolitis, bleeding of old peptic ulcer. **Hematologic:** Leukopenia, thrombocytopenia and anemia. **Skin:** *Alopecia (reversible),* vesiculation, photosensitivity, phlebitis, cellulitis, and sloughing following extravasation (at injection site). **Urogenital:** Urinary retention, *hyperuricemia,* aspermia. **Respiratory:** Bronchospasm.

INTERACTIONS Drug: Mitomycin may cause acute shortness of breath and severe bronchospasm; may decrease **phenytoin** levels; ALFA INTERFERONS, **erythromycin, itraconazole,** may increase vinblastine toxicity; may impair immune response to VACCINES.

PHARMACOKINETICS Distribution: Concentrates in liver, platelets, and leukocytes; poor penetration of blood–brain barrier. **Metabolism:** Partially metabolized in liver. **Elimination:** Excreted in feces and urine. **Half-Life:** 24 h.

NURSING IMPLICATIONS

Assessment & Drug Effects

- Lab tests: Monitor WBC count. Recovery from leukopenic nadir occurs usually within 7–14 days. With high doses, total leukocyte count may not return to normal for 3 wk.
- Do not administer drug unless WBC count has returned to at least 4000/mm^3, even if 7 days have passed.
- Be alert for and report signs of infection such as respiratory infections, aching, rashes, gastrointestinal distress, etc. Assess immunization status prior to beginning therapy in order to be alert for disease that poses risk.
- Monitor for unexplained bruising or bleeding, which should be promptly reported, even though thrombocyte reduction seldom occurs unless patient has had prior treatment with other antineoplastics.
- Adverse reactions seldom persist beyond 24 h with exception of epilation, leukopenia, and neurologic adverse effects.
- Monitor bowel elimination pattern and bowel sounds to recognize severe constipation or paralytic ileus. A stool softener may be necessary.
- Inspect skin surfaces over pressure areas daily if patient is not ambulating. Note condition of skin of older adults especially.
- Stop drug if oral tissues break down.
- Do not give IM or subcutaneously; very irritating to tissues. Intrathecal injections may cause death.

Patient & Family Education

- Keep all appointments so that course of treatment is not interrupted.
- Be aware that temporary mental depression sometimes occurs on second or third day after treatment begins.
- Inform patient that alopecia may occur.

- Avoid exposure to infection (crowds and other ill children), injury to skin or mucous membranes, and excessive physical stress, especially during leukocyte nadir period. Report signs of infection.
- Notify physician promptly about onset of symptoms of agranulocytosis (see Appendix D-1). Do not delay seeking appropriate treatment.
- Avoid exposure to sunlight unless protected with sunscreen lotion (SPF >12) and clothing.
- Do not get pregnant.
- Do not breast feed while taking this drug.

VINCRISTINE SULFATE ☻
(vin-kris′teen)
Oncovin, VCR
Classifications: ANTINEOPLASTIC; MITOTIC INHIBITOR
Pregnancy Category: D

AVAILABILITY 1 mg/mL injection

ACTIONS Cell-cycle-specific vinca alkaloid (obtained from periwinkle plant *Vinca rosea*); analog of vinblastine. Arrests mitosis at metaphase, thereby, inhibiting cell division. Antineoplastic mechanism unclear.
THERAPEUTIC EFFECTS In contrast to vinblastine, exhibits relatively low toxic effect on normal cells and thus produces minimal myelosuppression; however, neurologic and neuromuscular effects are more severe.

USES Acute lymphoblastic and other leukemias, Hodgkin's disease, lymphosarcoma, neuroblastoma, Wilms' tumor, lung and breast cancer, reticular cell carcinoma, and osteogenic and other sarcomas.
UNLABELED USES Idiopathic thrombocytopenic purpura, alone or adjunctively with other antineoplastics.

CONTRAINDICATIONS Obstructive jaundice; pregnancy (category D), lactation, men and women of childbearing potential; patient with demyelinating form of Charcot-Marie-Tooth syndrome.
CAUTIOUS USE Leukopenia; preexisting neuromuscular disease; hypertension; infection; patients receiving drugs with neurotoxic potential.

ROUTE & DOSAGE

Antineoplastic
Child: **IV** ≤10 kg or body surface <1 m², 0.05 mg/kg/dose at weekly intervals (max single dose 2 mg); >10 kg or body surface ≥1 m², 1–2 mg/m² at weekly intervals (max single dose 2 mg)
Adult: **IV** 1.4 mg/m² (max 2 mg/dose) at weekly intervals

STORAGE
Store powder in refrigerator in light-resistant containers. Refrigerate reconstituted solution up to 14–30 days without loss of potency (check manufacturer's recommendations).

ADMINISTRATION

Must be given under care and direction of pediatric oncology specialist. Use recommended handling techniques for hazardous medications (see Part I).

Intravenous

PREPARE Direct: Reconstitute with provided solution (bacteriostatic NaCl), sterile water, or NS to concentrations of 0.01 to 1.0 mg/mL. Note: Vincristine is available in solution form, which does not require reconstitution. Avoid contact with eyes. Severe irritation and persisting corneal changes may occur. Flush immediately and thoroughly with copious amounts of water. Wash both eyes; do not assume one eye escaped contamination.

ADMINISTER Direct: Drug is usually injected into tubing of running infusion over a 1-min period. Stop injection promptly if extravasation occurs. Use applications of moderate heat and local injection of hyaluronidase to help disperse extravasated drug. Restart infusion in another vein. Observe injection site for sloughing.

INCOMPATIBILITIES Solution/Additive: Furosemide. Y-Site: Cefepime, furosemide, idarubicin, sodium bicarbonate.

ADVERSE EFFECTS CNS: *Peripheral neuropathy,* neuritic pain, *paresthesias, especially of hands and feet;* foot and hand drop, sensory loss, athetosis, ataxia, loss of deep tendon reflexes, muscle atrophy, dysphagia, weakness in larynx and extrinsic eye muscles, ptosis, diplopia, mental depression. **Special Senses:** Optic atrophy with blindness; transient cortical blindness, ptosis, diplopia, photophobia. **GI:** Stomatitis, pharyngitis, anorexia, nausea, vomiting, diarrhea, abdominal cramps, *severe constipation (upper-colon impaction), paralytic ileus, (especially in children),* rectal bleeding; hepatotoxicity. **Urogenital:** Urinary retention, polyuria, dysuria, SIADH (high urinary sodium excretion, hyponatremia, dehydration, hypotension); uric acid nephropathy. **Skin:** Urticaria, rash, *alopecia,* cellulitis and phlebitis following extravasation (at injection site). **Body as a Whole:** Convulsions with hypertension, malaise, fever, headache, pain in parotid gland area, weight loss. **Metabolic:** Hyperuricemia, hyperkalemia. **CV:** Hypertension, hypotension. **Respiratory:** Bronchospasm.

INTERACTIONS Drug: Mitomycin may cause acute shortness of breath and severe bronchospasm; may decrease **digoxin, phenytoin** levels; may impair immune response to VACCINES.

PHARMACOKINETICS Distribution: Concentrates in liver, platelets, and leukocytes; poor penetration of blood–brain barrier. **Metabolism:** Partially metabolized in liver. **Elimination:** Excreted primarily in feces. **Half-Life:** 10–155 h.

NURSING IMPLICATIONS

Assessment & Drug Effects

- Be alert for report signs of infection such as respiratory infections, aching, rashes, gastrointestinal distress, etc. Assess immunization status prior to beginning therapy in order to be alert for diseases that pose risk.

- Monitor I&O ratio and pattern, BP, and temperature daily.
- Weigh patient under standard conditions weekly or more often if ordered. In the presence of edema or ascites, patient's ideal weight is used to determine dosage. Report a steady gain or sudden weight change to physician.
- Lab tests: Monitor serum electrolytes and CBC with differential. Complete bone marrow remission in leukemia varies widely and may not occur for as long as 100 days after therapy is started.
- Be aware that neuromuscular adverse effects, most apt to appear in the patient with preexisting neuromuscular disease, usually disappear after 6 wk of treatment. Children are especially susceptible to neuromuscular adverse effects.
- Assess for hand muscular weakness, and check deep-tendon reflexes (depression of Achilles reflex is the earliest sign of neuropathy). Also observe for and report promptly: Mental depression, ptosis, double vision, hoarseness, paresthesias, neuritic pain, and motor difficulties.
- Provide special protection against infection or injury during leukopenic days. Leukopenia occurs in a significant number of patients; leukocyte count in children usually reaches nadir on fourth day and begins to rise on fifth day after drug administration.
- Avoid use of rectal thermometer or intrusive tubing to prevent injury to rectal mucosa.
- Do not give IM or subcutaneously; very irritating to tissues. Intrathecal injections may cause death.
- Check patient's ability to ambulate and supply support if necessary. Walking may be impaired.
- Take care to distinguish between the depression associated with realization of neoplastic disease and that which is drug induced.

Patient & Family Education
- Avoid exposure to persons with infectious diseases. Report signs of infection.
- Notify physician promptly of stomach, bone, or joint pain, and swelling of lower legs and ankles.
- Start a prophylactic regimen against constipation and paralytic ileus (adequate fluids, high-fiber diet, laxatives) at beginning of treatment and report changes in bowel habit to health care providers as soon as manifested (paralytic ileus is most likely to occur in young children).
- Reversible hair loss is reportedly the most common adverse reaction and may persist for the duration of therapy. Regrowth may start before end of treatment. This is a distressing adverse effect because the scalp hair will drop out in large clumps.
- Do not get pregnant.
- Do not breast feed while taking this drug.

VITAMIN A
(vye′ta-min A)
Aquasol A, Del-Vi-A
Classification: VITAMIN
Pregnancy Category: A (X if dose exceeds RDA recommendations)

AVAILABILITY 5,000 international units tablets; 10,000 international units, 15,000 international units, 25,000 international units capsules; 50,000 international units/mL injection

ACTIONS Essential for normal growth and development of bones and teeth, for integrity of epithelial and mucosal surfaces, and for synthesis of visual purple necessary for visual adaptation to the dark. Synthetic fat-soluble vitamin available for clinical use as retinol or retinol esters. Formulation includes vitamin A as well as its precursors.
THERAPEUTIC EFFECTS Replacement therapy using Aquasol A. Used also to stimulate healing of cortisone-retarded wounds when applied topically.

USES Vitamin A deficiency and as dietary supplement during periods of increased requirements, such as pregnancy, lactation, infancy, and infections. Used as replacement therapy in conditions that affect absorption, mobilization, or storage of vitamin A (e.g., steatorrhea, severe biliary obstruction, liver cirrhosis, total gastrectomy). Used in skin disorders (e.g., folliculosis keratosis [Darier's disease], psoriasis); however, other retinoids are being preferentially selected. Also used as a screening test for fat malabsorption.

CONTRAINDICATIONS History of sensitivity to vitamin A or to any ingredient in formulation, hypervitaminosis A, oral administration to patients with malabsorption syndrome. Safe use in amounts exceeding 6000 international units during pregnancy (category A [category X if >RDA]) is not established.
CAUTIOUS USE Women on oral contraceptives, avoid use in neonates lactation (high doses).

ROUTE & DOSAGE

Severe Deficiency

Child: **PO/IM** *>1–8 y,* 5000 international units/kg/day × 5 days or until recovery occurs
Child 8 y/Adult: **PO** 500,000 international units/day for 3 days followed by 50,000 international units day for 2 wk, then 10,000–20,000 international units/day for 2 mo **IM** 50,000–100,000 international units/day for 3 days followed by 50,000 international units/day for 2 wk

Dietary Supplement

Infants/Child <6 mo: **PO** 1500 international units daily, *>6 mo–3 y* 1500–2000 international units daily, *4–6 y* 2500 international units daily, *7–10 y* 3300–3500 international units daily
Adult: 4000–5000 international units daily

STORAGE
Store at 15°–30° C (59°–86° F) in tightly closed, light-resistant containers.

ADMINISTRATION
Oral
- Give on an empty stomach or following food or milk if GI upset occurs.

V

ADVERSE EFFECTS CNS: Irritability, headache, intracranial hypertension (pseudotumor cerebri), increased intracranial pressure, <u>bulging fontanelles</u>, papilledema, exophthalmos, miosis, nystagmus, Visual disturbances. **Metabolic:** Hypervitaminosis A syndrome (malaise, lethargy, abdominal discomfort, anorexia, vomiting), hypercalcemia. **Musculoskeletal:** Slow growth; deep, tender, hard lumps (subperiosteal thickening) over radius, tibia, occiput; migratory arthralgia; retarded growth; premature closure of epiphyses. **Skin:** Gingivitis, lip fissures, excessive sweating, drying or cracking of skin, pruritus, increase in skin pigmentation, massive desquamation, brittle nails, alopecia. **Urogenital:** Hypomenorrhea, **GI:** Hepatosplenomegaly, vomiting, diarrhea, jaundice. **Endocrine:** Polydipsia, polyurea. **Hematologic:** Leukopenia, hypoplastic anemias, vitamin A plasma levels >1200 international units/dL, elevations of sedimentation rate and prothrombin time. **Body as a Whole:** <u>Anaphylaxis, death</u> (after IV use).

DIAGNOSTIC TEST INTERFERENCE Vitamin A may falsely increase *serum cholesterol* determinations *(Zlatkis-Zak reaction);* may falsely elevate *bilirubin* determination (with *Ehrlich's reagent*).

INTERACTIONS Drug: Mineral oil, cholestyramine may decrease absorption of vitamin A.

PHARMACOKINETICS Absorption: Readily absorbed from GI tract in presence of bile salts, pancreatic lipase, and dietary fat. **Distribution:** Stored mainly in liver; small amounts also found in kidney and body fat; distributed into breast milk. **Metabolism:** Metabolized in liver. **Elimination:** Excreted in feces and urine.

NURSING IMPLICATIONS

Assessment & Drug Effects

- Evaluate dosage with consideration of patient's average daily intake of vitamin A. Take dietary and drug history (e.g., intake of fortified foods, dietary supplements, self-administration or prescription drug sources). Women taking oral contraceptives tend to have significantly high plasma vitamin A levels.
- Monitor therapeutic effectiveness. Vitamin A deficiency is often associated with protein malnutrition as well as other vitamin deficiencies. It may manifest as night blindness, restriction of growth and development, epithelial alterations, susceptibility to infection, abnormal dryness of skin, mouth, and eyes (xerophthalmia) progressing to keratomalacia (ulceration and necrosis of cornea and conjunctiva), and urinary tract calculi.

Patient & Family Education

- Avoid use of mineral oil while on vitamin A therapy.
- Notify prescriber of symptoms of overdosage (e.g., nausea, vomiting, anorexia, drying and cracking of skin or lips, headache, loss of hair).
- Do not get pregnant while taking doses >RDA.
- Do not breast feed while taking this drug in high doses without consulting physician.
- Store this medication out of reach of children.

Common adverse effects in *italic;* life-threatening effects <u>underlined</u>; generic names in **bold;** drug classifications in SMALL CAPS; ♣ Canadian drug name; ❷ Prototype drug.

VITAMIN B$_1$
See Thiamine HCl.

VITAMIN B$_2$
See Riboflavin.

VITAMIN B$_3$
See Niacin.

VITAMIN B$_6$
See Pyridoxine.

VITAMIN B$_9$
See Folic acid.

VITAMIN B$_{12}$
See Cyanocobalamin.

VITAMIN B$_{12a}$
See Hydroxocobalamin.

VITAMIN C
See Ascorbic acid.

VITAMIN D
See Calcitriol.

VITAMIN E (TOCOPHEROL)
(vye′ta-min E)
Aquasol E, Vita-Plus E, Vitec
Classification: VITAMIN
Pregnancy Category: A

AVAILABILITY 100 international units, 200 international units, 400 international units, 500 international units, 800 international units tablets; 100 international units, 200 international units, 400 international units, 1000 international units capsules; 15 international units/0.3 mL, 15 international units/30 mL liquid

ACTIONS A group of naturally occurring fat-soluble substances known as tocopherols. Alpha tocopherol, comprising 90% of the tocopherols, is the most biologically potent and has been synthesized. An antioxidant, it prevents peroxidation, a process that gives rise to free radicals (highly reactive chemical structures that damage cell membranes and alter nuclear proteins). **THERAPEUTIC EFFECTS** Prevents cell membrane and protein damage and is essential to the digestion and metabolism of polyunsaturated fats. Maintains the integrity of cell membranes, protects against blood clot formation by decreasing platelet aggregation, enhances vitamin A utilization, and promotes normal growth, development, and tone of muscles. Deficiency causes no specific disease in humans but has been associated with increased susceptibility of RBC to hemolysis.

USES To treat and prevent hemolytic anemia due to vitamin E deficiency in premature neonates; to prevent retrolental fibroplasia secondary to oxygen treatment in neonates, and in treatment of diseases with secondary erythrocyte membrane abnormalities (e.g., sickle cell anemia, and G6PD deficiency and as supplement in malabsorption syndromes). Those with cystic fibrosis. Used in patients on diets containing large amounts of polyunsaturated fats for long periods and in the patient who abruptly discontinues such a diet. Also used topically for dry or chapped skin and minor skin disorders.

UNLABELED USES Muscular dystrophy and a number of other conditions with no conclusive evidence of value. A component of many multivitamin formulations and of topical deodorant preparations as an antioxidant.

CONTRAINDICATIONS No clinically significant contraindications established.

CAUTIOUS USE Large doses may exacerbate iron deficiency anemia.

ROUTE & DOSAGE

1 unit Vitamin E is equal to 1 mg dL alpha-tocopherol acetate.

Recommended Daily Requirement for Healthy Individual

Infant: **PO** *0–6 mo, 4 mg/day; 7–12 mo, 6 mg/day*
Child: **PO** *>1–3 y, 6 mg/day; 4–8 y, 7 mg/day; 9–13 y, 11 mg/day; 14–18 y, 15 mg/day*

Vitamin E Deficiency

Child: **PO** 1 international unit/kg/day (some clinicians recommend for malabsorptive syndromes) given to raise serum tocopherol concentrations to normal ranges in 2 mo
Adult: **PO/IM** 60–75 international units/day

Prophylaxis for Vitamin E Deficiency

Neonate: **PO** 5 international units/day
Child: **PO** 7–10 international units/day
Adult: **PO** 12–15 international units/day

Vitamin E for Cystic Fibrosis

Child: **PO** 5–10 international units/kg/day (max dose 400 international units/day)

STORAGE
Store in tightly closed, light-containers.

ADMINISTRATION

V

Oral

- Give on an empty stomach or following food or milk if GI upset occurs.

ADVERSE EFFECTS Body as a Whole: Skeletal muscle weakness, headache, fatigue (with excessive doses). **GI:** Nausea, diarrhea, intestinal cramps. **Urogenital:** Gonadal dysfunction. **Metabolic:** Increased serum creatine kinase, cholesterol, triglycerides; decreased serum thyroxine and triiodothyronine; increased urinary estrogens, androgens; creatinuria. **Skin:** Sterile abscess, thrombophlebitis, contact dermatitis. **Special Senses:** Blurred vision.

INTERACTIONS Drug: Mineral oil, cholestyramine may decrease absorption of vitamin E; may enhance anticoagulant activity of **warfarin.** Iron may increase levels of vitamin E.

Common adverse effects in *italic;* life-threatening effects underlined; generic names in **bold;** drug classifications in SMALL CAPS; ✦ Canadian drug name; ⦿ Prototype drug.

PHARMACOKINETICS Absorption: 20–60% absorbed from GI tract if fat absorption is normal; enters blood via lymph. **Distribution:** Stored mainly in adipose tissue; crosses placenta. **Metabolism:** Metabolized in liver. **Elimination:** Excreted primarily in bile.

NURSING IMPLICATIONS

Patient & Family Education

- If taking a large dose of iron, the RDA of vitamin E may be increased. Oral doses >200 units/day have been associated with necrotizing entercolitis in low-birth-weight infants.
- Natural sources of vitamin E are found in wheat germ (the richest source) as well as in vegetable oils (sunflower, corn, soybean, cottonseed), green leafy vegetables, nuts, dairy products, eggs, cereals, meat, and liver.
- Store this medication out of reach of children.

WARFARIN SODIUM

(war′far-in)
Coumadin Sodium, Panwarfin, Warfilone ♣
Classifications: BLOOD FORMERS, COAGULATORS, AND ANTICOAGULANTS; ORAL ANTICOAGULANT
Pregnancy Category: D

AVAILABILITY 1 mg, 2 mg, 2.5 mg, 3 mg, 4 mg, 5 mg, 6 mg, 7.5 mg, 10 mg tablets; 5 mg injection product available in the U.S.

ACTIONS Indirectly interferes with blood clotting by depressing hepatic synthesis of vitamin K-dependent coagulation factors: II, VII, IX, and X.
THERAPEUTIC EFFECTS Deters further extension of existing thrombi and prevents new clots from forming. Unlike heparin, its action is cumulative and more prolonged. Warfarin is not cross allergenic with other coumarin derivatives. Does not reverse ischemic tissue damage and has no effect on platelets. Has no effect on already synthesized circulating coagulation factors or on circulating thrombi.

USES Prophylaxis and treatment of deep-vein thrombosis and its extension, pulmonary embolism; treatment of atrial fibrillation with embolization. Also used as adjunct in treatment of coronary occlusion, cerebral transient ischemic attacks (TIAs), and as a prophylactic in patients with prosthetic cardiac valves and atrial fibrillation. Used extensively as rodenticide.

CONTRAINDICATIONS Hemorrhagic tendencies, vitamin C or K deficiency, hemophilia, coagulation factor deficiencies, dyscrasias; active bleeding; open wounds, active peptic ulcer, visceral carcinoma, esophageal varices, malabsorption syndrome; hypertension (diastolic BP >110 mm Hg), cerebral vascular disease; pregnancy (category D); pericarditis with acute MI; severe hepatic or renal disease; continuous tube drainage of any orifice; subacute bacterial endocarditis; recent surgery of brain, spinal cord, or eye; regional or lumbar block anesthesia; threatened abortion; unreliable patients.
CAUTIOUS USE Alcoholism, allergic disorders, during menstruation, lactation, debilitated patients. Endogenous factors that may increase

prothrombin time response (enhance anticoagulant effect): carcinoma, CHF, collagen diseases, hepatic and renal insufficiency, diarrhea, fever, pancreatic disorders, malnutrition, vitamin K deficiency. Endogenous factors that may decrease prothrombin time response (decrease anticoagulant response): edema, hypothyroidism, hyperlipidemia, hypercholesterolemia, chronic alcoholism, hereditary resistance to coumarin therapy.

ROUTE & DOSAGE

Anticoagulant
Child: **PO** 0.1–0.3 mg/kg/day, adjust to maintain INR of 2–3
Adult: **PO/IV** 10–15 mg/day for 2–5 days, then 2–10 mg once/day with dose adjusted to maintain a PT 1.2–2 times control or INR of 2–3

STORAGE

Store at 15°–30° C (59°–86° F). Discard discolored or precipitated solutions. Protect all preparations from light and moisture. Reconstituted solutions are stable at room temperature; discard after 4 h.

ADMINISTRATION

Note: Antidote for bleeding—anticoagulant effect usually is reversed by omitting 1 or more doses of warfarin and by administration of specific antidote phytonadione (vitamin K_1) 2.5–10 mg orally. Physician may advise patient to carry vitamin K_1 at all times, but not to take it until after consultation. If bleeding persists or progresses to a severe level, vitamin K_1 5–25 mg IV is given, or a fresh whole blood transfusion may be necessary.

Oral
- Give tablet whole or crushed with fluid of patient's choice.

Intravenous

PREPARE **Direct:** Add 2.7 mL of sterile water for injection to 5-mg vial, which gives a solution of 2 mg/mL warfarin powder.
ADMINISTER **Direct:** Give immediately by direct IV 2 mg/mL over 1–2 min.
INCOMPATIBILITIES **Solution/Additive: Ammonium chloride, 5% dextrose, Ringer's lactate,** AMINOGLYCOSIDES, **ascorbic acid, cimetidine, ciprofloxacin, epinephrine, metaraminol, metronidazole, oxytocin, promazine, tetracycline, vancomycin, vitamin B complex with C.**

ADVERSE EFFECTS Body as a Whole: <u>Major</u> or minor <u>hemorrhage</u> from any <u>tissue or organ</u>; hypersensitivity (dermatitis, urticaria, pruritus, fever). **GI:** Anorexia, nausea, vomiting, abdominal cramps, diarrhea, steatorrhea, stomatitis. **Other:** Increased serum transaminase levels, hepatitis, jaundice, burning sensation of feet, transient hair loss. **Overdosage:** <u>Internal</u> or <u>external bleeding, paralytic ileus; skin necrosis</u> of toes (purple toes syndrome), tip of nose, buttocks, thighs, calves, female breast, abdomen, and other fat-rich areas.

DIAGNOSTIC TEST INTERFERENCE Warfarin (coumarins) may cause alkaline urine to be red-orange; may enhance ***uric acid*** excretion, cause

Common adverse effects in *italic;* life-threatening effects <u>underlined;</u> generic names in **bold;** drug classifications in SMALL CAPS; ✤ Canadian drug name; ⊘ Prototype drug.

elevation of *serum transaminases,* and may increase *lactic dehydrogenase* activity.

INTERACTIONS Drug: In addition to the drugs listed below, many other drugs have been reported to alter the expected response to warfarin; however, clinical importance of these reports has not been substantiated. The addition or withdrawal of any drug to an established drug regimen should be made cautiously, with more frequent INR determinations than usual and with careful observation of the patient and dose adjustment as indicated. ▪ The following may enhance the anticoagulant effects of warfarin: **Acetohexamide, acetaminophen,** ALKYLATING AGENTS, **allopurinol,** AMINOGLYCOSIDES, **aminosalicylic acid, amiodarone,** ANABOLIC STEROIDS, ANTIBIOTICS (ORAL), ANTIMETABOLITES, ANTIPLATELET DRUGS, **aspirin, asparaginase, capecitabine, celecoxib, chloramphenicol, chlorpropamide, chymotrypsin, cimetidine, clofibrate, co-trimoxazole, danazol, dextran, dextrothyroxine, diazoxide, disulfiram, erythromycin, ethacrynic acid, fluconazole, glucagons, guanethidine,** HEPATOTOXIC DRUGS, **influenza vaccine, isoniazid, itraconazole, ketoconazole,** MAO INHIBITORS, **meclofenamate, mefenamic acid, methyldopa, methylphenidate, metronidazole, miconazole, mineral oil, nalidixic acid, neomycin (oral),** NONSTEROIDAL ANTI-INFLAMMATORY DRUGS, **plicamycin,** POTASSIUM PRODUCTS, **propoxyphene, propylthiouracil, quinidine, quinine, rofecoxib, salicylates, streptokinase, sulindac,** SULFONAMIDES, SULFONYLUREAS, TETRACYCLINES, THIAZIDES, THYROID DRUGS, **tolbutamide, tricyclic antidepressants, urokinase, vitamin E, zileuton.** ▪ The following may increase or decrease the anticoagulant effects of warfarin: **Alcohol** (acute intoxication may increase, chronic alcoholism may decrease effects), **chloral hydrate,** DIURETICS. ▪ The following may decrease the anticoagulant effects of warfarin: **barbiturates, carbamazepine, cholestyramine,** CORTICOSTEROIDS, **corticotropin, ethchlorvynol, glutethimide, griseofulvin,** LAXATIVES, **mercaptopurine,** ORAL CONTRACEPTIVES, **rifampin, spironolactone, vitamin C, vitamin K. Herbal:** Capsicum, celery, chamomile, clove, Devil's claw, Dong quai, echinacea, fenugreek, feverfew, garlic, ginger, ginkgo, horse chestnut, licorice root, passion flower herb, tumeric, willow bark may increase risk of bleeding; ginseng, green tea, St. John's wort may decrease effectiveness of warfarin. **Food:** Effects of warfarin may be decreased by diet high in vitamin K-containing foods.

PHARMACOKINETICS Absorption: Well absorbed from GI tract. **Onset:** 2–7 days. **Peak:** 0.5–3 days. **Distribution:** 97% protein bound; crosses placenta. **Metabolism:** Metabolized in liver. **Elimination:** Excreted in urine and bile. **Half-Life:** 0.5–3 days.

NURSING IMPLICATIONS

Assessment & Drug Effects

▪ Determine PT/INP prior to initiation of therapy and then daily until maintenance dosage is established.

▪ Obtain a CAREFUL medication history prior to start of therapy and whenever altered responses to therapy require interpretation; extremely IMPORTANT because many drugs interfere with the activity of anticoagulant drugs (see INTERACTIONS).

- Adjust dose to maintain PT at 1-½–2-½ times the control (12–15 sec), or 15–35% of normal prothrombin activity, or an INR of 2–4 depending on diagnosis.
- Lab tests: For maintenance dosage, PT/INR determinations at 1–4-wk intervals depending on patient's response; periodic urinalyses, stool guaiac, and liver function tests. Blood samples should be drawn at 12–18 h after last dose (optimum).
- Note: Patients at greatest risk of hemorrhage include those whose PT/INR are difficult to regulate, who have an aortic valve prosthesis, who are receiving long-term anticoagulant therapy, and older adult and debilitated patients.

Patient & Family Education

- Understand that bleeding can occur even though PT/INR are within therapeutic range. Stop drug and notify physician immediately if bleeding or signs of bleeding appear: Blood in urine, bright red or black tarry stools, vomiting of blood, bleeding with tooth brushing, blue or purple spots on skin or mucous membrane, round pinpoint purplish red spots (often occur in ankle areas), nosebleed, bloody sputum; chest pain; abdominal or lumbar pain or swelling, profuse menstrual bleeding, pelvic pain; severe or continuous headache, faintness or dizziness; prolonged oozing from any minor injury (e.g., nicks from shaving, use electric razor while on this drug).
- Stop drug and report immediately any symptoms of hepatitis (dark urine, itchy skin, jaundice, abdominal pain, light stools) or hypersensitivity reaction (see Appendix D-1).
- Avoid brand interchange, take drug at same time each day, and do NOT alter dose.
- Notify physician if there is an unusual increase in menstrual bleeding (slightly increased or prolonged). Note: PT/INR are checked at least monthly in menstruating women.
- Risk of bleeding is increased for up to 1 mo after receiving the influenza vaccine.
- Fever, prolonged hot weather, malnutrition, and diarrhea lengthen PT/INR (enhanced anticoagulant effect).
- A high-fat diet, sudden increase in vitamin K-rich foods (cabbage, cauliflower, broccoli, asparagus, lettuce, turnip greens, onions, spinach, kale, fish, liver), coffee or green tea (caffeine), or by tube feedings with high vitamin K content shorten PT/INR.
- Maintain a well-balanced diet and avoid excess intake of alcohol.
- Inform dentist or any new physician about anticoagulant therapy and duration of treatment.

- Use a soft toothbrush and to floss teeth gently with waxed floss.
- Use barrier contraceptive measures; if you become pregnant while on anticoagulant therapy the fetus is at great potential risk of congenital malformations.
- Do not take any other prescription or OTC drug unless specifically approved by physician or pharmacist. Carry medical identification at all times. It needs to indicate medical diagnosis, medication(s), physician's name, address, and telephone number.
- Do not breast feed while taking this drug without consulting physician.
- Store this medication out of reach of children.

XYLOMETAZOLINE HYDROCHLORIDE
(zye-loe-met-az'oh-leen)
Neo-Synephrine II, Otrivin, Otrivin Pediatric Nasal
Classifications: NASAL DECONGESTANT; VASOCONSTRICTOR
Prototype: Naphazoline
Pregnancy Category: C

AVAILABILITY 0.05%, 0.1% nasal solution

ACTIONS Markedly constricts dilated arterioles of nasal membrane. Has little or no beta-adrenergic activity. Structurally related to naphazoline.
THERAPEUTIC EFFECTS Decreases fluid exudate and mucosal engorgement associated with rhinitis and may open up obstructed eustachian ostia in patient with ear inflammation.

USES Temporary relief of nasal congestion associated with common cold, sinusitis, acute and chronic rhinitis, and hay fever and other allergies.

CONTRAINDICATIONS Sensitivity to adrenergic substances; angle-closure glaucoma; concurrent therapy with MAO inhibitors or tricyclic antidepressants; lactation, and infants. Safe use during pregnancy (category C) is not established.
CAUTIOUS USE Hypertension; hyperthyroidism; heart disease, diabetes mellitus, and children.

ROUTE & DOSAGE

Nasal Congestion
Child: Nasal <*6 mo,* 1 drop of 0.05% solution in each nostril q6h (max 3 doses/day); *6 mo–2 y,* 2–3 drops of 0.05% solution in each nostril q8–10h (max 3 doses/day); *2–12 y,* 1 spray or 2–3 drops of 0.05% solution in each nostril q8–10h (max 3 doses/day)
Adult: >*12 y,* nasal 1–2 sprays or 1–2 drops of 0.1% solution in each nostril q8–10h (max 3 doses/day)
Recommended: Do not use longer than 3–5 days.

STORAGE
Store at 15°–30° C (59°–86° F) in a tightly closed, light-resistant container.

ADMINISTRATION
Instillation
- Have patient clear each nostril gently before administering spray or drops.
- For younger child, use a bulb syringe to clear nostrils as necessary prior to administration.
- May use normal saline drops to clear dried mucus from nares prior to this drug's usage.
- Spray: Only use if child can follow directions for usage. Do not shake container. Hold tube vertically (spray end up) so that solution is delivered in a fine spray. Head should be erect; spray into each nostril; 3–5 min later, clear (blow) nose thoroughly.

- Drops: Patient should be in a lateral, head-low position to permit application of drops to lower nostril surface. Have patient remain in this position for 5 min, then apply drops to opposite nostril surface in same manner; or drops may be instilled with patient in reclining position with head tilted back as far as possible. Refer to Techniques of Administration section in Part I on how to give nasal medications to children.

ADVERSE EFFECTS All: Usually mild and infrequent; local stinging, burning, dryness and ulceration, sneezing, headache, insomnia, drowsiness. **With excessive use:** *Rebound nasal congestion* and vasodilation, tremulousness, hypertension, palpitations, tachycardia, arrhythmia, somnolence, sedation, coma.

INTERACTIONS Drug: May cause increase BP with **guanethidine, methyldopa,** MAO INHIBITORS; PHENOTHIAZINES may decrease effectiveness of nasal decongestant.

PHARMACOKINETICS Onset: 5–10 min. **Duration:** 5–6 h.

NURSING IMPLICATIONS

Assessment & Drug Effects
- Evaluate for development of rebound congestion (see ADVERSE EFFECTS).

Patient & Family Education
- Teach parents proper nasal instillation for the age of their child. Nasal instillation of drops may produce sensations of difficulty breathing or tickling, or cause a bad taste.
- Prevent contamination of nasal solution and spread of infection by rinsing dropper and tip of nasal spray in hot water after each use; restrict use to the individual patient
- Note: Prolonged use can cause rebound congestion and chemical rhinitis. Do NOT exceed prescribed dosage and report to physician if drug fails to provide relief within 3–4 days.
- Do NOT self-medicate children with OTC drugs, sprays, or drops without physician's prescriptions.
- Only use sprays with a child >2–5 y who can cooperate with usage instructions.
- Note: Excessive use by a child may lead to profound CNS depression and nasal irritation
- Do not breast feed while taking this drug.
- Store this medication out of reach of children.

ZAFIRLUKAST 🅟🅡
(za-fir-lu′kast)
Accolate
Classifications: BRONCHODILATOR (RESPIRATORY SMOOTH MUSCLE RELAXANT); LEUKOTRIENE RECEPTOR ANTAGONIST
Pregnancy Category: B

Z

AVAILABILITY 10 mg, 20 mg tablets

ACTIONS Selective peptide leukotriene receptor antagonist (LTRA) of leukotriene D_4 and E_4, thus inhibiting bronchoconstriction. Leukotriene production and receptor affinity have been correlated with the pathogenesis of asthma.

THERAPEUTIC EFFECTS Zafirlukast helps to prevent the signs and symptoms of asthma including airway edema, smooth muscle constriction, and altered cellular activity due to inflammation.

USES Only used as prophylaxis and chronic treatment of asthma in children >5. Used in combination with short acting inhaled bronchodilator and inhaled corticosteroid.

CONTRAINDICATIONS Hypersensitivity to zafirlukast, lactation, acute asthma attacks.
CAUTIOUS USE Hepatic impairment, pregnancy (category B). Safety and effectiveness in children <5 y are not established.

ROUTE & DOSAGE

Asthma
Child: **PO** *5–11 y,* 10 mg twice daily; *>12 y,* 20 mg twice daily

STORAGE
Store at 20°–25° C (68°–77° F); protect from light and moisture.

ADMINISTRATION
Oral
- Give 1 h before or 2 h after meals.

ADVERSE EFFECTS Body as a Whole: Generalized pain, asthenia, myalgia, fever, back pain. **CNS:** *Headache,* dizziness. **GI:** Nausea, diarrhea, abdominal pain, vomiting, dyspepsia; liver dysfunction, increased liver function tests. **Other:** <u>Churg-Strauss syndrome</u> (fever, muscle aches and pains, weight loss).

INTERACTIONS Drug: May increase prothrombin time (PT) in patients on **warfarin; erythromycin,** decreases bioavailability of zafirlukast; **aspirin** increases plasma levels of zafirlukast. **Food:** Food decreases bioavailability.

PHARMACOKINETICS Absorption: Rapidly absorbed from GI tract, bioavailability significantly reduced by food. **Onset:** 1 wk. **Peak:** 2.5 h. **Distribution:** >99% protein bound; secreted into breast milk. **Metabolism:** Metabolized in liver via cytochrome P-450 2C9 (CYP2C9) and possibly CYP3A4. **Elimination:** 90% excreted in feces, 10% in urine. **Half-Life:** 10 h.

NURSING IMPLICATIONS

Assessment & Drug Effects
- Assess respiratory status and airway function regularly.
- Lab tests: Periodic liver function tests.

Z

- Monitor closely phenytoin level with concurrent phenytoin therapy.
- Monitor closely PT and INR with concurrent warfarin therapy.

Patient & Family Education

- Taking medication as directed, even during symptom-free periods.
- Note: Drug is not intended to treat acute episodes of asthma.
- Report S&S of hepatic toxicity or flu-like symptoms to physician. Follow-up lab work is very important.
- Notify physician immediately if condition worsens while using prescribed doses of all antiasthmatic medications.
- Do not breast feed while taking this drug.
- Store this medication out of reach of children.

ZALCITABINE (DDC, DIDEOXYCYTIDINE)

(zal-cit'a-been)
Hivid
Classifications: ANTI-INFECTIVE; ANTIVIRAL
Prototype: Zidovudine
Pregnancy Category: C

AVAILABILITY 0.375 mg, 0.75 mg tablets; 0.1 mg/mL oral solution available from manufacturer's compassionate use program

ACTIONS A synthetic pyrimidine nucleotide that inhibits the replication of HIV by inhibition of viral DNA synthesis. It appears to act by becoming incorporated into the DNA chains of the HIV virus during viral replication.

THERAPEUTIC EFFECTS Zalcitabine is able to decrease the HIV viral load by its antiviral properties.

USES Combination therapy with triple-drug antiviral therapy for AIDS. Second-line monotherapy for AIDS.
UNLABELED USES Can be used in children.

CONTRAINDICATIONS Hypersensitivity to zalcitabine.
CAUTIOUS USE Moderate to severe neuropathy; history of pancreatitis; CHF, cardiomyopathy; renal impairment, hepatic impairment, alcohol abuse; pregnancy (category C). It is not known if zalcitabine is excreted in breast milk. Safety and effectiveness in HIV-infected children <13 y are not established.

ROUTE & DOSAGE

Combination Therapy for HIV

Child: >6 mo – 13 y, given under protocol conditions: **PO** 0.015–0.04 mg/kg q8h for 8 wk, after 8 wk of monotherapy an alternating regimen of zalcitabine and zidovudine is begun (4-wk cycle of zidovudine for 3 wk and zalcitabine for 1 wk)
Adult: >13 y, **PO** 0.75 mg q8h given with zidovudine 200 mg q8h

STORAGE
Store at 15°–30° C (59°–86° F) in tightly closed container.

ADMINISTRATION

Oral

- Give on an empty stomach. Tablet can be crushed.

ADVERSE EFFECTS CV: May exacerbate existing CHF and cardiomyopathy. **CNS:** _Peripheral neuropathy,_ numbness. **GI:** Diarrhea, mouth and esophageal ulcers, pancreatitis, may exacerbate existing hepatic dysfunction. **Hematologic:** Neutropenia, thrombocytopenia. **Skin:** _Transient symptom complex of cutaneous eruptions (maculovesicular in nature), fever, malaise, and aphthous mouth ulcers,_ arthralgia, urticaria, anaphylaxis.

INTERACTION Drug: May cause additive peripheral neuropathy with **didanosine.** Other drugs have the potential to cause peripheral neuropathy: **chloramphenicol, cisplatin, dapsone, disurlfiram, ethionamide, glutethimide, gold, hydralazine, isoniazide, metronidazole, nitrofurantoin, phenytoin, ribavirin, vincristine.** Bioavailability of drug may be decreased with use of **antacids** containing **aluminum** and **magnesium.** Because **aminoglycosides, amphotericin B** and **foscarnet** decrease renal clearance, these drugs could contribute to peripheral neuropathy. **Pentamidine** and other drugs associated with pancreatitis should not be used concomitantly with this drug.

PHARMACOKINETICS Absorption: Readily absorbed from GI tract. **Onset:** 2 wk. **Half-Life:** 1.2–1.8 h. **Distribution:** Distributes somewhat into CSF. **Metabolism:** Does not appear to be metabolized. **Elimination:** 62% excreted unchanged in urine.

NURSING IMPLICATIONS

Assessment & Drug Effects

- Discontinue drug and promptly notify physician if patient experiences numbness, tingling, burning, or pain in extremities (especially in the feet or shooting pains in legs lasting >1 h).
- Lab tests: Baseline and periodic tests for CBC, differential, CD_4+ T-cell counts, serum amylase, serum glucose, triglycerides, and serum calcium levels. Monitor closely in patients with history of pancreatitis or elevated serum amylase.
- Report vague abdominal pain, nausea, and vomiting especially if serum glucosides and triglycerides are elevated; may indicate pancreatitis.

Patient & Family Education

- Report to physician promptly S&S of pancreatitis and peripheral neuropathy (see Appendix D-1). These can be life threatening.
- Drug absorption decreased by food; give on an empty stomach.
- Do not use OTC drugs or alcohol while on this drug.
- Monitor for signs of infections.
- Understand that this drug is not a cure for, but may relieve, the symptoms of HIV.
- Use contraception while taking zalcitabine and practice safe sex.

Z

- Do not breast feed while taking this drug without consulting physician.
- Store this medication out of reach of children.

ZANAMIVIR
(zan'a-mi-vir)
Relenza
Classifications: ANTI-INFECTIVE; ANTIVIRAL
Prototype: Acyclovir
Pregnancy Category: B

AVAILABILITY 5 mg/Rotadisk blister

ACTIONS Inhibitor of influenza A and B viral enzyme; does not permit the release of newly formed viruses from the surface of the infected cells.
THERAPEUTIC EFFECTS Indicated by relief of flu-like symptoms. The inhibition of the viral neuroaminidase enzyme prevents the viral spread across the mucous lining of the respiratory tract, and inhibits the replication of influenza A and B virus.

USES Uncomplicated acute influenza in patients symptomatic <2 days.

CONTRAINDICATIONS Hypersensitivity to zanamivir.
CAUTIOUS USE Concurrent use of inhaled medication with inhaled zanamivir; asthma or underlying respiratory disease, pregnancy (category B), lactation. Safety and efficacy in children <7 y are unknown.

ROUTE & DOSAGE

Acute Influenza
Child >7 y/Adult: **Inhaled** 2 inhalations (one 5 mg blister/inhalation) b.i.d. (approximately 12 h apart) times 5 days

STORAGE
Store at 25° C (77° F).

ADMINISTRATION
Inhalation
- Initiate within 48 h of onset of flu-like symptoms.
- See Techniques of Administration section in Part I for use of disk inhaler.
- Give scheduled inhaled bronchodilator before zanamivir.

ADVERSE EFFECTS Body as a Whole: Headache. **CNS:** Dizziness. **GI:** Nausea, diarrhea, vomiting. **Respiratory:** Nasal symptoms, bronchitis, cough, sinusitis; ear, nose, throat infection.

INTERACTIONS Drug: No clinically significant interactions established.

PHARMACOKINETICS Absorption: 4–17% of inhaled dose is systemically absorbed. **Peak:** 1–2 h. **Distribution:** <10% protein bound. **Metabolism:** Not metabolized. **Elimination:** Excreted in urine. **Half-Life:** 2.5–5.1 h.

Z

NURSING IMPLICATIONS

Patient & Family Education

- Start within 48 h of onset of flu-like symptoms for most effective response.
- Bronchospasm may occur with underlying respiratory disease.
- Use any scheduled inhaled bronchodilator first; then use zanamivir.
- Can only be used with child who can follow directions for diskhaler's usage. Instruct family how to use diskhaler.
- This drug does not reduce risk of influenza virus transmission.
- Do not breast feed while taking this drug.
- Store this medication out of reach of children.

ZIDOVUDINE (AZIDOTHYMIDINE, AZT) ⓟⓡ
(zye-doe′vyoo-deen)
Retrovir, Apo-Zidovudine ♣ , Novo-AZT ♣
Classifications: ANTI-INFECTIVE; ANTIVIRAL
Pregnancy Category: C

AVAILABILITY 300 mg tablets; 100 mg capsules; 50 mg/5 mL syrup; 10 mg/mL injection

ACTIONS Analog of thymidine (a major nucleoside in DNA). On entering host cell, zidovudine is converted to a triphosphate (the active form) by endogenous thymidine kinase and other cellular enzymes. Appears to act by being incorporated into growing DNA chains by viral reverse transcriptase, thereby terminating viral replication.
THERAPEUTIC EFFECTS Zidovudine has antiviral action against HIV (human immunodeficiency virus), the causative agent of AIDS (acquired immune deficiency syndrome), LAV (lymphadenopathy-associated virus), and ARV (AIDS-associated retrovirus).

USES Patients who are HIV positive and have a CD_4 count ≤500/mm^3, asymptomatic HIV infection, early and late symptomatic HIV disease, prevention of perinatal transfer of HIV during pregnancy.
UNLABELED USES Pediatric patients, postexposure chemoprophylaxis.

CONTRAINDICATIONS Life-threatening allergic reactions to any of the components of the drug. Safe use during pregnancy (category C), lactation is not established.
CAUTIOUS USE Impaired renal or hepatic function, bone marrow depression.

ROUTE & DOSAGE

Symptomatic HIV Infection
Neonate: **PO** 2 mg/kg/dose q6h **IV** 1.5 mg/kg q6h, start within 12 h postdelivery and continute for 6 wk
Child: 3 mo–12 y, **PO** 160 mg/m^2/dose q8h (maximum dosage 200 mg q8h) **Intermittent IV:** 120 mg/m^2 q6h **Continuous IV Infusion:** 20 mg/m^2/h

Z

Adolescent: Some clinicians suggest that adolescents experiencing puberty be dosed as follows. Tanner Stages I–II: Dosed at child (3 mo–12 y) levels; Tanner Stage III females and IV males: Dosed at child (3 mo–12 y) or adult (>12 y) levels; Tanner Stage V: Dosed at adult (>12 y) levels
Adult: **PO** >12 y, 200 mg t.i.d. or 300 mg b.i.d. (600 mg/day)
IV 1 mg/kg q4h

Asymptomatic HIV Infection, Postexposure Prophylaxis

Child >12 y/Adult: **PO** 100 mg q4h while awake, 5 times/day

Prevention of Maternal–Fetal Transmission

Neonate: **PO** 2 mg/kg q6h for 6 wk beginning within 6–12 h after birth
IV 1.5 mg/kg/dose q6h over 60 min, started within 6–12 h after birth, continued until 6 wk of age; protocols are available for premature infants

STORAGE

Store at 15°–25° C (59°–77° F); protect from light unless otherwise directed.

ADMINISTRATION

Oral

- Do not expose capsules and syrup to light during drug preparation.

Intravenous

PREPARE **Intermittent:** Withdraw required dose from vial and dilute with D5W to a concentration not to exceed 4 mg/mL.
ADMINISTER **Intermittent:** Give calculated dose at a constant rate over 60 min; avoid rapid infusion. ■ Do not add drug to colloidal or biological fluids. ■ Dilute drug according to manufacturer's recommendation (4 mg/mL or less), stable for 48 h if refrigerated at 2°–8° C (36°–45° F) or 24 h at 15°–25° C (59°–77° F).

ADVERSE EFFECTS Body as a Whole: *Fever,* dyspnea, *malaise,* weakness, *myalgia,* myopathy. **CNS:** *Headache,* insomnia, dizziness, paresthesias, mild confusion, anxiety, restlessness, agitation. **GI:** *Nausea,* diarrhea, *vomiting, anorexia,* GI pain, lactose acidosis. **Hematologic:** <u>Severe bone marrow depression,</u> <u>granulocytopenia, anemia.</u> **Respiratory:** *Cough, wheezing.* **Skin:** *Rash,* itching, diaphoresis.

INTERACTIONS Drug: Acetaminophen ganciclovir, interferon-alfa may enhance bone marrow suppression; **amphotericin B, aspirin, atovaquone, dapsone, doxorubicin, fluconazole, flucytosine, indomethacin, interferon-alfa, methadone, pentamidine, vincristine, valproic acid** may increase risk of AZT toxicity; **probenecid** will decrease AZT elimination, resulting in increased serum levels and thus toxicity. **Phenytoin** decreases zidovudine clearance and alters **phenytoin** concentrations; **nelfinavir, rifampin, ritonavir** may decrease zidovudine (AZT) concentrations; other ANTIRETROVIRAL AGENTS may cause lactic acidosis and severe hepatomegaly with steatosis; **doxorubicin, ribavarin, stavudine** may antagonize AZT effects.

PHARMACOKINETICS Absorption: Readily absorbed from GI tract; 60–70% reaches systemic circulation (first-pass metabolism). **Peak:** 0.5–1.5 h.

Distribution: Crosses blood–brain barrier and placenta. **Metabolism:** Metabolized in liver. **Elimination:** 63–95% excreted in urine. **Half-Life:** 1 h.

NURSING IMPLICATIONS

Assessment & Drug Effects

- Evaluate patient at least weekly during the first month of therapy.
- Lab tests: Baseline and frequent (at least q2wk) blood counts, CD_4 (T_4) lymphocyte count, Hgb, and granulocyte count to detect hematologic toxicity.
- Myelosuppression results in anemia, which commonly occurs after 4–6 wk of therapy, and granulocytopenia in 6–8 wk. Frequently, both respond to dosage adjustment. Significant anemia (Hgb <7.5 g/dL or reduction >25% of baseline value), or granulocyte count <750/mm^3 (or reduction >50% of baseline) may require temporary interruption of therapy and transfusions.
- Monitor for common adverse effects, especially severe headache, nausea, insomnia, and myalgia.

Patient & Family Education

- Take drug as prescribed around the clock.
- Contact physician promptly if health status worsens or any unusual symptoms develop.
- Understand that this drug is not a cure for HIV infection; you will continue to be at risk for opportunistic infections.
- Do not share drug with others; take drug exactly as prescribed.
- Drug does NOT reduce the risk of transmission of HIV infection through body fluids.
- Do not breast feed while taking this drug; it is not known if the drug is secreted in human milk.
- Store this medication out of reach of children.

ZILEUTON

(zi-leu′ton)

Leutrol, Zyflo

Classifications: BRONCHODILATOR (RESPIRATORY SMOOTH MUSCLE RELAXANT); LEUKOTRIENE RECEPTOR ANTAGONIST

Prototype: Zafirlukast

Pregnancy Category: C

AVAILABILITY 600 mg tablets

ACTIONS Inhibits 5-lipoxygenase, the enzyme needed to start the conversion of arachidonic acid to leukotrienes. Leukotrienes are considered more important than prostaglandins as inflammatory agents; they induce bronchoconstriction and mucous production. Elevated sputum and blood levels of leukotrienes have been documented during acute asthma attacks.

Z

THERAPEUTIC EFFECTS Zileuton helps to prevent the signs and symptoms of asthma, including airway edema, smooth muscle constriction, and altered cellular activity due to inflammation.

USES Prophylaxis and chronic treatment of asthma; in adults and children >12 y.

CONTRAINDICATIONS Hypersensitivity to zileuton or zafirlukast, active liver disease, lactation, pregnancy (category C).
CAUTIOUS USE Hepatic insufficiency. Safety and effectiveness in children >12 y are not established.

ROUTE & DOSAGE

Asthma
Child >12 y/Adult: **PO** 600 mg q.i.d.

STORAGE
Store at 15°–30° C (59°–86° F); protect from light.

ADMINISTRATION
Oral
- Give at meals and bedtime. Can be given with or without food.

ADVERSE EFFECTS Body as a Whole: Pain, asthenia, myalgia, arthralgia, fever, malaise, neck pain/rigidity. **CNS:** *Headache,* dizziness, insomnia, nervousness, somnolence. **CV:** Chest pain. **GI:** Abdominal pain, *dyspepsia,* nausea, constipation, flatulence, vomiting, elevated liver function tests, asymptomatic hepatitis. **Skin:** Pruritus. **Other:** Conjunctivitis, hypertonia, lymphadenopathy, vaginitis, UTI, leukopenia.

INTERACTIONS Drug: May double **theophylline** levels and increase toxicity. Increases hypoprothrombinemic effects of **warfarin.** May increase levels of BETA-BLOCKERS (especially **propranolol**), leading to hypotension and bradycardia. May increase **terfenadine** levels, leading to prolongation of QT_c interval. May increase effects of **alprazolam, clozapine, digoxin.**

PHARMACOKINETICS Absorption: Rapidly absorbed from GI tract. **Peak:** 1.7 h. **Duration:** 5–8 h. **Distribution:** 93% protein bound; secreted in the breast milk of rats. **Metabolism:** Metabolized in liver primarily via glucuronide conjugation. **Elimination:** Excreted primarily in urine (94%). **Half-Life:** 2.5 h.

NURSING IMPLICATIONS

Assessment & Drug Effects
- Assess respiratory status and airway function regularly.
- Lab tests: Periodic CBC and routine blood chemistry; monthly liver function tests for 3 mo, then every 2–3 mo for rest of first year, then periodically.
- Instructions for CONCURRENT THERAPIES: Reduce theophylline dose and closely monitor theophylline levels; closely monitor PT and INR

Z

with warfarin therapy; closely monitor phenytoin level with phenytoin therapy; closely monitor HR and BP for excessive beta blockade with propranolol therapy.

Patient & Family Education

- Take medication regularly even during symptom-free periods.
- Drug is not intended to treat acute episodes of asthma.
- Report to prescriber promptly S&S of hepatic toxicity (see Appendix D-1) or flu-like symptoms. Follow-up lab work is very important.
- Notify prescriber if condition worsens while using prescribed doses of all antiasthmatic medications.
- Do not breast feed while taking this drug.
- Store this medication out of reach of children.

Z

APPENDIXES

APPENDIX A–1
<u>U.S. SCHEDULES OF CONTROLLED SUBSTANCES</u>

Schedule I

High potential for abuse and of no currently accepted medical use. Examples: Heroin, LSD, marijuana, mescaline, peyote. Not obtainable by prescription but may be legally procured for research, study, or instructional use.

Schedule II

High abuse potential and high liability for severe psychological or physical dependence. Prescription required and cannot be renewed.[a] Includes opium derivatives, other opioids, and short-acting barbiturates. Examples: Amphetamine, cocaine, meperidine, morphine, secobarbital.

Schedule III

Potential for abuse is less than that for drugs in Schedules I and II. Moderate to low physical dependence and high psychological dependence. Includes certain stimulants and depressants not included in the above schedules and preparations containing limited quantities of certain opioids. Examples: Chlorphentermine, glutethimide, mazindol, paregoric, phendimetrazine. Prescription required.[b]

Schedule IV

Lower potential for abuse than Schedule III drugs. Examples: Certain psychotropics (tranquilizers), chloral hydrate, chlordiazepoxide, diazepam, meprobamate, phenobarbital. Prescription required.[a]

Schedule V

Abuse potential less than that for Schedule IV drugs. Preparations contain limited quantities of certain narcotic drugs; generally intended for antitussive and antidiarrheal purposes and may be distributed without a prescription provided that:

1. Such distribution is made only by a pharmacist.
2. Not more than 240 mL or not more than 48 solid dosage units of any substance containing opium, nor more than 120 mL or not more than 24 solid dosage units of any other controlled substance may be distributed at retail to the same purchaser in any given 48-hour period without a valid prescription order.
3. The purchaser is at least 18 years old.
4. The pharmacist knows the purchaser or requests suitable identification.
5. The pharmacist keeps an official written record of name and address of purchaser, name and quantity of controlled substance purchased, date of sale, initials of dispensing pharmacist. This record is to be made available for inspection and copying by U.S. officers authorized by the Attorney General.
6. Other federal, state, or local law does not require a prescription order.

Under jurisdiction of the Federal Controlled Substances Act.

ᵃExcept when dispensed directly by a practitioner, other than a pharmacist, to an ultimate user, no controlled substance in Schedule II may be dispensed without a written prescription, except that in emergency situations such drug may be dispensed upon oral prescription and a written prescription must be obtained within the time frame prescribed by law. No prescription for a controlled substance in Schedule II may be refilled.
ᵇRefillable up to 5 times within 6 mo, but only if so indicated by physician.
Source: Reprinted with permission from Wilson BA, Shannon MT, Stang CL. *Nurse's Drug Guide 2005,* pages 1718–1719. Upper Saddle River, NJ: Pearson/Prentice Hall, © 2005.

APPENDIX A–2
FDA PREGNANCY CATEGORIES

The FDA requires that all prescription drugs absorbed systemically or known to be potentially harmful to the fetus be classified according to one of five pregnancy categories {A, B, C, D, X}. The identifying letter signifies the level of risk to the fetus and is to appear in the precautions section of the package insert. The categories described by the FDA are as follows:

Category A

Controlled studies in women fail to demonstrate a risk to the fetus in the first trimester (and there is no evidence of risk in later trimesters), and the possibility of fetal harm appears remote.

Category B

Either animal-reproduction studies have not demonstrated a fetal risk but there are no controlled studies in pregnant women, or animal-reproduction studies have shown an adverse effect (other than a decrease in fertility) that was not confirmed in controlled studies in women in the first trimester (and there is no evidence of a risk in later trimesters).

Category C

Either studies in animals have revealed adverse effects on the fetus (teratogenic or embryocidal effects or other) and there are no controlled studies in women, or studies in women and animals are not available. Drugs should be given only if the potential benefit justifies the potential risk to the fetus.

Category D

There is positive evidence of human fetal risk, but the benefits from use in pregnant women may be acceptable despite the risk (e.g., if the drug is needed in a life-threatening situation or for a serious disease for which safer drugs cannot be used or are ineffective). There will be an appropriate statement in the "warnings" section of the labeling.

Category X

Studies in animals or human beings have demonstrated fetal abnormalities or there is evidence of fetal risk based on human experience, or both, and the risk of the use of the drug in pregnant women clearly outweighs any possible benefit. The drug is contraindicated in women who are or may become pregnant. There will be an appropriate statement in the "contraindications" section of the labeling.

Source: Reprinted with permission from Wilson BA, Shannon MT, Stang CL. *Nurse's Drug Guide 2005,* page 1720. Upper Saddle River, NJ: Pearson/Prentice Hall, © 2005.

Some oral dosage forms should not be crushed or chewed. These dosage forms have been specially designed to release the drug slowly over several hours, to protect the drug from the low pH of the stomach, and/or to protect the stomach from the irritating effects of the drug.

Drugs may have an **enteric coating,** which is designed to allow the drug to pass through the stomach intact with the drug being released in the intestines. This protects the stomach from the irritating effects of the drug, protects the drug from being destroyed by the acid pH of the stomach, and can delay the onset of action.

Extended-release (slow release, SR) formulations are designed to release the drug over an extended period of time. These formulations can include multiple-layer compressed tablets where drug is released as each layer dissolves, mixed-release pellets that dissolve at different time intervals, and special tablets that are themselves inert but are designed to release drug slowly from the formulation. Some extended-release dosage forms are scored and may be broken in half without affecting the release mechanism but still should not be crushed or chewed. Some mixed-release capsule formulations can be opened and the contents sprinkled on food. However, the pellets should not be crushed or chewed. Some extended-release formulations can be identified by common abbreviations used in their brand names. These abbreviations include CR (controlled release), CRT (controlled-release tablet), LA (long acting), SR (sustained release), TR (time release), SA (sustained action), and XL or XR (extended release).

Occasionally, drugs should not be crushed because they are oral mucosa irritants, are extremely bitter, or contain dyes that may stain teeth or mucosal tissue.

The table contains a list of drugs found in the Guide that should not be crushed or chewed. A liquid dosage form may be available for many of these drugs. However, the dose or frequency of administration may be different from the slow-release product. Check with your pharmacist for liquid availability and dosing conversions.

	Generic Name	Comments
Accutane	isotretinoin	mucous membrane irritant
Acutrim	phenylpropanolamine	slow release
Adalat CC	nifedipine	slow release
Allerest 12 Hour	chlorpheniramine, phenylpropanolamine	slow release
Artane Sequels	trihexyphenydil	slow release; capsules may be opened and contents taken without chewing or crushing
Azulfidine Entabs	sulfasalazine	enteric coated

	Generic Name	Comments
Bayer Caplet	aspirin, enteric coated	enteric coated
Bayer Extra Strength Enteric 500	aspirin, enteric coated	enteric coated; slow release
Bayer Low Adult 81 mg	aspirin, enteric coated	enteric coated
Biphetamine	amphetamine, dextro-amphetamine	slow release
Bisacodyl	bisacodyl	enteric coated
Bisco-Lax	bisacodyl	enteric coated
Bromfed, Bromfed-PD	brompheniramine, pseudoephedrine	slow release
Calan SR	verapamil	slow release
Cama Arthritis Strength	aspirin, magnesium oxide, aluminum hydroxide	special table formulation
Cardizem, Cardizem CD, Cardizem SR	diltiazem	slow release; capsules may be opened and contents taken without chewing or crushing
Chloral Hydrate	chloral hydrate	liquid-filled capsule
Chlor-Trimeton Repetab	chlorpheniramine	slow release
Choledyl SA	oxytriphylline	slow release
Compazine Spansule	prochlorperazine	slow release; capsules may be opened and contents taken without chewing or crushing
Constant T	theophylline	slow release; capsules may be opened and contents taken without chewing or crushing
Contac	chlorpheniramine, phenylpropanolamine	slow release; capsules may be opened and contents taken without chewing or crushing
Cotazym S	pancrelipase	enteric coated; capsules may be opened and contents taken without chewing or crushing
Covera-HS	verapamil	slow release

	Generic Name	Comments
Deconamine SR	chlorpheniramine, pseudoephedrine	slow release
Depakene	valproic acid	slow release; mucous membrane irritant
Depakote	valproate disodium	enteric coated
Desoxyn Gradumets	methamphetamine	slow release
Dexatrim Max Strength	phenylpropanolamine	slow release
Dexedrine Spansule	dextroamphetamine	slow release
Diamox Sequels	acetazolamide	slow release
Dilacor XR	diltiazem	slow release
Dilatrate-SR	isosorbide dinitrate	slow release
Dimetane Extentab	brompheniramine, phenylephrine	slow release
Disophrol Chronotab	dexbrompheniramine, pseudoephedrine	slow release
Donnatol Extentab	atropine, scopolamine, hyoscyamine, phenobarbital	slow release
Donnazyme	pancreatin, pepsin, bile salts, atropine, scopolamine, hyoscyamine, phenobarbital	slow release
Drixoral	dexbrompheniramine, pseudoephedrine	slow release
Dulcolax	bisacodyl	enteric coated
Easprin	aspirin	enteric coated
Ecotrin	aspirin	enteric coated
E.E.S. 400	erythromycin ethylsuccinate	enteric coated
Elixophyllin SR	theophylline	slow release; capsules may be opened and contents taken without chewing or crushing
E-Mycin	erythromycin	enteric coated
Ergostat	ergotamine	sublingual tablet
Eryc	erythromycin	enteric coated; capsules may be opened and contents taken without chewing or crushing

	Generic Name	Comments
Ery-tab	erythromycin	enteric coated
Erythrocin Stearate	erythromycin	enteric coated
Erythromycin Base	erythromycin	enteric coated
Eskalith CR	lithium	slow release
Fedahist Timecaps	chlorpheniramine, pseudoephedrine	slow release
Feldene	piroxicam	mucous membrane irritant
Feosol	ferrous sulfate	enteric coated
Feosol Spansule	ferrous sulfate	slow release; capsules may be opened and contents taken without chewing or crushing
Fergon	ferrous gluconate	slow release; capsules may be opened and contents taken without chewing or crushing
Ferro-Sequels	ferrous fumarate, docusate	slow release
Fero-Gradumet	ferrous sulfate	slow release
Festal II	pancrelipase	enteric coated
Glucotrol XL	glipizide	slow release
Gris-Peg	griseofulvin ultramicrosize	crushing may result in precipitation of drug as larger particles
Ilotycin	erythromycin	enteric coated
Inderal LA	propranolol	slow release
Inderide LA	propranolol, hydro-chlorothiazide	slow release
Indocin SR	indomethacin	slow release; capsules may be opened and contents taken without chewing or crushing
Iso-Bid	isosorbide dinitrate	slow release
Isoptin SR	verapamil	slow release
Isordil Tembid	isosorbide dinitrate	slow release
Isosorbide dinitrate SR	isosorbide dinitrate	slow release
Isuprel Glossets	isoproterenol	sublingual

APPENDIX B   ORAL DOSAGE FORMS THAT SHOULD NOT BE CRUSHED

	Generic Name	Comments
Kaon CL 10	postassium chloride	slow release
Klor-Con	postassium chloride	slow release
Klotrix	postassium chloride	slow release
K-Tab	postassium chloride	slow release
Levsinex Timecaps	hyoscyamine	slow release
Lithobid	lithium	slow release
Meprospan	meprobamate	slow release; capsules may be opened and contents taken without chewing or crushing
Mestinon Timespan	pyridostigmine	slow release
Micro K	postassium chloride	slow release
MS Contin	morphine	slow release
Naldecon	phenylephrine, phenyl-propanolamine, chlorpheniramine, phenyltoloxamine	slow release
Nico-400	niacin	slow release
Nicobid	niacin	slow release
Nitro Bid	nitroglycerin	slow release; capsules may be opened and contents taken without chewing or crushing
Nitroglyn	nitroglycerin	slow release; capsules may be opened and contents taken without chewing or crushing
Nitrong SR	nitroglycerin	slow release
Nolamine	phenylpropanolamine, chlorpheniramine, phenindamine	slow release
Norflex	orphenadrine	slow release
Norpace CR	disopyramide	slow release
Novafed A	pseudoephedrine, chlorpheniramine	slow release
Oramorph SR	morphine	slow release
Ornade Spansule	phenylpropanolamine, chlorpheniramine	slow release
Pancrease	pancrelipase	enteric coated

	Generic Name	Comments
Papaverine Sustained Action	papaverine	slow release
Pavabid	papaverine	slow release
Pavabid Plateau	papaverine	slow release; capsules may be opened and contents taken without chewing or crushing
PBZ-SR	tripelennamine hydrochloride	slow release
Perdiem	psyllium hydrophilic mucioid	wax coated
Peritrate SA	pentaerythritol tetranitrate	slow release
Permitil Chronotab	fluphenazine	slow release
Phazyme, Phazyme 95	simethicone	slow release
Phyllocontin	aminophylline	slow release
Plendil	felodipine	slow release
Polaramine Repetabs	dexchlorphenir-amine	slow release
Prevacid	lansoprazole	slow release; capsules may be opened and contents taken without chewing or crushing
Prilosec	omeprazole	slow release
Procainamide HCl SR	procainamide	slow release
Procan SR	procainamide	slow release
Procardia XL	nifedipine	slow release
Pronestyl SR	procainamide	slow release
Proventil Repetabs	albuterol	slow release
Prozac	fluoxetine	slow release; capsules may be opened and contents taken without chewing or crushing
Quibron-T SR	theophylline	slow release
Quinaglute Dura Tabs	quinidine gluconate	slow release
Quinidex Extentabs	quinidine sulfate	slow release

	Generic Name	Comments
Respid	theophylline	slow release
Ritalin SR	methylphenidate	slow release
Robimycin Robitab	erythromycin	enteric coated
Rondec TR	pseudoephedrine, carbinoxamine	slow release
Roxanol SR	morphine	slow release
Sinemet CR	levodopa, carbidopa	slow release; tablet is scored and may be broken in half
Slo-Bid Gyrocaps	theophylline	slow release; capsules may be opened and contents taken without chewing or crushing
Slo-Phyllin Gyrocaps	theophylline	slow release; capsules may be opened and contents taken without chewing or crushing
Slow-Fe	ferrous sulfate	slow release
Slow-K	potassium chloride	slow release
Sorbitrate SA	isosorbide dinitrate	slow release
Sudafed 12 hour	pseudoephedrine	slow release
Tavist-D	phenylpropanolamine, clemastine	multiple compressed tablet
Teldrin	chlorpheniramine	slow release; capsules may be opened and contents taken without chewing or crushing
Tepanil Ten-Tab	diethylpropion	slow release
Tessalon Perles	benzonatate	slow release
Theo-24	theophylline	slow release
Theobid, Theobid Jr.	theophylline	slow release
Theo-Dur	theophylline	slow release
Theo-Dur Sprinkle	theophylline	slow release; capsules may be opened and contents taken without chewing or crushing
Theolair SR	theophylline	slow release
Thorazine Spansule	chlorpromazine	slow release

	Generic Name	Comments
Toprol XL	metoprolol	slow release
Trental	pentoxifylline	slow release
Triaminic	phenylpropanolamine, chlorpheniramine	enteric coated
Triaminic 12	phenylpropanolamine, chlorpheniramine	slow release
Triaminic TR	phenylpropanolamine, pyrilamine, pheniramine	multiple compressed tablet
Trilafon Repetabs	perphenazine	slow release
Triptone Caplets	scopolamine	slow release
Uniphyl	theophylline	slow release
Valrelease	diazepam	slow release
Verelan	verapamil	slow release; capsules may be opened and contents taken without chewing or crushing
Volmax	albuterol	slow release
Welbutrin SR	bupropion	slow release
Wyamycin S	erythromycin stearate	slow release
ZORprin	aspirin	slow release

Source: Reprinted with permission from Wilson BA, Shannon MT, Stang CL. *Nurse's Drug Guide 2005,* pages 1721–1728. Upper Saddle River, NJ: Pearson/Prentice Hall, © 2005.

Classifications	Prototype
ANTIGOUT AGENT	Colchicine

ANTIHISTAMINES
   ANTIHISTAMINES (H_1-RECEPTOR

ANTAGONIST).	Diphenhydramine HCl
NON-SEDATING	Loratidine
ANTIPRURITIC	Hydroxyzine HCl
ANTIVERTIGO AGENT	Meclizine HCl

ANTI-INFECTIVES

ANTIBIOTICS	
AMEBICIDE	Paromomycin Sulfate
ANTHELMINTIC	Mebendazole
AMINOGLYCOSIDES	Gentamicin Sulfate
ANTIFUNGALS	Amphotericin B
AZOLE ANTIFUNGAL	Fluconazole
BETA-LACTAM	Imipenem-Cilastatin
CEPHALOSPORIN	
FIRST GENERATION	Cefazolin Sodium
SECOND GENERATION	Cefonicid Sodium
THIRD GENERATION	Cefotaxime Sodium
CLINDAMYCIN	Clindamycin HCl
MACROLIDES	Erythromycin
PENICILLIN	
AMINOPENICILLIN	Ampicillin
ANTIPSEUDOMONAL PENICILLIN . .	Mezlocillin Sodium
NATURAL PENICILLIN	Penicillin G Potassium
QUINOLONES	Ciprofloxacin HCl
SULFONAMIDES	Sulfisoxazole
TETRACYCLINE	Tetracycline HCl
ANTILEPROSY (SULFONE) AGENT	Dapsone
ANTIMALARIAL	Chloroquine HCl
ANTIPROTOZOAL	Metronidazole
ANTITUBERCULOSIS AGENTS	Isoniazid
ANTIVIRAL AGENTS	
ANTIVIRAL AGENTS	Acyclovir
ANTIRETROVIRAL AGENTS	
NUCLEOSIDE REVERSE	
TRANSCRIPTASE INHIBITOR	Zidovudine
NONNUCLEOSIDE REVERSE	
TRANSCRIPTASE INHIBITOR	Nevirapine
PROTEASE INHIBITOR	Saquinavir
URINARY TRACT ANTI-INFECTIVE	Trimethoprim
VACCINE	Hepatitis B

*Based on the American Hospital Formulary Service Pharmacologic–Therapeutic Classification.

†Prototype drugs are highlighted in tinted boxes in this book.

Complete list of drugs for each classification found in Index starting on p. 1299.

Classifications	Prototype

ANTINEOPLASTICS

ALKYLATING AGENT . . . . Cyclophosphamide
ANTIBIOTIC . . . . Doxorubicin HCl
ANTIMETABOLITE . . . . Fluorouracil
CAMPTOTHECIN . . . . Topotecan HCl
AROMATASE INHIBITOR . . . . Anastrozole
HORMONE, ANTIESTROGEN . . . . Tamoxifen Citrate
MITOTIC INHIBITOR . . . . Vincristine Sulfate
NITROGEN MUSTARD . . . . Mechlorethamine HCl
TAXANE . . . . Paclitaxel

ANTITUSSIVES, EXPECTORANTS, & MUCOLYTICS

ANTITUSSIVE . . . . Benzonatate
EXPECTORANT . . . . Guaifenesin
MUCOLYTIC . . . . Acetylcysteine

AUTONOMIC NERVOUS SYSTEM AGENTS

ADRENERGIC AGONISTS
  (SYMPATHOMIMETICS)
  ALPHA-ADRENERGIC AGONIST . . . . . . Methoxamine HCl
  ALPHA- & BETA-ADRENERGIC
    AGONIST . . . . Epinephrine
  BETA-ADRENERGIC AGONIST . . . . Albuterol
ADRENERGIC ANTAGONISTS
  (SYMPATHOLYTICS)
  ALPHA ANTAGONISTS (BLOCKING
    AGENT) . . . . Prazosin HCl
  BETA ANTAGONISTS . . . . Propranolol HCl
  ERGOT ALKALOID . . . . Ergotamine Tartrate
  5-HT$_1$ SEROTONIN AGONISTS . . . . Sumatriptan
ANTICHOLINERGICS
  (PARASYMPATHOLYTICS)
  ANTIPARKINSON AGENTS . . . . Levodopa
  CATECHOLAMINE O-METHYL
    TRANSFERASE (COMT)
      INHIBITOR . . . . Tolcapone
  ANTIMUSCARINIC,
    ANTISPASMODIC . . . . Atropine Sulfate
CHOLINERGICS (PARASYMPATHOMIMETICS)
  CHOLINESTERASE INHIBITOR . . . . Neostigmine
  CENTRAL-ACTING . . . . Donepezil
  DIRECT-ACTING CHOLINERGIC . . . . . . Bethanechol Chloride

BENZODIAZEPINE ANTAGONIST . . . . Flumazenil

BIOLOGIC RESPONSE MODIFIERS

FUSION PROTEIN . . . . Alefacept
IMMUNOGLOBULIN . . . . Immune Globulin
IMMUNOSUPPRESSANT . . . . Cyclosporine
MONOCLONAL ANTIBODY . . . . Basiliximab

Classifications	Prototype
TUMOR NECROSIS FACTOR MODIFIER	Etanercept
BISPHOSPHONATE (REGULATOR, BONE METABOLISM)	Etidronate Disodium
BLOOD DERIVATIVE, PLASMA VOLUME, EXPANDER	Normal Serum Albumin
BLOOD FORMERS, COAGULATORS, & ANTICOAGULANTS	
ANTICOAGULANT	Heparin Sodium
DIRECT THROMBIN INHIBITOR	Lepirudin
LOW MOLECULAR WEIGHT HEPARIN	Enoxaparin
ANTIPLATELET AGENTS	Ticlopidine
GLYCOPROTEIN IIb/IIIa INHIBITOR	Abciximab
HEMATOPOIETIC GROWTH FACTOR	Epoetin Alpha
HEMOSTATIC	Aminocaproic Acid
IRON PREPARATION	Ferrous Sulfate
THROMBOLYTIC ENZYME	Alteplase
BRONCHODILATORS (RESPIRATORY SMOOTH MUSCLE RELAXANT)	
BETA-ADRENERGIC AGONIST	Isoproterenol HCl
LEUKOTRIENE INHIBITOR	Zafirlukast
XANTHINE	Theophylline
CARDIOVASCULAR AGENTS	
ANGIOTENSIN II RECEPTOR ANTAGONISTS	Losartan Potassium
ANGIOTENSIN-CONVERTING ENZYME INHIBITORS	Captopril
ANTIARRHYTHMIC AGENTS	
CLASS IA	Procainamide HCl
CLASS IB	Lidocaine HCl
CLASS IC	Flecainide
CLASS II	Propranolol HCl
CLASS III	Amiodarone HCl
ANTILIPEMICS	
BILE ACID SEQUESTRANT	Cholestyramine
FIBRATES	Clofibrate
HMG-CoA REDUCTASE INHIBITOR (STATIN)	Lovastatin
CALCIUM CHANNEL BLOCKER	Nifedipine
CARDIAC GLYCOSIDE	Digoxin
CENTRAL-ACTING ANTIHYPERTENSIVE	Methyldopa
INOTROPIC AGENT	Inamrinone
NITRATE VASODILATOR	Nitroglycerin
NONNITRATE VASODILATOR	Hydralazine HCl
RAUWOLFIA ALKALOID	Reserpine

Classifications	Prototype

CENTRAL NERVOUS SYSTEM AGENTS

ANALGESICS, ANTIPYRETICS
   NARCOTIC (OPIATE) AGONISTS . . . . . Morphine
   NARCOTIC (OPIATE)
     AGONIST-ANTAGONIST . . . . Pentazocine HCl
   NARCOTIC (OPIATE)
     ANTAGONIST . . . . Naloxone HCl
   NONNARCOTIC ANALGESICS . . . . . . Acetaminophen
   NONSTEROIDAL
     ANTI-INFLAMMATORY
       DRUGS (NSAID) COX-1 . . . . Ibuprofen
          COX-2 . . . . Celecoxib
   SALICYLATE . . . . Aspirin
ANESTHETIC
   GENERAL . . . . Thiopental Sodium
   LOCAL (AMIDE TYPE) . . . . Lidocaine HCl
   LOCAL (ESTER TYPE) . . . . Procaine HCl
ANTICONVULSANTS
   BARBITURATE . . . . Phenobarbital
   BENZODIAZEPINE . . . . Diazepam
   GABA INHIBITOR . . . . Valproic Acid Sodium
   HYDANTOIN . . . . Phenytoin
   SUCCINIMIDE . . . . Ethosuximide
   SULFONAMIDE . . . . Zonisamide
   TRICYCLIC . . . . Carbamazepine
ANXIOLYTICS, SEDATIVE-HYPNOTICS
   BARBITURATE . . . . Secobarbital
   BENZODIAZEPINE . . . . Lorazepam
   NONBENZODIAZEPINE . . . . Zolpidem
   CARBAMATE . . . . Meprobamate
CEREBRAL STIMULANT
   AMPHETAMINE . . . . Amphetamine Sulfate
   XANTHINE . . . . Caffeine
PSYCHOTHERAPEUTIC
   ANTIDEPRESSANTS
     SELECTIVE SEROTONIN-REUPTAKE
       INHIBITORS (SSRI) . . . . Fluoxetine HCl
     SEROTONIN NOREPINEPHRINE
       REUPTAKE INHIBITORS . . . . Venlafaxine
     MONOAMINE OXIDASE (MAO)
       INHIBITORS . . . . Phenelzine Sulfate
     TETRACYCLIC ANTIDEPRESSANTS . . Mirtazapine
     TRICYCLIC ANTIDEPRESSANTS . . . . . Imipramine HCl
   ANTIMANIC AGENT . . . . Lithium Carbonate
   ANTIPSYCHOTIC AGENT
     BUTYROPHENONE . . . . Haloperidol
     PHENOTHIAZINE . . . . Chlorpromazine
     ATYPICAL . . . . Clozapine

Classifications	Prototype

ELECTROLYTIC & WATER BALANCE AGENTS

DIURETIC
    LOOP . . . . Furosemide
    OSMOTIC . . . . Mannitol
    POTASSIUM-SPARING . . . . Spironolactone
    THIAZIDE . . . . Hydrochlorothiazide
PHOSPHATE BINDER . . . . Sevelamer HCl
REPLACEMENT SOLUTION . . . . Calcium Gluconate

ENZYMES

ENZYME INHIBITOR . . . . Alpha$_1$-Proteinase Inhibitor
ENZYME REPLACEMENT . . . . Pancrealipase

EYE, EAR, NOSE, & THROAT (EENT) PREPARATIONS

ANTIHISTAMINE, OCULAR . . . . Levocabastine HCl
CARBONIC ANHYDRASE INHIBITOR . . . . Acetazolamide
CYCLOPLEGIC . . . . Cyclopentolate HCl
MIOTIC (ANTIGLAUCOMA AGENT) . . . . . Pilocarpine HCl
MYDRIATIC . . . . Homatropine HBr
PROSTAGLANDIN . . . . Latanoprost
VASOCONSTRICTOR, DECONGESTANT Naphazoline HCl

GASTROINTESTINAL AGENTS

ANORECTANT . . . . Diethylpropion HCl
ANTACID, ADSORBENT . . . . Aluminum Hydroxide
ANTIDIARRHEAL . . . . Diphenoxylate HCl with
                               Atropine Sulfate
ANTIEMETIC . . . . Prochlorperazine
ANTIEMETIC (5-HT$_3$ ANTAGONIST) . . . . . Ondansetron HCl
ANTISECRETORY (H$_2$-RECEPTOR
    ANTAGONIST) . . . . Cimetidine
BULK LAXATIVE . . . . Psyllium Hydrophilic
                               Mucilloid
MUCOUS MEMBRANE
    ANTI-INFLAMMATORY . . . . Mesalamine
PROKINETIC AGENT (GI STIMULANT) . . . . Metoclopramide HCl
PROTON PUMP INHIBITORS . . . . Omeprazole
SALINE CATHARTIC . . . . Magnesium Hydroxide
STIMULANT LAXATIVE . . . . Bisacodyl
STOOL SOFTENER . . . . Docusate Calcium

GOLD COMPOUND . . . . Aurothioglucose

HORMONES & SYNTHETIC SUBSTITUTES

ADRENAL CORTICOSTEROID
    GLUCOCORTICOSTEROID . . . . Prednisone
    MINERALOCORTICOID . . . . Fludrocortisone Acetate
ANDROGEN/ANABOLIC STEROIDS . . . . Testosterone

Classifications	Prototype

ANTIANDROGENS
　5-ALPHA REDUCTASE INHIBITORS . . . . Finasteride
ANTIDIABETIC AGENTS
　ALPHA-GLUCOSIDASE INHIBITOR . . . . Acarbose
　BIGUANIDES . . . . Metformin
　INSULIN . . . . Insulin injection
　MEGLITINIDES . . . . Repaglinide
　SULFONYLUREAS . . . . Glyburide
　THIAZOLIDINEDIONES . . . . Rosiglitazone
ESTROGENS . . . . Estradiol
GONADOTROPIN-RELEASING
　HORMONE ANALOGS . . . . Leuprolide Acetate
GROWTH HORMONE . . . . Somatropin
OXYTOCIC . . . . Oxytocin Injection
PITUITARY (ANTIDIURETIC) . . . . Vasopressin Injection
PROGESTINS . . . . Progesterone
THYROID AGENTS
　ANTITHYROID AGENT . . . . Propylthiouracil
　THYROID . . . . Levothyroxine Sodium
VITAMIN D ANALOG . . . . Calcitriol

IMMUNOMODULATORS

INTERFERONS . . . . Interferon Alfa-2a

LUNG SURFACTANT . . . . Beractant

MAST CELL STABILIZER . . . . Cromolyn Sodium

PROSTAGLANDIN . . . . Dinoprostone

SKIN & MUCOUS MEMBRANE AGENTS

ANTIACNE (RETINOID) . . . . Isotretinoin
ANTI-INFLAMMATORY STEROID . . . . Hydrocortisone
PEDICULICIDE . . . . Permethrin
PSORALEN . . . . Methoxsalen
SCABICIDE . . . . Lindane

SOMATIC NERVOUS SYSTEM AGENTS

SKELETAL MUSCLE RELAXANTS
　CENTRAL-ACTING . . . . Cyclobenzaprine HCl
　DEPOLARIZING . . . . Succinylcholine Chloride
　NONDEPOLARIZING . . . . Tubocurarine Chloride

VASODILATOR

PHOSPHODIESTERASE INHIBITOR . . . . . . Sildenafil

Source: Reprinted with permission from Wilson BA, Shannon MT, Stang CL. *Nurse's Drug Guide 2005,* pages x–xvi. Upper Saddle River, NJ: Pearson/Prentice Hall, © 2005.

acute dystonia extrapyramidal symptom manifested by abnormal posturing, grimacing, spastic torticollis (neck torsion), and oculogyric (eyeball movement) crisis.

adverse effect unintended, unpredictable, and nontherapeutic response to drug action. Adverse effects occur at doses used therapeutically or for prophylaxis or diagnosis. They generally result from drug toxicity, idiosyncrasies, or hypersensitivity reactions caused by the drug itself or by ingredients added during manufacture, e.g., preservatives, dyes, or vehicles.

afterload resistance that ventricles must work against to eject blood into the aorta during systole.

agranulocytosis sudden drop in leukocyte count; often followed by a severe infection manifested by high fever, chills, prostration, and ulcerations of mucous membrane such as in the mouth, rectum, or vagina.

akathisia extrapyramidal symptom manifested by a compelling need to move or pace, without specific pattern, and an inability to be still.

analeptic restorative medication that enhances excitation of the CNS without affecting inhibitory impulses.

anaphylactoid reaction excessive allergic response manifested by wheezing, chills, generalized pruritic urticaria, diaphoresis, sense of uneasiness, agitation, flushing, palpitations, coughing, difficulty breathing, and cardiovascular collapse.

anticholinergic actions inhibition of parasympathetic response manifested by dry mouth, decreased peristalsis, constipation, blurred vision, and urinary retention.

bioavailability fraction of active drug that reaches its action sites after administration by any route. Following an IV dose, bioavailability is 100%; however, such factors as first-pass effect, enterohepatic cycling, and biotransformation reduce bioavailability of an orally administered drug.

blood dyscrasia pathological condition manifested by fever, sore mouth or throat, unexplained fatigue, easy bruising or bleeding.

cardiotoxicity impairment of cardiac function manifested by one or more of the following: hypotension, arrhythmias, precordial pain, dyspnea, electrocardiogram (ECG) abnormalities, cardiac dilation, congestive failure.

cholinergic response stimulation of the parasympathetic response manifested by lacrimation, diaphoresis, salivation, abdominal cramps, diarrhea, nausea, and vomiting.

circulatory overload excessive vascular volume manifested by increased central venous pressure (CVP), elevated blood pressure, tachycardia, distended neck veins, peripheral edema, dyspnea, cough, and pulmonary rales.

CNS stimulation excitement of the CNS manifested by hyperactivity, excitement, nervousness, insomnia, and tachycardia.

CNS toxicity impairment of CNS function manifested by ataxia, tremor, incoordination, paresthesias, numbness, impairment of pain or touch sensation, drowsiness, confusion, headache, anxiety, tremors, and behavior changes.

congestive heart failure (CHF) impaired pumping ability of the heart manifested by paroxysmal nocturnal dyspnea, cough, fatigue or dyspnea on exertion, tachycardia, peripheral or pulmonary edema, and weight gain.

Cushing's syndrome fatty swellings in the interscapular area (buffalo hump) and in the facial area (moon face), distention of the abdomen, ecchymoses following even minor trauma, impotence, amenorrhea, high blood pressure, general weakness, loss of muscle mass, osteoporosis, and psychosis.

dehydration decreased intracellular or extracellular fluid manifested by elevated temperature, dry skin and mucous membranes, decrease tissue turgor, sunken eyes, furrowed tongue, low blood pressure, diminished or irregular pulse, muscle or abdominal cramps, thick secretions, hard feces and impaction, scant urinary output, urine specific gravity above 1.030, an elevated hemoglobin.

disulfiram-type reaction Antabuse-type reaction manifested by facial flushing, pounding headache, sweating, slurred speech, abdominal cramps, nausea, vomiting, tachycardia, fever, palpitations, drop in blood pressure, dyspnea, and sense of chest constriction. Symptoms may last up to 24 hours.

enzyme induction stimulation of microsomal enzymes by a drug resulting in its accelerated metabolism and decreased activity. If reactive intermediates are formed, drug-mediated toxicity may be exacerbated.

first-pass effect reduced bioavailability of an orally administered drug due to metabolism in GI epithelial cells and liver or to biliary excretion. Effect may be avoided by use of sublingual tablets or rectal suppositories.

fixed-drug eruption drug-induced circumscribed skin lesion that persists or recurs in the same site. Residual pigmentation may remain following drug withdrawal.

half-life (t$_{1/2}$) time required for concentration of a drug in the body to decrease by 50%. Half-life also represents the time necessary to reach steady state or to decline from steady state after a change (i.e., starting or stopping) in the dosing regimen. Half-life may be affected by a disease state and age of the drug user.

heat stroke a life-threatening condition manifested by absence of sweating; red, dry, hot skin; dilated pupils; dyspnea; full bounding pulse; temperature above 40C (105F); and mental confusion.

hepatic toxicity impairment of liver function manifested by jaundice, dark urine, pruritus, light-colored stools, eosinophilia, itchy skin or rash, and persistently high elevations of alanine amino-transferase (ALT) and aspartate aminotransferase (AST).

hyperammonemia elevated level of ammonia or ammonium in the blood manifested by lethargy, decreased appetite, vomiting, asterixis (flapping tremor), weak pulse, irritability, decreased responsiveness, and seizures.

hypercalcemia elevated serum calcium manifested by deep bone and flank pain, renal calculi, anorexia, nausea, vomiting, thirst, constipation, muscle hypotonicity, pathologic fracture, bradycardia, lethargy, and psychosis.

hyperglycemia elevated blood glucose manifested by flushed, dry skin, low blood pressure and elevated pulse, tachypnea, Kussmaul's respirations, polyuria, polydipsia; polyphagia, lethargy, and drowsiness.

hyperkalemia excessive potassium in blood, which may

produce life-threatening cardiac arrhythmias, including bradycardia and heart block, unusual fatigue, weakness or heaviness of limbs, general muscle weakness, muscle cramps, paresthesias, flaccid paralysis of extremities, shortness of breath, nervousness, confusion, diarrhea, and GI distress.

hypermagnesemia excessive magnesium in blood, which may produce cathartic effect, profound thirst, flushing, sedation, confusion, depressed deeptendon reflexes (DTRs), muscle weakness, hypotension, and depressed respirations.

hypernatremia excessive sodium in blood, which may produce confusion, neuromuscular excitability, muscle weakness, seizures, thirst, dry and flushed skin, dry mucous membranes, pyrexia, agitation, and oliguria or anuria.

hypersensitivity reactions excessive and abnormal sensitivity to given agent manifested by urticaria, pruritus, wheezing, edema, redness, and anaphylaxis.

hyperthyroidism excessive secretion by the thyroid glands, which increases basal metabolic rate, resulting in warm, flushed, moist skin; tachycardia, exophthalmos; infrequent lid blinking; lid edema; weight loss despite increased appetite; frequent urination; menstrual irregularity; breathlessness; hypoventilation; congestive heart failure; excessive sweating.

hyperuricemia excessive uric acid in blood, resulting in pain in flank; stomach, or joints, and changes in intake and output ratio and pattern.

hypocalcemia abnormally low calcium level in blood, which may result in depression; psychosis; hyperreflexia; diarrhea; cardiac arrhythmias; hypotension;

muscle spasms; paresthesias of feet, fingers, tongue; positive Chvostek's sign. Severe deficiency (tetany) may result in carpopedal spasms, spasms of face muscle, laryngospasm, and generalized convulsions.

hypoglycemia abnormally low glucose level in the blood, which may result in acute fatigue, restlessness, malaise, marked irritability and weakness, cold sweats, excessive hunger, headache, dizziness, confusion, slurred speech, loss of consciousness, and death.

hypokalemia abnormally low level of potassium in blood, which may result in malaise, fatigue, paresthesias, depressed reflexes, muscle weakness and cramps, rapid, irregular pulse, arrhythmias, hypotension, vomiting, paralytic ileus, mental confusion, depression, delayed thought process, abdominal distention, polyuria, shallow breathing, and shortness of breath.

hypomagnesemia abnormally low level of magnesium in blood, resulting in nausea, vomiting, cardiac arrhythmias, and neuromuscular symptoms (tetany, positive Chvostek's and Trousseau's signs, seizures, tremors, ataxia, vertigo, nystagmus, muscular fasciculations).

hypophosphatemia abnormally low level of phosphates in blood, resulting in muscle weakness, anorexia, malaise, absent deeptendon reflexes, bone pain, paresthesias, tremors, negative calcium balance, osteomalacia, osteoporosis.

hypothyroidism condition caused by thyroid hormone deficiency that lowers basal metabolic rate and may result in periorbital edema, lethargy, puffy hands and feet, cool, pale skin, vertigo, nocturnal cramps, decreased GI motility, constipation, hypotension, slow pulse, depressed muscular activity, and enlarged thyroid gland.

hypoxia insufficient oxygenation in the blood manifested by dyspnea, tachypnea, headache, restlessness, cyanosis, tachycardia, dysrhythmias, confusion, decreased level of consciousness, and euphoria or delirium.

international normalizing ratio measurement that normalizes for the differences obtained from various laboratory readings in the value for thromboplastin blood level.

leukopenia abnormal decrease in number of white blood cells, usually below 5000 per cubic millimeter, resulting in fever, chills, sore mouth or throat, and unexplained fatigue.

liver toxicity manifested by anorexia, nausea, fatigue, lethargy, itching, jaundice, abdominal pain, dark-colored urine, and flu-like symptoms.

metabolic acidosis decrease in pH value of the extracellular fluid caused by either an increase in hydrogen ions or a decrease in bicarbonate ions. It may result in one or more of the following: lethargy, headache, weakness, abdominal pain, nausea, vomiting, dyspnea, hyperpnea progressing to Kussmaul breathing, dehydration, thirst, weakness, flushed face, full bounding pulse, progressive drowsiness, mental confusion, combativeness.

metabolic alkalosis increase in pH value of the extracellular fluid caused by either a loss of acid from the body (e.g., through vomiting) or an increased level of bicarbonate ions (e.g., through ingestion of sodium bicarbonate). It may result in muscle weakness, irritability, confusion, muscle twitching, slow and shallow respirations, and convulsive seizures.

microsomal enzymes drug-metabolizing enzymes located in the endoplasmic reticulum of the liver and other tissues chiefly responsible for oxidative drug metabolism, e.g., cytochrome P-450.

myopathy any disease or abnormal condition of striated muscles manifested by muscle weakness, myalgia, diaphoresis, fever, and reddish-brown urine (myoglobinuria) or oliguria.

nephrotoxicity impairment of the nephrons of the kidney manifested by one or more of the following: oliguria, urinary frequency, hematuria, cloudy urine, rising BUN and serum creatinine, fever, graft tenderness or enlargement.

neuroleptic malignant syndrome (NMS) potentially fatal complication associated with antipsychotic drugs manifested by hyperpyrexia, altered mental status, muscle rigidity, irregular pulse, fluctuating BP, diaphoresis, and tachycardia.

orphan drug (as defined by the Orphan Drug Act, an amendment of the Federal Food, Drug, and Cosmetic Act which took effect in January 1983): drug or biological product used in the treatment, diagnosis, or prevention of a rare disease. A rare disease or condition is one that affects fewer than 200,000 persons in the United States, or affects more than 200,000 persons but for which there is no reasonable expectation that drug research and development costs can be recovered from sales within the United States.

ototoxicity impairment of the ear manifested by one or more of the following: headache, dizziness or vertigo, nausea and vomiting with motion, ataxia, nystagmus.

prodrug inactive drug form that becomes pharmacologically active through biotransformation.

protein binding reversible interaction between protein and drug resulting in a drug–protein complex (bound drug) which is in equilibrium with free (active) drug in plasma and tissues. Because only free drug can diffuse to action sites, factors that influence drug-binding (e.g., displacement of bound drug by another drug, or decreased albumin concentration) may potentiate pharmacological effect.

pseudomembranous enterocolitis life-threatening superinfection characterized by severe diarrhea and fever.

pseudoparkinsonism extrapyramidal symptom manifested by slowing of volitional movement (akinesia), mask facies, rigidity and tremor at rest (especially of upper extremities); and pill rolling motion.

pulmonary edema excessive fluid in the lung tissue manifested by one or more of the following: shortness of breath, cyanosis, persistent productive cough (frothy sputum may be blood tinged), expiratory rales, restlessness, anxiety, increased heart rate, sense of chest pressure.

renal insufficiency reduced capacity of the kidney to perform its functions as manifested by one or more of the following: dysuria, oliguria, hematuria, swelling of lower legs and feet.

serotonin syndrome manifested by restlessness, myoclonus, mental status changes, hyperreflexia, diaphoresis, shivering, and tremor.

Somogyi effect rebound phenomenon clinically manifested by fasting hyperglycemia and worsening of diabetic control due to unnecessarily large p.m. insulin doses. Hormonal response to unrecognized hypoglycemia (i.e., release of epinephrine, glucagon, growth hormone, cortisol) causes insensitivity to insulin. Increasing the amount of insulin required to treat the hyperglycemia intensifies the hypoglycemia.

superinfection new infection by an organism different from the initial infection being treated by antimicrobial therapy manifested by one or more of the following: black, hairy tongue; glossitis, stomatitis; anal itching; loose, foul-smelling stools; vaginal itching or discharge; sudden fever; cough.

tachyphylaxis rapid decrease in response to a drug after administration of a few doses. Initial drug response cannot be restored by an increase in dose.

tardive dyskinesia extrapyramidal symptom manifested by involuntary rhythmic, bizarre movements of face, jaw, mouth, tongue, and sometimes extremities.

vasovagal symptoms transient vascular and neurogenic reaction marked by pallor, nausea, vomiting, bradycardia, and rapid fall in arterial blood pressure.

water intoxication (dilutional hyponatremia) less than normal concentration of sodium in the blood resulting from excess extracellular and intracellular fluid and producing one or more of the following: lethargy, confusion, headache, decreased skin turgor, tremors, convulsions, coma, anorexia, nausea, vomiting, diarrhea, sternal fingerprinting, weight gain, edema, full bounding pulse, jugular vein distention, rales, signs and symptoms of pulmonary edema.

Source: Reprinted with permission from Wilson BA, Shannon MT, Stang CL. *Nurse's Drug Guide 2005,* pages 1748–1752. Upper Saddle River, NJ: Pearson/Prentice Hall, © 2005.

ABGs	arterial blood gases
a.c.	before meals (*ante cibum*)
ACD	acid–citrate–dextrose
ACE	angiotensin-converting enzyme
ACh	acetylcholine
ACIP	Advisory Committee on Immunization Practices
ACLS	advanced cardiac life support
ACS	acute coronary syndrome
ACT	activated clotting time
ACTH	adrenocorticotropic hormone
ADD	attention deficit disorder
ADH	antidiuretic hormone
ADLs	activities of daily living
ad lib	as desired (*ad libitum*)
ADP	adenosine diphosphate
ADT	alternate-day drug (administration)
AIDS	acquired immunodeficiency syndrome
ALT	alanine aminotransferase (formerly SGPT)
AML	acute myelogenous leukemia
AMP	adenosine monophosphate
ANA	antinuclear antibody(ies)
ANC	acid neutralizing capacity; absolute neutrophil count
aPTT	activated partial thromboplastin time
ARC	AIDS-related complex
ARDS	adult respiratory distress syndrome
ASHD	arteriosclerotic heart disease
AST	aspartate aminotransferase (formerly SGOT)
AT$_1$	angiotensin II receptor subtype I
AT$_2$	angiotensin II receptor subtype II
ATP	adenosine triphosphate
AV	atrioventricular
b.i.d.	two times a day (*bis in die*)
BM	bowel movement
BMD	bone mineral density
BMR	basal metabolic rate
BP	blood pressure
bpm	beats per minute
BSA	body surface area
BSE	breast self-exam
BSP	bromsulphalein
BT	bleeding time
BUN	blood urea nitrogen
C	centigrade, Celsius
CAD	coronary artery disease
cAMP	cyclic adenosine monophosphate
CBC	complete blood count
cc	cubic centimeter

CDC	Centers for Disease Control and Prevention
CF	cystic fibrosis
CHF	congestive heart failure
Cl_{cr}	creatinine clearance
cm	centimeter
CMV	cytomegalovirus-I
CMVIG	cytomegalovirus immune globulin
CNS	central nervous system
Coll	collyrium (eye wash)
COMT	catecholamine-*o*-methyl transferase
COPD	chronic obstructive pulmonary disease
COX-2	cyclooxygenase-2
CPK	creatinine phosphokinase
CPR	cardiopulmonary resuscitation
CRF	chronic renal failure
C&S	culture and sensitivity
CSF	cerebrospinal fluid
CSP	cellulose sodium phosphate
CT	clotting time
CTZ	chemoreceptor trigger zone
CV	cardiovascular
CVA	cerebrovascular accident
CVP	central venous pressure
D5W	5% dextrose in water
D&C	dilation and curettage
DIC	disseminated intravascular coagulation
DKA	diabetic keto-acidosis
dL	deciliter (100 mL or 0.1 liter)
DM	diabetes mellitus
DNA	deoxyribonucleic acid
DTRs	deep-tendon reflexes
DVT	deep-venous thrombosis
ECG, EKG	electrocardiogram
ECT	electroconvulsive therapy
EEG	electroencephalogram
EENT	eye, ear, nose, throat
e.g.	for example (*exempli gratia*)
ENT	ear, nose, throat
EPS	extrapyramidal symptoms (or syndrome)
ER	estrogen receptor
ESR	erythrocyte sedimentation rate
F	Fahrenheit
FBS	fasting blood sugar
FDA	Food and Drug Administration
FSH	follicle-stimulating hormone
FTI	free thyroxine index
5-FU	5-fluorouracil
FUO	fever of unknown origin
g	gram
G6PD	glucose-6-phosphate dehydrogenase
GABA	gamma-aminobutyric acid
G-CSF	granulocyte colony-stimulating factor

GFR	glomerular filtration rate
GH	growth hormone
GI	gastrointestinal
GPIIb/IIIa	glycoprotein IIb/IIIa
GU	genitourinary
h	hour
HbA$_{1c}$	glycosylated hemoglobin
HCG	human chorionic gonadotropin
Hct	hematocrit
HDL	high density lipoprotein
HDL-C	high-density-lipoprotein cholesterol
HER	human epidermal growth factor
Hgb	hemoglobin
5-HIAA	5-hydroxyindoleacetic acid
HIT	heparin-induced thrombocytopenia
HIV	human immunodeficiency virus
HMG-CoA	3-hydroxy-3-methyl-glutaryl coenzyme A
HPA	hypothalamic-pituitary-adrenocortical (axis)
HPV	human papillomavirus
HR	heart rate
HSV-1	herpes simplex virus type 1
HSV-2	herpes simplex virus type 2
5-HT	5-hydroxytryptamine (serotonin receptor)
I&O	intake and output
IBW	ideal body weight
IC	intracoronary
ICP	intracranial pressure
ICU	intensive care unit
ID	intradermal
IDDM	insulin-dependent diabetes mellitus (Type I diabetes)
IFN	interferon
Ig	immunoglobulin
IL	interleukin
IM	intramuscular
INR	international normalizing ratio
IOP	intraocular pressure
IPPB	intermittent positive-pressure breathing
IV	intravenous
kg	kilogram
17-KGS	17-ketogenic steroids
17-KS	17-ketosteroids
KVO	keep vein open
L	liter
LDH	lactic dehydrogenase
LDL	low density lipoprotein
LDL-C	low-density-lipoprotein cholesterol
LE	lupus erythematosus
LFT	liver function test
LH	luteinizing hormone
LSD	lysergic acid diethylamide
LTRA	leukotriene receptor antagonist

M	molar (strength of a solution)
m²	square meter (of body surface area)
MAO	monoamine oxidase
MAOI	monoamine oxidase inhibitor
MBD	minimal brain dysfunction
MCH	mean corpuscular hemoglobin
MCHC	mean corpuscular hemoglobin concentration
mCi	millicurie
μg, mcg	microgram (1/1000 of a milligram)
μm	micrometer
MDI	metered-dose inhaler
MDR	minimum daily requirements
mEq	milliequivalent
mg	milligram
min	minute
MI	myocardial infarction
MIC	minimum inhibitory concentration
mL	milliliter (0.001 liter)
mm	millimeter
mo	month
MRSA	methicillin-resistant *Staphylococcus aureus*
MS	multiple sclerosis
N	normal (strength of a solution)
NADH	reduced form of nicotine adenine dinucleotide
NAPA	*N*-acetyl procainamide
nb	note well (*nota bene*)
ng	nanogram (1/1000 of a microgram)
NIDDM	non-insulin-dependent diabetes mellitus (Type II diabetes)
NMS	neuroleptic malignant syndrome
NNRTI	nonnucleoside reverse transcriptase inhibitor
NPN	nonprotein nitrogen
NPO	nothing by mouth
NS	normal saline
NSAID	nonsteroidal anti-inflammatory drug
NSR	normal sinus rhythm
OC	oral contraceptive
17-OHCS	17-hydroxycorticosteroids
OTC	over the counter (nonprescription)
PABA	*para*-aminobenzoic acid
PAS	*para*-aminosalicylic acid
PAWP	pulmonary artery wedge pressure
PBI	protein-bound iodine
PBP	penicillin-binding protein
p.c.	after meals (*post cibum*)
PCI	percutaneous coronary intervention
PERLA	pupils equal, react to light and accommodation
PG	prostaglandin
pH	hydrogen ion concentration
PID	pelvic inflammatory disease

PKU	phenylketonuria
PND	paroxysmal nocturnal dyspnea
PO	by mouth or orally (*per os*)
PPM	parts per million
PR	rectally (*per rectum*)
prn	when required (*pro re nata*)
PSA	prostate-specific antigen
PSP	phenolsulfonphthalein
PSVT	paroxysmal supraventricular tachycardia
PT	prothrombin time
PTH	parathyroid hormone
PTT	partial thromboplastin time
PUD	peptic ulcer disease
PVC	premature ventricular contraction
PVD	peripheral vascular disease
PZI	protamine zinc insulin
q	every
q.i.d.	four times daily
RA	rheumatoid arthritis
RAI	radioactive iodine
RAST	radioallergosorbent test
RBC	red blood (cell) count
RDA	recommended (daily) dietary allowance
RDS	respiratory distress syndrome
REM	rapid eye movement
rem	radiation equivalent man
RIA	radioimmunoassay
RNA	ribonucleic acid
ROM	range of motion
RSV	respiratory syncytial virus
RT$_3$U	total serum thyroxine concentration
sec	second
S&S	signs and symptoms
SA	sinoatrial
SBE	subacute bacterial endocarditis
SC	subcutaneous
S$_{cr}$	serum creatinine
SGGT	serum gamma-glutamyl transferase
SGOT	serum glutamic-oxaloacetic transaminase (*see* AST)
SGPT	serum glutamic-pyruvic transaminase (*see* ALT)
SIADH	syndrome of inappropriate antidiuretic hormone
SI Units	International System of Units
SK	streptokinase
SL	sublingual
SLE	systemic lupus erythematosus
SMA	sequential multiple analysis
SOS	if necessary (*si opus cit*)
sp	species
SPF	sun protection factor

sq	square
SR	sedimentation rate
SRS-A	slow-reactive substance of anaphylaxis
SSRI	selective serotonin-reuptake inhibitor
stat	immediately
STD	sexually transmitted disease
$t_{1/2}$	half-life
T_3	triiodothyronine
T_4	thyroxine
TCA	tricyclic antidepressant
TG	total triglycerides
TIA	transient ischemic attack
t.i.d.	three times a day *(ter in die)*
TNF	tumor necrosis factor
tPA	tissue plasminogen activator
TPN	total parenteral nutrition
TPR	temperature, pulse, respirations
TSH	thyroid-stimulating hormone
TT	thrombin time
URI	upper respiratory infection
USP	United States Pharmacopeia
USPHS	United States Public Health Service
UTI	urinary tract infection
UV-A, UVA	ultraviolet A wave
VDRL	venereal disease research laboratory
VLDL	very low density lipoprotein
VMA	vanillylmandelic acid
VS	vital signs
wk	week
WBC	white blood (cell) count
WBCT	whole blood clotting time
y	year

APPENDIX F–1
COMMON TOXIC EFFECTS OF ANTINEOPLASTICS:

Drug	Common Toxic Effects
ARA-C	Myelosuppression: megaloblastosis, reticulocytosis, leukopenia, thrombocytopenia, anemia High-dose: Neurologic: cerebral and cerebellar dysfunction GI: severe ulceration Pulmonary: respiratory distress, pulmonary edema
Asparaginase	Hypersensitivity: rash, urticaria, hypotension, dyspnea, arthralgia, anaphylaxis Hyperglycemia: severe vomiting
Bleomycin	Pulmonary: interstitial pneumonitis, pulmonary fibrosis, toxicity
Busulfan	Bone marrow failure, acute renal failure, pulmonary fibrosis
Carboplatin	Nausea, vomiting, thrombocytopenia, leukopenia, neutropenia, anemia, hyponatremia, hypomagnesemia, hypocalcemia, hypokalemia
Carmustine	Delayed myelosuppression, pulmonary infiltration or fibrosis, eye infarctions, nausea, vomiting
Chlorambucil	Hepatotoxicity, bone marrow depression, leukopenia, sterility
Cisplatin	Renal: increased serum creatinine, BUN, uric acid; decreased creatinine clearance, glomerular filtration rate Electrolyte imbalance: hypomagnesemia, hypocalcemia, hypokalemia, hypophosphatemia, hyponatremia GI: servere nausea and vomiting Ototoxicity: tinnitus, hearing loss Myelosuppression: less severe than with other agents
Cyclophosphamide	Myelosuppression: leukopenia, thrombocytopenia, anemia Hypothrombinemia GU: hemorrhagic cystitis, hematuria
Cytosine arabinoside (cytarabine)	Nausea, vomiting, leukopenia, thrombocytopenia, neurotoxicity
Dacarbazine	Myelosuppression: leukopenia, thrombocytopenia GI: nausea and vomiting

Drug	Common Toxic Effects
Dactinomycin	Myelosuppression: leukopenia, thrombocytopenia; less often anemia, pancytopenia, reticulopenia, agranulocytosis, aplastic anemia GI: stomatitis, diarrhea
Daunorubicin	Myelosuppression: leukopenia, thrombocytopenia, anemia Cardiac: congestive heart failure
Dexamethasone	Nasal irritation, increased ICP, hyperglycemia, cataract, peptic ulcer, bowel perforation, impaired wound healing, long bone and vertebral fractures, muscle weakness and wasting
Doxorubicin	Myelosuppression: leukopenia, thrombocytopenia, anemia Cardiac: congestive heart failure, cardiorespiratory decompensation; dose-related cardiotoxicity
Etoposide	Myelosuppression: leukopenia, granulocytopenia, thrombocytopenia, anemia, pancytopenia Cardiac: delayed hypotension
Fluorouracil	GI: stomatitis (day 5 to 8 of therapy), GI hemorrhage Myelosuppression: leukopenia, granulocytopenia, thrombocytopenia, anemia
Hydroxyurea	Myelosuppression: leukopenia, thrombocytopenia, anemia GI: severe nausea and vomiting
Ifosfamide	Confusion, hallucinations, nausea, vomiting, neutropenia, thrombocytopenia, hemorrhagic cystitis, nephrotoxicity
Irinotecan	Asthenia, fever, pain, diarrhea, dehydration, nausea, vomiting, weight loss, leukopenia, neutropenia, anemia, dyspnea
Lomustine	Delayed myelosuppression: leukopenia (6 weeks after therapy), thrombocytopenia (4 weeks after therapy), anemia (4–7 weeks after therapy), pancytopenia
Mechlorethamine	Myelosuppression: leukopenia, anemia, thrombocytopenia, delayed hemorrhage GI: severe nausea and vomiting
Melphalan	Leukopenia, agranulocytosis, thrombocytopenia, pulmonary fibrosis
Mercaptopurine	Myelosuppression: leukopenia, anemia, thrombocytopenia, agranulocytosis, pancytopenia, hypoplastic bone marrow Hepatic: jaundice, ascites, elevated liver enzymes, cholestasis

Drug	Common Toxic Effects
Methotrexate	GI: oral ulcers Myelosuppression: leukopenia, thrombocytopenia, anemia, hemorrhage
Paclitaxel	Bradycardia, peripheral neuropathy, nausea, vomiting, mucositis, neutropenia, anemia, thrombocytopenia, hypersensitivity reaction, arthralgia, myalgia
Prednisone	Muscle weakness and wasting, osteoporosis, growth suppression, hyperglycemia, hypokalemia, delayed wound healing
Prednisolone	Growth suppression, hypotension, muscle weakness and wasting, osteoporosis, delayed wound healing
Procarbazine	Myelosuppression: leukopenia, reticulocytopenia, thrombocytopenia, eosinophilia, anemia, blood cell hemolysis Neurologic: neuropathy, paresthesia, depression, tremors, confusion, seizures GI: stomatitis, diarrhea
Teniposide	Myelosuppression: neutropenia, diarrhea; nausea, vomiting, transient hypotension, hypersensitivity, neurotoxicity, fever
Thioguanine	Myelosuppression: leukopenia, thrombocytopenia, anemia Hepatic: jaundice, elevated liver enzymes GI: stomatitis, diarrhea
Thiotepa	Leukopenia, thrombocytopenia, anemia, pancytopenia
Vinblastine	Myelosuppression: leukopenia, granulocytopenia, thrombocytopenia, anemia Neurologic: numbness, paresthesia, peripheral neuropathy, depression
Vincristine	Neurologic: peripheral neuropathy with Achilles tendon reflex, depression, then loss of other deep tendon reflexes Myelosuppression: less severe than with other agents

Note: Drugs cause various responses in the body. Antineoplastic agents are expected to cause toxicity because of their potency and desired action on abnormal body cells. The symptoms listed here are the most common and earliest toxic effects. They require dosage lowering or temporary cessation of the drug. Generally, the highest dose possible is given that allows for absence of toxic effects but maximum therapeutic effects in the body. Toxic effects can lead to serious, life-threatening, and sometimes permanent damage in the body. They, therefore, require dosage adjustment, in contrast to other less threatening side effects. Each drug has unique toxic effects that indicate need for dosage adjustment.

These drugs have potentially severe toxic effects and should be given only under the supervision of a physician with training and experience in cancer chemotherapy. The drug's potential for toxic effects on healthcare personnel, as well as patients, necessitates careful handling during preparation and administration.

COMMONLY USED ANTINEOPLASTIC DRUG COMBINATIONS:

Acronym	Drug Combination
ABVD	Adriamycin (doxorubicin) + bleomycin + vinblastine + dacarbazine
ABVE	Adriamycin (doxorubicin) + bleomycin + vincristine + etoposide
ABVE-PC	Adriamycin (doxorubicin) + bleomycin + vincristine + etoposide + prednisone + cyclophosphamide
ACE	Adriamycin (doxorubicin) + cyclophosphamide + etoposide
A-COPP	Adriamycin (doxorubicin) + cyclophosphamide + vincristine (oncovin) + procarbazine + prednisone
APE	Adriamycin (doxorubicin) + procarbazine + etoposide
BEACOPP	bleomycin + etoposide + Adriamycin (doxorubicin) + cyclophosphamide + vincristine + procarbazine + prednisone
CAF	cyclophosphamide + doxorubicin + fluorouracil
CAMP	cyclophosphamide + doxorubicin + methotrexate + procarbazine
CAVe	lomustine + doxorubicin + vinblastine
CAVE, ECHO, CAPO, EVAC, or VOCA	etoposide + cyclophosphamide + doxorubicin + vincristine
CHOP	cyclophosphamide + doxorubicin + vincristine + prednisone
CHOR	cyclophosphamide + doxorubicin + vincristine
CISCA	cisplatin + cyclophosphamide
CMF	cyclophosphamide + methotrexate + fluorouracil
COPP	cyclophosphamide + vincristine + procarbazine + prednisone
CY-VA-DIC	cyclophosphamide + vincristine + doxorubicin + dacarbazine
EBVP	etoposide + bleomycin + vinblastine + prednisone
FAC	fluorouracil + doxorubicin + cyclophosphamide
MACC	methotrexate + doxorubicin + cyclophosphamide + lomustine
MOPP	mechlorethamine + vincristine + procarbazine + prednisone
MTX + MP + CTX	methotrexate + mercaptopurine + cyclophosphamide
OEPA	vincristine + etoposide + prednisone + Adriamycin (doxorubicin)
OPPA	vincristine + prednisone + procarbazine + Adriamycin (doxorubicin)

PVB or VBP	vinblastine + bleomycin + cisplatin
T-2	dactinomycin + doxorubicin + vincristine + cyclophosphamide
VAMP	vinblastine + Adriamycin (doxorubicin) + methotrexate + prednisone
VAP	vincristine + dactinomycin + cyclophosphamide
VEPA	vinblastine + etoposide + prednisone + Adriamycin (doxorubicin)
VP-L-asparaginase	vincristine + prednisone + L-asparaginase

APPENDIX G–1
PEDIATRIC ADVANCED LIFE SUPPORT MEDICATIONS FOR CARDIAC ARREST AND SYMPTOMATIC ARRHYTHMIAS:

Drug	Dosage (Pediatric)	Remarks
Adenosine	0.1 mg/kg	Rapid IV/IO bolus
	Repeat dose: 0.2 mg/kg	Rapid flush to central circulation
	Maximum single dose: 12 mg	Monitor ECG during dose.
Amiodarone for pulseless VF/VT	5 mg/kg IV/IO	Rapid IV bolus IV over 20 to 60 minutes
Amiodarone for perfusing tachycardias	Loading dose: 5 mg/kg IV/IO	Routine use in combination with drugs prolonging QT interval is *not* recommended.
	Maximum dose: 15 mg/kg per day	Hypotension is most frequent side effect.
Atropine sulfate*	0.02 mg/kg	May give IV, IO or ET.
	Minimum dose: 0.1 mg	Tachycardia and pupil dilation may occur but *not* fixed dilated pupils.
	Maximum single dose: 0.5 mg in child, 1.0 mg in adolescent. May repeat once.	
Calcium chloride 10% = 100 mg/mL (=27.2 mg/mL elemental Ca)	20 mg/kg (0.2 mL/kg) IV/IO	Give slow IV push for hypocalcemia, hypermagnesemia, calcium channel blocker toxicity, preferably via central vein. Monitor heart rate; bradycardia may occur.
Calcium gluconate 10% = 100 mg/mL (= 9 mg/mL elemental Ca)	60–100 mg/kg (0.6–1.0 mL/kg) IV/IO	Give slow IV push for hypocalcemia, hypermagnesemia, calcium channel blocker toxicity, preferably via central vein.
Epinephrine for symptomatic bradycardia*	IV/IO: 0.01 mg/kg (1:10 000, 0.1 mL/kg) ET: 0.1 mg/kg (1:1000, 0.1 mL/kg)	Tachyarrhythmias, hypertension may occur.
Epinephrine for pulseless arrest*	First dose: IV/IO: 0.01 mg/kg (1:10 000, 0.1 mL/kg) ET: 0.1 mg/kg (1:1000, 0.1 mL/kg)	

	Subsequent doses: Repeat initial dose or may increase up to 10 times (0.1 mg/kg, 1:1000, 0.1 mL/kg) Administer epinephrine every 3–5 minutes. IV/IO/ET doses as high as 0.2 mg/kg of 1:1000 may be effective.	
Glucose (10% or 25% or 50%)	IV/IO: 0.5–1.0 g/kg ▪ 1–2 mL/kg 50% ▪ 2–4 mL/kg 25% ▪ 5–10 mL/kg 10%	For suspected hypoglycemia; avoid hyperglycemia.
Lidocaine* Lidocaine infusion (start after a bolus)	IV/IO/ET: 1 mg/kg IV/IO: 20–50 μg/kg per minute	Rapid bolus 1–2.5 mL/kg per hour of 120 mg/100 mL solution or use "Rule of 6" (see Table 3)
Magnesium sulfate (500 mg/mL)	IV/IO: 25–50 mg/kg, Maximum dose: 2 g per dose	Rapid IV infusion for torsades or suspected hypomagnesemia; 10- to 20-minute infusion for asthma that responds poorly to β-adrenergic agonists.
Naloxone*	≤5 years or ≤20 kg: 0.1 mg/kg >5 years or >20 kg: 2.0 mg	For total reversal of narcotic effect. Use small repeated doses (0.01–0.03 mg/kg) titrated to desired effect.
Procainamide for perfusing tachycardias (100 mg/mL and 500 mg/mL)	Loading dose: 15 mg/kg IV/IO	Infusion over 30–60 minutes; routine use in combination with drugs prolonging QT interval is *not* recommended.
Sodium bicarbonate (1 mEq/mL and 0.5 mEq/mL)	IV/IO: 1 mEq/kg per dose	Infuse slowly and only if ventilation is adequate.

IV indicates intravenous; IO, intraosseous; ET, endotracheal.
*For endotracheal administration, use higher doses (2 to 10 times the IV dose); dilute medication with normal saline to a volume of 3–5 mL and follow with several positive-pressure ventilations.

APPENDIX G–2
PEDIATRIC ADVANCED LIFE SUPPORT MEDICATIONS TO MAINTAIN CARDIAC OUTPUT AND FOR POSTRESUSCITATION STABILIZATION:

Medication	Dose Range	Comment	Preparation*
Amrinone	IV/IO loading dose: 0.75–1.0 mg/kg IV over 5 minutes; may repeat 2 times IV/IO infusion: 5–10 mcg/kg per minute	Inodilator	6 × body weight (in kg) = No. of mg diluted to total 100 mL; then 1 mL/h delivers 1 mcg/kg per minute
Dobutamine	IV/IO infusion: 2–20 mcg/kg per minute	Inotrope; vasodilator	6 × body weight (in kg) = No. of mg diluted to total 100 mL; then 1 mL/h delivers 1 mcg/kg per minute
Dopamine	IV/IO infusion: 2–20 mcg/kg per minute	Inotrope; chronotrope; renal and splanchnic vasodilator in lower doses; pressor in higher doses	6 × body weight (in kg) = No. of mg diluted to total 100 mL; then 1 mL/h delivers 1 mcg/kg per minute
Epinephrine	IV/IO infusion: 0.1–1.0 mcg/kg per minute	Inotrope; chronotrope; vasodilator in lower doses and pressor in higher doses	0.6 × body weight (in kg) = No. of mg diluted to total 100 mL; then 1 mL/h delivers 0.1 mcg/kg per minute
Lidocaine	IV/IO loading dose: 1 mg/kg IV/IO infusion: 20–50 mcg/kg per minute	Antiarrhythmic, mild negative inotrope. Use lower infusion rate if poor cardiac output or poor hepatic function.	60 × body weight (in kg) = No. of mg diluted to total 100 mL; then 1 mL/h delivers 10 mcg/kg per minute or alternative premix 120 mg/100 mL at 1 to 2.5 mL/kg per hour
Milrinone	IV/IO loading dose: 50–75 mcg/kg IV/IO infusion: 0.5–0.75 mcg/kg per minute	Inodilator	0.6 × body weight (in kg) = No. of mg diluted to total 100 mL; then 1 mL/h delivers 0.1 mcg/kg per minute

Medication	Dose Range	Comment	Preparation*
Norepinephrine	IV/IO infusion: 0.1–2.0 mcg/kg per minute	Vasopressor	0.6 × body weight (in kg) = No. of mg diluted to total 100 mL; then 1 mL/h delivers 0.1 mcg/kg per minute
Prostaglandin E$_1$	IV/IO infusion: 0.05–0.1 mcg/kg per minute	Maintains patency of ductus arteriosus in cyanotic con-genital heart disease. Monitor for apnea, hypotension, and hypoglycemia.	0.3 × body weight (in kg) = No. of mg diluted to total 50 mL; then 1 mL/h delivers 0.1 mcg/kg per minute
Sodium nitroprusside	IV/IO infusion: 1–8 mcg/kg per minute	Vasodilator Prepare only in dextrose in water	6 × body weight (in kg) = No. of mg diluted to total 100 mL; then 1 mL/h delivers 1 mcg/kg per minute

IV indicates intravenous; IO, intraosseous.
*Most infusions may be calculated on the basis of the "Rule of 6" as illustrated in the table. Alternatively, a standard concentration may be used to provide more dilute or more concentrated drug solution, but then an individual dose must be calculated for each patient and each infusion rate as follows: Infusion rate (mL/h) = [weight (kg) × dose (mcg/kg per minute) × 60 min/h]/concentration (mcg/mL). Diluent may be 5% dextrose in water, 5% dextrose in half-normal saline, normal saline, or Ringer's lactate unless noted otherwise.

Reproduced with permission, *Guidelines 2000 for Cardiopulmonary Resuscitation and Emergency Cardiovascular Care,* © 2000, American Heart Association.

APPENDIX H–1
RECOMMENDED CHILDHOOD IMMUNIZATION SCHEDULE—UNITED STATES, JULY–DECEMBER, 2004:

Vaccines are listed under the routinely recommended ages. Bars indicate range of acceptable ages for vaccination. Shaded bars indicate *catch-up vaccination*. (Centers for Disease Control and Prevention, National Immunization Program).

FIGURE. Recommended childhood and adolescent immunization schedule[1] — United States, July–December 2004

1. Indicates the recommended ages for routine administration of currently licensed childhood vaccines, as of April 1, 2004, for children through age 18 years. Any dose not given at the recommended age should be given at any subsequent visit when indicated and feasible. [█] Indicates age groups that warrant special effort to administer those vaccines not given previously. Additional vaccines may be licensed and recommended during the year. Licensed combination vaccines may be used whenever any components of the combination are indicated and the vaccine's other components are not contraindicated. Providers should consult the manufacturers' package inserts for detailed recommendations. Clinically significant adverse events that follow vaccination should be reported to the Vaccine Adverse Event Reporting System (VAERS). Guidance about how to obtain and complete a VAERS form is available at http://www.vaers.org/ or by telephone, 800-822-7967.

2. **Hepatitis B vaccine (HepB).** All infants should receive the first dose of HepB vaccine soon after birth and before hospital discharge; the first dose also may be given by age 2 months if the infant's mother is HBsAg-negative. Only monovalent HepB vaccine can be used for the birth dose. Monovalent or combination vaccine containing HepB may be used to complete the series; 4 doses of vaccine may be administered when a birth dose is given. The second dose should be given at least 4 weeks after the first dose except for combination vaccines, which cannot be administered before age 6 weeks. The third dose should be drawn at least 16 weeks after the first dose and at least 8 weeks after the second dose. The last dose in the vaccination series (third or fourth dose) should not be administered before age 24 weeks. **Infants born to HBsAg-positive mothers** should receive HepB vaccine and 0.5 mL hepatitis B immune globulin (HBIG) within 12 hours of birth at separate sites. The second dose is recommended at age 1–2 months. The last dose in the vaccination series should not be administered before age 6 months. These infants should be tested for HBsAg and anti-HBs at age 9–15 months. **Infants born to mothers whose HBsAg status is unknown** should receive the first dose of the HepB vaccine series within 12 hours of birth. Maternal blood should be drawn as soon as possible to determine the mother's HBsAg status; if the HBsAg test is positive, the infant should receive HBIG as soon as possible (no later than age 1 week). The second dose is recommended at age 1–2 months. The last dose in the vaccination series should not be administered before age 24 weeks.

3. **Diphtheria and tetanus toxoids and acellular pertussis vaccine (DTaP).** The fourth dose of DTaP may be administered at age 12 months provided that 6 months have elapsed since the third dose and the child is unlikely to return at age 15–18 months. The final dose in the series should be given at age ≥4 years. Tetanus and diphtheria toxoids (Td) is recommended at age 11–12 years if at least 5 years have elapsed since the last dose of tetanus and diphtheria toxoid-containing vaccine. Subsequent routine Td boosters are recommended every 10 years.

4. **Haemophilus influenzae type b (Hib) conjugate vaccine.** Three Hib conjugate vaccines are licensed for infant use. If PRP-OMP (PedvaxHIB® or ComVax® [Merck]) is administered at ages 2 and 4 months, a dose at age 6 months is not required. DTaP/Hib combination products should not be used for primary vaccination in infants at ages 2, 4, or 6 months but can be used as boosters after any Hib vaccine. The final dose in the series should be given at age ≥12 months.

5. **Measles, mumps, and rubella vaccine (MMR).** The second dose of MMR is recommended routinely at age 4–6 years but may be administered during any visit, provided at least 4 weeks have elapsed since the first dose and both doses are administered beginning at or after age 12 months. Those who have not received the second dose previously should complete the schedule by the visit at age 11–12 years.

6. **Varicella vaccine (VAR).** Varicella vaccine is recommended at any visit at or after age 12 months for susceptible children (i.e., those who lack a reliable history of chickenpox). Susceptible persons aged ≥13 years should receive 2 doses given at least 4 weeks apart.

7. **Pneumococcal vaccine.** The heptavalent pneumococcal conjugate vaccine (PCV) is recommended for all children aged 2–23 months and for certain children aged 24–59 months. The final dose in the series should be given at age ≥12 months. Pneumococcal polysaccharide vaccine (PPV) is recommended in addition to PCV for certain high-risk groups. See MMWR 2000;49(No. RR-9);1–35.

8. **Influenza vaccine.** Influenza vaccine is recommended annually for children aged ≥6 months with certain risk factors (including but not limited to asthma, cardiac disease, sickle cell disease, HIV, and diabetes), health care workers, and other persons (including household members) in close contact with persons in groups at high risk (see MMWR 2004;53[RR][in press]) and can be administered to all others wishing to obtain immunity. In addition, healthy children aged 6–23 months and close contacts of healthy children aged 0–23 months are recommended to receive influenza vaccine, because children in this age group are at substantially increased risk for influenza-related hospitalizations. For healthy persons aged 5–49 years, the intranasally administered live, attenuated influenza vaccine (LAIV) is an acceptable alternative to the intramuscular trivalent inactivated influenza vaccine (TIV). See MMWR 2003;52(No. RR-13);1–8. Children receiving TIV should be administered a dosage appropriate for their age (0.25 mL if age 6–35 months or 0.5 mL if age ≥3 years). Children aged ≤8 years who are receiving influenza vaccine for the first time should receive 2 doses (separated by at least 4 weeks for TIV and at least 6 weeks for LAIV).

9. **Hepatitis A vaccine.** Hepatitis A vaccine is recommended for children and adolescents in selected states and regions and for certain high-risk groups. Consult your local public health authority and MMWR 1999;48(No.RR-12);1–37. Children and adolescents in these states, regions, and high-risk groups who have not been immunized against hepatitis A can begin the hepatitis A vaccination series during any visit. The 2 doses in the series should be administered at least 6 months apart.

Reprinted from Centers for Disease Control and Prevention, National Immunization Program.
Additional information about vaccines, including precautions and contraindications for vaccination and vaccine shortages is available at http://www.cdc.gov/nip or from the National Immunization Information Hotline, 800-232-2522 (English) or 800-232-0233 (Spanish). Approved by the Advisory Committee on Immunization Practices (http://www.cdc.gov/nip/acip), the **American Academy of Pediatrics** (http://www.aap.org) and the **American Academy of Family Physicians** (http://www.aafp.org).

TABLE. Catch-up immunization schedule for children and adolescents who start late or who are >1 month behind

Catch-up schedule for children aged 4 months–6 years

Dose 1 (minimum age)	Minimum interval between doses			
	Dose 1 to dose 2	Dose 2 to dose 3	Dose 3 to dose 4	Dose 4 to dose 5
DTaP (6 wk)	4 wk	4 wk	6 mo	6 mo
IPV [1] (6 wk)	4 wk	4 wk	4 wk [2]	
HepB [3] (birth)	4 wk	8 wk (and 16 wk after 1st dose)		
MMR (12 mo)	4 wk [4]			
VAR (12 mo)				
Hib [5] (6 wk)	4 wk: if 1st dose given at age <12 mo 8 wk (as final dose): if 1st dose given at age 12–14 mo No further doses needed: if 1st dose given at age ≥15 mo	4 wk [6]: if current age <12 mo 8 wk (as final dose) [6] : if current age ≥12 mo and 2nd dose given at age <15 mo No further doses needed: if previous dose given at age ≥15 mo	8 wk (as final dose): this dose only necessary for children aged 12 mo–5 y who received 3 doses before age 12 mo	
PCV [7] (6 wk)	4 wk: if 1st dose given at age <12 mo and current age <24 mo 8 wk (as final dose): if 1st dose given at age ≥12 mo or current age 24–59 mo No further doses needed: for healthy children if 1st dose given at age ≥24 mo	4 wk: if current age <12 mo 8 wk (as final dose): if current age ≥12 mo No further doses needed: for healthy children if previous dose given at age ≥24 mo	8 wk (as final dose): this dose only necessary for children aged 12 mo–5 y who received 3 doses before age 12 mo	

Catch-up schedule for children aged 7–18 years

	Minimum interval between doses		
	Dose 1 to dose 2	Dose 2 to dose 3	Dose 3 to booster dose
Td:	4 wk	Td: 6 mo	Td [8]: 6 mo: if 1st dose given at age <12 mo and current age <11 y 5 y: if 1st dose given at age ≥12 mo and 3rd dose given at age <7 y and current age ≥11 y 10 y: if 3rd dose given at age ≥7 y
IPV [9]:	4 wk	IPV [9]: 4 wk	IPV [2, 9]
HepB:	4 wk	HepB: 8 wk (and 16 wk after 1st dose)	
MMR:	4 wk		
VAR [10]:	4 wk		

Note: A vaccine series does not require restarting, regardless of the time that has elapsed between doses.

1. **Diphtheria and tetanus toxoids and acellular pertussis vaccine (DTaP):** The fifth dose is not necessary if the fourth dose was given after the fourth birthday.
2. **Inactivated polio vaccine (IPV):** For children who received an all-IPV or all-oral poliovirus (OPV) series, a fourth dose is not necessary if third dose was given at age ≥4 years. If both OPV and IPV were given as part of a series, a total of 4 doses should be given, regardless of the child's current age.
3. **Hepatitis B vaccine (HepB):** All children and adolescents who have not been vaccinated against hepatitis B should begin the hepatitis B vaccination series during any visit. Providers should make special efforts to immunize children who were born in, or whose parents were born in, areas of the world where hepatitis B virus infection is moderately or highly endemic.
4. **Measles, mumps, and rubella vaccine (MMR):** The second dose of MMR is recommended routinely at age 4–6 years, but may be given earlier if desired.
5. *Haemophilus influenzae* **type b (Hib) conjugate vaccine:** Vaccine generally is not recommended for children aged ≥5 years.
6. **Hib:** If current age is <12 months and the first 2 doses were PRP-OMP (PedvaxHIB® or ComVax® [Merck]), the third (and final) dose should be given at age 12–15 months and at least 8 weeks after the second dose.
7. **Pneumococcal conjugate vaccine (PCV):** Vaccine generally is not recommended for children aged ≥5 years.
8. **Tetanus and diphtheria toxoids (Td):** For children aged 7–10 years, the interval between the third and booster dose is determined by the age when the first dose was given. For adolescents aged 11–18 years, the interval is determined by the age when the third dose was given.
9. **IPV:** Vaccine generally is not recommended for persons aged ≥18 years.
10. **Varicella vaccine (VAR):** Give 2-dose series to all susceptible adolescents aged ≥13 years.

Reporting adverse reactions. Clinically significant adverse events that follow vaccination should be reported to the Vaccine Adverse Event Reporting System (VAERS). Guidance on completing a VAERS form is available at http://www.vaers.org or at telephone, 800-822-7967. **Disease reporting.** Suspected cases of vaccine-preventable diseases should be reported to state or local health departments. Additional information about vaccines, including precautions and contraindications for vaccination and vaccine shortages, is available at http://www.cdc.gov/nip or at the National Immunization Information hotline, telephone 800-232-2522 (English) or 800-232-0233 (Spanish).

APPENDIX H–2
RECOMMENDATIONS FOR IMMUNIZATION OF CHILDREN AND ADOLESCENTS WITH PRIMARY AND SECONDARY IMMUNE DEFICIENCIES:

Category	Specific Immunodeficiency	Vaccine Contraindications	Effectiveness and Comments
Primary			
B-lymphocyte (humoral)	X-linked and common variable agammaglobulinemia	OPV,[1] vaccinia, and live bacterial; consider measles and varicella	Effectiveness of any vaccine dependent on humoral response is doubtful; IGIV interferes with measles and possibly varicella response.
	Selective IgA deficiency and selective subclass IgG deficiency	OPV[1]; other live vaccines seem to be safe, but caution is urged	All vaccines probably effective. Vaccine response may be attenuated.
T-lymphocyte (cell-mediated and humoral)	Severe combined	All live vaccines[2,3]	Effectiveness of any vaccine dependent on humoral or cellular response is doubtful.
Complement	Deficiency of early components (C1, C4, C2, C3)	None	All routine vaccines probably effective. Pneumococcal and meningococcal vaccines recommended.
	Deficiency of late components (C5–C9), properdin, factor B	None	All routine vaccines probably effective. Meningococcal vaccine recommended.
Phagocytic function	Chronic granulomatous disease Leukocyte adhesion defect Myeloperoxidase deficiency	Live bacterial vaccines[3]	All routine vaccines probably effective. Inactivated influenza vaccine should be considered to decrease secondary infection.

Category	Specific Immunodeficiency	Vaccine Contraindications	Effectiveness and Comments
Secondary			
	HIV/AIDS	OPV,[1] vaccinia, BCG; withhold MMR and varicella in severely immunocompromised children	MMR, varicella, and all inactivated vaccines, including influenza, may be effective.[4]
	Malignant neoplasm, transplantation, immunosuppressive or radiation therapy	Live viral and bacterial, depending on immune status[2,3]	Effectiveness of any vaccine depends on degree of immune suppression.

OPV indicates oral poliovirus; IGIV, Immune Globulin Intravenous; Ig, immunoglobulin; HIV, human immunodeficiency virus; AIDS, acquired immunodeficiency syndrome; BCG, bacille Calmette-Guérin; MMR, measles-mumps-rubella.

[1] OPV vaccine no longer is recommended for routine use in the United States.

[2] Live viral vaccines: MMR, OPV, varicella, vaccinia (smallpox). Smallpox vaccine is not recommended for children.

[3] Live bacterial vaccines: BCG and Ty21a *Salmonella typhi* vaccine.

[4] HIV-infected children should receive IG after exposure to measles and may receive varicella vaccine if CD4+ lymphocyte count = 25%.

Source: Reprinted with permission from Committee on Infectious Diseases. (2003). *Redbook.* Elk Grove Village, IL: American Academy of Pediatrics.

APPENDIX H–3
SUGGESTED INTERVALS BETWEEN IMMUNE GLOBULIN ADMINISTRATION AND MEASLES IMMUNIZATION (MMR OR MONOVALENT MEASLES VACCINE):

Indication for Immunoglobulin	Route	Dose Units or mL	Dose mg IgG/kg	Interval, mo[1]
Tetanus (as TIG)	IM	250 units	approx 10	3
Hepatitis A prophylaxis (as IG)				
Contact prophylaxis	IM	0.02 mL/kg	3.3	3
International travel	IM	0.06 mL/kg	10	3
Hepatitis B prophylaxis (as HBIG)	IM	0.06 mL/kg	10	3
Rabies prophylaxis (as RIG)	IM	20 units/kg	22	4
Measles prophylaxis (as IG)				
Standard	IM	0.25 mL/kg	40	5
Immunocompromised host	IM	0.50 mL/kg	80	6
Varicella prophylaxis (as VZIG)	IM	125 units/10 kg (maximum 625 units)	20–39	5
RSV prophylaxis (palivizumab monoclonal antibody)	IM	. . .	15 mg/kg	None
Blood transfusion				
Washed RBCs	IV	10 mL/kg	Negligible	0
RBCs, adenine-saline added	IV	10 mL/kg	10	3
Packed RBCs	IV	10 mL/kg	20–60	5
Whole blood	IV	10 mL/kg	80–100	6
Plasma or platelet products	IV	10 mL/kg	160	7
Replacement (or therapy) of immune deficiencies (as IGIV)	IV	. . .	300–400	8
ITP (as IGIV)	IV	. . .	400	8
RSV-IGIV	IV	. . .	750	9
ITP	IV	. . .	1000	10
ITP or Kawasaki syndrome	IV	. . .	1600–2000	11

MMR indicates measles-mumps-rubella; IgG, immunoglobulin G; TIG, Tetanus Immune Globulin; IG, Immune Globulin; IM, intramuscular; HBIG, Hepatitis B IG; RIG, Rabies IG; VZIG, Varicella-Zoster IG; RBCs, Red Blood Cells; IV, intravenous; IGIV, IG intravenous; ITP, immune (formerly termed "idiopathic") thrombocytopenic purpura; RSV-IGIV, Respiratory Syncytial Virus IGIV.

[1]These intervals should provide sufficient time for decreases in passive antibodies in all children to allow for an adequate response to measles vaccine. Physicians should not assume that children are fully protected against measles during these intervals. Additional doses of IG or measles vaccine may be indicated after exposure to measles (see text).

From Committee on Infectious Diseases. (2003). *Redbook*. Elk Grove Village, IL: American Academy of Pediatrics.

APPENDIX H–4
TABLE OF REPORTABLE EVENTS FOLLOWING IMMUNIZATION:

Vaccine	Events	Interval from Vaccination
Tetanus in any combination DT, Td, TT, DTaP	A. Anaphylaxis or anaphylactic shock B. Brachial neuritis C. Any sequelae of A or B above D. Events described in manufacturer's package insert as contraindications to additional doses of vaccine	7 days 28 days not applicable See package insert[2]
Pertussis in any combination DTaP, DTP-HIB, P	A. Anaphylaxis or anaphylactic shock B. Encephalopathy or encephalitis C. Any sequelae of A or B above D. Events described in manufacturer's package insert as contraindications to additional doses of vaccine	7 days 28 days not applicable See package insert
Measles, mumps, rubella In any combination, MMR, MR, M, R	A. Anaphylaxis or anaphylactic shock B. Encephalopathy or encephalitis C. Any sequelae of A or B above D. Repeat D above	7 days 28 days not applicable See package insert
Rubella	A. Chronic Arthritis B. Any sequelae of above events C. Repeat D above	42 days not applicable See package insert
Measles in any combination MMR, MR, M	A. Thrombocytopenia purpura B. Vaccine-strain measles in immunodeficient viral infection C. Any sequelae of A and B above D. Repeat D above	7–30 days 6 months not applicable See package insert
Inactivated polio	A. Anaphylaxis or anaphylactic shock B. Any sequelae of above events C. Repeat D above	7 days not applicable See package insert
Hepatitis B	A. Anaphylaxis or anaphylactic shock B. Any sequelae of above events C. Repeat D above	7 days not applicable See package insert
Haemophilus influenzae, Type b (conjugate)	A. Early-onset HiB disease B. Any sequelae of above events C. Events described in manufacturer's package insert as contraindications to additional doses of vaccine	7 days not applicable See package insert
Varicella	Events described in manufacturer's package insert as contraindications to additional doses of vaccine	See package insert
Pneumococcal conjugate	Events described in manufacturer's package insert as contraindications to additional doses of vaccine	See package insert

From Centers for Disease Control & Prevention, National Immunization Program. http://www.cdc.gov.nip/publications/surv-manual/chap18_vaers.pdf

APPENDIX H–5
REPORTING EVENTS OCCURRING AFTER IMMUUNIZATION:

	Vaccine Purchased with Public Money	Vaccine Purchased with Private Money
Who reports:	Health care provider who administered the vaccine	Health care provider who administered the vaccine
What products to report:	DTP, P, DTaP, MMR, DT, Td, T, OPV, IPV, and DTaP, DTP/Polio Combined	DTP, P, DTaP, MMR, DT, Td, T, OPV, IPV, and DTaP, DTP/Polio Combined
What reactions to report:	Events listed in Appendix H–4 including contraindicating reactions specified in manufacturers' package inserts	Events listed in Appendix H–4 including contraindicating reactions specified in manufacturers' package inserts
How to report:	Initial report taken by local, county, or state health department. State health department completes CDC form 71.19	Health care provider completes Adverse Reaction Report-FDA form 1639 (include interval from vaccination, manufacturer, and lot number on form)
Where to report:	State health departments send CDC form 71.19 to: MSAEFI/IM (E05) Centers for Disease Control Atlanta, GA 30333	Completed FDA form 1639 is sent to: Food and Drug Administration (HFN-730) Rockville, MD 20857
Where to obtain forms:	State health departments	FDA and publications such as *FDA Drug Bulletin*

http://www.vaers.org

APPENDIX H–6
VACCINE ADVERSE EVENT REPORTING SYSTEM:

WEBSITE: www.vaers.org   E-MAIL: info@vaers.org   FAX: 1-877-721-0366

VACCINE ADVERSE EVENT REPORTING SYSTEM
24 Hour Toll-Free Information 1-800-822-7967
P.O. Box 1100, Rockville, MD 20849-1100
PATIENT IDENTITY KEPT CONFIDENTIAL

For CDC/FDA Use Only
VAERS Number _____
Date Received _____

Patient Name:

Last   First   M.I.

Address

City   State   Zip

Telephone no. (____) _____

Vaccine administered by (Name):

Responsible
Physician _____
Facility Name/Address

City   State   Zip

Telephone no. (____) _____

Form completed by (Name):

Relation   ☐ Vaccine Provider ☐ Patient/Parent
to Patient ☐ Manufacturer   ☐ Other
Address (if different from patient or provider)

City   State   Zip

Telephone no. (____) _____

| 1. State | 2. County where administered | 3. Date of birth mm dd yy | 4. Patient age | 5. Sex ☐ M ☐ F | 6. Date form completed mm dd yy |

7. Describe adverse events(s) (symptoms, signs, time course) and treatment, if any

8. Check all appropriate:
☐ Patient died   (date ___ / ___ / ___)
                          mm   dd   yy
☐ Life threatening illness
☐ Required emergency room/doctor visit
☐ Required hospitalization (_____days)
☐ Resulted in prolongation of hospitalization
☐ Resulted in permanent disability
☐ None of the above

9. Patient recovered   ☐ YES ☐ NO ☐ UNKNOWN

12. Relevant diagnostic tests/laboratory data

10. Date of vaccination
___ / ___ / ___
mm   dd   yy
Time _____ AM PM

11. Adverse event onset
___ / ___ / ___
mm   dd   yy
Time _____ AM PM

13. Enter all vaccines given on date listed in no. 10

Vaccine (type)	Manufacturer	Lot number	Route/Site	No. Previous Doses
a.				
b.				
c.				
d.				

14. Any other vaccinations within 4 weeks prior to the date listed in no. 10

Vaccine (type)	Manufacturer	Lot number	Route/Site	No. Previous doses	Date given
a.					
b.					

15. Vaccinated at:
☐ Private doctor's office/hospital   ☐ Military clinic/hospital
☐ Public health clinic/hospital   ☐ Other/unknown

16. Vaccine purchased with:
☐ Private funds   ☐ Military funds
☐ Public funds   ☐ Other/unknown

17. Other medications

18. Illness at time of vaccination (specify)

19. Pre-existing physician-diagnosed allergies, birth defects, medical conditions (specify)

20. Have you reported this adverse event previously?
☐ No
☐ To doctor
☐ To health department
☐ To manufacturer

Only for children 5 and under

22. Birth weight
_____ lb. _____ oz.

23. No. of brothers and sisters

21. Adverse event following prior vaccination (check all applicable, specify)

	Adverse Event	Onset Age	Type Vaccine	Dose no. in series
☐ In patient				
☐ In brother or sister				

Only for reports submitted by manufacturer/immunization project

24. Mfr./imm. proj. report no.

25. Date received by mfr./imm.proj.

26. 15 day report?
☐ Yes ☐ No

27. Report type
☐ Initial ☐ Follow-Up

Health care providers and manufacturers are required by law (42 USC 300aa-25) to report reactions to vaccines listed in the Table of Reportable Events Following Immunization.
Reports for reactions to other vaccines are voluntary except when required as a condition of immunization grant awards.

Form VAERS-1(FDA)

From Centers for Disease Control & Prevention, National Immunization Program, VAERS

NO POSTAGE
NECESSARY
IF MAILED
IN THE
UNITED STATES
OR APO/FPO

BUSINESS REPLY MAIL
FIRST-CLASS MAIL   PERMIT NO. 1895   ROCKVILLE, MD

POSTAGE WILL BE PAID BY ADDRESSEE

VAERS
P.O. Box 1100
Rockville MD 20849-1100

DIRECTIONS FOR COMPLETING FORM
(Additional pages may be attached if more space is needed.)

GENERAL

- Use a separate form for each patient. Complete the form to the best of your abilities. Items 3, 4, 7, 8, 10, 11, and 13 are considered essential and should be completed whenever possible. Parents/Guardians may need to consult the facility where the vaccine was administered for some of the information (such as manufacturer, lot number or laboratory data.)
- Refer to the Reportable Events Table (RET) for events mandated for reporting by law. Reporting for other serious events felt to be related but not on the RET is encouraged.
- Health care providers other than the vaccine administrator (VA) treating a patient for a suspected adverse event should notify the VA and provide the information about the adverse event to allow the VA to complete the form to meet the VA's legal responsibility.
- These data will be used to increase understanding of adverse events following vaccination and will become part of CDC Privacy Act System 09-20-0136, "Epidemiologic Studies and Surveillance of Disease Problems". Information identifying the person who received the vaccine or that person's legal representative will not be made available to the public, but may be available to the vaccine or legal representative.
- Postage will be paid by addressee. Forms may be photocopied (must be front & back on same sheet).

SPECIFIC INSTRUCTIONS

Form Completed By: To be used by parents/guardians, vaccine manufacturers/distributors, vaccine administrators, and/or the person completing the form on behalf of the patient or the health professional who administered the vaccine.

Item 7:   Describe the suspected adverse event. Such things as temperature, local and general signs and symptoms, time course, duration of symptoms, diagnosis, treatment and recovery should be noted.

Item 9:   Check "YES" if the patient's health condition is the same as it was prior to the vaccine, "NO" if the patient has not returned to the pre-vaccination state of health, or "UNKNOWN" if the patient's condition is not known.

Item 10:   Give dates and times as specifically as you can remember. If you do not know the exact time, please
and 11:   indicate "AM" or "PM" when possible if this information is known. If more than one adverse event, give the onset date and time for the most serious event.

Item 12:   Include "negative" or "normal" results of any relevant tests performed as well as abnormal findings.

Item 13:   List ONLY those vaccines given on the day listed in Item 10.

Item 14:   List any other vaccines that the patient received within 4 weeks prior to the date listed in Item 10.

Item 16:   This section refers to how the person who gave the vaccine purchased it, not to the patient's insurance.

Item 17:   List any prescription or non-prescription medications the patient was taking when the vaccine(s) was given.

Item 18:   List any short term illnesses the patient had on the date the vaccine(s) was given (i.e., cold, flu, ear infection).

Item 19:   List any pre-existing physician-diagnosed allergies, birth defects, medical conditions (including developmental and/or neurologic disorders) for the patient.

Item 21:   List any suspected adverse events the patient, or the patient's brothers or sisters, may have had to previous vaccinations. If more than one brother or sister, or if the patient has reacted to more than one prior vaccine, use additional pages to explain completely. For the onset age of a patient, provide the age in months if less than two years old.

Item 26:   This space is for manufacturers' use only.

APPENDIX I-1
INHALED CORTICOSTEROIDS (ORAL AND NASAL INHALATION):

CORTICOSTEROID, ANTI-INFLAMMATORY **Prototype for classification:**
Hydrocortisone Use: Oral inhalation to treat steroid-dependent asthma, nasal inhalation for the management of the symptoms of seasonal or perennial rhinitis.

Beclomethasone diproprionate Beclovent, Beconase Nasal Inhaler, QVAR, Vancenase Nasal Inhaler, Vanceril, Vanceril D, Vancenase AQ	**Asthma:** *Adult:* **Oral inhaler** 2 inhalations t.i.d. or q.i.d. up to 20 inhalations/day; may try to reduce systemic steroids after 1 wk of concomitant therapy; QVAR 40–80 mcg b.i.d. (max 320 mcg/day). *Child: 6–12 y.* **Oral inhaler** 1–2 inhalations t.i.d. or q.i.d. up to 10 inhalations/day; QVAR 5–11 y, 40–80 mcg b.i.d. (max 160 mcg/day). **Allergic Rhinitis:** *Adult:* **Nasal inhaler** 1 spray in each nostril b.i.d. to q.i.d. *Child >6 y:* 1 spray daily
Budesonide Pulmicort, Turbuhaler, Pulmicort, Respules, Rhinocort, Rhinocort Aqua, Rhinocort, Turbuhaler	**Asthma, Maintenance Therapy:** *Adult:* **Oral inhalation** 1 or 2 inhalations (200 mcg/inhalation) daily-b.i.d. (max 800 mcg b.i.d). *Child ≥6 y:* **Oral inhalation** 1 inhalation (200 mcg/inhalation) daily-b.i.d. (max 400 mcg b.i.d.) *Child 12 mo–8 y:* **Nebulization** 0.5 mg/day in 1–2 divided doses. **Rhinitis:** *Adult, Child ≥6 y:* **Intranasal** 2 sprays in each nostril in the morning and evening or 4 sprays in each nostril in the morning. Each actuation releases 32 mg from the nasal adapter.
Dexamethasone Aeroseb-Dex, Decadron, Decaspray	*Adult:* **Oral Inhalation** Up to 3 inhalations t.i.d. or q.i.d. (max 12 inhalations/day). **Intranasal** 2 sprays in each nostril b.i.d. or t.i.d. (max 12 sprays/day). *Child:* **Oral Inhalation** Up to 2 inhalations q.i.d. (max 8 inhalations/day). **Intranasal** 1 or 2 sprays in each nostril b.i.d. (max 8 sprays/day).
Flunisolide AeroBid, Nasalide, Nasarel	**Allergic Rhinitis:** *Adult:* **Inhaled/Intranasal** 2 sprays orally, or intranasally in each nostril, b.i.d.; may increase to t.i.d., if needed. *Child:* **Inhaled/Intranasal** 6–14 y, 1 spray orally, or intranasally in each nostril t.i.d. *or* 2 sprays b.i.d.
Fluticasone Flonase, Flovent	**Seasonal Allergic Rhinitis:** *Adult:* **Intranasal** 100 mcg (1 inhalation) in each nostril 1–2 times daily (max 4 times daily). **Inhalation** 1–2 inhalations b.i.d. *Child ≥4 y:* **Intranasal** 1 spray in each nostril once daily. May increase to 2 sprays in each nostril once daily if inadequate response, then decrease to 1 spray in each nostril once daily when control is achieved.

Mometasone furoate monohydrate Nasonex	*Adult:* **Intranasal** 2 sprays (50 mcg each) in each nostril once daily. *Child:* ≥2 y **Intranasal** 1 spray in each nostril once daily.
Triamcinolone acetonide Azmacort, **Tri-Nasal**	*Adult:* **Inhalation** 2 puffs 3–4 times/day (max 16 puffs/day) or 4 puffs b.i.d. **Nasal spray** 2 spray/nostril once daily (max 8 sprays/day) *Child: 6–12 y:* **Inhalation** 1–2 sprays t.i.d. or q.i.d. (max 12 sprays/day) or 2–4 sprays b.i.d.

Contraindicated in: Nonasthmatic bronchitis, primary treatment of status asthmaticus, acute attack of asthma. **Cautious use in:** Patients receiving systemic corticosteroids; use with extreme caution if at all in respiratory tuberculosis, untreated fungal, bacterial, or viral infections, and ocular herpes simplex; nasal inhalation therapy for nasal septal ulcers, nasal trauma, or surgery. **Adverse Effects: Oral inhalation:** *Candidal infection of oropharynx* and occasionally larynx, hoarseness, dry mouth, sore throat, sore mouth. **Nasal (inhaler):** *Transient nasal irritation, burning, sneezing,* epistaxis, bloody mucous, nasopharyngeal itching, dryness, crusting, and ulceration; headache, nausea, vomiting. **Other:** With excessive doses, symptoms of hypercorticism. **Clinical Implications:** Note that oral inhalation and nasal inhalation products are not to be used interchangeably. **Oral inhaler:** Emphasize the following: (1) Shake inhaler well before using. (2) After exhaling fully, place mouthpiece well into mouth with lips closed firmly around it. (3) Inhale slowly through mouth while activating the inhaler. (4) Hold breath 5–10 sec, if possible, then exhale slowly. (5) Wait 1 min between puffs. Clean inhaler daily. Separate parts as directed in package insert, rinse them with warm water, and dry them thoroughly. Rinsing mouth and gargling with warm water after each oral inhalation removes residual medication from oropharyngeal area. Mouth care may also delay or prevent onset of oral dryness, hoarseness, and candidiasis. **Nasal inhaler:** Directions for use of nasal inhaler provided by manufacturer should be carefully reviewed with patient. Emphasize the following points: (1) Gently blow nose to clear nostrils. (2) Shake inhaler well before using. (3) If 2 sprays in each nostril are prescribed, direct one spray toward upper, and the other toward lower part of nostril. (4) Wash cap and plastic nosepiece daily with warm water; dry thoroughly. Inhaled steroids do not provide immediate symptomatic relief and are not prescribed for this purpose.

APPENDIX I–2
TOPICAL CORTICOSTEROIDS:

CORTICOSTEROID, ANTI-INFLAMMATORY   Prototype for classification: Hydrocortisone Use: As a topical corticosteroid, the drug is used for the relief of the inflammatory and pruritic manifestations of corticosteroid-responsive dermatoses.

Hydrocortisone Aeroseb-HC, Alphaderm, Cetacort, Cortaid, Cort-Dome, Cortenema, Cortril, DermaCort, Dermolate, Hydrocortone, Hytone, Proctocort, Rectocort, Synacort Anusol HC, CaldeCort **Hydrocortisone acetate** Carmol HC, Colifoam, Cortaid, Cortamed, Cort-Dome, Cortef Acetate, Corticaine, Cortifoam, Cortiment A Epifoam, Hydrocortone Acetate	*Adult:* **Topical** Apply a small amount to the affected area 1–4 times/day. **PR** Insert 1% cream, 10% foam, 10–25 mg suppository, or 100 mg enema nightly.
Alclometasone diproprionate Alclovate	*Adult:* **Topical** 0.05% cream or ointment applied sparingly b.i.d. or t.i.d.; may use occlusive dressing for resistant dermatoses.
Amcinonide Cyclocort	*Adult:* **Topical** Apply thin film b.i.d. or t.i.d.
Betamethasone dipropionate Diprolene, Diprolene AF, Doprosone, Maxivate, Alphatrex, Teladar	*Adult:* **Topical** Apply sparingly b.i.d.

Betamethasone valerate
Betatrex, Luxiq, Valisone, Psorion, Beta-Val

Clobetasol propionate
Dermovate, Temovate

Adult: **Topical** Apply sparingly b.i.d. (max 50 g/wk), or b.i.d. 3 day/wk or 1–2 times/wk for up to 6 mo.

Clocortolone pivalate
Cloderm

Adult: **Topical** Apply thin layer 1–4 times/day.

Desonide
DesOwen, Tridesilon

Adult: **Topical** Apply thin layer b.i.d. to q.i.d.

Desoximetasone
Topicort, Topicort-LP

Adult: **Topical** Apply thin layer b.i.d.

Dexamethasone
Decaderm, Decadron

Adult: **Topical** Apply thin layer t.i.d. or q.i.d.

Diflorasone diacetate
Florone, Florone E, Maxiflor, Psorcon

Adult: **Topical** Apply thin layer of ointment 1–3 times/day or cream 2–4 times/day.

Fluocinolone acetonide
Fluoderm, Fluolar, Fluonid, Flurosyn, Synalar, Synalar-HP, Synemol

Adult: **Topical** Apply thin layer b.i.d. to q.i.d.

Fluocinonide
Lidemol, Lidex, Lidex-E, Lyderm, Topsyn

Adult: **Topical** Apply thin layer b.i.d. to q.i.d.

Flurandrenolide
Cordran, Cordran SP, Drenison

Adult: **Topical** Apply thin layer b.i.d. or t.i.d.; apply tape 1–2 times/day at 12 h intervals. *Child:* **Topical** Apply thin layer 1–2 times/day; apply tape once/day.

Fluticasone
Cutivate

Adult, Child >3 mo: **Topical** Apply a thin film of cream or ointment to affected area once or twice daily.

Halcinonide
Halog

Adult: **Topical** Apply thin layer b.i.d. or t.i.d. *Child:* **Topical** Apply thin layer once/day

| **Mometasone furoate** Elocon | *Adult:* **Topical** Apply a thin film of cream or ointment or a few drops of lotion to affected area once/day. |
| **Triamcinolone** Aristocort, Atolone, Kenacort, Kenalog, Kenalog-E | *Adult:* **Topical** Apply sparingly b.i.d. or t.i.d. |

Contraindicated in: Topical steroids contraindicated in presence of varicella, vaccinia, on surfaces with compromised circulation, and in children <2y. **Cautious use in:** Children; diabetes mellitus; stromal *herpes simplex;* glaucoma, tuberculosis of eye; osteoporosis; untreated fungal, bacterial, or viral infections. **Adverse Effects: Skin:** Skin thinning and atrophy, *acne, impaired wound healing;* petechiae, ecchymosis, easy bruisings; suppression of skin test reaction; hypopigmentation or hyperpigmentation, hirsutism, acneiform eruptions, subcutaneous fat atrophy; allergic dermatitis, urticaria, angioneurotic edema, increased sweating. **Clinical Implications:** Administer retention enema preferably after a bowel movement. The enema should be retained at least 1 h or all night if possible. If an occlusive dressing is to be used, apply medication sparingly, rub until it disappears, and then reapply, leaving a thin coat over lesion. Completely cover area with transparent plastic or other occlusive device or vehicle. Avoid covering a weeping or exudative lesion. Usually, occlusive dressings are not applied to face, scalp, scrotum, axilla, and groin. Inspect skin carefully between applications for ecchymotic, petechial, and purpuric signs, maceration, secondary infection, skin atrophy, striae or milaria; if present, stop medication and notify physician. Warn patient not to self-dose with OTC topical preparations of a corticosteroid more than 7 days. They should not be used for children <2 y. If symptoms do not abate, consult physician. Usually, topical preparations are applied after a shower or bath when skin is damp or wet. Cleansing and application of prescribed preparation should be done with extreme gentleness because of fragility, easy bruisability, and poor-healing skin. Hazard of systemic toxicity is higher in small children because of the greater ratio of skin surface area to body weight. Apply sparingly. Urge patient on long-term therapy with topical corticosterone to check expiration date.

Source: Reprinted with permission from Wilson BA, Shannon MT, Stang CL. *Nurse's Drug Guide 2005,* pages 1714–1717. Upper Saddle River, NJ: Pearson/Prentice Hall, © 2005.

BIBLIOGRAPHY

American Academy of Pediatrics. *Red book: Report of the Committee on Infectious Diseases.* 26th ed. Elk Grove Village, IL: Author. 2003.

American Hospital Formulary System. *AHFS Drug Information.* Bethesda, MD: American Society of Hospital Pharmacists. 2004.

Nechyba C, Gunn V, Eds. *Harriet Lane Handbook.* 16th ed. Baltimore, MD: Johns Hopkins University Press. 2002.

Physicians' Desk Reference. 58th ed. Oradell, NJ: Medical Economics Co. 2004.

Takemoto CK, Hodding JH, Kraus DM. *Pediatric Dosage Handbook.* 11th ed. Hudson, OH: Lexi-Comp. 2004.

USPDI: Advice to Patients. Rockville, MD: US Pharmacopeial Convention. 2004.

USPDI: Drug Information for the Health Care Professional. Rockville, MD: US Pharmacopeial Convention. 2004.

INDEX

Drug categories are in SMALL CAPS. Prototypes in **bold.**
Generic drug names are given in parentheses.

1299

Drug categories are in SMALL CAPS. Prototypes in **bold.**
Generic drug names are given in parentheses.

Drug categories are in SMALL CAPS. Prototypes in **bold.**
Generic drug names are given in parentheses.
1301

Drug categories are in SMALL CAPS. Prototypes in **bold.**
Generic drug names are given in parentheses.

1303

Drug categories are in SMALL CAPS. Prototypes in **bold.**
Generic drug names are given in parentheses.

Drug categories are in SMALL CAPS. Prototypes in **bold.**
Generic drug names are given in parentheses.

1305

Drug categories are in SMALL CAPS. Prototypes in **bold**.
Generic drug names are given in parentheses.

Drug categories are in SMALL CAPS. Prototypes in **bold.**
Generic drug names are given in parentheses.

Drug categories are in SMALL CAPS. Prototypes in **bold.**
Generic drug names are given in parentheses.

Drug categories are in SMALL CAPS. Prototypes in **bold.**
Generic drug names are given in parentheses.

1309

Drug categories are in SMALL CAPS. Prototypes in **bold.**
Generic drug names are given in parentheses.

Drug categories are in SMALL CAPS. Prototypes in **bold.**
Generic drug names are given in parentheses.

1311

INDEX

Drug categories are in SMALL CAPS. Prototypes in **bold.**
Generic drug names are given in parentheses.

Drug categories are in SMALL CAPS. Prototypes in **bold.**
Generic drug names are given in parentheses.

1313

Drug categories are in SMALL CAPS. Prototypes in **bold.**
Generic drug names are given in parentheses.

Drug categories are in SMALL CAPS. Prototypes in **bold.**
Generic drug names are given in parentheses.

1315

Drug categories are in SMALL CAPS. Prototypes in **bold.**
Generic drug names are given in parentheses.

Drug categories are in SMALL CAPS. Prototypes in **bold**.
Generic drug names are given in parentheses.

1317

Drug categories are in SMALL CAPS. Prototypes in **bold.**
Generic drug names are given in parentheses.

Drug categories are in SMALL CAPS. Prototypes in **bold.**
Generic drug names are given in parentheses.

1319

Drug categories are in SMALL CAPS. Prototypes in **bold.**
Generic drug names are given in parentheses.

Drug categories are in SMALL CAPS. Prototypes in **bold.**
Generic drug names are given in parentheses.

Drug categories are in SMALL CAPS. Prototypes in **bold.**
Generic drug names are given in parentheses.

Drug categories are in SMALL CAPS. Prototypes in **bold.**
Generic drug names are given in parentheses.

1323

Drug categories are in SMALL CAPS. Prototypes in **bold.**
Generic drug names are given in parentheses.

Drug categories are in SMALL CAPS. Prototypes in **bold.**
Generic drug names are given in parentheses.

1325

Drug categories are in SMALL CAPS. Prototypes in **bold.**
Generic drug names are given in parentheses.

1327

Drug categories are in SMALL CAPS. Prototypes in **bold.**
Generic drug names are given in parentheses.

Drug categories are in SMALL CAPS. Prototypes in **bold.**
Generic drug names are given in parentheses.

1329

Drug categories are in SMALL CAPS. Prototypes in **bold.**
Generic drug names are given in parentheses.

Drug categories are in SMALL CAPS. Prototypes in **bold.**
Generic drug names are given in parentheses.
1331

Drug categories are in SMALL CAPS. Prototypes in **bold.**
Generic drug names are given in parentheses.

1333

1334

Drug categories are in SMALL CAPS. Prototypes in **bold.**
Generic drug names are given in parentheses.

Drug categories are in SMALL CAPS. Prototypes in **bold.**
Generic drug names are given in parentheses.

1335

1336
Drug categories are in SMALL CAPS. Prototypes in **bold.**
Generic drug names are given in parentheses.

N

Drug categories are in SMALL CAPS. Prototypes in **bold.**
Generic drug names are given in parentheses.

1337

Drug categories are in SMALL CAPS. Prototypes in **bold.**
Generic drug names are given in parentheses.

1339

Drug categories are in SMALL CAPS. Prototypes in **bold.**
Generic drug names are given in parentheses.

1341

Drug categories are in SMALL CAPS. Prototypes in **bold.**
Generic drug names are given in parentheses.

Drug categories are in SMALL CAPS. Prototypes in **bold.**
Generic drug names are given in parentheses.

1343

Drug categories are in SMALL CAPS. Prototypes in **bold.**
Generic drug names are given in parentheses.

1345

Drug categories are in SMALL CAPS. Prototypes in **bold.**
Generic drug names are given in parentheses.

Drug categories are in SMALL CAPS. Prototypes in **bold.**
Generic drug names are given in parentheses.

1347

Drug categories are in SMALL CAPS. Prototypes in **bold.**
Generic drug names are given in parentheses.

Drug categories are in SMALL CAPS. Prototypes in **bold.**
Generic drug names are given in parentheses.

1349

Drug categories are in SMALL CAPS. Prototypes in **bold.**
Generic drug names are given in parentheses.

Drug categories are in SMALL CAPS. Prototypes in **bold.**
Generic drug names are given in parentheses.

Drug categories are in SMALL CAPS. Prototypes in **bold.**
Generic drug names are given in parentheses.

1353

Drug categories are in SMALL CAPS. Prototypes in **bold.**
Generic drug names are given in parentheses.

Drug categories are in SMALL CAPS. Prototypes in **bold.**
Generic drug names are given in parentheses.

1355

Drug categories are in SMALL CAPS. Prototypes in **bold.**
Generic drug names are given in parentheses.

ANTIBIOTIC DRUG IV-SITE COMPATIBILITY CHART

	AMINO-PHYLLINE	DOBUTA-MINE	DOPAMINE	HEPARIN	MEPERIDINE	MORPHINE	NITRO-GLYCERIN	ONDAN-SETRON	POTASSIUM IN D5W OR NS
acyclovir					C	I/C		—	C
alteplase		—	—	—	—	—	—	C	
amikacin	C			C	C	C		C	
amino acids (TPN)	C	C	C	—	C	C	C	—	C
aminophylline	C	—	—	—	C	C	C	—	C
amiodarone	—	C	C	C	—	C	C	—	C
ampicillin	C			C	C	C			C
ampicillin/sulbactam					C	C		C	
amrinone	C	C	C	C	C	C	C	C	C
aztreonam					C	C			
bretylium	C	C	C	C	C	C	C	C	C
bumetanide	—	—					C		
calcium chloride	C	C	C						C
cefamandole	C				C	C		C	C
cefazolin	C	—		C	—	C		—	
cefoperazone					C	C		C	
cefotaxime	C			C	—	C		C	
cefotetan	C		C		C	C		C	C
cefoxitin	C			C	C	C		C	C
ceftazidime	C				C	C		C	
ceftizoxime	C			C	C	C		C	C
ceftriaxone	C		C	C	C	C		C	C
cefuroxime	C		C	C	C	C		C	C
cephalothin	—	C	C	—	C	C		C	C
chloramphenicol		C	C	C	C	C			C
cimetidine	C	C	C	C	C	C		C	C
ciprofloxacin	—				C				
clindamycin	—	C		C	C	C		C	C
dexamethasone	C	C		C	C	C		C	C

	AMINO-PHYLLINE	DOBUTA-MINE	DOPAMINE	HEPARIN	MEPERIDINE	MORPHINE	NITRO-GLYCERIN	ONDAN-SETRON	POTASSIUM IN D5W OR NS
diazepam									I/C
digoxin	C	I/C		–	–	C			C
diltiazem	–	C	C	C	C	C	C	C	C
diphenhydramine	–		C	C	C	C			C
dobutamine	–	C	C	I/C	C	C	C		C
dopamine	–	C	–	–	C	C	C	C	C
doxycycline		C	C	C	C	C	C		
enalapril/enalaprilat	C	C	C	C		C		C	C
epinephrine	–			C		C			C
eptifibatide									
erythromycin	–			–	C	C			
esmolol	C	C	C	C	C	C	C	C	C
famotidine	C	C	C	C	C	C	C	C	C
filgrastim	C			C	C	C		C	C
fluconazole	C	C	C	–	C	C	C	C	
foscarnet	C	–		C		C			
fosphenytoin									
furosemide	C	I/C	C	C	I/C	–	C	–	C
ganciclovir	C			–				–	
gentamicin	C		C	C	C	C		C	
heparin	C	I/C	C	C	C	C	–	C	C
hydrocortisone	C		C	C	C	C		C	C
hydromorphone				C	C	C		C	
imipenem/cilastatin				C				C	
insulin		C		C	–	C		C	C
isoproterenol		C		C	C	C		C	C
labetolol	C	C	C	C	C	C	C		C
lidocaine	C	C	C	C	C	C	C	–	C
lorazepam								C	
magnesium		C		C	C	C		C	C

meperidine

methylprednisolone

metoclopramide

metoprolol

metronidazole

mezlocillin

midazolam

milrinone

morphine

moxalactam

nafcillin

nitroglycerin

nitroprusside

norepinephrine

ondansetron

penicillin G

phenylephrine

phenytoin

piperacillin

piperacillin/tazobactam

potassium Cl in D5W or NS

procainamide

propofol

ranitidine

sargramostim

sodium bicarbonate

ticarcillin

tobramycin

trimethoprim/sulfa-
methoxazole

vancomycin

C = compatible; I = incompatible; I/C = conflicting data